Evidence Based Cardiology

EVIDENCE BASED CARDIOLOGY

Edited by:

Salim Yusuf
Heart and Stroke Foundation of Ontario Research Chair, Medical Council of Canada Scientist

Director of Cardiology and Professor of Medicine, McMaster University, Hamilton General Hospital, Hamilton, Canada

John A Cairns
Dean, Faculty of Medicine, University of British Columbia, Vancouver, Canada

A John Camm
Professor of Clinical Cardiology and Chief, Department of Cardiological Sciences, St George's Hospital Medical School, London, UK

Ernest L Fallen
Professor, Department of Medicine, McMaster University, Hamilton, Canada

Bernard J Gersh
W Proctor Harvey Teaching Professor of Cardiology and Chief, Division of Cardiology, Georgetown University Medical Center, Cardiology Division, Washington DC, USA

First published in 1998
by BMJ Books, BMA House, Tavistock Square,
London WC1H 9JR

British Library Cataloguing in Publication Data

A catalogue record for this book is available from the British Library

ISBN 0-7279-1171-6

Typeset, printed and bound by Latimer Trend & Company Ltd, Plymouth, Devon.

Contents

Part III 353
Specific cardiovascular disorders
i: Stable coronary artery disease

Bernard J Gersh, Editor

Part III 393
ii: Acute ischemic syndromes

John A Cairns and Bernard J Gersh, Editors

Part III 417
iii: Acute myocardial infarction

John A Cairns and Bernard J Gersh

CONTENTS

Contributors

Sonia S Anand
Preventive Cardiology, HGH-McMaster Clinic, Hamilton, Canada

Jeffrey L Anderson
Division of Cardiology, LDS Hospital, Cardiology Division, Salt Lake City, USA

Bert Andersson
Wallenberg Laboratory for Cardiovascular Research, Sahlgrenska University Hospital, Goteborg University, Goteborg, Sweden

Samira Asma
Office on Smoking and Health, National Center for Chronic Disease Prevention, Atlanta, USA

Donald S Baim
Beth Israel Hospital, Cardiovascular Division, Boston, USA

Adrian P Banning
Department of Cardiology, John Radcliffe Hospital, Oxford, UK

Henry J M Barnett
Robarts Research Institute, London, Canada

David G Benditt
Cardiovascular Division, University of Minnesota Medical School, Minneapolis, USA

C R Benedict
Department of Internal Medicine, University of Texas Medical School, Houston, USA

John A Boone
Burrard Medical Building, Vancouver, Canada

Johannes Brachmann
Abt Innere Medizin III, Medizinische Klinik, Universität Heidelberg, Heidelberg, Germany

Jeffrey A Breall
Georgetown University Medical School, Washington, USA

Edmund A W Brice
Cardiac Clinic, University of Cape Town, Cape Town, South Africa

John D Brunzell
Women's Health Initiative, Fred Hutchinson Cancer Reseach Center, Seattle, USA

R W F Campbell
Academic Cardiology, Freeman Hospital, University of Newcastle Upon Tyne, Newcastle Upon Tyne, UK

Blase A Carabello
Department of Medicine, Medical University of South Carolina, Charleston, USA

John F Carlquist
Department of Medicine, University of Utah, Salt Lake City, Utah, USA

Joseph P Carrozza Jr
Harvard Medical School and Cardiovascular Division, Beth-Israel Deaconess Hospital, Boston, USA

David J Cohen
Harvard Medical School and Cardiovascular Division, Beth-Israel Deaconess Hospital, Boston, USA

Patrick J Commerford
University of Cape Town, Cardiac Clinic, Groote Schuur Hospital, Cape Town, South Africa

Stuart J Connolly
Hamilton General Hospital, McMaster University, Hamilton, Canada

Deborah Cook
St Joseph's Hospital, Hamilton, Canada

Harry J G M Crijns
Academische Ziekenhuis Groningen, Groningen, Netherlands

Jeffrey A Cutler
National Heart, Blood and Lung Institute, Bethesda, USA

Joseph M Delahanty
University of Rochester Medical Center, Rochester, New York, USA

Allan S Detsky
Departments of Health Administration and Medicine, University of Toronto, Toronto, Canada

Brian Dias
Hamilton General Hospital, Hamilton, Canada

Dan Diver
Cardiac Catheterization Laboratory, Georgetown University Medical Centre, Washington, USA

David T Durack
Becton Dickinson Microbiological Systems, Sparks, USA

M Eliasziw
Robarts Research Institute, London, Canada

Perry M Elliott
St George's Hospital Medical School, London, UK

Andrew E Epstein
Division of Cardiovascular Diseaes, University of Alabama, Birmingham, USA

Michael P Eriksen
Office on Smoking and Health, National Center for Chronic Disease Prevention, Atlanta, USA

Nathan R Every
Division of Cardiology, University of Washington, Washington, USA

William H Fabian
Cardiac Arrhythmia Center, University of Minnesota Medical School, Minneapolis, USA

Gerald F Fletcher
Emory School of Medicine, Center for Rehabilitation Medicine, Atlanta, USA

Godfrey Fowler
General Practice Research Group, Radcliffe Infirmary, Oxford, UK

John K French
Green Lane Hospital, Auckland, New Zealand

Erika S Froelicher
University of California, San Francisco School of Nursing, Department of Psychological Nursing, San Francisco, USA

Curt D Furberg
Department of Public Health Sciences, Bowman Gray School of Medicine, Winston-Salem, USA

Jacques Genest Jr
Cardiovascular Genetics Laboratory, Clinical Research Institute of Montreal, Montreal, Canada

Hertzel C Gerstein
McMaster University HSC, Hamilton, Canada

Raymond J Gibbons
Nuclear Cardiology Laboratory, Mayo Medical School, Mayo Clinic, Rochester, Minn, USA

Jeffrey S Ginsberg
Department of Medicine, McMaster University, Hamilton, Canada

Henry A Glick
Division of General Internal Medicine, University of Pennsylvania, USA

Brian Gribbin
John Radcliffe Hospital, Oxford, UK

Gordon H Guyatt
Clinical Epidemiology and Biostatistics, McMaster University, Hamilton, Canada

R Brian Haynes
Health Information Research Unit, McMaster University, Hamilton, Canada

Harry Hemingway
Department of Epidemiology and Public Health, University College London Medical School, and Kensington, Chelsea and Westminster Health Authority, London, UK

Brenda Hemmelgarn
McMaster University, Hamilton, Canada

Thomas Hilbel
Abt Innere Medizin III, Medizinische Klinik, Universität Heidelberg, Heidelberg, Germany

Jack Hirsh
Hamilton Civic Hospitals Research Centre, Hamilton, Canada

Mark A Hlatky
Health Research and Policy, Stanford University School of Medicine, Stanford, USA

Douglas A Holder
Hamilton General Hospital, Hamilton, Canada

David R Holmes Jr
Division of Cardiovascular Diseases, Mayo Clinic, Rochester, Minn, USA

William B Hood Jr
University of Rochester Medical Center, Rochester, New York, USA

Dereck L Hunt
Health Information Research Unit, McMaster University, Hamilton, Canada

Gohar Jamil
Division of Cardiovascular Disease, University of Alabama, Birmingham, USA

Desmond G Julian
British Heart Foundation, London, UK

G Neal Kay
Division of Cardiovascular Disease, University of Alabama, Birmingham, USA

Clive Kearon
McMaster University, Hamilton, Canada

Allan Kitching
Division of Cardiology, McMaster University, Hamilton, Canada

Michael D Klein
Cardiology Department, University Hospital, Boston, USA

Roberto Latini
Department of Cardiovascular Research, Mario Negri Institute, Milan, Italy

Malcolm Law
St Bartholomew's Medical College, London, UK

Herbert J Levine
New England Medical Center, Boston, USA

Eva M Lonn
Preventive Cardiology, McMaster University, HGH-McMcMaster Clinic, Hamilton, Canada

Keith G Lurie
Cardiac Arrhythmia Center, University of Minnesota Medical School, Minneapolis, USA

Benedito Carlos Maciel
Division of Cardiology, Medical School of Ribeirão Preto, University of São Paulo, Ribeirão Preto, Brazil

Aldo P Maggioni
Department of Cardiovascular Research, Mario Negri Institute, Milan, Italy

David J Malenka
Cardiac Ultrasound, Dartmouth–Hitchcock Medical Center, Lebanon, USA

José Antonio Marin-Neto
University of São Paulo, Ribeirão-Preto, Brazil

Daniel B Mark
Duke University Medical Center, Durham, USA

Michael Marmot
Department of Epidemiology and Public Health, University College School of Medicine, London, UK

Bongani M Mayosi
Cardiac Clinic, University of Cape Town, Cape Town, South Africa

Robert S McKelvie
HGH-McMaster Clinic, McMaster University, Hamilton, Canada

William J McKenna
Department of Cardiological Sciences, St George's Hospital, London, UK

K Ann McKibbon
Health Information Research Unit, McMaster University, Hamilton, Canada

H E Meldrum
Robarts Research Institute, London, Canada

L Brent Mitchell
Foothills Hospital, Division of Cardiology, University of Calgary, Calgary, Canada

C David Naylor
Sunnybrook HSC, University of Toronto, Toronto, Canada

Jim Nishikawa
McMaster University, Hamilton, Canada

Gerald T O'Connor
Center for Evaluative Clinical Science, Dartmouth Medical School, Hanover, USA

Celia M Oakley
Royal Postgraduate Medical School, Hammersmith Hospital, London, UK

Roberta K Oka
School of Nursing, University of California, San Francisco, USA

Lionel H Opie
Heart and Research Unit and Hypertension Clinic, Department of Medicine, Medical School, Observatory, Cape Town, South Africa

Jan Östergren
Section of Cardiovascular Medicine, Department of Internal Medicine, Karolinska Hospital, Stockholm, Sweden

Akbar A Panju
McMaster University, Hamilton, Canada

Paul J Pearson
Division of Thoracic and Cardiovascular Surgery, Mayo Clinic and Mayo Foundation, Rochester, Minn, USA

Terry F Pechacek
Office on Smoking and Health, National Center for Chronic Disease Prevention and Health Promotion, Atlanta, USA

Barbara A Pisani
Loyola University Medical Center, Maywood, USA

Jeffrey L Probstfield
Women's Health Initiative, Fred Hutchinson Cancer Research Center, Seattle, Washington, USA

Bruce M Psaty
Cardiovascular Health Research Unit, Seattle, USA

Shahbudin H Rahimtoola
University of Southern California, Los Angeles, USA

K Srinath Reddy
Department of Cardiology, Cardiothoracic Centre, All India Institute of Medical Sciences, New Delhi, India

Charanjit S Rihal
Division of Cardiovascular Diseases and Internal Medicine, Mayo Clinic, Rochester, Minn, USA

Jacques E Rossouw
Women's Health Initiative, National Heart, Lung and Blood Institute, Bethesda, USA

David L Sackett
Nuffield Department of Clinical Medicine, John Radcliffe Hospital, Headington, Oxford, UK

Giuseppe Sangiorgi
Division of Cardiovascular Diseases, Mayo Clinic, Rochester, Minn, USA

Hartzell V Schaff
Division of Thoracic and Cardiovascular Surgery, Mayo Clinic and Mayo Foundation, Rochester, Minn, USA

Kevin A Schulman
Economics Research Unit, Washington, USA

Robert S Schwartz
E-16 Cardiology, Mayo Clinic, Rochester, Minn, USA

Sanjay Sharma
St George's Hospital Medical School, London, UK

Marcus Vinícius Simões
Division of Cardiology, Medical School of Ribeirão Preto, University of São Paulo, Ribeirão Preto, Brazil

Maarten Simoons
Erasmus University, Rotterdam, Netherlands

Peter Sleight
University Department of Cardiovascular Medicine, John Radcliffe Hospital, Oxford, UK

Peter C Spittell
Mayo Clinic, Rochester, Minn, USA

Karl B Swedberg
Department of Internal Medicine, Ostra Hospital, Goteborg, Sweden

Jesper Swedenborg
Department of Surgery, Division of Vascular Surgery, Karolinska Hospital, Stockholm, Sweden

David O Taylor
University of Utah, Salt Lake City, USA

Pierre Théroux
Clinical Research, Montreal Heart Institute, Montreal, Canada

Robert G Tieleman
Thorax Center, Department of Cardiology, University Hospital, Groningen, Netherlands

William D Toff
Cardiology Department, Glenfield Hospital, Leicester, UK

Gianni Tognoni
Department of Cardiovascular Research, Mario Negri Institute, Milan, Italy

Michael L Towns
Becton Dickinson Microbiology Systems, Sparks, USA

Sanjeev Trehan
Department of Medicine, University of Utah, Salt Lake City, USA

Chen Y Tung
Duke University Medical Center, Durham, USA

Zoltan G Turi
Harper Hospital, Detroit USA

Alexander G G Turpie
HGH-McMaster Clinic, McMaster University, Hamilton, Canada

L Ronald van der Wieken
Onze Lieve Vrouwe Gasthuis, Amsterdam, Netherlands

Isabelle C Van Gelder
Thorax Center, Department of Cardiology, University Hospital, Groningen, Netherlands

Wiek H Van Gilst
Department of Clinical Pharmacology, University of Groningen, Groningen, Netherlands

James A Volmink
South African Cochrane Centre, Cape Town, South Africa

David Waters
Department of Cardiology, Hartford Hospital, Hartford, USA

W Douglas Weaver
Cardiovascular Medicine, Henry Ford Heart and Vascular Institute, Detroit, USA

Harvey D White
Cardiology Department, Greenlane Hospital, Auckland, New Zealand

Preface

"... if a man declares to you that he has found facts that he has observed and confirmed with his own experience, be cautious in accepting what he says. Rather, investigate and weigh this opinion or hypothesis according to requirements of pure logic, without paying attention to this contention that he affirms empirically."

MOSES MAIMONIDES, *ca.* 1195

Thus did the great physician Maimonides make a plea for an evidence based approach to medicine by admonishing his followers to seek common ground between objectivism and empiricism. If Maimonides had lived in the year 1785, he would likely have read William Withering's *An Account of the Foxglove*; a compendium of Withering's personal observations on the clinical effect of the digitalis leaf. At first blush, Maimonides would cry foul at such flagrant empiricism, demanding to know the whole of the inception cohort. It turns out that Withering, instead of selecting specific cases which would have "... spoken strong in favour of the medicine, and perhaps been flattering to my own reputation" went on to say in his Preface "I have therefore mentioned every case in which I have prescribed the foxglove, proper or improper, successful or otherwise ..." thus heralding a genuine, albeit retrospective, cohort study. It took 212 years before Withering was ultimately vindicated by the results of the first large scale randomised placebo controlled trial of digoxin (*N Engl J Med* 1997; **336**: 526). Sixty-eight hundred patients with congestive heart failure, in sinus rhythm, were randomized to receive digoxin (avg dose 0·25 mg/day) or placebo in addition to ACE inhibitors and diuretics. Over a three-year period there was no statistical difference in overall mortality but digoxin proved to be effective in reducing hospitalizations due to worsening heart failure.

The advent of large scale prospective randomized clinical trails has strengthened the external evidence upon which management decisions can be made with some confidence. We have come to rely on so-called external best evidence as critical guideposts for establishing minimal criteria for treatment of many cardiovascular disorders. In the process, some myths based on putative mechanisms have been dispelled while insights into the efficacy of new treatments have been more rapidly facilitated. On the other hand there is a danger of righteous complacency which, if unchecked, could lead to a slavish dependency on statistical bottom lines and, ultimately, to "cook book" medicine. It is the intent of this textbook to present a proper balance between "objectivism and empiricism". In this regard, the very first chapter by Kitching, Sackett and Yusuf begins by defining the practice of evidence based cardiology as "... integrating individual clinical expertise with the best available external clinical evidence from systematic research".

The textbook has four principal components. An introductory general section addresses important topics in clinical epidemiology, as applied both to the bedside and to a population. This section includes: critical appraisal of data; clinical trials methodology; quality of life measurements; health economics; and methods of decision analysis, all in the context of current clinical practice. Next follows a section on preventive strategies based on evidence that should enable the practicing physician to advise, with confidence, on risk factor modification and quality of life issues for selected patients. There follows a section on a broad range of specific cardiovascular disorders that highlight management issues based on current best evidence, Finally, the section on clinical applications is an attempt to put a clinical face on evidence derived from population statistics through the use of "live" clinical cases. Here, an attempt is made judiciously to couple external evidence with clinical expertise and a sound knowledge of cardiovascular pathophysiology. There is understandably a wide range of the kinds of evidence available to support different practices and treatments. The editors have chosen not to constrain the authors into rigid and uniform formats for each chapter. While several of the chapters have the level of evidence/recommendations graded, or key messages highlighted, a uniform format would not have been appropriate for every chapter.

This textbook is designed for a wide audience. Since cardiovascular disease comprises more than fifty percent of adult medicine, there is something here for everyone in clinical practise and at all levels of medical undergraduate and postgraduate training. Its emphasis on practical applications of research methodology and critical appraisal of data covering a cross-section of clinical topics should invite interest among those engaged in population studies, biostatistics, clinical epidemiology and health economics as well as those involved in healthcare decision analysis, quality assurance committees and stakeholders responsible for healthcare planning.

Because this textbook relies so heavily on current best evidence, it is by nature threatened with impending obsolescence. To ensure that this does not happen, the editors, in concert with the publisher, have agreed to issue up-dates periodically in the form of special supplements or updated editions, so that the text can be continually revised in accordance with emerging relevant data. In this context, it is well to bear in mind that good science always proceeds hesitantly through a series of tenuous conclusions. And so any recommendation made on the basis of available best evidence is subject to revision as we probe deeper into the mysterious nature of disease processes. One may ask of the large scale clinical trial "Why did it require more than 10,000 patients to show incontrovertible evidence that the experimental drug is effective?" Aye, there is the scientific question!

The editors wish to acknowledge the herculean efforts of Catherine Wright and Karin Dearness who kept everyone on track and offer a special appreciation to Mary Banks for her editorial expertise, patience and support.

Salim Yusuf
John A Cairns
A John Camm
Ernest L Fallen
Bernard J Gersh

Glossary

ABBREVIATIONS COMMONLY USED IN THIS BOOK

ACE	angiotensin converting enzyme (I = inhibitors)
AF	atrial fibrillation
AGE	advanced glycoprotein end product
AMI	acute myocardial infarction
APSAC	anisoylated plasminogen streptokinase activator complex; anistreplase
aPTT	activated partial thromboplastin time
AV	atrioventricular
BBB	bundle branch block
BMI	body mass index
BP	blood pressure (DBP – diastolic . . .; SBP – systolic . . .)
bpm	beats per minute
CABG	coronary artery bypass graft
CAD	coronary artery disease
CBVD	cerebrovascular disease
CCU	coronary care unit
CHD	coronary heart disease
CHF	congestive heart failure
CI	cardiac index
CI	confidence interval
COAD	chronic obstructive airways disease
COPD	chronic obstructive pulmonary disease
CVD	cardiovascular disease
CVP	central venous pressure
DALY	disability-adjusted life years
DHP	dihydropyridines
DVT	deep vein thrombosis/thrombi
ECG	electrocardiogram
ECM	encephalomyocarditis
EDD	end-diastolic dimension
EF	ejection fraction
EMS	emergency medical service
EP	electrophysiologic (studies)
ESD	end-systolic dimension
GP	glycoprotein
HDL	high density lipoprotein
HDL-C	high density lipoprotein cholesterol

HMG-CoA	3-hydroxy-3-methylglutaryl coenzyme A
HRQL	health-related quality of life
HSP	heat shock protein
IC	intracoronary
ICD	implantable cardiac defibrillator
IDC	idiopathic dilated cardiomyopathy
IFN	interferon
IL	interleukin
IM	intramuscular
INR	international normalized ratio
IR	instant release
IV	intravenous
LAD	left anterior descending (coronary artery)
LAE	left atrial enlargement
LAHB	left anterior hemiblock
LDL	low density lipoprotein
LDL-C	low density lipoprotein cholesterol
LV	left ventricular
LVEDP	left ventricular end-diastolic pressure
LVEF	left ventricular ejection fraction
LVH	left ventricular hypertrophy
MHC	major histocompatibility complex
MI	myocardial infarction/infarct
OR	odds ratio
PAI	plasminogen activator inhibitor
PCR	polymerase chain reaction
PPCM	peripartum cardiomyopathy
PTCA	percutaneous transluminal coronary angioplasty
QALY	quality-adjusted life years
RCT	randomized controlled trial
rPA	reteplase plasminogen activator
rtPA	recombinant tissue plasminogen activator
RR	relative risk/risk reduction (ratio)
RV	right ventricular
SC	subcutaneous
scuPA	single chain urokinase-type plasminogen activator
SFA	superficial femoral artery
SHF	severe heart failure
SK	streptokinase
TGF-β	transforming growth factor beta
TIA	transient ischemic attack
tPA	tissue plasminogen activator
UK	urokinase
VF	ventricular fibrillation
VLDL	very low density lipoprotein
VSD	ventricular septal defect
VTE	venous thromboembolism
VUI	venous ultrasound imaging
WPW	Wolff–Parkinson–White syndrome

TRIAL GROUPS, INDEX MEASURES, SCALES, SOCIETIES

ACIP	Asymptomatic Cardiac Ischemia Pilot
ACP	American College of Physicians
ASSET	Anglo-Scandinavian Study of Early Thrombolysis
BARI	Bypass Angioplasty Revascularization Investigation
CASS	Cardiac Artery Surgery Study
CAST	Cardiac Arrhythmia Suppression Trial
CCS	Canadian Cardiovascular Society
CHQ	Chronic Heart Failure Questionnaire
DUCCS	Duke University Clinical Cardiology Study
ECSS	European Coronary Surgery Study
FTT	Fibrinolytic Therapy Trialists' (Collaborative Group)
GISSI	Gruppo Italiano per lo Studio della Streptokinasi nell'Infarto Miocardico
GUSTO-1	Global Utilization of Streptokinase and Tissue Plasminogen Activator for Occluded Coronary Arteries
GUSTO-2(...)	Global Use of Strategies to Open Occluded Coronary Arteries
INJECT	International Joint Efficacy Comparison of Thrombolytics
ISIS	International Study of Infarct Survival
NRMI	National Registry of Myocardial Infarction
NYHA	New York Heart Association
RAPID	Reteplase vs Alteplase Patency Investigation During myocardial infarction
RITA	Randomized Intervention Treatment of Angina
SAS	Specific Activity Scale
SAVE	Survival and Ventricular Enlargement (trial)
SIP	Sickness Impact Profile
SOLVD	Studies of Left Ventricular Dysfunction
TIMI	Thrombolysis in Myocardial Infarction
TREND	Trial on Reversing Endothelial Dysfunction
WOSCOPS	West of Scotland Coronary Prevention Study

Grading of recommendations and levels of evidence used in *Evidence Based Cardiology*

GRADE A

Level 1a   Evidence from large randomized clinical trials (RCTs) or systematic reviews (including meta-analyses) of multiple randomized trials which collectively has at least as much data as one single well-defined trial.

Level 1b   Evidence from at least one "All or None" high quality cohort study; in which ALL patients died/failed with conventional therapy and some survived/succeeded with the new therapy (eg chemotherapy for tuberculosis, meningitis, or defibrillation for ventricular fibrillation); or in which many died/failed with conventional therapy and NONE died/failed with the new therapy (eg penicillin for pneumococcal infections).

Level 1c   Evidence from at least one moderate sized RCT or a meta-analysis of small trials which collectively only has a moderate number of patients.

Level 1d   Evidence from at least one RCT.

GRADE B

Level 2   Evidence from at least one high quality study of non-randomized cohorts who did and did not receive the new therapy.

Level 3   Evidence from at least one high quality case control study.

Level 4   Evidence from at least one high quality case series.

GRADE C

Level 5   Opinions from experts without reference or access to any of the foregoing (eg argument from physiology, bench research or first principles).

A comprehensive approach would incorporate many different types of evidence (eg RCTs, non-RCTs, epidemiologic studies, and experimental data), and examine the architecture of the information for consistency, coherence and clarity. Occasionally the evidence does not completely fit into neat compartments. For example, there may not be an RCT that demonstrates a reduction in mortality in individuals with stable angina with the use of beta-blockers, but there is overwhelming evidence that mortality is  reduced following MI. In such cases, some may recommend use of beta-blockers in angina patients with the expectation that some extrapolation from post-MI trials is warranted. This could be expressed as Grade A/C. In other instances (e.g. smoking cessation or a pacemaker for complete heart block), the non-randomized data are so overwhelmingly clear and biologically plausible that it would be reasonable to consider these interventions as Grade A.

Recommendation grades appear either in a shaded margin box with an 'R' logo as shown, or within the text, for example Grade A.

Part I
General concepts and critical appraisal

SALIM YUSUF, Editor

Grading of recommendations and levels of evidence used in *Evidence Based Cardiology*

GRADE A

Level 1a   Evidence from large randomized clinical trials (RCTs) or systematic reviews (including meta-analyses) of multiple randomized trials which collectively has at least as much data as one single well-defined trial.

Level 1b   Evidence from at least one "All or None" high quality cohort study; in which ALL patients died/failed with conventional therapy and some survived/succeeded with the new therapy (eg chemotherapy for tuberculosis, meningitis, or defibrillation for ventricular fibrillation); or in which many died/failed with conventional therapy and NONE died/failed with the new therapy (eg penicillin for pneumococcal infections).

Level 1c   Evidence from at least one moderate sized RCT or a meta-analysis of small trials which collectively only has a moderate number of patients.

Level 1d   Evidence from at least one RCT.

GRADE B

Level 2   Evidence from at least one high quality study of non-randomized cohorts who did and did not receive the new therapy.

Level 3   Evidence from at least one high quality case control study.

Level 4   Evidence from at least one high quality case series.

GRADE C

Level 5   Opinions from experts without reference or access to any of the foregoing (eg argument from physiology, bench research or first principles).

A comprehensive approach would incorporate many different types of evidence (eg RCTs, non-RCTs, epidemiologic studies, and experimental data), and examine the architecture of the information for consistency, coherence and clarity. Occasionally the evidence does not completely fit into neat compartments. For example, there may not be an RCT that demonstrates a reduction in mortality in individuals with stable angina with the use of beta-blockers, but there is overwhelming evidence that mortality is reduced following MI. In such cases, some may recommend use of beta-blockers in angina patients with the expectation that some extrapolation from post-MI trials is warranted. This could be expressed as Grade A/C. In other instances (e.g. smoking cessation or a pacemaker for complete heart block), the non-randomized data are so overwhelmingly clear and biologically plausible that it would be reasonable to consider these interventions as Grade A.

Recommendation grades appear either in a shaded margin box with an 'R' logo as shown, or within the text, for example Grade A.

Approaches to evaluating evidence

ALLAN KITCHING,
DAVID SACKETT,
SALIM YUSUF

As physicians, whether serving individual patients or populations, we always have sought to base our decisions and actions on the best possible evidence. The ascendancy of the randomized clinical trial and similarly rigorous strategies for determining the efficacy of therapeutic interventions, the accuracy of diagnostic tests, and the validity of prognostic decision rules have created a fundamental shift in the way that we establish the clinical bases for diagnosis, prognosis, and therapeutics. In selecting a treatment, previously it had been considered sufficient to understand the pathophysiological process in a disorder and to prescribe drugs or other treatments that had been shown to interrupt or otherwise modify this process. However, there is increasing awareness that such approaches are insufficient and must be complemented by demonstration of clinical benefit in humans before new therapies are accepted as being worthwhile. Thus, the observation that patients with frequent ventricular ectopic beats following myocardial infarction were at high risk of sudden death,[1] coupled with the demonstration that these extra beats could be suppressed by specific drugs, formed a sufficient rationale for the initial widespread prescription of these drugs to postinfarction patients with unstable cardiac rhythms.[2] However, subsequent randomized clinical trials examined outcomes, not processes, and showed that several of these drugs increased, rather than decreased, the risk of death in such patients, and their use for this purpose is now strongly discouraged.[3]

On the other hand, clinicians refused to be swayed by equally persuasive pathophysiological arguments favouring the use of thrombolytic drugs in suspected myocardial infarction, and insisted on evidence from rigorous randomized clinical trials of sufficient size to determine whether this intervention could reduce deaths. Furthermore, these data were sufficiently large to quantify both the degree of benefit and risk. Now, after a series of landmark trials involving over 50 000 patients, these interventions are being applied both in and out of hospitals all over the world.[4]

The irony in this pair of examples is underscored when we recognize that the number of impending-infarction patients we need to treat with thrombolytics to save a life is the same as the number of unstable postinfarction patients we need to treat with encainide and flecainide to lose a life! The need for valid, objective evidence, generated among suitable patients through the application of both best medical thought and best research methods, has led to the development of evidence based cardiology.

WHAT IS EVIDENCE BASED CARDIOLOGY?

By "evidence based cardiology" we mean the conscientious, explicit, and judicious use of current best evidence in making decisions about the care of individual patients with cardiac problems.[5] The practice of evidence based cardiology requires integrating individual clinical expertise with the best available external clinical evidence from systematic research. By individual clinical expertise we mean the proficiency and judgment that we individual clinicians acquire through clinical experience and clinical practice. Our increased expertise is reflected in many ways, but especially in more effective and efficient diagnosis and in the more thoughtful identification and compassionate consideration of individual patients' predicaments, rights, and preferences in making clinical decisions about their care. By best available external clinical evidence we mean clinically relevant research, often from the basic sciences of cardiology, but especially from patient centred clinical research into the accuracy and precision of diagnostic tests (including the clinical examination), the power of prognostic markers, and the efficacy and safety of therapeutic, rehabilitative, and preventive regimens.

Good doctors use both individual clinical expertise and the best available external evidence, and neither alone is enough. Without clinical expertise, practice risks becoming tyrannized by external evidence, for even excellent external evidence may be inapplicable to or inappropriate for an individual patient. Without current best external evidence, even the most compassionate and skilled of us risks becoming rapidly out of date, to the detriment of patients. Thus, the practice of evidence based cardiology is a process of lifelong, self-directed learning in which caring for our own patients creates the need for clinically important information about diagnosis, prognosis, therapy, and other clinical and health care issues, and in which we:

1. convert these information needs into answerable questions;
2. track down, with maximum efficiency, the best evidence with which to answer them;
3. critically appraise that evidence for its validity (closeness to the truth) and usefulness (clinical applicability);
4. integrate that appraisal with our clinical expertise and apply the results in our clinical practice; and
5. evaluate our performance.

Evidence based medicine is one of several disciplines that has evolved from clinical epidemiology and critical appraisal. Parallel developments, still with the individual patient as the focus of attention, are occurring in other clinical disciplines (evidence based surgery, evidence based nursing, evidence based dentistry, etc.). Other evidence based disciplines consider the community as the focus of attention rather than the individual patient (evidence based public health), or add an explicit economic element and seek to purchase or provide that mix of health care that will maximize some group or public benefit (evidence based purchasing). An appropriate global term for all of these is "evidence based health care", or EBHC.

AND WHAT IS IT NOT?

This description of what evidence based cardiology can properly be said to be, also helps clarify what evidence based cardiology is *not*. Evidence based cardiology is neither old hat nor so esoteric and theoretical that it is impossible to practice. The argument that "everyone is doing it already" falls before evidence of striking variations in both the integration of patient values into our clinical behavior[6] and in the varying rates with which we provide effective cardiovascular interventions to our patients. The argument that evidence based cardiology can be conducted only from ivory towers and armchairs is refuted by audits in the front lines of clinical care, where an inpatient clinical team in general medicine in the United Kingdom (where a major proportion of patients present with cardiovascular disorders) provided evidence based care to the vast majority of their patients,[7] by the striking increase in the rates of use of proven therapies and decrease in unproven therapies in selected coronary care units in Canada,[8] and by the use of evidence based approaches to the management of acute myocardial infarction in a registry of 14 hospitals in South India.[9] Such studies show that busy clinicians who devote their scarce reading time to selective, efficient, patient-driven searching, appraisal and incorporation of the best available evidence can practice evidence based cardiology.

External clinical evidence can inform, but can never replace, individual clinical expertise, and it is this expertise that decides whether the external evidence applies to the individual patient at all and, if so, how it should be integrated into a clinical decision. Similarly, any external guideline must be integrated with individual clinical expertise in deciding whether and how it matches the patient's clinical state, predicament, and preferences, and thus whether it should be applied.

Some fear that evidence based cardiology will be hijacked by purchasers and managers to cut the costs of health care. This confuses evidence based cardiology with the related discipline (described above) of evidence based purchasing. Doctors practicing evidence based cardiology will identify and apply the most efficacious interventions to maximize the quality and quantity of life for individual patients; this may raise rather than lower the cost of their care. In practicing evidence based cardiology, clinicians work in concert with colleagues engaged in evidence based purchasing, adopting strategies that benefit both individual patients and society at large (by abandoning useless procedures, employing less expensive but equally beneficial interventions, and adopting effective interventions that lower future costs), by agreeing to follow guidelines which are scientifically based, accepting waiting lists when these are based on sound economic analyses and do not put patients at undue risks, and by openly addressing situations in which pursuing the interests of individual patients is balanced with broader societal goals. With an evidence based approach the most appropriate and rational decision can be made.

Evidence based cardiology is not restricted to randomized clinical trials and meta-analyses. It involves tracking down the best external evidence with which to answer our clinical questions. The next section of this chapter will summarize the key clinical and methodological factors that characterize the best evidence.

EVIDENCE IN CARDIOLOGY

Our opening paragraphs provide examples and reasons of why we need valid evidence from methodologically rigorous human investigations when drawing conclusions about how we should care for patients (especially when we do so as members of expert panels or consensus groups who are making general recommendations or creating guidelines). In subsequent sections, we approach different kinds of problems that are encountered in practice and suggest ways of seeking "Level 1" evidence for each type of problem. We summarize the general approach in several displays. These "user's guides" have a common format regardless of the type of clinical problem (etiology, diagnosis, prognosis, therapy or prevention) and in each case three broad questions must be asked: *Are the study results valid? What are the study results?* and, *How will the study results help me care for my patient?* From these broad questions one must ask more detailed questions about the particular study design and analysis of results.

Although for interventions we generally advocate a rigorous point of view and prefer reliable and high level evidence from a systematic review (ideally, of individual patient data) of all relevant randomized clinical trials that include a sufficiently large number of patients (or remain silent when we lack such evidence), often we settle for less (for example, smaller trials, trials with surrogate outcomes and occasionally observational databases or case series) when making immediate decisions about the management of individual patients.

Evidence about etiology

You and your colleagues would like to know the commonest cause for congestive heart failure. Based on your hospital practice in a cardiology unit you believe that it is coronary artery disease and you set out to verify this by asking the question "What is the most likely predisposing factor for the development of congestive heart failure?" A quick search of the local library's computerized medical database reveals a report by Levy *et al.*[10] which appears to answer the question.

Are the study results valid? Assessment of the validity of a study of disease etiology requires a basic knowledge of study design, which will be reviewed here briefly.

A common study design to investigate etiology of disease is the case–control study. In this study design the investigators identify individuals who have developed the outcome of interest – in this case congestive heart failure – and a second group of individuals without the outcome of interest, and enquire into possible risk factors that may have led to this condition, such as hypertension. Such a study is useful in the sense that the outcome of interest is already present and therefore an answer can be obtained in a relatively short period of time. The disadvantages of the study design are that the direction of enquiry is not forward in time and therefore it is sometimes hard to make inferences about the cause and effect relationship between the factor of interest and outcome. In addition, the search for possible causal factors is made difficult as you are searching into the patient's past, relying on the completeness of the patient's memory or medical records. Finally, it is possible that the condition or a treatment may affect the risk factor of interest requiring care in the interpretation of the cause and effect relationship. For example, a myocardial infarction may lower blood pressure and so, if high blood pressure causes myocardial infarctions this will only be obvious if blood pressure is recorded before and not after the myocardial infarction.

A stronger study design is the cohort study. In this study design the investigators divide patients into two groups based on whether or not the individuals have been exposed to the putative causal factor and then followed to determine the frequency of the outcome of interest. The advantages of this study design are that the direction of enquiry is forward in time and the risk factors are usually measured with less confounding. However, if the disease is rare or takes a long time to develop, this study would be impractical.

A third potential study design would be that often called an analytic survey or ecologic study in which different populations (for example, blacks versus white Europeans or those in different countries) with known differences in a key risk factor are compared for the incidence of the outcome of interest. Such studies have the advantage that wider differences in a risk factor usually exist between populations but the disadvantage is that of additional confounders which may be hard to measure.

The final possible study design is that of the randomized clinical trial. In this case a group of individuals who have not developed the outcome of interest and have not been exposed, would be randomly allocated to two groups, with one group being exposed to the putative causal agent (or treatment) and the other group not exposed. Although this is one of the few forms of true experiments in clinical studies, it would be generally impractical and unethical purposely to expose a group of patients to something that could potentially be harmful. An alternative to inducing hypertension in one group of patients would be to take a group of hypertensive patients and randomly allocate them to two treatment groups, one group which has its hypertension treated and the other group not, and again looking for the outcome of interest, in this case frequency of congestive heart failure. However, it would again be considered unethical to withhold treatment from a group of individuals when it is known to be beneficial.

The study by Levy *et al.* is a cohort study. Two groups of individuals, initially free of congestive heart failure, were prospectively followed and the incidence of congestive heart failure determined. One group is hypertensive (SBP >139 mmHg or DBP >89 mmHg or use of medications for treatment of hypertension at beginning of the study) and the other group is normotensive. Ideally, the two study groups should be similar other than exposure to the putative causal agent. A review of important demographic and clinical characteristics of the hypertensive and normotensive patients in the study by Levy *et al.* reveals that the hypertensive group is older, more likely to have other risk factors for coronary artery disease and more likely to have manifest coronary artery disease. Adjustment of these prognostic factors left hypertension as a strong independent predictor for the development of congestive heart failure.

Questions that must be asked when considering the validity of study results (Figure 1.1) include whether exposures and outcomes were measured the same way in both study groups. In case-control studies bias may be introduced during the process of ascertaining exposures. Individuals with the outcome of interest may be more likely to recall an exposure than control subjects or admit to an exposure when probed by an interviewer. In cohort studies or randomized clinical trials bias can be introduced during the process of ascertaining outcomes. An investigator may search more thoroughly for a disease in an individual known to have been exposed to a putative causal factor. In the study by Levy *et al.* objective criteria for the diagnosis of congestive heart failure were constructed and applied equally to the hypertensive and normotensive patients in an effort to minimize bias. Follow-up of study patients must be of appropriate duration

Are the results of the study valid?
1 Were there clearly defined groups of patients, similar in all important ways other than exposure to the putative cause? If not, were these differences accounted for in a stratified or adjusted analysis?
2 Were exposures and clinical outcomes measured the same ways in both groups?
3 Was the follow-up of study patients complete and long enough?
4 Do the results satisfy some "diagnostic tests for causation"?
  • Is it clear that the exposure preceded the onset of the outcome?
  • Is there a dose–response gradient?
  • Is the association consistent from study to study?
  • Does the association make biological sense?

What are the study results?
Levy D, Larson MG, Vasan RS *et al.* The progression from hypertension to congestive heart failure. *JAMA* 1996;**275**:1557–62.

An inception cohort study of the original Framingham Heart Study and Framingham Offspring Study participants aged 40 to 89 years and originally free of congestive heart failure. Those with (2502) and those without (2641) a diagnosis of hypertension were followed for a mean of 14.1 years and the subsequent development of congestive heart failure.

		Congestive heart failure		Totals
		Present (Case)	Absent (Control)	
Hypertension	Yes (Cohort)	357 a	2145 b	a+b 2502
	No (Cohort)	c 35	d 2606	c+d 2641
	Totals	a+c 392	b+d 4751	a+b+c+d 5143

In a cohort study: Relative Risk (RR)=[a/(a+b)]/[c/(c+d)]=11

Figure 1.1 Approaches to evaluating evidence about etiology.

and completeness as well. The duration of follow-up must fit with the expected natural history of disease linking exposure and outcome. It is important to account for the outcome of as many of the patients who started in the study as possible as the outcomes of individuals who are unavailable for follow-up are likely to be different from those who remain in the study. If more individuals are missing from follow-up from one exposure group than the other, then the validity of the study results may be questioned.

The study of Levy *et al.* also finds that the exposure (hypertension) preceded the onset of the outcome (congestive heart failure), there was a dose–response gradient, with individuals with a higher systolic or diastolic blood pressure at the beginning of the study having a greater frequency of congestive heart failure than individuals with lower systolic or diastolic blood pressures, the association between hypertension and the development of congestive heart failure is consistent with that found in other investigations[11–13] and the association makes biologic sense with increasing evidence that left ventricular hypertrophy and diastolic dysfunction play an additional role in the development of symptoms of congestive heart failure.

What are the study results? The results of the study by Levy *et al.* investigating the progression from hypertension to congestive heart failure are presented in Figure 1.1. One useful measure of expressing the degree of association between an exposure and outcome is the relative risk ratio. The relative risk ratio is the rate of the risk of the outcome of interest in the exposed group divided by the risk of the outcome in the unexposed group. Because the risk of developing the outcome of interest is the same as the incidence of the outcome, the relative risk reduction is only appropriately applied to the results of prospective studies. The odds ratio, which provides an approximation of the relative risk reduction, is employed to present the results of retrospective studies such as the case–control study. The data presented in Figure 1.1. indicate that there were 357 cases of congestive heart failure among 2502 hypertensives (14.3%) compared to 35 cases of congestive heart failure among 2641 normotensives (1.3%). The relative risk ratio $[a/(a+b)]/[c/(c+d)]$ is 11. That is, the risk of developing congestive heart failure is 11 times as great for those with a history of hypertension than for those without such a history of hypertension. Using more sophisticated multivariable mathematical techniques which allow one to better describe the relationship between two or more variables the authors were able to adjust for differences in age and other risk factors for congestive heart failure between the two study groups and find that the risk of developing congestive heart failure was about two-fold in men and three-fold in women with a history of hypertension in comparison to normotensive study subjects. We now know that hypertension is a strong independent risk factor for the development of congestive heart failure but this does not tell us whether it is the most important risk factor. This requires assessing the proportion of all cases of congestive heart failure in a population that is attributable to hypertension. The absolute attributable risk is calculated by subtracting the risk of developing congestive heart failure for individuals without a history of hypertension from the risk of developing congestive heart failure in individuals with a history of hypertension and dividing this by the risk of developing congestive heart failure for individuals without a history of hypertension. Multivariable analyses in the study by Levy *et al.* indicate that hypertension is responsible for 39% of cases of congestive heart failure in men and 59% in women, placing it as the leading known cause for the disease in western society.

How will the study results help me care for my patient? The study of Levy *et al.* indicates that asymptomatic individuals need to be screened for hypertension, appropriately diagnosed and treated in order to prevent congestive heart failure as well as stroke.

Evidence about diagnosis

You are asked to see a young man on the internal medicine ward service with a clinical diagnosis of bacterial endocarditis. A transthoracic echocardiogram is performed which shows independently mobile masses, consistent with vegetations, associated with a bicuspid aortic valve. The infectious disease consultant requests a transesophageal echocardiogram. You review the transthoracic study with your colleague and there is general agreement that the study is of good quality and that the clinical and echocardiographic diagnosis is correct. However, the infectious disease consultant feels that a transesophageal echocardiogram may provide more useful information with respect to the patient's clinical course. Specifically, he is concerned that a transthoracic echocardiographic study alone may miss perivalvular abscesses which are known to increase the rate of major morbid and mortal events in these patients. The transesophageal study is arranged and you visit the library in an effort to find an answer to the question "What is the incremental value of performing a transesophageal echocardiogram, in addition to a transthoracic echocardiogram, in detecting perivalvular abscesses associated with endocarditis?" A search of the literature uncovers what appears to be a useful report by Daniel et al.[14]

Are the results of the study valid? The accuracy of a diagnostic test can only be determined by comparing it to the "truth". This is usually performed by comparing the results of a diagnostic test to a "gold standard" of diagnosis. A diagnostic test worthy of consideration as a gold standard for the presence of a target disorder is defined as a definitive test as determined by biopsy, autopsy, or surgery. A gold standard for the absence of a target disorder may be defined as a benign clinical course in the absence of active therapy. The diagnostic test under investigation should be applied both to patients that have been found to have the disorder of interest and to those patients found not to have the disorder of interest as determined by the gold standard. In the study of Daniel et al., patients were categorized as having endocarditis with abscesses or without abscesses as determined by surgical exploration or direct inspection and histopathological examination at autopsy (gold standard).

Transthoracic and transesophageal echocardiography were applied to both groups of patients. Ideally, the results of the diagnostic test under investigation should be interpreted by physicians who do not know whether a specific patient does or does not have the disorder of interest. Investigators in this study were "blind" to the outcome of interest (the presence or absence of abscesses) as the echocardiographic examinations were performed before surgery or death and autopsy (the gold standard of diagnosis). Other considerations include whether the diagnostic test under investigation was applied to patients generally seen in clinical practice. That is, did the study include an appropriate spectrum of patients with mild and severe and treated and untreated disease and similar conditions that may be confused with the target disorder. Finally, one should determine whether the diagnostic test under investigation influenced the decision to perform the gold standard diagnostic test thus allowing verification or work-up bias. In the study by Daniel et al. the criteria for cardiovascular surgery (gold standard) was clinical and no patient went on to valve replacement because of echocardiographic detection of perivalvular abscesses.

What are the results? The results of the study of Daniel et al. are outlined in Figure 1.2. The simplest way to analyse the data in display would be to calculate the accuracy of the diagnostic test examined and this would be performed by adding the number of true positives and the number of true negatives $(a+d)$ and dividing this by the total number of observations made $(a+b+c+d)$, which in this case is about 93% for transesophageal echocardiography. A similar table can be constructed with the data presented in the study report for transthoracic echocardiography and the calculated accuracy is about 77%. The problem with reporting only the overall accuracy of a diagnostic test is that valuable information regarding the rate of false positives and

Are the study results valid?
1   Was there an independent, blind comparison (or unbiased comparison) with a reference ("gold") standard of diagnosis?
2   Was the diagnostic test evaluated in an appropriate spectrum of patients (like those in whom it would be used in practice)?
3   Was the reference standard applied regardless of the diagnostic test result?

What are the results?
Daniel WG, Mugge A, Martin RP *et al.* Improvement in the diagnosis of abscesses associated with endocarditis by transesophageal echocardiography. *N Engl J Med* 1991;**324**:795–800.

Prospective examination, by transthoracic and transesophageal echocardiography, of 118 consecutive patients with infective endocarditis of 137 native or prosthetic valves documented at surgery or autopsy.

Results for transesophageal echocardiography:

		Number of patients with perivalvular abscesses		Totals
		Present	Absent	
Transesophageal echocardiography	Positive	40 a	4 b	44 a+b
	Negative	c 4	d 70	c+d 74
		a+c	b+d	a+b+c+d
	Totals	44	74	118

See text for complete definitions of terms.

Accuracy = $(a+d)/(a+b+c+d) = (40+70)/(40+4+4+70) = 0.93$
Sensitivity = $a/(a+c) = 40/(40+4) = 0.91$
Specificity = $d/(b+d) = 70/(70+4) = 0.95$
Likelihood Ratio (positive result) = sens/(1−spec) = $0.91/(1−0.95) = 18$
Likelihood Ratio (negative result) = (1−sens)/spec = $(1−0.91)/0.95 = 0.1$
Prevalence = $(a+c)/(a+b+c+d) = (40+4)/(40+4+4+70) = 0.37$
Positive Predictive Value = $a/(a+b) = 40/(40+4) = 0.91$
Negative Predictive Value = $d/(c+d) = 70/(4+70) = 0.95$

Figure 1.2   Approaches to evaluating evidence about diagnosis.

negatives is lost. It is common to calculate two basic additional descriptors of the results of a diagnostic test and this includes the sensitivity and the specificity. The sensitivity, or the rate of a true positive result in individuals with the disease of interest (cardiac abscess), is calculated using $a/(a+c)$ and is about 93% for transesophageal echocardiography and 41% for transthoracic echocardiography. The specificity, or the rate of a true negative result in individuals without the disease of interest $(d/(b+d))$, is 91% for transesophageal echocardiography and 99% for transthoracic echocardiography. In other words, if an abscess is seen by transthoracic or transesophageal echocardiography you can say with a high degree of certainty (high specificity) that an abscess is present. If an abscess is not seen by transthoracic echocardiography you are not as confident (low sensitivity) of ruling it out as you would be when an abscess is not visualized by transesophageal echocardiography (high sensitivity).

The use of sensitivity and specificity may seem a little odd to some since these measures are derived from knowledge of the results of applying the results of a gold standard. If the results of a gold standard are available then why get involved with the use of other less definitive diagnostic tests? However, in many situations the results of a gold standard of diagnosis are not available, or if applied would place the patient at undue risk. To get around this problem some prefer to use positive and negative predictive values. The positive predictive value is determined by dividing the number of true positives by the total number of individuals in which a positive result was found $(a/(a+b))$. The negative predictive value is likewise calculated by dividing the number of true negatives by the total number of individuals in which a negative result was found $(d/(c+d))$. For transesophageal echocardiography the values for positive and negative predictive values are 91% and 95%. For transthoracic echocardiography the values for positive and negative predictive values are 95% and 74%. Therefore in all patients with perivalvular abscesses visualized by transesophageal or transthoracic echocardiography approximately the same proportion (91–95%) truly have abscesses as determined by surgery or autopsy. However, the superiority of transesophageal echocardiography over transthoracic echocardiography is demonstrated by the higher negative predictive value (95% vs 74%), in which a number of abscesses were missed by the transthoracic approach. These measures may be more helpful in that they tell you what proportion of individuals with a positive or negative test result are truly likely to have the disease of interest but the validity of these values is dependent on the prevalence of the disease in the population of interest. It is the stable properties of the sensitivity and specificity that make these measures appealing in evaluating and comparing the use of different diagnostic tests.

The sensitivity and specificity can be manipulated to calculate likelihood ratios for positive and negative test results that may be more useful to clinicians. Likelihood ratios indicate to what degree the results of a diagnostic test raise or lower the pretest probability of a target disorder. For transesophageal echocardiogram the likelihood ratio for a positive test result is 18 in comparison to about 4 for that generated by a transthoracic echocardiogram. The likelihood ratio for a negative test result is 0.1 and 0.07 for transesophageal and transthoracic echocardiography respectively. A likelihood ratio of 1 indicates that the post-test probability of disease is no different from that of the pretest probability of disease. In general, a likelihood ratio of greater than 10 and less than 0.1 indicate conclusive changes from pretest to post-test probability of disease.

How will the study results help me care for my patient? A number of additional questions must be asked in order to assist the clinician in applying the results of a diagnostic test to a specific patient. In the case of transesophageal echocardiography, which appears to have incremental value in the evaluation of the patient with endocarditis in the identification of abscesses, one must determine whether the procedure is readily available and performed by someone with the proper training and ability to interpret the results. It is generally a well tolerated procedure, with little risk to the patient. The likelihood ratios generated by both a positive or negative test result would be in the range that would assist the clinician in making a definitive diagnosis and likely should be performed in patients with a diagnosis of endocarditis by transthoracic echocardiography. In general, transthoracic echocardiograms are performed first in the evaluation of an individual with suspected endocarditis. This approach is safe, readily available, and provides standardized views to best assess overall cardiac structure and function as well as endocardial surfaces for evidence of endocarditis. The results of the study by Daniel *et al.* indicate that there is incremental value in then performing a transesophageal echocardiogram. The transesophageal approach is an invasive procedure but is quite safe in the hands of an experienced operator. The chance of identifying by transesophageal echocardiogram abscesses that were missed by the transthoracic approach is greater if the aortic valve is involved and the organism isolated is a *Staphylococcus* species.

Evidence about prognosis

A running argument on your clinical service concerns whether you should be seeking and treating depression in patients recovering from myocardial infarction. You decide to put the discussion on an evidence base by examining the data yourself. You formulate the question: "Among survivors of myocardial infarction, does co-existent depression worsen survival?" A few minutes spent searching the prognosis section of Best Evidence[15] (with the free text terms "depression and infarction") yields a useful cohort study, and you study both the abstract[16] and the original article.[17]

Are the results of the study valid? Assessing a study investigating the role of one or more prognostic factors for a disease requires an understanding of the clinical course of the disease. The clinical course of a disease begins at the time of correct diagnosis and is a component of the natural history of the disease that begins at the time of biologic onset, which may be years before the time of possible diagnosis or usual diagnosis. As most diseases have some form of treatment, some more successful than others, the clinical course of disease is often modified by the treatments applied. It is important, in studying the clinical course of a disease and the factors that may influence prognosis, to make sure that the individuals being studied are all at the same approximate point in the clinical course of the disease. For example, if you studied a group of individuals who had been diagnosed many years previously and were presumably late in the clinical course of their disease you may miss the opportunity to study those individuals with recent diagnoses. In some of these individuals the disease may have taken a different form, resulting in a cure or early death and the exclusion of these patients would prevent one from determining the factors that predict a good or poor outcome. It is for this reason that it is suggested that studies of prognosis use an inception cohort of study subjects with all individuals at the same point in the clinical course of the disease, such as at first diagnosis.

Knowledge of the clinical course of disease is also helpful in determining whether the follow-up period used in the study is sufficiently long. Too short a follow-up period in a disease with a long clinical course may result in the identification of too few outcome events of interest, making the results of the study less useful. The clinical course of disease usually results in complete cure, death or one or more morbid events resulting in some degree of disability. It is important that all outcome criteria are determined in an unbiased way as possible and with the use of predefined objective criteria. Vague criteria for outcomes applied in a haphazard way would allow outcome assessors the

---

Is this evidence about prognosis valid?
1 Was a defined, representative sample of patients assembled at a common point in the course of their disease?
2 Was the patient follow-up sufficiently long and complete?
3 Were objective outcome criteria applied in an unbiased fashion?
4 If subgroups with different prognoses are identified, was there adjustment for other important prognostic factors?
5 Was there validation of any prognostic factors in an independent group "test-set" of patients?

Is this valid evidence about prognosis important?
1 How likely are the outcomes over time?
2 How precise are the prognostic estimates?

Can you apply this valid, important evidence about prognosis in caring for your patient?
1 Were the study patients similar to your own?
2 Will this evidence make a clinically important impact on your conclusions about what to offer or tell your patient?

Figure 1.3 Approaches to evaluating evidence about prognosis.

opportunity to consciously or unconsciously assign better or worse outcomes to patients with different prognostic factors, thus rendering the results of the study useless by providing an erroneous picture of the disease's clinical course. Individuals with a specific disease can also be categorized into different subgroups which may have a different prognosis independent of the prognostic factors under study. For example, age is often linked with a worse prognosis in many diseases. Therefore in the final analysis it is often important to assess the relationship between the prognostic factor(s) and the outcome of the disease by adjusting for other important prognostic factors.

Applying these guides (Figure 1.3), you decide that in the study conducted by Frasure-Smith et al.[17] they assembled an appropriate sample of infarction survivors (with explicit criteria, and excluding other serious illnesses and infarctions following surgery), characterized them carefully both for depression (using an accepted standard interview) and a series of other risk factors for mortality (previous MI, left ventricular ejection fraction, Killip class, frequency of premature ventricular contractions, thrombolytic therapy, and beta-blockade and angiotensin converting enzyme inhibitor prescriptions at discharge), and followed them for at least 18 months. In addition, all deaths were reviewed independently by three cardiologists.

What are the results? Data presented by Frasure-Smith et al. indicate that 35 of 222 patients (15.8%) included in their study were diagnosed with major inhospital depression after myocardial infarction. The mortality rate among those with a diagnosis of depression was 20% (7 deaths among 35 patients) in comparison to a mortality rate of 6.4% among those without a diagnosis of depression (12 deaths among 187 patients), a result that is statistically significant. In a "simple" analysis (not taking the other prognostic factors into account), depressed patients were three times as likely to die as non-depressed patients over the 18 month follow-up, and after the investigators "corrected" the analysis by controlling for previous myocardial infarctions, Killip class, and premature ventricular contractions, depressed patients were still at greater risk of dying of cardiac causes.

How will the study results help me care for my patient? Although it may be difficult to distinguish some of the symptoms of depression from those of low cardiac output, these results impress you enough to conclude that depression is a predictor of or is associated with a poor prognosis following myocardial infarction. This does not necessarily mean that treating depression will lead to an improved outcome. It has yet to be determined whether treating depression in survivors of a myocardial infarction has a beneficial effect.

Evidence about therapy or prevention

Your colleague is concerned about the safety of digoxin in patients with congestive heart failure based on the results of a published study. The study to which your colleague refers is the study by Moss *et al.*[18] which suggested that digoxin was dangerous in patients with congestive heart failure. This study reported on 972 patients who were retrospectively identified and followed-up after suffering a myocardial infarction. Four months after their myocardial infarction 21 of the 189 patients (11%) treated with digoxin for signs or symptoms of heart failure had died in comparison to the 24 deaths among 783 patients (3%) not treated with digoxin.

Are the results of the study valid? Careful examination of the study by Moss *et al.* reveals a number of methodologic concerns. First and foremost the patients in the study of Moss *et al.* were not allocated to digoxin or no digoxin treatment in any systematic way. Analysis of the report finds that patients subsequently treated with digoxin were likely to be more ill, with greater frequency of signs or symptoms of more severe left ventricular dysfunction and ventricular and/or supraventricular tachyarrhythmias or other markers of poor prognosis, such as previous myocardial infarction or diabetes. It is therefore unfair to compare mortality between these two very different groups. The authors therefore "adjusted" the results using statistical methods to account for these differences in markers of prognosis. Such statistical adjustments have questionable value because they depend on a number of contestable assumptions. These assumptions include that all important prognostic factors are known (which is usually unlikely), that information on these prognostic factors has been obtained in a reasonably standardized manner and is complete (rarely the case in a retrospective database), that these prognostic factors have been measured precisely (because errors in the measurement of these prognostic factors tend to underestimate its relationship with the outcome of interest), that the statistical "model" describing the relationship between the prognostic factors and the outcome derived from the current data set will hold true for future data sets (very unlikely) and that complex interactions between risk factors are accounted for. These considerations would make us skeptical about the reliability of such approaches. Most importantly, no degree of statistical modeling can fully capture the complex reasoning that a clinician uses to decide why he/she prescribed digoxin to a specific patient and not to another. These considerations led to the development of the randomized trial as the gold standard for the evaluation of treatments.

It is generally agreed that a randomized clinical trial is the best method of determining the value of a particular therapeutic agent or maneuver. A randomized clinical trial compares outcomes in a group of patients to which a test treatment has been applied with those observed in a comparable group of patients receiving a control treatment. For example, the control treatment may be no treatment, a placebo or an established drug considered part of standard therapy. Ideally the patients in the treatment and control groups would be identical in every way (both utilizing known and unknown risk factors) and therefore any differences in the rate of outcomes between the two groups could be attributed to the different treatments. However, in real life, patients differ in severity of their illness and other comorbid conditions (both known and unknown), all of which can affect prognosis. It is for this reason that a proper clinical trial must randomly allocate patients to the treatment and control groups in an effort to balance known, as well as potentially unknown, determinants of outcome. Other important methodologic features that you should carefully look for include unbiased assessment of the outcome(s) of interest and appropriate and complete follow-up of study patients. Knowledge of treatment assignment may potentially cause some physicians and patients to consciously or subconsciously alter treatment or their reporting of treatment outcomes. Blinding of patients, physicians and others to treatment assignment should minimize this threat to study validity. In some situations (trials evaluating a surgical procedure or trials of lifestyle modification) blinding may not be possible. In such cases, unbiased and blinded evaluation of the outcome(s) of interest is practicable and is usually valid. The validity of the conclusions of a study are also enhanced if every patient allocated to either treatment or control group is accounted for at the study conclusion. Missing patients often have a different prognosis, either better or worse, from the patients who have stayed in the study and an imbalance in the distribution of these patients may seriously undermine your confidence in the study results and conclusions. Furthermore, the reasons for omission may differ between the two comparison groups (side effects in one group and lack of efficacy in another group). Study results should be presented using a management or intention-to-treat analysis in which all outcomes that occur after randomization are attributed to the group assigned at the time of randomization. This method helps to minimize the threats to study validity that may be introduced by any post-randomization decisions made by patients or their physicians. You therefore decide to base your judgment on the impact of a large trial which was specifically designed to address the impact of digoxin on mortality.

The effect of digoxin on mortality and morbidity in patients with congestive heart failure was tested in a proper randomized clinical trial performed and reported by the Digitalis Investigation Group.[19] A total of 3397 patients with a documented left ventricular ejection fraction less than or equal to 45%, were randomly allocated to treatment with digoxin 0.25 mg each day while 3403 patients with similar baseline characteristics were allocated to placebo therapy. Allocation of patients to treatment groups was blinded as were outcome assessors and patients. Patients were followed for an average of 37 months with a minimum of loss to follow-up. Mortality and major morbid outcomes were described in a standardized way.

What were the results? There were 1181 deaths among 3397 patients (34.8%) assigned to digoxin therapy and 1194 deaths among 3403 patients (35.1%) assigned to placebo. The difference was not statistically significant. However, treatment with digoxin did result in a significant reduction in the rate of hospitalization for symptoms of congestive heart failure (Figure 1.4). There was a significant decrease in risk of death and hospitalization due to worsening congestive heart failure.

A simple method of evaluating the efficacy of a therapy tested in a randomized clinical trial would be to calculate and compare the risks of the outcome of interest occurring between the two or more treatment groups (such as those that did and did not receive digoxin). As outlined in Figure 1.4, the risk of hospitalization for worsening congestive heart failure was 26.8% in those treated with digoxin and 34.7% for those not treated

Are the results of this single therapeutic trial valid?

The main questions to answer

1   Was the assignment of patients to treatments randomized?
    – and was the randomization list concealed?
2   Aside from the experimental treatment, were the groups generally similar?
3   Were all patients who entered the trial accounted for at its conclusion?
    – and were they analysed in the groups to which they were randomized?
4   Were outcomes assessed without bias?
5   Was the study large enough to reliably detect or exclude a clinically important
    difference?

Are the results of this valid trial important?

The Digitalis Investigation Group. The effect of digoxin on mortality and morbidity in
    patients with heart failure. *N Engl J Med* 1997;**336**:525–33.

Randomized clinical trial in which patients with left ventricular ejection fractions of
    45% or less were randomaly allocated to digoxin (3397) or placebo (3403) in
    addition to diuretics and angiotensin converting enzyme inhibitors and were
    followed on average for 37 months. Primary outcome was all-cause mortality.
    Secondary outcomes were cardiovascular mortality, death due to worsening heart
    failure, hospitalization for worsening heart failure and hospitalization for other
    causes such as digitalis toxicity.

	Hospitalization for worsening congestive heart failure		Risk	Absolute risk reduction (ARR)	Relative risk reduction (RRR)
	Yes	No			
Digoxin	910	2487	26.8%	7.9%	22.8%
Placebo	1180	2223	34.7%		

Are these valid, potentially useful trial results applicable to your patient?

1   Do these results apply to your patient?
    (a) Is your patient so different from those in the trial that its results can't help you?
    (b) How great would the potential benefit of therapy actually be for your individual
        patient?
    (c) Are the benefits sufficiently large (or "major") to outweigh any adverse effects?
2   Are your patient's values and preferences satisfied by the regimen and its
    consequences?
    (a) Do your patient and you have a clear assessment of their values and
        preferences?
    (b) Are they met by this regimen and its consequences?

Figure 1.4 Approaches to evaluating evidence about therapy or prevention.

with digoxin. The size of this apparent benefit to digoxin therapy can be quantified by determining the absolute risk reduction (ARR) calculated by subtracting the risk of the outcome event in patients receiving the therapy under investigation (digoxin) from the risk of the outcome event in patients receiving the control therapy (placebo). The ARR in this example is 7.9%. The ARR is valuable in describing the overall number of events prevented by treating 100 patients but is weighted by the inherent risk of the patients and is less generalizable to patients at varying risks.

Another method of measuring treatment effect is to determine the relative risk reduction (RRR) which is calculated by dividing the ARR by the risk of the outcome of interest in the control (placebo) group. In our example the RRR is calculated by 7.9%/34.7% and equals 22.8%. The RRR allows one to examine the difference between two treatment groups with respect to an outcome of interest independent of the patient's inherent risk. At a single glance the physician can see that the risk of hospitalization for worsening congestive heart failure has been reduced by almost one-quarter with digoxin therapy. In general, RRRs of about 25% are almost always of clinical significance unless the inherent risk of the patient population is extremely low (less than 1%) or there is significant cost or toxicity to offset benefit.

A third option for quantifying the benefits of treatment is the determination of the number needed to treat (NNT). The NNT is calculated as the reciprocal of the ARR. In our example the NNT is approximately 13. That is, 13 patients needed to be treated with digoxin to avoid one admission to hospital with worsening congestive heart failure. There are advantages and disadvantages to each of these measures and there is no single measure of treatment effect at a single time that provides a comprehensive picture.[20]

How will the study results help me care for my patient? Once issues regarding the design, conduct and analysis of a clinical trial have been evaluated and you are confident that the results are true and the conclusions valid, then you must decide whether you can infer the conclusions from the trial to an individual patient. This is easy if your patient has the same demographic and prognostic characteristics as the patients in the clinical trial that you have just assessed. If the difference in the outcomes between the treatment and control groups, in favour of the new treatment for example, were clearly statistically significant (e.g. $P<0.001$), then presumably if the clinical trial were repeated, with your patient as a participant, the results should be generally the same. However, if your patient is different in some way then the task of applying the results becomes more involved.[21] Your patient may have the same disorder as those in the clinical trial but differ by being at greater risk of a morbid or mortal event. If the treatment effect was sufficiently large then it may be reasonable to generalize the results to your patient. Even if a significant rate of adverse effects has been reported the chance of a benefit would likely outweigh the risk in a patient already at high risk. Alternatively, your patient may differ by being at less risk than those enrolled in the clinical trial. If the treatment effect is small and the risk of an adverse event significant then you may choose not to try the new therapy on your patient until it has been properly tested on patients like yours and the benefits outweigh the risks. You may find yourself in the situation in which a clinical trial reports no overall significant clinical or statistical difference between the treatment groups but a subgroup analysis, which includes patients like yours, provides evidence for efficacy, or lack of efficacy, of the new treatment. Interpretation of subgroup analyses adds a further set of complexities and the reader is referred to two comprehensive essays on this.[22,23] Alternatively, you may have found the report of a meta-analysis combining the results of several negative clinical trials that also identifies a subgroup of patients, sufficiently similar to your own, that may benefit from a new therapy. If the difference in outcome between the treatment and control groups is clinically important and clearly statistically significant and the hypothesis tested in the subgroup of patients was stated prior to the analysis then you may be confident in applying the results of the subgroup analysis to your patient. The information that a clinician needs is whether the results observed in a subgroup analysis of a clinical trial are likely to be replicated. This depends on the statistical significance

(P<0.05 has only a 50% chance of replication whereas P<0.001 has a 90% chance of replication), how the P value was derived if the study were repeated using the same design (prospectively stated hypothesis, versus data derived or selected from several comparisons), and whether the results are supported by external evidence (e.g. other trials).

Evidence concerning overviews of interventions

Each month you and your colleagues meet to discuss matters regarding the function of your local cardiology service. Attempts are made at each meeting to review an important development in cardiology in an attempt to incorporate new findings in the diagnosis, prognosis, treatment or prevention of cardiovascular disease into current practice within the service. You also recognize that there are often several studies that address the same question. It would be useful to bring all these studies together to provide an overall judgment. This could be a qualitative review or a quantitative, systematic overview (meta-analysis). Meta-analyses of almost any kind of data are possible (e.g. meta-analysis of observational data or of randomized trials). Everyone agrees that the reporting of evidence concerning prevention and therapy in the form of a meta-analysis is an extremely valuable tool, but they are unsure as to how the validity of a meta-analysis should be determined. You are elected to provide some insights to your group as to how to interpret meta-analyses of randomized clinical trials.

In reviewing the literature you find numerous guidelines on how to assess the validity and generalizability of individual randomized clinical trials. Although evolving, there appears to be some general agreement about what makes the results of a randomized clinical trial valid. A strength of a well conducted randomized clinical trial is that all aspects are developed prospectively – a hypothesis, the intervention, the outcomes, the follow-up and the method of analysis, all of these are captured in a prospective protocol. In general, a valid and reliable systematic overview or meta-analysis needs to adhere to the same kind of guidelines regarding validity and generalizability, as do individual randomized clinical trials. It is strongly suggested that like a randomized clinical trial, a meta-analysis has a prospective protocol and identifies at least one primary medically important question. One major difference, though, which should be kept in mind, is that the question for a randomized clinical trial is always formulated before the data is collected. In contrast to this prospective approach, the hypothesis or question asked in a meta-analysis is often determined after at least some of relevant data have been examined. This process of asking the question in a retrospective manner is prone to bias as investigators could manipulate the data that is included in their meta-analysis or how it is analyzed in order to consciously or subconsciously support or refute their particular hypothesis. A key aspect of a meta-analysis is that all relevant randomized clinical trials of a question are included. Selective omissions/inclusions of certain trials could bias the results of the meta-analysis. Therefore the authors of the meta-analysis should describe in a reasonable amount of detail what criteria were established to include or reject randomized clinical trials, and how they identified the trials that they included, and why any trials were excluded. It is also important that the overview include randomized trials of comparable treatments. Although there will be a greater degree of heterogeneity in the patients, specifics of treatment and such things as follow-up, in comparison to that of a single randomized clinical trial, judgment must be used

---

Are the results of this overview valid and reliable?
1   Is it an overview of randomized trials of treatments?
2   Does it include a methods section that describes:
    (a) finding and including all the relevant trials?
    (b) assessing their individual validity?
    (c) using valid statistical methods that compared "like with like" stratified by
         study?
3   Were the results consistent from study to study?
4   Are the conclusions based on sufficiently large amounts of data to exclude a
    spurious difference (type I error) or missing a real difference (type II error).

Are these applicable to your patient?
Differences between subgroups should only be believed if you can say "yes" to all of
the following:
1   Was it hypothesised before the study began (rather than the product of dredging
    the data), and has it been confirmed in other, independent studies?
2   Was it one of just a few subgroups analyses carried out in this study?
3   Is the difference both clinically (beneficial for some but useless or harmful for
    others) and statistically significant?
4   Does it really make biologic and clinical sense?

Figure 1.5   Approaches to evaluating evidence concerning overviews.

to ensure that the combining of therapies towards a treatment of a common disorder makes clinical and biologic sense. Also, it is strongly recommended that all trials included truly allocate patients to treatment groups with random assignment. In addition, other design elements such as unbiased assessment of outcomes, that you would expect to find in individual randomized clinical trials, you would also expect to find in randomized clinical trials included in the meta-analysis. The stronger the design of the individual clinical trials, the less likely that the meta-analysis will be subject to bias.

It is essential that combination of the results of individual clinical trials should use valid methods that are primarily based on comparisons between treatment groups within a trial. The quality of data within each randomized clinical trial should be assessed by (a) exploring the integrity of the randomization process and by examining the balance of baseline characteristics between the patients in the treatment and control groups, (b) the completeness of follow-up, (c) compliance to the protocol, and (d) unbiased evaluation of outcomes. In a meta-analysis in which data are extracted from the reports of individual clinical trials, often information on all patients randomized is not available. In these cases one would hope that the authors of the meta-analysis would attempt to obtain as much of this information as possible from the authors of the individual trials. Another more involved and rigorous method is actually to combine data on individual patients. This process involves close cooperation between leaders of individual clinical trials and the statistical combination of the data tapes of individual patient data from the clinical trials into one large database. This process allows one to look for inconsistencies in the data that would normally occur if it were an individual clinical trial. Such a method will also allow one to assess the completeness of follow-up, which may also be difficult to do by simply obtaining information from the published reports of clinical trials.

You summarize by showing a list of recommended guidelines in assessing an overview of an intervention (Figure 1.5). In addition to providing an overall idea of the efficacy of a therapy, a meta-analysis can also provide a better estimate of the treatment effect with a higher degree of precision. A meta-analysis includes a larger number of patients than individual trials alone, and consequently the confidence interval around a treatment effect should be narrower, giving the clinician a better estimate of the true treatment effect. Finally, a meta-analysis, through the process of providing data on a larger number of patients, will often provide more information regarding specific subgroups of patients. Additional important questions must be asked if the results found in some of these subgroup analyses can be applied to your individual patient (Figure 1.5).

Integrating information from trials and observational data

In your attempt to find out if treatment of hypertension reduces the risk of congestive heart failure, you have examined the results of the Systolic Hypertension in the Elderly Program (SHEP) trial,[24] which showed that indeed lowering blood pressure reduced the risk of developing congestive heart failure. Although the results of this trial were convincing, you would like to examine whether the results were replicated consistently in other studies. You could peruse the few commonly quoted papers or you might decide that you wanted to know more about the totality of the data based on a quantitative overview of all relevant trials. You search the literature and discover two relevant overviews.[25,26]

On reviewing the meta-analyses by Garg and Yusuf[25] and Psaty et al.,[26] it is clear that lowering blood pressure using different drugs (diuretics, beta-blockers or angiotensin converting enzyme (ACE) inhibitors) reduces the risk of congestive heart failure, that the effect sizes are large (greater than or equal to a 50% risk reduction), estimated with substantial precision and replicated in many different trials and across a range of initial blood pressure levels. These findings are coherent with the findings from observational cohort studies where the risk of congestive heart failure in relation to blood pressure levels was continuous. You therefore extrapolate that as long as a patient has an appropriate level of risk for congestive heart failure (either due to elevated blood pressure or due to other factors or its combination), lowering blood pressure could possibly lower the risk of congestive heart failure. Some limited data supporting this come from one trial[27], the Studies of Left Ventricular Dysfunction trial (SOLVD) utilizing ACE inhibitors and therefore you prefer to use these drugs if the goal of therapy is reducing the risk of congestive heart failure.

The example above is fairly straightforward. Often the results of trials or their meta-analyses are more complex. Prior to 1991, the impact of cholesterol lowering on total mortality was much debated. Trials of primary or secondary prevention had not consistently demonstrated a reduction in total mortality. Although a meta-analysis indicated a reduction in cardiovascular mortality, this appeared to be counterbalanced by an excess of non-cardiovascular mortality. A more indepth analysis indicated that the reduction in cardiovascular deaths was paralleled by a reduction in non-fatal myocardial infarction. These benefits were related to both the degree of cholesterol lowering (trials with larger cholesterol lowering in the active versus control groups had greater benefit) and the duration of cholesterol lowering (greater benefits in longer term trials). The reduction in coronary heart disease was consistent with a vast body of experimental data, several observational cohort studies and a couple of randomized angiographic studies which demonstrated retardation of the development or progression of atherosclerosis. By contrast, the excess of non-coronary heart disease deaths did not indicate a dose–response relationship and was not supported either by strong experimental or epidemiologic data. Under the circumstances, the reduction in cardiovascular disease deaths observed in trials was considered to be more plausible than the excess of non-coronary heart disease deaths (which was more likely due to the play of chance), although the levels of statistical significance were similar in the overviews. This judgment was later proven to be valid by the future large trials evaluating "statins" in which treatment produced substantial reductions in both cholesterol and coronary heart disease mortality with little impact on non-coronary heart disease mortality. Therefore, there was a clear overall reduction in total mortality.

This discussion provides the reader with practical examples of integrating information from multiple sources and relying on the coherence of evidence from multiple methodologies. Such an integrated approach combined with good clinical skills and judgement will lead to the best practise of evidence based cardiovascular medicine.

CONCLUSIONS

In the sections above we have tried to provide the reader with approaches as to how to deal with relevant clinical problems. Different kinds of problems require different approaches. By utilizing a range of methodologic approaches and relevant information which are then coupled with good clinical judgment, the cardiologist will be well equipped to deal with problems, utilizing an evidence based approach. The remaining chapters in Part I of this book describe a number of methodologies that will be useful to clinicians as they evaluate evidence of different kinds. In Parts II and III expert clinicians and epidemiologists provide useful summaries about the state of knowledge in each area using an evidence based framework. These chapters are a fusion of both extensive "content" knowledge and indepth methodologic expertise. Part IV provides a number of case studies demonstrating practical applications of the principles of evidence based cardiology.

REFERENCES

1 Ruberman W, Weinblatt E, Goldberg JD et al. Ventricular premature beats and mortality after myocardial infarction. N Engl J Med 1977;297: 750–7.

2 Morganroth J, Bigger JT Jr, Anderson JL. Treatment of ventricular arrhythmia by United States cardiologists: a survey before the Cardiac Arrhythmia Suppression Trial results were available. Am J Cardiol 1990;65:40–8.

3 Echt DS, Liebson PR, Mitchell B et al. Mortality and morbidity in patients receiving encainide, flecainide, or placebo: the Cardiac Arrhythmia Suppression Trial. N Engl J Med 1991;324:781–8.

4 Fibrinolytic Therapy Trialists Collaborative Group. Indications for fibrinolytic therapy in suspected acute myocardial infarction: collaborative overview of early mortality and major morbidity results from all randomised trials of more than 1000 patients. Lancet 1994;343:311–22.

5 Sackett DL, Richardson WS, Rosenberg WMC, Haynes RB. Evidence-Based Medicine: How to Practise and Teach EBM. London: Churchill-Livingstone, 1997.

6 Weatherall DJ. The inhumanity of medicine. Br Med J 1994;308:1671–2.

7 Ellis J, Mulligan I, Rowe J, Sackett DL. Inpatient general medicine is evidence based. Lancet 1995; 346:407–10.

8 Tsuyuki RT, Teo KK, Ikuta RM et al. Mortality risk and patterns of practice in 2,070 patients with acute myocardial infarction, 1987–92. Relative importance of age, sex, and medical therapy. Chest 1994;105:1687–92.

9 Pais P et al. Personal communication.

10 Levy D, Larson MG, Vasan RS, Kannel WB, Ho KKL. The progression from hypertension to congestive heart failure. JAMA 1996;275: 1557–62.

11 Kannel WB, Castelli WP, McNamara PM, McKee PA, Feinleib M. Role of blood pressure in the development of congestive heart failure: the

Framingham Study. *N Engl J Med* 1972;**287**: 781–7.

12 Eriksson H, Svaldsudd K, Caidahl K *et al*. Early heart failure in the population. The study of men born in 1913. *Acta Med Scand* 1988;**223**: 197–209.

13 Remes J, Reunanen A, Alomaa A, Pyorala K. Incidence of heart failure in eastern Finland: a population-based surveillance study. *Eur Heart J* 1992;**13**:588–93.

14 Daniel WG, Mugge A, Martin RP *et al*. Improvement in the diagnosis of abscesses associated with endocarditis by transesophageal echocardiography. *N Engl J Med* 1991;**324**: 795–800.

15 Best Evidence. *Linking Medical Research to Practice*. American College of Physicians. PO Box 7777, Philadelphia, PA, USA, 19175–0980.

16 Depression predicted cardiac death within 18 months after myocardial infarction (Abstract). *Evidence-Based Medicine*, 1995; Nov-Dec:1:24. (Abstract of) Frasure-Smith N, Lesperance F, Talajic M. Depression and 18-month prognosis after myocardial infarction. *Circulation* 1995;**91**: 999–1005.

17 Frasure-Smith N, Lesperance F, Talajic M. Depression and 18-month prognosis after myocardial. *Circulation* 1995;**91**:999–1005.

18 Moss AJ, Davis HT, Conrad DL, DeCamilla JJ, Odoroff CL. Digitalis associated cardiac mortality after myocardial infarction. *Circulation* 1981;**65**: 1150–5.

19 The Digitalis Investigation Group. The effect of digoxin on mortality and morbidity in patients with heart failure. *N Engl J Med* 1997;**336**: 525–33.

20 Kitching AD, Yusuf S. From journal to bedside: quantifying the benefits of treatment. *Evidence-Based Cardiovascular Medicine* 1997;**1**:57–8.

21 Guyatt GH, Sackett DL, Cook DJ for the Evidence-Based Medicine Working Group. Users' guides to the medical literature II. How to use an article about therapy or prevention: B. What were the results and will they help me in caring for my patients? *JAMA* 1994;**271**:59–63.

22 Yusuf S, Wittes J, Probstfield J, Tyroler HA. Analysis and interpretation of treatment effects in subgroups of patients in randomized clinical trials. *JAMA* 1991;**266**:93–8.

23 Oxman AD, Guyatt GH. A consumer's guide to subgroup analysis. *Ann Intern Med* 1992;**116**: 78–84.

24 SHEP Cooperative Research Group. Prevention of stroke by antihypertensive drug treatment in older persons with isolated systolic hypertension: final results of the systolic hypertension in the elderly program (SHEP). *JAMA* 1991;**265**: 3255–64.

25 Garg R, Yusuf S. Overview of randomized trials of angiotensin-converting enzyme inhibitors on mortality and morbidity in patients with heart failure. Collaborative group on ACE inhibitor trials. *JAMA* 1995;**273**:1450–6.

26 Psaty BM, Smith NL, Siscovick DS *et al*. Health outcomes associated with anti-hypertensive therapies used as first-line agents. A systematic review and meta-analysis. *JAMA* 1997;**277**: 739–45.

27 The SOLVD Investigators. Effect of Enalapril on mortality and the development of heart failure in asymptomatic patients with reduced left ventricular ejection fractions. *N Engl J Med* 1992; **327**:685–91.

2 A critical appraisal of the cardiovascular history and physical examination

AKBAR PANJU,
BRENDA HEMMELGARN,
JIM NISHIKAWA,
DEBORAH COOK,
ALLAN KITCHING

There have been numerous technological advances made in the diagnosis and treatment of cardiovascular disease. In spite of this progress, a carefully conducted clinical examination remains the cornerstone in the initial assessment of the patient with known or suspected cardiovascular disease. Before conducting further laboratory or radiologic diagnostic tests, clinicians implicitly consider each piece of historical information and each finding from the physical examination as a diagnostic test that increases or decreases the probability of the possible diagnoses. The competency and accuracy of the clinical examination therefore is crucial, for it serves as the basis for our judgment not only regarding diagnosis, but prognosis and therapy as well.

This chapter is not intended to provide details of the technique, or the "how to", in performing a cardiovascular history and physical examination, and should be read in conjunction with standard textbooks on cardiology to obtain such information. Instead, we will provide the reader with the tools to identify those features of the history and physical examination reported in the literature which are the most reliable and valid in assessing a patient with cardiovascular disease. We will focus on strategies to locate literature on the clinical examination, as well as guidelines to assess the quality of these studies. These techniques will then be applied to three common features of the cardiovascular history, namely chest pain, dyspnea, and syncope, as well as common features of the physical examination, including assessment of the apical impulse, central venous pressure, systolic murmurs, blood pressure, and arterial pulse. The following topics will be covered:

1. Strategies used to locate literature on clinical examination.
2. How to critically appraise this literature.

Table 2.1   Search strategy for clinical skills articles using MEDLINE

Group One terms

Term(s) for clinical entity of interest (e.g. syncope, myocardial infarction)
  combined with (AND)[a]

Group Two terms

- Physical examination (exploded; in title, abstract or subject heading)
- Medical history taking (exploded)
- Professional competence (exploded)
- Diagnostic tests, routine
    combined with (OR)[a]

Group Three terms

- Sensitivity and specificity (textword; exploded)
- Reproducibility of results
- Observer variation
- Decision support techniques
- Bayes theorem

---

[a] AND and OR represent Boolean terms (symbolic representation of relationships between sets) for combining items.

3. Application of (1) and (2) above in the cardiovascular history (chest pain, dyspnea, syncope).
4. Application of (1) and (2) above in the cardiovascular physical examination (apical impulse, central venous pressure, systolic murmurs, blood pressure, arterial pulse).

STRATEGIES USED TO LOCATE LITERATURE ON CLINICAL EXAMINATION

There are no validated strategies for locating precise and accurate information on obtaining a cardiovascular history and conducting a physical examination. A proposed strategy for searching the MEDLINE database is summarized in Table 2.1. This strategy is the method suggested for authors of the Rational Clinical Examination series appearing in the *Journal of the American Medical Association*.[1] The first terms capture the clinical topic of interest by specifying the disease or presentation or function/dysfunction being sought. The second group of terms seeks clinical skills articles. The third group of terms is intended to find articles of high methodologic quality. An efficient strategy to locate high quality articles would be to combine the first two groups of terms with "diagnosis (pre-exploded)" to maximize sensitivity, or with "sensitivity (textword)" to maximize specificity. This is an extension of the method suggested by the ACP Journal Club for finding high quality articles on diagnostic tests in general.[2]

Any comprehensive search for relevant articles should include a review of reference lists from the articles found and review articles on the topic, as well as textbooks on clinical examination, and advice from clinicians interested in clinical examination.

HOW TO CRITICALLY APPRAISE THE LITERATURE ON CLINICAL EXAMINATION STUDIES

Having located articles on the cardiovascular clinical examination, one must carefully review each study to establish its validity, or accuracy, prior to deciding whether the results obtained will aid in establishing or ruling out a particular diagnosis. We propose a strategy for evaluating the literature on clinical examination based on a framework developed for the Users' Guides to the Medical Literature series.[3] In assessing the validity of the study, and interpreting the results, the following points should be considered.

Are the results of the clinical examination study valid?

1. Was there an independent blind comparison with a reference (gold) standard of diagnosis?
2. Was the clinical feature evaluated in an appropriate spectrum of patients (like those in whom it would be used in clinical practice)?
3. Was the reference standard applied regardless of the result of the clinical feature?
4. Were the methods of performing the clinical features described in sufficient detail to permit replication?
5. Was there a description of the experience of the individuals doing the examination?

What were the results?

1. Are likelihood ratios for the results presented, or data necessary for their calculation provided?
2. Has there been consideration given to reproducibility, precision, and disagreement?

The application of the initial five guides will help the reader determine whether the results of the study are likely to be valid. If the results are deemed to be valid, the reader can then go on to interpret the results presented, of which the likelihood ratio (LR) is the most important index in determining how good a particular diagnostic test is. The likelihood ratio is the probability that the results of a test would be expected in a patient with, as opposed to one without, the target disorder.

The application of these techniques for critically appraising the cardiovascular history and physical examination will now be described.

CLINICAL FEATURES IN THE CARDIOVASCULAR HISTORY

Chest pain

There are many causes of chest pain, including both cardiac and non-cardiac conditions, as outlined in Figure 2.1. Elucidating the cause of the chest pain is important for purposes of both management and prognosis. To ensure that the appropriate intervention

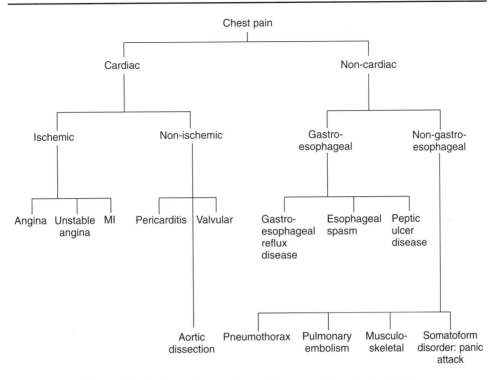

Figure 2.1 Cardiac and non-cardiac conditions presenting with chest pain.

is undertaken in the clinical setting, it is useful to classify patients presenting with chest pain into three categories:

1. Patients with myocardial infarction.
2. Patients with myocardial ischemia but no infarction.
3. Patients with non-cardiac chest pain.

Characteristics of the chest pain may help differentiate patients into the appropriate category. To identify features of the chest pain that may aid in classifying patients into category (1), myocardial infarction, we undertook a review of the literature using a search strategy similar to that outlined in the first section above. Relevant articles identified from this search were critically appraised using criteria outlined in the previous section. For the sake of relevance and clarity we have chosen to present only the results of those features in which a likelihood ratio of at least 2.0 or greater, or 0.5 or less, was obtained. The five studies which meet this criteria provide the best available evidence for identifying features of chest pain which aid in the diagnosis of myocardial infarction.

As outlined in Table 2.2, features of the chest pain that increased the probability of a myocardial infarction included chest pain radiation, pain in the chest or left arm, and chest pain described as the most important symptom. Chest pain radiation was the clinical feature which increased the probability of a myocardial infarction the most, with a widespread distribution of pain associated with the highest likelihood ratios. In particular, chest pain radiating to the left arm was twice as likely to occur in patients with, as opposed to those without, an acute myocardial infarction, while radiation to the right shoulder was three times, and radiation to both the left and right arm seven

27

Table 2.2 Features of chest pain that increase the probability of a myocardial infarction

Clinical feature	References	LR (95% CI)
Chest pain radiation:		
(R) shoulder	Tierney et al.[5]	2.9 (1.4–6.0)
(L) arm	Berger et al.[4]	2.3 (1.7–3.1)
both (L) and (R) arm	Berger et al.[4]	7.1 (3.6–14.2)
Pain in chest or (L) arm	Pozen et al.[6]	2.7[a]
Chest pain most important symptom	Pozen et al.[6]	2.0[a]

LR, likelihood ratio; CI, confidence interval.
[a] Data not available to calculate CIs.

Table 2.3 Features of chest pain that decrease the probability of a myocardial infarction

Clinical feature	References	LR (95% CI)
Pleuritic chest pain	Tierney et al.,[5] Lee et al.,[7] Solomon et al.[8]	0.2 (0.2–0.3)
Chest pain sharp or stabbing	Tierney et al.,[5] Lee et al.[7]	0.3 (0.2–0.5)
Positional chest pain	Lee et al.,[7] Solomon et al.[8]	0.3 (0.2–0.4)
Chest pain reproduced by palpation	Tierney et al.,[5] Lee et al.,[7] Solomon et al.[8]	0.2–0.4[a]

LR, likelihood ratio; CI, confidence interval.
[a] In heterogenous studies the likelihood ratios are reported as ranges.

times as likely to occur in such patients. The quality of the chest pain, including pain described as squeezing or pressure, added little to establishing a diagnosis of myocardial infarction, with likelihood ratios of less than 2.

Features of the chest pain that decrease the probability of myocardial infarction, and therefore would be useful in ruling out a myocardial infarction, are outlined in Table 2.3. Pleuritic or positional chest pain, as well as chest pain described as sharp or stabbing, all decrease the likelihood of a myocardial infarction. In addition, chest pain reproduced by palpation on physical examination was also associated with a low probability of myocardial infarction.

The precision in obtaining a chest pain history was addressed by Hickman and colleagues,[9] who assessed the interobserver agreement in chest pain histories obtained by general internists, nurse practitioners, and self-administered questionnaires for 197 inpatients and 112 outpatients with chest pain. The agreement between two internists for seven of the 10 items, including location and description of the pain, as well as aggravating and relieving factors, was substantial (kappa, a measure of chance-corrected agreement, was 0.50–0.89). Agreement was slightly lower between internist and questionnaire, and between the nurse practitioners and internist, with the lowest level of agreement between nurse and questionnaire. Features of the chest pain associated with a lower probability of myocardial infarction, namely pleuritic, positional, and sharp chest pain, were typically associated with a modest level of agreement for all comparisons (kappa 0.26–0.62).

Although cardiac catheterization remains the definitive diagnostic procedure for allocating patients into category two, that is the presence of myocardial ischemia or coronary artery disease, the character of the patient's chest pain has also been identified as one of the most important clinical features in establishing the diagnosis of coronary artery disease.[10] The combination of typical angina and a long duration of symptoms was particularly predictive of severe disease. Although this study was undertaken in a very select group of patients, those who underwent cardiac catheterization, similar results were obtained from outpatients referred for non-invasive testing.[11] After smoking, typical angina was the variable most strongly associated with significant coronary disease (defined as $\geq 75\%$ luminal narrowing of at least one major coronary artery). Subjects with typical angina were 13 times more likely to have significant coronary disease than those without.

There are many causes of non-cardiac chest pain, as outlined in Figure 2.1, and each condition has its own characteristic features and associated symptoms. It is beyond the scope of this chapter to identify all these conditions.

Dyspnea

Dyspnea, defined as an uncomfortable awareness of breathing, is a common complaint of both in- and outpatients. Cardiac and pulmonary causes of dyspnea are most common, with congestive heart failure, asthma, and chronic obstructive pulmonary disease accounting for most patients' complaints.[12] However, standard textbooks of internal medicine list over 30 different etiologies for dyspnea,[13] often with multiple etiologies explaining a patient's symptoms. It is often taught that the cause of dyspnea, either that of the heart or lungs, can be differentiated at the bedside by thorough history taking. Unfortunately, such strategies to diagnose a cardiac cause for the breathless patient have been incompletely studied.

Zema and coworkers[14] looked at the value of patients' symptoms as predictors of left ventricular systolic dysfunction in 37 patients with the clinical diagnosis of chronic obstructive pulmonary disease (COPD). Eliciting a symptom of dyspnea on exertion predicted depressed left ventricular systolic function with a sensitivity of 100% and a specificity of 20%. The symptom of orthopnea generated a sensitivity and specificity of 71% and 65%, paroxysmal nocturnal dyspnea 47% and 75%, and ankle edema 41% and 75% respectively. All features were associated with a likelihood ratio of 2 or less. In general, the study was well conducted, but the value of the results to the practicing clinician must be questioned. First, the symptoms of shortness of breath attributed to the heart were only considered in the context of impaired left ventricular (LV) systolic function. It is now generally agreed that abnormalities in LV diastolic function also cause symptoms of dyspnea. A better gold standard would perhaps have been radionuclide ventriculographic evidence of both LV systolic and diastolic dysfunction. The generalizability of the results are also lessened by the fact that their definition of heart failure was a left ventricular ejection fraction (LVEF) <50%, when in fact the target for treatment of patients with heart failure is most often an LVEF of <40%. Finally, the study was performed in patients who first had a clinical diagnosis of COPD, when patients present with many causes of shortness of breath, not just COPD.

In summary, therefore, specific features when elicited in a patient presenting with a complaint of dyspnea are of limited usefulness in making a definitive diagnosis of impaired LV function.

Syncope

Little detailed evidence exists for either individual or clusters of clinical examination findings in the evaluation of syncope. In a prospective study of 433 syncopal patients presenting in a university setting (emergency, in- and outpatients), the history and physical examination was found to identify 55% (140) of the 254 causes ultimately found.[15] Many of the non-cardiac causes of syncope in this study were defined in clinical terms and so provided the "diagnostic standard" for classification. The three most common non-cardiac causes of syncope were "orthostatic hypotension" (systolic drop of more than 25 mmHg, or drop of more than 10 mmHg to less than 90 mmHg with symptoms), "situational" (situations included cough, micturition and defecation and required appropriate timing and no other identifiable cause), and "vasovagal" (requiring a precipitating event and premonitory symptoms), representing 31%, 26% and 25% of identifiable causes of syncope overall.

Follow-up of the cohort demonstrated a 5-year mortality of 50.5% for cardiac versus 30% for non-cardiac or 24% for unknown causes. This provides some independent validation for the clinical classification criteria.

There is a need for further work in this area, particularly in developing and validating practical clinical tools to screen for psychiatric causes, to distinguish patients who will benefit from electrophysiologic testing, and to predict patients who will have a positive tilt-table test.

CLINICAL FEATURES IN THE CARDIOVASCULAR PHYSICAL EXAMINATION

Apical impulse

The apical impulse was first described by William Harvey in 1928[16] and is one of a number of palpable precordial pulsations reflecting underlying movement of the heart and great vessels. Many criteria exist defining the normal location, size, and character of the apical impulse, and many generations of medical students have been taught that an "abnormal" apical impulse may assist with the diagnosis of left ventricular enlargement and/or hypertrophy. It has only been recently that evidence has been published in the literature to support these claims.

The relationship between the location and size of the apical impulse and LV size, as determined by two-dimensional echocardiography (gold standard), was evaluated by Eilen and colleagues.[17] An apical impulse lateral to the midclavicular line, defined as half the distance between the tip of the acromion process and the sternal notch, was a sensitive (100%), but not specific (18%), indicator for LV enlargement, with a likelihood ratio of only 1.2. Identification of the apical impulse >10 cm from the midsternal line was just as sensitive (100%), but only marginally more specific (33%). An apical diameter of >3 cm was a good indicator of LV enlargement, with a sensitivity of 92% and a specificity of 75%, and was almost four times as likely to occur in patients with, as opposed to those without, LV enlargement (LR = 3.7).

O'Neill and coworkers[18] examined the relationship between the location of the apical impulse and the presence or absence of cardiomegaly on chest X-ray (defined as a cardiothoracic ratio greater than 50%). An apical impulse lateral to the midclavicular line had a sensitivity of 57%, a specificity of 76%, and a likelihood ratio of 2.4 for identifying cardiomegaly. Identification of the apical impulse >10 cm from the midsternal line was slightly more sensitive (78%), but considerably less specific (28%), and added little to establishing the diagnosis (LR = 1.1). The results of this investigation must be accepted with caution as the gold standard used in this case was chest X-ray which is not a sensitive or specific marker of LV enlargement. Therefore, the validity of this gold standard must be questioned. This was, however, one of the few studies which also evaluated the variation between observers (interobserver variation) in the clinical assessment of the apical impulse, and reported good agreement on apex palpability (kappa = 0.72) and moderate agreement on degree of apex displacement (kappa = 0.56) between two physicians.

Eagle and coworkers[19] examined multiple clinical features in 125 inpatients with a variety of cardiac and non-cardiac diagnoses in an attempt to determine which features best predicted LVEF. In general, physician estimates of LVEF were good, with 56% being accurate within 7.5% of measured value; 27% of physicians overestimated and 17% underestimated the LVEF. Multiple regression analysis identified three clinical features most predictive of LVEF, including S_3 gallop, hypotension, and sustained LV apical impulse (defined as a palpable impulse greater than two-thirds the ventricle systole).

In summary, the location, size, and character of the apical impulse may be used to assess LV size, LV function, and cardiomegaly, either alone or in combination with other clinical features or simple diagnostic tests. However, a number of limitations exist, including the fact that a palpable impulse may only be found in approximately 50% of patients. In addition, the high sensitivity but low specificity associated with determining the location and size of the apical impulse makes it a better test for ruling out rather than ruling in LV enlargement, which is good for screening, but has limited usefulness at the bedside.

Central venous pressure

The right internal jugular vein lies directly in line with the right atrium, and acts as a manometer displaying changes in blood flow and pressure caused by right atrial filling, contraction, and emptying. Elevated jugular venous pressure reflects an increase in central venous pressure (CVP).

The reliability and validity of the clinical assessment of CVP have been assessed in a limited number of studies. In one study, medical students, residents, and attending physicians examined the same 50 ICU patients and estimated these patients' CVP as low (<5 cm), normal (5–10 cm) or high (>10 cm).[20] Agreement between students and residents was substantial (kappa 0.65), agreement between students and attending physicians was moderate (kappa 0.56), and agreement between residents and staff was modest (kappa 0.30). Possible causes for disagreement include positioning of patients, poor lighting, difficulty in distinguishing carotid from venous pulsations, and variation in pressure with respiration.

As regards the relation between clinical assessments of CVP and the gold standard of simultaneous pressure measurements through a central venous catheter, one study[21] used an attending physician, a fellow, a medical resident, an intern, and a student to predict whether four hemodynamic variables, including CVP, were low, normal, high,

31

Table 2.4 Features of the clinical examination that increase the probability of aortic stenosis

Clinical feature	LR[a]
Slow rate of rise of carotid pulse	2.8–130
Late peaking murmur	8–101
Soft or absent second heart sound	3.1–50

[a] LR, likelihood ratio: range of point estimates from original studies cited.
Data from Etchells *et al*.[26]

or very high. The sensitivity of the clinical exam at identifying low (<0 mmHg), normal (0–7 mmHg), or high (>7 mmHg) CVP was 33%, 33%, and 49% respectively. The specificity of the clinical exam at identifying low, normal, or high CVP was 73%, 62%, and 76% respectively. In another study, Eisenberg and colleagues[22] compared clinical assessments with pulmonary artery catheter readings in 97 critically ill patients. Physicians correctly predicted CVP only 55% of the time, with CVP more frequently underestimated (27%) than overestimated (17%).

Clinical assessments of a high CVP increase the likelihood by about four fold that the measured CVP will be high; conversely, clinical assessments of a low CVP make the probability of finding a high measured CVP extremely unlikely (LR = 0.2).[20] The data demonstrate that clinical assessments of a normal CVP are truly indeterminate, with likelihood ratios approaching 1; such estimates provide no information because they neither increase nor decrease the probability of an abnormal CVP. Aside from less observer variation, CVP estimates are most accurate among patients breathing spontaneously.

The precision of the abdominojugular reflux test has not been reported, but its results will vary with the force of abdominal compression. Although the abdominojugular reflux is an insensitive way to diagnose congestive heart failure, the specificity of this test is high.[23,24] Moreover, the positive likelihood ratios (6.4 when diagnosis was based on a clinical–radiographic score, and 6.0 when diagnosis was based on emergency room physician judgment) indicate that this is a useful bedside test.[25]

Systolic murmurs

Etchells and colleagues have published a thorough review of the clinical examination for systolic murmurs.[26] This included a systematic review of the literature and grading of the quality of the original articles. Quality was assessed by the sample size and recruitment (consecutive versus convenience) and whether comparison with the diagnostic standard was done independently and blindly.

Useful data for ruling in or out aortic stenosis are given in Tables 2.4 and 2.5. The reliability of the exam by cardiologists for late peaking murmur shape is good (kappa 0.74), for the presence of murmurs is fair to moderate (kappa 0.29–0.48),[26] but for other maneuvers may be poorer.[27]

Studies of the clinical examination for other etiologies of systolic murmur were also reviewed but tended to be of lesser quality than those addressing aortic stenosis.

Etchells and his colleagues[26] point out that the majority of studies of this topic have used cardiologists as observers. The performance of non-cardiologists appears to be less

Table 2.5 Features of the clinical examination that decrease the probability of aortic stenosis

Clinical feature	LR[a]
Absence of a murmur	0
No radiation to right carotid artery	0.05–0.10

[a] LR, likelihood ratio: range of point estimates from original studies cited. Data from Etchells et al.[26]

accurate when studied. Further work using a broader range of clinicians and patients is needed to know the value of the clinical examination in more general settings.

Blood pressure

An extensive review of the technique, reliability, and validity of blood pressure (BP) measurement has been provided by Reeves.[28] As outlined in the review, two important sources of variation in BP measurement include the patient and the examiner. Random fluctuation in BP over time has been documented by the SD of readings, with a minute-to-minute variation of about 4 mmHg systolic and 2–3 mmHg diastolic, and day-to-day variation of 5–12 mmHg systolic and 6–8 mmHg diastolic. With respect to the examiner as the source of variability, differences of 10–8 mmHg by both physicians and nurses in routine medical practices have been noted.

Intra-arterial blood pressure measurement has been used as the gold standard to assess the accuracy of indirect BP measurement. With the indirect BP the phase I Korotkoff, or first audible sound, appears 15–4 mmHg below the direct systolic BP, while phase V, or disappearance of all sounds, appears 3–6 mmHg above the true diastolic BP in adults. Other factors which affect the accuracy of the indirect BP measurement, resulting in both an increase or decrease in systolic and/or diastolic measurements, are outlined in Tables 2.6 and 2.7.

Arterial pulse

Few studies have been undertaken to assess the reliability and validity of features of the arterial pulse in the cardiovascular examination, despite numerous descriptive accounts of its variability in different clinical conditions. Case series indicate that details regarding the presence and quality of the arterial pulse are more sensitive markers of coarctation of the aorta than aortic dissection. Absent femoral pulses or a femoral/brachial pulse discrepancy in patients was associated with a sensitivity of 88% in the diagnosis of coarctation of the aorta in patients less than 6 months of age.[29] Similar results were obtained for patients diagnosed with coarctation after one year of age, where weak or absent femoral pulses were associated with a sensitivity of 85%.[30]

The sensitivity of the presence and quality of the carotid, subclavian, and femoral pulses in establishing a diagnosis of both proximal (primary tear in the ascending aorta with or without involvement of the arch, De Bakey classification type I and II) and distal (primary tear in the descending thoracic aorta, De Bakey classification type III)

Table 2.6 Factors associated with an increase in blood pressure

Factor	Magnitude, SBP/DBP (mmHg)
Examinee	
Pseudohypertension	2–98/3–49
"White coat reaction" to physician	11–28/3–15
"White coat reaction" to non-physician	1–12/2–7
Paretic arm (due to stroke)	2/5
Pain, anxiety	May be large
Acute smoking	6/5
Acute caffeine	11/5
Acute ethanol ingestion	8/8
Distended bladder	15/10
Talking, sighing	7/8
Setting, equipment	
Leaky bulb valve	≥2 DBP
Blocked manometer vents	2 to 10
Examination	
Cuff too narrow	−8 − +10/2–8
Cuff not centered	4/3
Cuff over clothing	5–50
Elbow too low	6
Back unsupported	6–10
Arm unsupported	1–7/5–11
Too slow deflation	−1 − +2/5–6
Too fast deflation	DBP only
Parallax error	2–4
Using phase IV (adult)	6 DBP
Too rapid remeasure	1/1
Cold season (vs warm)	6/3–10

SBP, systolic blood pressure; DBP, diastolic blood pressure.
Data from Reeves *et al*.[28]

aortic dissections are outlined in Table 2.8. Proximal dissections were primarily associated with an absence or decrease in the brachiocephalic vessels, while distal dissections had almost exclusive involvement of the femoral arteries.

Features of the arterial pulse may also be used to determine the presence of valvular heart disease. As reported by Etchells *et al.*,[26] features of the arterial pulse, including rate of rise of the carotid pulse, apical carotid delay, and brachioradial delay, all increase the likelihood of establishing the diagnosis of aortic stenosis (Table 2.9).

Heart rate is another important component of the cardiovascular examination. The accuracy of the assessment of heart rate may be affected by both the site (apical or radial) as well as the counting interval (15, 30, or 60 seconds). With a regular rhythm, radial 15 second counts were the least accurate for both resting and rapid heart rates, while the 30 second counts were found to be the most accurate and efficient for rapid rates.[34] With the irregularly irregular rhythm of atrial fibrillation, however, the apical method and 60 second count have been reported to be the most accurate, with site being a more important source of error than counting interval.[35] Using the ECG as the

Table 2.7 Factors associated with a decrease in blood pressure

Factor	Magnitude, SBP/DBP (mmHg)
Examinee	
Recent meal	−1 − 1/1−4
Missed auscultatory gap	10–50 SBP
High stroke volume	Phase V can = 0
Habituation	0–7/2–12
Shock (additional pseudohypotension)	33 SBP
Setting, equipment	
Faulty aneroid device	Can be >10
Leaky bulb	≥2 SBP
Examiner	
Reading to next lowest 5 or 10 mmHg or expectation bias	Probably ≤10
Impaired hearing	SBP only
Examination	
Left vs right arm	1/1
Resting for too long (25 min)	10/0
Elbow too high	5/5
Too rapid deflation	SBP only
Excess bell pressure	≥9 DBP
Parallax error (aneroid)	2–4

SBP, systolic blood pressure; DBP, diastolic blood pressure.
Data from Reeves et al.[28]

Table 2.8 Sensitivity of the arterial pulse in the diagnosis of aortic dissection

| References | Aortic dissection | |
	Proximal[a]	Distal[b]
Lindsay and Hurst[31c]	62.5%	10.5%
Slater and De Sanctis[32c]	50.9%	15.5%
Spittell et al.[33d]	9.0%	2.4%

[a] De Bakey Classification type I and II.

[b] De Bakey Classification type III.

[c] Absence or decrease in amplitude of carotid, subclavian or femoral pulse(s).

[d] Absence of palpable carotid, subclavian or femoral pulse(s).

measure of true heart rate, the mean radial error for all counting intervals was 19.5 beats per minute, which was significantly higher than the mean apical error of 9.7 beats per minute.

Although the pulse in atrial fibrillation is typically described as "irregularly irregular", Rawles and Rowland,[36] using computerized analysis of R–R intervals and pulse volumes among patients with atrial fibrillation, disputed this assumption. In an assessment of 74 patients with atrial fibrillation, they reported a non-random sequence of R–R intervals in 30%, and the presence of pulsus alternans in less than half (46%). The authors

Table 2.9 Features of the arterial pulse that increase the probability of aortic stenosis

Clinical feature	LR[a]
Slow rate of rise of carotid pulse	2.8–130
Apical carotid delay	∞
Brachioradial delay	6.8

[a] LR, likelihood ratio: range of point estimates from original studies cited. Data from Etchells *et al*.[26]

concluded that patterns of regularity of the pulse are common in patients with atrial fibrillation.

SUMMARY

Despite the frequency with which details of the history and physical examination are used to establish or rule out a particular cardiovascular condition, there is a very limited amount of data available to support the reliability and validity of these features. The one component of the cardiovascular history which has been studied is that of chest pain in the diagnosis of myocardial infarction. Features of chest pain, particularly pain that has a wide distribution of radiation, increase the probability of myocardial infarction, while chest pain that is pleuritic, sharp or stabbing, positional, or reproduced by palpation all decrease the probability of myocardial infarction.

The reliability and validity of various features of the cardiovascular physical examination have also received little attention in the literature. Of those which have been studied, the apical impulse has been shown to be a sensitive but non-specific marker of LV size, which makes it useful for ruling out, rather than ruling in, LV enlargement. Clinical assessment of elevated CVP has been shown to be associated with a four-fold likelihood that the measured CVP will be high, with the abdominojugular reflex a useful bedside test to assist in the diagnosis of congestive heart failure.

Of the cardiac murmurs, aortic stenosis has been studied the most thoroughly. Features of the clinical examination which increase the probability of aortic stenosis include slow rate of rise of the carotid pulse, late peaking murmur, and soft or absent second heart sound. Conversely, absence of a murmur or no radiation to the right carotid artery were features associated with a decreased probability of aortic stenosis.

A number of features have been shown to influence the accuracy of the indirect assessment of BP, including those related to the examinee, the examiner, the setting and equipment, and the examination itself. Assessment of the arterial pulse in diagnosing coarctation of the aorta and aortic dissection have been limited to case series, therefore estimates of sensitivity only are available. Features of the arterial pulse have been shown to be relatively sensitive markers for coarctation of the aorta, and less so for aortic dissection. Finally, both counting interval and site (radial versus apical) have important implications on the accuracy of heart rate assessment.

As is evident from the information presented, unfortunately, for a variety of reasons, research on clinical examination has lagged behind compared to basic science and therapeutic research. So far, clinical examination is identified as the "art" of medicine and by incorporating an evidence based approach, one can make clinical examination the "art and science" of medicine.

REFERENCES

1 Simel D (Section editor, Rational Clinical Examination, *JAMA*). Personal communication, December 1996.

2 McKibbon KA, Walker-Dilks CJ. Beyond ACP Journal Club: How to harness MEDLINE for diagnostic problems (Editorial). *ACP J Club.* 1994; **121**:A10–A12.

3 Oxman AD, Sackett DL, Guyatt GH. Users' Guides to the Medical Literature: 1. How to get started. *JAMA* 1993;**270**:2093–5.

4 Berger JP, Buclin R, Haller E, Van Melle G, Yersin B. Right arm involvement and pain extension can help to differentiate coronary diseases from chest pain of other origin: a prospective emergency ward study of 278 consecutive patients admitted for chest pain. *J Intern Med* 1990;**227**:165–72.

5 Tierney WM, Fitzgerald D, McHenry R *et al*. Physicians' estimates of the probability of myocardial infarction in emergency room patients with chest pain. *Med Decis Making* 1986;**6**:12–17.

6 Pozen MW, D'Agostino RB, Selker HP, Sytkowski PA, Hood WB. A predictive instrument to improve coronary-care-unit admission practices in acute ischemic heart disease. *N Engl J Med* 1984;**310**: 1273–8.

7 Lee TH, Cook EF, Weisberg M *et al*. Acute chest pain in the emergency room. *Arch Intern Med* 1985;**145**:65–9.

8 Solomon CG, Lee TH, Cook EF *et al*. Comparison of clinical presentation of acute myocardial infarction in patients older than 65 years of age to younger patients: the multicenter chest pain study experience. *Am J Cardiol* 1989;**63**:772–6.

9 Hickman DH, Sox HC, Sox CH. Systematic bias in recording the history in patients with chest pain. *J Chron Dis* 1985;**38**:91–100.

10 Pryor DB, Shaw L, Harrell FE *et al*. Estimating the likelihood of severe coronary artery disease. *Am J Med* 1991;**90**:553–62.

11 Pryor DB, Shaw L, McCants CB. Value of the history and physical in identifying patients at increased risk for coronary artery disease. *Ann Intern Med* 1993;**118**:81–90.

12 Mulrow CD, Lucey CR, Farnett LE. Discriminating causes of dyspnea through clinical examination. *J Gen Intern Med* 1993;**8**:383–92.

13 Ingram RH Jr, Braunwald E. Dyspnea and pulmonary edema. In: Wilson JD *et al.*, eds. *Harrison's principles of internal medicine*, 12th edn. New York: McGraw-Hill. 1991.

14 Zema MJ, Masters AP, Malgouleff D. Dyspnea: the heart or the lungs? Differentiation at bedside by use of the simple valsalva maneuver. *Chest* 1984; **85**:59–64.

15 Kapoor WN. Evaluation and outcome of patients with syncope. *Medicine* 1990;**69**:160–75.

16 Harvey W. *An anatomical disquisition on the motion of the heart and blood in animals*, London, 1928. (Translated from the Latin by Robert Willis, Barnes, Surrey, England, 1847). In: Willius FA, Key TE. *Classics of cardiology*, vol. 1, Malabar, Florida: Robert E. Krieger, 1983.

17 Eilen SD, Crawford MH, O'Rourke RA. Accuracy of precordial palpation for detecting increased left ventricular volume. *Ann Intern Med* 1983;**99**: 628–30.

18 O'Neill TW, Barry M, Smith M, Graham IM. Diagnostic value of the apex beat. *Lancet* 1989;**i**: 410–11.

19 Eagle KA, Quertermous T, Singer DE *et al*. Left ventricular ejection fraction. Physician estimates compared with gated blood pool scan measurements. *Arch Intern Med* 1988;**148**: 882–5.

20 Cook DJ. The clinical assessment of central venous pressure. *Am J Med Sci* 1990;**299**:175–8.

21 Connors AF, McCaffree DR, Gray BA. Evaluation of right heart catheterization in the critically ill patient without acute myocardial infarction. *N Engl J Med* 1983;**308**:263–7.

22 Eisenberg PR, Jaffe AS, Schuster DP. Clinical evaluation compared to pulmonary artery catheterization in the hemodynamic assessment of critically ill patients. *Crit Care Med* 1984;**12**: 549–53.

23 Marantz PR, Kaplan MC, Alderman MH. Clinical diagnosis of congestive heart failure in patients with acute dyspnea. *Chest* 1990;**97**:776–81.

24 Maisel AS, Atwood JE, Goldberger AL. Hepatojugular reflux: useful in the bedside diagnosis of tricuspid regurgitation. *Ann Intern Med* 1984;**101**:781–2.

25 Cook DJ, Simel DL. Does this patient have abnormal central venous pressure? *JAMA* 1996; **275**:630–4.

26 Etchells E, Bell C, Robb K. Does this patient have an abnormal systolic murmur? *JAMA* 1997;**277**: 564–71.

27 Spodick DH, Sugiura T, Doi Y, Paladion D, Jaffty BG. Rate of rise of the carotid pulse: an investigation of observer error in a common clinical measurement. *Am J Cardiol* 1982;**49**: 159–62.

28 Reeves RA. Does this patient have hypertension? *JAMA* 1995;**273**:1211–18.

29 Ward KE, Pryor RW, Matson JR *et al*. Delayed detection of coarctation in infancy: implications for timing of newborn follow-up. *Pediatrics* 1990; **86**:972–6.

30 Strafford MA, Griffiths SP, Gersony WM. Coarctation of the aorta: a study in delayed detection. *Pediatrics* 1982;**69**:159–63.

31 Lindsay J, Hurst JW. Clinical features and prognosis in dissecting aneurysm of the aorta. *Circulation* 1967;**35**:880–8.

32 Slater EE, DeSanctis RW. The clinical recognition of dissecting aortic aneurysm. *Am J Med* 1976; **60**:625–33.

33 Spittell PC, Spittell JA, Joyce JW *et al*. Clinical features and differential diagnosis of aortic dissection: experience with 236 cases (1980 through 1990). *Mayo Clin Proc* 1993;**68**: 642–51.

34 Hollerbach AD, Sneed NV. Accuracy of radial pulse assessment by length of counting interval. *Heart Lung* 1990;**19**:258–64.

35 Sneed NV, Hollerbach AD. Accuracy of heart rate assessment in artial fibrillation. *Heart Lung* 1992; **21**:427–33.

36 Rawles JM, Rowland E. Is the pulse in artial fibrillation irregularly irregular? *Br Heart J* 1986; **56**:4–11.

Obtaining incremental information from diagnostic tests

3

Raymond J. Gibbons

INTRODUCTION

Consider the following case history. A 75-year-old male presents with a history of exertional chest pain. The patient describes substernal chest pain that he perceives as a "pressure sensation" that occurs when he walks too fast, uphill, or in the cold. It is relieved by rest within a few minutes. On two recent occasions, he tried a friend's nitroglycerin tablets, and obtained even more rapid relief of his symptoms. His symptoms have never occurred at rest. The patient has a history of diabetes mellitus, hypertension, and hypercholesterolemia. He smokes one pack of cigarettes a day. Several male family members died of coronary artery disease before the age of 60. The patient underwent carotid artery surgery a year ago for treatment of transient ischemic attacks.

On the basis of his age, gender, chest pain description, and risk factors, this patient is highly likely to have significant obstructive coronary artery disease. The added, or incremental, value of any stress test for the diagnosis of the presence of disease in such a situation is very small. Out of 100 patients with this presentation, perhaps only one or two will not have obstructive coronary artery disease. The potential contribution of stress testing is therefore restricted to only these one or two patients.

This example demonstrates the importance of the concept of incremental value for diagnostic tests. In the current era of health care reform, it is no longer sufficient that a test simply provide "more information". The more appropriate current questions are: (1) how much information does the test provide? and (2) at what cost? Increasingly, tests are also required to have a demonstrable impact on critical nodal, or decision, points with respect to patient management.

The demonstration of the incremental value of diagnostic tests requires rigorous methodology. The principles of the required methodology should be credited primarily to Dr George Diamond and his colleagues at Cedar Sinai Medical Center in Los Angeles.[1–3] First and foremost, such an analysis should reflect clinical decision making. Since clinical assessment is performed before any diagnostic tests, and usually at lower cost, parameters

39

available from this assessment should be considered separately without any information from subsequent testing. The analysis should preferably focus on hard, demonstrable endpoints such as significant obstructive coronary artery disease, severe (three vessel or left main) coronary artery disease, myocardial infarction, or death. Although alternative endpoints, such as functional impairment, unstable angina, and the need for revascularization, are often included to increase statistical power, such endpoints have major limitations with respect to reversibility, subjectivity, and definite impact on patient outcome. The analysis should create appropriate models which include all available important variables. An experienced clinician always takes the patient's age, gender, and history into account in making his or her clinical decision regarding patient management, even when testing results are available. These important clinical parameters must therefore be included in any final model that reflects the clinical decision making process. The analysis must demonstrate that the additional information is statistically significant in an appropriate patient population. Analyses that demonstrate additional information in older, "sicker" inpatient populations should not be casually extrapolated to younger, "less sick" outpatients in whom testing is customarily performed. Finally, the test must provide information that is clinically significant and cost effective. In very large patient samples, differences that have little if any clinical significance for individual patient management may emerge as statistically significant. The potential impact on patient management in *some* patients must compare favorably with the incremental cost of the test in *all* the patients who must be tested.

This chapter will attempt to elucidate this methodology using the published data with respect to the diagnosis of significant obstructive coronary artery disease, non-invasive screening for severe coronary artery disease, and patient outcome. All of these examples are drawn from the arena of ischemic heart disease, because this entity is a predominant feature of clinical practice in cardiology, and the published literature is voluminous and extensive. However, the same principles apply to other disease entities, both cardiac and non-cardiac.

CLINICAL ASSESSMENT

As outlined above, the initial step in any analysis designed to demonstrate incremental value is the consideration of all the information available prior to performance of the test. This will always include the results of the history and physical examination, and may sometimes include the results of other tests already performed. This section focuses on the information available from clinical assessment.

Diagnosis of coronary disease

As demonstrated by the earlier example, clinicians often encounter patients with chest pain and suspected coronary artery disease. The ability of clinical assessment to predict the likelihood of significant obstructive coronary artery disease has been demonstrated in numerous studies. The likelihood of significant disease based on clinical assessment is appropriately labeled the "pretest probability", in statistical terms.

Age, gender, and the patient's chest pain description are the most important clinical parameters for estimating the likelihood of coronary artery disease.[4] Older patients, men,

Table 3.1 Pretest probability of coronary artery disease

Age (yr)	Pretest probability (%)							
	Asymptomatic		Non-anginal chest pain		Atypical angina		Typical angina	
	F	M	F	M	F	M	F	M
30–39	<1	2	1	5	4	22	26	70
40–49	1	6	3	14	13	46	55	87
50–59	4	9	8	22	32	59	79	92
60–69	8	11	19	28	54	67	91	94

From Diamond and Forrester.[4] Reprinted by permission of the *New England Journal of Medicine* and Diamond GA. A clinically relevant classification of chest discomfort. *J Am Coll Cardiol* 1983;**1**:547–75.

and patients with chest pain that is typical, or classic, for angina pectoris are more likely to have coronary disease. Although multiple different systems have been used to classify chest pain, the simplest and easiest was proposed by Diamond.[5] He suggested a classification based on three elements – substernal location, precipitation by exertion, and relief by rest or nitroglycerin. If all three elements are present, the chest pain is classified as "typical angina". If two elements are present, the chest pain is classified as "atypical angina". If only one or none is present, the chest pain is classified as "non-anginal chest pain".

Table 3.1 shows published estimates of pretest probability on the basis of age, gender, and chest pain description.[4] It is obvious that there is a very wide range of pretest probability, ranging from 1% for a 35-year-old woman with non-anginal chest pain to 94% for a 65-year-old man with typical angina. Note that a 50-year-old man with atypical angina has about a 50% probability of disease.

A more comprehensive attempt to consider all clinical characteristics, including risk factors for atherosclerosis, was published from the Duke University Medical Center databank.[6] In addition to the three parameters previously discussed, this analysis found that evidence for previous infarction, smoking, hyperlipidemia, ST and T wave changes on the resting electrocardiogram, and diabetes were all highly significant predictors of the presence of coronary artery disease. Figure 3.1 shows a published nomogram for men that incorporates all of these parameters. Careful inspection of this figure demonstrates that the impact of the clinical parameters other than age, gender, and chest pain is variable. ECG and historical evidence of previous infarction has a major impact, diabetes and ECG ST-T changes have a modest impact, and lipids and smoking have a minimal impact. For example, a 50-year-old male with atypical angina has a 46% pretest probability of disease in the absence of smoking, hyperlipidemia, or diabetes, a 48% pretest probability in the presence of both smoking and hyperlipidemia, and a 65% pretest probability if he has diabetes as well. In the presence of ECG Q waves and a history of MI, his pretest probability exceeds 90%.

Non-invasive screening for severe coronary artery disease

Not surprisingly, clinical parameters are also very important in estimating the likelihood of severe (three vessel or left main) coronary artery disease.[7] The same parameters that

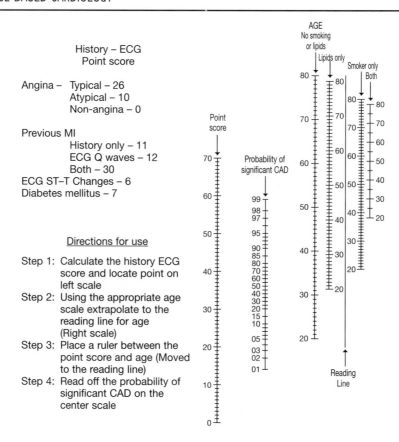

Figure 3.1 Nomogram for predicting the probability of significant coronary artery disease (CAD) in men. ECG, electrocardiographic; MI, myocardial infarction. (After Pryor *et al.*[6]) Example: A 50-year-old, white male with atypical angina and diabetes mellitus, but no ECG ST changes, previous MI, smoking, or hyperlipidemia. Point score on left scale = 10+7 = 17. Appropriate reading line on right labelled "no smoking or ↑ lipids". Connect age 50 on this reading line to point score of 17 with a straight edge. This intersects the middle line at 60, indicating that this is the percentage probability of significant CAD.

are most important for predicting the presence of disease – age, gender, and chest pain description – remain important. In addition, diabetes mellitus and history or electrocardiographic evidence of myocardial infarction are also very important. The simplest approach for estimating the likelihood of severe disease was published by Hubbard *et al.*[8] They assigned one point each for: male gender; typical angina; history and ECG evidence of myocardial infarction; diabetes; and insulin use. Thus, the point score had a minimum value of 0 and a maximum value of 5. Figure 3.2 shows a nomogram for the probability of severe coronary artery disease based on age and this point score. It is quickly apparent that age is an extremely important parameter for predicting severe disease.

A more comprehensive analysis on a larger number of patients was published from the Duke University Medical Center databank.[9] In addition to the five parameters already mentioned, these workers found that the duration of chest pain symptoms, other risk

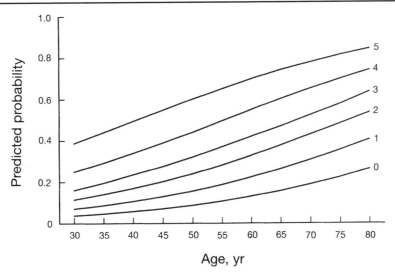

Figure 3.2 Nomogram showing the probability of severe (three vessel or left main) coronary artery disease based on a 5-point score. One point is awarded for each of the following variables – male gender, typical angina, history, and electrocardiographic evidence of MI, diabetes, and use of insulin. Each curve shows the probability of severe coronary disease as a function of age. (From Hubbard *et al.*,[8] with permission.)

factors (blood pressure, hyperlipidemia, and smoking), a carotid bruit, and chest pain frequency were also important determinants of the likelihood of severe coronary artery disease. However, the magnitude of their additional effect was modest.

Prediction of patient outcome

The ability of clinical assessment to predict patient outcome has been demonstrated in numerous previous studies. The largest and most important of these came from the Duke University databank[10] and the Coronary Artery Surgical Study Registry.[11] Many of the same parameters which predict the presence of disease and the presence of severe disease are also associated with adverse patient outcome. Age, gender, chest pain description, and previous myocardial infarction all have independent value in predicting patient outcome. In addition, history and physical examination evidence for congestive heart failure, history and physical examination evidence of vascular disease, unstable chest pain characteristics, and other electrocardiographic findings, such as ST–T wave changes, left bundle branch block, and intraventricular conduction delay, all have prognostic value. It is not generally appreciated how well clinical parameters perform in this regard. The Duke group reported that 37% of the patients undergoing stress testing at their institution had a predicted average annual mortality of 1% or less over the next 3 years, on the basis of clinical assessment.[11]

Several studies have shown that a normal resting electrocardiogram, and the absence of a history of prior infarction, predict a normal ejection fraction with $\geq 90\%$ confidence,[12,13] and therefore a favorable prognosis.[14–16]

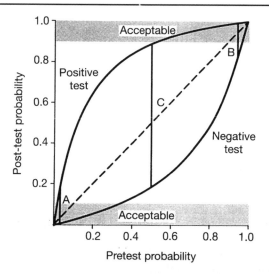

Figure 3.3 Relationship between pretest probability and post-test probability. The solid curves for positive and negative tests are plotted for a test with 80% sensitivity and a 90% specificity. Post-test probabilities that are acceptable for diagnosis ($\geq 90\%$ and $\leq 10\%$) are shown in the shaded zones. Line A represents a patient with a very low pretest probability; line B, a patient with a high pretest probability; line C, a patient with an intermediate probability. (Modified from Berman DS, Garcia EV, Maddahi J. Thallium-201 scintigraphy in the detection and evaluation of coronary artery disease. In: Berman DS, Mason DT, eds. *Clinical nuclear cardiology.* New York: Grune and Stratton, 1981, with permission.)

APPROACHES TO THE ASSESSMENT OF INCREMENTAL VALUE

Once the information available from clinical assessment (and other tests already performed) has been considered, these are a variety of conceptual and statistical approaches that can be employed to assess the incremental value of the test in question. This section will present examples of three such approaches.

Diagnosis of coronary artery disease

The application of multiple different stress tests for the diagnosis of coronary artery disease has been extensively studied. The most common approach used in this setting to demonstrate the incremental value of a new test employs Bayes' theorem.[17] This theorem indicates that the likelihood of disease following testing (post-test probability) can be calculated from the test characteristics (sensitivity and specificity) and the pretest probability. This calculated post-test probability is often plotted graphically as a function of pretest probability (Figure 3.3).

In Figure 3.3, the pretest probability is shown on the X-axis and the post-test probability is shown on the Y-axis. The dotted line represents the line of identity. The vertical distance from this line to the upper solid curve represents the increase in the probability of disease as a result of positive test. In analogous fashion, the vertical distance from this dotted line to the lower solid curve represents the decrease in probability as a result of a negative test. The solid vertical lines describe three different clinical situations.

Line A represents a patient with a very low pretest probability, such as a 40-year-old woman with non-anginal pain. A negative test changes probability very little. A positive test increases probability somewhat, but the post-test probability remains well under 50%, and the test is most likely a "false positive".

Line B represents a patient with a high pretest probability of disease, such as a 65-year-old man with typical angina. A positive test will increase the probability only slightly. A negative test will decrease the probability of disease somewhat, but the post-test probability remains substantially greater than 50%, so that the test is most likely a "false negative".

The final situation (line C) represents a patient with an intermediate probability of disease, such as a 50-year-old male with atypical angina. A positive test in such a patient would increase the probability of disease substantially to near 90%. On the other hand a negative test would decrease the probability of disease substantially to approximately 18%.

Thus, it is evident that the incremental value of diagnostic testing is greater in patients with an intermediate probability of disease, a principle that is broadly recognized.[17]

However, it is also recognized that this kind of analysis has a number of limitations. The single curves for positive and negative tests do not take into account the degree of test abnormality. The test results are therefore better displayed for a whole range of values for a parameter that helps distinguish normal from abnormal. The best known example of this would be the magnitude of ST segment depression on treadmill exercise testing.[18] In addition, multiple other parameters are reported during a treadmill exercise test which help to distinguish severely abnormal tests from only mildly abnormal tests.[19] Ideally, all of these parameters would be incorporated into a single "score" and a series of curves would be plotted.

Next, construction of such curves relies on the premise that the sensitivity of tests will be identical for any population of patients with disease regardless of disease prevalence. This assumption is usually invalid. As demonstrated in the previous section, those parameters which help to identify the presence of disease also help to identify the presence of severe disease. In general, the sensitivity of most tests is greater in patients with more severe disease. It is therefore quickly evident that sensitivity would be expected to vary with the prevalence of disease. This point has been demonstrated by several investigators,[20] and provides justification for the use of logistic regression analysis for diagnostic purposes.[21] Despite these limitations, Bayesian analysis serves as a useful framework for understanding the potential incremental value of diagnostic tests.

Non-invasive screening for severe coronary artery disease

The incremental value of testing for the diagnosis of severe coronary artery disease has been studied using both Bayesian analysis and logistic regression analysis. When the latter analysis is conducted properly, all of the previously discussed clinical parameters that are associated with severe coronary disease are incorporated into a model that is used to predict the probability of severe coronary artery disease. The output of such a model is a probability that ranges between 0 and 1. It is critically important that these candidate variables be "forced" into the model, even if they are statistically insignificant in the population under study. Most study populations are too small to have adequate power to detect the true significance of these variables, which has been demonstrated

Table 3.2 Logistic regression multivariate analysis: prediction of three vessel or left main (coronary artery) disease

Model	Direction	Odds ratio (95% CI)	P value
Clinical			
Diabetes mellitus	Present	2.0 (1.3–3.1)	0.001
Typical angina	Present	2.3 (1.4–3.9)	0.001
Sex	Male	3.2 (1.4–4.0)	0.007
Age[a]	Older	1.4 (1.1–1.9)	0.01
$\chi^2 = 31.3$			
Clinical and exercise			
Diabetes mellitus	Present	1.9 (1.2–3.0)	0.005
Typical angina	Present	1.9 (1.1–3.3)	0.02
Sex	Male	2.3 (0.9–5.3)	0.07
Age[a]	Older	1.2 (0.9–1.7)	0.16
Magnitude of ST depression	More	1.5 (1.3–1.8)	<0.001
Peak heart rate × peak systolic blood pressure[b]	Lower	0.9 (0.86–0.95)	<0.001
$\chi^2 = 65.0$			
Clinical, exercise, and thallium-201			
Diabetes mellitus	Present	1.9 (1.2–3.0)	0.004
Typical angina	Present	1.8 (1.1–3.2)	0.03
Sex	Male	2.2 (0.9–5.3)	0.07
Age[a]	Older	1.2 (0.9–1.7)	0.17
Peak heart rate × peak systolic blood pressure[b]	Lower	0.9 (0.86–0.95)	<0.001
Magnitude of ST depression	More	1.4 (1.2–1.7)	0.001
Global TI-201 score (delayed – after exercise)	Higher	1.1 (1.0–1.1)	0.02
$\chi^2 = 70.4$			

[a] Increments of 10 years (each 10-year increase in age increases the odds of severe disease 1.4-fold).
[b] Increments of 1000 units.
From Christian TF *et al.*,[16] with permission.

in very large subsets. For example, age should always be forced into such models, even if it does not appear to be significant in the particular population in question, because there is abundant evidence that it should always be considered (and indeed usually is by clinicians).

Using this approach, a second model should then be constructed which includes all of the clinical parameters, as well as pertinent new parameters from the test in question. If these parameters have statistical significance independent of the clinical parameters, the test has incremental value. This approach is demonstrated in Table 3.2, which shows the improvement in the logistic regression model for severe coronary artery disease reported by Christian *et al.*,[16] when the exercise test was added to clinical parameters, and when thallium imaging parameters were added to clinical and exercise parameters. An alternative approach is to construct the receiver operating characteristic (ROC) curves which display sensitivity and specificity as a function of the predicted probability of severe disease (the output of a logistic regression model). The area under the ROC curve can then be compared between the model that incorporates clinical parameters, and the model that incorporates clinical parameters and the new test parameters. Methods are available for determining the statistical significance of changes

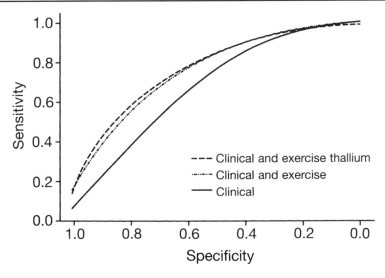

Figure 3.4 Receiver operator characteristic curves for three logistic regression multivariate models for the prediction of severe coronary disease. (From Christian *et al.*,[16] with permission.)

in the area under these two ROC curves.[22] An example of this approach is shown in Figure 3.4, taken from Christian *et al.*[16] The clinical significance of these differences in the models (assessed by either χ^2 analysis or ROC curves) is discussed later.

Prediction of patient outcome

The demonstration of incremental prognostic value for diagnostic tests is obviously extremely important for clinical decision making. It requires strict adherence to the rigorous standards that were outlined previously. In general, very few of the published studies demonstrating prognostic value of diagnostic tests meet the strict criteria necessary to demonstrate *incremental* prognostic value for these tests. The statistical model most often used for this purpose is a linear proportional hazards, or Cox, model.[23] When strictly applied, all the previous information available to the clinician, either from clinical assessment or previous testing, should be incorporated into a linear proportional hazards model that predicts time to an event. Once again, parameters that have been clearly demonstrated in larger populations to be significant must be "forced" into such models to make sure that their contribution is not neglected. The events in question should preferably be hard endpoints such as death and myocardial infarction. As previously mentioned, unstable angina and the need for revascularization are alternative endpoints that are often included to enhance statistical power, but these have major limitations.

One of the best examples of a rigorously constructed analysis demonstrating incremental prognostic value was published by Pollock *et al.* in 1992.[24] They tested the association between various combinations of variables, and time to death or myocardial infarction, in a linear proportional hazards model using the χ^2 statistic. Clinical and exercise variables were significantly better than clinical variables alone. Similarly, a model which added thallium redistribution to clinical and exercise variables was significantly better than the combination of clinical and exercise variables.

Another example of such a rigorous analysis was that reported by Christian et al.,[6] in patients with a normal resting electrocardiogram. Using a similar approach, these investigators reported that a model that added thallium variables to clinical and exercise variables did not add significantly to the model using clinical and exercise variables. Thus, in the subset of patients with a normal resting ECG, Christian et al.[16] were unable to confirm the findings of Pollock et al.[24]

CLINICAL SIGNIFICANCE AND COST-EFFECTIVENESS

Even when statistically significant incremental value has been demonstrated for a diagnostic test using appropriate rigorous methodology, the clinical significance of the findings must be equally rigorously examined. The two fundamental issues that should be addressed are the actual impact of this incremental value on clinical decision making and, where possible, cost-effectiveness. The principles of decision analysis which are pertinent to the first criterion will be presented in much greater detail in Chapter 7. The available published data on diagnostic testing in coronary disease that will be presented here use only rudimentary concepts with respect to decision analysis. Formal cost analysis also requires understanding of a much greater body of published knowledge, which will not be presented here. The examples presented will again be very rudimentary, but demonstrate the principle.

Diagnosis of coronary artery disease

The clinical significance of diagnostic testing can best be understood in terms of decision making thresholds. From the standpoint of diagnosis, a test will be useful primarily if it moves a significant number of patients from an "uncertain" pretest probability to an "acceptably certain" post-test probability. The exact criteria, or threshold, to be used in these classifications are clearly a matter of judgment; many investigators have chosen post-test probabilities of less than 10% and greater than 90% as criteria for definitive diagnosis.[25] Thus, non-invasive testing will be useful for diagnosis if it moves a reasonable number of patients into the shaded zone shown in Figure 3.3.

Although treadmill testing has clear incremental value for diagnosis, particularly in patients with intermediate pretest probability, as discussed earlier, its ability to move patients across such thresholds of probability appears to be very limited. Goldman et al.[26] examined the ability of treadmill exercise variables to classify 329 patients with coronary artery disease. Their results are summarized in Table 3.3. The pretest model was very powerful, as it classified 84% of the patients correctly. Table 3.3 shows the number of additional patients classified correctly for given thresholds of probability. For example, if 10% was considered an acceptable threshold to "rule out" CAD, 8 of 324 patients were moved across this threshold, but only 6 were moved correctly. Similarly, for a 90% threshold to "rule in" CAD, 53 patients were moved across this threshold but only 33 were moved across correctly. As a result, the net total number of patients who were correctly moved into the diagnostic zone in Figure 3.3 was only 17, or 5% of the patient population. Thus, the clinical significance of the incremental value provided by the treadmill test appears to be very limited.

Table 3.3 Effect of treadmill exercise test results in moving patients across various diagnostic thresholds

Threshold probability	No. of patients moved across	Correctly moved	Incorrectly moved	Net increase in diagnoses (correct–incorrect)
0.10	8	6	2	4
0.90	53	33	20	13
Either 0.10 or 0.90	61	39	22	17 (5%)

From Goldman *et al.*,[26] by permission of the American Heart Association, Inc.

Similar rigorous analyses have been published for radionuclide angiography.[27] The results of one of these are displayed in Figure 3.5. The study group excluded men with typical angina over the age of 40 in order to eliminate most patients with a high pretest probability. Logistic regression models developed on a retrospective population were applied prospectively to a group of 76 patients. As demonstrated in Figure 3.5, 8 (11%) of the 76 patients could be classified with 90% certainty on the basis of clinical variables alone. Following radionuclide angiography, 24 patients (32%) could be classified directly. Thus, the incremental value of exercise radionuclide angiography in moving patients across clinically meaningful decision thresholds appeared to be much greater than for the treadmill exercise test, as 21% of the patients were correctly classified using the radionuclide angiogram.

Similar findings have been reported for planar thallium imaging.[28,29] Unfortunately, no rigorous analyses are available for either SPECT imaging or sestamibi imaging, primarily because post-test selection bias has greatly limited the feasibility of such studies in the current era.

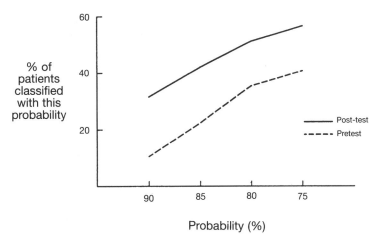

Figure 3.5 Percentage of patients classified with a given probability of coronary disease before and after exercise radionuclide angiography. The prospective study group of 76 patients excluded males of 40 years or older with typical angina. (From Gibbons *et al.*,[27] with permission.)

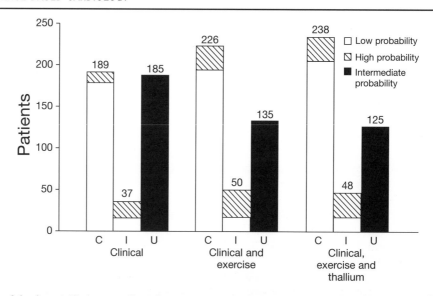

Figure 3.6 Correct (C), incorrect (I), and uncertain (U) classification of patients with three vessel or left main coronary artery disease by the use of logistic regression multivariate models. Low, intermediate, and high probability defined using: clinical variables only; clinical and exercise variables; clinical, exercise, and thallium-201 variables. (From Christian et al.,[16] with permission.)

Non-invasive screening for severe coronary artery disease

The same threshold approach has been applied to the non-invasive identification of severe coronary artery disease. Here the ability of tests to move patients across somewhat different thresholds of probability, as assessed by logistic regression models, has been tested. Christian et al.[16] defined a low probability group for severe coronary artery disease as less than 0.15, a high risk group as >0.35, and an intermediate group as 0.15–0.35. These thresholds were chosen to correspond to earlier work from Duke University reporting on the utility of the early positive treadmill test.[30] Figure 3.6 shows the results that were obtained using this approach. Using clinical parameters alone, 189 patients (46% of the study group) were correctly classified as low or high probability. Thirty-seven patients (9%) were incorrectly classified as low or high probability. The remaining 185 patients (45% of the study group) had an intermediate probability, and were therefore in an uncertain category. The addition of exercise parameters correctly classified an additional 37 patients at the expense of 13 additional incorrect classifications, for a net of 24 additional correct classifications (6% of the study group). The addition of thallium parameters led to 12 additional correct classifications, and two fewer incorrect classifications for a net increase of 14 correct classifications (3% of the study group). These workers then used Medicare reimbursement figures to calculate the cost per additional correct classification. For exercise testing, the cost per additional correct patient classification was $1524. For thallium scintigraphy, the cost was $20 550 per additional correct classification.

Thus, this analysis demonstrated that the clinical impact was modest, and the cost was high, when thallium imaging was used in patients with a normal resting electrocardiogram to try to non-invasively identify patients with severe coronary artery disease. Although thallium scintigraphy clearly had statistically significant incremental value, it did not appear to be cost-effective for this purpose.

Prediction of patient outcome

The issues of clinical significance and cost-effectiveness are particularly pertinent to the application of diagnostic tests for the prediction of the patient outcome. These applications often involve relatively low risk patient groups with few subsequent events. Tests applied to the entire population may identify a subset of patients who are at considerably increased risk.[31,32] These results will be highly statistically significant, and generate very impressive P values and risk ratios. However, it must be recognized that the absolute rate of events often remains too low in the high risk patient subgroup to be clinically meaningful, and the cost of this identification is often therefore prohibitive when viewed on a per event basis.

This concept was nicely demonstrated in a study by Berman et al.[33] on patients with a low clinical likelihood of coronary artery disease studied by SPECT sestamibi. During 20 months of follow-up, only patients with an abnormal sestamibi study suffered death or myocardial infarction. This difference was statistically highly significant ($P = 0.007$). However, this increment in prognostic value was clearly not cost-effective, as noted by the authors. Although the cost analysis by the authors was quite detailed, the cost-ineffectiveness of this approach is readily apparent with very simple analysis. The 107 patients in the high risk group suffered only three events during 20 months of follow-up. In order to identify the high risk group, testing was required of 548 patients. Using a Medicare reimbursement figure of $700 per test,[16] more than $383 000 of testing would be required to identify the high risk cohort. The cost of testing alone would therefore exceed $127 000 per possible event prevented. This simple analysis ignores the additional costs that would accrue from the subsequent cardiac catheterizations and coronary revascularizations that would be necessary in the high risk group in order to attempt to prevent the three events. (There is obviously no certainty that the three events could actually be prevented by revascularization.)

Similar analyses have been published for screening in asymptomatic individuals. As a general principle, it should be recognized that non-invasive testing for the assessment of prognosis is far less cost-effective in subsets of patients at intrinsically low risk.

CONCLUSION

Clinicians should recognize that an evidence based approach to the evaluation of the incremental value of diagnostic tests is not simple or straightforward. Unfortunately, it is far easier for both clinicians and investigators to use simple, less rigorous, approaches which appear to demonstrate important incremental value for each new diagnostic test. Although convenient, such approaches lead to incorrect conclusions, and generally overestimate the added value of each new testing modality. The examples presented in this chapter will hopefully provide a framework for thinking clinicians to better evaluate new publications on new diagnostic tests. However difficult these analyses may be, and however disappointing the results, the escalating costs of health care demand an approach of rigorous methodology and thoughtful analysis to make certain that the *incremental* value of a diagnostic test is not only statistically significant, but clinically significant and cost-effective.

REFERENCES

1 Diamond G. Penny wise. *Am J Cardiol* 1988;**62**: 806–8.

2 Bobbio M, Pollock BH, Cohen I, Diamond GA. Comparative accuracy of clinical tests for diagnosis and prognosis of coronary artery disease. *Am J Cardiol* 1988;**62**:896–900.

3 Ladenheim ML, Kotler TS, Pollock BH, Berman DS, Diamond GA. Incremental prognostic power of clinical history, exercise electrocardiography and myocardial perfusion scintigraphy in suspected coronary artery disease. *Am J Cardiol* 1987;**59**:270–7.

4 Diamond GA, Forrester JS. Analysis of probability as an aid in the clinical diagnosis of coronary artery disease. *N Engl J Med* 1979;**300**:1350–8.

5 Diamond GA. Letter: a clinical relevant classification of chest discomfort. *J Am Coll Cardiol* 1983;**1**:574–5.

6 Pryor DB, Harrell FE Jr, Lee KL, Califf RM, Rosati RA. Estimating the likelihood of significant coronary artery disease. *Am J Med* 1983;**75**: 771–80.

7 Weiner DA, McCabe CH, Ryan TJ. Identification of patients with left main and three vessel coronary disease with clinical and exercise test variables. *Am J Cardiol* 1980;**46**:21–7.

8 Hubbard BL, Gibbons RJ, Lapeyre AC, Zinsmeister AR, Clements IP. Identification of severe coronary artery disease using simple clinical parameters. *Arch Intern Med* 1992;**152**:309–12.

9 Pryor DB, Shaw L, Harrell FE Jr *et al.* Estimating the likelihood of severe coronary artery disease. *Am J Med* 1991;**90**:553–62.

10 Pryor DB, Shaw L, McCants CB *et al.* Value of the history and physical in identifying patients at increased risk for coronary artery disease. *Ann Intern Med* 1993;**118**:81–90.

11 Weiner DA, Ryan TJ, McCabe CH *et al.* The role of exercise testing in identifying patients with improved survival after coronary artery bypass surgery. *J Am Coll Cardiol* 1986;**8**:741–8.

12 O'Keefe JH Jr, Zinsmeister AR, Gibbons RJ. Value of electrocardiographic findings in predicting rest left ventricular function in patients with chest pain and suspected coronary artery disease. *Am J Med* 1989;**86**:658–62.

13 Rihal CS, Davis KB, Kennedy JW, Gersh BJ. The utility of clinical, electrocardiographic, and roentgenographic variables in the prediction of left ventricular function. *Am J Cardiol* 1995;**75**: 220–3.

14 Connolly DC, Elveback LR, Oxman HA. Coronary heart disease in residents of Rochester, Minnesota. IV. Prognostic value of the resting electrocardiogram at the time of initial diagnosis of angina pectoris. *Mayo Clin Proc* 1984;**59**: 247–50.

15 Gibbons RJ, Zinsmeister AR, Miller TD, Clements IP. Supine exercise electrocardiography compared with exercise radionuclide angiography in noninvasive identification of severe coronary artery disease. *Ann Intern Med* 1990;**112**: 743–9.

16 Christian TF, Miller TD, Bailey KR, Gibbons RJ. Exercise tomographic thallium-201 imaging in patients with severe coronary artery disease and normal electrocardiogram. *Ann Intern Med* 1994; **121**:825–32.

17 Epstein SE. Implications of probability analysis on the strategy used for noninvasive detection of coronary artery disease. *Am J Cardiol* 1980;**46**: 491–9.

18 Rifkin RD, Hood WB Jr. Bayesian analysis of electrocardiographic exercise stress testing. *N Engl J Med* 1977;**297**:681–6.

19 Cohn K, Kamm B, Feteih N, Brand R, Goldschlager N. Use of treadmill score to quantify ischemic response and predict extent of coronary disease. *Circulation* 1979;**59**:286–96.

20 Currie PJ, Kelly MJ, Harper RW *et al.* Incremental value of clinical assessment, supine exercise electrocardiography, and biplane exercise radionuclide ventriculography in the prediction of coronary artery disease in men with chest pain. *Am J Cardiol* 1983;**52**:927–35.

21 Morise AP, Detrano R, Bobbio M, Diamond GA. Development and validation of a logistic regression-derived algorithm for estimating the incremental probability of coronary artery disease before and after exercise testing. *J Am Coll Cardiol* 1992;**20**:1187–96.

22 Wieand S, Gail M, James K, James B. A family of non-parametric statistics for comparing diagnostic tests with paired or unpaired data. *Biometrika* 1989;**76**:585–92.

23 Cox DR. Regression models and life tables. *J R Stat Soc B* 1972;**34**:197–220.

24 Pollock SG, Abbott RD, Boucher CA, Beller GA, Kaul S. Independent and incremental prognostic

value of tests performed in hierarchical order to evaluate patients with suspected coronary artery disease. Validation of models based on these tests. *Circulation* 1992;**85**:237–48.

25 Diamond GA, Forrester JS, Hirsch M *et al.* Application of conditional probability analysis to the clinical diagnosis of coronary artery disease. *J Clin Invest* 1980;**65**:1210–21.

26 Goldman L, Cook EF, Mitchell N *et al.* Incremental value of the exercise test for diagnosing the presence or absence of coronary artery disease. *Circulation* 1982;**66**:945–53.

27 Gibbons RJ, Lee KL, Pryor DB *et al.* The use of radionuclide angiography in the diagnosis of coronary artery disease: a logistic regression analysis. *Circulation* 1983;**68**:740–6.

28 Detrano R, Yiannikas J, Salcedo EE *et al.* Bayesian probability analysis: a prospective demonstration of its clinical utility in diagnosing coronary disease. *Circulation* 1984;**69**:541–7.

29 Melin JA, Wijns W, Vanbutsele RJ *et al.* Alternative diagnostic strategies for coronary artery disease in women: demonstration of the usefulness and efficiency of probability analysis. *Circulation* 1985; **71**:535–42.

30 McNeer JF, Margolis JR, Lee KL *et al.* The role of the exercise test in the evaluation of patients for ischemic heart disease. *Circulation* 1978;**57**: 64–70.

31 Rautaharju PM, Prineas RJ, Eifler WJ *et al.* Prognostic value of exercise electrocardiogram in men at high risk of future coronary heart disease: multiple risk factor intervention trial experience. *J Am Coll Cardiol* 1986;**8**:1–10.

32 Giagnoni E, Secchi MB, Wu SC *et al.* Prognostic value of exercise EKG testing in asymptomatic normotensive subjects: a prospective matched study. *N Engl J Med* 1983;**309**:1085–9.

33 Berman DS, Hachamovitch R, Hosen K *et al.* Incremental value of prognostic testing in patients with known or suspected ischemic heart disease: a basis for optimal utilization of exercise technetium-99m sestamibi myocardial perfusion single-photon emission computed tomography. *J Am Coll Cardiol* 1995;**26**: 639–47.

4 Finding current best evidence to practice evidence based cardiology

Dereck L. Hunt,
K. Ann McKibbon,
R. Brian Haynes

INTRODUCTION

Staying current with new diagnostic tests, treatments and other clinically useful new knowledge in a rapidly evolving field such as cardiology requires effort. Fortunately, this once daunting task is becoming more feasible because of new evidence based information resources and the steady advance of information technology into clinical settings. This chapter will review ways to find current best evidence for the care of patients with cardiac problems, including both solving patient problems as they arise, and keeping up with new evidence that is ready for application in clinical practice.

The patients whom we see on a daily basis provide the best stimulus to staying current. They may have clinical problems that we are unfamiliar with, or that we have not recently reviewed. They may also present us with information from the media or friends to evaluate or ask us questions that we need to research before answering. Depending on the type of center in which we work, our colleagues, teachers, and students may also ask questions or provide suggestions that make us realize that our knowledge may be "time-challenged".

To become proficient in responding to such challenges (also known as "learning opportunities"), we can make use of a growing array of specialized information resources, aided by information technology that can bring access to our fingertips, almost wherever we may be. To illustrate how patient contacts can provide us with the stimulus to keep up to date and be aware of new evidence, consider the following scenarios.

1. During your outpatient clinic, you see a 56-year-old woman who recently became your patient after she moved to your community. She has been diagnosed as having idiopathic dilated cardiomyopathy and had an echocardiogram 6 months ago which revealed a diffusely enlarged left ventricle with no segmental abnormalities. The ejection fraction was estimated to

be less than 30%. You review her current condition and note that her symptoms are controlled on an angiotensin converting enzyme (ACE) inhibitor, digoxin, and a diuretic. Still she complains of fatigue and dyspnea on moderate exertion. Before leaving, she asks if you can recommend any other medications that would help.

2. Later that day, you visit the intensive care unit. Another of your patients, a 76-year-old man with a history of stable angina, recently had an elective repair of an abdominal aortic aneurysm. After the surgery, he developed congestive heart failure, but now is improving after diuresis. An electrocardiogram shows non-specific changes, and while the creatine kinase is elevated, the MB fraction is not diagnostic of an acute myocardial infarction. You still consider myocardial infarction to be the most likely diagnosis, and the house staff ask you whether one of the new markers of myocardial injury, such as troponin, would be helpful in establishing a firm diagnosis.

3. Finally, as you are leaving the hospital, you pass through the emergency department where an emergency physician happens to notice you. She has been working up a 65-year-old man who presented with a swollen left calf. He had an ultrasound that confirmed the presence of a deep venous thrombosis. The patient is anxious to return home because his wife is ill and requires care. The emergency physician is interested in your opinion on the use of low molecular weight heparin for the treatment of deep venous thrombosis in outpatients.

These questions are consistent with the common information needs of physicians. For internists, questions arise at a rate of two questions for every three outpatients seen[1] and five questions on average for every inpatient.[2] No one knows whether cardiologists confront similar numbers of questions, but no professional discipline studied to date is immune from the need to address unanswered questions to keep up with the advance of knowledge. And being able to find the best evidence to answer clinical questions appropriately and efficiently is becoming all the more important these days with shrinking budgets and increasing demands for financial and legal accountability.

How would you address each of the questions raised by the clinical scenarios? The possibilities include, but are not limited to, using an electronic bibliographic database such as MEDLINE, specialized abstract journals like *ACP Journal Club* or *Evidence-Based Cardiovascular Medicine*, current textbooks, and new electronic resources such as *Best Evidence*, The Cochrane Library and the Internet. We will consider the strengths and weaknesses of each of these resources and apply them to the clinical problems.

MEDLINE

MEDLINE is a huge, multipurpose database of medical literature citations and abstracts produced by the US National Library of Medicine (NLM). It includes citations to almost all important clinical studies, and also a much larger volume of non-clinical studies and articles. Few other resources currently rival this scope. Accessing MEDLINE is relatively easy.[3–5] CD-ROM based systems, online systems, and Internet versions are all available. Examples of CD-ROM systems include OVID, Aries and SilverPlatter. Online access by modem is available through several vendors, including the NLM (Grateful Med), DIALOG, PaperChase, and HealthGate systems.[6] Internet access is readily available (see Medical Matrix [http://www.slackinc.com/matrix] and Dr Felix's Free MEDLINE Page [http://www.netlink.co.uk/users/Sharkli/medline-html] sites for links to locations that currently offer MEDLINE access). Some of these MEDLINE systems have user fees but, at least at present, free access is available from some, led by the NLM with two free internet sites,

Internet Grateful Med [http://www.igm.nlm.nih.gov/] and PubMed [http://www.ncbi.nlm.nih.gov/PubMed/clinical.htm]. The latter features earliest MEDLINE access to newly published articles and point-and-click search strategies that improve the yield of clinically useful studies on the cause, course, diagnosis and treatment of clinical problems.

If ready access is one of MEDLINE's strengths, the skills needed to rapidly and dependably locate high quality articles that specifically address a clinical question are a weakness. A working knowledge of MEDLINE searching terminology and searching strategies is essential. Luckily, most hospital and university libraries offer training courses for MEDLINE. The NLM has also established a set of eight regional medical libraries that are charged with providing access and training for all US health personnel (+1-800-272-4787). Physicians in the United Kingdom can call the Health Care Information Service (+44 171 412 7477) for similar information, while Canadians can call the Canada Institute for Scientific and Technical Information (+1-800-668-1222).

Turning to our initial scenario, we are interested in locating information about new medical therapies for patients with idiopathic dilated cardiomyopathy. Also, it would be wise to focus initially on treatments that already have been adequately tested in well designed clinical trials.[7] While it may be interesting to read about new medications that are being designed and tested at the laboratory level, or are undergoing early human testing, this information will not be immediately applicable in our clinical practices.

Turning to MEDLINE for assistance, it would be reasonable to begin searching by using a medical subject heading (MeSH) for congestive heart failure. MEDLINE indexers choose appropriate terms from a thesaurus of 14 000 specific terms and 18 000 synonyms for content and methodology. Unfortunately, these terms are not always intuitive (e.g., beta-blockers indexed as adrenergic beta-antagonists). Therefore, it is often necessary to search through the MeSH vocabulary before carrying out a search. The software for all search systems includes MeSH, so it is quite easy to search for appropriate terms. For our topic, a search for CONGESTIVE HEART FAILURE leads to HEART FAILURE, CONGESTIVE.

Depending on the topic and the scope that you are interested in covering, you may also want to take advantage of two additional features of MeSH headings. Because many articles deal predominantly with two or three topics, the NLM will indicate these topics for each citation by designating them as major subjects of the article. Some MEDLINE searching systems use the term MAJORING to designate this, while others use the asterisk (*) symbol before the MeSH heading. Limiting your search to articles in which the search term has been designated as the major subject heading will be beneficial if you retrieve too many citations from using the search term without "majoring" it, although sometimes you can miss important studies this way, because they have not been properly indexed. A trial and error approach may be needed to retrieve the best studies.

"Exploding" is another useful feature of MEDLINE MeSH indexing. When articles are indexed, they are classified according to the most specific MeSH heading available. Thus, if you wish to identify all articles that deal with congestive heart failure, including those with more specific MeSH terms such as congestive cardiomyopathy, then you can do so by searching with the term EXPLODE HEART FAILURE, CONGESTIVE. This search retrieves 6577 citations (using the 1992 to December 1996 MEDLINE database)!

If you are searching for a topic that has not been well indexed, you may want to take advantage of textword searching. Using this approach, you are simply asking MEDLINE to search the titles and abstracts of all the citations for any occurrences of a certain sequence of letters, such as "dilated". This approach is particularly useful for new drugs, such as carvedilol, or concepts (such as ventilator-associated or nosocomial pneumonia) that have not yet been incorporated into MeSH. MeSH is updated annually, but the lag can be considerably longer for new terms.

If several different endings to a word may have been used, and you wish to identify them all, you can use "truncation", using the ":" symbol. For example, if you asked for RANDOM:, MEDLINE would search for RANDOM, RANDOMIZATION, RANDOMIZED, RANDOMISATION, RANDOMISED, and RANDOMLY. Be careful with truncation. The term "salmon:" retrieves not only the fish but salmonella as well! Some systems may use symbols other than ":", such as "?".

Returning to identifying new therapies for patients with significant left ventricular dysfunction, EXPLODE HEART FAILURE, CONGESTIVE is a good start, but we need to narrow in on treatments that have been tested in well designed studies. Luckily, a number of methodological search strategies have been tested and validated for retrieving sound studies for questions relating to therapy, prognosis, etiology or cause, and diagnosis[8,9] (Table 4.1). Alternatively, you can search for a systematic review of studies. Research is currently ongoing to establish the best approach to identify systematic reviews and meta-analyses.[10] For our current search, limiting the 6577 citations to systematic reviews and meta-analyses seemed like a reasonable first step. A simple, but not fully validated strategy to identify systematic reviews and meta-analyses is to identify all citations in which the publication type is designated as meta-analysis (note that in addition to indexing articles according to subject, the NLM also indexes citations according to "publication type". Over 40 publication types are recognized, including "meta-analysis", "randomized controlled trial", and "review"), as well as citations that include the phrase "meta-anal:" as a textword, and citations that are designated as reviews in the publication type section, but also have the textword "MEDLINE" in their abstract. Putting this all together yielded the following search strategy using an OVID search system:

1. exp heart failure, congestive	6577	(exp indicates explode)
2. meta-analysis.pt.	1670	(pt indicates publication type)
3. meta-anal:.tw.	1817	(tw indicates textword)
4. review.pt. and medline.tw.	861	
5. 2 or 3 or 4	3311	(the "or" means that all citations in either #2 or #3 or #4 will be included)
6. 1 and 5	32	(the "and" means that only citations that occur in both #1 and #5 will be identified)

Many hospital and library MEDLINE systems also permit citations to be limited to journals that the library currently receives (*limit to local holdings*), as well as limiting the results to articles in the English language (*limit to English language*), articles that have an abstract (*limit to abstracts*) (this gets rid of letters and editorials), and many other features such as the publication date, age groups, etc.

7. limit 6 to local holdings	30
8. limit 7 to English language	27
9. limit 8 to abstracts	24

Table 4.1 Optimal search strategies for identifying studies relating to treatment, diagnosis, prognosis, or etiology using MEDLINE

Treatment	
Best single term:	clinical trial.pt. ("pt" indicates publication type)
Combination of terms with best specificity:	placebo:.tw. ("tw" indicates textword)
	OR double.tw. AND blind:.tw.
Combination of terms with best sensitivity:	randomized controlled trial.pt.
	OR random:.tw.
	OR drug therapy (as a subheading of the subject)
	OR therapeutic use (as a subheading of the subject)
Diagnosis	
Best single term:	explode diagnosis
Combination of terms with best specificity:	explode "sensitivity and specificity"
	OR predictive.tw. AND value:.tw.
Combination of terms with best sensitivity:	explode "sensitivity and specificity"
	OR explode diagnosis (as a subheading of the subject)
	OR sensitivity.tw.
	OR specificity.tw.
	OR diagnostic use (as a subheading of the subject)
Prognosis	
Best single term:	explode cohort studies
Combination of terms with best specificity:	prognosis
	OR survival analysis
Combination of terms with best sensitivity:	incidence
	OR explode mortality
	OR follow-up studies
	OR prognos:.tw.
	OR predict:.tw.
	OR course:.tw.
	OR mortality (as a subheading of the subject)
Etiology or cause	
Best single term:	risk.tw.
Combination of terms with best specificity:	cohort studies
	OR case-control studies
Combination of terms with best sensitivity:	explode cohort studies
	OR explode risk
	OR odds.tw. AND ratio:.tw.
	OR relative.tw. AND risk.tw.
	OR case.tw. AND control:.tw.

Based on Haynes *et al.*[8] and Wilczynski *et al.*[9]

Looking at the titles and abstracts of these 24 articles, you see that eight discuss ACE inhibitors, 14 relate to a range of topics including the epidemiology of idiopathic cardiomyopathy and the role of diuretics, anticoagulation, and revascularization in congestive heart failure, and two relate to the use of beta-blockers in patients with left ventricular dysfunction. One of these two articles on beta-blockers is a meta-analysis and the abstract suggests that these medications may be beneficial. You decide to go to the library to retrieve this paper[11] and then to critically appraise it using the guidelines for a systematic review.[12] This article may well answer your question relating to your first patient, or you may decide to do another search specifically on the role of beta-blockers in patients with congestive heart failure.

Many alternative ways exist for conducting a MEDLINE search for many topics, including the one just displayed. Unfortunately, because no perfect recipe exists, what works well in one situation may not work as well in another. Combining an appropriate content term (HEART FAILURE, CONGESTIVE, in this case) with methods terms for reviews (above) or for sound study designs (as in Table 4.1) will usually result in better search results. It also has to be considered, however, that such searches are bound to take some time. This is because of the general nature of this huge biomedical research database: it is so big and comprehensive that even the extensive indexing and care that is taken in preparing it are insufficient to guarantee quick and accurate retrieval for clinical uses. Fortunately, many vendors have developed specialized subsets of MEDLINE for clinical use in cardiology. For example, Aries (www.ariessys.com) offers a cardiovascular disease subset (CardLine) on compact disk that you can subscribe to yourself. Instead of having one full year of MEDLINE on each CD-ROM disk, these subsets provide journals and citations relating to a specific field for inclusion. For example, CardLine has cardiology citations from MEDLINE for the 10 most recent years on one disk.

SPECIALIZED CLINICAL INFORMATION RESOURCES

While large electronic bibliographic databases such as MEDLINE can be very helpful, they can also be very frustrating or overwhelming because of the different ways that articles can be indexed and because of the vast array of pre-clinical and non-clinical literature that is included. MEDLINE serves many user groups besides clinicians (basic scientists and other researchers, educators, librarians, journalists, etc.). An alternative is to use a resource that includes only methodologically sound and clinically relevant articles, such as *ACP Journal Club* (American College of Physicians (ACP)), for internal medicine and its subspecialties, *Evidence-Based Medicine* (for all major specialties; from ACP and from the BMJ Publishing Group), and a new cardiology journal *Evidence-Based Cardiovascular Medicine* (published by Churchill Livingstone). These are available in paper form and the first two have been combined into an electronic version known as *Best Evidence* (from ACP and the BMJ Publishing Group) that includes studies from over 75 medical journals, beginning in 1991. In addition to including only methodologically sound articles[13] and presenting the results using a structured abstract format, these journals also include a commentary written by a clinical expert that is designed to put the study findings into clinical context.

Searching *Best Evidence* using the terms HEART FAILURE and BLOCK*, limited to articles on Therapeutics and Prevention yields 30 items in a few seconds, including recent studies on carvedilol and other new beta-blockers. Recalling the second scenario at the beginning of this chapter, searching *Best Evidence* using the term "troponin" retrieves two citations. One of these deals with the diagnosis of myocardial infarction out of the context of perioperative care.[14] The second appears to be directly on target[15] but is from the "Other Articles Noted" section of the database, that is, studies that meet methodologic criteria but which were not abstracted because of space limitations in the print publications. Again, this search takes only a few seconds, certainly faster than any MEDLINE search. You already have one potentially useful reference from *Best Evidence* but may want more. Trying MEDLINE once again, you conduct a search using the MeSH term TROPONIN and cross this with a diagnostic test methodology search strategy with high specificity.

1.	*troponin	497
2.	myocardial infarction	11265
3.	1 and 2	92
4.	exp "Sensitivity and Specificity"	30304
5.	predictive.tw. AND value:.tw.	6845
6.	4 or 5	33487
7.	3 and 6	27
8.	limit 7 to local holdings	18
9.	limit 8 to English language	17
10.	limit 9 to abstracts	14

This yields 14 citations, including an article entitled "Troponin T as a marker for myocardial ischemia in patients undergoing major noncardiac surgery".[16] The abstract looks promising. You retrieve the full article for this study and the study by Adams and colleagues to review and appraise.[17,18] It appears that troponin is a valid marker for perioperative myocardial infarction. For the time being, however, you decide against ordering the test. Even if the test indicated that your patient had not suffered a recent myocardial infarction, you would still wish to have him in a monitored setting for another 1–2 days.

This leaves the question posed in relation to your third patient unanswered. Can either of the resources that you have just familiarized yourself with guide you in advising your patient on the wisdom of outpatient heparinization for deep venous thrombosis? Searching *Best Evidence* using the text phrase "low molecular weight heparin" you locate several relevant references, including one directly on target.[19] This report summarizes the findings of two randomized controlled trials comparing intravenous heparin administered in hospital with subcutaneous low molecular weight heparin administered at home, and both found that outpatient therapy was as safe and effective as inhospital management. Having located sufficient information, you decide that you do not need to turn to MEDLINE in this case.

OTHER RESOURCES

The Cochrane Library is a new and increasingly valuable source of evidence summaries and trials of health care interventions. This new electronic database is updated quarterly and contains the collected work of the Cochrane Collaboration, an international voluntary organization that prepares, maintains, and disseminates systematic reviews of randomized trials of health care interventions. Available on disk and CD-ROM, and via the Internet (http://www.medlib.com), the Cochrane Library consists of four sections: the Cochrane Database of Systematic Reviews (CDSR), the Database of Abstracts of Reviews of Effectiveness (DARE), the Cochrane Controlled Trials Registry (CCTR), and the Cochrane Review Methodology Database (CRMD). The CDSR consists of the full reports of Cochrane Collaboration systematic reviews as well as protocols for ongoing systematic reviews. DARE is produced by the UK National Health Services Centre for Reviews and Dissemination located at the University of York. It contains citations to many non-Cochrane systematic reviews, and includes structured abstracts for many of them. The CCTR is a growing collection of over 150 000 citations to therapeutic intervention trials.

Searching the Cochrane Library is relatively easy and only requires entering a word or short phrase. The Library automatically searches all four sections for any relevant reviews or citations. Applying this to our scenarios, searching using the term "congestive heart failure" in Cochrane Library 1997, Issue 4, yields numerous citations: seven citations to completed reviews in the CDSR, 18 citations in the DARE, and 864 citations in the CCTR. None of the Cochrane reviews addresses our question; the structured abstracts within the DARE relate to the role of exercise, phosphodiesterase inhibitors, revascularization, anticoagulation, and ACE inhibitors in patients with left ventricular dysfunction as well as including a meta-analysis of hypertension treatment trials. An *ACP Journal Club* reference discusses the role of the physical examination in patients with dyspnea. Sixteen more citations to systematic reviews are included under the DARE section. Doing a similar search using the term "low molecular weight heparin" locates numerous references including an abstract in the DARE that addresses the safety of low molecular weight heparin in comparison with unfractionated heparin.[20] While these reports are interesting, the studies that were identified using *Best Evidence* are more current and are more relevant to the clinical question.

TEXTBOOKS

At this point, you may be thinking about your textbooks. What role do these have in clinical practice and in particular with respect to staying current? Textbooks remain an important resource for clinicians in terms of anatomy and pathophysiology, the basics of practice that usually do not change very quickly, except perhaps for molecular biology. They also provide descriptions of the classical presentations of numerous disease conditions and review important aspects of the history, physical examination, and diagnostic testing. By reviewing conditions that may present with similar findings, a good textbook can also help to broaden the differential diagnosis in more complex cases. These references may also describe medication side effects and pharmacokinetics, and may include historical perspectives and practical suggestions to assist in patient management.

As an example of a textbook that is relatively up-to-date, consider the 1997 edition of *Heart disease: a textbook of cardiovascular medicine*.[21] This book devotes several pages to discussing the role of beta-blockers in the management of patients with heart failure, and reviews the role of cardiac-specific troponin assays in the diagnosis of a myocardial infarction. Unfortunately, there is often a passage of three or more years between updates of specialty textbooks, and many new studies will be published in the interval. For example, in the third edition of *Hemostasis and thrombosis*, edited by Colman and colleagues,[22] four paragraphs are devoted to discussing the role of low molecular weight heparins for the treatment of deep venous thrombosis. Several randomized controlled trials comparing standard heparin with low molecular weight heparin are reviewed. At the time of publication, however, no trials had been conducted to compare standard heparin administered in hospital with outpatient management of deep venous thrombosis using low molecular weight heparin.

Textbooks are also seldom explicit about the quality or currency of evidence used in recommendations for management. Particularly for rapidly evolving aspects of management such as laboratory diagnosis and therapeutics, print textbooks simply cannot be trusted. Fortunately, we are beginning to see the emergence of CD-ROM textbooks with regular updates, such as *Scientific American Medicine* (SAM),[23] and texts are starting to appear on the Internet.

THE INTERNET

This brings us to the World Wide Web, an increasingly useful resource for locating current information, and one that our patients are accessing at an increasing rate. We have already mentioned how MEDLINE can be accessed over the Web. Additionally, a growing number of journals are available online. A few examples include the *New England Journal of Medicine* (http://www.nejm.org), *Annals of Internal Medicine* (http://acponline.org), *JAMA* (http://www.ama-assn.orrg), *British Medical Journal* (*BMJ*) (http://www.bmj.com), and *The Lancet* (http://www.thelancet.com). These sites provide online access to the editorials, letters, narrative review articles, and abstracts to original studies that appeared in these journals during the past few years. Some of the journals also provide search engines to locate articles on a particular topic. The complete text versions of a growing number of studies are also becoming available.

If you do not have ready access to a comprehensive medical library, online access to complete articles is especially helpful. Despite the growing number of full text articles, however, many journals do not yet offer this service. Instead, they may offer to send complete copies of articles to you for a fee. In a similar fashion, several websites (including HealthGate's site at http://www.healthgate.com) that provide MEDLINE searching facilities also allow users to order print versions of articles of interest.

Finally, a growing number of sites on the Internet contain information relevant to clinical medicine. Some cardiology textbooks are available online, as are many clinical practice guidelines. And while many of these sources currently contain information that is less current than some of the articles indexed by MEDLINE, this may well change with the rapid rate of development of the Internet. One example of a healthcare website worth exploring is the Medical Matrix (http://www.slackinc/com/matrix).

JOURNALS AND BROWSING TO KEEP UP TO DATE

We have focused to this point on looking for evidence when it is needed. If the search is successful, the evidence can be applied immediately and this can be a powerful learning experience. But what if we don't search for evidence because we don't know that we are out of date? A complementary strategy is needed, browsing the medical literature regularly in one way or another. The difficulty is that so many journals include articles relevant to cardiology that it is impracticable to review them all. The best solution to this is to subscribe to a journal such as *Evidence-Based Cardiovascular*

Medicine that continuously scans a wide range of journals in a systematic way (according to explicit criteria) and includes structured abstracts and commentaries on methodologically sound and clinically relevant studies.

CONCLUSION

In summary then, while the time that we devote to updating ourselves with new developments is limited, a growing number of easy-access resources are available so that we can use this time effectively. MEDLINE is more readily available now than it ever has been before and is seeding the development of specialty-specific collections. Journals that abstract only high quality, clinically relevant articles are appearing, and systematic reviews are becoming the norm. Applying these resources to clinical care on an ongoing basis after appraising the quality of information and considering how it relates to our individual patients can improve the quality of care we provide.

- New resources are rapidly emerging that make keeping up to date with clinically significant developments in cardiology easier than ever.
- Large bibliographic databases, such as MEDLINE, are becoming more accessible to practicing physicians, and search strategies for locating high quality studies are now available.
- Specialty journals, such as *Evidence-Based Cardiovascular Medicine*, that identify and abstract methodologically sound and clinically relevant studies, also facilitate the ongoing process of staying current.

REFERENCES

1 Covell DG, Uman GC, Manning PR. Information needs in office practice: are they being met? *Ann Intern Med* 1985;**103**:596–9.

2 Osheroff JA, Forsythe DE, Buchanan BG *et al.* Physicians' information needs: analysis of questions posed during clinical teaching. *Ann Intern Med* 1991;**114**:576–81.

3 McKibbon KA, Walker-Dilks CJ. Beyond ACP. Journal Club: How to harness MEDLINE to solve clinical problems (Editorial). *ACP J Club* 1994; **120**:A10–A12.

4 Haynes RB, Walker CJ, McKibbon KA, Johnston M, Willan A. Performance of 27 MEDLINE systems tested by searches on clinical questions. *J Am Med Informatics Assoc* 1994;**1**:285–95.

5 Engstrom P. MEDLINE free-for-all spurs questions about search value: who pays? *Medicine on the NET* 1996;**2**:1–5.

6 Haynes RB, McKibbon KA, Walker CJ *et al.* Online access to MEDLINE in clinical settings. A study of use and usefulness. *Ann Intern Med* 1990;**112**: 78–84.

7 Sackett DL, Richardson SR, Rosenberg W, Haynes RB. *Evidence-based medicine: how to practise and teach EBM*. London: Churchill Livingstone, 1997.

8 Haynes RB, Wilczynski N, McKibbon KA, Walker CJ, Sinclair JC. Developing optimal search strategies for detecting clinically sound studies in MEDLINE. *J Am Med Informatics Assoc* 1994;**1**: 447–58.

9 Wilczynski NL, Walker CJ, McKibbon KA, Haynes RB. Assessment of methodological search filters in MEDLINE. *Proc Annu Symp Comp Appl Med Care* 1994;**17**:601–5.

10 Hunt DL, McKibbon KA. Locating and appraising systematic reviews. *Ann Intern Med* 1997;**126**: 532–8.

11 Zarembski DG, Nolan PE Jr, Slack MK, Lui CY. Meta-analysis of the use of low-dose beta-adrenergic blocking therapy in idiopathic or ischemic dilated cardiomyopathy. *Am J Cardiol* 1996;**77**:1247–50.

12 Oxman A, Cook D, Guyatt G. Users' guides to the medical literature. VI. How to use an overview. *JAMA* 1994;**272**:1367–71.

13 Haynes RB. The origins and aspirations of ACP Journal Club (Editorial). *ACP J Club* 1991;**114**: A18.

14 Bedside serum cardiac troponin T analysis was sensitive for myocardial infarction (Abstract). *ACP J Club* 1995;**123**:72. [Abstract of Antman EM, Grudzien C, Sacks DB. Evaluation of a rapid

bedside assay for detection of serum cardiac troponin T. *JAMA* 1995;**273**:1279–82.]

15 Adams JE 3rd, Sicard GA, Allen BT *et al.* Diagnosis of perioperative myocardial infarction with measurement of cardiac troponin I. *N Engl J Med* 1994;**330**:670–4.

16 Lee TH, Thomas EJ, Ludwig LE *et al.* Troponin T as a marker for myocardial ischemia in patients undergoing major noncardiac surgery. *Am J Cardiol* 1996;**77**:1031–6.

17 Jaeschke R, Guyatt G, Sackett DL. Users' guides to the medical literature. III. How to use an article about a diagnostic test. A. Are the results of the study valid? *JAMA* 1994;**271**:389–91.

18 Jaeschke R, Guyatt G, Sackett DL. Users' guides to the medical literature. III. How to use an article about a diagnostic test. B. What were the results and will they help me in caring for my patients? *JAMA* 1994;**271**:703–7.

19 Low-molecular-weight heparin at home was as effective as unfractionated heparin in the hospital in proximal DVT (Abstracts). *ACP J Club* 1996; **125**:2–3. [Abstracts of Koopman MM, Prandoni P, Piovella F *et al.* Treatment of venous thrombosis with intravenous unfractionated heparin administered in the hospital as compared with subcutaneous low-molecular-weight heparin administered at home. *N Engl J Med* 1996;**334**: 682–7; and Levine M, Gent M, Hirsh J *et al.* A comparison of low-molecular-weight heparin administered primarily at home with unfractionated heparin administered in the hospital for proximal deep-vein thrombosis. *N Engl J Med* 1996;**334**:677–81.]

20 Leizorovicz A, Simonneau G, Decousus H, Boissel JP. Comparison of efficacy and safety of low molecular weight heparins and unfractionated heparin in initial treatment of deep venous thrombosis: a meta-analysis. *Br Med J* 1994;**309**: 299–304.

21 Braunwald E, ed. *Heart disease: a textbook of cardiovascular medicine*, 5th edn. Philadelphia: WB Saunders, 1997.

22 Colman RW *et al.*, eds. *Hemostasis and thrombosis*, 3rd edn. Philadelphia: Lippincott, 1994.

23 Dale DC, Federman DD, eds. *Scientific American Medicine*. New York: Scientific American Medicine; 1978–97.

Understanding concepts related to the quality of life

5

GORDON H. GUYATT

This chapter relies largely on a previous formulation of concepts related to measurement of health-related quality of life (HRQL),[1] focussing on issues relevant to cardiology. The chapter describes general aspects of measurement of HRQL and then focusses on instruments available for heart failure, and more briefly on measurement of HRQL in angina, myocardial infarction, and hypertension.

WHAT IS HEALTH-RELATED QUALITY OF LIFE?

Health status, *functional status*, and *quality of life* are three concepts often used interchangeably to refer to the same domain of "health".[2] The health domain ranges from negatively valued aspects of life, including death, to positively valued aspects such as role function or happiness. I will use the term *health-related quality of life* (HRQL) because there are widely valued aspects of life that are not generally considered as "health", including income, freedom, and quality of the environment.

WHY MEASURE HRQL?

The important role of HRQL in measuring the impact of chronic disease is increasingly acknowledged.[3] Physiological measures provide important information to clinicians but are of limited interest to patients, and often correlate poorly with functional capacity and wellbeing, the areas in which patients are most interested and familiar. In patients with chronic heart disease exercise capacity in the laboratory is only weakly related to exercise capacity in day-to-day life.[4] These considerations explain why patients, clinicians, and health care administrators are all keenly interested in the effects of medical interventions on HRQL.[5]

THE STRUCTURE OF HRQL MEASURES

Some HRQL measures consist of a single question, which essentially asks, "How is your quality of life?"[6] More commonly, HRQL instruments are questionnaires made up of a number of *items*, or questions. These items are added up in a number of *domains* (also sometimes called *dimensions*). A domain or dimension refers to the area of behavior or experience that we are trying to measure. For some instruments, investigators have undertaken rigorous valuation exercises in which the importance of each item is rated in relation to the others. More often, items are equally weighted, implying that their value is equal.

WHAT MAKES A GOOD HRQL INSTRUMENT?

Measuring at a point in time vs measuring change

The goals of HRQL measures include differentiating between people who have a better HRQL and those who have a worse HRQL (a *discriminative instrument*), and measuring how much HRQL has changed (an *evaluative instrument*).[7] The properties that make useful discriminative and evaluative instruments are summarized in the box below.

What makes a good HRQL measure?

	Evaluative instruments	Discriminative instruments
● Instrument property	(measuring differences within patients over time)	(measuring differences between patients at a point in time)
● High signal to noise ratio	Responsiveness	Reliability
● Validity	Correlations of changes in measures over time consistent with theoretically derived predictions	Correlations between measures at a point in time consistent with theoretically derived predictions
● Interpretability	Differences within subjects over time can be interpreted as trivial, small, moderate, or large	Differences between subjects at a point in time can be interpreted as trivial, small, moderate, or large

---

Signal and noise

Instruments will be useful in so far as we can detect the signal (whatever we are trying to measure) from the associated noise. For discriminative instruments, the way of quantitating the signal to noise ratio is called *reliability*. If the variability in scores between patients (the *signal*) is much greater than the variability within patients (the *noise*), an instrument will be deemed reliable. Reliable instruments will generally demonstrate that stable patients show more or less the same results on repeated administration.

For evaluative instruments, those designed to measure changes within individuals over time, the way of determining the signal to noise ratio is called *responsiveness*. Responsiveness refers to an instrument's ability to detect change. If a treatment results in an important difference in HRQL, investigators wish to be confident they will detect that difference, even if it is small. Responsiveness will be directly related to the magnitude of the difference in score in patients who have improved or deteriorated (the signal) and the extent to which patients who have not changed obtain more or less the same scores (the noise).

Validity

Validity has to do with whether the instrument is measuring what it is intended to measure. When there is no gold or criterion standard, HRQL investigators have borrowed validation strategies from clinical and experimental psychologists who have for many years been dealing with the problem of deciding whether questionnaires examining intelligence, attitudes, and emotional function are really measuring what they are supposed to measure. The types of validity that psychologists have introduced include face, content, and construct validity. *Face validity* refers to whether an instrument appears to be measuring what it is intended to measure and *content validity* refers to the extent to which the domain of interest is comprehensively sampled by the items, or questions, in the instrument. Quantitative testing of face and content validity are rarely attempted.

The most rigorous approach to establishing validity is called *construct validity*. A construct is a theoretically derived notion of the domain(s) we wish to measure. An understanding of the construct will lead to expectations about how an instrument should behave if it is valid. Construct validity therefore involves comparisons between measures, and examination of the logical relationships that should exist between a measure and characteristics of patients and patient groups.

The first step in construct validation is to a establish a "model" or theoretical framework, which represents an understanding of what investigators are trying to measure. That theoretical framework provides a basis for understanding how the system being studied behaves, and allows hypotheses or predictions about how the instrument being tested should relate to other measures. Investigators then administer a number of instruments to a population of interest, and examine the data. Validity is strengthened or weakened according to the extent the hypotheses are confirmed or refuted.

The principles of validation are identical for evaluative instruments, but their validity is demonstrated by showing that *changes* in the instrument being investigated correlate with *changes* in other related measures in the theoretically derived predicted direction and magnitude. For instance, the validity of the "emotions" domain of measure of HRQL for patients after myocardial infarction was supported by the finding of moderate correlations between changes in the instrument's and changes in established emotional function questionnaires.[8]

Interpretability

A final key property of an HRQL measure is *interpretability*. For a discriminative instrument, we could ask whether a particular score signifies that a patient is functioning normally, or has mild, moderate, or severe impairment of HRQL. For an evaluative instrument we might ask whether a particular change in score represents a trivial, small but important, moderate, or large improvement or deterioration.[9,10]

TYPES OF HRQL MEASURES

Generic instruments – health profiles

Two basic approaches characterize the measurement of HRQL: *generic instruments* (including single indicators, health profiles, and utility measures) and *specific instruments*.[11]

Taxonomy of measures of HRQL		
Approach	**Strengths**	**Weaknesses**
● Generic instruments		
Health profile	Single instrument	May not focus adequately on area of interest
	Detects differential effects on different aspects of health status	May not be responsive
	Comparison across interventions, conditions possible	
Utility measurement	Single number representing net impact on quantity and quality of life	Difficulty determining utility values
		Does not allow examination of effect on different aspects of quality of life
	Cost–utility analysis possible	May not be responsive
	Incorporates death	
● Specific instruments	Clinically sensible	Does not allow cross-condition comparisons
Disease-specific	May be more responsive	May be limited in terms of populations and interventions
Population-specific		
Function-specific		
Condition- or problem-specific		

Health profiles are instruments that attempt to measure all important aspects of HRQL. The Sickness Impact Profile (SIP) is an example of a health profile, and includes a *physical* dimension (with categories of ambulation, mobility, and body care and movement), a *psychosocial* dimension (with categories including social interaction, alertness behavior, communication, and emotional behavior), and five independent categories including eating, work, home management, sleep and rest, and recreations and pastimes. Advantages of health profiles include the fact that they deal with a wide variety of areas and can be used in virtually any population, irrespective of the underlying condition. Because generic instruments apply to a wide variety of populations, they allow for broad comparisons of the relative impact of various health care programs. Generic profiles may, however, be less responsive to changes in specific conditions.

Generic instruments – utility measures

The other type of generic instruments, *utility measures* of quality of life, are derived from economic and decision theory, and reflect the preferences of patients for treatment process and outcome. The key elements of utility measures are that they incorporate preference measurements, and relate health states to death. This allows them to be used in *cost–utility analyses* which combine duration and quality of life. In utility measures HRQL is summarized as a single number along a continuum that usually extends from death (0.0) to full health (1.0) (although scores less than zero, representing states worse than death, are possible).[12] Utility scores reflect both the health status and the *value* of that health status to the patient. The usefulness of utility measures in economic analysis is increasingly important in an era of cost constraints.

Utility measures provide a single summary score of the net change in HRQL – the HRQL gains from the treatment effect minus the HRQL burdens of side effects. Utility measures are therefore useful for determining whether patients are on net better off as the result of therapy, but may fail to reveal the dimensions of HRQL on which patients improved versus those on which they worsened.

The preferences in utility measurements may come directly from individual patients who are asked to rate the value of their health state. Alternatively, patients can rate their health status using a multiattribute health status classification system (such as the Quality of Well-Being scale). A previously estimated scoring function derived from results of preference measurements from groups of other patients, or from the community, is then used to convert health status to a utility score.[13]

Specific instruments

The second approach to HRQL measurement focusses on aspects of health status that are specific to the area of primary interest. The rationale for this approach lies in the potential for increased responsiveness that may result from including only important aspects of HRQL that are relevant to the patients being studied. The instrument may be specific to the disease (such as heart failure or coronary artery disease), to a population of patients (such as the frail elderly), to a certain function (such as sleep or sexual function) or to a problem (such as pain). In addition to the likelihood of improved responsiveness, specific measures have the advantage of relating closely to areas routinely explored by clinicians.

USE OF DISEASE-SPECIFIC MEASURES IN HEART FAILURE – THE CHRONIC HEART FAILURE QUESTIONNAIRE

I will use the example of our own instrument to illustrate how disease-specific measures can be developed and tested in the setting of controlled clinical trials. Through a review of the literature, consultation with cardiac nurse specialists and cardiologists, and unstructured interviews with patients, we generated 123 items of possible importance to heart failure patients.[14] We asked 88 patients with heart failure if the 123 items represented ways in which their lives were affected by their heart problem, and selected the most important items, which fell into domains of dyspnea, fatigue, and emotional function, for the final questionnaire. Patients rate their degree of impairment on each item using a seven-point scale.

We used the resulting Chronic Heart Failure Questionnaire (CHQ) in a double-blind crossover study of digoxin in heart failure patients in sinus rhythm.[15] Measures of outcome included a clinical heart failure score (including findings from history, physical examination, and chest radiograph);[16] a 6-minute walk test;[17] the CHQ global ratings of change in dyspnea, fatigue, and emotional function; the Specific Activity Scale (SAS);[18] and the New York Heart Association (NYHA) functional classification.

The study showed digoxin to be of benefit. Seven patients required shortened periods because of increasing heart failure; all seven treatment failures occurred while patients were taking placebo ($P=0.016$). The CHQ showed trends favoring digoxin which were found in all three domains. However, the digoxin-induced changes in dyspnea were small, and in fatigue and emotional function very small. Only for the dyspnea domain did the difference between digoxin and placebo reach conventional levels of statistical significance ($P=0.04$).

The results suggest that either digoxin did not make any difference to fatigue and emotional function (and only a small difference in dyspnea), or digoxin had an important effect that the CHQ failed to detect. To elucidate this issue we examined changes in scores in patients whose global ratings of change suggested improvement or deterioration between study visits, irrespective of what treatment they were receiving. Eleven of the 20 patients reported an improvement in their global rating of dyspnea at some time during the study; in these 11, CHQ dyspnea domain scores improved over these visits, and a paired t-test showed the differences to be statistically significant ($P<0.01$). The findings for each of the three domains were similar, despite the small number of patients who reported improvement at some time during the study. These results suggest the CHQ is responsive to improvement in health status. The findings in patients who deteriorated also show substantial differences which were statistically significant ($P<0.01$).

To explore the instrument's construct validity, we made the following predictions about how the CHQ should behave if it is really measuring HRQL. The predictions are followed by the results actually observed.

1. Change in the three CHQ domains should bear a close relation ($r \geq 0.5$) to changes in patient's corresponding global ratings of change. The correlation between change in CHQ dyspnea and the global rating of change in dyspnea was 0.65 ($P<0.001$); between change in CHQ fatigue and the global rating of change in fatigue was 0.62 ($P<0.001$); and between change in CHQ emotional function and the global rating of change in emotional function 0.34 ($P<0.001$).

2. Change in CHQ dyspnea score should relate closely ($r \geq 0.5$) to change in walk test score. The correlation observed was 0.60.

3. Change in CHQ dyspnea score should bear a moderate correlation ($r>0.4$) with change in heart failure score. The correlation observed was 0.42.

The strong correlations support the validity of the questionnaire. It would be worthwhile knowing how other functional status measures used in heart failure patients compare with the CHQ. Since the NYHA and SAS are measures of dyspnea on daily activity in patients with heart failure, the appropriate comparison is with the CHQ dyspnea score, and if these other instruments are valid then predictions regarding dyspnea should also apply. We examined correlations between changes in CHQ dyspnea, the NYHA functional class, and the SAS on the one hand, and global rating of change in dyspnea, change in walk test score, and change in heart failure score on the other hand. The correlations were consistently higher with the CHQ dyspnea score than with the other instruments, suggesting the CHQ is a more valid measure of changes in shortness of breath in heart failure patients.

HEART FAILURE: OTHER INSTRUMENTS

There are a number of instruments other than the CHQ available for measuring HRQL in heart failure patients. Blackwood and colleagues[19] used visual analog scales which addressed areas of breathlessness, anxiety, depression, irritability, tiredness, energy, concentration, sleep, and limitation of activities in a controlled trial of xamoterol and digoxin in heart failure. The trial failed to show differences between the treatments and placebo either in exercise capacity or HRQL, though both exercise capacity and health-related quality of life improved in all groups. Tandon and colleagues examined the performance of a nine-item disease-specific Self-rating Scale and three generic measures (the QL Index,[20] the Sickness Impact Profile (SIP),[21] and the Quality of Well-Being Index[22]) in a randomized trial in which patients received "standard therapy" or "placebo replacement for standard therapy". The Self-rating Scale and the QL Index were able to differentiate the two conditions, whereas the other two instruments were not. This suggests that the former two instruments may be more responsive than the latter two.

Rector and colleagues[23] have developed a specific questionnaire which they have called the Minnesota Living with Heart Failure Questionnaire. The instrument consists of 21 items focussed on patient perceptions concerning the effects of congestive heart failure on their physical, psychologic, and socioeconomic lives. Response options are presented as six-point scales. In initial testing, these investigators found that the instrument is reproducible (weighted kappa upon readministration at 7–21 days 0.84). In addition, they obtained initial evidence of validity (correlation with global rating 0.80 and with the NYHA functional scale 0.60).

They used the SIP and their specific questionnaire in a before–after study of an experimental inotrope. Despite lack of change in arterial pressure, pulmonary wedge pressure, cardiac index, or exercise capacity, patients scores on both questionnaires improved, and the difference reached conventional levels of statistical significance. The design could not show whether these changes had anything to do with the experimental intervention.[24]

The Minnesota Living with Heart Failure Questionnaire performed in an impressive fashion in a double-blind, randomized, multicenter trial of pimobendan in patients with moderate to severe heart failure. Patients were randomized to receive either placebo or three different doses of pimobendan (2.5, 5.0, and 10 mg). Approximately 50 patients were randomized to each of the four treatment regimens. The questionnaire was self-administered under supervision. Trends were seen in favor of active drug versus placebo in both exercise capacity and health-related quality of life on all three doses, but the largest differences were seen with the 5 mg dose. The statistical power of the exercise test and the questionnaire were comparable (P value associated with changes in the 5 mg group versus placebo were <0.01 for both measures).[25]

The investigators also examined the validity of the questionnaire in the context of the trial. Changes in questionnaire score were not related to changes in ejection fraction.

However, changes in total score and physical function score (but not emotional function) showed weak to moderate correlations with changes in exercise time (0.33 and 0.35 respectively). The Minnesota Living with Heart Failure questionnaire was able to distinguish patients whose global ratings of dyspnea and fatigue showed improvement or deterioration from those who reported no change.[26] The overall pattern of correlations (higher correlations for variables more closely related to quality of life, lower correlations for ejection fraction) supports the validity of the questionnaire.

Further evidence for the responsiveness of the Minnesota Living with Heart Failure Questionnaire comes from the Studies of Left Ventricular Dysfunction (SOLVD) trial. Data from 37 patients with overt heart failure receiving enalapril and 40 such patients who received placebo were available. Both the physical function dimension and the total score (but not the emotional function dimension) showed improvements relative to placebo ($P<0.001$ and $P<0.01$ respectively).[27]

Taken together, these results provide strong evidence that the Minnesota Living with Heart Failure Questionnaire is responsive to the sort of changes in health-related quality of life that follow from the administration of effective medication. The questionnaire has the advantage of being self-administered. Determination of the changes that constitute small, medium, and large effects would be helpful.

One other instrument has demonstrated responsiveness in the context of multicenter randomized trials. The "Yale scale" examines patients' dyspnea and fatigue by aggregating three components: the specific physical task that causes dyspnea and fatigue, the effort or pace with which the task is performed and the patient's general functional capacity.[28] The instrument provides guides for questions asked by health personnel, rather than a specific sequence of questions. The instrument proved responsive in two different clinical trials, demonstrating greater improvement with lisinopril than captopril or placebo. In addition, the investigators found moderate correlations of change in the Yale scale and changes in global ratings of dyspnea and fatigue, and exercise capacity.

Wiklund and colleagues used quite similar methodology to our own to develop their Quality of Life Questionnaire in Severe Heart Failure (QLQ–SHF).[29] A 90-item questionnaire was administered to 51 heart failure patients. Twenty-six items were chosen for the final questionnaire on the basis of the number of patients who identified the item as a significant problem, the extent to which a cardiologist thought they were important problems, and loaded high on the appropriate component of a factor analysis. The final questionnaire has somatic, psychological, life dissatisfaction, and physical limitation domains. The test–retest reliability of the domains after one week was 0.75 to 0.85. Validity was demonstrated by correlations of 0.42 to 0.72 with appropriate domains of the SIP, the Mood Adjective Check List, and a cardiologist's rating of the patients' function.

CORONARY ARTERY DISEASE

The New York Heart Association functional classification was designed to apply to both heart failure and angina. While it has proved useful as a simple means for physicians to communicate the extent to which patients are limited by their cardiac disease, the vagueness of the description of activity thresholds, and the fact that it has only four categories, limits it use as a measure for clinical trials. The Canadian Cardiovascular Society Grading Scale suffers similar limitations.[30]

Recent trials in angina patients that have examined HRQL have used generic measures,[31] a battery of function-specific measures,[32] or a combination.[33] Investigators now also have the option of selecting a disease-specific instrument. Wilson and colleagues have developed a "Summary Index" for angina[34] which they used successfully in a controlled trial of nitrate administration.[35] Investigators have translated a modified version of this questionnaire into French and shown expected correlations with a generic index and the clinical severity of angina pectoris.[36]

An American group has developed another disease-specific measure which they call the Seattle Angina Questionnaire (SAQ)[37] and found that all five domains correlate with other measures of diagnosis and patient function (0.31 to 0.70). Scores from stable patients remained unchanged over 3 months while improvements were noted in patients undergoing angioplasty. Subsequently, the SAQ proved more responsive than a generic measure.[38]

Our group has developed an instrument specifically directed at patients who have had a myocardial infarction, and provided preliminary evidence of responsiveness and validity.[8] The measure has proved useful in one randomized trial of cardiac rehabilitation[39] and a modified, self-administered version[40] demonstrated quality of life improvement with rehabilitation in a second trial of patients after myocardial infarction.[41] We have also developed an instrument to measure quality of life in spouses of those post myocardial infarction,[42] though it has seen little use thus far.

HYPERTENSION

Hypertension, if symptomatic at all, causes only relatively minor non-specific symptoms. Investigators' primary interest in HRQL in hypertension has been examining the impact of alternative treatment regimens. To do this, they have used a battery of function and problem-specific instruments. This approach has succeeded in demonstrating differences in HRQL in randomized trials in hypertensive patients offered alternative drug therapy.[43,44]

CONCLUSION

Through advances in methodology we now have tools available to measure HRQL in a valid and responsive manner. Results of HRQL measurement can inform both clinicians and health care policy makers. HRQL measurement should form part of any trial that includes effects on patient well-being as one of the important endpoints.

REFERENCES

1 Guyatt GH, Feeny DH, Patrick DL. Measuring health-related quality of life: Basic Sciences Review. *Ann Intern Med* 1993;**70**:225–30.

2 Patrick D, Bergner M. Measurement of health status in the 1990s. *Annu Rev Publ Hlth* 1990; **11**:165–83.

3 Patrick DL, Erickson P. *Health status and health policy: quality of life in health care evaluation and resource allocation.* New York: Oxford University Press, 1992.

4 Guyatt GH, Thompson PJ, Berman LB *et al.* How should we measure function in patients with chronic heart and lung disease? *J Chron Dis* 1985; **38**:517–24.

5 Wennberg JE. Outcomes research, cost containment, and the fear of health care rationing. *N Engl J Med* 1990;**323**:1202–4.

6 Torrance GW. Measurement of health state utilities for economic appraisal. *J Hlth Economics* 1986;**5**:1–30.

7 Kirshner B, Guyatt GH. A methodologic framework for assessing health indices. *J Chron Dis* 1985;**38**:27–36.

8 Hillers T, Guyatt GH, Oldridge N *et al*. Quality of life after myocardial infarction. *J Clin Epidemiol* 1994;**47**:1287–96.

9 Guyatt GH, Feeny D, Patrick D. Proceedings of the international conference on the measurement of quality of life as an outcome in clinical trials: postscript. *Controlled Clin Trials* 1991;**12**: 266S–269S.

10 Jaeschke R, Guyatt G, Keller J, Singer J. Measurement of health status: ascertaining the meaning of a change in quality-of-life questionnaire score. *Controlled Clin Trials* 1989; **10**:407–15.

11 Patrick DL, Deyo RA. Generic and disease-specific measures in assessing health status and quality of life. *Medical Care* 1989;**27**:F217–32.

12 Boyle MH, Torrance GW, Sinclair JC, Horwood SP. Economic evaluation of neonatal intensive care of very-low-birth-weight infants. *N Engl J Med* 1983;**308**:1330–7

13 Feeny D, Barr RD, Furlong W *et al*. A comprehensive multiattribute system for classifying the health status of survivors of childhood cancer. *J Clin Oncol* 1992;**10**:923–8.

14 Guyatt GH, Nogradi S, Halcrow S *et al*. Development and testing of a new measure of health status for clinical trials in heart failure. *J Gen Intern Med* 1989;**4**:101–7.

15 Guyatt GH, Sullivan MJJ, Fallen E *et al*. A controlled trial of digoxin in congestive heart failure. *Am J Cardiol* 1988;**61**:371–5.

16 Lee DC, Johnson RA, Bingham JB *et al*. Heart failure in outpatients: a randomized trial of digoxin versus placebo. *N Engl J Med* 1982;**306**: 699–705.

17 Guyatt GH, Sullivan MJ, Fallen EL *et al*. The six minute walk: a new measure of exercise capacity in patients with chronic heart failure. *Can Med Assoc J* 1985;**132**:919–23.

18 Goldman L, Hashimoto D, Cook EF. Comparative reproducibility and validity of systems for assessing cardiovascular functional class: advantages of a new Specific Activity Scale. *Circulation* 1981;**64**:1227–34.

19 Blackwood R, Mayou RA, Garnham JC *et al*. Exercise capacity and quality of life in the treatment of heart failure. *Clin Pharmacol Ther* 1990;**48**:325–32.

20 Spitzer WO, Dobson AJ, Hall J *et al*. Measuring the quality of life of cancer patients. *J Chron Dis* 1981;**34**:585–97.

21 Bergner M, Bobbitt RA, Carter WB, Gilson BS. The Sickness Impact Profile: development and final revision of a health status measure. *Medical Care* 1981;**19**:787–805.

22 Kaplan RM, Bush JW. Health-related quality of life measurement for evaluation research and policy analysis. *Hlth Psychol* 1982;**1**:61–80.

23 Rector TS, Kubo SH, Cohn JN. Patients' self-assessment of their congestive heart failure: II: Content, reliability and validity of a new measure – the Minnesota Living with Heart Failure Questionnaire. *Heart Failure* 1987;**3**:198–209.

24 Kubo SH, Rector TS, Strobeck JE, Cohn JN. OPC-8212 in the treatment of congestive heart failure: results of a pilot study. *Cardiovasc Drugs Ther* 1988;**2**:653–60.

25 Kubo SH, Gollub S, Bourge R *et al*. Beneficial effects of pimobendan on exercise tolerance and quality of life in patients with heart failure. *Circulation* 1992;**85**:942–9.

26 Rector TS, Cohn JN. Assessment of patient outcome with the Minnesota Living with Heart Failure Questionnaire: reliability and validity during a randomized, double-blind, placebo controlled trial of pimobendan. *Am Heart J* 1992; **124**:1017–25.

27 Rector TS, Kubo SH, Cohn JN. Validity of the Minnesota Living with Heart Failure Questionnaire as a measure of therapeutic response: to enalapril and placebo. *Am J Cardiol* 1993;**71**:1106–7.

28 Feinstein AR, Fisher MB, Pigeon JG. Changes in dyspnea-fatigue ratings as indicators of quality of life in the treatment of congestive heart failure. *Am J Cardiol* 1989;**64**:50–5.

29 Wiklund I, Lindvall K, Swedberg K, Zupkis RV. Self-assessment of quality of life in severe heart failure. *Scand J Psychol* 1987;**28**:220–5.

30 Cox J, Naylor CD. The Canadian Cardiovascular Society Grading Scale for angina pectoris: is it time for refinements? *Ann Intern Med* 1992;**117**: 677–83.

31 Pocock SJ, Henderson RA, Seed P, Treasure T, Hampton JR. Quality of life, employment status, and anginal symptoms after coronary angioplasty or bypass surgery. *Circulation* 1996;**94**:135–42.

32 Rehnqvist N, Hjemdahl P, Billing E *et al*. Effects of metoprolol vs verapamil in patients with stable angina pectoris. *Eur Heart J* 1996;**17**:76–81.

33 O'Neill C, Normand C, Cupples M, McKnight A. A comparison of three measures of perceived distress: results from a study of angina patients in general practice in Northern Ireland. *J Epidemiol Commun Hlth* 1996;**50**:202–6.

34 Wilson A, Wiklund I, Lahti T, Wahl M. A summary index for the assessment of quality of life in angina pectoris. *J Clin Epidemiol* 1991;**44**:981–8.

35 Nissinen A, Wiklund I, Lahti T *et al*. Anti-anginal therapy and quality of life. *J Clin Epidemiol* 1991; **44**:989–97.

36 Marquis P, Fayol C, Joire, Leplege A. Psychometric properties of a specific quality of life questionnaire in angina pectoris patients. *Quality Life Res* 1995; **4**:540–6.

37 Spertus JA, Winder JA, Dewhurst TA *et al*. Development and evaluation of the Seattle Angina Questionnaire. *J Am Coll Cardiol* 1995;**25**: 333–41.

38 Spertus JA, Winder JA, Dewhurst TA, Deyo RA, Fihn SD. Monitoring the quality of life in patients with coronary artery disease. *Am J Cardiol* 1994; **15**:1240–4.

39 Oldridge N, Guyatt GH, Jones N *et al*. Effects on quality of life with comprehensive rehabilitation after acute myocardial infarction. *Am J Cardiol* 1991;**67**:1084–89.

40 Lim L, Valenti LA, Knapp JC *et al*. A self-administered quality of life questionnaire after acute myocardial infarction. *J Clin Epidemiol* 1993;**46**:1249–56.

41 Heller RF, Knapp JC, Valenti LA, Dobson AJ. Secondary prevention after acute myocardial infarction. *Am J Cardiol* 1993;**72**:759–62.

42 Ebbesen LS, Guyatt GH, McCartney N, Oldridge NB. Measuring quality of life in cardiac spouses. *J Clin Epidemiol* 1990;**43**:481–7.

43 Croog SH, Levine S, Testa MA *et al*. The effects of antihypertensive therapy on the quality of life. *N Engl J Med* 1986;**314**:1657–64.

44 Testa MA, Anderson RB, Nackley JF *et al*. Quality of life and antihypertensive therapy in men. A comparison of captopril with enalapril. The Quality-of-Life Hypertension Study Group. *N Engl J Med* 1993;**328**:907–13

6 Understanding concepts related to health economics

MARK A. HLATKY

INTRODUCTION

Economics is concerned with how to allocate scarce resources among alternative uses efficiently and effectively. It is a fundamental principle of economics that resources are limited relative to human wants, and that those resources have alternative uses.[1] Consequently, when people say that the cost of health care has grown too high, they mean that the quantity of resources flowing towards medical care has grown to the point where additional funds cannot be spent on other things that society values, such as education, public safety, environmental protection, public works, pensions for the retired or disabled, or assistance to the poor. The fact that most people put a very high value on health does not mean that they are willing to provide limitless resources to medical care. Indeed, even the goal of improving health and longevity may also be served by non-medical expenditures on programs such as nutritional supplements, a safe and clean water supply, police and fire protection, or safety improvements to roads, as well as by medical expenditures.

The cost of medical care has been rising steadily for the past 50 years, but it has only been in the past decade that the level of expenditures became so large as to cause alarm among policy makers, payers, and the general public (Table 6.1). The steady expansion of health care has now begun to meet substantial resistance in the large industrial countries, and new policies and payment mechanisms have been introduced to contain the rising cost of medical care. As a consequence, physicians must now consider cost as they design programs to prevent, diagnose, and treat disease. Cardiovascular diseases consume a large share of health care resources (Table 6.2), so cardiovascular specialists must be particularly knowledgeable about health economics. This chapter will attempt to outline the major principles of health economics relevant to cardiovascular medicine. First, some general concepts of health economics will be presented. Second, methods to identify and compare the costs of cardiovascular interventions will be described. Finally, the principles of cost-effectiveness analysis will be discussed.

Table 6.1 US national health care expenditures, 1994

Category	US$ ($\times 10^9$)	Percentage
Hospital care	338.5	36
Physician services	189.4	20
Other professionals	91.8	10
Drugs, supplies	78.6	8
Nursing home	72.3	8
Home health care	26.2	3
Durable equipment	13.1	1
Other personal health care	21.8	2
Administration	58.7	6
Public health	28.8	3
Research	15.9	2
Construction	14.3	2
Total	949.4	100

Data from *Health Affairs* 1996; **15**: 130–44.

Table 6.2 Resources devoted to cardiovascular care in the United States

Category	No. (thousands)		Percentage (of total)
Deaths[a]	951		41
Hospital admissions[b]	5779		19
Myocardial infarction		759	
Heart failure		874	
Cerebrovascular disease		885	
Operations and procedures[b]	4653		11
Cardiac catheterization		1048	
CABG		318	
PTCA		428	
Pacemaker-related		328	
Physician office visits[c]	51 613		7
EKGs		13 673	
Stress tests		1767	
Prescriptions[c]	132 356		14

CABG, coronary artery bypass graft; PTCA, percutaneous transluminal coronary angioplasty.
[a] NCHS Monthly Vital Statistics Report 1997; 45(11): Suppl 2.
[b] NCHS Advance Data 1996 (No. 278).
[c] NCHS Advance Data 1997 (no. 286).

GENERAL CONCEPTS

Various societies have adopted different systems to pay for health care, and these systems reflect societal values and the historical experience within each country. The United Kingdom has a national health service, Canada has national health insurance, France and Germany have public/private financing for health care, and the United States has a perplexing and rapidly evolving patchwork of public and private health insurance systems. These are very different systems to finance health care, and yet each is faced

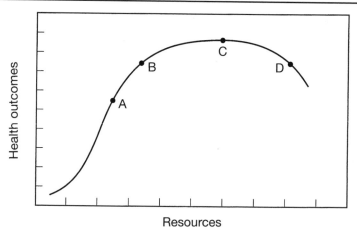

Figure 6.1 General relationship between increasing health care resources (horizontal axis) and health outcomes (vertical axis). At Point A, outcomes are improving rapidly with increased resources and treatment is cost-effective. At Point B, outcomes are still improving with increased resources, but at a rate that is not cost-effective. At Point C, increased resources are no longer improving outcome (i.e., "flat at the curve"), and at Point D increased resources actually lead to worse outcomes, through iatrogenic complications and overtreatment.

with the same issues of how to allocate the limited resources available to best provide health care. Each country is also facing the same steady rise of health care costs, despite the wide differences in the ways they finance health care.

Provision of cardiovascular services requires resources in all societies, irrespective of the method of financing or delivering health care. Coronary bypass surgery, for example, is very resource-intensive, with the operation requiring cardiac surgeons, a cardiac anesthesiologist or anesthetist, a perfusionist, several nurses, and considerable quantities of specialized supplies and equipment. Postoperative care also requires skilled nurses and physicians, with support from specialized supplies, equipment, and facilities. Each health professional involved in cardiac surgery spends the scarce resource of time to care for the patient – time that could be put to other valuable uses, such as care for other patients. The drugs used, the disposable supplies, the operating room equipment, even the hospital building, all cost money. All of these are true costs to the system, even if the coronary bypass operation is performed "for free", i.e., without charge to the patient. The scene in the operating room, the postoperative recovery areas, and the hospital wards is much the same in the United Kingdom, Canada, France, Germany, and the United States despite the different ways these societies pay for medical care. The resources used in the care of patients, and the increasing sophistication of that care, drives health care costs up in each of these countries, irrespective of the way such care is paid for.

Another basic concept of economics is the so-called "law of diminishing returns". This concept is illustrated in Figure 6.1, in which the quantity of resources used in health care is plotted on the horizontal axis, and the resulting health benefits on the vertical axis. In the case of the patient with an acute myocardial infarction, for example, survival would be improved as more resources are applied, such as prehospital transportation, electrocardiographic monitoring, access to defibrillation, and a competent team to deliver coronary care. Outcomes might be further improved by reperfusion therapy, but with a greater increment in survival from using a cheaper, basic approach (e.g., streptokinase) relative to no therapy, than from more expensive alternatives (e.g., tissue plasminogen activator (tPA) or PTCA). The extra benefit from adding even more aggressive care will be smaller still, and at some point the patient may be harmed by overly aggressive care. Helping physicians define the optimal point on this curve (Figure 6.1) is one of the goals of economic analysis.

DETERMINATION OF COSTS

The cost of producing a particular health care service can be defined in a variety of ways. The cost of performing a coronary angiogram can be used as a specific example that will illustrate the various aspects of cost and how the cost might be measured. Performing a coronary angiogram requires a variety of resources, including radiographic equipment, trained personnel (including an angiographer and technical assistants), and specialized supplies such as catheters, radiographic contrast, and sterile drapes. The equipment needed is very expensive to purchase, and the health care facility where it is installed may require special renovations to assure proper radiation shielding and adequate electrical power. The capital cost for a coronary angiography laboratory will be considerable, perhaps $2–3 million, depending on the type of equipment purchased. The laboratory will have a physical lifespan of perhaps 7–10 years, although technologic innovations may lead to replacement of the equipment before the end of its physical lifespan. The cost of building an angiography suite represents a large *fixed cost* for coronary angiography, a cost that is roughly the same whether the laboratory performs 250 or 2500 angiograms per year. The cost per case is lower in the high volume laboratory, however, because the fixed equipment costs can be spread over more cases. Thus, if the equipment costs $2.5 million and has a useful life of 10 years, the prorated share of fixed costs for each patient in the low volume laboratory performing 200 cases per year is

$$\text{fixed costs/case} = \frac{\$2\,500\,000}{(200 \text{ cases/yr})(10 \text{ years})} = \$1250/\text{case}$$

whereas in the high volume laboratory (2000 cases per year) the prorated share of fixed costs per case would be

$$\text{fixed costs/case} = \frac{\$2\,500\,000}{(2000 \text{ cases/yr})(10 \text{ years})} = \$125/\text{case}.$$

Procedures that have high fixed costs will be performed with greater economic efficiency in centers that have sufficient volume to spread those fixed costs over a larger number of individual patients. (There may be additional advantages to larger procedure volumes as well, since the technical proficiency is higher and clinical outcomes of many procedures are usually better when performed in higher volume clinical centers.)[2–4] Procedures with lower fixed costs will have a smaller effect of volume on costs.

In contrast to the fixed equipment costs, the cost of supplies consumed in performing coronary angiography varies directly with the volume of cases performed, and the supply cost per case will be fairly constant irrespective of the volume of cases performed (apart from the small effect of discounts available to large volume purchasers). The cost of laboratory staff falls in between these two extremes, in that the hours worked in the

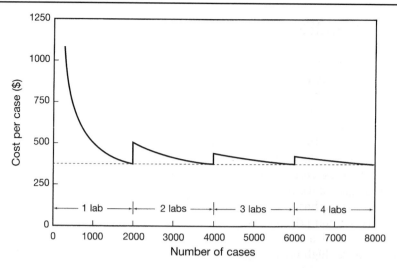

Figure 6.2 Cost per case for coronary angiography as a function of clinical volume. Assumes fixed costs per laboratory of $250 000 per year, and marginal (i.e., variable) costs of $250 per case. When volume reaches 2000 cases per year in a laboratory, the model assumes an additional laboratory will be built. The dotted line indicates the "long run average" cost per case of $375.

catheterization laboratory by technical staff can be varied somewhat according to the volume of cases performed, but some staff effort is required regardless of patient volumes, such as supervisors.

Hospital overhead is also a real cost, but one that is less directly linked to any one medical service or procedure. Hospitals must pay for admitting offices, the medical records department, central administration, the laundry service, the cafeteria, housekeeping and utilities, to name just a few areas. These costs cannot be tied easily to the coronary angiography procedure in the same way as the cost of the catheters or radiographic contrast. Most facilities assign a share of these costs to patient care services according to a formula such as the step down method. Discussion of specific methods to allocate hospital overhead is beyond the scope of this chapter, but can be found in several articles and books.[5,6]

The overall effect of procedure volume on the cost per case is illustrated in Figure 6.2. In general, the cost per case declines as more cases are performed, up to the limit of the facility's capacity (e.g., 2000 cases). If volume increases further, more facilities must be built, increasing the cost per case, as more fixed costs are spread over a few more patients. Figure 6.2 also illustrates the distinction between concepts of "marginal cost" and long run "average cost". The marginal cost is the added cost of doing one more case. In an already equipped and staffed coronary angiography laboratory, the marginal cost of performing one more procedure is just the cost of the disposable supplies consumed in the case: the catheters, radiographic contrast, and other sterile supplies. In the example of Figure 6.2, the marginal cost is $250 per case. The marginal cost is lower than the average cost per case ($375 per case), which also includes a prorated share of the salaries of the laboratory staff, depreciation of the laboratory equipment costs, and the facility's overhead costs.

COSTS vs CHARGES

Costs and charges are related but distinct concepts. The cost of a medical service represents the value of the resources required to produce it. The charge for a service is a specific form of reimbursement to health care providers in a fee-for-service health care system. The cost and charge for providing a service should be quite close to one another in a competitive economic market. The reason is simple: if one provider charged an amount much higher than it actually cost to provide a service, a competitor could offer the same service at a lower price and still come out ahead. Conversely, if a provider charged less than the costs of production, the provider would lose money. These basic economic principles have not applied very well to medical care, at least until recently, because medical care has not had significant competition on prices.

In regulated or non-price competitive health care systems, the charge (price) for a service need not bear a close relationship to the cost of producing a service. Hospitals might choose to set high prices for some services, such as coronary bypass surgery, and use the excess revenues to subsidize other services that were less well reimbursed, such as the emergency department or, in academic centers, medical education and research. With greater price sensitivity on the part of health care payers, the subsidization of one medical service with the proceeds of another service has been sharply curtailed. While this trend has had the positive effect of bringing an element of economic reality to medicine, it has also caused dislocations and considerable harm as worthwhile endeavors have lost the funding they previously enjoyed from cross-subsidization. In the long run, medical education, clinical research, and services to uninsured or poorly insured patients will no doubt receive direct funding to replace the indirect funding by cross-subsidies, but in the transition these endeavors have been threatened due to loss of a traditional funding base.

ESTIMATION OF COSTS

The cost of providing a specific service, such as coronary bypass surgery, can be established in several alternative ways. In principle, one valid way to measure cost would be to identify a competitive market for medical service, and note the charge (price) for coronary bypass surgery in that market. While competitive market pricing might work well for commodities such as consumer electronic devices or farm products, it is not well suited to medical care, where there are few competitive markets. An alternative method to measure cost is to take note of the charge for a service, and apply correction factors to estimate cost more accurately. A third method to estimate costs is to examine in detail the resources used to provide a service, and apply price weights to the resources used; i.e.,

$$\text{Cost}_j = \sum_i (\text{Quantity})_{ij} \times (\text{Price})_{ij}.$$

The use of these different approaches to cost determination is illustrated by a study that estimated the costs savings achievable by substituting coronary angioplasty for coronary bypass surgery.[7] In that study, hospital billing records were used to construct resource consumption profiles for patients undergoing either angioplasty or bypass surgery for the treatment of stable angina. A microcosting approach was then applied

Table 6.3 Effect of different definitions of cost on the savings possible by substitution of coronary angioplasty for bypass surgery

Definition of cost	PTCA cost ($)	CABG cost ($)	Difference ($)	PTCA/CABG ratio (%)
Variable cost only	2672	4 607	1 935	58
Average direct cost				
By microcosting	4073	8 666	4 593	47
By ratio of cost-to-charges	4935	10 281	5 346	48
Average cost + overhead	7530	15 367	7 837	49
Charges	9556	19 644	10 088	49

Adapted from Hlatky *et al.*[7]

to the resource consumption profiles, with the cost of a specific resource (e.g., an electrocardiogram) defined either as the cost of supplies only (marginal cost or variable cost) or as the cost of supplies, personnel and equipment, but omitting overhead (average direct cost). Charges on the billing record for a service were also converted to costs by two different correction factors, also known as ratios of cost to charges. One cost–charge ratio included all direct costs of providing a service (supplies, personnel, and equipment), but omitted hospital overhead (e.g., medical records, laundry, utilities, administration). The second cost–charge ratio allocated a share of hospital overhead to each service in addition to its direct costs.

As shown in Table 6.3, the cost savings attributable to substitution of angioplasty for bypass surgery varied considerably according to how costs were defined. The lowest cost savings are evident when only marginal costs are included, and fixed cost and overhead excluded. The average direct cost difference is intermediate in value, and comparable estimates of this cost savings were obtained from the use of resource consumption profiles and cost weights (Method 2) or the cost-to-charge ratio method that omitted overhead (Method 3). Finally, the inclusion of overhead (Method 4) led to the highest absolute difference in costs.

The differences in cost as estimated using these methods is directly related to the issue of how the information is to be used or, put another way, depends on the answer to the question, "cost to whom?" A hospital manager might be most interested in the marginal cost of procedures (Method 1) in looking at the effect of adding or subtracting a small number of cases to the volume performed in an institution. Under a fixed budget for cardiac services, for instance, the effect of substituting angioplasty for bypass surgery may be small, given that the personnel, equipment and overhead are largely fixed. Performing a few extra procedures with existing facilities adds very little cost from the perspective of the head of a clinical service or a hospital manager. They may even be willing to perform a modest number of additional cases at a reimbursement level below their actual average cost, but above marginal cost, in order to increase volume and spread their fixed costs over more patients. Thus, marginal or variable costs are quite relevant to decision makers within the institution providing a service.

The perspective of a policy maker or health planner includes a longer time horizon and the possibility of adding or subtracting substantial volumes of clinical services. From this perspective, no cost is truly fixed, for personnel needs can be adjusted, and the number of facilities providing a service can be altered. This perspective is a broader

Table 6.4 Effect of differences in medical prices on costs of alternative treatments

	Country 1		Country 2	
	TxA	TxB	TxA	TxB
Drug	$2000	$200	$1500	$150
Nursing hours	50	54	50	54
Nursing wages	$30	$30	$35	$35
Total	$3500	$1820	$3250	$2040
Cost savings (A − B)	$1680		$1210	
Cost ratio B/A	52%		63%	

one, and the costs considered are therefore more inclusive. For most policy level discussions, long run average cost is the most relevant measure.

INTERNATIONAL PERSPECTIVES

With the advent of large multicenter clinical trials that enroll patients from several countries, interest has developed in cost comparisons between countries for the same service. Cost estimation as part of large randomized trials will enhance clinical decision making, for the randomized design is the strongest way to compare all outcomes of therapeutic alternatives, including cost. Extension of cost comparisons across national borders introduces a number of technical and conceptual issues that deserve discussion.

Different countries measure cost in their respective national currencies, so that readers in another country need to convert between units (e.g., pounds sterling or German marks to US dollars). These conversions can be done using currency exchange rates, or the closely related purchasing power parity factors. The differences between countries in units of measurement are important, but this issue is fairly simple to address.

A more thorny issue in international comparisons is differences in the relative prices of the resources used to provide a service and differences in resource profiles used to provide a service. Thus, if the cost of service j is defined as

$$\text{Cost}_j = \sum_i (\text{Quantity})_{ij} \times (\text{Price})_{ij}$$

then cost may differ among countries due to either differences in the quantity of resources used to provide a service, price differentials for the same resources, or both. A specific example will help illustrate these concepts (Table 6.4). Care of a patient with acute myocardial infarction given thrombolysis includes the cost of the drug, the cost of basic hospital care, and the cost of additional tests and treatments in the convalescent phase. Table 6.4 presents hypothetical costs of basic care in two countries, with monetary values expressed in dollar units for simplicity. The costs of drugs in Country 1 are higher than in Country 2, where drug prices are strictly regulated. The time spent by the hospital staff to care for the patient are quite similar in Country 1 and Country 2 (50 hours per patient for Treatment A and 54 for Treatment B, a difference due to lower complication rates with Treatment A). The average hourly compensation for hospital staff is, however, higher in Country 2, so that total personnel costs are higher as well. Thus, both cost savings and the relative costs of Treatment A and B are different in

Table 6.5 Effect of differences in resource utilization on costs of alternative treatments

	Country 1		Country 2	
	TxA	TxB	TxA	TxB
Drug/nursing	$3500	$1820	$3250	$2040
Coronary angiography	40%	60%	10%	15%
Angio cost	$1000	$1000	$1000	$1000
Total	$3900	$2420	$3350	$2190
Cost savings (A − B)	$1480		$1160	
Cost ratio (B/A)	62%		65%	

these two health care systems, due to different prices for the same resources used to care for a myocardial infarct patient.

There may also be differences in the level of resource use between countries, especially for discretionary procedures such as coronary angiography. Suppose that the use of Treatment A cuts the use of coronary angiography by one-third, partially offsetting the higher cost of the drug. If, however, the baseline rates of angiography are different between countries, the cost implications of reducing angiography by one-third in each country will be quite different (Table 6.5). A reduction by one-third in the high rate of angiography in Country 1 (from 60% to 40%) provides a $200 cost offset per patient, whereas a reduction by one-third in the low rate of angiography in Country 2 (from 20% to 15%) provides only a $50 cost offset per patient.

International comparisons of the cost of therapies can thus be affected by (a) differences in resource use patterns that reflect differences in practice style and the organization of medical care, and (b) by differences between countries in the prices attached to specific resources, such as health care wages, drugs, and supplies. Data from cost studies can be most readily applied in different practice environments if the study provides information on both resource consumption patterns and price weights attached to the specific resources used, as well as a summary cost measure. This detail is needed for readers to understand the applicability of the cost findings to their own practice settings.

COST-EFFECTIVENESS ANALYSIS

The cost of providing a particular medical service can be measured, but determination of whether the service provides good value for the money spent is a more difficult judgment. Cost-effectiveness analysis is a method of weighing the cost of a service in light of the health effects it confers in an attempt to facilitate the ultimate value judgment about whether the service is "worth" the cost.

Cost-effectiveness analysis is one of several alternative analytic methods, each with its own strengths and limitations.[5] If two alternative therapies are either known to yield identical results or can be shown to be clinically equivalent, they can be compared on the basis of cost alone. This form of analysis, which is termed "cost-minimization analysis", is particularly appropriate to commodities such as drugs, supplies and equipment that can be expected to yield equivalent results when applied clinically. In such situations, the relative costs of the alternatives become the predominant consideration.

Many alternative therapies are known to differ both in clinical outcomes and in cost. In this situation, both the difference in cost and the difference in effectiveness of the therapeutic alternatives must be measured and weighed against each other. When the effectiveness on intervention is measured in clinical terms (e.g., lives saved, years of life added), the analysis is termed "cost-effectiveness". If the clinical measures of effectiveness are translated into monetary units, the term "cost–benefit analysis" is applied. Cost–benefit analysis has been used to guide public policy in areas outside of medicine, such as in the construction of transportation systems or whether to remove or reduce environmental exposures. Cost–benefit analysis measures the effects of programs in monetary terms, so that net cost (in dollars) can be compared with net benefits (in dollars). Since there is great reluctance on the part of physicians and health policy makers to assign a dollar value to saving a life or improving a patient's function, cost-effectiveness analysis rather than cost–benefit analysis has been applied predominantly to medical problems.

Cost-effectiveness analysis was first applied to medical programs only 20 years ago[8,9] and has since been widely used.[10–12] The principles of cost-effectiveness analysis for medical programs have recently been examined in detail by a Task Force convened by the United States Public Health Service.[13–15] A group of experts attempted to establish consensus on a number of methodologic issues, with the goal of standardizing the technical aspects of cost-effectiveness analysis among studies, thereby enhancing their comparability. The principles articulated by this group are reasonable, and should guide this important field in its next 20 years.

A basic principle of cost-effectiveness analysis is that the analysis should compare alternative programs, and not look at any single program in isolation. Thus, a drug to treat life-threatening arrhythmias might be compared with placebo, or an implantable cardioverter defibrillator might be compared with a drug. In essence, cost-effectiveness analysis must always answer the question, "cost-effective compared with what?"

Another principle is that the costs included in cost-effectiveness analysis should be comprehensive. The cost of a specific therapy should include the cost of the intervention itself (e.g., thrombolytic therapy for acute myocardial infarction) and the costs of any complications the therapy induced (e.g., bleeding), any cost savings due to reduction of complications (e.g., heart failure). The need for other concomitant therapy should also be included, which is particularly important when assessing the cost-effectiveness of screening programs or diagnostic testing strategies. The length of follow-up should be sufficient to include all relevant costs and benefits – such as readmissions to the hospital due to treatment failures. Non-monetary costs directly related to the medical intervention should also be included, such as the cost of home care by the patient's family, since omission of these costs would bias assessments toward programs that rely on unpaid work by family members or volunteers. Other costs not directly related to the intervention, however, such as the patient's lost wages or pension costs, are omitted by convention from the measured costs in a cost-effectiveness analysis.

Another important issue in cost-effectiveness analysis is the perspective taken by the analysis. There is general agreement that the analysis should include all relevant costs, regardless of who pays them. This principle is known as "taking the societal perspective", and it assures a complete accounting of costs in the analysis. A hospital, for instance, may not care about the out-of-pocket costs paid directly by the patient, but these are real costs and should be considered in the analysis.

Medical costs may accrue over long periods of time, especially in preventive programs or the treatment of chronic disease. Time scales of more than a year or so bring up two related but distinct issues – inflation and discounting. The nominal value of any currency changes over time; a dollar in 1977 had more purchasing power than a dollar in 1997. Studies conducted over long time periods will need to correct for the changing value of currencies, typically by application of the Consumer Price Index (or the GDP deflator). Application of the Consumer Price Index removes the effect of inflation, but does not address the separate issue of time preference for money. Even in a country free of inflation, citizens would prefer to receive $100 today than a promise they will be paid $100 in a year. One might have to promise to pay more money in a year, say $103, to compensate for the delay. The same is true in health programs: we would prefer to be paid today instead of in the future, and we would also prefer to pay our obligations in the future, and we would also prefer to pay our obligations in the future rather than today. Use of a discount rate provides a way to correct for the lower value of future costs relative to current costs. The technical experts' consensus is that future costs should be discounted at a rate equivalent to the interest paid on safe investments such as government bonds in an inflation-free environment, or about 3% per year. The effect of alternative discount rates between 0% and 5–10% per year should also be checked to document the sensitivity of the analysis to future costs.

In summary, a cost-effectiveness analysis should include all medical costs, including those of complications of therapy and adverse effects prevented. The study should be of sufficient duration to measure all relevant costs and benefits of the treatment. All costs and benefits should be included, regardless of who bears or receives them. In studies covering more than a year or so, corrections should be made for inflation, and 3% per year discount rate should be applied to follow-up costs.

MEASURING EFFECTIVENESS

The effectiveness of an intervention in practice can be measured in a variety of ways, with different outcome measures most appropriate for specific application. Physiologic endpoints are often used in clinical trials, with the result of therapy assessed by a laboratory measure such as millimeters of mercury for blood pressure or episodes of non-sustained ventricular tachycardia on an electrocardiographic monitor. Laboratory measures are useful in judging the physiologic effects of therapy and its mechanism of action, but these surrogate markers may not predict the ultimate effect of therapy on mortality and morbidity, as vividly illustrated by the results of the Cardiac Arrhythmia Suppression Trial (CAST).[16] Physiologic endpoints are also tied closely to one specific disease, making comparisons against other benchmark therapies difficult. The patient and public are most concerned with the effect of therapy on survival and on their ability to function; i.e., upon the length of life and the quality of life. A common denominator measure of effectiveness is thus the life years of expected survival, or the quality-adjusted life years (QALYs). This measure is relevant to patients and to the public and can be applied to virtually any therapy.

Mortality is a common endpoint in clinical trials, and leads directly to the measure of life years of survival. The mean life expectancy of a cohort of patients is equal to the area under a standard survival curve. The difference in life expectancy between two therapies is therefore equal to the difference in the areas under their respective survival curves. Since many clinical studies do not follow patient cohorts long enough to observe complete survival times for all patients, some assumptions and modeling of long term survival may be needed to estimate the full survival benefit of therapy for a cost-effectiveness analysis.[17]

Improvement in quality of life is often as important to patients as reducing mortality, and it is often the main goal of therapies, such as the relief of disabling angina or improvement in exercise tolerance. A quality of life measure can be translated into a scale that ranges from a low of 0.0 (the worst possible health state, usually taken as death) to 1.0 (perfect health). This quality of life measure is multiplied by the length of time a patient spends in the health state to yield a quality-adjusted life year (QALY). Thus,

$$QALY = \sum_i Q_i \times t_i$$

when $QALY =$ the quality-adjusted life years, $Q_i =$ the quality factor for follow-up period "i" and $t_i =$ the length of time spent in period "i". This equation shows that the effectiveness of a treatment, as measured in QALYs, can be improved by either enhancing the patient's quality of life (Q_i) or the patient's length of life (t_i), or both.

CALCULATION OF COST-EFFECTIVENESS

After the costs of therapy and the medical effectiveness of therapy have been assessed, cost-effectiveness (CE) can be calculated as:

$$CE\ Ratio = \frac{Cost_2 - Cost_1}{QALY_2 - QALY_1}$$

where $Cost_i$ represents the total medical cost of program "i", and $QALY_i$ represents the effectiveness of program "i" measured in quality-adjusted life years.

There are several implications of using this formula. First, cost-effectiveness ratios that are positive (i.e., >0) result if and only if one alternative has both higher cost and greater effectiveness; i.e., $Cost_2 > Cost_1$ and $QALY_2 > QALY_1$ (or the reverse: $Cost_2 < Cost_1$ and $QALY_2 < QALY_1$). Cost-effectiveness ratios of <0 are not generally important for decision making, since they arise only when one alternative has both lower costs and greater clinical effectiveness than the other (e.g., $Cost_2 > Cost_1$, and $QALY_2 < QALY_1$). In this case, Program 1 is superior in all respects: it has better outcomes and lower cost than Program 2, and thus is said to "dominate" the alternative. The decision of which program to recommend is therefore simple.

Another important implication of the formula used to calculate cost-effectiveness is that the ratio is undefined when the two alternatives provide equal outcomes, since when $QALY_2 = QALY_1$, the denominator in the cost-effectiveness ratio is equal to zero. The implication is that when the difference in outcomes between two programs is negligible, cost-effectiveness analysis is unnecessary, and the choice between two alternatives can be based on cost alone (i.e., cost minimization analysis is more appropriate than cost-effectiveness analysis).

Most commonly, one of two therapeutic alternatives has higher costs and greater effectiveness, and use of the formula yields a cost-effectiveness ratio greater than zero. One treatment may have a cost-effectiveness ratio of $5000 per year of life saved, and another might have a ratio of $75 000 per year of life saved. Since it is problematic to assign a dollar value to life, interpretation of these ratios is best made by consideration of benchmarks – other generally accepted therapies that serve as a rough gauge to an "acceptable" cost-effectiveness ratio. Renal dialysis is a form of therapy that most people would consider expensive, and yet dialysis is an intervention that the United States and most other industrialized countries provide as a life saving therapy. The endstage renal disease program in the United States costs about $35 000 a year per patient, and if this therapy were withdrawn the patient would die. Thus, renal dialysis has a cost-effectiveness ratio of $35 000 per year of life saved (or if one considers the reduced quality of life for a dialysis patient, perhaps $50 000 per quality-adjusted year of life saved). Therapies with cost-effectiveness ratios considerably more favorable than renal dialysis (i.e., <$20 000) would be considered very cost-effective, whereas therapies with cost-effective ratios much higher (say >$75 000) would be considered too expensive.

Different societies may come to different conclusions about the level of cost-effectiveness they consider a good value. Wealthy countries with high per capita incomes are more willing to pay for expensive therapies than are poor countries. For instance, the percentage of gross domestic product and per capita health spending in Eastern Europe is much less than in Western Europe or North America, and these countries have not chosen to provide expensive services such as bypass surgery as readily or as frequently.

Decisions about funding programs might be more equitable and rational when guided by the relative cost-effectiveness of programs. When studies use similar methods to measure cost and effectiveness, cost-effectiveness ratios can be compared to rank the economic attractiveness of alternatives. Tables comparing various treatments, such as Table 6.6, have been termed "league tables" because of their similarity to the athletic league standings published in newspapers. Given the uncertainly inherent in measuring cost and effectiveness of medical interventions, and the methodologic variations among studies, only relatively large differences in cost-effectiveness ratios should be considered significant. Thus, a program with a cost-effectiveness ratio of $5000 per life year added is much better than one with a ratio of $30 000. Programs with ratios of $25 000 and $30 000 are so close that no firm conclusion about the relative values should be drawn.

PATIENT SELECTION AND COST-EFFECTIVENESS

Drugs and procedures in medicine are applied to different patient groups for different clinical indications. The medical effectiveness of therapies varies considerably according to patient selection. Cholesterol lowering therapy, for instance, will extend the life expectancy of a patient with multiple cardiac risk factors more than it will for a patient with the same cholesterol level and no other cardiac risk factors. Coronary bypass surgery provides greater life extension to a patient with left main coronary artery obstruction than it does to a patient with single vessel disease.[18] The cost-effectiveness ratio for these therapies will therefore vary among patient subgroups due to the impact of patient characteristics on the clinical effectiveness of therapy, which forms the denominator of the cost-effectiveness ratio. Similarly, the cost of a particular therapy may also vary according to patient characteristics, since the therapy itself may be more or less expensive according to different patient subgroups, or the likelihood of costly complications may be higher or lower in different groups of patients.

The clinical effectiveness of a therapy is generally the most important factor determining cost-effectiveness. The reason for this importance is (a) that clinical effectiveness of a therapy generally varies more among patients than does the cost of

Table 6.6 Cost-effectiveness of selected cardiovascular therapies

Strategy	Patient group	Cost-effectiveness[a]
Lovastatin	Post MI Men 45–54 Chol ≥ 250	Saves dollars and lives
Enalapril	CHF EF $<35\%$	Saves dollars and lives
Radio frequency ablation	WPW, post cardiac arrest	Saves dollars and lives
Physician counselling	Smoking	$1300
Beta-blocker	Post MI High risk	$3600
CABG	Left main CAD Severe angina	$9200
Beta-blocker	Post MI Low risk	$20 200
Lovastatin	Primary prevention Men 55–64 Chol >300 3 risk factors	$20 200
tPA	Acute MI	$32 800
CABG	Two vessel CAD Angina	$42 500
Lovastatin	Primary prevention Men 55–64 Chol >300 No other risk factors	$78 300
Exercise ECG	Asymptomatic 40-year-old men	$124 400
CABG	Single vessel CAD Mild angina	$1142 000
Lovastatin	Primary prevention 35–44-year-old women Chol >300 No other risk factors	$2024 800

[a] $ values = dollars per year of life added.
Adapted from Kupersmith *et al.*[10–12]

therapy, and (b) the value of the cost-effectiveness ratio is more sensitive to changes in the denominator (effectiveness) than to changes in numerator (cost). In the last analysis, a therapy must be clinically effective before it can be cost-effective. Cost-effectiveness analysis relies more on the assessment of medical effectiveness than it does on determination of cost.

DIAGNOSTIC TESTS AND COST-EFFECTIVENESS

Cost-effectiveness analysis has been applied primarily to assess specific therapies or therapeutic strategies, for which it is natural to measure effectiveness in terms of patient outcome. The principles of cost-effectiveness can be extended to analyze screening tests and diagnostic strategies as well, but some additional factors must also be considered.

Therapies are expected to improve patient outcome *directly*, by intervening in the pathophysiology of disease processes. In contrast, a diagnostic test is expected to provide the physician with information about the patient, which in turn is expected to improve management and thereby *indirectly* improve patient outcome. The value of a test is therefore linked closely with patient selection for therapy, and the value of testing may well change as new therapies are developed, or alternative tests become available.

The information provided by a test may be used in different decisions, and the test may be more or less useful in these different settings. An exercise electrocardiogram, for example, can be used as a diagnostic test for coronary disease, a prognostic test for patients with recent myocardial infarction, a monitoring test to assess the effect of anti-ischemic therapy, or even as a way to establish target heart rates for an exercise training program. The efficacy and cost-effectiveness of applying the exercise electrocardiogram will be different for these varied uses of the information provided by the test. The value of the test will depend on the indication for which it is used, much as the value of a beta-blocker will vary whether it is used to treat hypertension or as secondary prevention after a myocardial infarction.

The same test (e.g., the exercise EKG) applied for the same purpose (e.g., diagnosis of coronary disease) will provide more information in some groups of patients than in others. As discussed in detail in Chapter 3, a diagnostic test provides more value if used when the pretest probability of disease is intermediate than when the pretest probability is either very high or very low. The test has the most value when the result is likely to change the estimated probability of disease such that clinical management is changed. Tests that never change patient management cannot change patient outcome, which is the "bottom line" in assessing cost-effectiveness.

CONCLUSIONS

Economic analysis is designed to assist decisions about the allocation of scarce resources. Physicians now must address the cost implications of clinical decisions, and be aware of the effects on scarce resources. Economic efficiency is but one of many goals, however, and issues of fairness and humaneness are also central to medical care, and must be considered as well.

REFERENCES

1 Fuchs VR. *Who shall live? Health, economics and social choice.* New York: Basic Books, 1974.
2 Jollis JG, Peterson ED, DeLong ER *et al.* The relation between the volume of coronary angioplasty procedures at hospitals treating Medicare beneficiaries and short-term mortality. *N Engl J Med* 1994;**331**:1625–9.
3 Kimmel SE, Berlin JA, Laskey WK. The relationship between coronary angioplasty procedure volume and major complications. *JAMA* 1995;**274**:1137–42.
4 Hannan EL, Racz M, Ryan TJ *et al.* Coronary angioplasty volume–outcome relationships for hospitals and cardiologists. *JAMA* 1997;**279**: 892–8.
5 Drummond MF, Stoddart GL, Torrance GW. *Methods for the economic evaluation of health care programmes.* Oxford: Oxford University Press, 1987.
6 Finkler SA. The distinction between costs and charges. *Ann Intern Med* 1982;**96**:102–10.
7 Hlatky MA, Lipscomb J, Nelson C *et al.* Resource use and cost of initial coronary revascularization. Coronary angioplasty versus coronary bypass surgery. *Circulation* 1990;**82**(Suppl IV): IV-208–IV-213.
8 Weinstein MC, Stason WB. Foundations of cost-effectiveness analysis for health and medical practices. *N Engl J Med* 1977;**296**:716–21.

9 Detsky AS, Naglie IG. A clinician's guide to cost-effectiveness analysis. *Ann Intern Med* 1990;**113**: 147–54.

10 Kupersmith J, Holmes-Rovner M, Hogan A, Rovner D, Gardiner J. Cost-effectiveness analysis in heart disease, Part I: general principles. *Prog Cardiovasc Dis* 1994;**37**:161–84.

11 Kupersmith J, Holmes-Rovner M, Hogan A, Rovner D, Gardiner J. Cost-effectiveness analysis in heart disease, Part II: preventive therapies. *Prog Cardiovasc Dis* 1995;**37**:243–71.

12 Kupersmith J, Holmes-Rovner M, Hogan A, Rovner D, Gardiner J. Cost-effectiveness analysis in heart disease, Part III: ischemia, congestive heart failure, and arrhythmias. *Prog Cardiovasc Dis* 1995;**37**:307–46.

13 Russell LB, Gold MR, Siegel JE, Daniels N, Weinstein MC. The role of cost-effectiveness analysis in health and medicine. *JAMA* 1996; **276**:1172–7.

14 Weinstein MC, Siegel JE, Gold MR, Kamlet MS, Russell LB. Recommendations of the panel on cost-effectiveness in health and medicine. *JAMA* 1996;**276**:1253–8.

15 Siegel JE, Weinstein MC, Russell LB, Gold MR. Recommendations for reporting cost-effectiveness analyses. *JAMA* 1996;**276**:1339–41.

16 Echt DS, Liebson PR, Mitchell LB *et al*. Mortality and morbidity in patients receiving encainide, flecainide, or placebo: the Cardiac Arrhythmia Suppression Trial. *N Engl J Med* 1991;**324**:781–8.

17 Mark DB, Hlatky MA, Califf RM *et al*. Cost effectiveness of thrombolytic therapy with tissue plasminogen activator as compared with streptokinase for acute myocardial infarction. *N Engl J Med* 1995;**332**:1418–24.

18 Yusuf S, Zucker D, Peduzzi P *et al*. Effect of coronary artery bypass graft surgery on survival: overview of 10-year results from randomised trials by the Coronary Artery Bypass Graft Surgery Trialists Collaboration. *Lancet* 1994;**344**:563–70.

7 Introduction to decision analysis

KEVIN A. SCHULMAN,
HENRY A. GLICK,
ALLAN S. DETSKY

The concept of evidence based medicine challenges physicians to improve their use of the medical literature to guide their decision making in specific clinical settings. The concept is discussed extensively throughout this book. However, there are circumstances in which clinical trials do not address all of the issues of interest to a clinician. This may be because the trials do not compare the risks and benefits of all relevant treatment alternatives or because the trials are missing important data on the outcomes and costs of therapy. In these cases, researchers and clinicians are developing analytic strategies to improve their ability to synthesize the available information from the clinical literature and to help resolve these unanswered questions. One method of achieving this synthesis is the use of decision analysis, a set of mathematical strategies for aggregating information, making issues related to clinical decisions explicit, and solving for an optimal strategy under the constraints of the analysis. This decision analysis is a framework that can be used in the analysis of clinical problems as well as in economic analysis (see Chapter 6).

Decision analysis has been available to cardiologists for over 20 years.[1–3] In that time, the techniques of decision analysis have become more sophisticated and begun to address a broader range of questions.[4–6]

The goal of this chapter is to introduce the reader to some of the basic concepts of decision analysis and to review the use of decision analysis in the cardiovascular literature. For more specific information about the concepts or methods of decision analysis, the reader is referred to several excellent summary articles[2,7–11] or to one of the major texts in the field.[12–14]

EXAMPLES OF DECISION ANALYSIS

In this section, we present two examples of the use of decision analysis – a clinical example and an economic example. These examples are provided to demonstrate the steps involved in developing a decision analysis. As will be clearly demonstrated, decision-analytic models must simplify reality in order to structure the problem and analysis.

While our examples are extremely simplified to illustrate the steps involved in decision analysis, many models in the clinical literature offer more complex depictions of clinical reality.[16–24,33,37,38,50–55]

Steps in decision analysis

1 Identify the strategic options.
2 Draw the tree (structure of outcomes).
3 Determine the probabilities.
4 Determine the relevant outcome measures (effects, utility, survival, costs).
5 Evaluate the tree.
6 Make a structured analysis of the problem.
7 Develop a conclusion.

A comparative clinical analysis: warfarin vs aspirin for atrial fibrillation

For patients with non-valvular atrial fibrillation, both warfarin and aspirin have been shown to reduce the risk of stroke.[25–32] However, the effectiveness and side effects of these two treatments can vary substantially. Since there has been no randomized trial of aspirin and warfarin for stroke prevention, decision analysis has been used to identify the clinical outcomes resulting from treatment with each medication.[33]

Step 1: Identify the strategic options

In terms of therapeutic benefit, patients who receive either warfarin or aspirin experience a reduction in the risk of stroke. However, patients receiving these therapies also experience risk of bleeding complications. Both stroke and hemorrhage can be either fatal or non-fatal.

Step 2: Draw the tree

Based on these facts, we can graphically depict the issue using a decision tree (Figure 7.1). The tree is displayed so that the decision of interest is on the left side of the diagram, while the strategies to be compared are in the center, and the outcomes of those strategies are on the right. There are several pieces of information included in this simple figure.

In the decision tree, a choice is represented by a square, also called a "decision node". In this example, the decision node represents a choice between warfarin and aspirin. Once a decision is made, patients experience the potential for different clinical events (stroke or hemorrhage). These decisions and their subsequent clinical events are represented by lines or "pathways" running through the tree diagram. Figure 7.1 contains six possible pathways: warfarin with stroke; warfarin with neither stroke nor hemorrhage; warfarin with hemorrhage but without stroke; aspirin with stroke; aspirin with neither stroke nor hemorrhage; and aspirin with hemorrhage but without stroke.

After the initial treatment decision between warfarin and aspirin has been made, subsequent outcomes occur with a defined probability such that all of the potential

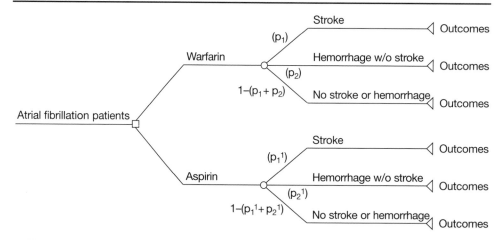

Figure 7.1 A decision tree for a comparative clinical analysis: warfarin vs aspirin for atrial fibrillation.

treatment outcomes are represented by the treatment pathways. The individual patient's achievement of a given treatment outcome (e.g., stroke or no stroke) is not a decision; it is, instead, a chance occurrence, where the "chance" event is represented by a circle in the decision tree.

The final treatment outcomes for each pathway are represented by triangles. These figures represent the outcomes of each treatment strategy. One, two, or more outcomes can be expressed for each pathway (survival, quality-adjusted survival, or costs).

Step 3: Determine the probabilities

Once a tree has been developed to depict a clinical problem, the next step is to begin to develop the data required to complete the analysis. In our example, we must identify the probability of stroke for patients in our two treatment categories and identify the potential risk of bleeding complications associated with each therapy.

Rates of stroke without therapy, outcomes of stroke, and stroke risk reduction with prophylaxis with aspirin or warfarin can be estimated from clinical trials or epidemiologic studies.[33] Rates of major hemorrhage associated with warfarin and aspirin therapy, and the outcomes of such an event, can be estimated in the same fashion.[33] However, in pooling these various data sources, investigators are left with a degree of uncertainty around these estimates. Sensitivity analysis, a method for assessing the impact of uncertainty in data analysis of clinical problems, will be discussed later, but it is an integral component of most well constructed decision-analytic models.

Step 4: Determine the relevant outcome measures (effects, utility, survival, costs)

For this analysis, quality-adjusted survival will be the primary outcome measure. Other possible outcome measures include event-free survival or simple survival. Analysis of quality-adjusted survival uses estimates of patient preferences for a variety of possible health states for patients with stroke. Patient preferences are a measure of health-related quality of life, or utility, as defined on a 0–1 scale, in which 0.0 represents the worst imaginable health state, and 1.0 denotes the best imaginable health state. Quality-adjusted survival is the product of the expected survival of patients and their preferences for the different health states resulting from a stroke or hemorrhage. These data can be estimated from expert opinion as reported in the medical literature or derived from patient interviews.[34] Calculation of quality-adjusted life years (QALYs) is described in greater detail elsewhere.[9]

Step 5: Evaluate the tree

Once data have been compiled for the specified model parameters, the next step is to analyze the tree. This step requires the calculation of the expected value for each pathway of the tree. For both warfarin and aspirin therapies, the expected value of the outcome (effects, utility, survival, or costs) is a weighted average of all possible treatment outcomes. This weighted average is calculated as the product of the value of each terminal node and the probabilities of the occurrence of that node (the product of the probabilities of achieving that node). The value of each node is then summed to result in the weighted average value for the treatment (e.g., the outcome for warfarin would be the weighted average of the products of the probability of no stroke and the outcome for no stroke, the probability of a stroke while taking warfarin and the outcome for stroke, the probability of no hemorrhage while taking warfarin and the outcome for no hemorrhage, and the probability of a hemorrhage and the outcome for hemorrhage).

A more complicated decision analysis proceeds in stepwise fashion for each set of probabilities and outcomes. This is called folding back the tree. The net result is an assessment of the outcomes for the two treatments, warfarin and aspirin. Other techniques can be used to solve more complicated problems for which there are many branches of each tree – for example, when the risk of stroke or hemorrhage is related to the duration of treatment. (These methods are based on the probability of moving between health states over time. Analysis can also be based on "state transition models" or Markov models.)

For clinical analyses, decision trees allow an incremental analysis of the treatment benefits of one medical therapy compared to another. They are used to compare the expected utility for each branch of the tree to pick the best treatment option. The best option is the one with the highest value in terms of clinical effects (survival or utility) or the one with the smallest value in terms of cost. An incremental analysis assesses the additional benefits gained from one treatment and, thus, differs from a calculation of the absolute benefit of a treatment.

Step 6: Structured analysis of the problem

Finally, the primary analysis having been completed, investigators should examine uncertainty in their estimates using a technique called "sensitivity analysis". By recognizing that a decision tree can suffer from uncertainty in the probability of each treatment strategy, investigators can ask how the results might change were the possibilities of stroke or hemorrhage to increase or decrease by 10% for each treatment arm. In a sensitivity analysis, the investigator recalculates the results of the model to address the robustness of the analysis to changes in the model specification.

Step 7: Conclusion

This decision analysis was structured to compare the outcomes of two strategies for the treatment of stroke prophylaxis – warfarin and aspirin. Such an analysis allows for an assessment of the clinical benefits of the two strategies, incorporating both the differences in risk reduction of stroke and the differences in hemorrhage resulting from the prophylactic treatment. The analysis would end with an estimate of the quality-adjusted survival resulting from each treatment strategy. The results could reveal that warfarin is superior to aspirin, that aspirin is superior to warfarin, that the treatments are comparable, or that there is not enough information available from which to draw a firm conclusion. The analysis would also address how sensitive the analysis was to differing model parameters. This sensitivity analysis could help define areas for further research to resolve outstanding issues in the clinical assessment.

A cost-effectiveness analysis: implantable cardiac defibrillators

At present, there is a great deal of debate about the most appropriate treatment of patients with arrhythmias, especially about whether implantable cardiac defibrillators (ICDs) will reduce cost and mortality for high risk patients. Early clinical trial results address mortality issues related to the use of ICDs in high risk populations.[35] However, there remains a great deal of concern about the findings of the study and the robustness of its results.[36] While decision analysis cannot answer the clinical questions regarding ICD use, these techniques have been used to model the costs and effects of ICD insertion to estimate the potential cost-effectiveness of this clinical therapy given current estimates of ICD clinical effectiveness.[37,38] To understand the decision analysis approach to this question, we will review the clinical issues and then build a decision-analytic model to formalize the question.

High risk patients experience an increased incidence of sudden cardiac death.[39] One new technology, the ICD, has been proposed as a means of reducing the incidence of sudden death in cardiac patients.[35,40–45] Should a patient choose to receive this therapy, he or she must undergo a surgical procedure and maintain the device over the remainder of their lifetime.

Step 1: Identify the strategic options

In terms of treatment benefit, patients who receive an ICD have the potential for different survival probability than patients who do not receive an ICD. From a cost perspective, patients receiving an ICD bear the additional cost of the device itself, as well as the future costs of maintaining the device.

Step 2: Draw the tree

Based on this discussion, we can graphically depict the issue using a decision tree (Figure 7.2). There are four possible pathways in this figure: ICD with sudden death; ICD without sudden death; no ICD with sudden death; and no ICD without sudden death. In this simple model, we consider only two health states: sudden death and no sudden death.

Step 3: Determine the probabilities

Estimates of the possibility of sudden cardiac death for high risk patients are available in the medical literature and in trials of ICDs.[40–46] Estimates of the probability of sudden

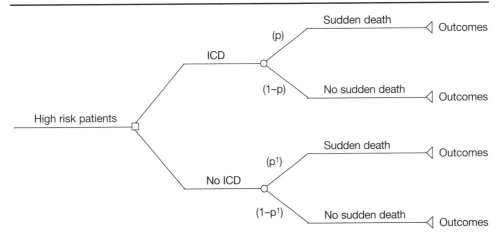

Figure 7.2 A decision tree for a cost-effective analysis: ICD to reduce incidence of sudden death in cardiac patients.

death for patients receiving an ICD are available from the MADIT Study[35] or may be estimated based on clinical trial protocols for expected treatment benefits.[38] The quality of the evidence from these data sources can vary. Data from the literature on non-ICD patients, the probability of sudden death without an ICD, come from observational studies, while data on ICD patients come from a controversial randomized controlled trial. Thus, there exists some uncertainty around these estimates.[10]

Step 4: Determine the relevant outcome measures (effects, utility, survival, costs)

Treatment benefits can be expressed in terms of survival (years of life gained) or in terms of quality-adjusted survival (QALYs). Calculation of these benefits proceeds as outlined in the stroke example.

Estimates of treatment costs often must be developed from primary sources (e.g., hospital accounting departments), from standard price lists for specific costs,[47] from literature reviews, or from expert opinion. Costs included in these models can include direct medical costs (the costs of medical care, such as hospital or physician costs), direct non-medical costs (the costs patients incur in receiving medical care services, such as the cost of transportation to a physician's office), indirect costs (the costs of morbidity or mortality related to disease), or intangible costs (the costs of pain and suffering related to disease).[48,49]

Step 5: Evaluate the tree

Once the data are available for all of these model parameters, the next step is to analyze the tree. For economic analyses, decision trees allow an incremental analysis of the treatment costs and benefits of one medical therapy compared to another in a cost-effectiveness analysis. The incremental cost-effectiveness of therapy A compared to therapy B is defined by the following formula:

$$\text{Cost-effectiveness of Treatment A} = \frac{(\text{Cost}_A - \text{Cost}_B)}{(\text{Effects}_A - \text{Effects}_B)}$$

Table 7.1 Use of decision analysis in cardiovascular literature

Clinical issue	Efficacy data	Cost data	Sensitivity analysis	Source	Evidence[a] grade
New technologies					
Inpatient ICD placement	Observational study; utility not assessed	Hospital charges; literature review for resource use data	Yes	Kupersmith et al.[16]	B/C
Outpatient ICD placement	Literature review for survival and utility estimates	Hospital and claims data; literature review for resource use data	Yes	Owens et al.[38]	B/C
Treatment strategies for WPW syndrome	Literature review; expert opinion; authors' estimates for utility data	Cost-accounting data for 13 patients at one study center	Yes	Hogenhuis et al.[17]	B/C
Specific products					
Low vs high osmolality contrast media	Literature review; authors' estimates for utility data; patient survey for intangible cost estimates	Resource use from a clinical trial; literature review; costs from Canadian hospital	Yes	Barrett et al.[18]	A/B
Simvastatin, high cholesterol	Clinical trial data; utility not assessed	Resource use from clinical trial; costs from hospitals in Sweden; employment status from clinical trial	Yes	Johannesson et al.[19]	A
Pravastatin, high cholesterol	Clinical trial data from 2 studies; utility not assessed	Literature review and expert opinion for resource use data; costs from aggregate US hospital data	Yes	Ashraf et al.[20]	B/C
Captopril, acute MI	Clinical trial data; utility data from 82 patients	Resource use from subset of study patients; costs from US Medicare reimbursement rates	Yes	Tsevat et al.[21]	A
Estrogen replacement	Literature review; utility not assessed	Not assessed	Yes	Zubialde et al.[22]	A/B

continued

Table 7.1 *continued*

Streptokinase vs tPA, suspected MI	Literature review, including utility data	Resource use estimated; drug and hospital cost data from Ireland	Yes	Kellett et al.[23] — B
Warfarin vs quinidine vs amiodarone, acute atrial fibrillation	Literature review and expert opinion, including utility data	Not assessed	Yes	Dirsch et al.[24] — B/C
Warfarin vs aspirin, stroke prophylaxis	Literature review; utility data from study of 74 patients	Resource use estimated; costs from literature review, Medicare data, and survey of pharmacies	Yes	Gage et al.[33] — A
Preoperative coronary angiography and revascularization, non-cardiac vascular surgery	Literature review; utility not assessed	Literature review	Yes	Mason et al.[52] — B
Treatment strategies				
CCU admission	Cohort study; utility not assessed	Hospital charges from the cohort adjusted to costs	Yes	Tosteson et al.[53] — B
Emergency medical services	Literature review; utility not assessed	Analysis of existing EMS program in Canada	Yes	Nichol et al.[54] — B
Cardiac transplantation selection	Transplant registries	Not assessed	Yes	Stevenson et al.[55] — B/C
Aortic valve replacement				Wong et al.[56] — B

[a] Evidence grades for decision analyses are complicated by the many different sources of data used in constructing the analysis. Evidence grades here are based on the data for the most important component of the analysis for the clinical portion of the decision tree. Where sources of evidence for the analysis were from a variety of sources, two grades were assigned to reflect the differing quality of data available for the analysis. (See Owens et al.[38] for an example of grades of evidence for data incorporated into a decision analysis.)
Grade A: Decision trees with the primary effect estimate from a large, high quality study (a randomized controlled trial with greater than 500 patients) or decision trees with a formal meta-analysis for the primary effect estimate.
Grade B: Decision trees with the primary effect estimate based on literature review but without a formal meta-analysis for primary effect estimate, includes evidence from case series and randomized controlled trials with fewer than 500 patients.
Grade C: Decision trees with the primary effect estimate based on expert opinion.

where Cost$_A$ is the cost of Treatment A, Cost$_B$ is the cost of Treatment B, Effects$_A$ are the effects of Treatment A, and Effects$_B$ are the effects of Treatment B.[49] Decision trees may also allow enumeration of the costs and consequences of different treatments without comparing the costs and effects of treatment in a cost-effectiveness ratio.

Step 6: Structured analysis of the problem

Sensitivity analysis would be conducted to assess the impact of uncertain values on the model. For example, because there was uncertainty in the probability of each treatment strategy, how would the results change if the possibilities of sudden death were increased or decreased by 10% for each treatment arm? Similarly, how would the results differ if ICD costs were increased or decreased by 10%? In a sensitivity analysis, the investigator recalculates the results of the model to address the robustness of the analysis to changes in the model specification.

Step 7: Conclusion

This decision analysis was structured to assess the cost-effectiveness of a new therapy for the treatment of patients at high risk for sudden cardiac death. It would conclude with an estimate of the incremental effects of ICD therapy in years of life gained per patient, the incremental costs of ICD treatment per patient, and an estimate of the cost-effectiveness of ICD therapy for patients evaluated in the model. The paper would also address how sensitive the analysis was to different model parameters. This sensitivity analysis could help define areas for further research to resolve outstanding issues in the clinical assessment.

APPLICATIONS OF DECISION ANALYSIS TO CARDIOLOGY

The above examples offer a simplified explanation of some of the basic components of decision analysis. They also illustrate the issues that must be addressed before using the results of a decision analysis to guide clinical decision making. As when reviewing clinical trials, clinicians must assess whether the population considered in the decision analysis model is relevant to the clinician's population. The reader must consider the strength of the evidence available to the investigator in developing the model to understand the strength of the recommendations resulting from the model. This not only includes whether the evidence was based on randomized controlled trials or on observational studies, but also whether the original studies included detailed information required by the model (for example, in the stroke analysis, whether the clinical studies reported both hemorrhage and stroke rates for the study's patients). Finally, the reader should consider the model used by the investigator to determine whether the investigator constructed the model appropriately and considered all relevant comparisons.[1,5]

Decision analysis has been used extensively in cardiology over the past several years (Table 7.1). These examples include articles from a MEDLINE search of decision analysis and cardiology from 1993 to 1997. Issues addressed using decision analysis have included the use of specific technologies, such as ICDs for patients at risk for sudden death, as well as specific diagnostic or pharmacologic products for defined populations of patients (e.g., treatment of high blood cholesterol), and the assessment of patient management strategies for defined populations of patients (e.g., selection of patients for placement on a cardiac transplant list). Each of the analyses listed in Table 7.1 will be reviewed in this section.

Decision analysis evaluating new technologies

ICD PLACEMENT

Over the past several years, investigators have attempted to calculate the cost-effectiveness of the ICD in patients at high risk for sudden cardiac death. Recent evidence from the Antiarrhythmics versus Implantable Defibrillators Trial indicates a decrease of 27 per cent in two-year mortality with ICD.[15] Kupersmith et al.[16] assessed ICD placement on an inpatient basis for patients with and without prior electrophysiologic (EP) studies. The investigators assumed an 84% improvement in life expectancy for patients undergoing ICD therapy based on a case series of 218 non-randomized patients who received an ICD when it was assumed that the patients would have died at the time of the first event (first shock or death). In this analysis, ICD patients had a mean life expectancy of 3.78 years, while EP-guided drug therapy patients had a mean life expectancy of 2.06 years. Total charges for these treatments were $146 797 for ICD patients and $93 340 for the EP-guided patients. The investigators found that the cost of ICD placement, including the cost of the device and the hospitalization, would range between $27 200 and $44 000 per year of life saved.

R
Grade A

The investigators conducted an extensive sensitivity analysis around their cost data and around the period of replacement of the ICD generator. They found that the cost-effectiveness of the therapy was sensitive to the magnitude of the clinical benefit of the therapy (this included the efficacy of the therapy as well as the estimated life expectancy for the underlying population, as represented by ejection fraction). The model was less sensitive to the cost of ICD therapy. The authors concluded that ICD use was economically attractive, especially using endocardial lead placement (based on preliminary estimates of the cost of this new procedure).*

Owens et al.[38] assessed implantation of ICDs on an outpatient basis using a decision-analytic model. In this analysis, the investigators modeled the potential cost-effectiveness of therapy, assuming in their principal analysis that the ICD led to a 20–40% reduction

---

* There are four possible outcomes of a cost-effectiveness analysis: (1) the intervention will save money and be more effective than the comparison; (2) the intervention will cost money and be more effective than the comparison; (3) the intervention will save money and be less effective than the comparison; and (4) the intervention will cost money and be less effective than the comparison.[48] The first outcome is the most preferred, and the intervention will always be adopted. The last outcome is never preferred, and the intervention will never be adopted. The second and third outcomes may be preferred at times, and the interventions may be adopted, depending on the relationship between the costs and effects of the intervention (the cost-effectiveness ratio). The second outcome may be adopted if the intervention yields a great enough benefit for the additional cost (in the USA, an economically attractive intervention may be one that costs less than $50 000 per year of life gained, whereas some Canadian authors have suggested that therapies that cost less than CDN$100 000 might be economically attractive).[32,50] The third outcome may be adopted if the intervention yields a small enough reduction in outcomes for the reduction in cost (e.g., the same Canadian authors suggested an economically attractive intervention may be one that saves more than CDN$100 000 per year of life forgone).[32,49]

in mortality. The investigators found that the cost of patients receiving ICD therapy would be $88 400, and the cost of patients receiving amiodarone therapy alone would be $51 000. For high risk patients, the investigators reported that ICD patients would have an estimated survival of 4.18 QALYs, whereas patients treated with amiodarone alone could expect a survival of 3.68 QALYs. Investigators found that the cost-effectiveness of therapy ranged from $37 300 per QALY saved for high risk patients, assuming a 40% reduction in mortality for patients treated with the ICD compared to those treated with amiodarone alone, to $138 900 QALYs saved for intermediate risk patients and assuming a 20% reduction in mortality for patients treated with the ICD compared to amiodarone alone. They concluded that the use of an ICD will not be economically attractive unless all-cause mortality is reduced by 30% or more compared to amiodarone.

ALTERNATIVE THERAPIES FOR WPW SYNDROME

Hogenhuis et al.[17] determined which of five management strategies should be used for the treatment of patients with Wolff–Parkinson–White (WPW) syndrome – observation, observation until cardiac arrest-driven therapy, initial drug therapy guided by non-invasive monitoring, initial radiofrequency ablation, and initial surgical ablation. The model included the risks of cardiac arrest, arrhythmia, drug side effects, procedure-related complications, and mortality, and assumed that radiofrequency ablation had an overall efficacy of 92% in preventing cardiac arrest and arrhythmia. For survivors of a cardiac arrest, radiofrequency ablation offered additional survival at reduced cost compared to all other treatment strategies.

For patients with arrhythmia without hemodynamic compromise, radiofrequency ablation resulted in a cost of $6600 per QALY gained in 20-year-old patients and $19 000 per QALY gained in 60-year-old patients without hemodynamic compromise. For asymptomatic patients, radiofrequency ablation costs from $33 000 per QALY gained in 20-year-old patients to $540 000 per QALY gained for 60-year-old patients. The authors conclude that their analysis supports the practice of radiofrequency ablation in patients with WPW syndrome who survive cardiac arrest, but their findings also support the current practice of merely observing asymptomatic patients, given that radiofrequency ablation was economically unattractive in this population of patients.

Decision analysis in the evaluation of specific products

Decision analysis has been used extensively in the evaluation of specific clinical products, including contrast media and pharmaceutical products.

CONTRAST MEDIA

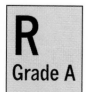

Barrett et al.[18] developed a decision-analytic model to assess the economic impact of low and high osmolality contrast media for cardiac angiography. Investigators assumed that low osmolality contrast media reduced the risk of myocardial infarction and stroke. Reduction in the risk of specific clinical events with low osmolality contrast media was assumed to be 0% in fatal events, 25% in severe events, 80% in moderate events, and 10% in minor events. The investigators found that the incremental cost per QALY gained with these media is $17 264 in high risk patients and $47 874 in low risk patients for a third party payer. From a societal perspective, the corresponding costs are $649 and $35 509. The authors report that these estimates were sensitive to cost of the contrast media and the total cost of contrast media used per patient. The authors also suggest that the model is extremely sensitive to changes in assumptions regarding the efficacy of low osmolality contrast media for prevention of severe reactions. To allow the reader to better understand the inputs of this model, the authors include a cost-consequence analysis of the program as a separate presentation in the results. The authors concluded that, in the context of restricted budgets, limiting the use of low osmolality contrast media to high risk patients is justifiable. The recommendation to limit use of this media was also justified by the lack of clinical evidence that low osmolality contrast media prevents severe or fatal reactions.

CHOLESTEROL REDUCTION

Several authors have used decision analysis to investigate the cost-effectiveness of therapies designed to reduce high blood cholesterol.[51] Two recent studies use clinical trial data to assess the cost-effectiveness of cholesterol reduction in secondary prevention of coronary artery disease. Johanneson et al.[19] developed an analysis based on the Scandinavian Simvastatin Survival Study, which reported that, in patients with preexisting coronary disease, reduction in blood cholesterol resulted in a 30% reduction in overall mortality based on a median follow-up of 5.4 years. The authors modeled the effects of 5 years of cholesterol-reducing therapy on patients' outcomes, using a model based on data reported from the trial. The costs of therapy were based on the assumption that the use of cholesterol-reducing agents would not entail any additional costs for patients with preexisting coronary disease other than the cost of medication itself and then used data on hospitalizations to estimate the direct medical costs incurred for the treatment of cardiovascular disease.

Interestingly, this model also included the indirect costs of medical care based on the employment status of patients in the trial. The investigators found that simvastatin treatment for 5 years in 59-year-old patients with a history of heart disease and a pretreatment total cholesterol level of 261mg/dl would have a net cost of $1524 with 0.28 years of life gained, resulting in a cost per year of life gained of $5400 for men and a net cost of $1685 with 0.61 years of life gained, resulting in a cost of per year life gained of $10 500 for women. An analysis that included direct and indirect costs showed that cholesterol reduction leads to an additional $1065 decrease in associated morbidity cost for men and an $876 reduction in associated morbidity cost for women. The analysis was somewhat sensitive to baseline cholesterol level and patient age at the initiation of treatment, to follow-up and screening costs and to the price of simvastatin. However, treatment remained economically attractive in all of these analyses. The model was somewhat sensitive to reduction in cardiovascular risk and the risk of mortality after coronary events. The authors concluded that, in patients with coronary artery disease, simvastatin therapy is economically attractive among both men and women at the ages and cholesterol levels studied.

Ashraf et al.[20] assessed the cost-effectiveness of cholesterol reduction based on 3 year data from the Pravastatin Limitation of Atherosclerosis in the Coronary Arteries (PLAC I) and Pravastatin, Lipids and Atherosclerosis in the Carotids (PLAC II) studies. These trials reported no statistically significant decrease in all-cause mortality but did report

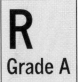

a decrease in the number of coronary events in men in the group receiving drug therapy to reduce high blood cholesterol. Therapy was estimated using a Markov model based on data from the Framingham Heart Study to estimate subsequent annual morbidity and mortality rates for patients with non-fatal myocardial infarction. Costs of therapy were based on the costs of drug therapy, and hospitalization costs were derived from the cost of treatment of myocardial infarction and from expert opinion on frequency of medical events. Investigators found that cost per year of life saved for patients from secondary prevention was sensitive to a number of risk factors but ranged from $7124 per year of life saved for a male patient with three risk factors to $12 665 per year of life saved for a male patient with one risk factor. The model was sensitive to assumptions about efficacy of therapy and cost of services. The model was also sensitive to patient characteristics such as the number of risk factors of patients receiving secondary prevention. The authors conclude that pravastatin is economically attractive compared to other widely accepted medical interventions.

POSTMYOCARDIAL INFARCTION TREATMENT

R

Grade A

Tsevat et al.[21] used decision analysis to assess the cost-effectiveness of captopril therapy after acute myocardial infarction (MI). In this paper, the investigators used data from the Survival and Ventricular Enlargement (SAVE) trial, which demonstrated that captopril therapy reduced mortality in patients who survived MI. The effectiveness of therapy was modeled using a decision-analytic model based on all-cause mortality within the clinical trial observation period and the projected clinical benefits over a patient's lifetime. This paper also incorporated data on quality of life from a subset of patients in the SAVE trial. Cost estimates for the model were based on a subset of 123 study patients for whom hospital data were obtained for all hospitalizations in the subset. The investigators used two projection methods, a limited-benefit model and a persistent-benefit model. The limited-benefit model was more conservative in that it assumed similar annual mortality rates between captopril and control patients beyond the clinical trial period. This analysis resulted in an estimated cost-effectiveness for captopril therapy ranging from $60 800 per QALY for 50-year-old patients to $3600 per QALY for 80-year-old patients. The persistent-benefit model was more optimistic in that it assumed that the clinical benefits observed in the trial persisted throughout each patient's lifetime. In this analysis, the cost-effectiveness ratios were similar to those in the limited-benefit model for patients aged 60–80 years, but they were substantially better for 50-year-old patients. In the sensitivity analysis, the models were most sensitive to the annual cost of captopril therapy, and the persistent-benefit model appeared to be more stable than the limited-benefit analysis. The investigators concluded that angiotensin converting enzyme inhibitor therapy with captopril was not only effective in improving survival after MI but also moderately economically attractive.

HORMONE REPLACEMENT THERAPY

R

Grade B

Zubialde et al.[22] used a decision-analytic model to assess gains in life expectancy resulting from the use of estrogen replacement therapy for postmenopausal women. Efficacy data for this analysis were obtained from a review of the literature that suggested that risk reduction with estrogen therapy for coronary artery disease was between 40 and 50%. The model did not assume an increased incidence in breast cancer in the principal analysis, but it did include an increased incidence of endometrial cancer. Results of the analysis suggested that the benefit of estrogen and progesterone therapy in average-risk women aged 50 years at the time of therapy initiation was 0.86 years with a range of 0.41–1.19 years, while therapy in average-risk women aged 65 years at the time of therapy initiation was 0.47 years with a range of 0.21–0.66 years. The authors reported that the benefits of estrogen and progesterone therapy were similar to gains from cholesterol reduction to 200 mg/dl and smoking cessation. The authors concluded that significant potential benefits in life expectancy in coronary artery disease reduction combined with the osteoporosis prevention in symptom relief would point to greater emphasis on postmenopausal estrogen use in appropriate patients.

THROMBOLYTIC THERAPY

Kellett et al.[23] presented a paper on the use of thrombolytic therapy for patients with suspected MI. This paper assessed the use of two types of thrombolytic therapy – streptokinase and accelerated tissue plasminogen activator (tPA) – on patients with suspected MI. The efficacy of the two therapies was based on reports from the medical literature. The authors assessed the clinical benefits of thrombolytic therapies for patients presenting with different likelihoods of MI given their clinical and ECG findings, different age groups, and different probabilities of death given MI. Data on clinical efficacy for the two strategies were based on the GISSI-2, ISIS-3, and GUSTO trials. The authors suggested that, for patients with a 26% probability of MI (a group with chest pain and a history of coronary artery disease but a normal ECG), thrombolytic therapy would only be beneficial if the probability of death given an MI was 20% or greater. In contrast, for patients presenting with a probability of MI of 78% (chest pain plus ST or T wave changes), thrombolytic therapy would be beneficial for all patients except for patients greater than 80 years of age who had a probability of death given an MI of 2.5% or less. The authors conclude that, for a typical 60-year-old man presenting 4 hours after the onset of symptoms with definite acute MI, treatment with streptokinase in addition to aspirin would gain 150 quality-adjusted life days, while treatment with aspirin and accelerated tPA would result in 255 quality-adjusted life days compared to no thrombolytic therapy. Thrombolytic therapy is preferred over no thrombolytic therapy as long as the probability of stroke is less than 5% for streptokinase and 8% for accelerated tPA. The cost per QALY was estimated based on the probability of acute MI, the extra days of quality-adjusted life, and the probability of death given an MI. The analysis was sensitive to estimates of efficacy for both streptokinase and accelerated tPA as well as the probability of death given thrombolytic therapy. The authors conclude that decision analysis can be a useful bedside tool to guiding thrombolytic therapy.

R
Grade A

MANAGEMENT OF ATRIAL FIBRILLATION

Dirsch et al.[24] developed a decision-analytic model to assess the outcomes of four treatment strategies for patients with acute atrial fibrillation undergoing cardioversion – warfarin therapy, quinidine therapy, and low-dose amiodarone therapy. Efficacy was based on a review of the literature, including randomized controlled trials, observational studies, and expert clinical opinion when necessary. Investigators found that all four treatment strategies differed by 0.2 QALYs over patients' lifetimes, with 4.55 expected QALYs for patients who undergo no treatment after cardioversion and 4.75 expected

R
Grade A/B/C

QALYs for patients who undergo cardioversion with amiodarone. Use of warfarin and quinidine therapies yielded expected quality-adjusted life benefits between amiodarone and no treatment. The model was sensitive to the annual rate of bleeding on warfarin, the annual rate of stroke for patients on warfarin, the annual rate of stroke for patients with atrial fibrillation, the decrement in quality of life associated with taking warfarin, and the excess mortality of quinidine and amiodarone. The authors conclude that cardioversion followed by low dose amiodarone to maintain normal sinus rhythm appears to be a relatively safe and effective treatment for patients with chronic atrial fibrillation for a hypothetical cohort of patients with atrial fibrillation.

PROPHYLAXIS OF STROKE

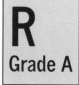

Gage et al.[33] developed a decision-analytic model to assess the cost-effectiveness of warfarin and aspirin treatment for prophylaxis of stroke in patients with non-valvular atrial fibrillation. The clinical efficacy of the treatment strategies was obtained from the published literature. The quality-of-life estimates for this study were obtained by interviewing patients with atrial fibrillation. Costs were also estimated from a literature review and from a survey of national pharmacies and laboratories. The authors found that, for patients with non-valvular atrial fibrillation and no additional risk factors for stroke, warfarin would minimally affect quality-adjusted survival but increase costs significantly. For patients with non-valvular atrial fibrillation and one additional risk factor, warfarin therapy resulted in a cost of $8000 per QALY saved compared to aspirin. The model was most sensitive to the rate of stroke if no therapy was prescribed, the effectiveness of aspirin, the rates of major hemorrhage, and the disutility of taking warfarin. The authors conclude that treatment with warfarin is economically attractive (has a low cost-effectiveness ratio) in patients with non-valvular atrial fibrillation and one or more additional risk factors for stroke. However, in patients with non-valvular atrial fibrillation without other risk factors for stroke, use of warfarin instead of aspirin would add significantly to costs with minimal additional clinical benefit.

PREOPERATIVE CARDIAC REVASCULARIZATION

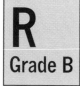

Mason et al.[52] developed an analysis to determine whether preoperative coronary angiography and revascularization improved short term outcomes in patients undergoing non-cardiac vascular surgery with three strategies. The first was to proceed directly to vascular surgery, the second was to perform coronary angiography followed by selective coronary revascularization prior to surgery and to cancel vascular surgery in patients with severe inoperable coronary disease, and the third was to perform coronary angiography followed by selective coronary revascularization and to perform vascular surgery in patients with inoperable coronary artery disease. The literature was scrutinized for data on the efficacy of all three strategies. The authors found that proceeding directly to vascular surgery led to a lower morbidity and cost in the base-case analysis. The coronary angiography strategy led to a higher mortality of vascular surgery in patients with inoperable coronary disease but led to a lower mortality in operable patients who did not proceed to vascular surgery. The model was sensitive to the surgical mortality rates for both catheterization and the vascular surgical procedure. The authors conclude that decision analysis indicates that vascular surgery without preoperative angiography generally leads to better outcomes and that preoperative coronary angiography should be reserved for patients whose estimated mortality for vascular surgery is substantially higher than average.

Use of decision analysis in treatment strategies

CCU ADMISSION

Tosteson *et al.*[53] used a decision-analytic model to identify cost-effective guidelines for admission to a coronary care unit (CCU) for uncomplicated patients without other indications for intensive care. The probabilities of death and minor, major, and life-threatening complications were based on 12 139 emergency department patients who were enrolled in a multicenter chest pain study. Cost data were available from a subset of patients in the study admitted to one study center. Under the assumption that there is a 15% relative increase in mortality when patients with acute MI are admitted to the intermediate care unit instead of an intensive CCU, the authors found that costs per year of life saved for triage to the CCU varied markedly depending on the age of the patient and the probability of MI. For 55 to 64-year-old patients with an emergency department probability of infarction of 1%, the cost per year of life saved was $1.4 million. But when the probability of infarction was 99%, the cost per year of life saved was $15 000. Admission to the intensive care unit was generally more costly for younger patients, and use of the CCU had a cost-effectiveness ratio of less than $50 000 per year of life saved when the initial probability of acute MI was greater than 57% among patients 30–44 years of age and greater than 21% among patients 65–74 years of age. The model was sensitive to the reduction of mortality associated with the use of the intensive care unit and was sensitive to costs of the intensive care unit. The authors conclude that the CCU should generally be reserved for patients with a moderate or high probability of acute MI, unless patients need intensive care for other reasons.

EMERGENCY MEDICAL SERVICES

Nichol *et al.*[54] used a decision-analytic model to assess the cost-effectiveness of potential improvements to emergency medical services (EMS) for patients with out-of-hospital cardiac arrest. The authors developed their analysis based on a review of the effectiveness of various emergency systems from an extensive meta-analysis, costing of each component of the EMS, and community characteristics and response times for EMS. The authors also modeled a one-tier system versus a two-tier system. In the one-tier response system, the response team is trained in advanced life support, and in the two-tier response system, the first response team is trained in basic life support and the second response team is trained in advanced life support. The authors found that the fixed cost of the first tier of a two-tier EMS system was $651 129 for Hamilton, Ontario, with estimates of survival of 5.2% in the one-tier response system and 10.5% in the two-tier response system. They found that a 1 minute decrease in response time improved survival by 0.4% in a one-tier system and by 0.7% in a two-tier system. The authors found that a change from a one-tier system to a two-tier system will result in 0.19 QALYs saved and an incremental cost of $7700 per patient, or a cost per QALY of $40 000. Improvement in a one-tier EMS system by the addition of more basic life support providers in the first tier would result in an incremental survival benefit of 0.40 QALYs with an incremental cost of $2400 or cost per QALY of $53 000. An improvement

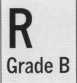

in response time in a one-tier system by the addition of more providers and ambulances would achieve an incremental survival benefit of 0.2 QALYs for a cost per QALY of $368 000. The authors performed an extensive sensitivity analysis based on a combination of the model's parameters. The authors concluded that the most attractive options in terms of incremental cost-effectiveness ratios for an EMS program would be improved response time in a two-tier EMS system or a change from a one-tier EMS system to a two-tier system. However, the authors were concerned about the poor quality of the data available for their analysis.

HEART TRANSPLANTATION

Stevenson et al.[55] used a decision-analytic model to determine optimal strategies for selecting patients for cardiac transplantation. The authors developed a model based on data from cardiac transplantation data bases. The decision-analytic model was developed to determine the size and outcomes of the waiting list population, depending upon different strategies for listing heart transplant candidates. They found that, if current practices continue, all hearts will be transplanted to hospitalized candidates and newly listed urgent candidates, and 3700 outpatient transplant candidates would be listed with virtually no transplantation unless they deteriorate to an urgent status. Decrease in the upper age limit to 55 years for transplantation will reduce the number listed each month by 30%. If this strategy were to be adopted, the waiting list would reduce to one-third the current size, with 50% of all hearts available for outpatient candidates. The authors conclude that immediate provisions should be made to limit candidate listing and revise expectations to reflect the diminishing likelihood of transplantation for outpatient candidates.

SURGERY FOR AORTIC STENOSIS

Wong et al.[56] used decision analysis to assess whether to recommend cardiac surgery for elderly women with aortic stenosis. This analysis was based on a specific case of assessing the treatment choice for an 87-year-old patient with severe aortic stenosis, three vessel coronary disease, depressed left ventricular function, and moderately severe heart failure. Data for this analysis were based on the medical literature. Specific data elements included in the analysis were life expectancy with and without surgery for an octogenarian, morbidity and mortality associated with surgery, and quality of life with congestive heart failure. Sensitivity analysis assessed the sensitivity of the model to assumptions used in developing the analysis and assessed the impact of patients' risk preferences regarding treatment choice. The authors also modeled valvuloplasty compared to surgery. They found that life expectancy with surgery (5.0 QALYs) was greater than that for medical therapy (1.1 QALYs).* In sensitivity analysis, surgery still had the highest life expectancy until mortality from the procedure was greater than 70%. Valvuloplasty was the best strategy if the patient was not the best candidate for surgery or, perhaps, in cases in which the perioperative mortality rate was greater that

---

* These gains in life expectancy are substantial. Most interventions reported in the medical literature yield incremental gains in life expectancy from 0.167 to 1.2 years of life.[57]

50%. They conclude that even in the upper decades of life, aortic valve surgery wins out substantially over medical therapy.

SUMMARY

Decision analysis offers powerful techniques to better understand uncertain clinical decisions in cardiology. Increasing use of these techniques has already shown them to be very valuable in clinical and policy decision making in a variety of settings. Decision analysis may be most useful when clinical trial data do not clearly answer the clinical issue, when the clinical trial concludes that there are differences in risks and benefits across two treatment groups, when the relevant outcomes were not collected as part of the clinical trial, or when the decision maker is concerned with both clinical benefits and costs. Readers of a decision analysis paper should consider the strength of the evidence underlying the analysis, whether the model was constructed appropriately from a clinical perspective, and whether all relevant comparisons were included in the model.[5,6]

Key points
- Decision analysis may be most useful when clinical trial data do not clearly answer the clinical issue, when the clinical trial concludes that there are differences in risks and benefits across two treatment groups, when the relevant outcomes were not collected as part of the clinical trial, or when the decision maker is concerned with both clinical benefits and costs.
- Sensitivity analysis is used to assess the impact of uncertainty on decision-analytic models.
- In reviewing a decision analysis paper, the reader must assess whether the population considered in the decision-analytic model is relevant to the clinician's population, the strength of the evidence available to the investigator in developing the model, and whether the model used by the investigator is constructed appropriately by including all relevant comparisons.
- Decision analysis has been used to assess a wide variety of clinical issues in cardiology.

REFERENCES

1 Paulker SA. Coronary artery surgery: the use of decision analysis. *Ann Intern Med* 1976;**85**:8–18.

2 Detsky AS, Naglie G, Krahn MD, Naimark D, Redelmeier DA. Primer on medical decision analysis: part 1 – getting started. *Medical Decision Making* 1997;**17**:123–5.

3 Stason WB, Weinstein MC. Allocation of resources to manage hypertension. *N Engl J Med* 1977;**296**:732–9.

4 Kassirer JP, Moskowitz AJ, Lau J, Pauker SG. Decision analysis: a progress report. *Ann Intern Med* 1987;**106**:275–91.

5 Richardson WS, Detsky AS. User's guide to the medical literature: VII. How to use a clinical decision analysis: A. Are the results of the study valid? *JAMA* 1995;**273**:1292–5.

6 Richardson WS, Detsky AS. User's guide to the medical literature: VII. How to use a clinical decision analysis: B. What are the results and will they help me in caring for my patients? *JAMA* 1995;**273**:1610–13.

7 Greenberg ML, Malenka DJ, Disch DL. Therapeutic strategies for atrial fibrillation: the value of decision analysis. *Cardiol Clin* 1996;**14**:623–40.

8 Detsky AS, Naglie G, Krahn MD, Redelmeier DA, Naimark D. Primer on medical decision analysis: part 2 – building a tree. *Medical Decision Making* 1997;**17**:126–35.

9 Naglie G, Krahn MD, Naimark D, Redelmeier DA, Detsky AS. Primer on medical decision analysis: part 3 – estimating probabilities and utilities. *Medical Decision Making* 1997;**17**:136–41.

10 Krahn MD, Naglie G, Naimark D, Redelmeier DA, Detsky AS. Primer on medical decision analysis: part 4 – analyzing the model and interpreting the results. *Medical Decision Making* 1997;**17**:142–51.

11 Naimark D, Krahn MD, Naglie G, Redelmeier DA, Detsky AS. Primer on medical decision analysis: part 5 – working with Markov processes. *Medical Decision Making* 1997;**17**:152–9.

12 Weinstein MC, Fineberg HV et al. *Clinical decision analysis*. Philadelphia: WB Saunders, 1980.

13 Sox HC, Blatt MA, Higgins MC, Marton KI. *Medical decision making*. Boston: Butterworth–Heinemann, 1988.

14 Petitti DB, Sidney S, Quesenberry CP Jr, Bernstein A. Incidence of stroke and myocardial infarction in women of reproductive age. *Stroke* 1997;**28**:280–3.

15 The Antiarrhythmics versus Implantable Defibrillators (AVID) Investigators. A comparison of antiarrhythmic-drug therapy with implantable defibrillators in patients resuscitated from near-fatal ventricular arrhythmias. *N Engl J Med* 1997;**337**:1576–83.

16 Kupersmith J, Hogan A, Guerrero P et al. Evaluating and improving the cost-effectiveness of the implantable cardioverter-defibrillator. *Am Heart J* 1995;**130**:507–15.

17 Hogenhuis W, Stevens SK, Wang P et al. Cost-effectiveness of radiofrequency ablation compared with other strategies in Wolff–Parkinson–White syndrome. *Circulation* 1993;**88**:437–46.

18 Barrett BJ, Parfrey PS, Foley RN, Detsky AS. An economic analysis of strategies for the use of contrast media for diagnostic cardiac catheterization. *Medical Decision Making* 1994;**14**:325–35.

19 Johannesson M, Jönsson B, Kjekshus J et al. Cost-effectiveness of simvastatin treatment to lower cholesterol levels in patients with coronary heart disease. *N Engl J Med* 1997;**336**:332–6.

20 Ashraf T, Hay JW, Pitt B et al. Cost-effectiveness of pravastatin in secondary prevention of coronary artery disease. *Am J Cardiol* 1996;**78**:409–14.

21 Tsevat J, Duke D, Goldman L et al. Cost-effectiveness of captopril therapy after myocardial infarction. *J Am Coll Cardiol* 1995;**26**:914–19.

22 Zubialde JP, Lawler F, Clemenson N. Estimated gains in life expectancy with use of postmenopausal estrogen therapy: a decision analysis. *J Family Pract* 1993;**36**:271–80.

23 Kellett J, Clarke J. Comparison of accelerated tissue plasminogen activator with streptokinase for treatment of suspected myocardial infarction. *Medical Decision Making* 1995;**15**:297–310.

24 Dirsch DL, Greenberg ML, Holzberger PT, Malenka DJ, Birkmeyer J. Managing chronic atrial fibrillation: a Markov decision analysis comparing warfarin, quinidine, and low-dose amiodarone. *Ann Intern Med* 1994;**120**:449–57.

25 The European Atrial Fibrillation Trial Study Group. Secondary prevention in non-rheumatic atrial fibrillation after transient ischæmic attack or minor stroke. *Lancet* 1993;**342**:1255–62.

26 Connolly SJ. Canadian Atrial Fibrillation Anticoagulation (CAFA) Study. *J Am Coll Cardiol* 1991;**18**:349–55.

27 Ezekowitz MD, Bridgers SL, James KE et al. Warfarin in the prevention of stroke associated with nonrheumatic atrial fibrillation. *N Engl J Med* 1992;**327**:1406–12.

28 Stroke Prevention in Atrial Fibrillation Investigators. Stroke Prevention in Atrial Fibrillation (SPAF) Study: final results. *Circulation* 1991;**84**:527–39.

29 Stroke Prevention in Atrial Fibrillation Investigators. Warfarin versus aspirin for prevention of thromboembolism in atrial fibrillation: Stoke Prevention in Atrial Fibrillation II Study. *Lancet* 1994;**343**:687–91.

30 Petersen P, Boysen G, Godtfredsen J, Andersen ED, Andersen B. Placebo-controlled, randomised trial of warfarin and aspirin for prevention of thromboembolic complications in chronic atrial fibrillation: the Copenhagen aFASAK Study. *Lancet* 1989;**i**:175–9.

31 The Boston Area Anticoagulation Trial for Atrial Fibrillation Investigators. The effect of low-dose warfarin on the risk of stroke in patients with nonrheumatic atrial fibrillation. *N Engl J Med* 1990;**323**:1505–11.

32 Laupacis A, Feeny D, Detsky AS, Tugwell PX. How attractive does a new technology have to be to warrant adoption and utilization? Tentative guidelines for using clinical and economic evaluations. *Can Med Assoc J* 1992;**146**:473–81.

33 Gage BF, Cardinalli AB, Albers GW, Owens DK. Cost-effectiveness of warfarin and aspirin for prophylaxis of stroke in patients with nonvalvular atrial fibrillation. *JAMA* 1995;**274**:1839–45.

34 Solomon NA, Glick HA, Russo CJ, Schulman KA. Patient preferences for stroke outcomes. *Stroke* 1994;**25**:1721–5.

35 Moss AJ, Jackson Hall W, Cannom DS for the Multicenter Automatic Defibrillator Implantation Trial (MADIT) Investigators. Improved survival with an implanted defibrillator in patients with coronary disease at high risk for ventricular arrhythmia. *N Engl J Med* 1996;**335**:1933–40.

36 Friedman PL, Stevenson WG. Unsustained ventricular tachycardia – to treat or not to treat? *N Engl J Med* 1996;**335**:1984–5.

37 Boyko W, Schulman KA, Tracy CM, Glick H, Solomon AJ. The economic impact of prophylactic defibrillators. *J Am Coll Cardiol* 1997;**29**(2 Supplement A):256A.

38 Owens DK, Sanders GD, Harris RA et al. Cost-effectiveness of implantable cardioverter defibrillators relative to amiodarone for prevention of sudden cardiac death. *Ann Intern Med* 1997;**126**:1–12.

39 Schatzkin A, Cupples LA, Heeren T et al. The epidemiology of sudden unexpected death: risk

factors for men and women in the Framingham Heart Study. *Am Heart J* 1984;**107**:1300–6.

40 Pinski SL, Trohman RG. Implantable cardio-verter-defibrillators: implications for the nonelectrophysiologist. *Ann Intern Med* 1995; **122**:770–7.

41 The Coronary Artery Bypass Graft (CABG) Patch Trial Investigators and Coordinators. The CABG Patch Trial. *Prog Cardiovasc Dis* 1993;**36**:97–114.

42 Cardiomyopathy Trial Investigators. The Cardiomyopathy Trial. *Pacing Clin Electrophysiol* 1993;**16**:576–81.

43 The DEFIBRILAT Study Group. Actuarial risk of sudden death while awaiting cardiac transplantation in patients with atherosclerotic heart disease. *Am J Cardiol* 1991;**68**:545–6.

44 AVID Trial Investigators. Antiarrhythmics Versus Implantable Defibrillators (AVID) – rationale, design, and methods. *Am J Cardiol* 1995;**75**: 470–5.

45 Connolly SJ, Gent M, Roberts RS *et al.* Canadian Implantable Defibrillator Study (CIDS): study design and organization. *Am J Cardiol* 1993;**72**: 103F–8F.

46 Hine LK, Laird NM, Hewitt P, Chalmers TC. Meta-analysis of empirical long-term atiarrhythmic therapy after myocardial infarction. *JAMA* 1989; **262**:3037–40.

47 Health Care Financing Administration. Revisions to payment policies and adjustments to the relative value units under the physician fee schedule for calendar year 1995; Final rule. *Federal Register*, December 2, 1995.

48 Eisenberg JM, Schulman KA, Glick H, Koffer H. Pharmacoeconomics: economic evaluation of pharmaceuticals. In: Strom BL, ed. *Pharmacoepidemiology*, 2nd edn. New York: John Wiley & Sons, 1994.

49 Detsky AS, Naglie IG. A clinician's guide to cost-effectiveness analysis. *Ann Intern Med* 1990;**113**: 147–54.

50 Naimark DM, Detsky AS. The meaning of life expectancy: what is a clinically significant gain? *J Gen Intern Med* 1994;**9**:702–7.

51 Glick H, Heyse JF, Thompson D *et al.* A model for evaluating the cost-effectiveness of cholesterol-lowering treatment. *Int J Technol Assessment Hlth Care* 1992;**8**:719–34.

52 Mason JJ, Owens DK, Harris RA, Cooke JP, Hlatky MA. The role of coronary angiography and coronary revascularization before noncardiac vascular surgery. *JAMA* 1995;**273**:1919–25.

53 Tosteson ANA, Goldman L, Udvarhelyi S, Lee TH. Cost-effectiveness of a coronary care unit versus an intermediate care unit for emergency department patients with chest pain. *Circulation* 1996;**94**:143–50.

54 Nichol G, Laupacis A, Stiell IG *et al.* Cost-effectiveness analysis of potential improvements to emergency medical services for victims of out-of-hospital cardiac arrest. *Ann Emerg Med* 1996; **27**:711–20.

55 Stevenson LW, Warner SL, Steimle AE *et al.* The impending crisis awaiting cardiac transplantation: modeling a solution based on selection. *Circulation* 1994;**89**:450–7.

56 Wong JB, Salem DN, Paulke SG. You're never too old. *N Engl J Med* 1993;**328**:971–5.

57 Naimark DM, Detsky AS. The meaning of life expectancy: what is a clinically significant gain? *Medical Decision Making* 1992;**12**:344.

8 Assessing and changing cardiovascular clinical practices

C. David Naylor

INTRODUCTION

Research into cardiovascular clinical practice has grown enormously in volume and sophistication since the turn of the century, driven by the worldwide prominence of atherosclerotic vascular diseases. The sheer volume of research literature has made it virtually impossible for even a subspecialist to stay abreast of her/his field. There is insufficient time for any evidence oriented practitioner to critically appraise the full array of individual studies relevant to practice, and a real risk that, as the years go by, his/her filtering of the literature will prove misleading.

One solution is for practitioners to rely increasingly on integrative reports. As documented throughout this volume, evidence on a particular clinical topic is often usefully compiled in published meta-analyses, decision analyses, or practice guidelines. These integrative reports synthesize the best evidence available from multiple research studies to help define what a practitioner ought to do when confronted with a particular clinical situation.

While information uptake from integrative reports is necessary to ensure that clinical care evolves in evidence driven directions, it may not be sufficient. For decades, researchers have shown that the rates of provision of various cardiovascular services vary inexplicably across regions and among nations. Some of this variation is random; some represents reasonable disagreement in the absence of definitive evidence about best practices. However, when practices are examined more closely using explicit criteria for appropriateness of care, it has become clear that actual practice sometimes differs sharply from what the evidence suggests ought to be done, raising concerns about quality of care. Quality concerns are further galvanized by evidence that technical skill and patient outcomes vary among procedural specialists.

Concerns with costs and quality of care have led a growing cadre of researchers, clinician leaders, facility managers, third party payers, and public policy makers to examine what clinicians do, and to seek ways to change clinical practice. Accordingly, this chapter provides an introduction to some methods in health services research as applied to the realm of cardiovascular medicine and surgery.

The nature of this material demands a different treatment than later chapters where it is possible to provide integrative summaries of evidence to inform contemporary practice or steer future research. Since our focus is on how evidence is translated into clinical action, it stands to reason that there will seldom be one "right answer". Instead, practice will inevitably be shaped not just by evidence, but by values and circumstances or context. Thus, it is important for the reader to suspend judgment as to whether there is one right health system, or one right profile of services for all populations with a given cardiovascular condition. A corollary of this point is that hundreds of descriptive and analytical studies have been published in cardiovascular health services research, many of which are context-specific. Our hope is to use a small number of these studies to heighten the reader's understanding of analytical principles and general lessons. For consistency, the examples will relate to clinical management of coronary artery disease, not to primary and secondary prevention. However, the conceptual frameworks are obviously applicable to all areas of cardiovascular care. It is hoped that the evidence oriented reader will be able to generalize the methodological insights from this chapter to his/her particular clinical and research context.

PRIMARY vs SECONDARY DATA SOURCES

Health services researchers use both primary and secondary data sources.[1] Primary data are detailed data collected by design to answer specific research questions. Secondary data are those collected for other purposes. For the purposes of this chapter, we are interested in two secondary data sources: databases designed for ongoing epidemiological surveillance of medical care, but not designed for addressing a specific hypothesis (for example, most clinical registries); or databases that were designed for administrative and managerial rather than research purposes, but are now being used for research (for example, administrative databases). Administrative data offer population coverage and low cost, but lack clinical detail and usually provide poor characterization of patients, services, and providers.[2] Partly in consequence, researchers often combine primary and secondary data collection. For example, a study may assess patients' short term outcomes using self-administered health status questionnaires, and then track their subsequent utilization of health services with administrative data.

PROCESS-OF-CARE STUDIES

Descriptive studies of practice variations

Health services research gained considerable momentum in the 1970s and 1980s from studies pioneered by Wennberg and Gittelsohn[3,4] that documented unexplained geographic variations in rates of services. Outcomes were not considered, and the focus was on service provision alone. These early studies were a population-wide extension of research done in single hospitals or in public and private prepayment plans starting in the 1930s that showed variations in how different physicians managed apparently similar patients. However, computerized systems of hospital discharge abstracts were coupled with census data to show that citizens living in one area were significantly more or less likely to undergo certain procedures than those living in other areas.

All such studies involve rates or proportions, with various numerators and denominators. Possible numerators include primary care visits or encounters, specialized diagnostic and therapeutic services, composite measures of utilization, such as overall numbers of hospital bed-days used per 1000 residents, or even mean expenditures per capita on health care for all types of services. Denominators may be institution- or practice-specific, defined by patient residency in a given geographic area, or a combination of the two as defined by hospital market shares (for example, the total population living in an area where a specified percentage of all patients receive their cardiac care at the hospital of interest).

In almost any jurisdiction and for almost any cardiovascular service where interpractitioner, interinstitutional, or interregional variations in service rates have been sought, they are demonstrable. Greater variation is demonstrable when procedures are more discretionary or elective, or where there is uncertainty about the indications for the procedure or service of interest.[5,6] In these instances, values and circumstances vie strongly with evidence in driving decisions about service provision.[7]

These descriptive studies raise the possibility that there may be a problem with quality or accessibility. Specifically, if the null hypothesis is that the rates of service should vary no more than would be expected on the basis of the play of chance alone, then significant variations lend themselves to two interpretations: some patients may be overserviced and put at risk of needless complications, with a concomitant waste of resources, while others may be denied beneficial treatment.

Several statistical summary measures are used in variations analyses.[8,9] Computational details and statistical properties of these measures are beyond the scope of this chapter. What matters is that the degree of variation should be both statistically significant and suggestive of meaningful differences from the standpoint of quality, accessibility, or efficiency of care provision. Thus, examination of the patterns of service and potential outcome implications is arguably more illuminating than focusing on specific summary measures.

In sum, descriptive variations studies are tantamount to screening tests in medical practice. They tend to raise more questions than they answer. Most studies do use direct or indirect standardization to control for differences in the age–sex profile of the populations being compared, but many other sources of variation must be considered (see Box). This leads logically to more analytical approaches to variations in processes of care.

Sources of regional/institutional variation in service profiles

- Age and sex composition
- Age/sex specific disease incidence
- Random variation with time and place
- Availability and practice organization, e.g.
  Primary care
  Specialist services
  Hospital services/bed provision
  Overall funding levels
  Methods of payment
  Alternative services
- Referral patterns
- Practice styles of service providers
- Variations in patient expectations, demands, health education/behaviors
- Rates of previous service (for example, organ removal where relevant)

Analytical studies of practice variations

More sophisticated studies of variations seek to isolate causes of variations in care, or at minimum to control for the effects of some of the more plausible confounders, as listed in the box on page 114, when variations are found. Survey/cross-sectional analyses as well as more formal cohort designs are used. On occasion, these analyses include "ecological variables", i.e. variables that are not specific to patients but instead are part of the context in which care is being provided, such as number of coronary care unit beds in a hospital, or the cardiovascular death rate of several regions.

As one example of this genre, Chen et al.[10] documented significant interhospital variations in length of stay after acute myocardial infarction (AMI) in Ontario. These variations persisted after adjusting for various factors such as coronary angiography on the index admission, patients' age and sex, and comorbidity as inferred from secondary diagnoses on discharge abstracts.

At times, cross-sectional and cohort methodologies can be combined in a single study. For example, Payne and Saul[11] undertook a mail survey of a random sample of 16 750 residents of the Sheffield (UK) region, and found that 4.0% of subjects had symptoms suggestive of angina pectoris. The prevalence of angina was significantly higher in neighborhoods with lower socioeconomic status, but these same areas had significantly lower rates of mechanical revascularization. In other words, area variations in service profiles were inversely related to ecological markers of both population need and population deprivation – obvious grounds for concern about access or equity of service utilization. The authors went further, however, and used data linkage methods to determine procedures actually provided to individuals identified as having angina. In so doing, they effectively shifted from a cross-sectional study reliant on ecological inferences to a cohort design. They found that among subjects reporting angina who lived in affluent neighborhoods, 11.2% had undergone procedures, as compared to 4.2% in less affluent areas ($P = 0.03$).

Such cohort methods have advantages in strengthening the evidentiary basis for inferences based on practice variations. For example, men are about four times as likely to undergo coronary artery bypass graft (CABG) as women, but this difference could be explained in part by differences in disease incidence. Ayanian and Epstein[12] used administrative data to define cohorts of patients hospitalized in 1987 with coronary heart disease-related diagnoses in Massachusetts ($n = 49\,623$) and Maryland ($n = 33\,159$). They compared the use of procedures in men and women, using multiple logistic regression to control for age, secondary diagnoses of congestive heart failure or diabetes mellitus, race, and insurance status. This approach effectively eliminated disease incidence as an explanation for gender differences in procedure use. They demonstrated significantly higher odds of undergoing angiography and revascularization for men in both jurisdictions, and confirmed this finding on a subgroup of men and women hospitalized with a principal diagnosis of AMI.

Other studies have since used administrative data on patients hospitalized with AMI and shown similar sex differences in the UK[13] and Canada.[14] The consistency of relative effects is striking since the baseline rate of post-MI revascularization varies dramatically across these nations. However, as Ayanian and Epstein[12] noted, "These differences may represent appropriate levels of care for men and women, but it is also possible that they reflect underuse in women or overuse in men." The debate about the gender gap in service intensity continues.

Let us turn now, however, to the issue suggested by Ayanian and Epstein's allusion to "appropriate levels of care". How and why do we measure appropriateness of processes of care?

Criteria-based utilization analyses

In assessing appropriateness of clinical processes, health services researchers (and managers) seek to determine whether the right service is provided to the right type of patient for the right reasons at the right time and place. This can be done by implicit reviews, relying on the individualized judgments of expert clinicians. Unfortunately, lack of standardization renders implicit reviews unreliable.[15,16] Explicit criteria, which form the basis for most process-of-care analyses in the literature, have the advantages of standardization and consistency, as well as transparency. Where necessary, trained staff can apply them retrospectively to medical records without a major time commitment from clinicians. These studies are described in America as "utilization reviews" and in the UK as "clinical audits".[17]

Process-of-care audits have the advantage of efficiency in comparison to outcomes studies as quality management tools. A focus solely on outcomes has the disadvantage that bad outcomes caused by negligence and incompetence are (happily) rare. Technical competence does not necessarily equate with good judgment and appropriateness of service provision. Moreover, bad outcomes from *under*treatment are hard to detect because much of what modern cardiovascular care does makes life only a little better or reduces the risk of otherwise-rare events. For example, from overviews of randomized placebo-controlled trials we know that beta-blockers confer about a 25% *relative* reduction in mortality in the first year after a myocardial infarction. For a cohort of medium risk patients, this equates to an *absolute* reduction in cumulative postdischarge mortality from 4% to 3%. To show such a mortality difference on a comparative *outcomes* audit of two practices (80% power, 2-sided alpha of 0.05), we require over 5000 patients per practice; but a 1% mortality difference presumes absolutely no use of beta-blockers in the practice with poorer outcomes. A more realistic assumption would be that about 70% of eligible patients receive beta-blockers in the practice with worse outcomes versus over 95% in the exemplary practice. Based on the randomized trials, this equates to perhaps a 0.2% increase in mortality. To detect such a small difference in mortality would require over 100 000 patients per practice! In contrast, one could simply examine charts to see whether patients were getting beta-blockers or not – a process-of-care audit. If a better practice had over 90% beta-blocker prescriptions, versus 70% in the other practice, one would only need to examine about 75 charts in each practice for a reliable assessment.

This latter audit is simple in another respect. We can basically use randomized trial inclusion and exclusion criteria to decide who should be getting the drug, make sure there are no obvious contraindications or medication intolerances documented on the medical record, and tally whether patients are getting the treatment that they ought to be getting. In general, however, audits require close attention to the validity, application, and applicability of the criteria chosen.[17]

User's guide to appraising and applying the results of a process-of-care audit

Are the criteria valid?

- Was an explicit and sensible process used to identify, select, and combine evidence for the criteria?
  What is the quality of the evidence used in framing the criteria?
  If necessary, was an explicit, systematic, and reliable process used to tap expert opinion?
  Was an explicit and sensible process used to consider the relative values of different outcomes?
- If the quality of the evidence used in originally framing the criteria was weak, have the criteria themselves been correlated with patient outcomes?

Were the criteria applied appropriately?

Was the process of applying the criteria reliable, unbiased, and likely to yield robust conclusions?
What is the impact of uncertainty associated with evidence and values on the criteria-based ratings of process of care?

Can you use the criteria in your own practice setting?

Are the criteria relevant to your practice setting?
Have the criteria been field-tested for feasibility of use in diverse settings, including settings similar to yours?

Adapted from Naylor and Guyatt.[17]

VALIDITY OF AUDIT CRITERIA

To be valid, the criteria must have a direct link either to improving health (as is obvious with beta-blockers for secondary prevention after AMI) or to lowering resource use without compromising health outcomes. There should be an explicit and sensible process to identify, select, and combine the relevant outcomes-based evidence.

The hierarchy of evidence outlined above by Kitching, Sackett and Yusuf applies here. Evidence from randomized trials is strongly preferred, but evidence from observational sources cannot be ignored. For example, from observational studies within trials, it is plain that the largest survival benefits with thrombolytic therapy are obtained when treatment is administered early.[18] It would be unethical to randomize patients to receive thrombolysis on a delayed or urgent basis to determine how large these effects are. Thus, guidelines now recommend that thrombolytic therapy be administered, wherever possible, within 30 minutes of a patient's arrival to hospital.[19] Studies from America,[20] Canada,[21] the UK,[22] Italy[23] and New Zealand[24] have all documented remediable problems with treatment delays in administering thrombolytic agents to eligible patients. All are classic examples of criteria-based audits.

If only some of the indications for a particular service under audit will be covered by high quality evidence, then weaker sources of evidence, inference, and expert opinion must often be brought into play, usually through formal panel processes. Such panels should include an explicit process for selecting panelists, and a sensible, systematic method for collating their judgments. In this respect, the RAND group has pioneered multispecialty panel methods that are widely emulated.[25-27] Scenarios are compiled that describe a potential indication for the procedure or clinical service in question. Each expert panelist independently rates hundreds of different case scenarios on a risk–benefit

Table 8.1 Categorization of appropriateness of indications for cardiovascular procedures based on actual audits in the field: cross-national differences in expert panel assessments

Procedure	Location/sample	Year	n	Panel nationality	Appropriate	Uncertain	Inappropriate
Coronary artery bypass graft	USA, 4 hospitals in Washington State	1979–80 1982	386	American British	62 41	25 24	13 35
	UK, 3 hospitals in Trent region	1987–8	319	American British	67 57	26 27	7 16
	Canada, 13 hospitals in Ontario and British Columbia	1989–90	556	American Canadian	88 85	9 11	3 4
	USA, 15 hospitals in New York State	1990	1336	American Canadian	91 85	7 10	2 6
Coronary angiography	USA, 4 hospitals in Washington State	1979–80 1982	376	American British	50 11	23 29	27 60
	USA, Medicare beneficiaries in 3 states	1981	1677	American British	74 39	9 19	17 42
	UK, 3 hospitals in Trent region	1987–8	320	American British	71 49	12 30	17 21
	Canada, 20 hospitals in Ontario and British Columbia	1989–90	533	American Canadian	77 58	18 33	5 9
	USA, 15 hospitals in New York State	1990	1333	American Canadian	76 51	20 39	4 10

Adapted from Naylor.[7]

scale. Scenarios are rerated at a panel meeting after patterns of interpanelist agreement and disagreement are shown anonymously and discussed. The final set of panelists' ratings then determines whether a given indication is deemed potentially appropriate, uncertain, or inappropriate.

With this method, it is not clear whether the appropriateness ratings for any given indication rest primarily on research evidence or inference, extrapolation and opinion. The relative values placed on different outcomes are also unclear. For example, in randomized trials of CABG versus percutaneous transluminal coronary angioplasty (PTCA),[28–31] PTCA has a slightly lower early mortality, along with lower initial costs and more rapid recovery from the procedure. Longer term mortality data are similar, but CABG patients appear to achieve better symptom relief, have decreased use of medication, and require fewer subsequent procedures. When an expert panel addresses the respective appropriateness of PTCA and CABG, the findings reflect these tradeoffs, but we cannot be sure that patients themselves would make the same choices. The conflation of facts and values in panel-based criteria is highlighted by studies showing that the nationality of a panel markedly affects the criteria and the results of applying them to cardiovascular procedures (see Table 8.1).[7,32] Nonetheless, the RAND methods compare very favorably with those used to create several utilization review tools now in widespread use.[17]

APPLICATION AND APPLICABILITY OF THE AUDIT CRITERIA

Application of explicit process-of-care criteria often rests on data derived from retrospective chart reviews by professional auditors. The audit process must therefore be reliable. Biases can be introduced through skewed sampling of practitioners, hospitals, and patients. Even a meticulous audit, however, may miss mitigating factors. Thus, in many instances, if the explicit review shows potential problems with the appropriateness of a service, the case is assessed by experienced clinicians to preclude "false-positives".

It is also crucial that enough cases be reviewed to draw robust conclusions. For example, in one study, RAND researchers used explicit criteria to assess the appropriateness of PTCA in 1990 for 1306 randomly selected patients in 15 randomly selected New York State hospitals.[33] The inappropriate utilization rate varied by hospital from 1% to 9% ($P = 0.12$). Differences of this magnitude, if real, could be important to patients, payers, and policy-makers. Thus, this sample size may have been insufficient for the investigators to confirm important differences in quality among hospitals.

Although the task is subjective, end-users must consider intangibles such as local medical culture and practice circumstances before accepting audit criteria that may not be relevant. The stronger the evidence on which the criteria are based, the less one needs to consider local factors; for example, few medical cultures would reject aspirin for AMI – a cheap and simple drug treatment that has been definitively proven to yield reductions in mortality. With weaker evidence and higher costs, however, the judgments are less straightforward.

Last, even if criteria are sufficiently valid and relevant, training times and other costs must be considered. Special logistical problems arise when criteria are used for concurrent case management rather than retrospective utilization review. Any errors associated with concurrent case management will have immediate consequences for individual patients and physicians. Nonetheless, many American hospitals already do a range of concurrent reviews.

USING PROCESS-OF-CARE AUDITS FOR POLICY INFERENCES

Table 8.1 shows the proportion of appropriate, inappropriate, and "uncertain" indications for cardiac procedures as randomly audited in the USA, UK, and Canada.[7,32,34,35] Since all the procedures shown are used many times more often in the USA than in the UK, it seems almost paradoxical that the proportions of inappropriate cases are not much higher in the USA. The literature has suggested that relationships between appropriateness of care and cardiovascular service intensity are similarly weak within nations.[6,36-38]

However, two recent studies shed a slightly different light on this issue. The rates of all major coronary procedures in New York State, USA are about twice as high as in Ontario, Canada.[39] Figure 8.1 shows the relative rate of isolated coronary artery bypass surgery for the two jurisdictions by age and anatomy. Overall, only 6% of CABG patients in Ontario versus 30% of patients in New York had limited coronary artery disease – one or two vessel disease without proximal left anterior descending (PLAD) involvement. However, more patients in New York had left mainstem disease (23% vs 16%, $P<0.001$). In relative terms, the differences are most dramatic among elderly persons (Figure 8.1). For example, New York brings 17 times as many persons over the age of 75 to surgery with anatomical patterns of coronary disease that are not associated with life expectancy

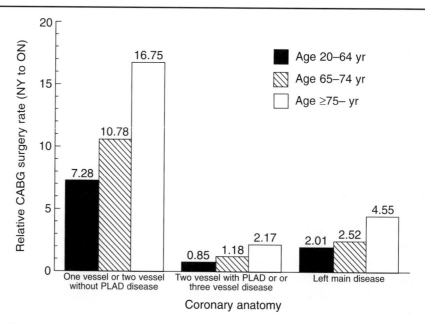

Figure 8.1 Relative rate of isolated coronary artery bypass surgery (CABG) for New York State (NY) and Ontario (ON) according to age and disease anatomy.[39]

gains after CABG. Nonetheless, much of this extra utilization could pass an appropriateness audit, since 90% of the persons with limited coronary anatomical disease in New York had moderate to severe angina before surgery.[39]

A reasonable inference is that major increases in capacity, and expansion of population-based service rates, are associated with *diminishing marginal returns*. The Canadian approach – fixed budgets in a universal health system, and "managed delay" with organized waiting lists[40,41] – seems to promote more efficient use of resources, with patients receiving surgery primarily if they are likely to have life expectancy gain. However, restricted use of coronary angiography leads to some implicit rationing that affects primarily the elderly, and a certain proportion of patients at all ages with left mainstem disease are not detected and/or do not undergo surgery.

A second study[42] of CABG develops this argument more strongly. Rather than using appropriateness criteria from an expert panel, Hux *et al.* based their case-specific assessment on a meta-analysis of randomized trials by Yusuf *et al.*[43] Whereas the broad category of "appropriate" care as defined by expert panels includes a range of risk–benefit ratios, a trials-based assessment allowed estimation of the *degree* of potential 10-year survival benefit conferred by CABG surgery among patients for whom, by and large, it was appropriate. Hux *et al.* found that only 6% of 5058 Ontario patients undergoing isolated CABG in 1992–3 fell in the low benefit category – that is, patients for whom there is no survival advantage from early CABG. However, the degree of anticipated benefit differed according to the center where surgery was provided. For instance, the proportion of patients in a high benefit category ranged from 65.2 to 79.9% ($P<0.001$). Significantly more patients were in a high benefit category in hospitals serving areas with lower population-based rates of CABG. Analyzing the data by site of residence, there was an inverse relationship between marginal degree of life expectancy gains and the surgical rates for each county.[42]

In sum, if one accepts that overtly inappropriate services are unlikely to be commonplace in any health system, the relationship between appropriateness of care and population-based services rates can be redefined. Rather than seeking to relate the prevalence of bad judgment to high service intensity, or decrying health systems with low service intensity for rationing care, researchers might better assess whether the marginal returns of other forms of cardiovascular care are indeed smaller in areas where those services are utilized more frequently. The policy decision then becomes one of tradeoffs: given competing demands on scarce health care resources, at what point do the marginal returns of particular cardiac services become low enough that further investment in those services cannot be justified?

Evidence oriented clinicians must be positioned to contribute to these debates by marshalling comparative utilization data that help decision-makers make explicit determinations of the likely yields from funding different sets of cardiovascular and non-cardiovascular services. Arguably, they must also use these evaluative tools to safeguard their patients against inappropriate underuse of necessary services.

Again, explicit process-of-care criteria can be helpful. For example, analytical variations studies using American data have repeatedly shown that black and uninsured patients have lower coronary angiography rates than those who are insured.[44–46] Laouri et al.[47] drew on audit data from four teaching hospitals in Los Angeles and assembled a cohort of 352 patients who met explicitly defined criteria for the necessity of coronary angiography as established by an expert panel. The patients were tracked forward for 3 months and, after adjustment for confounding factors, those managed in the public hospital system had a 35% rate of angiography versus 57% for private hospital patients ($P<0.005$). The lesson, simply put, is that evidence must be sought for both inappropriate overuse and underuse of cardiovascular services in any and all health care systems.

ASSESSING OUTCOMES

A cardiovascular service may pass scrutiny under process-of-care criteria, and yet be provided in a substandard fashion that leads to needlessly poor outcomes. Outcomes of interest, after Kerr White, can be conveniently remembered as the six "D's": death, disease, dysfunction, disability, distress, and dissatisfaction.[48] Unfortunately, many outcomes studies are flawed by a failure to consider the full range of outcomes relevant to patients.[49]

It is salient to distinguish observational studies aimed at determining efficacy from those aimed at elucidating quality of care. For efficacy assessments, randomized trials are usually possible and always preferable, given the unavoidable biases of observational studies.[50] A poorly conducted non-randomized outcomes comparison for quality management purposes may at worst mislead patients and tarnish the reputation of a number of capable cardiologists or cardiac surgeons. A poorly conducted non-randomized outcomes comparison of two treatments may, if taken seriously, misguide clinical practice worldwide.

Understanding and appraising non-randomized outcomes studies

Here we review the questions to be asked when assessing studies that compare outcomes of care between providers or institutions.[51]

User's guide to appraising an observational outcomes study

- Are the outcome measures accurate and comprehensive?
- Were there clearly identified, sensible comparison groups?
- Were all important determinants of outcome measured accurately and reliably?
- Were the comparison groups similar with respect to important determinants, other than the one of interest?
- Was multivariate analysis used to adjust for imbalances in patient prognostic factors and other outcome determinants?
- Did additional analyses (particularly in low risk subgroups) demonstrate the same results as the primary analysis?

Adapted from Naylor and Guyatt.[51]

ACCURACY AND COMPREHENSIVENESS OF OUTCOME MEASURES

The easiest outcomes for health services researchers to measure are those that are defined objectively and usually captured in large insurance databases or computerized hospital administrative data, for example, death, those inhospital complications of surgery that are routinely coded, or readmissions to hospital. Linkage to vital status registries is also performed to track out-of-hospital deaths. However, these crude databases may either mismeasure patients' outcomes or fail to capture outcomes, such as functional status or quality of life, that are important to patients and their physicians.

SALIENT COMPARISONS

Clinicians and health care managers usually focus on interpractitioner and interinstitutional differences in technical quality of care, as reflected in patient outcomes. Analytical attention is also focussed frequently on potential volume–outcome relationships, either at the centre level, or for individual practitioners. For example, several studies[52–55] have shown volume–outcome relationships for angioplasty mortality and complications at the level of the hospital, interventional cardiologist, or both. However, the greater the difference between service settings being compared, the more difficult it is to be sure that patients were similar, or to isolate which aspects, if any, of the process of care relate to the outcomes observed. This is especially true when comparisons are made on a broad geographic footing between regions or countries in which populations and processes of care differ in many ways. In these latter comparisons, we are obviously veering away from the use of non-randomized outcomes data to benchmark technical quality of care for homogeneous procedures, and entering a more complex realm in which inferences must be drawn with caution.

For example, three studies[56–58] have shown that Canadian patients have more symptoms or worse functional status after AMI than do American patients. None showed any survival differences. The largest and most comprehensive study[57] found that rates of revascularization were much higher in the USA, that Canadians drew their post-MI care more often from family physicians and general internists, and that Americans relied more on cardiologists and received more cardiac rehabilitation services. Determining the causes of the observed differences in outcomes becomes difficult when so many factors vary simultaneously. For that matter, some of the findings may be attributable to cross-cultural differences in rating behavior on health status instruments. As always, use of non-randomized outcomes data for comparing performance of complex systems plunges the researcher into a thicket of causes, effects, and epiphenomena.

DETERMINING PROGNOSTIC CONFOUNDERS

In the absence of randomization, there is uncertainty about whether outcome differences are due to patients' prognostic characteristics or technical competence. For frequently studied procedures such as CABG, major studies have tended to show relative consistency in the types of prognostic clinical factors that must be taken into account for risk adjustment purposes.[59] Nonetheless, researchers and quality-of-care evaluators are unlikely to know all the prognostic factors that interact with various treatment strategies and conditions to alter outcomes.

MEASURING CONFOUNDERS

Even if key prognostic confounders are known and measured, they may not have been measured or recorded accurately. Inaccurate measurement or recording is a particular concern when information comes from administrative databases. For instance, Jollis *et al.*[60] compared information about cardiac risk factors in an administrative database in patients undergoing angiography with information collected prospectively for a clinical database. A chance-corrected measure of agreement (kappa statistic) showed moderate to poor agreement as follows: hypertension (56%), heart failure (39%), and unstable angina (9%). Hannan *et al.*[61] found similar discrepancies in comparing a cardiac surgery registry to an administrative database in New York State. These inaccuracies mattered: the ability of evaluators to predict mortality was clearly higher with the detailed clinical data as opposed to the administrative database. Thus, the accuracy, reproducibility, and fairness of adjustments for differences in patients can be undermined by poor data quality.

The problem of limited or inaccurate data in insurance databases or computerized hospital discharge abstracts may be partly ameliorated by supplementing the information with chart audits. A much more efficient approach may be to establish specific registry mechanisms geared to measuring key patient characteristics, process-of-care elements, and relevant outcomes.

ADJUSTING FOR CONFOUNDERS

It is common for researchers to use some form of multivariate analysis wherein they adjust for imbalances in prognostic factors between the comparison groups of interest. Validated prognostic indices or risk adjustment algorithms are available for most cardiovascular procedures that provide some guidance as to how these analyses should be undertaken. However, other strategies should routinely be used to check the robustness of any results. For example, the consistency of the findings should be confirmed after restricting the analysis to a relatively *low* risk subgroup of the patients being examined.[50] Eliminating patients in higher risk categories associated with more widely varying physiological states increases the likelihood of a "level playing field" for comparisons. Other methods to reduce the impact of confounding, such as use of "propensity scores" and "instrumental variables", are beyond the scope of this chapter.

Outcomes measurement for quality management

In sum, given the relatively weak inferences possible from most observational studies of outcomes, alternative strategies for ensuring the quality of medical care should always be considered. It will often be feasible and more efficient to use randomized trials or meta-analyses of trials to establish optimal management strategies, and then ensure that quality of care is maintained by monitoring the process of care to ensure that well-proven practices are consistently applied to eligible patients. On the other hand, for high volume and technically demanding procedures where reasonable risk adjustment methods can be brought into play, outcomes measurement has merit and should be done routinely.

CHANGING PRACTICE PATTERNS

General considerations

Practices clearly change over time in response to published evidence. At times, these changes can be rapid and dramatic, particularly when an innovation is associated with overwhelmingly positive risk–benefit ratios and is feasible for large numbers of practitioners to adopt. This model of knowledge-based practice change is termed *passive diffusion*. Its impact is heightened by the extent to which the mass media pick up major medical advances, and by the marketing initiatives of drugs and devices manufacturers. However, as implied by studies showing unexplained and undesirable variations in practice patterns, the model of passive diffusion leads to inconsistent uptake of evidence into practice.

How, then, can evidence be incorporated into practice more consistently? And what happens when data are in hand showing either that practice departs sharply from what available evidence suggests should be the norm, or when technical competence is below standard? How can the gap between "is" and "ought" in medical care be closed? These questions relate to changing physician (and system) performance, and follow logically from work done to measure or assess practice processes and outcomes.

Although there is limited randomized evidence on this topic for specific aspects of cardiovascular care, a wealth of experience – some unhappy – has shown that direct incentives and disincentives, financial and otherwise, can have a major impact on practice. Bonuses are paid in American managed care organizations if practitioners meet certain financial and clinical performance targets. Within the UK National Health Service, meeting targets for prespecified preventive services leads to extra payments for general practitioners. System-wide funding mechanisms and budgetary latitude are also important. Simply shifting the mode of physician payment may be an effective way of modifying behavior. For example, exponents of fee-for-service remuneration of cardiovascular medicine and surgery argue that salary and capitation schemes impose a risk of underservicing. Critics of fee-for-service argue that it undervalues quality and cognitive services, and creates a conflict of interest that promotes the use of procedures. As to non-financial incentives and disincentives, the range of options include merit awards, disciplinary proceedings, and litigation.

Arguably more relevant to the evidence oriented practitioner is the available information on non-administrative mechanisms to improve physician performance that key on voluntary knowledge- or information-based change. Such initiatives have the advantage of calling forward the better instincts of health professionals who, with few exceptions, seek first to serve patients as competently as possible.

Exponents of clinical guidelines initially believed that dissemination of guidelines might prove a key component in catalyzing knowledge-based improvements in physician performance.[62] Guidelines would usefully compile the totality of relevant evidence on several related aspects of a clinical condition, treatment, or procedure. The evidence oriented practitioner would no longer have to comb through the clinical literature, critically appraise it, and keep the relevant materials at hand or in her/his memory. The guideline would instead provide a convenient source of definitive evidence. Furthermore, because inference and expert judgment could be brought into play in developing guidelines, and because values and circumstances could also be considered when framing guidelines, clinicians would be able to rely on regionally developed guidelines to navigate the many "grey zones" of clinical practice[7] where evidence alone is insufficient. Last, guidelines could be developed, endorsed and disseminated by authorities with clinical credibility, lending weight to evidence that might otherwise appear rather impersonally in clinical journals.

Lomas[63] termed this latter approach the model of *active dissemination*, and criticized its prospects for success on the grounds that it ignored other factors in the practice environment, and presupposed that information acquisition alone leads to behavior change. The available evidence does suggest that there is some impact from more active approaches to informing and educating physicians about relevant clinical advances or guideline content.[64] However, the more passive the educational process, and the more removed it is from the physicians' own practice context, the less likely it appears to succeed.

Researchers and administrators have accordingly developed an array of non-coercive interventions designed to improve physician performance (see Box on page 126). In 1995 Davis *et al.*[65] and Oxman *et al.*[66] conducted systematic reviews of all the available controlled studies of the effects of these strategies on physicians' and other health professionals' performance. They included any strategy designed to persuade physicians "to modify their practice performance by communicating clinical information". Purely administrative interventions or financial and similar applied incentives and disincentives were excluded.

There were 99 studies involving physicians and a further three on other health professionals' behavior. Most of the studies on physician performance focus on internists or family physicians, and specific cardiovascular studies are limited in number to date. Single-intervention studies had positive effects on process or outcome parameters in 49/ 81 (60%) of trials where they were applied. Short educational seminars or conferences and dissemination of educational materials (printed or in audiovisual format) were least effective of all the single-intervention modalities explored. This finding supports proponents of implementation as opposed to dissemination.

125

Simple audit-and-feedback studies had limited impact. However, it is important to distinguish the types of studies that fall into this category. For example, in randomized studies from the early 1980s, investigators showed that a computer-based monitoring system with reminders and feedback led to significantly better follow-up and blood pressure control for patients with hypertension.[67,68] Two controlled studies by Pozen et al.[69,70] showed that a point-of-service strategy to facilitate implementation of a predictive algorithm for chest pain diagnosis reduced inappropriate utilization of coronary care units. These studies can best be regarded as "reminder" studies because there is continuous feedback at point of service. Audit-and-feedback studies that appear to be ineffective are those where data are collected and cumulated about processes or outcomes, and fed back only intermittently to practitioners without mechanisms to ensure local buy-in, to address local barriers to change, or to rectify specific gaps in clinical knowledge that may be associated with aberrant practice patterns.

Some methods used to alter physician performance/behavior

- **Education materials:** Distribution of published or printed recommendations, including practice guidelines and audiovisual materials or electronic publications
- **Conferences:** Participation of health care providers in conferences, lectures, workshops, or traineeships outside their practice settings
- **Outreach visits:** Use of a trained person who meets with providers in their practice settings to provide information. The information given may include feedback on the provider's performance
- **Local opinion leaders:** Use of providers explicitly nominated by their colleagues to be "educationally influential"
- **Patient-mediated interventions:** Any intervention aimed at changing the performance of health care providers for which information was sought from or given directly to patients by others (for example, direct mailings to patients, patient counselling delivered by others, or clinical information collected directly from patients and given to the provider)
- **Audit and feedback:** Any summary of clinical performance of health care over a specified period, with or without recommendations for clinical action. The information may have been obtained from medical records, computerized databases or patients or by observation
- **Reminders:** Any intervention (manual or computerized) that prompts the health care provider to perform a clinical action. Examples include concurrent or inter-visit reminders to professionals about desired actions such as screening or other preventive services, enhanced laboratory reports or administrative support (for example, follow-up appointment systems or stickers on charts)
- **Marketing:** Use of personal interviewing, group discussion (focus groups) or a survey of targeted providers to identify barriers to change and the subsequent design of an intervention
- **Local consensus processes:** Inclusion of participating providers in discussion to ensure agreement that the chosen clinical problem is important and the approach to managing it appropriate

Modified from Oxman et al.[66]

The latter distinction also highlights the fact that feedback can occur concurrently with service provision, or retrospectively, that is, after the service has been provided. Concurrent audit and feedback arguably is taken to its administrative conclusion in utilization management programs that refuse to authorize payment for a cardiovascular procedure unless the patient meets certain criteria, or in mandatory second opinion programs. These types of programs were not included in the reviews by Davis et al.[65] and Oxman et al.[66]

The methods that had the most consistent effects were: outreach visits including formal academic detailing and opinion-leader studies where an educationally influential physician was nominated by local peers to be the vector for the information; physician reminder systems at point of service; and patient-mediated methods, including reminders or educational materials. If two or more modalities were combined, then the effects were greater. That is, combining two effective methods (for example, academic detailing with support from a local opinion leader) had more impact than combining two less effective methods (for example, audit-and-feedback combined with a one-day seminar). Multifaceted interventions showed the strongest effects, with 31 of 39 (79%) positively affecting processes or outcomes of care.

Davis et al.[65] noted that most interventions appear to have a greater impact on process of care measures and other indices of physician performance, than on patient outcomes. They postulated that this may be because the clinical interventions themselves have limited impact (a rationale for the power argument given earlier), and also because patients do not always accept physician recommendations. They also suggest that a recurring weakness in interventions designed to improve processes and outcomes of care is a failure to conduct a needs analysis that addresses barriers to change.

These systematic reviews of practice-change interventions do not provide definitive evidence about which behavior change interventions are most effective and efficient in particular contexts or clinical conditions. This is because the studies cover a wide range of clinical condition and provider groups, rendering inferences across studies difficult. As in any meta-analysis, cross-study inferences involve non-randomized comparisons with all their potential pitfalls. Furthermore, factorial designs in behavior change studies have been more the exception than the rule, and it is therefore usually unclear as to which element(s) in a multifactorial strategy was (were) truly effective. Nonetheless, the evidence from controlled trials does suggest that practice changes are best achieved by combining credible evidence or information with active local strategies of implementation using multifactorial methods.

The case of outcomes report cards

As noted above, the interest in outcomes measurement to assure technical competence has led to state-wide initiatives whereby all cardiac surgery centers in New York and Pennsylvania, USA, are mandated to provide clinical data to permit compilation of publicly released mortality "report cards" on their CABG patients. These report cards provide a final case study that bridges some of the material presented above on outcomes assessment and behavior change.

In New York between 1989 and 1992, inhospital postoperative mortality of CABG showed an unadjusted relative decline of 21%.[71,72] Patients were apparently becoming sicker in the same period, so that the risk adjusted mortality decline was computed as 41%. Exponents of outcomes reporting claim that this improvement was catalyzed by a reporting system that provided relevant data to patients, administrators, and referring physicians.[71,72]

There can be no doubt that the New York and Pennsylvania report cards have pinpointed problems with a few operators who had very poor technical outcomes. The key question is how much of the overall improvement in mortality can be attributed to public outcomes reportage. Some critics contend that the trends are confounded by two factors. More assiduous coding of risk factors would artefactually increase the overall expected mortality, and surgeons could generate better mortality profiles by selectively turning down high risk patients, even though such patients may have most to gain from CABG. There has indeed been a striking increase in the prevalence of various reported risk factors in the New York database since its inception. For example, prevalence of congestive heart failure rose from 1.7% in 1989 to 7.6% in 1991; renal failure rose from 0.4% to 2.8%, chronic obstructive pulmonary disease (COPD) from 6.9% to 17.4% and unstable angina from 14.9% to 21.8% in the same period.[73] As well, a survey[74] of randomly selected cardiologists and cardiac surgeons in Pennsylvania found that about 60% of cardiologists reported greater difficulty in finding surgeons who would operate on high risk patients; a similar number of surgeons reported that they were less willing to operate on such patients. However, this type of survey is weak evidence for harm done by untoward case selection, and internal New York data do not support such a trend in that state.[75]

A more telling criticism is the fact that ecological correlations between falling mortality and initiation of reportage are tantamount to a case series in medicine. They provide weak and uncontrolled evidence for causation. In fact, the above-noted survey[74] of randomly selected cardiologists in Pennsylvania showed that most referring physicians did not view the Pennsylvania guide as an important source of information because of concerns about inadequate risk adjustment, unreliable data, and the absence of indicators of quality other than mortality. Other factors, such as New York State's insistence on minimum case volumes before certifying any cardiac surgery program, have doubtless played an important role. Moreover, in the absence of any report cards, the drop in post-CABG mortality in neighboring Massachusetts[76] has rivalled that seen in New York and Pennsylvania. Technical improvements in surgery, together with closer quality monitoring at the institutional level, appear to be the primary reason for these improved outcomes.

Given what has been learned about physician behavior change, the controversy about the New York State and Pennsylvania programs is hardly surprising. These externally mandated experiments in outcomes assessment contrast with initiatives that involve influential professionals and promote local buy-in from the outset. O'Connor discusses elsewhere in this volume the successful regional collaboration for continuous quality improvement that was developed in northern New England by involving cardiac surgeons in a systematic examination and improvement of processes and outcomes of care.[77–79] In Canada, a similar cooperative venture exists through the Cardiac Care Network of Ontario which draws together representatives of all major cardiovascular referral centers in the province.[80] Confidential report cards on mortality and length of stay are generated for the chief of cardiac surgery and CEO at each center, using risk adjustment algorithms coauthored by leaders of the Cardiac Care Network itself.[59] CABG outcomes in Ontario are comparable to those in New York and Pennsylvania. Moreover, as in Massachusetts, the trend to improved outcomes antedates the report card system.[80,81]

In sum, the unresolved issues with public outcomes report cards include validity and reliability of the data and the risk adjustment algorithms, as well as inadvertent side effects (for example, avoidance of high risk patients, and consumers' or referring physicians' focus on point estimates rather than statistically reliable ranges). Potential harm to the public from substandard technical competence must be weighed against needless patient anxieties and confusion, along with harm to skilled health workers and fine institutions caused by poorly founded and widely publicized inferences about inferior outcomes. Debate continues, but it is untenable to assume that all hospitals or providers are equally technically competent, and the public has an unequivocal right to receive reliable and current data on physician and hospital performance. Thus, the trend must inexorably be toward greater public reporting of both process and outcome indicators of quality of care. The challenges for evidence oriented practitioners are to ensure that the right indicators are chosen, that reliable data are analyzed appropriately, and that responsible reporting mechanisms are developed.

CONCLUSIONS

Assessing cardiovascular practices involves observational methods that can focus on either processes or outcomes of care. Methodologies for process-of-care assessments range from simple descriptive studies revealing variations in practice, to highly sophisticated case-specific audits using explicit criteria. Process-of-care assessments are more efficient than outcomes assessments in many respects, and lend themselves to measuring both over- and underuse of necessary cardiovascular services, thereby shedding light on quality and accessibility of care.

The primary role of observational outcomes measurement is in assessing provider or institutional quality of care for high volume and relatively homogenous procedures where technical skill is a factor. These comparisons must be made with caution, given the inevitable influence of unrecognized confounding through selection biases inherent in routine practice. The use of well-validated risk adjustment algorithms is imperative to improve the chances that differences in outcomes arise from the technical quality of care provided, rather than from differences in prognostic characteristics of patients themselves.

To reduce general inconsistencies in the uptake of evidence into practice, and to redress instances where processes or outcomes of clinical care are measured and found overtly wanting, several proven strategies are available. First, while new evidence published in journals or distilled into educational materials and practice guidelines does change practice through passive diffusion, evidence is most likely to have an impact if actively disseminated and made relevant and salient locally to practitioners. Strategies to achieve this end include reminder systems, concurrent audit and feedback, local outreach through academic detailing, patient-mediated interventions, local involvement of an educationally influential practitioner, and a local needs assessment with a consensus among providers on the issues as well as barriers and facilitators to positive change.

As a new millennium looms, the greatest limitation of evidence based cardiovascular medicine and surgery is less and less the evidence itself, and increasingly the inability of any practitioner to stay abreast of the field. Information systems in practice can and will be re-engineered to be more conducive to evidence based clinical decision-making. However, it will also remain important to assess practice patterns on a systematic basis, to share that information with patients and providers, and, wherever necessary, take steps to improve physician performance with a view to optimizing the quality, accessibility, and efficiency of cardiovascular care.

REFERENCES

1 Huston P, Naylor CD. Health services research: reporting on studies using secondary data sources. *Can Med Assoc J* 1996;**155**:1697–1702.

2 Dans PE. Looking for answers in all the wrong places. *Ann Intern Med* 1993;**119**:855–7.

3 Wennberg JE, Gittelsohn A. Small area variations

in health care delivery. *Science* 1973;**182**: 1102–9.

4 Wennberg JE, Gittelsohn A. Variation in medical care among small areas. *Sci Am* 1982;**246**: 120–35.

5 Wennberg JE, Barnes BA, Zubkoff M. Professional uncertainty and the problem of supplier-induced demand. *Soc Sci Med* 1982;**16**:811–24.

6 Wennberg JE. Which rate is right? *N Engl J Med* 1986;**314**:310–11.

7 Naylor CD. Grey zones of clinical practice: some limits to evidence based medicine. *Lancet* 1995; **345**:840–2.

8 Diehr P, Cain KC, Kreuter W, Rosenkranz S. Can small-area analysis detect variation in surgery rates? The power of small-area variation analysis. *Med Care* 1992;**30**:484–502.

9 Diehr P, Cain K, Connell F, Volinn E. What is too much variation? The null hypothesis in small-area analysis. *Health Services Res* 1990;**24**: 741–71.

10 Chen E, Naylor CD. Variation in hospital length of stay for acute myocardial infarction in Ontario, Canada. *Med Care* 1994;**32**:420–35.

11 Payne N, Saul C. Variations in use of cardiology services in a health authority: comparison of coronary artery revascularisation rates with prevalence of angina and coronary mortality. *Br Med J* 1997;**314**:257–61.

12 Ayanian JZ, Epstein AM. Differences in the use of procedures between women and men hospitalized for coronary heart disease. *N Engl J Med* 1991; **325**:221–5.

13 Petticrew M, McKee M, Jones J. Coronary artery surgery: are women discriminated against? *Br Med J* 1993;**306**:1164–6.

14 Jaglal SB, Gael V, Naylor CD. Sex differences in the use of invasive coronary procedures in Ontario. *Can J Cardiol* 1994;**10**:239–44.

15 The Health Services Research Group. Quality of care: 1. What is quality and how can it be measured? *Can Med Assoc J* 1992;**146**:2153–60.

16 The Health Services Research Group. Quality of care: 2. Quality of care studies and their consequences. *Can Med Assoc J* 1992;**147**:163–7.

17 Naylor CD, Guyatt GH. Users' guides to the medical literature: XI. How to use an article about a clinical utilization review. *JAMA* 1996;**275**: 1435–9.

18 Anon. Indications for fibrinolytic therapy in suspected acute myocardial infarction: collaborative overview of early mortality and major morbidity results from all randomised trials of more than 1000 patients. Fibrinolytic Therapy Trialists' (FTT) Collaborative Group. *Lancet* 1994; **343**:311–22.

19 Anon. Recommendations for ensuring early thrombolytic therapy for acute myocardial

infarction. The Heart and Stroke Foundation of Canada, the Canadian Cardiovascular Society and the Canadian Association of Emergency Physicians for the Emergency Cardiac Care Coalition. *Can Med Assoc J* 1996;**154**:483–7.

20 Rogers WJ, Bowlby LJ, Chandra NC *et al.* Treatment of myocardial infarction in the United States (1990 to 1993). Observations from the National Registry of Myocardial Infarction. *Circulation* 1994;**90**:2103–114.

21 Cox JL, Lee E, Langer A, Armstrong PW, Naylor CD, for the Canadian GUSTO Investigators. Time to treatment with thrombolytic therapy: determinants and effect on short-term nonfatal outcomes of acute myocardial infarction. *Can Med Assoc J* 1997;**156**:497–505.

22 Birkhead JS. Time delays in provision of thrombolytic treatment in six district hospitals. Joint Audit Committee of the British Cardiac Society and a Cardiology Committee of Royal College of Physicians of London. *Br Med J* 1992; **305**:445–8.

23 Anon. Epidemiology of avoidable delay in the care of patients with acute myocardial infarction in Italy. A GISSI-generated study. GISSI – Avoidable Delay Study Group. *Arch Intern Med* 1995;**155**: 1481–8.

24 Porter G, Doughty R, Gamble G, Sharpe N. Thrombolysis in AMI: reducing in hospital treatment delay. *NZ Med J* 1995;**108**:253–4.

25 Park RE, Fink A, Brook RH *et al.* Physician ratings of appropriate indications for six medical and surgical procedures. *Am J Publ Health* 1986;**76**: 766–72.

26 Brook RH, Chassin MR, Fink A *et al.* A method for the detailed assessment of the appropriateness of medical technologies. *Int J Tech Assess Health Care* 1986;**2**:53–64.

27 Park RE, Fink A, Brook RH *et al.* Physician ratings of appropriate indications for three procedures: theoretical indications vs indications used in practice. *Am J Public Health* 1989;**79**:445–7.

28 Hamm CW, Reimers J, Ischinger T *et al.* A randomized study of coronary angioplasty compared with bypass surgery in patients with symptomatic multivessel coronary disease. German Angioplasty Bypass Surgery Investigation (GABI). *N Engl J Med* 1994;**331**: 1037–43.

29 King SB, 3rd, Lembo NJ, Weintraub WS *et al.* A randomized trial comparing coronary angioplasty with coronary bypass surgery. Emory Angioplasty versus Surgery Trial (EAST). *N Engl J Med* 1994; **331**:1044–50.

30 Anon. Coronary angioplasty versus coronary artery bypass surgery: the Randomized Intervention Treatment of Angina (RITA) trial. *Lancet* 1993;**341**:573–80.

31 Rodriguez A, Boullon F, Perez-Balino N *et al.* Argentine randomized trial of percutaneous transluminal coronary angioplasty versus coronary artery bypass surgery in multivessel disease (ERACI): in-hospital results and 1-year follow-up. ERACI Group. *J Am Coll Cardiol* 1993; **22**:1060–7.

32 Brook RH, Kosecoff JB, Park RE *et al.* Diagnosis and treatment of coronary disease: comparison of doctor's attitudes in the USA and UK *Lancet* 1988;**i**:750–753.

33 Hilborne LH, Leape LL, Bernstein SJ *et al.* The appropriateness of use of percutaneous transluminal coronary angioplasty in New York state. *JAMA* 1993;**269**:761–5.

34 McGlynn EA, Naylor CD, Anderson GM *et al.* Comparison of the appropriateness of coronary angiography and coronary artery bypass graft surgery between Canada and New York State. *JAMA* 1994;**272**:934–40.

35 Bernstein SJ, Kosecoff JB, Gray D, Hampton JR, Brook RH. The appropriateness of the use of cardiovascular procedures. *Int J Tech Assess Health Care* 1993;**9**:3–10.

36 Chassin MR, Kosecoff JB, Park RE *et al.* Does inappropriate use explain geographic variations in the use of health care services? A study of three procedures. *JAMA* 1987;**258**:2533–7.

37 Leape LL, Park RE, Solomon DH *et al.* Does inappropriate use explain small-area variations in the use of health care services? *JAMA* 1990; **263**:669–72.

38 Wennberg JE. The paradox of appropriate care. *JAMA* 1987;**258**:2568–9.

39 Tu JV, Naylor CD, Kumar D *et al.* Coronary artery bypass graft surgery in Ontario and New York State: Which rate is right? *Ann Intern Med* 1997; **126**:13–19.

40 Naylor CD. A different view of queues in Ontario. *Health Aff (Millwood)* 1991;**10**:110–28.

41 Naylor CD, Sykora K, Jaglal SB, Jefferson S. Waiting for coronary artery bypass surgery: population-based study of 8517 consecutive patients in Ontario, Canada. The Steering Committee of the Adult Cardiac Care Network of Ontario. *Lancet* 1995;**346**:1605–9.

42 Hux JE, Naylor CD, and the Steering Committee of the Provincial Cardiac Care Network of Ontario. Are the marginal returns of coronary artery surgery smaller in high rate areas? *Lancet* 1996; **348**:1202–7.

43 Yusuf S, Zucker D, Peduzzi P *et al.* Effect of coronary artery bypass graft surgery on survival: overview of 10-year results from randomised trials by the Coronary Artery Bypass Graft Surgery Trialists Collaboration. *Lancet* 1994;**344**:563–70.

44 Goldberg KC, Hartz AJ, Jacobsen SJ, Krakauer H, Rimm AA. Racial and community factors influencing coronary artery bypass graft surgery rates for all 1986 Medicare patients. *JAMA* 1992; **267**:1473–7.

45 Hadley J, Steinberg EP, Feder J. Comparison of uninsured and privately insured hospital patients. Condition on admission, resource use, and outcome. *JAMA* 1991;**265**:374–9.

46 Hannan EL, Kilburn H, Jr, O'Donnell JF, Lukacik G, Shields EP. Interracial access to selected cardiac procedures for patients hospitalized with coronary artery disease in New York State. *Med Care* 1991; **29**:430–41.

47 Laouri M, Kravitz RL, Bernstein SJ *et al.* Underuse of coronary angiography: application of a clinical method. *Int J Qual Health Care* 1997;**9**:15–22.

48 White K. Improved health statistics and health services systems. *Pub Health Rep* 1967;**82**: 847–54.

49 Health Services Research Group. Outcomes and the management of health care. *Can Med Assoc J* 1992;**147**:1775–80.

50 Wen SW, Hernandez R, Naylor CD. Pitfalls in non-randomized outcomes studies: the case of incidental appendectomy with open cholecystectomy. *JAMA* 1995;**274**:1687–91.

51 Naylor CD, Guyatt GH, for the evidence Based Medicine Working Group. Users' guides to the medical literature: X. How to use an article reporting variations in the outcomes of health services. *JAMA* 1996;**275**:554–8.

52 Hannan EL, Racz M, Ryan TJ *et al.* Coronary angioplasty volume-outcome relationships for hospitals and cardiologists. *JAMA* 1997;**277**: 892–8.

53 Ritchie JL, Phillips KA, Luft HS. Coronary angioplasty. Statewide experience in California. *Circulation* 1993;**88**:2735–43.

54 Jollis JG, Peterson ED, DeLong ER *et al.* The relation between the volume of coronary angioplasty procedures at hospitals treating Medicare beneficiaries and short-term mortality. *N Engl J Med* 1994;**331**:1625–9.

55 Kimmel SE, Berlin JA, Laskey WK. The relationship between coronary angioplasty procedure volume and major complications. *JAMA* 1995;**274**:1137–42.

56 Rouleau JL, Moye LA, Pfeffer MA *et al.* A comparison of management patterns after acute myocardial infarction in Canada and the United States. *N Engl J Med* 1993;**328**:779–84.

57 Mark DB, Naylor CD, Hlatky MA *et al.* Use of medical resources and quality of life after acute myocardial infarction in Canada and the United States. *N Engl J Med* 1994;**331**:1130–5.

58 Pilote L, Racine N, Hlatky MA. Differences in the treatment of myocardial infarction in the United States and Canada. A comparison of two university hospitals. *Arch Intern Med* 1994;**154**: 1090–6.

59 Tu JV, Jaglal SB, Naylor CD. Multicenter validation of a risk index for mortality, intensive care unit stay, and overall hospital length of stay after cardiac surgery. Steering Committee of the Provincial Adult Cardiac Care Network of Ontario. *Circulation* 1995;**91**:677–84.

60 Jollis JG, Ancukiewicz M, DeLong ER *et al.* Discordance of databases designed for claims payment versus clinical information systems. Implications for outcomes research. *Ann Intern Med* 1993;**119**:844–50.

61 Hannan EL, Kilburn H, Jr, Lindsey ML, Lewis R. Clinical versus administrative databases for CABG surgery. Does it matter? *Med Care* 1992;**30**: 892–907.

62 The Health Services Research Group. Standards, guidelines and clinical policy. *Can Med Assoc J* 1992;**146**:833–7.

63 Lomas J. Retailing research: increasing the role of evidence in clinical services for childbirth. *Milbank Q* 1993;**71**:439–75.

64 Grimshaw JM, Russell IT. Effect of clinical guidelines on medical practice: a systematic review of rigorous evaluations. *Lancet* 1993;**342**: 1317–22.

65 Davis DA, Thomson MA, Oxman AD, Haynes RB. Changing physician performance. A systematic review of the effect of continuing medical education strategies. *JAMA* 1995;**274**:700–5.

66 Oxman AD, Thomson MA, Davis DA, Haynes RB. No magic bullets: a systematic review of 102 trials of interventions to improve professional practice. *Can Med Assoc J* 1995;**153**:1423–31.

67 Barnett GO, Winickoff RN, Morgan MM, Zielstorff RD. A computer-based monitoring system for follow-up of elevated blood pressure. *Med Care* 1983;**21**:400–9.

68 Dickinson JC, Warshaw GA, Gehlbach SH *et al.* Improving hypertension control: impact of computer feedback and physician education. *Med Care* 1981;**19**:843–54.

69 Pozen MW, D'Agostino RB, Selker HP, Sytkowski PA, Hood WB Jr. A predictive instrument to improve coronary-care-unit admission practices in acute ischemic heart disease. A prospective multicenter clinical trial. *N Engl J Med* 1984;**310**: 1273–8.

70 Pozen MW, D'Agostino RB, Mitchell JB *et al.* The usefulness of a predictive instrument to reduce inappropriate admissions to the coronary care unit. *Ann Intern Med* 1980;**92**:238–42.

71 Hannan EL, Kilburn H Jr, Racz M, Shields E, Chassin MR. Improving the outcomes of coronary artery bypass surgery in New York State. *JAMA* 1994;**271**:761–6.

72 Hannan EL, Siu AL, Kumar D, Kilburn H Jr, Chassin MR. The decline in coronary artery bypass graft surgery mortality in New York State. *JAMA* 1995;**272**:209–13.

73 Green J, Wintfeld N. Report cards on cardiac surgeons. Assessing New York State's approach. *N Engl J Med* 1995;**332**:1229–32.

74 Schneider EC, Epstein AM. Influence of cardiac-surgery performance reports on referral practices and access to care. A survey of cardiovascular specialists. *N Engl J Med* 1996;**335**:251–6.

75 Hannan EL, Siu AL, Kumar D, Racz M, Pryor DB *et al.* Assessment of coronary artery bypass graft surgery performance in New York. Is there a bias against taking high risk patients? *Med Care* 1997; **35**:49–56.

76 Ghali WA, Ash AS, Hall RE, Moskowitz MA. Statewide quality improvement initiatives and mortality after cardiac surgery. *JAMA* 1997;**277**: 379–82.

77 O'Connor GT, Plume SK, Olmstead EM *et al.* A regional intervention to improve the hospital mortality associated with coronary artery bypass graft surgery. The Northern New England Cardiovascular Disease Study Group. *JAMA* 1996; **275**:841–6.

78 O'Connor GT, Plume SK, Olmstead EM *et al.* A regional prospective study of in-hospital mortality associated with coronary artery bypass grafting. The Northern New England Cardiovascular Disease Study Group. *JAMA* 1991;**266**:803–9.

79 Malenka DJ, O'Connor GT. A regional collaborative effort for CQI in cardiovascular disease. Northern New England Cardiovascular Study Group. *Jt Comm J Qual Improv* 1995;**21**: 627–33.

80 Tu JV, Naylor CD, and the Steering Committee of the Cardiac Care Network of Ontario. Coronary bypass mortality rates in Ontario: a Canadian approach to quality assurance in cardiac surgery. *Circulation* 1996;**94**:2429–33.

81 Ivanov J, Weisel RD, David TE, Naylor CD. Fifteen-year trends in risk severity and operative mortality in elderly patients undergoing coronary bypass surgery. *Circulation* 1997 (in press).

Learning from clinical practice 9

GERALD T. O'CONNOR,
DAVID J. MALENKA

INTRODUCTION

Learning from daily practice and using the lessons learned to continually improve the outcomes of health care is a goal shared by society, payers, and clinicians. It is essential for the public good that practitioners of medicine and surgery assume responsibility for improving the quality of clinical care. They have unique knowledge of clinical reasoning and processes, are most appropriate to render opinion on the adequacy of clinical care, and have traditionally assumed the role of patient advocates. The outcomes movement is based on creating the ability to learn from actual practice, believing that this knowledge will be most relevant to both practitioners and to patients.[1]

The task of capturing the lessons learned and using them to improve clinical care is daunting. It is hampered by factors which include: a lack of useful information on current and past outcomes; the insular nature of much of clinical practice; the rarity of adverse clinical events in the experience of individual practitioners; and lack of efficient methods to bring about change. Both office practices and hospitals are awash in data, yet these data often provide little useful information to guide improvement. While there are highly developed systems for billing and purchasing, there may not be clinical data systems available to guide change. Further, in the experience of an individual practitioner, even one with many years in practice, it may be difficult to recall the specific circumstances of the few cases of adverse events. The average cardiothoracic surgeon in northern New England does 140 cases of coronary artery bypass graft (CABG) surgery in a year and there are approximately four deaths. Different patient and disease characteristics and modes of death make it very difficult to reach robust conclusions and devise methods to improve care from this small number of events. Further, in our experience, much of clinical practice is quite insular, with little opportunity to critically compare clinical practices and the organization of clinical care with that practiced by colleagues. Lastly, much of cardiovascular care is provided in complex organizations with multiple professions and medical specialties and it is often difficult to create either a consensus for change or a series of processes to affect changes in clinical care.

The purpose of this chapter is to discuss methods for learning from the daily practice of clinical medicine and to present some examples of techniques that are currently in use for collecting, interpreting, and using clinical information to improve the outcomes of clinical care. Many of these examples will come from work that we have done with a regional research collaborative in northern New England, but we believe that these methods will also be useful in other settings.[2]

DATA COLLECTION IN CLINICAL PRACTICE

Thoughtful practice is made substantially more difficult without accurate data. Memory has been shown to be a poor substitute for data because of our tendency to remember selectively.[3] Adverse outcomes and specific clinical situations may provide clues for improvement or may only provide anecdotes. Systematic collection of data may be the difference between the two. Data from our actual practices also allow us to examine our beliefs about the relative efficacy of alternative treatments. Such data can help to inform clinical decision making, using past experience to improve current decisions. Variation in the practice of medicine is, at least in part, a consequence of uncertainty about outcomes.[4] There is uncertainty because: physicians may not remember the information correctly; the necessary information may not be available or may not be generalizable to the patient under care.

Three rules of data collection may seem obvious yet are often violated: keep it simple, get it right and have a basis for comparison. Data collection which occurs in daily clinical practice must not be overly burdensome or it will not occur. Data which are not valid will not provide a sound basis for the examination of outcomes and will not reliably lead to change in clinical practices. Results of data collection cannot be interpreted without reference to results obtained from other practices or other time periods in our own practice.

Keep it simple

The infinite variety of clinical practice and the large number of questions that we may wish to pose often result in a proliferation of possible data elements. Since 1987, the Northern New England Cardiovascular Disease Study Group has been collecting data on cardiac surgery outcomes. During these years we have collected data on approximately 30 000 consecutive CABG and valve operations and 35 000 PTCA procedures. The data collection forms are one page, one side. The CABG data form, as well as those developed by other groups, may be down loaded from the Internet site of the Society of Thoracic Surgeons (http://www.sts.org/). The discipline required by a one page form has necessitated careful scrutiny of each data element. The routine collection of 20–40 data elements has not been a significant burden. There is no issue that so threatens data collection as does the multiple page data collection form. It often results in calls for additional personnel or for automatic computerized data collection methods. Lack of resources then may halt the data collection effort. In our experience simple "paper and pencil" forms have been both inexpensive and flexible. Sometimes even pocket cards can provide a useful method for data collection.[5]

So where do you start? Start by establishing the most important outcomes for your practice. Often this means collecting data on your most commonly cared for condition or most frequently performed procedure. Unless there is a compelling reason to do so, it is probably not useful to attempt data collection on everything that you do. Capturing data on the dominant activities is often more useful than that collected on rarely performed procedures or rarely seen conditions. The data collection should benefit your practice; be sure that it captures those processes and events that you would like to monitor on a regular basis to be sure that care is being conducted in the manner that you wish.

As to what data you should collect, the rule is to collect what others have used and found to be important, and what you need to answer questions that are important to you and your practice. Allow yourself some flexibility to include a few data elements that are items of your curiosity. Learn from the work of others. In each specialty there is often a national consensus on the patient and disease characteristics most relevant to a particular condition.[6,7] These can be very useful in suggesting data elements and definitions.

It may be that it is more convenient for you to participate in a national data collection effort, such as that conducted by the Society of Thoracic Surgeons[8] or the American College of Cardiology.[9] These services provide professionally designed data forms, data entering, report generation, and a basis for comparison with other practitioners. The disadvantage is that data are reported only annually and that the process is somewhat driven by the interests of others. However, some customization, to reflect local interests, is possible with most major data services.

When possible, develop your data collection tool to have multiple purposes. Data collection forms may also provide the basis for letters to referring physicians or for discharge summaries.

Get it right

The inference achieved will never exceed the quality of the data. Incomplete or inaccurate data fields are very commonly encountered in virtually all clinical settings and they may render the entire effort useless. They occur because of lack of discipline, unavailability of the data element or because of flaws in the design of the data collection plan. The incorporation of routine data collection into the daily work requires both leadership and discipline. In our experience, the most commonly cited reasons for incomplete data forms are lack of time to complete the form or unavailability of the required information. For example, the cardiac surgery patient is transferred from another hospital with a cineangiogram film but without a formal catheterization report. The film is reviewed by the cardiologist and the surgeon but no record is made of the left ventricular ejection fraction. This is not fundamentally a time issue and the lack of information makes the outcome of this patient difficult to evaluate. Leadership and discipline are required to achieve accurate data collection.

Missing data and data elements forms occur for a number of reasons. The forms are misplaced or the patient arrives late at night, or in an emergency situation the available time is appropriately used to provide needed care rather than to complete a data form. In these situations we have found the routine comparison of our clinical data forms to the administrative records invaluable. Where hospitals and clinical practices send out requests for payment, these provide an easily accessible method to identify patients with missing data forms. These few forms can then be completed retrospectively. Data elements may also be unavailable because we are attempting to collect data elements which are not a part of routine clinical care. For example, if carotid ultrasound examinations of CABG patients are rarely done in your practice or your institution they will not provide very useful data. Either decide that they are important and order them, or do not attempt what will certainly be uninformative data collection efforts.

Most often the data forms must be entered into a computer file for statistical analysis. While occasional data entry may not be burdensome, large scale data entry is most efficiently done by professionals. If you collect large numbers of data forms, have them professionally keypunched. It is more accurate and less expensive than doing it yourself. We also suggest that you avoid text fields on data forms. These are data fields in which a written reply is required (e.g. diagnosis [specify]:————). Handwriting is often difficult to read and each text field must be examined by someone and interpreted and coded later. It is almost always better and more efficient to specify the responses that interest you on the data collection form. Lastly, the information in each data field is only as good as the definition that describes the field. If you are designing your own data collection form be sure that you know the definitions that have been used by others and be sure that you print the definition that you wish to use on the data form itself.

Provide a basis for comparison

Keep in mind that the data that you collect is to guide action. Too often databases are collected and never used to influence subsequent clinical practice. Interpretation of the data that you collect will often involve comparison with data collected by others. This may involve comparison to the national or regional databases or comparison to your past performance. Tracking clinic outcomes over time may often make good use of control charts as are used regularly by industry.[10]

Data collection in clinical settings
- Keep it simple
  Collect only those risk and outcome variables that are essential.
  Use a one page data form with printed definitions.
  Avoid text fields on data forms.
- Get it right
  Discipline and leadership will obtain complete data.
  Validate completeness using administrative data.
- Provide a basis for comparison
  Use regional or national comparison groups.
  Track time-related changes in processes or outcomes.

USES OF DATA IN CLINICAL PRACTICE

Accurate data are of fundamental importance to clinical practice. These data can answer simple but important questions. The patient asks: "What are my chances?" The physician asks: "How am I doing?" The health care system asks: "How can we improve?" Each of these topics – informing patients, monitoring clinical performance, and continuously adding value to health care – is current, important and data-dependent. Much of what we know about treatment effectiveness comes from clinical trials but most of what we know about actual clinical care is learned from observational studies. Much of the controversy that swirls around quality monitoring has to do with its methodology. Assessing the outcomes of clinical care is substantially difficult and must rely on the methods of observational epidemiology.

The primary threats to the validity of observational studies are chance, bias, and confounding.[11] Each plays a potentially important role in measuring the outcomes of clinical care. Chance is random variability and it may play an important role in the assessment of rare adverse outcomes. During a year an interventional cardiologist may perform 100 percutaneous transluminal coronary angioplasties (PTCA) and two patients will die. This observed 2% mortality rate has 95% confidence intervals from 0 to 7.0%. One solution to sparse data is to aggregate results over a longer time period, yet this may obscure important time-related effects. The use of control charts, which allow us to differentiate between sampling-related variability and actual process change, may advantage quality monitoring activities. Bias is systematic error in the data. Discipline and the enthusiastic participation of clinicians will be required to yield accurate data. Confounding is a distortion of the observed mortality rates brought about by differences in patient case mix. This is perhaps the most debated aspect of assessing the outcomes of clinical care. Although most debated, it may not deserve as much attention as the complex system of causation that produces a clinical outcome. Although chance, bias, and confounding are substantial issues, assessing the outcomes of commonly performed procedures like CABG surgery and PTCA rests largely on professional consensus and secure science.[6,7]

Informing patients

Patients request and deserve accurate information about the risks and benefits of invasive procedures. Yet, accurate estimation of their risk is a difficult task.[12] Its difficulty arises from the multiple factors which must be considered, weighted, and combined. The patient asks: "What are my chances?" The physician most accurately responds by using outcome data derived from other patients' characteristics similar to those of the current patient. Often these queries are answered qualitatively, e.g. "low risk", but if relevant outcome data are available then clinical prediction equations provide a simple, accurate method for obtaining a quantitative estimate of risk. Prediction rules are derived from multivariate analyses of the data which results in a risk equation which can be solved on a microcomputer or programmable calculator. They are based on sound science, and standards for their development and validation have been developed.[13,14] The prediction equation shown in Figure 9.1 estimates the risk of fatal and of non-fatal outcomes associated with PTCA. There are two regression models, one for each dependent variable. The coefficients of these equations are obtained from a large reference database and the patient and disease characteristics of the current patient are used to solve the equations yielding the conditional probability of a fatal or non-fatal adverse outcome. Prediction equations do not tell the physician or the patient what to do. They accurately summarize data from large numbers of patients in a manner that would be otherwise impossible and the product of that calculation provides an important piece of information for the consideration of physician and patient. A number of prediction equations have been developed for use in cardiovascular disease management; we have cited a few references as an introduction to this literature.[13,15–18]

Prediction of risk of fatal and non-fatal adverse outcome

Variables	adj. OR	P value	Coefficients
Fatal outcomes			
Age (per year)	1.07	<0.001	0.0712
Gender (1 = female, 0 = male)	1.72	0.011	0.5431
Previous MI (1 = yes, 0 = no)	1.90	0.004	0.6405
Cardiogenic shock (1 = yes, 0 = no)	9.33	<0.001	2.2337
Emergent priority (1 = yes, 0 = no)	6.22	<0.001	1.8284
Preop IABP (1 = yes, 0 = no)	7.78	<0.001	2.0522
Preop IV nitroglycerin (1 = yes, 0 = no)	2.01	0.002	0.6996
Preop salicylates (1 = yes, 0 = no)	0.50	0.001	−0.6941
LVEDP (per mmHg)	1.05	0.007	0.0456
Number of diseased vessels (>70% stenosis)	1.97	<0.001	0.6788
Proximal LAD (1 = yes, 0 = no)	1.87	0.008	0.6303
Intercept			−12.3268
Non-fatal outcomes			
Urgent priority (1 = yes, 0 = no)	1.50	0.001	0.4028
Emergent priority (1 = yes, 0 = no)	3.92	<0.001	1.3671
Preop IV nitroglycerin (1 = yes, 0 = no)	1.48	0.001	0.3928
Number of diseased vessels (>70% stenosis)	1.21	0.005	0.1887
LAD (1 = yes, 0 = no)	1.27	0.015	0.2382
Lesion type B (1 = yes, 0 = no)	2.48	<0.001	0.9088
Lesion type C (1 = yes, 0 = no)	3.04	<0.001	1.1109
Intercept			−4.7092

Fatal outcomes: model χ^2(11df)=405.1, P<0.0001; non-fatal outcomes: model χ^2(7df)=224.1, P<0.0001

Calculation of predicted risk using patient data and the logistic regression coefficients
Calculate the ODDS using the patient's values and the coefficients:

Fatal outcomes: ODDS=EXP(−12.3268 + [0.0712 × Age] + [0.5431 × Gender] + [0.6405 × Prev. MI] + [2.2337 × Card. Shock] + [1.8284 × Emergent] + [2.0522 × IABP] + [0.6996 × IV NTG] − [0.6941 × Salicylates] + [0.0456 × LVEDP] + [0.6788 × No. Dis. Vessels] + [0.6303 × Prox. LAD]

Non-fatal outcomes: ODDS=EXP(−4.7092 + [0.4028 × Urgent] + [1.3671 × Emergent] + [0.3928 × IVNTG] + [0.1887 × No. Dis. Vessels] + [0.2382 × LAD] + [0.9088 × Lesion type B] + [1.1109 × Lesion type C]

Use the ODDS to calculate the PREDICTED PROBABILITY: Predicted probability=ODDS/(1+ODDS)

Figure 9.1 Clinical prediction rule: fatal and non-fatal adverse outcomes associated with PTCA. MI, myocardial infarction; IABP, intra aortic balloon pump; LVEDP, left ventricular end-diastolic pressure; LAD, left anterior descending artery. Reproduced with permission from O'Connor GT, Malenka DJ, Levy DG, Disch DL, Quinton HB for the Northern New England Cardiovascular Disease Study Group. Multivariate prediction of adverse outcomes associated with percutaneous transluminal coronary angioplasty. *Circulation* 1993;**88**:1–300.

Monitoring clinical performance

The ability to use patient and disease data to calculate the conditional probability of an adverse event also allows the monitoring of clinical performance. If the prediction equation was calculated for all patients of a particular clinician or an institution, the sum of the conditional probabilities would yield the number of adverse outcomes that would be expected. For a decade we have been developing and using prediction equations as part of our regional cardiovascular collaborative in northern New England.[2,19] Reports are sent to all clinicians and to all institutions and discussed at regional meetings held three times per year. Part of a CABG outcomes report is shown in Figure 9.2. Each of these run charts shows both the observed and the expected rates of these adverse clinical outcomes by quarter. This is a regional report but similar reports are generated for each medical center and each surgeon. These reports are quite sophisticated in their science but are simple to interpret and allow the indentification of time-related trends. This use of prediction equations has been a topic of concern and debate in health care.[20,21]

The reports of adverse clinical outcomes are important to medical centers and to physicians but they are substantially incomplete as measures of the effectiveness of health care. A more comprehensive view is provided by an instrument panel which assesses multiple aspects of health care outcomes.[22] Shown in Figure 9.3 is an instrument panel describing the outcomes of isolated CABG surgery in a single institution. Four dimensions of care are shown (clinical outcomes, functional outcomes, patient satisfaction, and cost and utilization data). In addition, there is a summarization of patient case mix and selected clinical process variables during this quarter and during the past 2 years. This method is not yet implemented widely but is likely to become the method of choice for evaluating the outcomes of clinical care.

Continuously adding value to health care

Patients and physicians are well served by efforts to improve the outcomes and decrease the cost of clinical care. Improving processes of care requires data and organization and the use of techniques borrowed from industry.[23]

Between 1987 and 1989, members of the Northern New England Cardiovascular Disease Study Group collected risk and outcomes data on 3055 consecutive CABG procedures. The regional hospital mortality rate was 4.3%. The rate varied among centers (range: 3.1–6.3%) and among surgeons (range: 1.9–9.2%). A number of statistically significant predictors of mortality were identified (e.g. age, female gender, small body surface area, greater comorbidity, reoperation, poorer preoperative cardiac function, and emergent or urgent surgery). After adjusting for the effects of potentially confounding variables, substantial and statistically significant variability was observed among medical centers ($P=0.021$) and among surgeons ($P=0.025$).[15] The group concluded that the observed differences in inhospital mortality rates among institutions and among surgeons were not solely the result of differences in case mix as described by these variables and likely reflected differences in unknown aspects of patient care. This observed variability in outcomes provided the rationale to closely examine the processes of cardiac surgery and to attempt to learn from each other. This knowledge of variability and the comfort that grew during the early years of the consortium led the group to organize a regional effort to improve the clinical outcomes of cardiac surgery. We planned a three-part intervention consisting of: feedback of outcome data, training in continuous quality improvement techniques, and benchmarking site visits to other medical centers.[24] Monitoring of mortality rates continued and there were 74 fewer deaths during the 27-month postintervention period (24% reduction) than would have been expected based on historical data from this region. This reduction in mortality rate was temporally associated with the interventions, was similar across patient risk groups, and was not substantially influenced by surgeon migration. These improved outcomes were not significantly different for men and women or for elective and non-elective patients. A full report of the interventions and the outcomes has been published.[25]

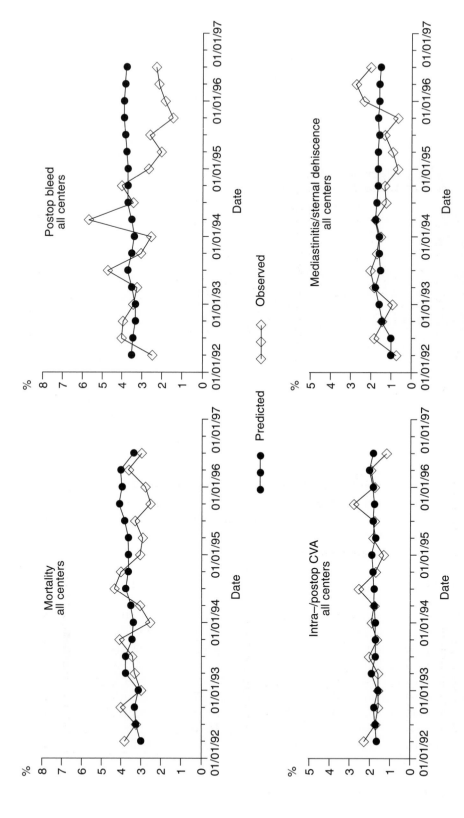

Figure 9.2 Reports of CABG clinical outcomes. Plots based on 12 988 consecutive isolated CABGs, 1 April 1992 and 30 September 1996.

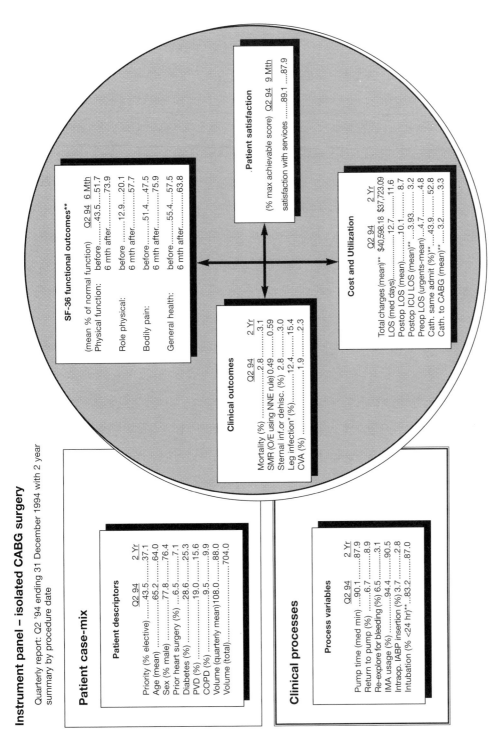

Instrument panel – isolated CABG surgery

Quarterly report: Q2 '94 ending 31 December 1994 with 2 year summary by procedure date

Patient case-mix

Patient descriptors

	Q2 94	2 Yr
Priority (% elective)	43.5	37.1
Age (mean)	65.2	64.0
Sex (% male)	77.8	76.4
Prior heart surgery (%)	6.5	7.1
Diabetes (%)	28.6	25.3
PVD (%)	19.0	15.6
COPD (%)	9.5	9.9
Volume (quarterly mean)	108.0	88.0
Volume (total)		704.0

Clinical processes

Process variables

	Q2 94	2 Yr
Pump time (med min)	90.1	87.9
Return to pump (%)	6.7	8.9
Re-explore for bleeding (%)	6.5	3.1
IMA usage (%)	94.4	90.5
Intraop. IABP insertion (%)	3.7	2.8
Intubation (% <24 hr)**	83.2	87.0

SF-36 functional outcomes**

(mean % of normal function)	Q2 94	6 Mth
Physical function:	before	43.5	51.7
	6 mth after		73.9
Role physical:	before	12.9	20.1
	6 mth after		57.7
Bodily pain:	before	51.4	47.5
	6 mth after		75.9
General health:	before	55.4	57.5
	6 mth after		63.8

Patient satisfaction

	Q2 94	9 Mth
(% max achievable score)		
satisfaction with services	89.1	87.9

Clinical outcomes

	Q2 94	2 Yr
Mortality (%)	2.8	3.1
SMR (O/E using NNE rule)	0.49	0.59
Sternal inf.or dehisc. (%)	2.8	3.0
Leg infection* (%)	12.4	15.4
CVA (%)	1.9	2.3

Cost and Utilization

	Q2 94	2 Yr
Total charges (mean)**	$40,598.18	$37,723.09
LOS (med days)	12.7	11.6
Postop LOS (mean)	10.1	8.7
Postop ICU LOS (mean)**	3.93	3.2
Preop LOS (urgents-mean)	4.7	4.8
Cath. same admit (%)**	43.9	52.8
Cath. to CABG (mean)**	3.2	3.3

Figure 9.3 CABG surgery value compass. * 21 months of data; ** 9 months of data. COPD, chronic obstructive pulmonary disease; IMA, internal mammary artery; IABP, intra-aortic balloon pump; LOS, low output syndrome.

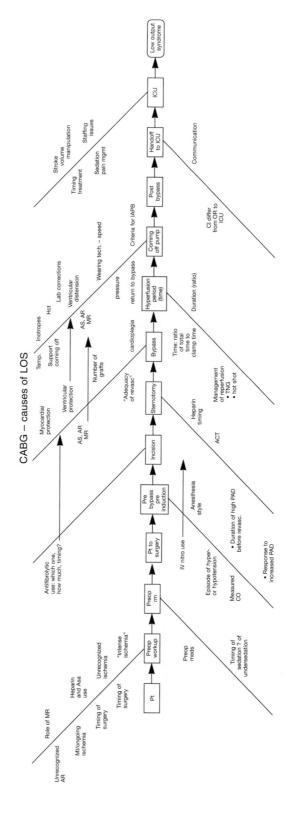

Figure 9.4 Process flow diagram for low cardiac output syndrome. From Camp RC (Ed). *Global Cases in Benchmarking: Best Practices from Organizations Around the World.* Milwaukee: ASQ Quality Press, 1998.

142

More recent quality improvement work has been focused on the low cardiac output syndrome. Multidisciplinary and specialty teams are attempting to understand the processes of cardiac surgery as they may relate to low cardiac output. This work makes use of process flow diagrams as a method of representing the temporal and causal relationships between process and outcome (Figure 9.4). This process has been very useful especially when combined with process improvement cycles.[26,27]

CONCLUSION

The efficient collection of reliable data and the use of these data to inform clinical decision making, to monitor processes and outcomes of clinical care, and to support the continual improvement of clinical care is an important idea in health care and is likely to become more important because of financial pressures. This approach holds great potential to save lives, improve functional health status, and increase the efficiency of clinical care.

The uses of data to learn from clinical practice

- Using data to inform clinical decisions
  Use of clinical prediction rules
- Monitoring clinical performance
  Risk adjusted run charts of clinical outcomes
  Value compass techniques for a comprehensive view of outcomes
- Adding value to health care
  Regional or national comparison groups
  Time-related changes in processes or outcomes

REFERENCES

1 Wennberg JE. What is outcomes research? In: Gelijns AC, ed. *Medical innovation at the crossroads: Modern methods of clinical investigation*, Vol. 1. Washington, DC: National Academy Press, 1990, pp 33–46.

2 O'Connor GT, Plume SK. Wenneberg JE. Regional organization for outcomes research. *Ann NY Acad Sci* 1993;**703**:44–51.

3 Taversky A, Kahnemann D. Judgement under uncertainty: heuristics and biases. 34. *Science* 1974;**185**:1124–31.

4 Wennberg JE, Freeman JL, Shelton RM, Bubolz TA. Hospital use and mortality among Medicare beneficiaries in Boston and New Haven. *N Engl J Med* 1989;**321**:1168–73.

5 Wasson JH, O'Connor GT, James DH, Olmstead EM, Group NNECDS, COOP DPC. A physician-completed patient registry system: pilot results for unstable angina in the elderly. *J Gen Intern Med* 1992;**7**:298–303.

6 Jones RH, Hannan EL, Hammermeister KE *et al.* Identification of preoperative variables needed for risk adjustment of short-term mortality after coronary artery bypass graft surgery. *J Am Coll Cardiol* 1996;**28**:1478–87.

7 Block PC, Peterson EC, Krone R *et al.* Identification of variables needed to risk adjust outcomes in coronary interventions: evidence-based guidelines for efficient data collection. *J Am Coll Cardiol.* In press.

8 Clark RE. The Society of Thoracic Surgeons National Database status report. *Ann Thorac Surg* 1994;**57**:20–6.

9 Weintraub WS, McKay CR, Riner R *et al.* The American College of Cardiology National Database: progress and challenges. *J Am Coll Cardiol* 1997;**29**:459–65.

10 Wheeler DJ, Chambers DS. *Understanding statistical process control*, 2nd edn. Knoxville, TN: SPC Press, Inc., 1992.

11 Hennekens CH, Buring JE. *Epidemiology in medicine*. Boston, MA: Little Brown & Co., 1988.

12 O'Connor GT, Plume SK, Beck JR *et al.* What are my chances? It depends on whom you ask. The

choice of a prosthetic heart valve. *Med Decis Making* 1988; 8.

13 Harrell FE, Jr, Lee KL, Mark DB. Multivariable prognostic models: issues in developing models, evaluating assumptions and adequacy, and measuring and reducing errors. *Stat Med* 1996; **15**:361–87.

14 Wasson J, Sox H, Neff R, Goldman L. Clinical prediction rules: applications and methodological standards. *N Engl J Med* 1985;**313**:793–9.

15 O'Connor GT, Plume SK, Olmstead EM *et al*. Multivariate prediction of inhospital mortality associated with coronary artery bypass graft surgery. *Circulation* 1992;**85**:2110–18.

16 Hannan EL, Kilburn H, O'Donnell JF, Lukacik G, Shields EP. Adult open heart surgery in New York State: an analysis of risk factors and hospital mortality rates. *JAMA* 1990;**264**:2768–74.

17 Pryor DB, Shaw L, Harrell FE, Jr *et al*. Estimating the likelihood of severe coronary artery disease. *Am J Med* 1991;**90**:553–62.

18 Ricotta JJ, Faggioli GL, Castilone A, Hassett JM. Risk factors for stroke after cardiac surgery: Buffalo Cardiac-Cerebral Study Group. *J Vasc Surg* 1995;**21**:359–63 (discussion 364).

19 Malenka DJ, O'Connor GT, Group NNECDS. A regional collaborative effort for continuous quality improvement. The Northern New England Cardiovascular Disease Study Group. *Jt Comm J Qual Improv* 1995;**21**:627–33.

20 Topol EJ, Califf RM. Scorecard cardiovascular medicine: its impact and future directions. *Ann Intern Med* 1994;**120**:65–70.

21 Berwick DM, Wald DL. Hospital leaders' opinions of the HCFA mortality data. *JAMA* 1990;**263**:247–9.

22 Nelson EC, Batalden PB. Patient-based quality measurement systems. *Qual Management Hlth Care* 1993;**2**:18–30.

23 Berwick DM. Continuous improvement as an ideal in health care [see Comments]. *N Engl J Med* 1989;**320**:53–6.

24 Kasper JF, Plume SK, O'Connor GT. A methodology for QI in the coronary artery bypass grafting procedure involving comparative process analysis. *Qual Rev Bull* 1992;**18**:129–33.

25 O'Connor GT, Plume SK, Olmstead EM *et al*. A regional intervention to improve the hospital mortality associated with coronary artery bypass graft surgery. The Northern New England Cardiovascular Disease Study Group [see Comments]. *JAMA* 1996;**275**:841–6.

26 Batalden PB, Nelson EC, Roberts JS. Linking outcomes measurement to continual improvement: the serial "V" way of thinking about improving clinical care. *Jt Comm J Qual Improv* 1994;**20**:167–80.

27 Nelson EC, Wasson, MD John H. Using patient-based information to rapidly redesign care. *Hlth Care Forum J* 1994;**37**:25–9.

Part II
Prevention of cardiovascular diseases

SALIM YUSUF, Editor

Grading of recommendations and levels of evidence used in *Evidence Based Cardiology*

GRADE A

Level 1a   Evidence from large randomized clinical trials (RCTs) or systematic reviews (including meta-analyses) of multiple randomized trials which collectively has at least as much data as one single well-defined trial.

Level 1b   Evidence from at least one "All or None" high quality cohort study; in which ALL patients died/failed with conventional therapy and some survived/succeeded with the new therapy (eg chemotherapy for tuberculosis, meningitis, or defibrillation for ventricular fibrillation); or in which many died/failed with conventional therapy and NONE died/failed with the new therapy (eg penicillin for pneumococcal infections).

Level 1c   Evidence from at least one moderate sized RCT or a meta-analysis of small trials which collectively only has a moderate number of patients.

Level 1d   Evidence from at least one RCT.

GRADE B

Level 2   Evidence from at least one high quality study of non-randomized cohorts who did and did not receive the new therapy.

Level 3   Evidence from at least one high quality case control study.

Level 4   Evidence from at least one high quality case series.

GRADE C

Level 5   Opinions from experts without reference or access to any of the foregoing (eg argument from physiology, bench research or first principles).

A comprehensive approach would incorporate many different types of evidence (eg RCTs, non-RCTs, epidemiologic studies, and experimental data), and examine the architecture of the information for consistency, coherence and clarity. Occasionally the evidence does not completely fit into neat compartments. For example, there may not be an RCT that demonstrates a reduction in mortality in individuals with stable angina with the use of beta-blockers, but there is overwhelming evidence that mortality is reduced following MI. In such cases, some may recommend use of beta-blockers in angina patients with the expectation that some extrapolation from post-MI trials is warranted. This could be expressed as Grade A/C. In other instances (e.g. smoking cessation or a pacemaker for complete heart block), the non-randomized data are so overwhelmingly clear and biologically plausible that it would be reasonable to consider these interventions as Grade A.

Recommendation grades appear either in a shaded margin box with an 'R' logo as shown, or within the text, for example Grade A .

Global perspective on cardiovascular disease

10

K. SRINATH REDDY

INTRODUCTION

Cardiovascular diseases (CVD) contributed 15.3 million deaths in 1996, accounting for 30% of the global death toll that year.[1] They accounted for 45.6% of all deaths in the developed countries and 24.5% of all deaths in the developing countries. In absolute numbers, the developing countries contributed 9.77 million deaths due to CVD, in contrast to 5.52 million in the developed countries (an excess of 76%).[1] Even in 1990, the developing countries had a relative excess of 70%.[2] Regional estimates of CVD mortality then indicated that the difference was even higher if the term "developed countries" is restricted to established market economies only and excludes the former socialist economies[2,3] (Tables 10.1, 10.2).

Table 10.1 Regional difference in burden of cardiovascular disease (1990)

Region	Population ($\times 10^6$)	CVD mortality ($\times 10^3$)	Coronary mortality ($\times 10^3$)	Cerebrovascular mortality ($\times 10^3$)	DALYs lost ($\times 10^3$)
Developed regions	**1144.0**	**5328.0**	**2678.0**	**1447.9**	**39 118**
Established market economies	797.8	3174.7	1561.6	782.0	22 058
Former socialist economies	346.2	2153.3	1116.3	665.9	17 060
Developing regions	**4123.4**	**9016.7**	**2469.0**	**3181.2**	**10 8802**
India	849.5	2385.9	783.2	619.2	28 592
China	1133.7	2566.2	441.8	1271.1	28 369
Other Asia and Islands	682.5	1351.6	589.2	350.4	17 267
Sub-Saharan Africa	510.3	933.9	109.1	389.1	12 252
Middle Eastern Crescent	503.1	992.3	276.6	327.4	12 782
Latin America	444.3	786.7	269.1	224.1	9538

DALY, disability adjusted life year.
Adapted from Murray and Lopez.[3]

Table 10.2 Regional contribution to mortality (1990): percentage of world total

Region	All causes (%)	CVD (%)
Established market economies	14	22
Former socialist economies	8	15
India	19	17
China	18	18
Other Asia and Islands	11	9
Sub-Saharan Africa	10	7
Middle Eastern Crescent	9	7
Latin America	6	5
World	100	100

Adapted from Murray and Lopez.[3]

Among the leading causes of mortality, coronary heart disease (CHD) and cerebrovascular disease (stroke) ranked first and second with 7.2 million and 4.6 million deaths respectively in 1996. Their relative importance, however, varied from country to country. For example, more than twice as many deaths from stroke occurred in the developing countries as in the developed countries.[1]

The rise and recent decline of the CVD epidemic in the developed countries have been well documented.[1,4–7] The identification of major risk factors through population based studies and effective control strategies combining community education and targeted management of high risk individuals have together contributed to the fall in CVD mortality rates (inclusive of coronary and stroke deaths) that has been observed in almost all industrialized countries. It has been estimated that, during the period 1965–90, CVD related mortality fell by 50% or so in Australia, Canada, France and the United States and by 60% in Japan.[2] Other parts of Western Europe reported more modest declines (20–25%).[2] The decline in stroke mortality has been more marked compared to the decline in coronary mortality. In the United States, the decline in stroke mortality commenced nearly two decades earlier than the decline in coronary mortality and maintained a sharper rate of decline.[5] During the period 1979–89, the age-adjusted mortality from stroke declined, in that country, by about one-third while the corresponding decline in coronary mortality was 22%.[6] Recent estimates indicate that in Canada, Japan, Switzerland and the United States, stroke mortality has declined by more than 50% in men and women aged 65–74 years since the 1970s.[1] In Japan, where stroke mortality outweighs coronary mortality, the impressive overall decline in CVD mortality is principally contributed by the former. The discordant trend of rising CVD mortality rates in Eastern and Central Europe, however, is in sharp contrast to the decline in Western Europe.[2] CHD mortality rates are now the highest in the world and are still rising in countries like Bulgaria and Hungary, in both men and women.[1] The average life expectancy in Russian males has rapidly fallen in recent years to below 60 years, a phenomenon to which rising CVD rates have contributed substantially.[8]

Rheumatic heart disease (RHD) is also a major burden in the developing countries. It is the most common CVD in children and young adults. Although it is rare in the develped countries, at least 12 million persons are presently estimated to be affected by RHD globally.[1] More than 2 million require repeated hospital admission and 1 million will need heart surgery over the next 20 years.[1] Annually 500 000 deaths occur as a result RHD and many poor persons, whom the disease preferentially affects, are disabled because of lack of access to the expensive medical and surgical care demanded by their disease. The prevalence of RHD in the developing countries ranges from 1 to 10 per 1000 and the incidence of rheumatic fever ranges from 10 to 100 per 100 000, with a high rate of recurrence.

Early age of CVD deaths in developing countries

While the present high burden of CVD deaths is in itself an adequate reason for attention, a greater cause for concern is the early age of CVD deaths in the developing countries compared to the developed countries. For example, in 1990, the proportion of CVD deaths occuring below the age of 70 years was 26.5% in the developed countries compared to 46.7% in the developing countries.[3] The contrast between the truly developed "established market economies" (22.8% of CVD deaths <70 years) and a large developing country like India (52.2%) was even sharper.[3] Therefore, the contribution of the developing countries to the global burden of CVD, in terms of disability adjusted years of life lost, was 2.8 times higher than that of the developed countries (Table 10.1).

EPIDEMIOLOGIC TRANSITION AND THE EVOLUTION OF THE CVD EPIDEMIC

What is the "transition"?

The health status and dominant disease profile of human societies have been historically linked to the level of their economic development and social organization at any given stage. The shift from nutritional deficiences and infectious diseases, as the major causes of death and disability, to degenerative disorders (chronic diseases like CVD, cancer, diabetes) has marked the economic ascent of nations as they industrialized. This shift has been called the epidemiologic transition.

The economic and social changes that propel this transition are related to a rise in per capita income; greater investments in public sanitation, housing and health care; assured availability of adequate nutrition and technological advances in medical care. Life expectancy rises as causes of childhood and early adult mortality decline. This, in turn, leads to a decline in fertility. The age profile of the population changes from a pyramidal distribution dominated by the young to a columnar structure where adults and the elderly progressively expand their numbers. This has been described as the demographic transition. Since the disease profile is also linked to the age profile of the population, the health transition encompasses the effects of the epidemiologic and demographic transitions.

CVD profile at different stages of the epidemiologic transition

The model of epidemiologic transition originally described by Omran[9] with three phases (the age of pestilence and famine; the age of receding pandemics; the age of degenerative and man-made diseases), was later modified to include a fourth phase (the age of delayed degenerative diseases).[10] Life expectancy progressively increases from around 30 years in the first phase to over 70 years in the fourth phase. The shift to a dominant chronic disease profile occurs in the third phase. As the average life expectancy exceeds 50–55 years, the proportionate mortality due to CVD begins to exceed that of infectious diseases.[11,12]

The transition not only occurs between the broad disease categories but also within them. The disease profile within CVD alters at each phase of the epidemiologic transition. In the first phase (the age of pestilence and famine), CVD accounts for 5–10% of deaths.[12] The major causes of CVD are, however, related to infectious and nutritional deficiences. Thus, RHD and cardiomyopathies (e.g., Chagas disease) are the main CVD in this phase. Even as countries emerge from this phase, the residual burden of chronic valvular heart disease and congestive heart failure often remains for some period. These effects are still evident in sub-Saharan Africa and parts of South America and South Asia.[12]

In the second phase (the age of receding pandemics), the decline in infectious disease which accompanies socioeconomic development ushers in changes in diet. As the subsistance nutrition changes to more complete diets, the salt content of the food increases. Hypertension and its sequelae (hypertensive heart disease and hemorrhagic stroke) now affect the population whose average age also has risen with increased life expectancy.[12] Some residual burden of RHD and cardiomyopathies is also evident. These non-atherosclerotic diseases contribute to 10–35% of deaths. This pattern currently prevails in parts of Africa, North Asia, and South America.[12]

In the third phase (the age of degenerative and man-made disease), accelerated economic development and increased per capita incomes promote lifestyle changes in diet, physical activity, stress, and addictions. A diet rich in calories, saturated fat and salt is accompanied by reduced physical activity through increased use of mechanized transport and sedentary leisuretime pursuits. The metabolic mismatch leads to obesity, increased blood lipids, diabetes, and elevated blood pressure. Tobacco consumption, especially cigarette smoking, starts as a pleasurable pastime and turns into a severe addiction. These factors result in the onset of clinically manifest atherosclerotic vascular disease (CHD, atherosclerotic stroke, and peripheral vascular disease) at around 55 years of age. Such patterns first occur in the upper socioeconomic classes who have disposable income to expend on rich diets, tobacco and transport vehicles. Several countries in South America and Asia currently manifest this pattern. As the epidemic advances further and involves all social strata, with homogenization of risk behaviors and risk factors across the population, the death toll of CVD rises to range between 35% and 65% of all deaths. This scenario is currently observed in Eastern Europe.

In the fourth phase (the phase of delayed degenerative disease), a number of changes occur in the society to modify risk behaviors and reduce risk factor levels in the population. Health research augments the knowledge of CVD risk factors. The desire to reduce the adverse impact of CVD on individuals as well as on the society steer the community as well as the policymakers to apply this knowledge for disease prevention and health promotion. Community awareness through education, as well as its ability to exercise healthy choices through supportive regulatory measures, empower its members to adopt healthier lifestyles. Saturated fat and salt consumption declines and leisuretime physical activity and exercise programs are avidly pursued. With concerns over the effects of active and passive smoking, tobacco consumption falls. Simultaneously, medical research makes available new technologies which are very effective in saving lives, modifying the course of disease, and reducing the levels of risk factors. All of these changes, in unison, delay the onset of disease, lower the age-standardized mortality rates and reduce the disability. The contribution of CVD to total mortality falls to 50% or below. These patterns are now established in most of North America, Western Europe, and New Zealand.[12]

Variations in the transition

There are, however, variations within this theme. Even within Europe, for example, Northern Europe and the Mediterranean countries have differences in CVD mortality rates which are better explained by cultural differences in diet than by the level of economic development.[13] Japan has, thus far, avoided the CHD epidemic. Whether recent changes in diet with a rise in mean plasma cholesterol levels of the population, combined with high smoking rates, will lead to a major CHD epidemic in the future remains to be seen.

The question of "arrested epidemiologic transition" is also raised with respect to some of the developing countries. If poverty continues to be a major problem for them, will they experience the CVD epidemic in its full fury or will the pretransitional diseases of nutrition and infection continue to occupy the centre-stage? Even now, there is evidence that the social gradient has begun to reverse for risk factor levels and even for morbidity measures in some populations in the developing world.[14] Unless economic development is greatly stunted in some countries, it is likely that the model of epidemiologic transition will be applicable to most of the developing countries.

Early and late adopters

The pace of epidemiologic transition will vary both among countries and within countries. Usually lifestyle changes towards risk-prone behaviors occur first in the higher socioeconomic groups and urban communities for whom the innovations of modernity are more easily accessible and affordable. As these innovations diffuse and become routinely available at prices amendable to mass consumption, the poorer sections and rural communities also join the CVD bandwagon. Soon the awareness of CVD risks as well as the economic independence to make healthy lifestyle choices in relation to diet and leisuretime exercise (along with the greater ability to access health care) moves the "early adopters" in the affluent and urban strata into a reduced risk zone. The burden of CVD then is largely concentrated in the lower socioeconomic groups and rural populations who continue to practice high risk behaviors and display elevated risk factor levels.[12] These "late adopter" groups also will slowly alter their behaviours, lower their levels of risk and reduce their burden of CVD, as healthcare responses to the CVD epidemic become universally effective.

This is the evolutionary profile of the CVD epidemic, as evident from the analysis of mature epidemics in industrial nations and the advancing epidemics in the developing countries. Differences within countries and between countries, suggested by cross-sectional views at any point in this evolution, should not obscure the longitudinal perspective of an evolving epidemic in which most countries will traverse similar paths, albeit at different times determined by their pace of development. Global shifts in CVD risk factors and their reflection in global CVD

Table 10.3 Contribution of cardiovascular disease to DALY loss (percentage of total)

Region	1990	2020
World	10.85%	14.7%
Developed countries	25.7%	22.0%
Developing countries	8.9%	13.8%

Adapted from Murray and Lopez.[3,15]

trends indicate that all countries and communities have far more in common in terms of disease causation than the differences which demarcate them. The challenge of epidemiologic transition is not whether it will happen in the developing countries, but whether we can apply the available knowledge to telescope the transition and abbreviate phase three of the model in these countries.

PROJECTIONS

The Global Burden of Diseases study estimates that annual mortality from non-communicable diseases will rise from an estimated 28.1 million deaths in 1990 to 49.7 million in 2020.[15] CVD, which accounts for a large proportion of these, will rise as a result of the accelerating epidemic in the developing countries. CHD will continue to be the leading cause of death in the world and, in terms of Disability Adjusted Life Years (DALY) lost, will rise from its fifth position in 1990 to top the DALY table in 2020.[15]

The profile of DALY loss attributable to CVD in 1990 in various regions of the world and the projected estimates for 2015 (Table 10.3) also indicate a large rise.[3,15] Among the developed countries, the sharp decline in the industrial nations is partly offset by the rise in the former socialist countries.

Deaths attributable to tobacco, a risk factor for CVD and other chronic diseases, are projected to rise from 3.0 million in 1990 to 8.4 million in 2020. The largest increases will be in India, China and other developing countries in Asia, where tobacco-attributable deaths will rise from 1.1 million to 4.2 million in 2020.[15]

MECHANISMS WHICH PROPEL A CVD EPIDEMIC IN DEVELOPING COUNTRIES

Demographic changes due to the epidemiologic transition

A major public health challenge, identified by recent analyses of global health trends, is the projected rise in both proportional and absolute CVD mortality rates in the developing countries, over the next quarter century. The reasons for this anticipated acceleration of the epidemic are many.[14] In the second half of the twentieth century, most developing countries experienced a major surge in life expectancy. This was principally as a result of a decline in deaths occuring in infancy, childhood and adolescence and was related to more effective public health responses to perinatal, infectious and nutritional deficiency disorders and to improved economic indicators like per-capita income and social indicators like female literacy in some areas. These demographic shifts have augmented the ranks of middle aged and older adults. The increasing longevity provides longer periods of exposure to the risk factors of CVD, resulting in greater probability of clinically manifest CVD events. The concomitant decline of infectious and nutritional disorders (competing causes of death) further enhances the proportional burden due to CVD and other chronic lifestyle-related diseases.

The ratio of deaths due to pretransitional diseases (related to infections and malnutrition) to those caused by post-transitional diseases (like CVD and cancer) varies among regions and between countries, depending on factors like the level of economic development and literacy as well as availability and access to healthcare. The direction of change towards a rising relative contribution of post-transitional diseases is, however, common to and consistent among the developing countries.[16] The experience of urban China, where the proportion of CVD deaths rose from 12.1% in 1957 to 35.8% in 1990, illustrates this phenomenon.[17]

Population expansion

Despite relative declines in fertility, the continuing growth of populations in the developing countries will also increase the absolute numbers at risk of CVD. World population is expected to rise from 5.71 billion in 1995 to 8.29 billion in 2025.[1] Combined with changes in the demographic profile, this will result in a large number of adults who are potentially vulnerable to CVD.

Presently, there are an estimated 380 million people aged 65 or more, including around 220 million in the developing countries. By 2020, the figures are projected to reach more than 690 million and 460 million respectively.[1]

In India, for example, the population is expected to rise from 683.2 million in 1981 to somewhere between 1253.8 and 1480.5 million in 2021. Simultaneously, the proportion of adults aged 35 years or above will rise from 28.4% of the population to 42.4%.[18]

Increased standard of living leading to deleterious health behaviors

A third reason to arouse concern is that, if population levels of CVD risk factors rise as a consequence of adverse lifestyle changes accompanying industrialization and urbanization, the rates of CVD mortality and morbidity could rise even higher than the rates predicted solely by demographic changes. Both the degree as well as the duration of exposure to CVD risk factors would increase as a result of higher risk factor levels coupled with a longer life expectancy. Increase in body weight (adjusted for height), blood pressure and cholesterol levels in Chinese population samples aged 35–64 years, between the two phases of the Sino-MONICA study (1984–86, 1988–89) and the substantially higher levels of most CVD risk factors in urban population groups compared to rural population groups in India, provide evidence of such trends.[17,18] The increasing use of tobacco in a number of developing countries will also translate into higher mortality rates of CVD, lung cancer and other tobacco related diseases, while undesirable alterations in diet and physical activity are also impacting adversely on cardiovascular health.

The global availability of cheap vegetable oils and fats has resulted in greatly increased fat consumption among low income countries in recent years.[19] The transition now occurs at lower levels of the gross national product than previously and is further accelerated by rapid urbanization. In China, for example, the proportion of upper income persons who were consuming a relatively high fat diet (>30% of daily energy intake) rose from 22.8% to 66.6% between 1989 and 1993. The lower and middle income groups too showed a rise (from 19% to 36.4% in the former and from 19.1% to 51.0% in the latter).[19] The Asian countries, traditionally high in carbohydrates and low in fat, have shown an overall decline in the proportion of energy from complex carbohydrates along with an increase in the proportion of fat.[19] The globalization of food production and marketing is also contributing to the increasing consumption of energy dense foods that are poor in dietary fiber and several micronutrients.[20]

The rising tobacco consumption patterns in most developing countries contrast sharply with the overall decline in the industrial nations.[21] Recent projections, from the World Health Organization, suggest that by the year 2020 tobacco will become the largest single cause of death accounting for 12.3% of global deaths.[22] India, China and countries in the Middle Eastern Crescent will by then have tobacco contributing to more than 12% of all deaths. In India alone, the tobacco-attributable toll will rise from 1.4% in 1990 to 13.3% in 2020.[22] A large component of this will be in the form of cardiovascular deaths.

Thrifty gene

A "programming" effect of factors promoting selective survival may also determine individual responses to environmental challenges and, thereby, the population differences in CVD. The "thrifty gene" has been postulated to be a factor in promoting selective survival, over generations, of persons who encountered an adverse environment of limited nutritional resources.[23] While this may have proved advantageous in surviving the rigours of a spartan environment over thousands of years, the relatively recent and rapid changes in environment may have resulted in a metabolic mismatch. Thus a salt-sensitive person whose forefathers thrived despite a limited supply of salt now reacts to a salt-enriched diet with high blood pressure. It has also been hypothesized that populations subjected to food scarcity have undergone selection of a gene which increases the efficiency of fat storage through an oversecretion of insulin in response to a meal. While this favors survival in a situation of low caloric availability, a current excess of caloric intake may lead to obesity, hyperinsulinemia, diabetes, and atherosclerosis.[12] Similarly, an insulin-resistant individual whose ancestors may have survived because a lack of insulin sensitivity in the skeletal muscle ensured adequate blood glucose levels for the brain in daunting conditions of limited calorie intake and demanding physical challenges, may now respond to a high-calorie diet and a sedentary lifestyle with varying degress of glucose intolerance and hyperinsulinemia. While such mechanisms seem plausible, their contribution to the acceleration of the CVD epidemic in the developing countries remains speculative.

Maternal–fetal exposures as a cause of midlife CVD

A recently reported association which, if adequately validated by the tests of causation, may have special relevance to the developing countries is the inverse relationship between birth size and CVD in later life.[24–27] The "foetal origins hypothesis" states that adverse intrauterine influences like poor maternal nutrition lead to impaired fetal growth resulting in low birth weight, short birth length, and a small head circumference. These adverse influences are postulated to also "program" the fetus to develop adaptive metabolic and physiologic responses which facilitate survival. These responses, however, may lead to disordered responses to environmental challenges as the child grows, with an increased risk of glucose intolerance, hypertension and dyslipidemia in later life, with adult CVD as a consequence. While some supportive evidence for the hypothesis has been provided by observational studies, it awaits further evaluation for a causal role. If it does emerge as an important risk factor for CVD, the populations of developing countries will be at an especially enhanced risk because of the vast numbers of poorly nourished infants who have been born in the past several decades. The steady improvement in child survival will lead to a higher proportion of such infants surviving to adult life when their hypothesized susceptibility to vascular disease may manifest itself.

Ethnic diversity

Although ethnic diversity in CVD rates, risk factor levels and risk factor interactions are evident from population studies, the extent to which genetic factors contribute is unclear. It is only after demographic profiles, environmental factors and possible programming factors are ascertained and adjusted for that differences in gene frequency or expression can be invoked as a probable explanation for interpopulation differences in CVD.[28] The extent to which chronic diseases, including CVD, occur within and amongst different populations is determined by genetic–environmental interaction which occurs in a wide and variable array, ranging from the essentially genetic to the predominantly environmental. This is perhaps best illustrated by the knowledge gained from studies in migrant groups, where environmental changes due to altered lifestyles are superimposed over genetic influences. These "natural experiments" have been of great value in enhancing the understanding of why CVD rates differ amongst ethnic groups. The classical Ni-Hon-San study of Japanese migrants revealed how blood cholesterol levels and CHD rates rose from Japan to Honolulu and further still to San Francisco, as Japanese communities in the three areas were compared.[29] The experience gleaned from the study of South Asians, Chinese and Pima Indians further elucidates the complexities of ethnic variations in CHD.[30–32] The comparison of Afro-Caribbeans, South Asians and Europeans in UK brought out the sharp differences in central obesity, glucose intolerance, hyperinsulinemia and related dyslipidemia between the three groups despite similar profiles of blood pressure, body mass index and total plasma cholesterol.[33] However, urban–rural comparisons within India,[18,30] as well as migrant Indian comparison with their non-migrant siblings,[34] reveal large differences in these conventional risk factors. Thus, where the environment is common but gene pools differ, the non-conventional risk factors appear to be explanatory of risk variance, while when the same gene pool is confronted with different environments, the conventional risk factors stand out as being of major importance.

155

To what extent ethnic diversity in response to CVD risk factors influences the course of the CVD epidemic in different developing countries remains to be studied. However the experience of some of the migrant groups (e.g., South Asians) portends severe epidemics in the home countries as they advance in their transition.

STRATEGIES TO DEAL WITH THE CORONARY EPIDEMIC

CVD prevention

EVOLVING CONCEPTS OF RISK FACTORS

Risk factor

Decades of research, embracing evidence from observational epidemiology and clinical trials, have demonstrated that CHD is multifactorial in causation. The term "risk factor" was first used in the context of CHD.[35] Several such risk factors have been identified, ranging from the established "major" factors like smoking, elevated blood cholesterol and hypertension to the recently investigated factors like homocysteine and lipoprotein "a". A risk factor must fulfill the criteria of causality: strength of association (high relative risk or odds ratio), consistancy of association (over many studies), temporal relationship (cause preceding the effect), dose–response relationship (greater the exposure higher the risk), biologic plausibility, experimental evidence and, very importantly, evidence from human studies.

"Clinical" vs "prevention" norms

The need for making "clinical" decisions related to the management of these risk factors led to definition of threshold levels of risk and practice guidelines based on those. These "clinical norms" erroneously came to be identified, by the health professionals as well as the community, to also represent the prevention norms. The former are defined by evidence of benefit exceeding risk when as intervention reduces a risk factor below a particular level (the net benefit being demonstrated in clinical trials specifically designed for that purpose). The latter, however, are usually identified from observational studies (long term longitudinal prospective studies of large cohorts) and denote the optimal values of the risk factor at which the risk of developing disease is minimal.

The targeting of individuals is promoted by the "clinical" approach of healthcare providers who seek to identify persons at "high risk" of disease or its outcomes for intensive investigation and intervention. Thus thresholds are defined to categorize persons with "high cholesterol" or "high blood pressure" and implement individualized control strategies. Attention and action above this threshold often contrast with indifference and inertia below it.

As trial evidence is gathered, the clinical norms may progressively move towards the prevention norms, as in the case of cholesterol or hypertension where the thresholds for intervention have been lowered dramatically in the last decade. They may, however, remain higher than the prevention norms, since clinical trials may be conducted at a stage in the natural history where the risks of prior exposure may not be completely reversible and also because the intervention may itself be associated with some adverse effects. Thus the benefits of lowering a risk factor may appear less than those that may occur by preventing its rise in the first place.

The continuum of risk

It is clear that even though lifestyle disorders afflict some individuals, they arise from causes that are widespread in the population as a whole. Risk factors like cholesterol and blood pressure operate in a continuum of progressively increasing risk rather than through an all-or-none relationship suggested by cut-off values. For example, a systolic blood pressure (SBP) in the range 130–139 mmHg carries a higher risk than values in the range 120–129 mmHg for both heart attacks and strokes. While a SBP of 180 mmHg carries a much higher risk for an individual than 140 mmHg the number of persons in any population who have SBP values in the range 130–139 mmHg is higher than those with values of 180 mmHg or higher. The Multiple Risk Factor Intervention Trial's cohort study in the United States (MRFIT) revealed that of all heart attacks which are attributable to SBP, 7.2% arise from the 0.9% segment of the population which represents the 180+ mmHg range, while 20.7% of all such heart attacks occur in the 22.8% segment of the population which has pressures in the range 130–139 mmHg[36] (Figure 10.1). Similarly, 57% of all excess deaths attributable to diastolic blood pressure occur in the range 80–95 mmHg compared to only 15% which occur in the high range of 105–130 mmHg.

This dichotomy is also clearly seen in the Framingham Study on coronary risk factors in a recent review.[38] People with a blood cholesterol level of 300 mg/dl run three to five times the risk of CHD as do people at a cholesterol level of 200 mg/dl. At cholesterol levels over 300 mg/dl, 90 out of 100 persons developed the disease in the next 16–30 years of followup in Framingham. At cholesterol levels under 200 mg/dl, the rate was 20 out of 100 during the same period. However, more than twice as many people developed CHD with cholesterol levels under 200 mg% all their lives as did those with cholesterol levels over 300 mg%. This is because a 20% fraction of a 45% segment of the population is a much larger number than a 90% fraction of a 3–5% segment of the population.[38]

Thus, for most causal factors, there is a "risk pyramid". Those at the top of the pyramid are at the highest individual risk of disease but those at the lower levels of the pyramid account for the largest number of cases in the community because they constitute the largest segment of the population. Any approach which targets only those at the highest risk produces limited gains for the community, despite conferring definite benefits to the individuals in that category.

The concept that "sick individuals arise from sick populations" was propounded and proved by Geoffrey Rose.[39,40] He demonstrated that risk factor "distributions" throughout the population are predictive of disease burden in that community. The mean (average) levels of a risk factor across different populations correlate with the proportions of high risk individuals in those populations, whatever be the cut-off value. Thus, as the average population blood pressure value rises amongst populations, the proportion of hypertensive individuals also rises. In each population, there are groups who represent the extremes of the risk profile (very low risk vs very high risk). However the proportion at 'high risk' would be determined by the average value of that risk factor in the population. This in turn is dependent on the dominant behaviors that characterize the society at each stage of its development.

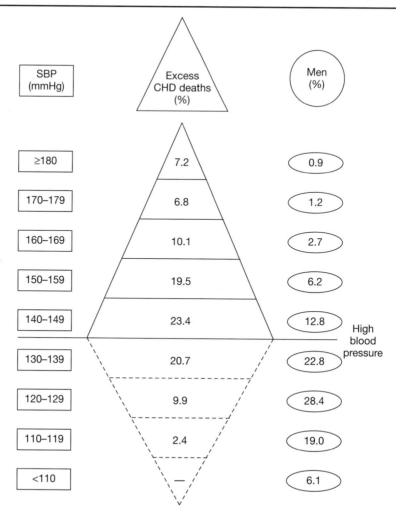

Figure 10.1 The risk pyramid for blood pressure and coronary heart disease (CHD): baseline SBP and CHD death rates for men screened in MRFIT.[37] (Adapted with permission from Stamler *et al.* 1993.[36])

Multiplicative risk

The process of identifying and estimating the independent risk associated with any single risk factor led to clinical and preventive strategies targeting it in isolation. However, observational studies like Framingham and MRFIT have clearly revealed that the coexistence of multiple risk factors confers a magnified risk which is multiplicative rather than merely additive. A smoker with modest elevations of cholesterol and diastolic or systolic blood pressure is at a greater risk of coronary death than a non-smoker with severe hypertension or marked hypercholesterolemia. In the MRFIT study, a non-smoker with SBP less than 118 mmHg and a total serum cholesterol level less than 182 mg% had a 20-fold lower risk of coronary death than a smoker with a SBP exceeding 142 mmHg and a serum cholesterol exceeding 245 mg% (age adjusted CHD mortality of 3.09 vs 62.11, per 10 000 person years). A smoker who has a SBP of 132–141 mmHg and a serum cholesterol of 203–220 mg% has a CHD mortality risk of 28.87 per 10 000 person years, compared to a risk of 12.36 in a non-smoker with a SBP below 118 mmHg but with a serum cholesterol exceeding 245 mg%.[41]

The demonstration of such multiplicative risk has led to the concept of "comprehensive cardiovascular risk" or "total risk", quantifying an individual's overall risk of CVD resulting from the confluence of risk factors.[37] Both clinical and preventive strategies are veering away from unifactorial risk reduction to multifactorial risk modification, to reduce this overall risk in individuals as well as in populations.

HIGH RISK APPROACH FOR PREVENTION

Having recognized that environmental risk factors do not affect only a few individuals in isolation but are spread across populations, with a continuous rather than a threshold relationship to disease, how should that influence disease control strategies? The health policy debate, until recently, was on whether to focus the control strategies on individuals at the highest risk of disease (in view of their markedly elevated risk factor levels) or on the population as a whole (aiming to achieve modest reductions in the risk of most members of that community). The high risk approach aims at identifying persons with markedly elevated risk factors and, therefore, at the highest risk of disease.[39] These individuals are then targeted by interventions which aim to reduce the risk factor levels. If successful, the benefits to individuals are large, because the individuals risks are large. However, since the number of persons in this high risk category is proportionately much smaller than those in the moderate risk group, the overall benefits to society are limited in terms of deaths or disability avoided. The strategy also does not minimize the risk for the individuals concerned. Although a fall of blood cholesterol from 300 mg% to 240 mg% does indeed reduce the risk, even this attained value poses greater risk than 200 mg%. Thus there is still a substantial residual risk, despite the impressive risk reduction due to the change from the initial cholesterol levels. Further, this strategy is behaviorally inappropriate.[39] An individual with high blood cholesterol levels may be advised to eat low fat food but can he stictly adhere to it if his family and friends consume a very different diet? The main advantage of the high risk approach, however, is that physicians as well as patients are highly motivated to act, because the projected risks compel attention and the benefits of reduction appear attractive.[39]

POPULATION APPROACH FOR PREVENTION

In contrast, the population approach aims at reducing the risk factor levels in the population as a whole, through community action.[39] Because there is a continuum of risk associated with most risk factors, this mass change will result in mass benefit across a wide range of risk. While individual benefits are relatively small, the cumulative societal benefits are large ("the prevention paradox"). The strategy is also behaviorally more appropriate.[39] If the eating habits in the community alter towards preferred consumption of foods with lower saturated fat and salt content and a greater daily intake of fresh fruit and vegetables, even the high risk individual on a prescribed diet will find a supportive ambience which does not mark him out as a deviant from social norms. If a new generation grows up in an environment where healthy behavior is considered common practice, its average blood cholesterol level may remain below

200 mg% rather than around 240 mg% and thus be at a lower risk than even the beneficiary of the high risk strategy. However, the risks and benefits of such a strategy are less obvious to those in the moderate risk range. The motivation for change is, therefore, not as strong as for those in the high risk group. The gratification of achieving readily identifiable success in high risk individuals, through drugs or other powerful interventions, is also denied to the physicians in the population strategy where the potential beneficiaries, though many, are faceless and nameless. Since such "anonymity of prevention" denies the pleasure of individual rescue acts, physician motivation for community counselling is neither strong nor sustained.[39] Policymakers can, however, ill afford to ignore the imperatives of investing in a population approach which will pay large long term dividends in the control of lifestyle diseases. Health professionals too must recognize the benefits of this strategy to play a strong advocacy role for health promoting behaviors in the community.

The success of the population strategy has been demonstrated both in developed countries (e.g., Finland)[42] and in some developing countries (e.g., Mauritius).[43] The North Karelia Project demonstrated large reductions in CVD mortality (50.1% in males and 63.5% in females), CHD mortality (53.4% and 59.8%) and all-cause mortality (39.5% and 40.4%) during the 20-year intervention period. These accompanied changes in CVD risk factors, following community based intervention programmes. Impressive reductions in cigarette smoking, prevalence of hypertension and mean population cholesterol levels, as well as increase in leisuretime physical activity were noted during the period 1987–92, consequent to lifestyle intervention programs in Mauritius.

The impact of the population strategy is likely to be large, as suggested by a recent estimate that if every American had a diastolic blood pressure value which is a mere 2 mmHg lower than his or her present value, the number of heart attacks that could be prevented would exceed those that could be avoided by effectively treating every person with a diastolic pressure of 95 mmHg or higher. The corresponding benefit for preventing paralytic strokes would be 93% of those avoided by drug therapy.[44] Such blood pressure changes can be effectively achieved and sustained through modest reductions in weight and salt intake or through exercise.

COMBINING THE STRATEGIES

Both of these strategies are not mutually exclusive but are synergistic, complementary and necessary. The risks and benefits demonstrated in high risk individuals serve to educate the community about risk factors, while the population approach makes it easier to achieve the desired level of lifestyle change in high risk individuals. The population based, lifestyle linked risk reduction approach is particularly relevant in the context of the developing countries, where it is necessary to ensure that communities currently at low risk are protected from acquisition or augmentation of risk factors ("primordial prevention"). This is true for adults in the rural regions of most developing countries as well as for children in all populations. It is also eminently applicable to moderate risk groups in urban areas, where lifestyle based risk modification will help avoid drug therapy, with its attendant economic and biologic costs. There will still be some persons who need such pharmacologic or technologic interventions because of their high risk status. However, their numbers too will decrease as the risk profile of the whole community gradually shifts.

Case management

Despite these preventive strategies, several individuals will manifest clinical disease because risks are not totally eliminated in the community or because genetic susceptibility is strongly expressed. The success of preventive efforts will reduce their number as well as delay the age of onset of clinical events. Those who develop disease will require optimal clinical care which can avert early death, reduce disability, and assure an adequate quality of life. This mandates early detection of disease.

The cost-effectiveness and safety of these diagnostic and therapeutic techniques would have to be established through appropriately designed clinical research. This scientific evidence has to be translated into practice guidelines which then need to be widely disseminated. The rapid diffusion of these guidelines across various levels of health care and their sustained impact on clinical practice will ensure that the burden of cardiovascular disease in the community is mitigated through appropriate application of available knowledge. Postmyocardial infarction risk reduction through thrombolytic agents, aspirin, beta-blockers, ACE inhibitors and statins is clearly illustrative of the benefits of such evidence based clinical care.[45–50]

The decline in CVD mortality rates in industrial countries is the collective result of population based prevention strategies improving the risk factor profile of communities, a high risk approach of targeted interventions to protect individuals with markedly elevated risk factor levels, and case-management strategies to salvage, support and sustain persons presenting with clinical problems. These strategies are not diverse and divisive but are continuous and complementary in the effort to control the incidence and impact of CVD.

THE ENORMOUS NEED FOR EVIDENCE-BASED MEDICINE IN DEVELOPED AND DEVELOPING COUNTRIES

CVD related expenditure in developed countries

The management of CVD is often technology intensive and expensive. Procedures for diagnosis or therapy, drugs, hospitalization and costs of frequent consultations with healthcare providers all contribute to high costs, both to affected persons and to society. In developed countries, they already account for about 10% of direct healthcare costs, equal to between 0.5% and 1% of a country's gross national product.[1] As life expectancy increases and the duration of the therapy gets prolonged, the costs may further escalate, until preventive strategies succeed in greatly reducing the incidence of CVD.

CVD related expenditure in developing countries

The costs of CVD related healthcare have not been clearly estimated in the developing countries. However, high expenditure on tertiary care in most of these countries has a likely large contribution from CVD. As the epidemic advances many more persons will be affected, escalating the costs of CVD related healthcare. This may divert scarce resources intersectorally from developmental activities and intrasectorally from the "unfinished agenda" of infectious and nutritional disorders. As the epidemic matures, the social gradient will reverse and many of the poor who are then afflicted will be unable to afford or access the expensive health care that CVD demands.

Need for evidence based medicine

The need for cost-effective prevention and case management is, therefore, urgent. These practices need to be based on the best available evidence which is generalized to the context of each developing country. Where such evidence is unavailable or insufficient to guide policy and practice, health research must quickly address those information needs. International cooperation can greatly further these efforts to acquire, appraise, analyse and apply such knowledge. *Evidence* from health research must do *justice* to the needs of public health! Evidence based cardiovascular medicine must pursue this advocacy to secure acquittal from CVD for countries under the trial of epidemiologic transition.

REFERENCES

1 *The World Health Report* 1997. Geneva: World Health Organization, 1997.

2 Lopez AD. Assessing the burden of mortality from cardiovascular disease. *Wld Hlth Stat Q* 1993;**46**: 91–6.

3 Murray CJL, Lopez AD. *Global comparative assessments in the health sector.* Geneva: World Health Organization, 1994.

4 Thom TJ, Epstein FH, Feldman JJ, Leaverton PE, Wolz M. *Total mortality and mortality from heart disease, cancer, and stroke from 1950 to 1987 in 27 countries: highlights of trends and their interrelationships among causes of death.* NIH Publ No 92–3088. Washington, DC: US DHHS PHS, National Institutes of Health, 1992.

5 Whelton PK, Brancati FL, Appel LJ, Klag MJ. The challenge of hypertension and atherosclerotic cardiovascular disease in economically developing countries. *High Blood Press* 1995;**4**: 36–45.

6 Feinleib M, Ingster L, Rosenberg H, Maurer J, Singh G, Kochanek K. Time trends, cohort effects and geographic patterns in stroke mortality. United States. *Ann Epidemiol* 1993;**3**:458–65.

7 Marmot M. Coronary heart disease: rise and fall of a modern epidemic. In: Marmot M, Elliott P, eds. *Coronary heart disease epidemiology. From aetiology to public health.* Oxford: Oxford University Press, 1992, pp 3–19.

8 Shkolniko V, Mesle F, Vallin J. Recent trends in life expectancy and causes of death in Russia (1970–1993). In: *Commission on Behaviour and Social Sciences and Education, Committee on Population.* New York: National Academy of Sciences, 1994.

9 Omran AR. The epidemiologic transition: a key of the epidemiology of population change. *Millbank Mem Fund Q* 1971;**49**:509–38.

10 Olshansky SJ, Ault AB. The fourth stage of the epidemiologic transition: the age of delayed degenerative diseases. *Millbank Mem Fund Q* 1986;**64**:355–91.

11 Pearson TA, Jamison DT, Trejo-Gutierrez H. Cardiovascular disease, In: Jamison DT, ed. *Disease control priorities in developing countries.* New York: Oxford University Press, 1993, pp 577–99.

12 Pearson TA. Global perspectives on cardiovascular disease. *Evidence Based Cardiovasc Med* 1997;**1**:4–5.

13 Verschuren WMM, Jacobs DR, Bloemberg BPM *et al.* Serum total cholesterol and long-term coronary heart disease mortality in different cultures: twenty-five year follow-up of the Seven Country Study. *JAMA* 1995;**274**:131–6.

14 Reddy KS, Yusuf S. The emerging epidemic of cardiovascular disease in developing countries. *Circulation* 1998 (in press).

15 Murray CJL, Lopez AD. Alternative projections of mortality and disability by cause 1990–2020: Global Burden of Disease Study. *Lancet* 1997;**349**: 1498–504.

16 Bulatao RA, Stephens PW. Global estimates and projections of mortality by cause 1970–2015. Pre-working paper 1007. Washington DC: Population Health and Nutrition Department, World Bank, 1992.

17 Yao C, Wu Z, Wu J. The changing pattern of cardiovascular diseases in China. *Wld Hlth Stat Q* 1993;**46**:113–18.

18 Reddy KS. Cardiovascular disease in India. *Wld Hlth Stat Q* 1993;**46**:101–7.

19 Drewnowski A, Popkin BM. The nutrition transition: new trends in the global diet. *Nutr Rev* 1997;**55**:31–43.

20 Lang T. The public health impact of globalisation of food trade. In: Shetty PS, McPherson K, eds. *Diet, nutrition and chronic disease. Lessons from contrasting worlds.* Chichester: Wiley, 1997, pp 173–87.

21 Peto R. Tobacco – the growing epidemic in China. *JAMA* 1996;**275**:1683–4.

22 *Tobacco or health: First global status report.* Geneva: World Health Organization, 1996.

23 Thrifty genotype rendered detrimental by progress (editorial). *Lancet* 1989;**ii**:839–40.

24 Barker DJP, Martyn CN, Osmond C, Haleb CN, Fall CHD. Growth *in utero* and serum cholesterol concentrations in adult life. *Br Med J* 1993;**307**:1524–7.

25 Martyn CN, Barker DJP, Jespersen S, Greenwald S, Osmond C, Berry C. Growth *in utero*, adult blood pressure and arterial compliance. *Br Heart J* 1995;**73**:116–21.

26 Law CM, Shiell AW. Is blood pressure inversely related to birth weight? The strength of evidence from a systematic review of the literature. *J Hyperten* 1996;**14**:935–41.

27 Joseph KS, Kramer MS. Review of evidence on fetal and early childhood antecedents of adult chronic disease. *Epidemiologic Rev* 1996;**18**:158–74.

28 Reddy KS, Coronary heart disease in different racial groups. In: Yusuf S, Wilhelmsen L, eds. *Advanced issues in prevention and treatment of atherosclerosis.* Surrey: Euromed Communications, 1996, pp 47–60.

29 Robertson TL, Kato H, Rhoads GG *et al.* Epidemiologic studies of coronary heart disease and stroke in Japanese men living in Japan, Hawai and California. Incidence of myocardial infarction and death from coronary heart disease. *Am J Cardiol* 1977;**39**:239–49.

30 Enas EA, Mehta JL. Malignant coronary artery disease in young Asian Indians: thoughts on pathogenesis, prevention and treatment. *Clin Cardiol* 1995;**18**:131–5.

31 Li N, Tuomilehto J, Dowse G *et al.* Prevalence of coronary heart disease indicated by electrocardiogram abnormalities and risk factors in developing countries. *J Clin Epidemiol* 1994;**47**:599–611.

32 Sievers ML, Nelson RG, Bennet PH. Adverse mortality experience of a southwestern American Indian community: overall death rates and underlying causes of death in Pima Indians. *J Clin Epidemiol* 1990;**43**:1231–42.

33 Chaturvedi N, McKeigue PM, Marmot MG. Relationship of glucose intolerance to coronary risk in Afro-Caribbeans compared with Europeans. *Diabetologia* 1994;**37**:765–72.

34 Bhatnagar D, Anand IS, Durrington PN *et al.* Coronary risk factors in people from the Indian Subcontinent living in West London and their siblings in India. *Lancet* 1995;**345**:404–9.

35 Kannel WB, Dawber TR, Kagan A, Revotskie N, Strokes III J. Factors of risk in the development of coronary heart disease – six-year follow-up experience. *Ann Intern Med* 1961;**55**:33–50.

36 Stamler J, Stamler R, Neaton JD. Blood pressure, systolic and diastolic, and cardiovascular risks: US population data. *Arch Intern Med* 1993;**153**:598–615.

37 *Hypertension control.* World Health Organization Technical Report No 862. Geneva: World Health Organization, 1996.

38 Castelli WP, Anderson K, Wilson PW, Levy D. Lipids and risk of coronary heart disease. The Framingham Study. *Ann Epidemiol* 1992;**2**(1–2):23–8.

39 Rose G, Sick individuals and sick populations. *Int J Epidemiol* 1985;**14**:32–8.

40 Rose G, Day S. The population mean predicts the number of deviant individuals. *Br Med J* 1990;**301**:1031–4.

41 Neaton JD, Kuller LH, Wentworth D, Borhani NO, for the Multiple Risk Factor Intervention Trial Research Group. Total and cardiovascular mortality in relation to cigarette smoking, serum cholesterol concentration, and diastolic blood pressure among black and white males followed for five years. *Am Heart J* 1984;**108**:759–69.

42 Puska P, Tuomilehto J, Aulikki N, Enkki V. *The North Karelia Project. 20 years results and experiences.* Helsinki: National Public Health Institute, 1995.

43 Dowsen GK, Gareeboo H, George K *et al.* Changes in population cholesterol concentrations and other cardiovascular risk factor levels after five years of non-communicable disease intervention programme in Mauritius. *Br Med J* 1995;**311**:1255–9.

44 Cook NR, Cohen J, Hebert PR, Taylor JO, Hennekens CH. Implications of small reductions in diastolic blood pressure for primary prevention. *Arch Intern Med* 1995;**155**:701–9.

45 Matching the Intensity of Risk Factors Management with the Hazard for Coronary Disease Events (27th Bethesda Conference). *J Am Coll Cardiol* 1996;**27**:957–1047.

46 Antiplatelet Trialists Collaboration. Collaborative overview of randomized trials of antiplatelet therapy. I. Prevention of death, myocardial infarction and stroke by prolonged antiplatelet therapy in various categories of patients. *Br Med J* 1994;**308**:235–46.

47 Yusuf S, Wittes J, Friedman L. Overview of results of randomized clinical trials in heart disease. I treatments following myocardial infarction. *JAMA* 1988;**260**:2088–93.

48 Walsh JT, Gray D, Keating NA *et al.* ACE for whom? Implictions for clinical practice of post-infarct trials. *Br Heart J* 1995;**73**: 470–4.

49 Scandinavian Simvastatin Survival Study Group. Randomised trial of cholesterol lowering in 4444 patients with coronary heart disease: the Scandinavian Simvastatin Survival Study (4S). *Lancet* 1994;**344**:1383–9.

50 Sacks FM, Pfeffer MA, Moye LA *et al.* The effect of Pravastatin on coronary events after myocardial infarction in patients with average cholesterol levels. *N Engl J Med* 1996;**335**: 1001–9.

Tobacco: global burden and community solutions

11

Terry F. Pechacek,
Samira Asma,
Michael P. Eriksen

While smoking is universally known to be deadly, few are aware of precisely how deadly. In the United States, smoking is the leading preventable cause of death, killing over 400 000 people each year, wasting 5 million years of potential life and costing over $50 billion in health expenditures. Since the first Surgeon General's Report on smoking in 1964, 10 million Americans have died from smoking. If current trends continue, an additional 25 million Americans alive today, including 5 million children, will die a painful and premature death caused by smoking. While the United States statistics are appalling, the global projections are even more dire. Globally, if current trends continue, the number of people killed by tobacco will more than triple to 10 million a year by the year 2025. The only ray of hope is that the precursors for the projected global tobacco epidemic are not yet all in place. While high smoking rates among men are nearly universal, the same cannot be said for women and teens. Thus, despite the unprecedented toll of tobacco and the gloomy projections, there is the potential for prevention.

This chapter will explore that potential, particularly for coronary heart disease, by (1) examining the current global burden of tobacco and future projections, (2) reviewing the mixed evidence for community-based tobacco control interventions, and (3) proposing a new and dynamic model for community-based tobacco control, based on state innovations, proven to be effective in the United States, and which may be able to be applied throughout the world.

CURRENT GLOBAL BURDEN OF TOBACCO AND FUTURE PROJECTIONS

Tobacco-related morbidity and mortality is the most important determinant of human health trends worldwide. The unprecedented rise in tobacco-related disease and death is a strong prediction because most of the tobacco-related mortality and disability in

Table 11.1   Estimated number of smokers in the world, early 1990s (millions)

	Males	Females	Total
Developed countries	200	100	300
Developing countries	700	100	800
World	900	200	1100

Source: WHO estimates.

2020 will be due to current levels of smoking. Tobacco products are estimated to have caused about 3 million deaths annually in the early 1990s, and the death toll is increasing. Unless current smoking trends are reversed, that figure is expected to increase to 10 million deaths annually by the 2020s or early 2030s; 70% of those deaths will occur in developing countries.[1]

Although there have been large decreases in the incidence of some chronic diseases, such as stomach cancer and stroke, there have been large increases in others, such as lung cancer and myocardial infarction. The causes of these chronic diseases are many, but at present one far exceeds all others: namely, the smoking of manufactured cigarettes.

This section quantifies the burden caused by tobacco. The term "burden" constitutes the years of life lost due to premature mortality and the years of life lived with disability. DALY (disability adjusted life years) is a measure of life lost due to disability or premature death cuased by disease or injuries.[2]

The World Health Organization estimates that there are approximately 1100 million smokers in the world, representing about one-third of the global population aged 15 years and over. The vast majority of the smokers are in developing countries (800 million), and most of these are men (700 million) (Table 11.1).

Globally, it is estimated that 47% of men and 12% of women smoke. In the developed countries, the corresponding figures are 42% for men and 24% for women and in developing countries, available data suggest that about 48% of men and 7% of women smoke. Smoking among women is most prevalent in the formerly socialist countries of Central and Eastern Europe (28%), in countries with established market economies (23%) and in Latin American and Caribbean countries (21%) (Table 11.2). People are beginning to smoke at younger and younger ages, with the median age of initiation under 15 in many countries. Starting to smoke at younger ages not only increases the risk of death from a smoking-related cause, but also lowers the age at which such risks will occur. Young people who begin smoking early in life often find it difficult to quit smoking. Among those who continue to smoke throughout their lives, about one-half can be expected to die from a smoking-related cause. Half of these deaths will occur in middle age (age 35–69), and the other half will occur in older age (70 and over).[3]

TOBACCO: A RISK FACTOR FOR CORONARY HEART DISEASE

Of all the diseases causally associated with smoking, lung cancer is the most well known simply because nearly all lung cancers deaths are due to smoking. However, smoking actually causes more deaths from diseases other than lung cancer. In 1995, there were 514 000 smoking-attributable lung cancer deaths in developed countries, compared to 625 000 smoking-attributable deaths from heart and vascular diseases in the same year.[3]

Table 11.2   Daily smoking prevalence, men and women aged 15 and over, early 1990s (%)

	Men	Women
More developed countries	42	24
Established market economies	37	23
Formerly socialist economies of Europe	60	28
Less developed countries	48	7
China (1984)	61	7
India (1980s)	40	3
Other Asia and Islands	54	7
Middle Eastern crescent[a]	41	8
Sub-Saharan Africa[b]	25	3
Latin America and the Caribbean	40	21
World	47	12

[a] Smoking prevalence estimates for Africa are based on very limited information and should be used with caution.
[b] Includes countries of Northern Africa, Western Asia and the Central Asian Republics of the former Soviet Union.

Source: WHO estimates.

The extent to which smoking is responsible for deaths from diseases other than lung cancer varies substantially from one population to another. For example, smoking is particularly cardiotoxic for people who already have other risk factors such as high blood cholesterol. The range of other diseases that are caused by smoking is so extensive that the influence of other specific risk factors may effectively average out even in different populations. For example, although in many developing countries, cholesterol levels are low (limiting the cardiotoxic effects of tobacco), a high prevalence of respiratory diseases may greatly increase the pulmonary vulnerability to tobacco.[4]

Smokers have twice the risk of heart attack compared with non-smokers. Smoking is also a major risk factor for sudden death from heart attack, with smokers having two to four times the risk of non-smokers. The risk increases with the number of cigarettes smoked. Overall, cigarette smokers have coronary heart disease (CHD) rates 70% higher than those of non-smokers, with heavy smokers dying from CHD at rate two to three times that of non-smokers.[1] In addition, recent epidemiologic evidence shows that never-smokers exposed to environmental tobacco smoke (ETS) have an increased risk not only for lung cancer but also for cardiovascular disease. Two recent prospective trials[5–7] and meta-analyses[8] estimate the relative risk for cardiovascular diseases at 1.2 to 1.3 individuals exposed to ETS. Of the deaths caused by ETS, the number of deaths from heart disease is about three times the number of non-cardiac deaths.[8]

Cardiovascular deaths account for a significant portion of adult deaths in all countries. Worldwide, slightly more than 50 million people are estimated to have died in 1990, 53% of whom were males. Ischemic heart disease (IHD) was the leading cause of death worldwide, accounting for just under 6.3 million deaths – 2.7 million in established market economies (EME) and formerly socialist economies of Europe (FSE); 3.6 million in the developing regions. Stroke was the next most common cause of death (4.38 million deaths, almost 3 million in developing countries), closely followed by acute respiratory infections.[9] Of the various coronary heart disease pathologies, IHD and stroke predominate in the developed regions, accounting for 75–80% of all cardiovascular deaths. Stroke is proportionately more important as a cause of cardiovascular disease death in FSE (31%) than in EME (25%). Rheumatic heart disease is estimated to cause

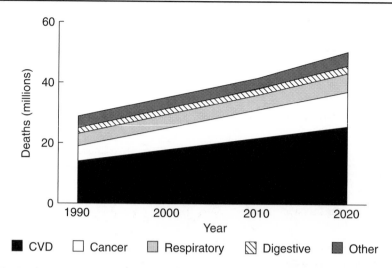

Figure 11.1 Baseline projections of deaths from group II causes, world, 1990–2020 (from Murray and Lopez, 1996,[10] with permission).

between 1% and 6% of all CHD deaths in the developing regions (and about 2.4% globally). The category labeled as inflammatory heart disease (pericarditis, endocarditis, myocarditis, and cardiomyopathies) accounts for similar proportions of CHD deaths, being highest in sub-Saharan Africa (SSA) (7.8%). It is also worth noting the substantial contribution of IHD in all developing regions, ranging from 52% of cardiovascular deaths in India to 26% in SSA. Stroke, on the other hand, is by far the leading cause of cardiovascular deaths in China and SSA, causing roughly half of all coronary heart disease deaths in 1990.[10]

FUTURE PROJECTIONS

Worldwide, a very large increase in deaths from non-communicable diseases (group 2) is expected, with a rise in annual mortality from an estimated 28.1 million deaths in 1990 to 49.7 million in 2020. Conversely, annual mortality from communicable maternal, perinatal, and nutritional disorders (group 1) is predicted to decline from 17.2 million in 1990 to 10.3 million in 2020 (Figure 11.1).

It is of interest to examine how DALYs from various leading causes are expected to change over the next three decades (Figure 11.2). Figure 11.3 shows the change in cause of mortality. IHD is projected to be the leading cause of disability and death by 2020. It has been plausibly predicted that the current global total of about 3 million deaths per year from tobacco (2 million developed, 1 million developing) would reach approximately 10 million deaths per year (3 million developed, 7 million developing) during the second quarter of next century (Figure 11.4). This would mean that over 200 million of today's children and teenagers will be killed by tobacco, as well as a comparable number of today's adults, predicting that a total of about half a billion of the world's population today will be killed by tobacco. About 250 million will die in middle age (35–69), with each person losing about 20 years of life.[1]

In the present century, most of the deaths from smoking have been in the developed countries, but in the next century the opposite will be true. The annual number of deaths from smoking is still increasing in developed population, but it will be increasing

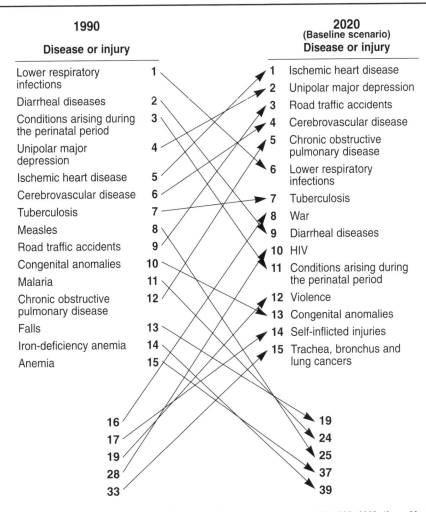

Figure 11.2 Change in rank order of DALYs for the 15 leading causes, world, 1990–2020 (from Murray and Lopez, 1996,[10] with permission).

even faster elsewhere. There has, over the past few decades, been a massive global increase in cigarette consumption, which will have its chief effects on mortality in the next century. However, worldwide mortality from tobacco is still rising rapidly (particularly in less developed countries), partly because of the population growth but chiefly because previous large increases in cigarette smoking by young adults will have caused large increases in mortality by the time the young adults of today are middle aged. In developed countries, 2 million deaths per year are tobacco-attributable. Tobacco is projected to cause about 20 million deaths during this decade. At present, most of these deaths from tobacco in developed countries are in males; however, in many countries female mortality from tobacco will increase substantially as well, due to the large increase in smoking over the past few decades. More than half the deaths from smoking occur between the ages of 35 and 69, making tobacco the most important cause of premature death in developed countries. In developing countries, cigarette sales have increased substantially in recent years. The male prevalence of smoking now exceeds 50% in many parts of the developing world (although the female prevalence is generally

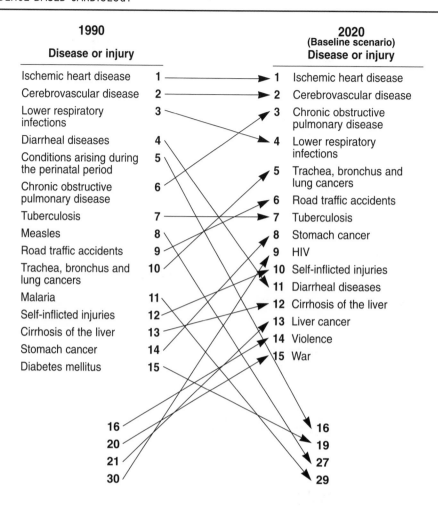

1990

Disease or injury

		2020 (Baseline scenario) **Disease or injury**
Ischemic heart disease	1	1 Ischemic heart disease
Cerebrovascular disease	2	2 Cerebrovascular disease
Lower respiratory infections	3	3 Chronic obstructive pulmonary disease
Diarrheal diseases	4	4 Lower respiratory infections
Conditions arising during the perinatal period	5	5 Trachea, bronchus and lung cancers
Chronic obstructive pulmonary disease	6	6 Road traffic accidents
Tuberculosis	7	7 Tuberculosis
Measles	8	8 Stomach cancer
Road traffic accidents	9	9 HIV
Trachea, bronchus and lung cancers	10	10 Self-inflicted injuries
Malaria	11	11 Diarrheal diseases
Self-inflicted injuries	12	12 Cirrhosis of the liver
Cirrhosis of the liver	13	13 Liver cancer
Stomach cancer	14	14 Violence
Diabetes mellitus	15	15 War
	16	16
	20	19
	21	27
	30	29

Figure 11.3   Change in rank order of deaths for the leading 15 causes, world, 1990–2020 (from Murray and Lopez, 1996,[10] with permission).

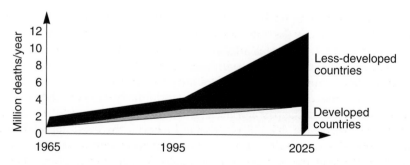

Figure 11.4   Annual deaths attributed to tobacco (WHO Program on Substance Abuse; WHO, 1995 A48/9).

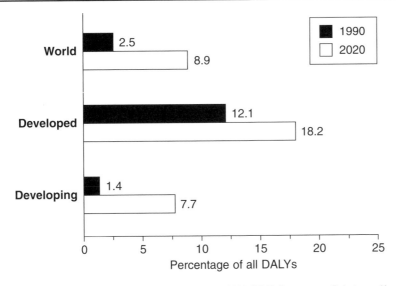

Figure 11.5 Tobacco as a cause of DALYs, 1990 and 2020 (WHO Program on Substance Abuse).

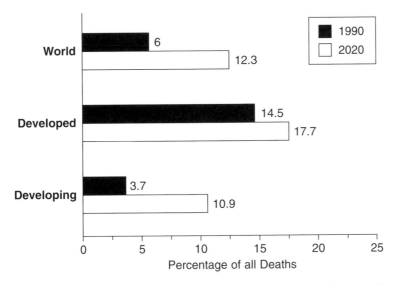

Figure 11.6 Tobacco as a cause of death, 1990 and 2020 (WHO Program on Substance Abuse).

low). This future burden from tobacco use is especially troubling because chronic disease mortality rates are already high in many parts of Asia and Latin America. Overall, in the 1990s the annual number of deaths from tobacco in the developing world was about one million, and is projected to be about 7 million by 2020.

In terms of DALYs, the contribution of tobacco is projected to increase to account for nearly 9% of worldwide burden (18.2% of burden in developed countries and 7.7% in developing countries) in 2020 (Figure 11.5). Tobacco is also projected to cause about 12% of deaths worldwide (17.7% of deaths) in developed countries and 10.9% in developing countries) by 2020 (Figure 11.6). DALYs from cancers are expected to rise from 5.1% to 9.9% of the worldwide total in 2020. The proportionate share of the global burden of disease due to cardiovascular diseases is projected to rise from 11.1%

171

to 14.75%.[11] In conclusion, tobacco is projected to be the leading cause of death and disability globally.

COMMUNITY SOLUTIONS

The relationship between smoking and cardiovascular morbidity and mortality has been extensively documented in the last half of this century. Therefore, the reduction of tobacco use within populations has been a recommended strategy in the primary and secondary prevention of cardiovascular diseases for many years.[12] However, the development and testing of specific strategies to implement this recommendation has proceeded more slowly. During this interval, there has been a paradigm shift from an individual or clinical approach to smoking prevention and cessation to a more public health or population-based approach.[13–15] Community-based cardiovascular prevention trials started in the early 1980s were conducted during this shift in paradigm.[16] Results from all of these trials showed significant declines in the prevalence of smoking overall; however, the declines in the intervention communities did not exceed the declines in the comparison communities by a statistically significant amount in several of the trials[17–20] nor in a joint analysis of the three US community trials.[21]

The community-based cardiovascular prevention trials initiated in the 1980s recognized that the critical behaviors related to cardiovascular risk (e.g. diet, exercise, smoking) all involved individual choices but also involved societal or cultural barriers and enticements, monetary and opportunity costs, local and regional policies, and other communitywide factors.[16] The intervention methods which were developed in these trials shared many common elements, but largely were restricted from applying an ecological and policy oriented health promotion approach that combines educational, political, regulatory, and organizational supports for changes in the target health behaviors.[22] Green and Richard posit that the early community-based cardiovascular prevention trials could rely on an expansion of the traditional health education models which would initiate change in early adopters in societies.[22] However, as the rate of diffusion of the adoption of heart-healthy lifestyle changes (including smoking cessation) accelerated, these more traditional approaches lost efficacy.

The smoking cessation results from the community-based cardiovascular prevention trials initiated in the 1980s must be viewed as modest at best. While the Stanford Five-City Project observed a significantly greater decline ($+13\%$) in smoking rates in the intervention communities among the cohort samples,[23,24] no effect on smoking rates was observed in the cross-sectional surveys by end of treatment[23,24] or at the follow-up during which the comparison communities were declining somewhat, but not significantly, more rapidly than the intervention communities.[25] In the Minnesota Heart Health Project, the long term smoking cessation results were mixed, with evidence of an intervention effect only for women in cross-sectional survey data.[17,26] Unexpectedly strong secular declines in smoking prevalence, especially among men, were observed in comparison communities. In the Pawtucket Heart Health Program, the prevalence of cigarette smoking declined slightly, but not significantly, more in the comparison community.[18]

More recently, the German Cardiovascular Prevention Study has reported more encouraging treatment effects for smoking, observing a 6.7% decline in smoking, with the strongest effect in men.[27] Among men, the prevalence of smoking among 25–69-

year-olds declined from 41.8% in 1985 to 39.2% in 1991 in the national reference sample, in comparison with the significantly greater decline from 44.5% to 37.4% in the intervention regions. This result is consistent with the diffusion model posited by Green[22,28] that the largely individually oriented health educational approaches applied in the community-based cardiovascular prevention trials initiated in the 1980s have their largest impact among populations who are at the earlier stages of adoption of the recommended preventive lifestyle.

In addition to the community-based cardiovascular prevention trials initiated in the 1980s, the Community Intervention Trial for Smoking Cessation (COMMIT) was started in the late 1980s. COMMIT focused solely on smoking cessation and built upon the initial experience in the ongoing cardiovascular prevention trials. Additionally, COMMIT was planned as a randomized community trial with 11 pairs of communities and had adequate power to detect relatively small intervention effects.[29] The modest effects observed in this trial were very sobering for the public health community. No cessation effect was observed for the "heavy" smokers (defined as smoking 25 or more cigarettes per day at baseline) for whom the trial was specifically designed. Among the evaluation cohorts of light-to-moderate smokers, a significantly greater quit rate (30.6% vs 27.5%) was observed over the four-year intervention period, with the effect strongest among the less educated residents of the communities.[19] Overall, the prevalence of smoking declined slightly, but non-significantly, more in the intervention communities (3.5 percentage points) than in the comparison communities (3.2 percentage points). While the COMMIT intervention protocol sought to apply the best smoking cessation strategies available, investigators were limited in their ability to be involved in many of the ecological and policy oriented health promotion strategies which Green and others[12,22] recommend due to the federal sources of funds for the study. While an intervention "receipt index" of the strategies applied significantly correlated with quit rate differences across the 11 community pairs among the light-to-moderate smokers, process data showed that implemented protocol did *not* change many important intermediate variables (e.g. MD/DDS counseling rates, worksite smoking bans, public attitudes toward smoking).

Several reviewers have provided some perspectives on the modest smoking cessation effects which have been observed in these community trials.[16,22,30–32] Common themes are (1) the difficulty in observing intervention effects relative to the large secular declines in cardiovascular risk factors, including smoking, occurring during the period when the trials were implemented, and (2) the need for a more ecological and policy oriented health promotion approach to be applied. Within this perspective, results from these trials in combination with more recent data from other large scale interventions, such as the excise tax funded efforts in the US (e.g., California and Massachusetts) and other countries, support a multicomponent population-based approach to tobacco control. This model includes six key elements:

1. Prevention.
2. Treatment and cessation.
3. Reduction of exposure to environmental tobacco smoke.
4. Counter-advertising and promotion.
5. Economic incentives.
6. Product regulation.

In many ways, this model is a refinement of the population-based approach first outlined in 1979 by the WHO Expert Committee on Smoking Control[12] and more recently updated.[33]

The scientific rationale for this population-based approach to controlling smoking and tobacco use in industrialized societies has been growing in recent years. Significant and sustained declines in population level measures of tobacco use have been demonstrated in many countries.[33] Initial data from California and Massachusetts[34] and some demonstration trials[27] also show that large scale public health actions on tobacco prevention and control can produce significant declines in tobacco use. Nevertheless, the partial application of the model has not been demonstrated to be effective in some controlled trials (i.e. COMMIT). Therefore, the data on individual elements in the model as well as the model overall will be discussed. Given the importance of reducing population levels of tobacco use in the primary prevention of cardiovascular diseases, as well as many other chronic diseases, efforts to apply and evaluate the full model more widely are needed.

Tobacco use is an individual behavior, and individually focused educational and clinical interventions have dominated the history of public health approaches to this problem. Too often, the interventions have focused on only a small segment of the overall societal problem of tobacco use. In the area of prevention of tobacco use among youth, this has been particularly true. Excellent social–psychological approaches were applied to school-based prevention programs in the past two decades.[38] School-based smoking prevention programs that identify social influences to smoke and teach skills to resist those influences have demonstrated consistent and significant reductions in adolescent smoking prevalence, and program effects have lasted between one and three years.[35] However, it has been noted that these effects have tended to attenuate over time and that the durability of the effect is enhanced by communitywide programs that involve parents, mass media, community organizations, and other elements of an adolescent's social environment.[35–37] Unfortunately, the full range of recommended communitywide efforts to modify the social environments of adolescents,[35] including removal of pervasive imagery-based pro-tobacco advertising, significant tobacco tax increases, enhanced enforcement of minors' access laws, and well financed and sustained youth oriented counter-advertising campaigns, need to be applied in conjunction with experimentally tested school-based tobacco use prevention curricula and tobacco-free school policies. This comprehensive approach to youth tobacco use prevention is only beginning to be applied in states such as Massachusetts and California. During the period of the 1990s when smoking rates among youth in the United States were consistently increasing, rates in Massachusetts and California appear to have risen more slowly[38] and even declined among 7–8 graders in Massachusetts.[39] If national efforts to limit the influence of pervasive imagery-based pro-tobacco advertising[40] can be applied, several states which have received recent funding for tobacco control, such as Oregon, Maine, Florida, and Mississippi, may be able to institute even more effective comprehensive youth prevention efforts.

In many ways, efforts to assist adult smokers to quit smoking have made the slowest progress in the paradigm shift from the clinical to the public health model. While most cessation still occurs outside formal treatment,[41] the focus of most cessation research has been on improvement of clinical preventive services. Dramatic improvements in these treatment modalities have been made,[42] especially related to Nicotine Replacement Therapies.[43,44] However, the most significant and sustained declines in population levels of cigarette consumption have been observed in California and Massachusetts where changes in the social environments rather than enhanced clinical services have been the focus of the programs.[34] One of the major elements of the programs in these states has been the focus on protection of non-smokers from environmental tobacco smoke

(ETS). Extensive smoking policy and environmental changes at worksites, public places, and in homes appear to have been significant factors, along with excise tax increases and mass media educational efforts, related to cigarette consumption rates declining two to three times faster than in the rest of the nation combined.[34]

The importance of the price of tobacco products on a society's level of tobacco use is now widely accepted.[33,35] Numerous econometric studies have confirmed that increases in cigarette excise taxes both decrease consumption and increase quitting among current smokers as well as discourage smoking initiation among youth.[35,45,46] The most recent research among youth indicates that for every 10% increase in price, youth smoking rates would decrease by 7%.[38] In Massachusetts, preliminary data suggest that rates of smokeless tobacco use among youths also are very price sensitive.[39] Data from California and Massachusetts, which are both states whose tobacco prevention and control programs were funded by raising the state excise tax, indicate that, while increasing excise taxes on cigarettes may be one of the most cost-effective short term strategies to reduce tobacco consumption among adults and prevent youth initiation of tobacco use, the ability to sustain this reduction in per capita consumption was greater when the tax increase was combined with population-based tobacco prevention campaign, including counter-advertising and environmental changes.[34]

Tobacco products have been largely unregulated in comparison to other consumer products. While the importance of nicotine addiction is now well recognized as a factor maintaining tobacco use behaviors,[47] regulatory efforts to decrease the addictiveness of the product are only now emerging.[48] Based upon the experience related to the widespread adoption of so called "light" cigarettes in recent decades, the need for public education related to the tobacco products they choose is now becoming recognized.[49]

The full multicomponent population-based approach to tobacco control, including the six key elements of prevention, treatment and cessation, reduction of exposure to environmental tobacco smoke, counter-advertising and promotion, economic incentives, and product regulation[50] has yet to be applied fully. In the states of Massachusetts and California where sufficient resources have been available from excise tax increases to fund comprehensive state-wide programs, initial results indicate that substantial effects on adult smoking consumption and prevalence are being observed. However, even in these states, all aspects of the recommendations have not been applied fully. Based upon the experience from these states, the latest states (i.e., Oregon, Maine, Florida, Mississippi) which are receiving funding for comprehensive tobacco prevention and control programs either from excise tax increases or other sources are developing what may be even more efficient and effective programs.

Following the passage of a voters' initiative in Oregon in November 1996, the State Health Division, with technical assistance from CDC, began developing and implementing a comprehensive tobacco-use prevention and education program incorporating components that have been effective in past research and other state-wide demonstration efforts.[51] The Oregon Tobacco Prevention and Education Program will have four major components:

1. **Local coalition and community-based activities program** operated through grants to local health departments. The 1995 Oregon Statewide Tobacco Prevention Plan will serve as a guidebook for the community prevention and education programs, including retailer education, youth prevention programs, reducing secondhand smoke exposure, and cessation programs. An innovative "Community-Based Best

Practices to Reduce Tobacco Use" Toolkit Manual has been developed to guide these local programs.

2. **Comprehensive school-based prevention programs** funded by grants to school districts to implement programs based upon the CDC's Guidelines for School Health Programs to Prevent Tobacco Use and Addiction.[52] To be awarded a grant, districts must contract to implement programs which include all of the following essential elements: no-tobacco school policies for youth and adults; effective prevention curriculum for grades 6–8; staff/teacher training; involvement of parents and families; links to community prevention work; cessation support throughout the school; and participation in statewide evaluation efforts.

3. **Statewide public awareness and education campaign** will deliver multimedia messages about the dangers of tobacco use and secondhand smoke, as well as the value of prevention and cessation programs. Additional elements of the campaign will include high viability prevention and recognition events, education materials and the use of role models to promote tobacco-free lives and communities.

4. **Statewide and regional projects program** will award grants for special populations for innovative and specially targeted tobacco prevention and education programs. These projects will include grants to Indian Tribes, a quitter's hotline, local training, conferences and technical assistance on the best practices for effective programs, and grants to other special populations, including multicultural groups.

The Oregon Health Division will guide the implementation of this program and coordinate the overall evaluation effort. This "Oregon Model" is viewed as an improved and more efficient statewide program model. It is now being quickly diffused out to Maine, Florida, and Mississippi and other States to guide the development of newly funded programs.

As results are obtained from these most recent states as well as continuing data from California and Massachusetts, our understanding of the potential effectiveness of the full multicomponent population-based approach to tobacco prevention and control will be known.

REFERENCES

1 Peto R, Lopez AD, Boreham J, Thun M, Heath C Jr. *Mortality from smoking in developed countries 1950–2000.* Indirect estimates from National Vital Statistics. Oxford: Oxford University Press (Oxford Medical Publication), 1994.

2 Murray CJL, Lopez AD (eds). *The global burden of disease. A comprehensive assessment of mortality and disability from diseases, injuries, and risk factors in 1990 and projected to 2020.* Cambridge, MA: Harvard University Press, 1996.

3 World Health organization. *Tobacco or health: global status report.* Geneva: WHO, 1997.

4 US Department of Health and Human Services. *The health consequences of smoking: cardiovascular disease.* (A Report of the Surgeon General.) DHHS publication PHS 84-50204. Rockville, MD: Public Health Service, Office on Smoking and Health; 1984.

5 Steenland K, Thun M, Lally C, Heath C. Environmental tobacco smoke and coronary heart disease in the American Cancer Society CPS-II cohort. *Circulation* 1996;**94**:622–8.

6 Kawachi I, Colditz GA, Speizer FE *et al.* A prospective study of passive smoking and coronary heart disease. *Circulation* 1997;**95**:2374–9.

7 Howard G, Wagenknecht LE, Burke GL *et al.* for the ARIC investigators. Cigarette smoking and progression of atherosclerosis: the Atherosclerosis Risk in Communities (ARIC) study. *JAMA* 1998;**279**:119–24.

8 Glantz SA, Parmley WW. Passive smoking and heart disease: epidemiology, physiology, and biochemistry. *Circulation* 1991;**83**:1–2.

9 Murray, CJL, Lopez A. Mortality by cause for eight regions of the world: Global Burden of Disease Study. *Lancet* 1997;**149**:1274.

10 Murray CJL, Lopez AD (eds). *The Global Burden of Disease. A comprehensive assessment of mortality*

and disability from diseases, injuries, and risk factors in 1990 and projected to 2020. Cambridge, MA: Harvard University Press, 1996.

11 Murray CJL, Lopez AD. Alternative projections of mortality and disability by cause 1990–2020: Global Burden of Disease Study. *Lancet* **349**;1997: 1502.

12 World Health Organization. *Report of the WHO Expert Committee on Smoking Control. Controlling the smoking epidemic.* WHO Technical Report Series No. 636; Geneva: WHO, 1979.

13 Jeffery TW. Risk behaviors and health. *Am Psychol* 1989;**44**:1194–202.

14 Lichtenstein E, Glasgow RE. Smoking cessation: what have we learned over the past decade? *J Consult Clin Psychol* 1992;**60**:518–27.

15 National Cancer Institute. *Strategies to control tobacco use in the United States: a blueprint for public health action in the 1990s.* Smoking and Tobacco Control Monographs No. 1. Rockville, MD: US Department of Health and Human Services, National Cancer Institute, 1991.

16 Luepker RV. Community trials. *Prev Med* 1994; **23**:602–5.

17 Luepker RV, Murray DM, Jacobs DR *et al.* Community education for cardiovascular disease prevention: risk factor changes in the Minnesota Heart Health Program. *Am J Publ Hlth* 1994;**84**: 1383–93.

18 Carleton RA, Lasater TM, Assaf AR *et al.* The Pawtucket Heart Health program: community changes in cardiovascular risk factors and projected disease risk. *Am J Publ Hlth* 1995;**85**: 777–85.

19 The COMMIT Research Group. Community intervention trial for smoking cessation: I. Cohort results from a 4-year community intervention. *Am J Publ Hlth* 1995;**85**:183–92.

20 The COMMIT Research Group. Community intervention trial for smoking cessation: II. Changes in adult cigarette smoking prevalence. *Am J Publ Hlth* 1995;**85**:193–200.

21 Winkleby MA, Feldman HA, Murray DM. Joint analysis of three US community intervention trials for reduction of cardiovascular disease risk. *J Clin Epidemiol* 1997;**50**:645–58.

22 Green LW, Richard L. The need to combine health education and health promotion: the case for cardiovascular disease prevention. *Promotion ET Education.* 1993; Special No. 11–8.

23 Farquhar JW, Fortmann, SP, Flora JA *et al.* Effects of community wide education on cardiovascular disease risk factors. *JAMA* 1990;**264**:359–65.

24 Fortmann SP, Taylor, CB, Flora JA, Jatulis DE. Changes in adult cigarette smoking prevalence after five years of community health education: the Stanford Five-City Project. *Am J Epidemiol* 1993;**137**:82–96.

25 Winkelby MA, Taylor CB, Jatulis D, Fortmann SP. The long-term effects of a cardiovascular disease prevention trial: the Stanford Five-City Project. *Am J Publ Hlth* 1996;**86**:1773–9.

26 Lando HA, Pechacek TF, Pirie PL *et al.* Changes in adult cigarette smoking in the Minnesota Heart Health Program. *Am J Publ Hlth* 1995;**85**:201–8.

27 Hoffmeister H, Mensink GBM, Stolzenberg H *et al.* Reduction of coronary heart disease risk factors in the German Cardiovascular Prevention Study. *Prev Med* 1996;**25**:135–45.

28 Green LW, Johnson JL. Dissemination and utilization of health promotion and disease prevention knowledge: theory, research, and experience. *Can J Publ Hlth* 1996;**87**:S11–17.

29 Gail MH, Byar DP, Pechacek TF, Corle DK, for the COMMIT Study Group. Aspects of statistical design for the community intervention trial for smoking cessation (COMMIT). *Control Clin Trials* 1992;**13**:6–21 [and erratum, *Control Clin Trials* 1993;**14**:253–4].

30 Susser M. Editorial: The tribulation of trials – intervention in communities. *Am J Publ Hlth* 1995;**85**:156–8.

31 Fisher EB: The results of the COMMIT Trial. *Am J Publ Hlth* 1995;**85**:159–60.

32 MA. The future of community-based cardiovascular disease intervention studies (Editorial). *Am H Publ Hlth* 1994;**84**:1369–72.

33 World Health Organization. Guidelines for controlling and monitoring the tobacco epidemic. Geneva: WHO Tobacco or Health Programme, 1996.

34 Centers for Disease Control and Prevention. Cigarette smoking before and after an excise tax increase and an antismoking campaign. *MMWR* 1996;**45**:966–70.

35 US Department of Health and Human Services. *Preventing tobacco use among young people.* (A Report of the Surgeon General). Rockville, MD: Public Health Service, Centers for Disease Control and Prevention, National Center for Chronic Disease Prevention and Health Promotion, Office on Smoking and Health, 1994.

36 Perry CL, Kelder SH, Murray DM, Klepp KI *et al.* Communitywide smoking prevention: long-term outcomes of the Minnesota Heart Health Program and the Class of 1989 Study. *Am J Publ Hlth* 1992;**82**:1210–16.

37 Flynn BS, Worden JK, Secker-Walker RH *et al.* Mass media and school interventions for cigarette smoking prevention: effects 2 years after completion. *Am J Publ Hlth* 1994;**87**:1148–50.

38 Chaloupka FJ, Grossman M. Price, tobacco control, policies and youth smoking. Working Paper Series No. 5740. Cambridge, MA: National Bureau of Economic Research, 1996.

39 Health and Addictions Research, Inc. *Adolescent tobacco use in Massachusetts: trends among public*

school students, 1984–1996. Boston, MA: The Commonwealth of Massachusetts, Department of Public Health, 1997.

40 Gostin LO, Arno PS, Brandt AM. FDA regulation of tobacco advertising and youth smoking: historical, social and constitutional perspectives. *JAMA* 1997;**277**:410–18.

41 Fiore MC, Novotny TE, Pierce JP *et al.* Methods used to quit smoking in the US: do cessation programs help? *JAMA* 1990;**263**:2760–5.

42 Consensus Statement. The Agency for Health Care Policy and Research Smoking Cessation Clinical Practice Guideline. *JAMA* 1996;**275**;1270–80.

43 Fiore MC, Smith SS, Jorenby DE, Baker TB. The effectiveness of the nicotine patch for smoking cessation. A meta-analysis. *JAMA* 1994;**271**:2–9.

44 Law M, Tang JL. An analysis of the effectiveness of interventions intended to help people stop smoking. *Arch Intern Med* 1995;**155**:1933–41.

45 US General Accounting Office. Teenage smoking; higher excise tax should significantly reduce the number of smokers. GAO/HRD-89-119, June 1989.

46 National Cancer Institute. *The impact of cigarette excise taxes on smoking among children and adults.* Summary Report of a National Cancer Institute Expert Panel. Bethesda, Maryland: National Cancer Institute, Division of Cancer Prevention and Control, Cancer Control Science Program, 1993.

47 US Department of Health and Human Services. *The health consequences of smoking: nicotine addiction.* (A Report of the Surgeon General). DHHS publication (CDC) 88-8406, Rockville, MD: Public Health Service, Centers for Disease Control, Center for Health Promotion and Education, 1988.

48 Warner KE, Slade J, Sweanor DT. The emerging market for long-term nicotine maintenance. *JAMA* 1997;**278**:1087–92.

49 Kozlowski LT, Goldberg ME, Yost BA *et al.* Smokers are unaware of the filter vents now on most cigarettes: results of a national survey. *Tobacco Control* 1996;**5;265–70.**

50 **Office on Smoking and Health.** *CDC's tobacco use prevention program: working toward a healthier future.* Rockville, MD: US Department of Health and Human Services, Public Health Services, Centers for Disease Control and Prevention, 1996.

51 Centers for Disease Control and Prevention. Tobacco tax initiative. *MMWR* 1997;**46**: 246–8.

52 Centers for Disease Control. Guidelines for school health programs to prevent tobacco use and addiction. *MMWR Recommendations and Reports* 1994;**43**:1–18, No. RR-2.

Tobacco and cardiovascular disease: achieving smoking cessation

12

GODFREY FOWLER

INTRODUCTION

Worldwide, there are about one billion current smokers and about three million die annually from their smoking, half before the age of 70. This includes about 150 000 annually in the UK and half a million in the USA.[1] Even in countries where the health hazards of smoking are widely acknowledged, it remains a common behavior: in the USA and Canada, for example, about a quarter of all adults smoke and in the UK, the situation is worse with about one third of adults smoking.

Cardiovascular disease, in particular ischemic heart disease, is the commonest smoking-related cause of death in developed countries.[2] This is because although the relative risk of death from cardiovascular disease in smokers, compared with non-smokers, is much lower than the relative risk from cancer (in particular lung cancer) and chronic obstructive lung disease, ischemic heart disease is much the commonest cause of death in these countries. Overall, the relative risk of death from cardiovascular disease in smokers compared with non-smokers is roughly doubled, though this varies with the different cardiovascular diseases and is greater at a younger age. Passive smoking also increases the risk of cardiovascular disease but the extent of this increase remains uncertain.[3,4]

STRATEGIES FOR TOBACCO CONTROL

Strategies for reducing the health consequences of smoking should aim to:

- reduce the uptake of smoking by young people;
- increase the numbers of smokers stopping smoking;
- encourage a shift to less harmful tobacco use;
- decrease exposure to environmental tobacco smoke.

Reducing the uptake of smoking by young people is a priority in many countries. Laws to ban tobacco sales to those below a certain age and to prohibit tobacco advertising and promotion are common in developed countries but are frequently contravened. Other measures include restrictions on smoking in public places, fiscal policies to increase the cost of smoking, and a variety of educational programs. In spite of these, smoking prevalence in teenagers has remained remarkably resistant to change over the last decade and in the UK about a quarter of young people are regular smokers by the age of 16 years.

Modification of cigarettes, particularly with regard to tar yield, over the last two or three decades has undoubtedly contributed to less harmful tobacco use but it should be emphasized that this is no substitute for tobacco avoidance. But although such changes have certainly contributed to a decline in lung cancer, possible benefits from these changes relating to cardiovascular disease have not yet been established with certainty.[5]

Decreased exposure to environmental tobacco smoke is a desirable objective in itself but, again, the contribution this might make to reducing cardiovascular disease risk is very difficult to estimate.

For established smokers, smoking cessation is the most important step to safeguarding future health and this chapter will consider evidence based methods of achieving this objective.

EVIDENCE OF BENEFITS FROM SMOKING CESSATION

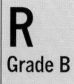

R
Grade B

Many observational epidemiological studies have investigated the effect of stopping smoking on smoking-related diseases and there is a wealth of evidence that not only is tobacco smoking a major risk factor for cardiovascular disease, but also stopping smoking reduces this risk. But there is less agreement about the rate at which the risk attenuates after smoking cessation. In the 20-year follow-up of the British Doctors Study, for example, excess risk was halved within two or three years of smoking cessation and by 10 years the risk had returned to that of a non-smoker[6] (Figure 12.1).

However, follow-up of the cohort men in the British Regional Heart Study indicates that attenuation of risk is much slower and even men who had given up smoking for more than 10 years still had an increased risk, compared with non-smokers[7] (Figure 12.2).

Following myocardial infarction, smoking cessation confers substantial benefits and is particularly important. In one observational study, stopping smoking halved both the number of non-fatal recurrences and the number of cardiovascular deaths[8] (Figure 12.3).

In another study, follow-up over 13 years of postmyocardial infarction patients showed a 37% mortality in those who had stopped smoking, compared with 82% mortality in those who continued smoking.[9] Furthermore, a UK trial of smoking cessation advice in smokers with evidence of ischemic heart disease showed a (non-significant) 13% difference in cumulative coronary heart disease deaths over 20 years in those given smoking cessation advice, compared with those who were not.[10]

The mechanisms through which tobacco smoking mediates its adverse cardiovascular effects are largely unknown and certainly multiple. There is evidence that smoking contributes to both the atherosclerotic and the thrombotic processes; free radical

180

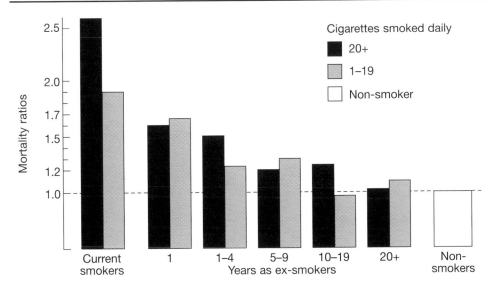

Figure 12.1 Diminished risk of death from coronary heart disease in former light and heavy smokers. Both light and heavy smokers show a steady decline in risk after stopping until, after 10–20 years, it is little different from the risk of non-smokers. (Source: Royal College of Physicians. *Smoking or health?* London: Pitman Medical, 1977.)

damage to vascular endothelium has been demonstrated, as have effects on platelet survival, platelet aggregation, and fibrinogen levels.[11-13]

THE NATURE OF TOBACCO SMOKING

Before considering individual smoking interventions and cessation methods, it is helpful to review briefly the nature of tobacco smoking and the consequent implications for interventions.

Tobacco smoking is a complex behavior to which psychological, social, and pharmacological factors contribute.[14] Its acquisition is almost invariably in adolescence, as the result of desire for experimental rebellious behavior which is perceived as adult and encouraged by peer group pressure. But pharmacological addiction usually then becomes a factor determining persistence of the behavior and making it difficult to stop because of the addictive effects of nicotine and the discomforts associated with withdrawal. Although the balance between psychological factors and pharmacological addiction varies from smoker to smoker, there is now increasing awareness of the importance of nicotine addiction in maintaining smoking behavior and the powerful nature of this addiction has been compared with addiction to heroin or cocaine.[15]

THE EVIDENCE BASIS FOR SMOKING CESSATION

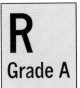

Emphasis on smoking cessation in individual established smokers is a vital component of any tobacco control strategy and should complement efforts to prevent the uptake of smoking by young people. But individual approaches to both cessation and avoidance

181

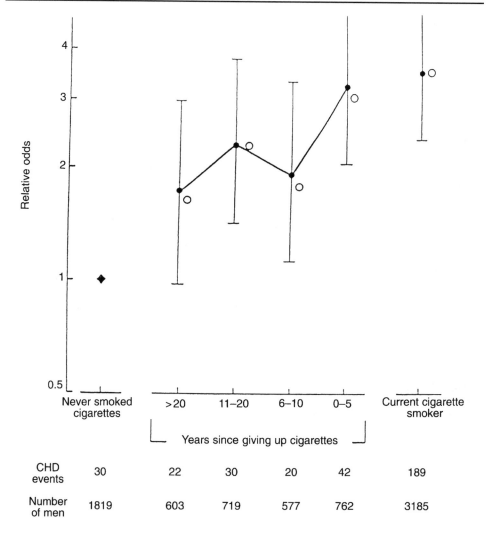

	Never smoked cigarettes	>20	11–20	6–10	0–5	Current cigarette smoker
CHD events	30	22	30	20	42	189
Number of men	1819	603	719	577	762	3185

Years since giving up cigarettes

Figure 12.2 Relative odds of a major CHD event in relation to years since stopping smoking cigarettes. (Source: Cook *et al*.[7])

can only be supplementary to "whole population" approaches, including legislation (banning sales to "minors" and controlling advertising promotion), restrictions on smoking, public information and campaigns, tax measures, and so on.

For many established smokers, stopping smoking is very difficult, for both behavioral and psychopharmacological reasons, and only a minority of established smokers ever succeed in stopping for good. Most of those who succeed in stopping find the process of stopping is a dynamic one rather than a single discrete event (Figure 12.4).

Relapses are common and eventual success is usually the outcome of many attempts. Motivation to stop and confidence in the ability to succeed are important predictors of success. Relapse in the first few weeks is a common pattern, but the tendency to relapse

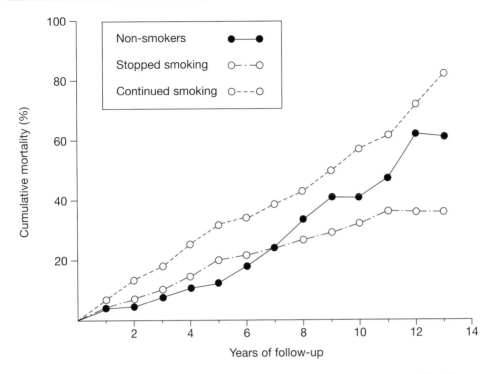

Figure 12.3 Cumulative mortality for 498 survivors of a coronary attack by smoking habit. Life table curves start 2 years after attack. Average annual mortality was 6.5% in non-smokers, 3.7% in those who stopped smoking, and 10.2% in those who continued smoking. (Source: Daly *et al.*[9])

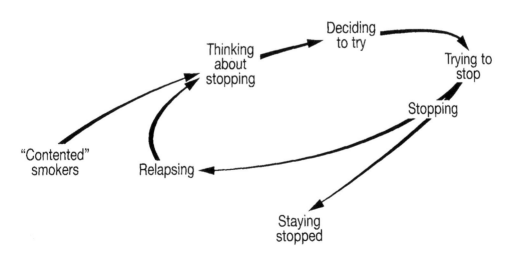

Figure 12.4 Stopping smoking is a process.

declines as time progresses and most of those who manage to avoid relapse for a year are then able to achieve sustained abstinence.

The great majority of those smokers who do achieve long term smoking cessation do so on their own without any special aids or assistance. But research has shown that smoking cessation advice and support from a health professional and the use of smoking cessation aids can enhance the chances of success.[16]

As already indicated, motivation to stop smoking is critical to success and this motivation may be determined by a variety of concerns – personal health, family health, financial anxieties, social pressures, and so on. The so-called Stages of Change model acknowledges different levels of motivation and activity, from precontemplation through contemplation, preparation and action, to maintenance or relapse.[17] Identification of the stage which an individual smoker is at can enable motivational or interventional methods to be targeted more appropriately (though the evidence basis for the effectiveness of such targeting is currently lacking).

A favorable factor is that the majority of smokers in many countries report that they want to quit smoking and have tried to do so, often many times. They also cite advice from a health professional as being important to them in influencing their motivation to quit. Surprisingly perhaps, only a minority of smokers say they have ever been asked by a doctor about smoking and advised to stop.[14]

COMMUNITY INTERVENTIONS

Community or population based smoking cessation interventions have been implemented in a number of settings. Typically, they involve use of mass media to promote public awareness and education and to encourage health professionals to raise smoking as an issue in consultations with patients and to offer self-help materials. Evaluation of the effectiveness of such programs is difficult and they are discussed in Chapter 11.

INDIVIDUAL ADVICE

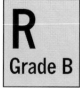

R

Grade B

Individual smoking interventions by health professionals have been extensively studied.[16] An early and influential trial in the UK was conducted by Russell and colleagues in general practices in London in the 1970s. In this study, over 2000 smokers attending their general practitioners for routine consultations were randomly allocated to a non-intervention control group and three intervention groups; these were (a) completion of a brief smoking questionnaire, (b) brief (1–2 minutes) smoking cessation advice, and (c) brief advice supplemented with a simple self-help smoking cessation leaflet. Smoking cessation rates achieved at 1 month and sustained for 1 year were 1.6%, 3.3%, and 5.1% respectively in three intervention groups compared with 0.3% in the control group[18] (Figure 12.5).

Many similar randomized controlled trials of simple, brief smoking cessation advice in medical settings have subsequently been conducted and this finding of a small percentage of biochemically validated long term smoking cessation, resulting from such interventions, has been replicated.[19]

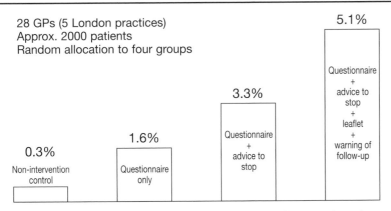

28 GPs (5 London practices)
Approx. 2000 patients
Random allocation to four groups

5.1%

Questionnaire
+
advice to
stop
+
leaflet
+
warning of
follow-up

3.3%

Questionnaire
+
advice to
stop

1.6%

0.3%

Questionnaire
only

Non-intervention
control

% = proportion who stopped smoking during the first month and
were still not smoking 1 year later (P< 0.001)
Equivalent to 25 long term successes per GP each year

Figure 12.5 Effect of GP's advice against smoking. (Based on Russell *et al.*[18])

NICOTINE REPLACEMENT

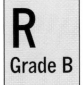

R

Grade B

The advent of nicotine chewing gum in the 1970s provided the first specific pharmacological "treatment" for smoking cessation. Subsequent development of transdermal nicotine patches, nicotine nasal sprays, and nicotine oral inhalers has increased the range of products available. The objective in using these "nicotine replacement" products is to provide a temporary alternative source of nicotine to allay withdrawal symptoms and so enhance the potential for smoking cessation. Large placebo-controlled trials have clearly demonstrated that the use of such products as an adjunct to advice from a health professional can approximately double smoking cessation rates, compared with placebo.[20,21] Several systematic reviews of the many trials which have now been conducted with them have confirmed the benefits and shown that all preparations are effective, but the evidence is particularly substantial for nicotine gum and nicotine patches.[22,23] Both appear to have similar effectiveness but, because of greater social acceptability, ease of use, and simpler compliance, transdermal patches have been found by many to be preferable, though gum appears more effective for the most dependent smokers. A summary of the effectiveness of nicotine replacement therapies and estimates of the number needed to treat (NNT) to achieve one success are provided in Table 12.1.

Table 12.1 Nicotine replacement therapy preparations and abstinence

NRT preparation (no. of trials)	% Quitting		OR (95% CI)	NNT
	Active	Control		
Gum (39)	18.2	10.6	1.6 (1.5–1.8)	13
Patches (9)	20.5	10.8	2.1 (1.6–2.6)	10
Nasal spray (1)	25.9	9.9	2.9 (1.5–5.7)	6
Inhaler (1)	15.2	5.0	3.0 (1.4–6.6)	10

NRT, nicotine replacement therapy; OR, odds ratio.

PATIENTS WITH CARDIOVASCULAR DISEASE

Concern has been expressed about the use of nicotine replacement products in patients with cardiovascular disease because of the potentially adverse effects of nicotine on the cardiovascular system. But in considering this issue, it is important to be aware that use of nicotine replacement is advocated only as a temporary substitute source of nicotine in those already self-administering this drug through tobacco smoking. It is also important to bear in mind that blood levels of nicotine achieved with nicotine replacement products are substantially lower than those achieved by moderate or heavy smoking. Furthermore, there is no evidence that nicotine itself contributes to the atherogenetic or thrombotic processes, unlike tobacco smoking.

In a placebo-controlled randomized trial specifically investigating the safety of transdermal nicotine patches in patients with cardiac disease, no increase was found in rates of arrhythmia, myocardial infarction or death in high risk patients (with a history of myocardial infarction or coronary revascularization procedure or of angina, heart failure, arrhythmia, peripheral vascular disease or cerebral vascular disease) in those using nicotine patches compared with those using placebo patches.[24]

REVIEW OF CESSATION STUDIES

In a comprehensive systematic review of 188 randomized controlled trials of the efficacy of a wide range of interventions aimed at helping people to stop smoking, it was concluded that simple advice, even on one occasion only, given by a doctor in general or family practice or in a hospital clinic to all smokers who consulted resulted in sustained cessation of about 2% and that additional encouragement and support (additional visits, exhaled CO measurement, letters, etc.) further enhances this effect.[25] Whether similar interventions delivered by nurses are equally effective remains uncertain,[26] though there is evidence that nurse support, subsequent to doctor advice, can enhance the effect of this.[27]

This comprehensive review[25] also endorsed the use of nicotine replacement therapy but concluded that a variety of other smoking cessation interventions – hypnosis, acupuncture, aversion therapy, and pharmacological agents other than nicotine, which are sometimes advocated – have not been shown by rigorous scientific evidence to be effective, though it must be acknowledged that the methodological problems associated with attempts to evaluate these have yet to be overcome. A summary of estimates of effectiveness is provided in Table 12.2.

SPECIALIST SMOKING CESSATION CLINICS

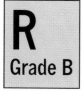

R
Grade B

Specialist smoking cessation clinics have been shown to deliver effective interventions and can make a useful contribution to the provision of individual interventions, usually by providing regular group treatments. There is some evidence that they can achieve enhanced attendance and abstinence rates as high as 20% or more. But interpretation of their success should take account of the fact that they recruit widely and participants are generally highly motivated to stop, compared with the majority of those expressing

Table 12.2 Summary estimates of randomized controlled trials of interventions to help people to stop smoking

Intervention	% estimate of efficacy (95% CIs)	Statistical significance	Number of subjects (trials)	Comment
Simple physician advice (once)	2 (1,3)	<0.001	14 438 (17)	Effective
Physician advice with additional encouragement/support	5 (1,8)	<0.01	6466 (10)	Effective
Nurse advice	1 (−1,3)	>0.10	3369 (2)	Unproven
Advice in infarct survivors	36 (23,48)	<0.001	223 (1)	Important
Advice in healthy men at high CHD risk	21 (10,31)	<0.001	13 205 (4)	Important
Hypnosis	24 (10,38)	<0.001	646 (10)	No trials with biochemical validation
Acupuncture	3 (−1,6)	>0.10	2759 (8)	No trials with biochemical validation

Adapted from Law *et al.*[25]

an intention to do so. When available, they offer a self-referral and secondary referral service and can provide valuable opportunities for smoking cessation research.[28] But as they are relatively few in number in relation to the huge need for such interventions, their overall contribution will inevitably be small.

PRACTICAL ASPECTS OF SMOKING CESSATION IN CLINICAL PRACTICE

The essential features of individual smoking cessation interventions in medical practice are to:

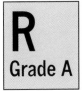

R
Grade A

- *assess* in any medical consultation the smoking status of the patient, whether a non-smoker, smoker or ex-smoker;
- *advise* all smokers about the desirability and importance of stopping smoking because of health hazards, especially those who already have smoking-related diseases;
- *assist* smokers to stop smoking, particularly those with smoking-related diseases and especially if expressing interest to do so;
- *follow up* at subsequent consultations to assess the outcome and, if necessary, further assist those trying to stop smoking while encouraging ex-smokers to maintain their non-smoking status.[29]

Assessment

The smoking status of all patients should be recorded in medical records in such a way that the information is easily accessible in future consultations. Assessment of smoking should include a brief history of the patient's smoking, including attempts to stop and their current tobacco consumption. Assessment of nicotine addiction should also be made by enquiring how soon after waking they smoke their first cigarette and some assessment of their motivation to stop smoking.

Advice

All patients with smoking-related diseases should be advised to stop smoking and any reasons that patients put forward for wanting to stop smoking should be strongly reinforced.

Assistance

Specific help with smoking cessation should be strongly influenced by patients' preferences and patients should themselves be active in deciding what to do. There is no set "prescription" for how to go about stopping smoking, but it is possible to provide

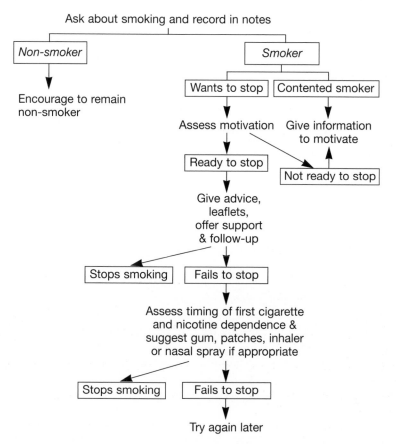

Figure 12.6   Smoking cessation protocol for doctor/nurse intervention.

guidance which experience has shown to be useful. It is important to adopt an individual approach but guidance might include:

- setting a target date for stopping;
- some preparation for stopping, review of motivation and reasons for stopping;
- awareness of times when a particular need is felt for a cigarette and attempts to change routines to avoid association of these times with smoking;
- eliciting support for cessation from friends and colleagues and, ideally, recruiting a fellow smoker (particularly a spouse) to join in the attempt to give up smoking.

Generally, sudden complete withdrawal is likely to be more successful than attempts to gradually reduce smoking. Strategies need to be planned for coping with withdrawal symptoms and other difficulties likely to be encountered immediately after cessation; avoidance of other smokers and smoking environments is likely to be important, particularly at "danger times", like teabreaks and after meals or when having a drink.

A number of self-help leaflets are available from a variety of sources to supplement and reinforce such simple guidance. These leaflets have particular value and effectiveness when handed out by health professionals as an adjunct to brief advice.

Use of nicotine replacement therapy should be encouraged in all those (except perhaps the lightest smokers) for whom advice and self-help are not enough. Assessment of nicotine dependence is most simply done by asking how soon after waking the first cigarette is smoked. If this is within half an hour, this is evidence of at least moderate dependence and suggests likely benefit from using nicotine replacement.

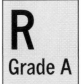

As already indicated, although there is debate about the safety of using nicotine replacement in patients with cardiovascular disease, evidence of harm from doing this is lacking and there is some evidence which suggests that it is safe. This is likely to be so if nicotine gum or patches are used (as they should be) as a temporary substitute for smoking. A combination of smoking and nicotine replacement may well be potentially harmful and should be strongly discouraged. A simple smoking cessation protocol is illustrated in Figure 12.6.

Key points

- Tobacco smoking is a critically important, modifiable cardiovascular risk factor (especially in those with established cardiovascular disease).
- Smoking cessation attenuates cardiovascular risk and early benefits accrue (again, especially in those with established cardiovascular disease).
- There is good evidence for the effectiveness of simple, brief smoking cessation advice and the use of nicotine replacement as an adjunct to this. Nicotine replacement products are effective and safe.
- Smoking and smoking cessation should be routinely addressed by health professionals in any consultations with patients who smoke.
- Simple cessation advice and support should be routinely offered by health care professionals in any consultations with patients who smoke.
- Nicotine replacement therapy (NRT) – chewing gum, transdermal patches, nasal spray or oral inhaler – should be recommended to all smokers trying to quit. Encouragement and support should accompany this and compliance for 2 or 3 months should be encouraged in those who achieve short term abstinence with it.

REFERENCES

1 Peto R, Lopez AD, Boreham J, Thun M, Heath C. *Mortality from smoking in developed countries 1950–2000*. Oxford: Oxford University Press, 1994.

2 Doll R, Peto R, Wheatley K, Gray R, Sutherland I. Mortality in relation to smoking: 40 years' observation on male British doctors. *Br Med J* 1994;**309**:901–11.

3 Fourth Report of Independent Scientific Committee on Smoking and Health. London: HMSO, 1988.

4 Glanz SA, Parmley WW. Passive smoking and heart disease: mechanisms and risk. *JAMA* 1995; **273**:1047–53.

5 Darby SC, Doll R, Stratton IM. Trends in mortality from smoking-related diseases in England and Wales. In: Wald N, Frogatt P. eds. *Nicotine, smoking and the low tar programme*. Oxford: Oxford University Press, 1989, pp 70–82.

6 Doll R, Peto R. Mortality in relation to smoking: 20 years' observation of British male doctors. *Br Med J* 1976;**4**:1525–36.

7 Cook DG, Pocock SJ, Shaper AG *et al.* Giving up smoking and the risk of heart attacks. *Lancet* 1986;**2**:1376–80.

8 Wilhelmssen C, Vedin J, Elmfeld D *et al.* Smoking and myocardial infarction. *Lancet* 1975;**1**: 415–17.

9 Daly LE, Mulcahy R, Graham IM, Hickey M. Long term effect on mortality of stopping smoking after unstable angina and myocardial infarction. *Br Med J* 1983;**287**:324–6.

10 Rose G, Colwell L. Randomised controlled trial of antismoking advice. *J Epidemiol Community Health* 1992;**46**:75–7.

11 Pittilo RM, Woolf N. Cigarette smoking, endothelial injury and atherosclerosis. *J Smoking-related Dis* 1993;**4**:17–25.

12 Hawkins RI. Smoking, platelets and thrombosis. *Nature* 1972;**263**:450–2.

13 Meade TW, Imeson J, Sterling Y. Effect of changes in smoking on clotting factors and on risk of ischaemic heart disease. *Lancet* 1987;**ii**:986–8.

14 Marsh A, Matheson J. *Smoking attitudes and behaviour*. London: HMSO, 1993.

15 US Department of Health and Human Services. *The health consequences of smoking and nicotine addiction*. Report of Surgeon General 1988. Washington DC: DHHS, 1989.

16 Kottke T, Battista R, DeFriese G, Brekke M. Attributes of successful smoking cessation interventions in medical practice: a meta-analysis of 39 controlled trials. *JAMA* 1988;**259**:2883–9.

17 Prochaska JO, DiClemete C. Towards a comprehensive model of change. In: Miller WR, Heather N. eds. *Treating addictive behaviours: processes of change*. New York: Plenum, 1986.

18 Russell MAH, Wilson C, Taylor C, Bales CD. Effect of general practitioner's advice against smoking. *Br Med J* 1979;**ii**:231–5.

19 Jamrozik K, Vessey M, Fowler G *et al.* Controlled trial of three different antismoking interventions in general practice. *Br Med J* 1984;**288**: 1499–1503.

20 Russell MAH, Merrium L, Stapleton J, Taylor W. Effect of nicotine chewing gum as an adjunct to general practitioners' advice against smoking. *Br Med J* 1983;**287**:1782–5.

21 Imperial Cancer Research Fund General Practice Research Group. Randomised trial of nicotine patches in general practice: results at one year. *Br Med J* 1994;**308**:1476–7.

22 Silagy C, Mant D, Fowler G, Lodge M. Meta-analysis of the efficacy of nicotine replacement in smoking cessation. *Lancet* 1994;**343**:139–42.

23 Tang TL, Law M, Wald N. How effective is nicotine replacement in helping people to stop smoking? *Br Med J* 1994;**308**:21–6.

24 Joseph AM, Norman SM, Ferry LH *et al.* The safety of transdermal nicotine as an aid to smoking cessation in patients with cardiac disease. *N Engl J Med* 1996;**335**:1792–8.

25 Law M, Tang TL, Wald N. An analysis of the effectiveness of interventions intended to help people stop smoking. *Arch Intern Med* 1995; **155**:1933–41.

26 Sanders D, Fowler G, Mant D *et al.* Randomised controlled trial of anti-smoking advice by nurses in general practice. *J Roy Coll Gen Pract* 1989; **39**:273–6.

27 Hollis J, Lichenstein E, Vogt T *et al.* Nurse-assisted counselling for smokers in primary care. *Ann Intern Med* 1993;**118**:521–5.

28 Sutherland G, Stapleton J, Russell MAH *et al.* Randomised controlled trial of nasal nicotine spray in smoking cessation. *Lancet* 1992;**340**: 324–9.

29 US Department of Health and Human Services. *1996 clinical practice guidelines no 18: smoking cessation*. Washington DC: DHHS, 1996.

Lipids and cardiovascular disease

13

Malcolm Law

Few issues in medicine have been so controversial and difficult to resolve as lipids and cardiovascular disease. Yet the high fat diet typical of many Western countries over the greater part of the 20th century has proven to be the major underlying factor in the epidemic of ischemic heart disease and modern cholesterol lowering drugs can reduce risk more than any other single intervention.[1]

SERUM TOTAL AND LOW DENSITY LIPOPROTEIN CHOLESTEROL

Typical values of serum total and low density lipoprotein (LDL) cholesterol in Western countries are high in comparison to those in agricultural and hunter-gatherer communities, because of the high saturated fat content of the Western diet. Average serum cholesterol concentration (in men aged 45–60) is about 3.0–3.5 mmol/l in hunter-gatherer societies and rural China (where heart disease is rare), 5.0 mmol/l in Japan, 5.4 mmol/ in Mediterranean populations, 5.7 mmol/l in the USA and 6.2 mmol/l in Britain and several other European countries.[2] Average levels of LDL cholesterol are about 2 mmol/l lower.[2] Use of the term "normal" in reference to usual or average Western cholesterol values may therefore be misleading.

Of the average total serum cholesterol in Western populations, two-thirds is low density lipoprotein (LDL) cholesterol and one-quarter is high density lipoprotein (HDL) cholesterol. The atherogenic properties lie in the LDL fraction (sometimes measured as its carrier protein, apolipoprotein B, with which it is highly correlated). Many of the large epidemiological studies and randomized trials measured only total serum cholesterol and results based on total serum cholesterol have been taken to estimate effects of LDL cholesterol. Fortuitously, the approximation is a good one. The absolute reduction in total serum cholesterol produced by diet and by most drugs is similar to the reduction in LDL cholesterol (simvastatin, for example, reduced total and LDL cholesterol by 1.8 mmol/l[1]). Observational differences between individuals in total cholesterol are close to the corresponding differences in LDL cholesterol, because HDL cholesterol is independent of total serum cholesterol.[3,4] This arises because the tendency for HDL

Table 13.1 Relative advantages of cohort studies and randomized trials in assessing the relation between serum cholesterol and ischemic heart disease

Objective	Advantage (comment)
Statistical power	Cohort studies (recorded about three times more ischemic heart disease events than the trials)
Dose–response relationship	Cohort studies (observation across wide range of cholesterol values)
Wide age range	Cohort studies (ischemic heart disease events at age 35–85, but mostly 55–65 in trials)
Long term effects of cholesterol differences	Cohort studies (on recruitment the serum cholesterol was the same in intervention and control groups)
Short term effects of cholesterol differences	Randomized trials (on recruitment serum cholesterol was the same in intervention and control groups)
Avoid bias	Randomized trials (not a major advantage – bias in cohort studies can be allowed for)

cholesterol to be positively associated with total cholesterol (as HDL cholesterol is part of total) is offset by the small inverse association between HDL and LDL cholesterol. Much epidemiological and clinical trial data are therefore available in estimating quantitatively the effect of lowering serum LDL cholesterol on the risk of ischemic heart disease.

SERUM CHOLESTEROL AND ISCHEMIC HEART DISEASE

Evidence from genetics, animal studies, experimental pathology, epidemiological studies, and clinical trials indicates conclusively that increasing serum cholesterol is an important cause of ischemic heart disease and that lowering serum cholesterol reduces the risk.[5] Three important practical questions arise: the nature of the dose–response relationship, the size of the effect, and the speed of the reversal of risk. To answer these questions data from both observational epidemiology (cohort studies) and randomized controlled trials are necessary. The two are complementary; examining trial data alone is misleading. Table 13.1 summarizes the advantages of each. In cohort (or prospective) studies serum cholesterol is measured in a large number of individuals and subsequent heart disease mortality (or incidence of myocardial infarction) is recorded. Cohort studies are easier to conduct than trials (since there is no intervention) and can therefore be much larger. Accordingly, their statistical power is greater and they can examine the association across a wider range of serum cholesterol values and a wider range of ages than trials have done.

Most of the cohort studies and trials of cholesterol and ischemic heart disease recruited men, for reasons of economy as ischemic heart disease is more common in men. The limited data from women indicate a similar effect as in men.[1,5,6]

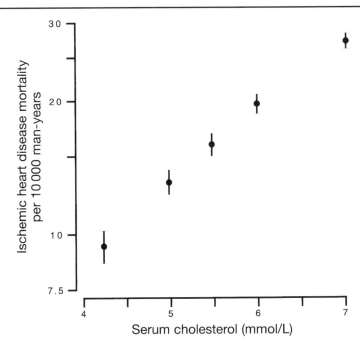

Figure 13.1 Mortality from ischemic heart disease (with 95% confidence intervals) according to serum cholesterol in a large cohort study.[7]

The nature of the dose–response relationship: is there a threshold?

Figure 13.1 shows mortality from ischemic heart disease plotted according to quintile groups (fifths) of the ranked serum cholesterol measurements in a large cohort study of serum cholesterol and ischemic heart disease (MRFIT Screenees).[7] With ischemic heart disease plotted on a logarithmic scale the relationship is described almost perfectly by a straight line linking the *proportional* change in ischemic heart disease to the *absolute* difference in serum cholesterol (r = 0.997). Other cohort studies show the same relationship.[6] The 95% confidence limits of the risk estimates in each quintile group do not overlap, establishing that there is no threshold below which a further decrease in serum cholesterol is not associated with a further decrease in risk of ischemic heart disease. The exponential relationship indicated by the straight line means that a given absolute difference in serum cholesterol concentration from *any* point on the cholesterol distribution is associated with a constant percentage difference in the incidence of ischemic heart disease.

This absence of a threshold has been contentious; many published guidelines on lowering cholesterol invoke one. Yet the evidence is firmly against any threshold. The data in Figure 13.1 (which alone are conclusive) are supported by data from other large cohort studies,[6] including one from China which shows that the continuous relationship extends below serum cholesterol values of 4 mmol/l.[8] In the "4S" trial serum cholesterol was lowered to about 4 mmol/l in the quarter of the patients with lowest total or LDL cholesterol on entry and the proportionate reduction in myocardial infarction and heart disease death in these patients was similar to that in patients with higher serum

Table 13.2   Estimates (from 10 cohort studies) of the percentage decrease in risk of ischemic heart disease according to extent of serum cholesterol reduction and age[6]

Age (years)	Estimated percentage decrease in risk for a serum cholesterol reduction (mmol/l) of:			
	0.3 (5%)	0.6 (10%)	1.2 (20%)	1.8 (30%)
40	32	54	79	90
50	22	39	63	77
60	15	27	47	61
70	11	20	36	49
80	10	19	34	47

cholesterol on entry,[9] again excluding a threshold above 4 mmol/l. The recent LIPID trial confirms this finding. Experimental data on the transfer of cholesterol from the blood into atheromatous lesions exclude a threshold as low as 1 mmol/l.[10]

The size of the effect

Cohort studies provide the best estimates because they cover a wide age range and have high statistical power and because the serum cholesterol differences between individuals recorded on entry to a cohort study will have been present on average for decades beforehand (so cohort studies show long term associations). Trials, on the other hand, show the effect of short term differences. Cohort studies are subject to bias but this can be corrected. The major bias is the so-called "regression dilution bias".[3] This is not specific to cholesterol; it affects all observational studies in which the explanatory (horizontal axis) variable is, like serum cholesterol, subject to random fluctuation over time in an individual. For example, in a group of men all selected because a single serum cholesterol reading was about 7 mmol/l (above average), the true (long term average) value will be closer to 6 mmol/l in some (in whom the single reading of 7 mmol/l was unusually high) and closer to 8 mmol/l in others (in whom the single reading of 7 mmol/l was unusually low). A long term average serum cholesterol of 6 mmol/l is common, however, and one of 8 mmol/l uncommon, so in the group as a whole the long term average serum cholesterol will be lower than 7 mmol/l. Correspondingly, in a group of men selected because a single cholesterol measurement was about 5 mmol/l (below average), the long term average will be greater than this. Random error thereby introduces bias. The range of serum cholesterol concentrations based on single measurements will be wider than that on long term average values. Both are associated with the same range of heart disease death rates, so a plot of heart disease mortality against serum cholesterol concentration will be steeper (by about 50%) if based on long term average values.

Table 13.2 shows estimates of the long term percentage decrease in the risk of ischemic heart disease according to the decrease in serum cholesterol concentration and age at death. The estimates are taken from an analysis of the 10 largest cohort studies, corrected for the regression dilution bias and for the minor distinction between differences in total and in LDL cholesterol discussed above.[3,6] A reduction in total or LDL cholesterol of 0.6 mmol/l (about 10%) is associated with a decrease in risk of

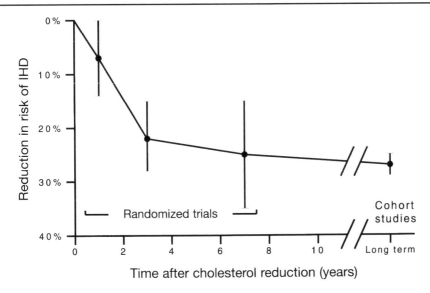

Figure 13.2   Reduction in the incidence of ischemic heart disease (IHD) per 0.6 mmol/l (about 10%) decrease in serum cholesterol as estimated from randomized trials according to time since entry and from cohort studies (which reflect the long term association).[6]

ischemic heart disease of about 50% at age 40, 40% at 50, 30% at 60, and 20% at 70–80. The *proportional* decrease in risk decreases with age, but the *absolute* benefit increases because the disease becomes more common with age. The increasing reduction in risk with greater reduction in serum cholesterol shown in Table 13.2 follows from the exponential relationship described above. For a 0.6 mmol/l cholesterol reduction at age 60, for example, the reduction in risk is 27% and the relative risk is therefore 0.73; with a serum cholesterol reduction three times as great (1.8 mmol/l), the relative risk is 0.73,[3] or 0.39, and the reduction in risk is 61%.

Speed of reversal and consistency of observational and trial data

Data have been analyzed from the "old generation" of 28 randomized trials in which the average serum cholesterol reduction was about 0.6 mmol/l (10%).[6] Figure 13.2 shows the reduction in incidence of ischemic heart disease in all trials combined according to time since entry. In the first 2 years there was little reduction in risk (in fact, none in the first year). From 2 to 5 years, the average reduction in risk was 22% and after 5 years the reduction was 25%. The ischemic heart disease events in these trials mostly occurred at an average age of about 60 and at this age the estimate of the long term effect from the cohort studies is 27% (Table 13.2). The similarity of the estimates of effect from the cohort studies and from the trial data from the third year onwards therefore indicate that the reversal of risk is near maximal after 2 years – a surprisingly rapid effect.

The trial data show that the proportionate reduction in risk from lowering serum cholesterol is similar in persons with and without previous myocardial infarction or other clinical evidence of coronary artery disease.[6]

Table 13.3 Serum cholesterol and dietary saturated fat in Japan and Britain. Data compiled from national surveys in each country[2]

Age	Japan	Britain	Difference
		Dietary saturated fat (% calories)	
All ages	6%	16%	10%
		Serum cholesterol (mmol/l)	
20–9	4.5	5.0	0.5
30–9	5.0	5.6	0.6
40–9	5.1	6.0	0.9
50–9	5.2	6.2	1.0
60–9	5.0	6.2	1.2

Recent large trials of "statin" drugs have attained a larger reduction in total and LDL cholesterol, of 0.9–1.8 mmol/l.[1,11–13] These too showed a relatively small reduction in heart disease in the first 2 years, but a reduction after 2 years that is close to the maximum indicated by cohort studies. The average age at which an ischemic heart disease event occurred was again about 60. In two of the trials the average reduction in serum total and LDL cholesterol was about 1.8 mmol/l, so the expected long term reduction in ischemic heart disease mortality is 61% (Table 13.2) and this was almost exactly the observed reduction from the third year onwards.[1,11] In the other trials, two published[12,13] and two at present unpublished (LIPID and AFCAPS), the average serum cholesterol reduction was about 1.0 mmol/l and the reduction in risk from the third year on was about 40%, as expected.

"Statin" drugs therefore can more than halve the risk of heart disease death after 2 years. The absolute effect of this can be expressed simply. Heart disease mortality approximately doubles with every 8 years of increasing age. An intervention that halves the risk of ischemic heart disease death therefore reduces risk to that of a person 8 years younger. Most survivors of myocardial infarction (a major target group for cholesterol lowering drugs) will eventually die of ischemic heart disease. Halving their ischemic heart disease death rates is equivalent to postponing this eventual ischemic heart disease death by about 8 years on average – a major gain.

DIETARY FAT AND SERUM CHOLESTEROL

The relationship between dietary saturated fat and serum cholesterol is shown by the data from Japan and Britain in Table 13.3. This comparison is a useful one because dietary saturated fat differs greatly yet dietary polyunsaturated fat and cholesterol are similar in the two countries. As in other situations (salt and blood pressure, for example), the size of the association varies with age yet there has been a tendency to generalize to older age groups the results of studies conducted in younger age groups. Most dietary trials, for example, have been conducted in people under 30. The few that have been conducted in people over 50 tend to support the above Japan–Britain comparison.[6] In older people a reduction in dietary saturated fat equivalent to 10% of calories will lower serum cholesterol by about 1 mmol/l, which in turn will reduce ischemic heart disease mortality in the long term by about 40%.

The chain lengths of saturated fatty acids influence the extent to which they increase blood cholesterol. Palmitic ($C_{16:0}$) and myristic ($C_{14:0}$) acids have the major effect, lauric acid ($C_{12:0}$) some effect, while stearic acid ($C_{18:0}$) and medium chain fatty acids have little or no effect.

Trans-unsaturated fatty acids are also important; randomized trials show that they increase serum total and LDL cholesterol by about as much as these longer chain saturated fatty acids.[14,15] They are scanty in naturally occurring fats but are generated by the hydrogenation of vegetable oils for use as hardening agents in manufactured foods. They constitute 6–8% of dietary fat, or 2% of calories, in Western diets.

Naturally occurring *cis*-unsaturated fatty acids reduce serum cholesterol by approximately half as much as longer chain saturated fatty acids increase it. Reduction in dietary cholesterol has a small effect on blood cholesterol concentration.[5] Substitution of *cis*-unsaturated for saturated fats in the Western diet is thus the most appropriate change in lowering the high levels of blood cholesterol in Western populations.

The reduction in serum total or LDL cholesterol that can easily be attained by individuals trying to alter their diet in isolation from family, friends, and workmates is relatively small (about 0.3 mmol/l or 5%). A larger serum cholesterol reduction, about 0.6 mmol/l (10%), is realistic on a community basis, since the availability of palatable low fat food increases when other family members or the community alter their diet and the dietary change is perceived more positively. A reduction by about 7% of calories, a realistic target for a high fat population, would lower serum cholesterol by 0.6 mmol/l, which in turn would reduce the mortality from ischemic heart disease at age 60 by 25–30%. Reductions in serum cholesterol of about 0.6 mmol/l through dietary change have occurred in entire Western communities, in the United States and Finland for example.[2] Measures that facilitate such a change include wider public education, labeling of foods sold in supermarkets, and provision of information on the fat content of restaurant meals. Most important is the implementation of national and international policies on food subsidies that are linked to health priorities.

SERUM CHOLESTEROL AND CIRCULATORY DISEASES OTHER THAN ISCHEMIC HEART DISEASE

Table 13.4 shows death rates from all circulatory diseases according to total serum cholesterol concentration, in the same cohort study (MRFIT Screenees[16]) as shown in Figure 13.1. Apart from ischemic heart disease, serum cholesterol is associated with stroke and with other circulatory diseases.

Stroke

The data from the large cohort study of the MRFIT Screenees (Table 13.4) are particularly useful because hemorrhagic and non-hemorrhagic stroke were distinguished. For non-hemorrhagic (mainly thrombotic) stroke the data are consistent with a continuous dose–response relationship with serum cholesterol, analogous to that shown for ischemic heart disease in Figure 13.1. For hemorrhagic stroke (intracranial and subarachnoid), there is no significant increase in risk with increasing serum cholesterol, nor any reason to expect such an association. There is an *excess* risk of intracranial hemorrhage in the

Table 13.4 Death rates per 100 000 man-years (number of deaths) from circulatory diseases according to serum cholesterol in a large cohort of men[16]

Cause of death (IDC-9 code)	Serum cholesterol (mmol/l) (% of all men):				
	<4.1 (6%)	4.1–5.1 (31%)	5.2–6.1 (39%)	≥6.2 (24%)	P (trend)
Ischemic heart disease (410–4)	65 (160)	98 (1239)	169 (2731)	289 (2804)	<0.001
Stroke:					
non-hemorrhagic (433–8)	6 (14)	6 (73)	8 (135)	13 (126)	<0.001
intracranial hemorrhage (431–2)	9 (22)	4 (55)	5 (86)	6 (57)	—
subarachnoid hemorrhage (430)	2 (5)	4 (46)	3 (55)	3 (33)	—
Other circulatory diseases	29 (72)	35 (437)	38 (615)	54 (523)	<0.001
All circulatory diseases (390–459)	110 (273)	147 (1850)	224 (3622)	365 (3543)	<0.001

lowest serum cholesterol group, an L-shaped rather than continuous association which is a common finding in observational studies recording sufficient numbers of deaths at very low cholesterol levels to detect it;[17] some studies report no association, however.[18] There may be an interaction with high blood pressure. Whether the association is cause and effect is uncertain. It is more difficult to see how a spurious (non-causal) association with intracranial hemorrhage might arise through the disease (or predisposition to the disease) lowering serum cholesterol than is the case with depression and suicide or cancer. Experimental data lend some support to an interpretation of a causal effect of low cholesterol in that the endothelium of intracerebral arteries might be weaker at very low serum cholesterol levels.[17] As Table 13.4 shows, however, the increased mortality from hemorrhagic stroke at very low cholesterol concentrations, even if cause and effect, is small compared to the lower mortality from ischemic heart disease and other circulatory diseases. Even at the lowest serum cholesterol concentrations in Western populations, the mortality from all circulatory diseases is substantially lower than in the next lowest group.

An analysis of pooled data from 45 cohort studies (recording 13 000 strokes) yielded a different result. There was no association between serum cholesterol and stroke mortality except in the youngest age group (<45 years).[18] Separate data on hemorrhagic and non-hemorrhagic stroke were unavailable, however, and it was acknowledged that a negative association with the former could offset a positive association with the latter.[18]

The older cholesterol lowering trials were uninformative on stroke because they recorded relatively few deaths and attained relatively small reductions in cholesterol. The large "statin" trials are more informative because they recorded non-fatal events (which are far more numerous) and attained larger cholesterol reductions. The results are shown in Table 13.5. Combining the relative risk estimates from the four trials yields an overall estimate of a 27% reduction in risk (95% confidence interval 11%, 40%; P=0.001). Including smaller trials does not alter this estimate,[19] and the LIPID

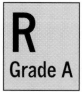

R
Grade A

Table 13.5 Incidence of stroke in four trials of "statin" drugs (cholesterol reduction 0.9–1.8 mmol/l, fatal and non-fatal events combined)

Trial	No. of events/no. of patients		Relative risk (95% CI)
	Treated	Placebo	
4S[1]	70/2221	98/2223	0.70 (0.52, 0.96)
Pravastatin intervention program[11]	5/995	13/936	0.38 (0.03, 1.09)
West of Scotland[12]	46/3302	51/3293	0.89 (0.60, 1.33)
CARE[13]	54/2081	78/2078	0.69 (0.48, 0.97)
All four trials			0.73* (0.60, 0.89)

* $P = 0.001$

trial recorded a similar result. This resolves the uncertainty from the observational studies, supporting the association shown in Table 13.4, of an increasing risk of non-hemorrhagic stroke as serum cholesterol increases above 4 mmol/l. As with heart disease, it is likely that a greater long term reduction in the trials is diluted by the absence of an early effect.[11] The starting levels of serum cholesterol in the four trials were such that few treated patients had cholesterol levels around 4 mmol/l, so the trials cannot test whether the excess hemorrhagic stroke was a causal association.

Peripheral arterial disease

Observational data show the expected association between peripheral arterial disease and serum cholesterol. In a large case-control study, the association was equivalent in magnitude to an increase in risk of intermittent claudication of about 24% for a 0.6 mmol/l increase in serum cholesterol[20] (uncorrected for regression dilution bias), similar in magnitude to the association of serum cholesterol with ischemic heart disease. In the 4S trial (serum cholesterol reduction 1.8 mmol/l) the incidence of intermittent claudication was reduced by 38% (95% confidence interval 12%, 56%; 52 v 81 cases).[21] Again, it is likely that a greater long term reduction is diluted by the absence of an effect in the first 1–2 years and that the observational and trial data are consistent.

Abdominal aortic aneurysm

The pathology of the condition is complex, but abdominal aortic aneurysms are associated with atheromatous disease and tend to coexist with coronary artery or peripheral arterial disease. Abdominal aortic aneurysms are associated with a higher serum LDL cholesterol and triglyceride and a lower HDL cholesterol.

Other circulatory diseases

Table 13.4 shows a strong association between serum cholesterol and all circulatory diseases other than ischemic heart disease and stroke. Deaths from peripheral arterial disease and abdominal aortic aneurysm are too infrequent to fully account for this association. It is probably attributable also to poorly certified ischemic heart disease: deaths certified due to atrial fibrillation, heart failure, myocardial degeneration, and atherosclerosis, for example, are in many cases due to ischemic heart disease.

SAFETY OF CHOLESTEROL REDUCTION

The uncertainty concerning the excess mortality from hemorrhagic stroke at very low serum cholesterol concentration is unresolved, as discussed above. This apart, there are no material grounds for concern about hazard. Trials of "statin" drugs, particularly informative on safety because of the large reduction in serum cholesterol that they attain, have resolved the issue of safety because they show no excess mortality from non-circulatory causes.[1,12,13] The excess mortality from cancer and accidents and suicide at very low serum cholesterol in observational studies is attributable to cancer or depression lowering serum cholesterol, not the reverse.[17] The excess mortality from accidents and suicide in two of the older cholesterol lowering trials (which was not statistically significant) occurred among men who had not taken the medication and was therefore attributable to chance.[22] Further reassurance on safety is provided by the condition of heterozygous familial hypobetalipoproteinemia, in which serum cholesterol levels are as low as 2–3 mmol/l. Life expectancy is prolonged because coronary artery disease is avoided and no adverse effects from the low cholesterol are recognized[23,24] – an important natural experiment.

WHY HAS CHOLESTEROL REDUCTION BEEN CONTENTIOUS?

Many clinicians regard serum cholesterol reduction with uncertainty or suspicion. Until recently, unfavorable evidence had been reported at regular intervals over the last 30 years. The earliest trials used toxic agents to lower serum cholesterol, notably estrogen (in men) and thyroxine. Some early trials were short in duration[25] and showed no reduction in risk because none occurs in the first year after lowering cholesterol. Cross-sectional studies of dietary saturated fat and serum cholesterol showed little or no relationship, an observation that was wrongly interpreted as indicating that lowering dietary saturated fat did not reduce cholesterol, until randomized trials established that it did. (The weak observational association arises because the inaccuracy in measuring individual dietary saturated fat is large in comparison to the small degree of variation between individuals in true saturated fat consumption.[26]) The notion that the average serum cholesterol in entire Western populations is high appeared counterintuitive, since the blood concentration of many nutrients is homeostatically controlled. The issue of safety caused concern, as discussed above. Lastly, it has seemed inconsistent that serum cholesterol is a poor screening test yet an important cause of heart disease, as discussed below. All these issues are now satisfactorily resolved.

DIETARY FAT AND COAGULATION

Dietary fat increases blood levels of coagulation factor VII and hence increases the risk of thrombosis, myocardial infarction, and cerebral thrombosis.[27,28] Saturated and unsaturated fat increase factor VII equally and the increase appears directly related to the extent of postprandial lipemia. The importance of this effect in increasing the risk of cardiovascular death is difficult to quantify. However, analyses of data on serum cholesterol and ischemic heart disease mortality across different populations (so-called "ecological" comparisons), such as the Seven Countries Study, yield significantly larger estimates of the relationship than obtained from the cohort studies and trials discussed above. At age 60, for example, the ecological estimate is a 38% difference in risk for a 0.6 mmol/l cholesterol difference, compared to a 27% difference in the cohort studies (Table 13.2).[3,6] Material confounding by other dietary variables is unlikely and this difference may partly be attributable to the effect of dietary fat on coagulation. While variation *between* populations in serum cholesterol is largely attributable to differences in saturated fat (unsaturated fat varies less), over half of the variation in serum cholesterol among individuals in a cohort is attributable to genetic factors. (The difference between population averages is reproduced in migration studies, confirming that genetic differences between populations are relatively small. Between individuals, however, genetic differences are large whereas differences in dietary saturated fat consumption are small because most of the individuals in a community eat similar foods.)

TRIGLYCERIDES

Serum triglyceride concentration was associated with the risk of ischemic heart disease in many cohort studies, but the association is subject to confounding by serum LDL and HDL cholesterol, diabetes, and other factors.[4,29] The effect of dietary fat increasing factor VII will also produce an indirect association between triglycerides and heart disease mortality. Whether an independent association exists is contentious. Very high serum levels of triglyceride caused by genetic defects (familial lipoprotein lipase deficiency, for example) are not associated with atheroma or coronary artery disease and this observation, together with the potential for confounding in cohort studies, suggests that a material cause and effect relationship between serum triglyceride and heart disease is unlikely.

HIGH DENSITY LIPOPROTEIN CHOLESTEROL

There is an inverse association between HDL cholesterol (or apolipoprotein A1) and ischemic heart disease. An absolute increase corresponding to 0.12 mmol/l (about 10% of the average value) is associated with about a 15% decrease in the risk of ischemic heart disease at age 60[4,29] or a 20% decrease with adjustment for the regression dilution bias.[29] The effect of alcohol in increasing HDL cholesterol is the major mechanism in its protective effect against heart disease.[30] The effect of smoking in decreasing HDL cholesterol contributes to the excess risk of heart disease in smokers. The "statin" cholesterol lowering drugs increase HDL cholesterol by about 5%,[1,12,13] which would be expected to reduce heart disease mortality by a further 10% beyond the large effect of the reduction in LDL cholesterol. Certain other cholesterol lowering drugs (such as fibrates and niacin) increase HDL cholesterol more than "statins", but even in persons with relatively low HDL cholesterol, the overall protective effect of these drugs is smaller because they reduce LDL cholesterol less.

LIPIDS AS SCREENING TESTS

Serum cholesterol reduction is important in reducing the risk of ischemic heart disease, but cholesterol and other lipids are poor population screening tests for ischemic heart disease. The reason for the apparent discrepancy is that the screening potential of a factor depends not only on the strength of its relationship with disease, but also on its variation in magnitude between individuals in a community. In the case of lipids, the high average values in Western societies place everyone at risk and the variation between individuals is too small for use in population screening. By analogy, if everybody smoked between 15 and 25 cigarettes per day, cases of lung cancer would not cluster in the minority who smoked 25 cigarettes a day to the extent that those who smoked 15 or 20 could be ignored.

Among men aged 35–64, the 5% with the highest serum total cholesterol experience only about 12% of all deaths from ischemic heart disease – their risk is little more than double the population average.[29] The 5% of men with highest LDL cholesterol (or its carrier protein apolipoprotein B) experience 17% of the heart disease deaths.[29] Including HDL cholesterol improves this poor detection by only about one percentage point. Lipids cannot identify a small minority of the population in whom the majority of future heart disease deaths will cluster.

APPROPRIATE POLICY

In a small proportion of the population (1% or so), notably persons with familial hypercholesterolemia, the absolute risk of death from ischemic heart disease at a young age is so great that affected persons should be identified and treated, even though the condition accounts for a fraction of all heart disease deaths in a population. The most appropriate screening strategy has not yet been devised; measuring lipids in relatives of known cases will not identify all cases.

Since screening cannot identify a group who would *not* benefit from a reduction in dietary fat and serum cholesterol, such measures should be directed at the entire population. Serum cholesterol reductions of 0.6 mmol/l (10%), as discussed above, have occurred in entire Western communities, facilitated by health education, the wider availability of healthy food in restaurants and supermarkets, and a positive image of healthy eating. A reduction of 0.6 mmol/l is less likely when an individual attempts dietary change in isolation. The most important measures to lower cholesterol in healthy people therefore involve wider public education and encouragement of labeling of the nutrient content of foods and the widespread availability of palatable low fat foods.

Clinicians need to direct their activities towards high risk patients and the most important high risk group (based on the proportion of all heart disease deaths that can be anticipated) are survivors of myocardial infarction. As a group, these patients face a risk of death from ischemic heart disease of about 5% per year (untreated), a risk that varies relatively little with age or sex. As in healthy people, serum cholesterol testing cannot identify a substantial group at either materially higher or materially lower than average risk of death. Also, the evidence strongly indicates that there is no threshold below which serum cholesterol reduction is not effective. It follows that serum cholesterol should be reduced in all survivors of myocardial infarction. "Statin" drugs, which can

R

Grade A

R

Grade A

lower serum cholesterol by 1.8 mmol/l (30%), are justified because of the high absolute risk of death of these patients; as discussed above, "statins" reduce mortality from heart disease by about 60% after 2 years, a substantially larger reduction in risk than can be attained by any other single intervention. Serum cholesterol measurements should not be used to impose artificial thresholds, only for purposes of monitoring the reduction in serum cholesterol attained with therapy.

After infarct survivors and familial hypercholesterolemia, the groups at next greatest risk of heart disease are patients with angina and diabetics. Whether to offer "statins" to those patients will depend primarily on cost-effectiveness calculations.

The "population" and "high risk" approaches are complementary – the first primarily a public health issue aimed at altering the population diet and hence the incidence of ischemic heart disease, the second primarily a clinical activity, identifying and treating with "statins" patients with coronary artery disease.

CONCLUSIONS

The high levels of serum cholesterol found in Western populations are a major cause of the high mortality from ischemic heart disease and, to a lesser extent, stroke and other circulatory diseases. Realistic dietary change in a community can lower serum cholesterol by 0.6 mmol/l (10%) and reduce heart disease mortality by about 25–30%. Cholesterol lowering drugs ("statins") can lower cholesterol by 1.8 mmol/l (30%) and reduce the risk of heart disease death by about 60% from the third year onwards and should be offered to all survivors of myocardial infarction. Despite the importance of lowering cholesterol, lipids are poor screening tests of individual risk, because the average risk is high and the range across a population is relatively narrow.

Serum cholesterol and ischemic heart disease

- The effect of serum cholesterol reduction on ischemic heart disease mortality is large and important.
- There is little reduction in risk in the first year, but most of the expected reduction in risk is attained from the third year on.
- There is no threshold across the range of cholesterol values in Western countries below which reducing serum cholesterol reduction is not worthwhile.
- The greater the reduction in serum cholesterol, the greater the reduction in risk.
- "Statin" drugs can lower cholesterol by 1.8 mmol/l (30%) and reduce the risk of heart disease death at age 60 by about 60% from the third year onwards.
- Realistic dietary change in a community can lower serum cholesterol by 0.6 mmol/l (10%) and reduce the risk of heart disease death by 25–30% at age 60. In an individual acting alone, the realistic change is half this.
- The benefits are similar in men and women.

R Grade A/B

Serum cholesterol and other circulatory diseases

- "Statin" drugs, lowering cholesterol by 1.0–1.8 mmol/l, reduce mortality from thrombotic stroke by at least 25%.
- There is excess mortality from hemorrhagic stroke at very low cholesterol levels. The interpretation is uncertain. The possible hazard, however, is greatly outweighed by the benefit of low mortality from heart disease at very low cholesterol levels.
- Serum cholesterol is associated with peripheral arterial disease and abdominal aortic aneurysm.

R Grade A/B

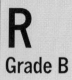

R

Grade B

Screening

- Lipids are poor screening tests in predicting heart disease death in an individual: it is not possible to identify a small minority in a community who will experience the majority of heart disease deaths.
- The 5% of men with highest total serum cholesterol experience about 12% of heart disease deaths.
- In the extremity of the distribution, familial hypercholesterolemia (top 1% or so of cholesterol levels) is important to detect because the absolute risk of heart disease death at a young age is high, even though the condition accounts for only a small proportion of heart disease deaths.

REFERENCES

1 Scandinavian Simvastatin Survival Study Group. Randomised trial of cholesterol lowering in 4444 patients with coronary heart disease: the Scandinavian Simvastatin Survival Study (4S). *Lancet* 1994;**344**:1383–9.

2 Law MR, Wald NJ. An ecological study of serum cholesterol and ischaemic heart disease between 1950 and 1990. *Eur J Clin Nutr* 1994; **48**: 305–25.

3 Law MR, Wald NJ, Wu T, Hackshaw A, Bailey A. Systematic underestimation of association between serum cholesterol concentration and ischaemic heart disease in observational studies: data from the BUPA study. *Br Med J* 1994;**308**: 363–6.

4 Pocock SJ, Shaper AG, Phillips AN. Concentrations of high density lipoprotein cholesterol, triglycerides, and total cholesterol in ischaemic heart disease. *Br Med J* 1989;**298**: 998–1002.

5 American Heart Association, National Heart, Lung, and Blood Institute. The cholesterol facts: a summary of the evidence relating dietary fats, serum cholesterol, and coronary heart disease. *Circulation* 1990;**81**:1721–33.

6 Law MR, Wald NJ, Thompson SG. By how much and how quickly does reduction in serum cholesterol concentration lower risk of ischaemic heart disease? *Br Med J* 1994;**308**:367–72.

7 Neaton JD, Wentworth D. Serum cholesterol, blood pressure, cigarette smoking, and death from coronary heart disease. *Arch Intern Med* 1992; **152**:56–64.

8 Chen Z, Peto R, Collins R *et al.* Serum cholesterol concentration and coronary heart disease in a population with low cholesterol concentrations. *Br Med J* 1991;**303**:276–82.

9 Scandinavian Simvastatin Survival Study Group. Baseline serum cholesterol and treatment effect in the Scandinavian Simvastatin Survival Study (4S). *Lancet* 1995;**345**:1274–5.

10 Smith EB, Slater RS. Relationship between low-density lipoprotein in aortic intima and serum-lipid levels. *Lancet* 1972;**i**:463–9.

11 Byington RP, Juhema JW, Salonen JT *et al.* Reduction in cardiovascular events during pravastatin therapy: pooled analysis of clinical events of the Pravastatin Atherosclerosis Intervention Program. *Circulation* 1995;**92**: 2419–25.

12 Shepherd J, Cobbe SM, Ford I *et al.* Prevention of coronary heart disease with pravastatin in men with hypercholesterolemia. *N Engl J Med* 1995; **333**:1301–7.

13 Sacks FM, Pfeffer MA, Moye LA *et al.* The effect of pravastatin on coronary events after myocardial infarction in patients with average cholesterol levels. *N Engl J Med* 1996;**335**:1001–9.

14 Mensink RP, Katan MB. Effect of dietary trans fatty acids on high-density and low-density lipoprotein cholesterol levels in healthy subjects. *N Engl J Med* 1990;**323**:439–45.

15 Nestel P, Noakes M, Belling B *et al.* Plasma lipoprotein lipid and Lp[a] changes with substitution of elaidic acid for oleic acid in the diet. *J Lipid Res* 1992;**33**:1029–36.

16 Neaton JD, Blackburn H, Jacobs D *et al.* Serum cholesterol level and mortality findings for men screened in the multiple risk factor intervention trial. *Arch Intern Med* 1992;**152**:1490–500.

17 Law MR, Wald NJ, Wu T, Bailey A. Assessing possible hazards of reducing serum cholesterol. *Br Med J* 1994;**308**:373–9.

18 Prospective Studies Collaboration. Cholesterol, diastolic blood pressure and stroke: 13 000 strokes in 450 000 people in 45 prospective cohorts. *Lancet* 1995;**346**:1647–53.

19 Crouse JR, Byington RP, Hoen HM, Furberg CD. Reductase inhibitor monotherapy and stroke prevention. *Arch Intern Med* 1977;**157**:1305–10.

20 Fowkes FGR, Housley E, Riemersma RA *et al.* Smoking, lipids, glucose intolerance, and blood pressure as risk factors for peripheral atherosclerosis compared with ischaemic heart disease in the Edinburgh Artery Study. *Am J Epidemiol* 1992;**135**:331–40.

21 Kjekshuj J, Pedersen TR, Pyorala K, Olsson AG. Effect of simvastatin on ischaemic signs and symptoms in the Scandanavian Simvastatin Survival Study (4S). *J Am Coll Cardiol* 1997; **29**(Suppl A):75A.

22 Wysowski DK, Gross TP. Deaths due to accidents and violence in two recent trials of cholesterol-lowering drugs. *Arch Intern Med* 1990;**150**: 2169–72.

23 Linton MF, Farese RV, Young SG. Familial hypobetalipoproteinemia. *J Lipid Res* 1993;**34**: 521–41.

24 Glueck CJ, Gartside P, Fallat RW, Sielski J, Steiner PM. Longevity syndromes: familial hypobeta and familial hyperalpha lipoproteinemia. *J Lab Clin Med* 1976;**88**:941–57.

25 Frantz ID, Dawson EA, Ashman PL *et al.* Test of effect of lipid lowering by diet on cardiovascular risk. The Minnesota coronary survey. *Arteriosclerosis* 1989;**9**:129–35.

26 Jacobs DR, Anderson JT, Blackburn H. Diet and serum cholesterol. *Am J Epidemiol* 1979;**110**: 77–87.

27 Miller GJ, Cruickshank JK, Ellis LJ *et al.* Fat consumption and factor VII coagulant activity in middle-aged men. An association between a dietary and thrombotic coronary risk factor. *Atherosclerosis* 1989;**78**:19–24.

28 Salomaa V, Rasi V, Pekkanen J *et al.* The effects of saturated fat and n-6 polyunsaturated fat on postprandial lipemia and hemostatic activity. *Atherosclerosis* 1993;**103**:1–11.

29 Wald NJ, Law M, Watt HC *et al.* Apolipoproteins and ischaemic heart disease: implications for screening. *Lancet* 1994;**343**:75–9.

30 Gaziano JM, Buring JE, Breslow JL *et al.* Moderate alcohol intake, increased levels of high-density lipoprotein and its subfractions, and decreased risk of myocardial infarction. *N Engl J Med* 1993; **329**:1829–34.

14 Use of lipid lowering agents in the prevention of cardiovascular disease

JEFFREY L. PROBSTFIELD,
JOHN D. BRUNZELL

INTRODUCTION

Coronary heart disease (CHD) has been declining by about 1% a year for the last three decades and CHD mortality by between 2% and 4% a year during the same period. However, it remains the most prevalent cause of death in Westernized countries, particularly in men aged over 45 years and women aged over 60 years. The associated morbidity, treatment of related conditions, and preventive approaches for CHD are reviewed in other chapters of this book.

A major risk factor for the development of CHD is hypercholesterolemia. Prospective epidemiologic studies have explored the CHD risks associated with other lipids and lipoproteins in only a limited fashion. An emerging story relates to the cluster of lipid abnormalities including elevated plasma levels of triglycerides in association with low plasma levels of high density lipoprotein cholesterol (HDL-C) and the presence of small dense low density lipoprotein (LDL) particles. This configuration may have relatively similar CHD risk to that of elevated plasma LDL cholesterol levels (LDL-C).[1] While previous risk factor analyses have suggested that only about half of prevalent CHD could be related to all known risk factors, a recent series of 152 patients aged less than 62 years who were catheterized as part of an evaluation for chest pain demonstrated that 75% with documented CHD had one or more of the following: increased plasma levels of LDL cholesterol, apolipoprotein B, Lp(a) or triglycerides, or a decrease in plasma HDL-C.

Recently completed trials have clearly demonstrated that decreases in LDL-C are associated with reductions in total mortality,[2,3] CHD mortality,[2,3] fatal and non-fatal CHD,[2,4] coronary artery atherosclerosis progression (in fact, regression),[5] carotid atherosclerosis progression (in fact, regression)[6] and progression and occlusion of atherosclerosis in saphenous vein bypass grafts.[7] Decreases in total and cause-specific mortality have been demonstrated both in primary[3] and secondary[2] coronary heart

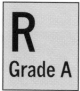

R

Grade A

disease prevention settings, and in those with elevated[2,3] and average[4] LDL-C levels. While we have the evidence associating plasma LDL-C reduction with CHD prevention, the implementation of strategies to realize the benefits of risk reduction is lacking. Review of hospital records, even in tertiary hospital settings, shows that the major risk factors of cigarette smoking, hypertension, and hypercholesterolemia are infrequently screened for and if found, are not uniformly treated. Dr William Roberts, Editor of the *American Journal of Cardiology*, has written about poor implementation of prevention strategies[8] and commented at the 1996 meeting of the American College of Cardiology that "The screening for and treatment of the major risk factors for CHD is a national disgrace (in the US)".

The development of safe and effective agents for the reduction of elevated lipid and lipoprotein plasma levels and for the reduction of associated morbidity and mortality has been a major scientific and medical care focus. The primary purpose of this chapter is to review the plasma lipid altering medications, their mechanism of action, dosage, and dosing schedules, results of administration on lipid and lipoprotein variables, adverse effects, and clinical use. Summary comments are included on evidence for cholesterol lowering in the elderly, women, diabetics, and in those with small dense LDL particles. Specific description and review of the clinical management of the inherited lipid disorders is discussed elsewhere.[9]

With the emergence of the HMG-CoA reductase inhibitor agents (statins) as highly effective and safe LDL-C lowering agents, the list of agents used for lipid and lipoprotein therapy has shortened. We will review only the statins, bile acid sequestering agents (resins), nicotinic acid (niacin), and fibrates. Many previously used lipid and lipoprotein altering agents have taken on the role of supplementary medications for LDL-C lowering because they are less effective or have more prevalent associated adverse reactions. Newer members of the statin family appear to be progressively more cost-effective. A careful review of the costs /1% LDL-C lowering/year is included.

Specific guidelines for initiating LDL-C lowering were originally developed as part of the National Cholesterol Education Program and have been revised.[10] These guidelines were developed on the basis of the patient's established baseline LDL cholesterol, presence or absence of CHD or its risk factors, and therapeutic goals for treatment and attainment of desired levels of plasma LDL-C. National Cholesterol Education Program guidelines developed by the US Public Health Service are summarized in Tables 14.1 and 14.2 for purposes of discussion. Guidelines by groups in other countries have also been adopted.[11–15]

USE OF INDIVIDUAL LIPID ALTERING AGENTS

In this short, evidence based overview we focus on documented activities of known lipid and lipoprotein altering drugs on lipid and lipoprotein variables and their related adverse effects. We identify those items which remain more speculative as such. The interested reader is referred to the following excellent and more complete reviews.[10,16,17]

HMG-CoA reductase inhibitors (statins)

These most powerful LDL-C lowering agents are considered to have a class effect. They differ only in their dose–response curves and unit cost. Mevastatin was first isolated in

Table 14.1 Guidelines for classification of plasma cholesterol concentrations and suggested therapeutic approaches

Total cholesterol[a] (mg/dl)	LDL-C (mg/dl)	Presence of CHD or CHD risk factors	Suggested treatment and follow-up
Desirable			
<200	<130	No	Repeat plasma cholesterol within 5 years
	<100	Yes	Further evaluation, diet therapy
Borderline			
200–239	130–159	No	Dietary therapy and annual follow-up
		Yes	Further evaluation, diet therapy, ?drug therapy
High			
>240	>160	No	Diet therapy, drug therapy considered, if LDL-C >190 mg/dl[b]
		Yes	Diet and drug therapy

[a] Total cholesterol values are not used as part of the NCEP Adult Treatment Panel Guidelines for therapy decision making. They are included here for general reference purposes.
[b] For men aged less than 35 years and premenopausal women who have no additional CHD risk factors, plasma LDL-C levels may be treated with hygienic measures.
CHD risk factors: males aged >45, females aged >55 or premenopausal without estrogen therapy, HDL-C <35 mg/dl, family history of premature CHD, cigarette smoking, hypertension (>140/>90 mmHg), diabetes mellitus. Negative risk factor: HDL-C >60 mg/dl.
Adapted from Witztum.[3]

1976 by Endo and colleagues as a natural product from *Penicillium* species. A related natural product, lovastatin, was approved by the Federal Drug Agency for cholesterol lowering in 1987. Subsequently, simvastatin, pravastatin, fluvastatin, and atorvastatin have been developed.

MECHANISM OF ACTION

Brown and colleagues demonstrated that lovastatin inhibits HMG-CoA reductase, the rate limiting enzyme in cholesterol biosynthesis.[18] Total body cholesterol synthesis is reduced by at least 20%. Ultimately, a critical reduction in cholesterol concentration occurs in the liver cell leading to an enhanced production of hepatic LDL receptors[19] and an increased cellular uptake of LDL-C. Further, reduced very low density lipoprotein (VLDL) biosynthesis occurs. Although speculative, it appears that the mechanism by which an increased removal of VLDL from the plasma occurs best fits with the upregulation of LDL receptors and an enhanced removal of VLDLs from the plasma due to an alteration in VLDL structure (specifically apo B-100).[20]

DOSAGE

The recommended dosages of these agents have been described.[21,22] Their effect on lipids and lipoproteins is shown in Figure 14.1. Statins are to be taken with the evening meal or, if they are taken b.i.d., with the morning and evening meals.

Table 14.2 Therapeutic goals for treatment of hypercholesterolemic patients by risk category

Therapeutic goal LDL-C (mg/dl)	Patient categories by risk
Low risk for CAD clinical events	
<220	Adult men <35 yr and premenopausal women with no family history of CAD and no other CAD risk factors
<190	Adult men <35 yr and premenopausal women with a family history of premature CAD or diabetes mellitus
<160	Adult men >35 yr and postmenopausal women with no family history of CAD and no other CAD risk factors
Moderate risk for CAD clinical events	
<130	Individuals with a family history of CAD or two or more CAD risk factors
High risk for CAD clinical events	
<100	Patients with existing CAD (including PTCA or stent placement or after coronary artery bypass graft surgery[a])

Abbreviation: CAD, coronary artery disease.
[a] Post-CABG Trial 1997.[7] Not part of NCEP guidelines.
Adapted from Witztum.[3]

RESULTS (FIGURE 14.1)

All of these agents except atorvastatin will lower plasma cholesterol by between 20% and 40% and LDL-C by 25% to 45% at maximum doses. Fluvastatin appears to lower cholesterol by up to 20% and LDL-C by 25% at maximum doses. To achieve 35–45% LDL-C lowering, daily doses of 40 mg of simvastatin or 80 mg of lovastatin are required. Triglycerides are reduced by between 10% and 30%. Patient HDL-C plasma levels are frequently increased by 5–10%, but the increases may be more modest or absent in those with inherently low levels. Lp(a) levels are little affected.[23] Statin therapy alters small dense LDL particles to a larger, more buoyant form and also normalizes the responsiveness of coronary vessels to vasoactive stimulus.[24] E-selectin, a cell adhesion molecule with increased expression in atherosclerotic states, is reduced with simvastatin or atorvastatin as monotherapy or in combination with colestipol.[25]

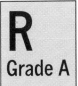

Atorvastatin, a newly approved agent, is considered separately only because it may represent a more powerful member of this class of agents. Reductions in total cholesterol of 45–50%, in LDL-C of up to 60%, and in triglycerides of 35–45% are seen at 80 mg/d doses. Reductions in apo B levels of 35–40% have been observed.[22] Changes in plasma levels of Lp(a) are small, if they occur.[26] Increases in HDL-C are inconsistent but may reach 12%.[27]

ADVERSE REACTIONS

Overall adverse effects occur in less than 2% of individuals. Increases in liver transaminase levels occur in 0.5% of patients. Liver function abnormalities are not dose dependent and more commonly occur after several months.[28] Therapy should be stopped if the transaminase levels exceed three times the upper limits of normal. Rare (less than 0.1%)

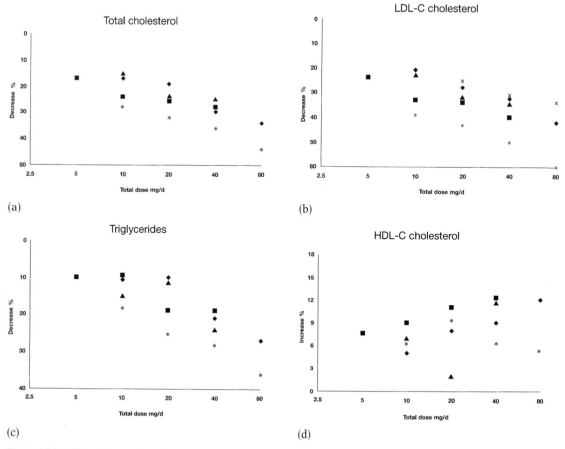

Figure 14.1. These four graphs (data taken from that submitted to the FDA and published in PDR or package insert) indicate the response between 2.5 and 80 mg/d of the five statin agents on plasma levels of total cholesterol, LDL-C, triglycerides and HDL-C with the following codes: ◆ lovastatin 10 mg q.d., all other doses b.i.d.; ■ simvastatin; ▲ pravastatin; ✕ fluvastatin; * atorvastatin.

and reversible increases of greater than 10-fold in Creatine Phosphokinase (CPK) levels have been described. Statins compete with other drugs for specific metabolic pathways of the cytochrome P450 system.[29] Caution is urged in those patients using statins with cyclosporin (a known inhibitor of CYP3A4), particularly when other inhibitors of the cytochrome P450 system are in use, such as erythromycin. Mild muscle enzyme elevations may occur in 5–10% of individuals. However, one should consider discontinuing therapy if CPK increases by more than three-fold. The cause of CPK elevation and myopathy remains unexplained.

CLINICAL USE

Although the biggest proportional reduction in LDL-C levels occurs at low doses (Figure 14.1), the clinical response to statins is a dose–response relationship and appears to be independent of patient characteristics such as age, gender, smoking status, and initial lipid and lipoprotein levels.[30] Initiation of LDL-C lowering therapy has been recommended only after a trial (up to 6 months) of dietary therapy.[10] A key issue in the prevention of clinical coronary events is stabilization of rapidly progressive plaques.[31] This appears

Table 14.3 Non-statin lipid altering agent summary

Agent	Lipid/ lipoprotein indication	Dosage and dosing	Response expected	Common adverse effects	Comments
Nicotinic acid	↑Triglyceride (TGs) ↑LDL-C ↓HDL-C ↑Lp(a)	1–3 g/d 6–8 g/d maximum dose 3–4 admin/d	↓TGs 20–80% ↓LDL-C 25–40% ↑HDL-C 25% ↓Lp(a) 10–30%	Cutaneous flushing, pruritis GI symptoms "Flu-like" syndrome	Start low dose advance slowly Relative contraindications ↑FBS, ↑Liver function test (LFTs)
Bile acid sequestrants	↑LDL-C	4–24 g cholestyramine 5–30 g colestipol	↓LDL-C 25–35% at maximum dose ↑TGs 15–20%	GI symptoms	Premix, slow admin Alters absorption of other drugs, e.g. glycosides, warfarin, etc.
	↓HDL-C	2 admin/d, 1 @ major meal	↑HDL-C 4–7%		Contraindicated in hypertriglyceridemia
Fibric acid derivatives	↑TGs	Clofibrate 1 g b.i.d. Gemfibrozil 0.6 g/b.i.d. Fenofibrate 0.4 g q.d.	↓LDL-C 10–20% ↓TGs 40–55% ↑HDL-C 15–20%	GI symptoms	Will ↑LDL-C in hypertriglyceridemic patients Contraindicated in those with gall stones Marked dose alteration in those with chronic renal failure

to occur with a minimum of 30 mg/dl or about 20% lowering of the plasma LDL-C levels.[32] While observance of a low fat diet is central to long term optimal lipid altering therapy, it may be judicious after a myocardial infarct to start medication as part of therapy earlier to encourage plaque stability. Initiating statin therapy for patients postinfarction without baseline and subsequent monitoring is inconsistent with best practice patterns.

Nicotinic acid (Table 14.3)

Profound reductions in plasma total cholesterol and triglyceride levels in association with administration of nicotinic acid-C were first noted by Attschult in the early 1950s. Nicotinic acid (NA) is known to have the most marked clinical effect on HDL[33] and is the only lipid altering agent to consistently lower Lp(a) plasma levels.[34]

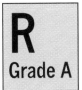

R

Grade A

MECHANISM OF ACTION

The predominant effect on plasma lipid levels is a reduced production of VLDL particles[35] with subsequently reduced production of intermediate density lipoprotein (IDL) and LDL particles. The major effect on VLDL metabolism results from an inhibition of hormone sensitive lipase-induced lipolysis in adipose tissue and decreased triglyceride esterification in the liver. HDL-C increases appear related to reduced apo A-I clearance and increased production of apo A-II. How Lp(a) levels are reduced is unknown, but it may be related to early NA-induced hepatotoxicity.

DOSAGE

Crystalline NA is available in 0.1 and 0.5 g tablets and the sustained release form in dosages of 0.125, 0.25, and 0.5 g. A common maximum dose is 3 g/day[36] (Table 14.3).

RESULTS

Regardless of the patient's clinical lipoprotein abnormality, dose dependent reductions in total and LDL-C and plasma triglycerides have been achieved. HDL-C levels may increase by 15–40%, but the response usually plateaus between 1.5 and 3.0 g/d with an average 25% increase. Reductions in Lp(a) of 25–30% are achieved.[37] Small dense LDL particles become larger and more buoyant during therapy.[38] Optimal responses of certain individuals may be formulation and dosing regimen dependent.[39]

ADVERSE REACTIONS

Even very low doses (0.05–0.10 g) cause cutaneous flushing (>80%) and pruritis (50%), gastrointestinal symptoms (5–20%), elevation of liver enzymes (3–10%), uric acid (5–10%), fasting blood sugar (FBS) or an abnormal glucose tolerance test (GTT) (5–10%). Blurred vision with macular edema occurs very rarely. Liver enzyme elevations occur more commonly with slow release preparations and rapid increases in dose. A "flu-like syndrome" may occur that can include a hepatitis-like picture on liver biopsy, a secretory defect with profound decreases in LDL-C, decreases in HDL-C, and an abnormality in the prothrombin time. This clinical picture is dose dependent and resolves with cessation of the agent.[40] Prednisone use with nicotinic acid is contraindicated and results in patients manifesting clinical diabetes.

CLINICAL USE

Many prescription and non-prescription forms of nicotinic acid are available in the US. Non-prescription forms are usually less expensive, but bioavailability may be a problem. Nicolar and Rugby brands are both highly effective and available by prescription and the latter also as a non-prescription medication. The larger crystalline form tablets are scored and allow easy tailoring of the therapeutic regimen, starting with a single low dose of either 0.1 or 0.25 g/d. Because of the biological half-time of the agent, frequent administrations are necessary.[41] Dosing with the crystalline form requires 3–4 administrations a day. No preparation or dosing regimen has been shown to be superior to multiples of 0.1 g crystalline tablets administered four times a day. Although recommended by the NCEP-II,[16] many patients will have little or no effect from two administrations a day, unless using sustained release preparations. Increases in the dosage are implemented only every few days.[39] Commonly physicians reduce the number of administrations to three times per day and use 0.5 g tablets, starting with 0.25 g q.d.

for the first week. Sustained release preparations should be used only in those patients with a documented response to immediate release forms.

Nicotinic acid should always be taken with food. Hot and alcoholic drinks should be avoided at administration and dosages should be reduced or perhaps restarted if several successive doses are missed. Cutaneous flushing and pruritis will occur routinely if the above precautions are not followed. In any case, if symptoms occur, they are most severe during the first administration. Although aspirin is thought to reduce symptoms of cutaneous flushing and pruritis, this was not demonstrated in a double-blind study.[42] The clinical picture of mild liver function abnormalities usually resolves with continued therapy or at reduced dose. Although nicotinic acid may profoundly alter glucose metabolism in some, many diabetics have had successful management of their lipid disorders with this agent. An FBS of >115 mg/dl predicts those who lose their acute insulin response as manifested during an IV glucose tolerance test.[43] An FBS level below 100 mg/dl should identify those who can be managed with nicotinic acid without the development of clinical diabetes.

Bile acid sequestering agents (resins) (Table 14.3)

This class of agents was first developed for the treatment of cholestasis-related pruritis by Carey and Williams in 1960. Hashim and van Itallie subsequently demonstrated that cholestyramine lowered plasma cholesterol. It was approved by the FDA in 1973.

R

Grade A

MECHANISM OF ACTION

The enterohepatic circulation of bile acids allows for only 6–7% of them to be excreted each day. These polymers with a molecular weight of over 10^6 are not absorbed and function by binding bile acids in the gastrointestinal lumen. Since bile acid excretion from the body and production in the liver increase, relative depletion of cholesterol from the liver cells occurs, inducing an increased level of hepatic LDL receptor activity.[44,45] The net effect is an increase in the catabolism of LDL-C and plasma levels are decreased.

DOSAGE

Resins are dispensed in individual packets and are also available in a cost-effective bulk formulation. Scoops, equivalent in size to the number of grams in one packet, are used to dispense from the parent container.

RESULTS

Resins are associated with significant reductions in plasma total and LDL-C and with small increases in plasma HDL-C levels.[46] Plasma triglycerides are inconsistently affected, but substantial increases may occur if used in those with already elevated plasma triglyceride levels.[47] In familial dysbetalipoproteinemia (type III or remnant removal disease) plasma triglyceride levels may increase by more than three-fold.

ADVERSE REACTIONS

No long-term adverse effects have been demonstrated.[46] Drugs that are highly charged, including the cardiac glycoside, coumarin anticoagulant, diuretic, and beta-blocker (unpublished data) classes, as well as thyroid hormone, will have their absorption affected,[48] if taken in close proximity to the administration of the resin. Regulation of coumarin therapy during concomitant resin therapy may present extremely challenging problems. If the effect of the resins on the absorption of a specific medication is not known, the resin should be taken at least 2 hours after or 4 hours before other medications. In clinical situations of existing gastrointestinal malabsorption, the absorption of fat soluble vitamins may also be reduced.

CLINICAL USE

The biggest proportional reduction in lipid levels occurs at low doses and in those who have moderately elevated levels of cholesterol.[49] Careful selection of the vehicle and logistics used in resin administration will promote long term participant adherence. While using cold water with premixing (taking advantage of the resin's hygroscopic nature) and slow oral intake is by far the most frequent and successful method of administration, the use of a heavily textured juice has proven effective for some. Pre-existing gastrointestinal symptoms should be dealt with before resin therapy is started. Bloating, belching, and increased flatus are related to rapid ingestion. Dyspepsia and increased stool consistency or frank constipation can be managed with increases in fluids or dietary fiber intake.

Fibric acid derivatives (Table 14.3)

R
Grade A

While clofibrate and gemfibrozil are the only members of this class currently marketed in the US, fibrates available in other countries include bezafibrate, fenofibrate, ciprofibrate, beclafibrate, etiofibrate, and clinofibrate. In the WHO study clofibrate was shown to reduce modestly ($P<0.05$) all cardiovascular events. However, an increase in non-cardiovascular morbidity and mortality and total mortality occurred.[50] Gemfibrozil in the Helsinki Heart Study was associated with a 35% reduction in myocardial infarctions, particularly in those with increases in plasma LDL-C and triglycerides and decreases in plasma HDL-C. Increases in non-cardiovascular deaths and no reduction in total mortality occurred[51] and led to concerns about the use of fibrates. Although the incidence of gastrointestinal symptoms and clinical gall bladder disease in the two studies was very similar, the use of clofibrate has decreased and the use of gemfibrozil has increased. These agents are approved for use primarily in those with hypertriglyceridemia.

MECHANISM OF ACTION

Decreased synthesis of VLDL with more efficient lipolysis and increased VLDL triglyceride catabolism has long been suggested as the mechanism of action of fibrates on lipid metabolism. Schoonjans and colleagues, in 1996, offered direct evidence that fibrates and fatty acids work as ligands for a class of compounds called peroxisome proliferator activated receptors (PPAR), of the nuclear receptor superfamily.[52] PPAR-α partially mediates the inductive effects of fibrates on HDL-C levels by regulating the transcription of HDL apolipoproteins, apo A-I and apo A-II. Four specific actions are noted:

1. increased hydrolysis of plasma triglycerides due to induction of LPL and reduction of apo-CIII expression;

2. stimulation of cellular fatty acid uptake and conversion to acyl-CoA derivatives due to increased expression of genes for fatty acid transport protein and acyl-CoA synthetase;
3. increased peroxisomal and mitochondrial beta-oxidation;
4. decreased synthesis of fatty acids and triglycerides with a concomitantly decreased production of VLDLs.

DOSAGE

See Table 14.3 for clofibrate and gemfibrozil (also available in sustained release form). Bezafibrate 0.2 g t.i.d. (0.4 g sustained q.d.), fenofibrate 0.3–0.4 g q.d., ciprofibrate 0.1–0.2 g q.d.

RESULTS

In patients with *familial combined hyperlipidemia*, LDL-C levels may be reduced by fibrates but, particularly in those with elevated baseline levels of plasma triglycerides, there will almost uniformly be an increase in LDL-C levels as VLDL-C levels decrease.[53] Gemfibrozil and clofibrate were found to give equivalent results in lipids and lipoproteins in a double-blind crossover study.[54] In patients with moderate to severe forms of hypertriglyceridemia reductions in plasma triglycerides of 40–60% may occur with concomitant increases of 12–30% in HDL-C levels, but 100% increases in LDL cholesterol may occur.[55]

ADVERSE REACTIONS

Fibrates are associated with adverse effects in 5–10% of patients. Gastrointestinal side effects (5%) are the most common, but only rarely are these sufficient to warrant discontinuation of the medication. The increased incidence of hepatobiliary disease (particularly gall stones) occurs with all agents in this class.[56] Minor alterations in several plasma biochemical values may occur, but these are dose dependent and usually transient. The effective non-toxic dose range is narrow and at high doses, fibrates cause myositis.

CLINICAL USE

The primary indication for the use of this class of agents has shifted to treatment of severe hypertriglyceridemia and, more specifically, familial dysbetalipoproteinemia or remnant removal disease. They are preferred by those who are less experienced in the use of nicotinic acid in clinical circumstances with increases in plasma LDL-C and reductions in HDL-C levels. Because of the long term adverse effects on hepatobiliary function and the potential for increases in LDL-C levels, liver function tests and LDL-C levels must be monitored closely. Chronic renal failure requires a reduction in fibric acid dosage (7.5% of clofibrate and 50% of gemfibrozil respective doses).[57]

Probucol

A definitive role for probucol in the treatment of hyperlipidemia was never identified.[17,58] Its effect on LDL-C lowering was substantially more modest than other

Table 14.4 Stepped approach to lipid medication altering therapies

	↑LDL-C	↑TG/LDL,↓HDL-C	↑Lp(a)	↑↑↑TGs*
1.	Statin	Niacin	Niacin	Fibrate/niacin
2.	Statin + resin	Niacin + Resin		
3.	↑Statin + resin	↑Niacin + resin		
4.	↑Statin + resin + niacin	↑Niacin + statin or Statin + fibrate		

* TGs >500 mg/dL.

agents. It was thought to have a beneficial effect on the development and progression of atherosclerosis through its antioxidant properties. The agent has a demonstrated regressive effect on xanthelasma and tendon xanthoma in those with familial hypercholesterolemia. A study has been published showing a 50% reduction in restenosis with probucol treatment following PTCA.[59] However, a long term benefit on CHD clinical events has yet to be demonstrated. This agent has recently been removed from the market in the US.

Combination therapy

Combination drug therapy should be used when diet and single drug therapy is inadequate to reduce LDL-C levels to the desired range. Verification of adherence to and the efficacy of a prescribed regimen should be made on at least two occasions at monthly intervals before adding to the regimen. Table 14.4 describes a stepped approach to combination therapy depending upon the lipid and/or lipoprotein variable(s) that are the objective of the treatment regimen. Remember that reduction in LDL-C is the only alteration in lipid(s) or lipoprotein(s) that has been demonstrated to reduce risks for CHD in clinical trials. Epidemiologic data do demonstrate an increased risk associated with reduced levels of HDL-C, an increased plasma Lp(a) (usually in association with increased LDL-C levels) and to a lesser extent increased plasma triglyceride levels (usually in association with other risk factors).

GUIDELINES FOR SELECTING COMBINATION THERAPY

Practitioners should review four questions before adding other agents to initial diet and lipid altering drug therapy regimens.[60]

1. Has adherence to and efficacy of the initial regimen been verified?
2. Does the patient have fasting hypertriglyceridemia? (Bile acid sequestering agents should be used as the second or third agent only.)
3. What contraindications exist to the addition of other lipid altering agents? (Other diseases or clinical conditions or other lipid altering agents.)
4. What are the total costs of additional drug therapy to the patient?

Table 14.5 Efficacy of selected combinations of hyperlipidemic drug therapy in modifying plasma concentrations of total, LDL and HDL cholesterol levels

Drug combination	% Change			Reference
	Total	LDL	HDL	
Cholestyramine				
+ Niacin	−26	−32	+23	Angelin *et al.*, 1986[61]
+ Lovastatin	−51	−61	+21	Leren *et al.*, 1988[67]
+ Pravastatin	−36	−43	+18	Jacob *et al.*, 1993[66]
Colestipol				
+ Niacin	−41	−48	+25	Packard *et al.*, 1980[69]
+ Lovastatin	−45	−54	−2	Illingworth *et al.*, 1981[64]
+ Niacin	−55	−66	+32	Malloy *et al.*, 1987[68]
+ Simvastatin	−41	−50	+9	Simons *et al.*, 1992[70]
+ Fenofibrate	−39	−54	+15	Heller *et al.*, 1981[63]
Lovastatin				
+ Gemfibrozil	−34	−40	+7	Illingworth *et al.*, 1989[65]
Simvastatin				
+ Gemfibrozil	−54	−58	+18	Feussner *et al.*, 1992[62]

EFFICACY OF VARIOUS COMBINATIONS

Selected examples of maximum lipid and lipoprotein alteration are given in Table 14.5.[61-70] Prior to the development of atorvastatin the maximum lowering of LDL-C was demonstrated with a combination of lovastatin (40 mg/d), colestipol (30 g/d), and nicotinic acid (5.5 g/d) at 70%. Triglyceride reductions of 80% can be effected with nicotinic acid alone with little to be gained in efficacy by adding another agent. Lp(a) levels are affected substantially only by nicotinic acid. HDL-C can be consistently raised by 25% with nicotinic acid alone with little further gained by adding other agents.

R

Grade A

ADVERSE EFFECTS

The important adverse effects of the single agents are described in Table 14.3. The most serious interaction is seen in organ transplant patients when one of the statins is used in combination with cyclosporin and myopathy develops. While cessation of the statin allows symptomatic myopathy and elevated muscle enzymes to resolve, continued therapy at the same dose may lead to frank rhabdomyolysis, necessitating hemodialysis. Statins have also been associated with myopathic syndromes in patients using erythromycin, niacin, and gemfibrozil. Reduced levels of any statin should be used in transplant patients in association with niacin and gemfibrozil with careful monitoring of muscle enzyme levels. Erythromycin use should be considered absolutely contraindicated in transplant patients already on cyclosporin and a statin. If erythromycin is used, the statin must be temporarily discontinued.

CLINICAL USE

Although single drug therapy offers a simple regimen, much interest has recently been shown in combination therapy with low dose statin and low dose bile acid sequestrant.[66,70] Since the largest portion of lipid alteration is effected at low doses of both of these classes of agents and they work by very different mechanisms, an additive or synergistic response may occur. Low dose combinations provide a good clinical alternative for patients who have symptoms at higher statin dosages and for organ transplant patients. They also appear to be more cost effective than using statin as a single agent.

INFORMED DECISIONS ABOUT "GRAY ZONES"

Indications for treatment of increased plasma levels of LDL-C in the following groups are sparse. Eligibility criteria for clinical trials are frequently arbitrary and may reflect a lack of risk information about the group(s) excluded. While implications for treatment of populations or individuals beyond those treated in trials must be carefully considered, those outside the populations studied are likely to obtain some therapeutic benefit. This concept is particularly relevant for continuous variables, such as age, blood pressure or serum cholesterol.

How and when do we treat the following groups?

The elderly

The average age of death for males and females in the US is 72 and 78 years respectively. If one lives until age 80, the average additional life expectancy is 8 years. Older individuals appear to be at least as responsive to cholesterol lowering agents as individuals in lower age groups. While some have suggested that risk attenuates for those who have hypercholesterolemia at older age, the absolute risk for developing CHD outcomes in the elderly over a short time interval is much higher than it is in younger individuals. Therefore the absolute risk attributable to high cholesterol actually increases with age.[10]

The West of Scotland Coronary Prevention Study (WOSCOPS)[5] (primary intervention or PI) included patients up to the age of 64 years, 4S[2] (secondary intervention or SI) up to the age of 70 years, Post-CABG[7] (SI) up to 74 years and CARE[4] (SI) up to 75 years. These studies showed benefit for CHD and CVD morbidity. All except Post-CABG showed benefit on CHD and CVD mortality. WOSCOPS and 4S showed benefit on total mortality, although statistical significance of the data from WOSCOPS was marginal. Limited analyses by age group included in these reports support benefit related to LDL-C lowering in the elderly.

Additional information will soon be available from the Heart Protection Study (HPS, 20 000 participants, completion 2000, simvastatin), the Women's Health Initiative (WHI, 48 000 participants, completion 2007, diet) and the Antihypertensive and Lipid Lowering Treatment to Prevent Heart Disease Trial (10 000 participants, completion 2002, pravastatin). These studies have upper age limits of 75 years, 79 years, and no upper age limit respectively.[71] While waiting for the completion of these studies, treatment of hypercholesterolemia in the elderly gives physicians an opportunity to craft therapy according to perceived risks and potential benefit for each individual.

Women

Women were not included in early cholesterol lowering trials because of concerns about confounding related to hormonal effects on lipids, specifically in premenopausal women. The "silent epidemic" of coronary heart disease in women and the clearly established relationship between increases in plasma cholesterol and coronary heart disease in women at any age dictate that therapeutic benefits of cholesterol lowering in women be established.

Women comprised the following respective proportions of the recently completed trials: 4S[2] 19%, Post-CABG[7] 8%, WOSCOPS[3] 0% and CARE[4] 14%. Although the numbers of women are modest, 35% and 46% reductions in major coronary events were observed in 4S and CARE respectively. Commensurate risk reductions for the men were 34% and 20% respectively.

LIPID with 17% GISSI Prevention with 20%, and AFCAPS/TEXCAPS with 15% women will report in either 1997 or 1998. HPS with 30%, ALLHAT with 45%, and WHI with 100% women will report in 2000, 2002, and 2007 respectively.[71] Current evidence suggests a comparable effect for cholesterol lowering on CHD outcomes and no evidence of harm in women.

Diabetics

While aggressive control of blood glucose levels in insulin-dependent diabetic patients has been shown to reduce microvascular clinical outcomes, its effect on macrovascular disease outcomes remains unknown. Other traditional CHD risk factors are believed to increase dramatically the risk for clinical CHD events in these patients. Inherent in the diabetic disease process is an abnormality of lipoprotein lipase activity that is partially but not completely corrected by optimal glucose control. Any additional lipid and lipoprotein disorder(s) present in diabetics because of either inherited or secondary causes (obesity, alcohol consumption, etc.) accelerate atherosclerotic progression and increase the risk of clinical CHD events. Treatment of lipid disorders in diabetics with commensurate lowering of blood cholesterol levels has given results suggestive of a similar treatment benefit in diabetics.[2,4] Cholesterol lowering and lipoprotein alteration in diabetics is currently under investigation in several trials.[71]

Peripheral vascular disease

Patients who have peripheral vascular disease have a substantially increased risk of dying of CHD. Criqui and colleagues have described this in a series of articles from the Rancho Bernardo Study. No specific clinical outcome trial of LDL-C reduction has been performed in these patients although the HPS will have an enriched population of these individuals.[71] More than 80% of these individuals have CHD although a number will manifest few symptoms. It is reasonable, but unsubstantiated, to treat these individuals as if they have CHD.

Table 14.6 Comparative cost, dose and LDL-C lowering of statins

Agent	Dose (mg)	LDL-C reduction	AWP (cost/d)	Cost/1%LDLR (dollars/yr)
Lovastatin	*20*	*−24*	*2.25*	*32.48*
	40	−30	4.05	46.77
	80	−40	7.77	70.16
Simvastatin	*10*	*−30*	*2.03*	*25.30*
	20	−35	3.54	36.40
	40	−40	3.68	31.85
Pravastatin	*20*	*−32*	*1.97*	*22.47*
	40	−34	3.32	35.64
Fluvastatin	*20*	*−22*	*1.22*	*19.71*
	40	−24	1.36	20.31
Atorvastatin	*10*	*−39*	*1.82*	*17.95*
	20	−43	2.82	25.10
	40	−50	3.40	24.80

LDL-C: Reductions according to PDR and atorvastatin brochure approved.
AWP: Average wholesale price according to Red Book® Update, February 1997.
COST/1%LDLR: Cost in $/yr/1% LDL reduction.
Common starting dose

Small dense LDL-C particles (Phenotype B)

The entire population may be generally divided into two categories on the basis of predominant LDL species present in plasma. People with a predominance of smaller, more dense LDL particles exhibit an increased propensity for oxidative susceptibility of these species.[72] These individuals demonstrate a higher risk for CHD.[73] This increased risk of CHD has been connected to some interrelated changes in plasma lipids, specifically an increase in triglycerides and reduced plasma levels of HDL. It has also been suggested that this pattern may be related to the insulin resistance syndrome or syndrome X with impaired glucose tolerance, increased insulin levels, hypertension, and abnormalities of coagulation factors. Treatment of those with small dense LDL particles with a successful shift to LDL particles of a larger, more buoyant size is predictive of those who demonstrate benefit on angiographic follow-up.[74]

COSTS AND COST EFFECTIVENESS OF LIPID ALTERATIONS FOR CHD PREVENTION

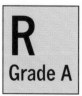

R

Grade A

True benefits for individuals and the public health have only been demonstrated for alteration of plasma LDL-C. One method for comparing the costs of cholesterol lowering is represented by the data in Table 14.6 where the cost of the various statins is given in terms of the number of dollars per percent of LDL-C lowering per year.

Until the release of results from the 4S study, reductions in CHD morbidity from plasma cholesterol-related CHD had been modest and reductions in CHD and total mortality had not been demonstrated. Since elevated plasma cholesterol is regarded as one of the major risk factors for CHD and since elevated plasma cholesterol is prevalent in Western countries, evaluation of the cost effectiveness of plasma cholesterol lowering is important because of the size of the potential population for intervention and the associated health care costs, with potentially lifelong medication intervention. Data from 4S demonstrate cost effectiveness, including sensitivity analysis,[75] of intervention for both men and women at ages from 35 to 70 years and at plasma cholesterol levels above 213 mg/dl. Similar findings, although with more limited indications, have been published by Goldman and colleagues using extrapolations from epidemiological data and a model of lovastatin therapy in secondary as well as primary prevention.[76] Data from the prospective randomized trial (4S) provide more rigorous information for this evaluation.

Standards for cost effective therapies have been previously published.[77] The estimates of treatment costs for benefits observed in both men and women and at all plasma cholesterol levels between 213 and 309 mg/dl fit well within the boundaries of what would be considered to be cost effective. Whether or not similar conclusions can be made concerning plasma cholesterol lowering for primary prevention of CHD is uncertain.

SUMMARY

Powerful and cost effective single and combination drug regimens for LDL-C reduction for the prevention of CHD and the prolongation of life are now available. Effective single and combination agent regimens for intervention on other plasma lipid and lipoprotein variables are also available. Indications for regimen use to manipulate lipid and lipoprotein variables other than LDL-C are limited by our incomplete knowledge concerning the impact of alteration of their respective plasma levels on CHD, CVD, and total mortality.

Cardinal issues for using lipid altering agents

- Is the diagnosis of hyperlipidemia certain?
- Are there currently medications in the patient's regimen that cause dyslipidemia or offer the potential for drug interactions with hypolipidemic therapy?
- ALWAYS start the therapeutic regimen with dietary modification.
- The statins act as a class of agents, but possess different dose–response curves.
- The statins have powerful lipid altering effects and a very low order of adverse effects.
- Nicotinic acid is a powerful agent which can be effective in many people when used carefully.
- Nicotinic acid is the most effective of any agent on HDL-C levels and the only one with a demonstrated effect on Lp(a).
- Resin therapy can be effective for lowering LDL-C plasma levels with careful attention to details of dosing and administration, particularly when added to low dose statin or low dose niacin.
- Fasting hypertriglyceridemia is a relative contraindication to primary or combination resin therapy.
- Fibrates are effective agents for lowering triglyceride and moderately raising HDL-C levels, but changes in LDL-C levels need to be monitored.
- Are there contraindications to the specific hypolipidemic drug combinations?
- Consider the direct and indirect costs before initiating primary lipid altering therapy and before the addition of each agent to the combined regimen.

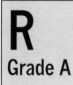

R

Grade A

Lipid and lipoprotein alteration for prevention of coronary heart disease

- Plasma cholesterol lowering is effective in both men and women.
- Plasma cholesterol lowering is effective for ages up to 75 years, particularly in women.
- Plasma cholesterol lowering is cost effective in men and women between 35 and 70 years of age and above a plasma cholesterol of 213 mg/dl (5.5 mmol).
- Plasma cholesterol lowering maintains the patency of coronary artery saphenous vein grafts.
- NIDDM, hypertension, increased plasma triglycerides, low plasma HDL-C, small dense LDL, and increased PAI-1 levels are components of the so-called "insulin resistance syndrome" which appears to be a marker for individuals with small dense LDLs.
- Alteration of plasma lipids (triglycerides) and other lipoproteins (VLDL-C, HDL-C) beyond total plasma cholesterol and LDL-C have not been demonstrated to affect CHD cause specific morbidity or mortality.

REFERENCES

1 Austin MA, Breslow JL, Hennekens CH *et al.* Low-density lipoprotein subclass patterns and risk of myocardial infarction. *JAMA* 1988;**260**: 1917–21.

2 Scandinavian Simvastatin Survival Study Group. Randomized trial of cholesterol lowering in 4444 patients with coronary heart disease: the Scandinavian Simvastatin Survival Study (4S). *Lancet* 1995;**344**:1383–9.

3 Shepherd J, Cobbe SM, Ford I *et al.* for the West of Scotland Coronary Prevention Study Group. Prevention of coronary heart disease with pravastatin in men with hypercholesterolemia. *N Engl J Med* 1995;**333**:1301–7.

4 Sacks FM, Pfeffer MA, Moye LA *et al.* for the Cholesterol and Recurrent Events Trial Investigators. The effect of pravastatin on coronary events after myocardial infarction in patients with average cholesterol levels. *N Engl J Med* 1996;**335**:1001–9.

5 Brown G, Albers JJ, Fisher LD *et al.* Regression of coronary artery disease as a result of intensive lipid-lowering therapy in men with high levels of apolipoprotein B. *N Engl J Med* 1990;**323**: 1289–98.

6 Furberg CD, Adams HP, Applegate WB *et al.* for the Asymptomatic Carotid Plaque Study (ACAPS) Research Group. Effect of lovastatin and warfarin on early carotid atherosclerosis and cardiovascular events. *Circulation* 1994;**90**: 1670–87.

7 The Post Coronary Artery Bypass Graft Trial Investigators. The effect of aggressive lowering of low-density lipoprotein cholesterol levels and low-dose anticoagulation on obstructive changes in saphenous-vein coronary-artery bypass grafts. *N Engl J Med* 1997;**336**:153–62.

8 Roberts WC. Preventing and arresting coronary atherosclerosis: poor implementation of risk factor interventions. *Am Heart J* 1995;**130**:580–600.

9 Brunzell JB. Disorders of lipoprotein metabolism. In: Wyngaarden JB, Smith LH, Bennett JC. Eds. *Cecil textbook of medicine*, 19th edn. Phidelphia: WB Saunders, 1992.

10 Expert Panel on Detection, Evaluation and Treatment of High Blood Cholesterol in Adults National Cholesterol Education Program. Summary of the second report of the expert panel. Detection, evaluation, and treatment of high blood cholesterol in adults (Adult Treatment Panel II). *Circulation* 1994;**89**:1329–445.

11 Pyorala K, DeBacker G, Graham I, Poole-Wilson P, Wood D on behalf of the Task Force of the European Society of Cardiology, European Atherosclerosis Society and the European Society of Hypertension. Prevention of coronary heart disease in clinical practice: recommendations of the task force. *Eur Heart J* 1994;**15**:1300–31.

12 National Cholesterin-Initiative. Ein Strategie-Papier zur Erkennung and Behandlung von Hyperlipidamen. *Dtsch Artztebl* 1990;**87**: A1358–82.

13 Irish Hyperlipidemia Association. *Guidelines for the management of hyperlipidemia*, 3rd edn. Dublin: Irish Hyperlipidemia Association, 1992.

14 Betteridge DJ, Dodson PM, Durrington PN *et al.* Management of hyperlipidemia: guidelines of the British Hyperlipidemia Association. *Postgrad Med J* 1993;**69**:359–69.

15 Mann J, Crooke M, Fear H *et al.* Guidelines for detection and management of dyslipidemia. *N Z Med J* 1993;**106**:133–41.

16 Rifkind BM. Ed. *Drug treatment of hyperlipidemia*. New York: Dekker, 1991.

17 Witztum J. Drugs used in the treatment of hyperlipoproteinemia In: Gilman AG, Rall TW, Nies AS, Taylor P. Eds. *Goodman and Gilman's the pharmacological basis of therapeutics*. Oxford: Pergamon Press, 1995.

18 Brown MS, Faust JR, Goldstein JL. Inhibition of 3-hydroxy-3-methylglutaryl coenzyme A reductase activity in human fibroblasts incubated with

compactin (ML-236B), a competitive inhibitor of the reductase. *J Biol Chem* 1978;**253**:1121–8.

19 Brown MS, Goldstein JL. A receptor-mediated pathway for cholesterol homeostasis. *Science* 1986;**232**:34–47.

20 Berglund LF, Beltz WF, Elam RL, Witztum JL. Altered apolipoprotein B metabolism in very low density lipoprotein from lovastatin-treated guinea pigs. *J Lipid Res* 1994;**35**:956–65.

21 Illingworth DR, Tobert JA. A review of clinical trials comparing HMG-CoA reductase inhibitors. *Clin Ther* 1994;**16**:366–85.

22 Atorvastatin calcium. Approved brochure and package insert. Warner Lambert-Pfizer, 1997.

23 Arky R. Ed. *Physicians' desk reference*. Montvale, NJ: Medical Economics, 1997.

24 Anderson TJ, Meredith IT, Yeung AC *et al*. The effect of cholesterol-lowering and antioxidant therapy on endothelium-dependent coronary vasomotion. *N Engl J Med* 1995; **332**:488–93.

25 Hackman A, Yasunori A, Insull Jr W *et al*. Levels of soluble cell adhesion molecules in patients with dyslipidemia. *Circulation* 1996;**93**:1334–8.

26 Nawrocki JW, Weiss SR, Davidson MH *et al*. Reduction of LDL cholesterol by 25% to 60% in patients with primary hypercholesterolemia by atorvastatin, a new HMG-CoA reductase inhibitor. *Arterioscler Thromb Vasc Biol* 1995;**15**: 678–82.

27 Bakker-Arkema RG, Davidson MH, Goldstein RJ *et al*. Efficacy and safety of a new HMG-CoA reductase inhibitor, atorvastatin, in patients with hypertriglyceridemia. *JAMA* 1996;**275**:128–33.

28 Bradford RH, Shear CL, Chremos AN *et al*. Expanded clinical evaluation of lovastatin (EXCEL) study results. I: Efficacy in modifying plasma lipoproteins and adverse event profile in 8245 patients with moderate hyper-cholesterolemia. *Arch Intern Med* 1991;**151**:43–9.

29 Neuvonen PJ, Jalava K-M. Itraconazole drastically increases plasma concentrations of lovastatin and lovastatin acid. *Clin Pharmacol Ther* 1996;**60**: 54–61.

30 Shear CL, Franklin FA, Stinnett S *et al*. Expanded clinical evaluation of lovastatin (EXCEL) study results: effect of patient characteristics on lovastatin-induced changes in plasma concentrations of lipids and lipoproteins. *Circulation* 1992;**85**:1293–303.

31 Brown BG, Zhao X-Q, Sacco DE, Albers JJ. Lipid lowering and plaque regression: new insights into prevention of plaque disruption and clinical events in coronary disease. *Circulation* 1993;**87**: 1781–91.

32 Rossouw JE. Lipid-lowering interventions in angiographic trials. [Meta-analysis] *Am J Cardiol* 1995;**76**:86C–92C.

33 Alderman JD, Pasternak RC, Sacks FM *et al*. Effect of modified, well tolerated niacin regimen on serum total cholesterol, high density lipoprotein cholesterol and the cholesterol to high density lipoprotein ratio. *Am J Cardiol* 1989;**64**:725–9.

34 Carlson LA, Hampsten A, Asplund A. Effects of hyperlipidemic drugs on serum levels of lipoprotein Lp(a) in hyperlipidemic subjects treated with nicotinic acid. *J Int Med* 1989;**226**: 271–6.

35 Grundy SM Mok HYI, Zech L, Berman M. Influence of nicotinic acid on metabolism of cholesterol and triglycerides in man. *J Lipid Res* 1981;**22**:24–36.

36 Illingworth DR, Stein EA, Mitchel YB *et al*. Comparative effects of lovastatin and niacin in primary hypercholesterolemia. *Arch Intern Med* 1994;**154**:1586–95.

37 Superko HR, Krauss RM. Differential effects of nicotinic acid in subjects with different LDL subclass patterns. *Atherosclerosis* 1992;**95**:69–76.

38 Zambon A, Brown BG, Hokanson JE, Brunzell JD. Hepatic lipase changes predict coronary artery disease progression/regression in familial atherosclerosis treatment study (FATS). *Circulation* 1997;**94**:1–539.

39 Probstfield JL, Hunninghake DB. Nicotinic acid as a lipoprotein-altering agent: therapy directed by the primary physician. *Arch Intern Med* 1994; **154**:1557–9.

40 Patterson DJ, Dew EW, Gyorkey F, Graham DY. Niacin hepatitis. *Southern Med J* 1983;**76**: 239–41.

41 Miller ON, Hamilton JG, Goldsmith GA. Investigation of the mechanisms of nicotinic acid on serum lipid levels in man. *Am J Clin Nutr* 1960;**8**:480–90.

42 Welan AM, Price SO, Fowler SF, Hainer BL. The effect of aspirin on niacin-induced cutaneous reaction. *J Fam Pract* 1992;**34**:165–8.

43 Brunzell JD, Robertson RP, Lerner RL *et al*. Relationships between fasting plasma glucose levels and insulin secretion during intravenous glucose tolerance tests. *J Clin Endocrinol Metabol* 1976;**42**:222–9.

44 Shepherd J, Packard CJ, Bicker S, Lawrie TD, Morgan HG. Cholestyramine promotes receptor-mediated low-density-lipoprotein catabolism. *N Engl J Med* 1980;**302**:1219–22.

45 Kovanen PT, Bilheimer DW, Goldstein JL, Jaramillo JJ, Brown MS. Regulatory role for hepatic low density lipoprotein receptors in vivo in the dog. *Proc Natl Acad Sci* 1981;**78**:1194–8.

46 Lipid Research Clinics Program. The Lipid Research Clinics Coronary Primary Prevention Trial results. I: Reduction in the incidence of coronary heart disease. *JAMA* 1984;**251**:351–64.

47 Levy RI (Moderator). Discussants: dietary and drug treatment of primary hyperlipoproteinemia, NIH Conference. *Ann Intern Med* 1972;**77**: 267–94.

48 Hunninghake DB. Bile acid sequestrants. In: Rifkind BM. Ed. *Drug Treatment of Hyperlipidemia*. New York: Dekker.

49 Superko HR, Greenland P, Manchester RA *et al*. Effectiveness of low dose colestipol therapy in patients with moderate hypercholesterolemia. *Am J Cardiol* 1992;**70**:135–40.

50 Committee of Principal Investigators. W.H.O. cooperative trial on primary prevention of ischemic heart disease with clofibrate to lower serum cholesterol: mortality follow-up. *Lancet* 1980;**ii**:279–385.

51 Frick MJ, Elo O, Haapa K *et al*. Helsinki Heart Study: primary prevention trial with gemfibrozil in middle-aged men with dyslipidemia: safety of treatment, changes in risk factors, and incidence of coronary heart disease. *N Engl J Med* 1987; **317**:1237–45.

52 Schoonjans K, Staels B, Auwrex J. Role of the peroxisome proliferator-activated receptors (PPAR), in mediating the effects of fibrates and fatty acids on gene expression. *J Lipid Res* 1996; **37**:907–25.

53 Hokanson JE, Austin ME, Zambon A, Brunzell JD. Plasma triglyceride and LDL heterogeneity in familial combined hyperlipidemia. *Arterioscler Thromb* 1993;**13**:427–34.

54 Rabkin SW, Hayden M, Frohlich J. Comparison of gemfibrozil and clofibrate on serum lipids in familial combined hyperlipidemia. A randomized placebo-controlled, double-blind, crossover clinical trial. *Atherosclerosis* 1988; **73**:233–40.

55 Illingworth DR. Fibric acid derivatives. In: Rifkind BM. Ed. *Drug treatment of hyperlipidemia*. New York: Dekker, 1991.

56 Palmer RH. Effects of fibric acid derivatives on biliary litogenicity. *Am J Med* 1987;**83**(suppl 5B): 37–43.

57 Goldberg AP, Sherrard DJ, Hass LB, Brunzell JD. Control of clofibrate toxicity in uremic triglyceride. *Clin Pharmacol Ther* 1977;**21**: 317–25.

58 Steinberg D, Witztum JL. Probucol. In: Rifkind Bm. Ed. *Drug treatment of hyperlipidemia*. New York: Dekker, 1991.

59 Tardif JD, Cote G, Lesperance J *et al*. for the Multivitamin and Probucol Study Group. Probucol and multivitamins in the prevention of restenosis after coronary angioplasty. *N Engl J Med* 1997;**337**:365–72.

60 Hoeg JM. Combination drug therapy. In: Rifkind BM. Ed. *Drug treatment of hyperlipidemia*. New York: Dekker, 1991.

61 Angelin B, Eriksson M, Einarsson K. Combined treatment with cholestyramine and nicotinic acid in heterozygous familial hypercholesterolemia: Effects on biliary lipid composition. *Eur J Clin Invest* 1986;**16**:391–96.

62 Feussner G, Eichinger M, Ziegler R. The influence of simvastatin alone or in combination with gemfibrozil on plasma lipids and lipoproteins in patients with type III hyperlipoproteinemia. *Clin Investig* 1992;**70**:1027–35.

63 Heller FR, Desager JP, Hervengt C. Plasma lipid concentration and lecithin: cholesterol acyltransferase activity in normolipidemic subjects given fenofibrate and colestipol. *Metabolism* 1981;**30**:67–71.

64 Illingworth DR, Bacon S. Influence of lovastatin plus gemfibrozil on plasma lipids and lipoproteins in patients with heterozygous familial hypercholesterolemia. *Circulation* 1989;**79**:590–96.

65 Illingworth DR, Phillipson BE, Rapp JH, Connor WE. Colestipol plus nicotinic acid in treatment of heterozygous familial hypercholesterolemia. *Lancet* 1989;**1**:296–98.

66 Jacob BG, Richter WO, Schwandt P. Long-term treatment (2 years) with the HMG CoA reductase inhibitors lovastatin or pravastatin in combination with cholestyramine in patients with severe primary hypercholesterolemia. *J Cardiovasc Pharmacol* 1993;**22**:396–400.

67 Leren TP, Hjermann I, Berg K, Leren P, Foss OP, Viksmoen L. Effects of lovastatin alone and in combination with cholestyramine on serum lipids and apolipoproteins in heterozygotes for familial hypercholesterolemia. *Atherosclerosis* 1988;**73**: 135–41.

68 Malloy MJ, Kane JP, Kunitake ST, Tun P. Complementarity of colestipol, niacin, and lovastatin in treatment of severe familial hypercholesterolemia. *Ann Intern Med* 1987;**107**: 616–23.

69 Packard CJ, Stewart JM, Morgan G, Lorimar AR, Shepherd J. Combined drug therapy for familial hypercholesterolemia. *Artery* 1980;**7**:281–89.

70 Simons LA, Simons J, Parfitt A. Successful management of primary hypercholesterolaemia with simvastatin and low-dose colestipol. *Med J Aust* 1992;**157**:455–9.

71 The Cholesterol Treatment Trialists' (CTT) Collaboration. Protocol for a prospective collaborative overview of all current and planned randomized trials of cholesterol treatment regimens. *Am J Cardiol* 1995;**75**:1130–4.

72 Chait A, Brazg RL, Tribble DL, Krauss RM. Susceptibility of small, dense low-density lipoproteins to oxidative modification in subjects with the atherogenic lipoprotein phenotype, pattern B. *Am J Med* 1993;**94**:350–6.

73 Lamarche B, Tchernof A, Moorjani S *et al*. Small, dense low-density lipoprotein particles as a predictor of the risk of ischemic heart disease in men: prospective results from the Quebec Cardiovascular Study. *Circulation* 1997;**95**: 69–75.

74 Miller BD, Alderman EL, Haskell WL, Fair JM, Krauss RM. Predominance of dense low-density lipoprotein particles predicts angiographic benefit of therapy in the Stanford Coronary Risk Intervention Project. *Circulation* 1996;**94**: 2146–53.

75 Weinstein MC, Stason WB. Foundations of cost effectiveness analysis for health and medical practices. *N Engl J Med* 1977;**296**:716–21.

76 Goldman L, Weinstein MC, Goldman PA, Williams LW. Cost-effectiveness of HMG CoA reductase inhibition for primary and secondary prevention of coronary heart disease. *JAMA* 1991;**265**: 1145–51.

77 Jacobson TA. Cost-effectiveness of 3-hydroxy-3-methylglutaryl-coenzyme A (HMG-CoA) reductase inhibitor therapy in the managed care era. *Am J Cardiol* 1996;**78**(S6A):32–41.

15 Blood pressure and cardiovascular disease

CURT D. FURBERG,
BRUCE M. PSATY,
JEFFREY A. CUTLER

DEFINITION

A new classification of elevated blood pressure that places greater emphasis on systolic blood pressure was introduced in the 1993 Fifth Report of the Joint National Committee on Detection, Evaluation and Treatment of High Blood Pressure (JNC V)[1] and slightly modified in the 1997 JNC VI.[2] Hypertension is defined as systolic blood pressure (SBP) 140 mmHg or greater and/or diastolic blood pressure (DBP) 90 mmHg or greater (Table 15.1). The new classification addresses the issue of severity or increased risk by defining three stages of hypertension, ranging from stage 1 (SBP 140–159 mmHg and/or DBP 90–99 mmHg) to stage 3 (SBP ≥ 180 mmHg and/or DBP ≥ 110 mmHg).

In middle aged populations, the most common type of elevated blood pressure is combined systolic-diastolic hypertension. A second type, isolated systolic hypertension, generally occurs in older persons, probably as a result of age-related stiffening of the arteries.

Hypertension is also classified as complicated or uncomplicated according to the presence or absence of target organ manifestations. These manifestations, which can be cardiac, cerebrovascular, peripheral vascular, renal or retinal, represent complications of hypertension and they also increase the risk of other hypertension-related complications (Table 15.2).

Thus, hypertension is classified by its type (combined systolic-diastolic or isolated systolic hypertension), its severity (stage 1–3), and by coexisting target organ manifestations (if present, complicated or uncomplicated). These classifications are clinically important, since they have risk as well as treatment implications.

Table 15.1 Classification of blood pressure for adults aged 18 years and older[a]

Category	Systolic (mmHg)		Diastolic (mmHg)
Optimal[b]	<120	and	<80
Normal	<130	and	<85
High normal	130–139	or	85–89
Hypertension			
Stage 1[c]	140–159	or	90–99
Stage 2[c]	160–179	or	100–109
Stage 3[e]	≥ 180	or	≥ 110

[a] Not taking antihypertensive drugs and not acutely ill. When systolic and diastolic blood pressures fall into different categories, the higher category should be selected to classify the individual's blood pressure status. For example, 160/92 mmHg should be classified as stage 2 hypertension and 174/120 mmHg should be classified as stage 3 hypertension. Isolated systolic hypertension is defined as SBP ≥ 140 mmHg and DBP <90 mmHg and staged appropriately (e.g. 170/82 mmHg is defined as stage 2 isolated systolic hypertension).

In addition to classifying stages of hypertension on the basis of average blood pressure levels, clinicians should specify presence or absence of target organ disease and additional risk factors. This specificity is important for risk classification and treatment.

[b] Optimal blood pressure with respect to cardiovascular risk is <120/80 mmHg. However, unusually low readings should be evaluated for clinical significance.

[c] Based on the average of two or more readings taken at each of two or more visits after an initial screening.

Adapted from JNC.[2]

Table 15.2 Components for cardiovascular risk stratification in patients with hypertension

Major risk factors
Smoking
Dyslipidemia
Diabetes mellitus
Age older than 60 years
Gender (men and postmenopausal women)
Family history of cardiovascular disease: women under age 65 or men under age 55

Target organ damage/clinical cardiovascular disease
Heart diseases
- Left ventricular hypertrophy
- Angina/prior myocardial infarction
- Prior coronary revascularization
- Heart failure

Stroke or transient ischemic attack
Nephropathy
Peripheral arterial disease
Retinopathy

Adapted from JNC.[2]

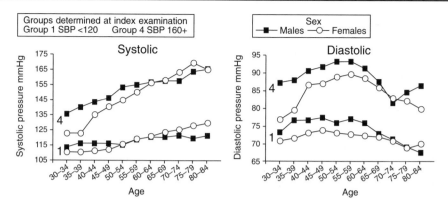

Figure 15.1 Arterial pressure components by age: group averaged data by sex. Averaged blood pressure levels from all available data for each subject with 5-year age intervals (30–34 through 80–84) by SBP groupings 1 vs 4. (Adapted from Franklin *et al*.[3])

PREVALENCE

In cohort analysis,[3] mean SBP increases gradually with age, regardless of initial blood pressure level (Figure 15.1). Mean DBP also increases until the age of 55–60 years, when it levels off.[3] Later in life there is a reduction in the mean DBP, especially in those with high initial levels (Figure 15.1). The age-related changes in blood pressure explain the increase in overall prevalence of hypertension with age and the increase in the prevalence of isolated systolic hypertension with advanced age. The prevalence of target organ manifestations also increases with age, as a result of the increasing prevalence and the longer duration of hypertension.

The prevalence of hypertension is greater for African-Americans than for non-Hispanic whites and Mexican-Americans[4] and for less educated than more educated people.

NATURAL HISTORY

Hypertension is one of the major risk factors for cerebrovascular disease (stroke), coronary heart disease (acute myocardial infarction), congestive heart failure (both systolic and diastolic dysfunction), and renal dysfunction. The risk is directly associated with the blood pressure level and with the presence of target organ manifestations and cardiovascular risk factors (Figure 15.2).[5] Thus, there is a substantial difference in the absolute risk of these hypertensive complications between a 55-year-old male non-smoker with normal serum cholesterol and blood glucose and a 55-year-old male smoker with hypercholesterolemia (8 mmol/l), glucose intolerance, and left ventricular hypertrophy regardless of blood pressure level. The number needed to treat to prevent a major complication within 8 years is much higher for low risk hypertensives than for high risk hypertensive persons.

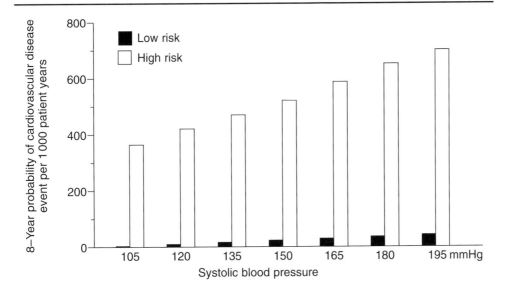

Figure 15.2 Absolute and relative risk for a cardiovascular disease event in a high and low risk 55-year-old man by systolic blood pressure. High risk = left ventricular hypertrophy, cigarette smoker, glucose intolerance, cholesterol 8.02 mmol/l. (Adapted from Alderman.[5])

DISEASE BURDEN

Hypertension is one of the most common medical conditions in the developed world. It has been estimated that as many as 43 million adult non-institutionalized Americans have hypertensive blood pressure levels or are taking antihypertensive medications. Another seven million persons may be controlling their hypertension using non-pharmacologic methods.[4]

Over the last two decades, the National High Blood Pressure Education Program has markedly raised the population's awareness concerning the high prevalence and complications of hypertension.[1] The number of patients taking antihypertensive medications and having their elevated blood pressures controlled has increased dramatically. The rates of awareness, treatment, and control for hypertension (defined as ≥ 160/95 mmHg) in a US population sample in 1988–91 were 84%, 73% and 55%, respectively.[6]

The annual cost of antihypertensive drugs in the US alone has been estimated at $8 billion. Among the 25 top selling medications in the US in 1995, six are prescribed predominantly for the indication of hypertension. Since approximately half of all hypertensives (defined as ≥ 140/90) remain untreated, the annual drug costs could easily double, unless we can change lifestyle more successfully or can be more efficient in allocating resources. During the late 1980s and early 1990s, the shift away from the less expensive, often generic diuretics and beta-blockers (with proven efficacy) to the newer, generally more expensive, ACE-inhibitors, calcium antagonists, alpha-blockers and angiotensin II blockers (with unproven efficacy) has been costly to society.[7]

PREVENTION OF HYPERTENSION

Despite the established benefits of antihypertensive treatment, concerns are often raised about the prospect of decades-long use of antihypertensive drugs by 20% or more of the adult population. All drugs have adverse effects and the cost of medical care for hypertension is considerable. Also, the 12-year follow-up of approximately 350 000 middle aged men screened for the Multiple Risk Factor Intervention Trial shows that 32% of the CHD deaths related to elevated blood pressure occurred below the level at which drug treatment would be considered.[8] Therefore, the prevention of hypertension is a desirable goal.

The multifactorial etiology of hypertension is reflected by the large number of non-pharmaceutical approaches that have been tested.[9–11] Two types of populations have been examined. In individuals with above optimal but non-hypertensive blood pressure levels, lifestyle interventions have been tested to determine their effect on blood pressure. The outcome has been either blood pressure reduction in short term trials or prevention of blood pressure elevation with age and reduction in the incidence of hypertension in long term trials. Trials have also been conducted in hypertensive patients with the objective of determining the blood pressure lowering effects of various non-pharmacologic interventions. One rationale has been that the findings are likely to be generalizable to non-hypertensive individuals. Another rationale has been to determine the efficacy of lifestyle modifications as definitive first line or adjuvant therapy for hypertension. All treatment guidelines recommend lifestyle modifications as the first therapeutic approach in newly diagnosed less severe hypertensive patients, with pharmacologic treatment to follow only in those who fail to respond adequately.

Cross-sectional or longitudinal observational studies have found the following factors to be associated with blood pressure and prevalence or incidence of hypertension: adiposity, physical inactivity, alcohol consumption, high intake of sodium, low intake of potassium, magnesium, calcium, and certain types of dietary fiber, intake of certain macronutrients and chronic stress.

Most of the more than 100 published randomized clinical trials evaluating hypertension prevention and treatment were small and short term, had follow-up periods of weeks or months, and focused on a single intervention. The interventions required varying amounts of involvement by the patients. Lifestyle modifications such as weight loss, exercise, reduced alcohol or sodium intake require substantial counseling and commitment on the part of patients. Short term changes may be accomplished, but whether these are sustained is often unknown. Other interventions have been based on supplementation (potassium, magnesium, calcium, fish oil or fiber) by taking pills, capsules or various forms of wheat brans, although some dietary trials have been conducted.

R

Grade A

Trial results on the efficacy of interventions for prevention of hypertension are summarized in Table 15.3. Based on literature reviews, including meta-analysis, evidence of efficacy is conclusive for weight loss, exercise and reduction in alcohol and sodium intake and potassium supplementation. A weight reduction of 10 lb (4.5 kg) can be expected to lower the blood pressure by approximately 4/3 mmHg. Since exercise, as part of efforts to achieve caloric balance, influences weight, distinguishing an exercise effect on blood pressure from the effect of weight loss can be difficult, but there is good evidence of blood pressure reduction from fitness training.[12] Low intensity/high frequency activity appears as effective as or more effective than high intensity exercise. A sodium

Table 15.3 Trial results on efficacy of interventions for primary prevention of hypertension

Intervention	Duration (months)	Change in targeted factors	Change in BP, mmHg (systolic/diastolic)
Sodium reduction	6[14]	−50 mmol/day	−2.9/−1.6
	18[14]	−43 mmol/day	−2.0/−1.2
	36[14]	−40 mmol/day	−1.2/−0.7
	0.5–36[10]	−76 mmol/day	−1.9/−1.1
Weight loss	6[14]	−4.5 kg	−3.7/−2.7
	18[14]	−2.7 kg	−1.8/−1.3
	36[14]	−1.9 kg	−1.3/−0.9
Exercise	1–16[13]	To 65% maximum exercise capacity	−2.1/−1.6
Alcohol reduction	1.5[13]	−2.6 drinks/day	−3.8/−1.4
Potassium increase	0.3–36[11]	+46 mmol/day	−1.8/−1.0
Dietary pattern	2[15]	Increased fruit, vegetables, low fat dairy, protein, lower saturated fat, dietary cholesterol	−3.5/−2.1

reduction of 80–100 mmol/day induces an average blood pressure reduction of 5/3 mmHg in hypertensives and 2/1 mmHg in non-hypertensives.[10] Similar blood pressure effects were observed in trials which accomplished alcohol reductions of about 85% (a mean consumption of three drinks/day reduced to three drinks/week).[13]

The blood pressure effects of lifestyle modifications are modest, but they appear to be additive under some circumstances.[14,15] A short-term study recently reported substantial blood pressure reductions in adults given a diet rich in fruits, vegetables, and low fat dairy foods and reduced saturated and total fat.[15] However, counseling, if required on an indefinite basis through a traditional clinical setting, may not be more cost effective than drugs. Therefore, interventions (such as reducing salt intake by modifying processed foods) that can potentially be accomplished on a population basis are attractive. The efficacy of supplementation with magnesium, fiber, fish oil or calcium has been judged to be limited or unproven at this time.[9] The trial findings are discordant and the effect sizes small. Potassium supplementation (50–100 mmol KCl or equivalent increase from food) moderately reduces blood pressure, especially in those who have a high sodium intake.[11]

Long term trials in individuals with high normal blood pressure have documented that the incidence of hypertension can be reduced by as much as 50%. The most impressive results are from a 5-year trial of a multifactorial intervention.[16] The cumulative incidence of hypertension was 19.2% in the control group and 8.8% in the intervention group. The main factors contributing to this blood pressure reduction were weight loss and sodium reduction.[14] Overweight adults with high normal blood pressure appear to be prime candidates for this intervention.

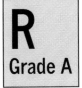

Lifestyle modification is an integral part of management of hypertension. The blood pressure lowering effects are on average modest. Some patients do not respond or are unable to modify their lifestyles, while others respond well. As a consequence, many patients do not have to be placed on antihypertensive drugs and if they are, lower drug doses or fewer drugs may be required. The challenge is to sustain the lifestyle modifications.

DRUG TREATMENT

Despite efforts at lifestyle modifications, many patients require pharmacologic treatment. In the US, almost 23 million civilian non-institutionalized adults are currently taking antihypertensive medications.[6] This high level of drug use to treat an asymptomatic condition has been justified by the high population burden of major morbidity and mortality causally related to untreated hypertension, and by strong evidence of treatment efficacy and safety from large, long term clinical trials. In SHEP,[17] which enrolled older adults with isolated systolic hypertension, the 5-year event rates for the combined endpoints of coronary heart disease and stroke per 100 patients were 13.6 in the placebo group and 9.4 in the active group. The risk difference of 4.2% means that about 24 older adults need to be treated for 5 years in order to prevent one coronary or cerebrovascular event. It must be recognized that calculating the number needed to treat in this manner from randomized clinical trials produces an underestimate for several reasons, chiefly the selection or self-selection of lower risk patients into trials and the dilution of effects due to drop-in to active treatment by patients in the control group. For middle-aged populations, which are at lower risk, the number needed to treat would be much higher. Because many people must receive therapy so that a few will benefit, even uncommon adverse effects may minimize or eliminate the blood pressure lowering benefits of antihypertensive therapy. Only with large, long term trials such as SHEP can we be assured that the health benefits actually outweigh the health risks of particular therapies.

In a recent meta-analysis,[18] the evidence from large, long term, controlled clinical trials of antihypertensive therapy was reviewed. The 18 randomized trials included 48 220 patients followed for an average of about 5 years. Clinical trials were classified according to the primary treatment strategy. While most studies used more than one drug, the agents were generally used in a stepwise fashion and it was usually easy to identify the first line therapy.

Compared with controls, beta-blocker therapy was effective in preventing stroke and congestive heart failure (Table 15.4). Similarly, high dose diuretic therapy, which typically started with the equivalent of 50 mg of hydrochlorothiazide and often went to 100 mg per day, was associated with a reduced risk of stroke and heart failure. Despite lowering blood pressure by an average of about 5–6 mmHg, neither beta-blocker therapy nor high dose diuretic therapy demonstrated significant reduction of coronary disease events (Table 15.4).

Compared with controls, low dose diuretic therapy prevented not only stroke and heart failure but also coronary heart disease and cardiovascular and total mortality (Table 15.4). In contrast to high dose diuretic therapy, the adverse metabolic effects of low dose diuretic therapy are minimal. The safety and proven effectiveness make low dose diuretic therapy the logical first line pharmacologic treatment for hypertension. Beta-blockers, which clearly prevent stroke and heart failure in hypertensive patients, are an alternative. The current US guidelines[1,2] appropriately identify low dose diuretics and beta-blockers as preferred first line agents in the treatment of hypertension.

It is not clear why low dose diuretic therapy prevents coronary heart disease, but neither high dose diuretic therapy nor beta-blocker therapy is associated with a reduced risk of coronary disease. The low dose trials (see[18] for references) were conducted mainly in older adults while the high dose trials were conducted largely in middle aged adults. Evidence from observational studies suggests that, compared with low dose diuretic

R

Grade A

Table 15.4 Meta-analysis of randomized, placebo-controlled clinical trials in hypertension according to first line treatment strategy

Outcome drug regimen	Dose	No. of trials	Events, active treatment/control	RR (95% CI)	RR (95% CI)
Stroke					
Diuretics	High	9	88/232	0.49 (0.39–0.62)	
Diuretics	Low	4	191/347	0.66 (0.55–0.78)	
Beta-blockers	High	4	147/335	0.71 (0.59–0.86)	
HDFP	High	1	102/158	0.64 (0.50–0.82)	
Coronary heart disease					
Diuretics	High	11	211/331	0.99 (0.83–1.18)	
Diuretics	Low	4	215/363	0.72 (0.61–0.85)	
Beta-blockers	High	4	243/459	0.93 (0.80–1.09)	
HDFP	High	1	171/189	0.90 (0.73–1.10)	
Congestive heart failure					
Diuretics	High	9	6/35	0.17 (0.07–0.41)	
Diuretics	Low	3	81/134	0.58 (0.44–0.76)	
Beta-blockers		2	41/175	0.58 (0.40–0.84)	
Total mortality					
Diuretics	High	11	224/382	0.88 (0.75–1.03)	
Diuretics	Low	4	514/713	0.90 (0.81–0.99)	
Beta-blockers	High	4	383/700	0.95 (0.84–1.07)	
HDFP	High	1	349/419	0.83 (0.72–0.95)	
Cardiovascular mortality					
Diuretics	High	11	124/230	0.78 (0.62–0.97)	
Diuretics	Low	4	237/390	0.76 (0.65–0.89)	
Beta-blockers	High	4	214/410	0.89 (0.76–1.05)	
HDFP	High	1	195/240	0.81 (0.67–0.97)	

Treatment better ← → Treatment worse

0.4   0.7   1.0

Trials indicate number of trials with at least 1 end point of interest. RR, relative risk; CI, confidence interval; HDFP, Hypertension Detection and Follow-up Program Study (5484 subjects in stepped care and 5455 in referred care). For these comparisons, the numbers of participants randomized to active therapy and placebo were 7768 and 12 075 for high dose diuretic therapy; 4305 and 5116 for low dose diuretic therapy; and 6736 and 12 147 for beta-blocker therapy. Because the Medical Research Council trial included 2 active arms, the placebo group is included twice in these totals, once for a diuretic comparison and again for a beta-blocker comparison. The total number of participants randomized to active therapy and control therapy were 24 294 and 23 926, respectively. Adapted from Psaty *et al.*[18]

233

therapy, high dose diuretic therapy is associated with an increased risk of sudden death.[19] For high dose diuretics, the most likely explanation is the dose of the diuretics rather than the age of patients. Abrupt withdrawal of beta-blocker therapy is associated with an increased risk of myocardial infarction in patients with high blood pressure.[20] It is possible that withdrawal reactions from non-compliance with beta-blockers may have minimized their ability to prevent coronary heart disease in hypertensive patients, who generally represent a low risk population group.

The findings for beta-blocker and high dose diuretic therapy provide direct evidence that blood pressure lowering alone is not adequate to predict the effect of an antihypertensive medication on important health outcomes. "In light of all previous cardiovascular trials . . ." Topol and colleagues remark, "surrogate end points cannot be considered authentic measures of true clinical efficacy and safety."[21]

Yet drug regulatory agencies currently approve antihypertensive medications on the basis of their ability to lower blood pressure. As a result, several commonly used classes of antihypertensive agents, including calcium-channel blockers and angiotensin converting enzyme (ACE) inhibitors, have not been adequately evaluated in large, long term clinical trials. A recently completed placebo-controlled trial of nitrendipine, which is not available in the US, in isolated systolic hypertension (Syst-Eur) found a statistically significant reduction in stroke risk and showed trends for reductions in risks of major coronary events and congestive heart failure.[22] Several large, long term randomized trials are currently evaluating these newer classes of agents. In the meantime, uncertainty about the validity of using blood pressure lowering as a proxy for the effect of drugs on health outcomes argues against the widespread use of calcium-channel blockers and ACE inhibitors as first line antihypertensive agents.

R

Grade B

For short acting calcium-channel blockers, several but not all observational studies have raised questions about their safety. The use of short acting calcium-channel blockers in hypertensive patients has been associated with increased risks of myocardial infarction,[23] congestive heart failure,[24] cardiovascular events,[24] total mortality,[24] gastrointestinal hemorrhage,[25] perioperative bleeding,[26] and cancer.[27,28] In a meta-analysis of the secondary prevention randomized trials, short acting nifedipine, especially in high doses, was associated with an increased risk of total mortality.[29] In the Multicenter Isradipine Diuretic Atherosclerosis Study, the use of intermediate acting isradipine was associated with a higher risk of cardiovascular events than low dose diuretic therapy (RR = 1.78; 95% CI = 0.94–3.38).[30] Besides the benefits seen in Syst-Eur noted above, the only observational study of long acting agents observed a non-significant higher risk of cardiovascular events (RR = 1.28; 95% CI = 0.76–2.16).[31] Because the observational studies serve to develop hypotheses regarding safety of medications (as well as being potentially useful for interim treatment guidelines), we urgently need evidence about the efficacy and safety of the major subclasses of calcium-channel blockers from additional large, long term trials.

The rationale for withholding therapies such as low dose diuretics, which are proven safe and effective, must be a compelling one. Clinical trial evidence of health benefits for another indication is a compelling rationale. In patients with heart failure or ventricular dysfunction, the use of ACE inhibitors is associated with a decreased risk of morbidity and mortality. While ACE inhibitors affect the progression of renal disease in patients with insulin-dependent diabetes, their role in patients with non-insulin dependent diabetes remains unclear. Indeed, the recent report from SHEP highlights the marked health benefits of low dose diuretic therapy in patients with non-insulin dependent diabetes.[32] The use of beta-blockers in patients with coronary heart disease

Table 15.5 Costs (US$) in wholesale medication prices to prevent a fatal or non-fatal CHD event, a fatal or non-fatal stroke, a death of any cause or any of these events in patients with uncomplicated mild to moderate hypertension assuming similar efficacy[a]

Event	Hydrochlorothiazide		Nifedipine GITS	
	Middle aged	Elderly	Middle aged	Elderly
CHD	21 374	3822	1 571 809	281 025
Stroke	7413	2453	545 141	180 372
Mortality	14 826	3931	1 090 281	289 078
Any of above	4730	1588	347 859	116 758

[a] The relative efficacy of calcium blockers compared to diuretics has not been reliably evaluated. These estimates assume similar impact of the two agents.
Adapted from Pearce *et al.*[37]

clearly reduces the risk of reinfarction and death.[33,34] In patients with established coronary disease, the non-dihydropyridine calcium-channel blockers appear to be associated with a reduced risk of reinfarction,[35] but the evidence in favor of beta-blockers as the primary therapy for patients with coronary disease is much more extensive, consistent, and persuasive.[36]

For patients who require drug treatment, low dose diuretic therapy is both safe and effective. With additional studies, we are discovering that low dose diuretic therapy also has special indications such as isolated systolic hypertension in non-insulin dependent diabetics.

COST EFFECTIVENESS

It has been estimated that medications account for 50–90% of the direct cost of hypertensive treatment.[37] The 1996 wholesale prices for starting doses of antihypertensive drugs may vary by at least 40-fold. Thus, the choice of drug(s) has a major effect on direct treatment costs.

The direct costs of routine outpatient physician visits and laboratory tests are also substantial. If one assumes three annual office visits (at $70 each) and two serum chemistry panels (at $29), these non-drug costs of hypertension management amount to $268 per patient per year. For every one million of the 20 million untreated patients in the US started on drug treatment, the total cost could be as low as $450 million or as high as $1 billion annually. The question from a cost effectiveness viewpoint is not whether treatment is effective, but whether the benefits justify the costs in light of competing health care needs.

Formal cost effectiveness analyses are not possible for the newer antihypertensive agents due to the lack of data on effectiveness. One has to make assumptions about the magnitude of effectiveness. If we assume that the newer agents are as effective as low dose diuretics, the wholesale medication costs to prevent a fatal or non-fatal coronary event, a fatal or non-fatal stroke, a death from any cause, and any of these complications among patients with uncomplicated mild to moderate hypertension are as shown in Table 15.5. The costs are given for low dose diuretics and a prototype of the newer unproven agents, nifedipine GITS.

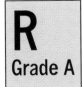

Grade A

235

In the context of health care systems in which priorities are being established (fixed budgets), the prime candidates for antihypertensive drug treatment are:

- elderly patients;
- patients with moderate to severe hypertension;
- patients with target organ manifestations.

These patient groups (among others) are at a higher risk of clinical hypertensive complications. Since clinical trials have demonstrated similar relative reductions in risk of stroke, acute myocardial infarction, congestive heart failure, and mortality in low risk compared to high risk patients, the absolute benefit expressed as number needed to treat to prevent one event or as number of events prevented per 100 patients treated is substantially greater in the high risk groups described above.

UNANSWERED QUESTIONS

- Are the newer (and more expensive) classes of antihypertensive agents – calcium antagonists, alpha-blockers, ACE inhibitors and angiotensin II blockers – effective in reducing the risk of hypertensive complications? This question would typically be answered by large, long term, randomized, placebo-controlled trials, but such trials are no longer ethical to conduct in patients with high blood pressure. The only exception is borderline isolated systolic hypertension, which has not been studied in placebo-controlled trials.
- Are the newer agents, in particular calcium antagonists,[23-31] safe for long term use? In the absence of sufficient data from long term clinical trials we have to settle for well designed and analyzed postmarketing studies.
- In terms of efficacy and safety, how do the new agents compare with the proven treatments, low dose diuretics and beta-blockers? Are they superior, the same or inferior? This question and the following one are the key clinical questions today. The answer to this question depends on large, long term trials that include an actively treated control group. ALLHAT is an excellent example.[38]
- Compared to the older proven drugs, are the newer agents cost effective? Regrettably, formal analysis cannot be conducted due to lack of efficacy data. If, in ongoing trials, they turn out to be superior, we have to decide whether the degree of superiority justifies the price differential and, if so, whether the newer drugs deserve to be considered as first line agents. If the newer agents are the same or inferior, their use should be restricted to second or third line agents and be limited to patients who do not respond to low dose diuretics and beta-blockers or who cannot tolerate them or to specific targeted populations.
- What is the optimal level of treated blood pressure? Should the goals be even lower than 140 mmHg (systolic) or 90 mmHg (diastolic)?
- How can we improve risk stratification, i.e. find better methods of identifying an individual's risk?
- What are the optimal method(s) for long term lifestyle modifications?
- How can we best reduce the incidence of hypertension?

Key points

- Hypertension should be classified by its type (diastolic/combined vs isolated systolic hypertension), its severity (stage 1–3) and by coexisting target organ manifestations (complicated vs uncomplicated).
- If choices must be made, high risk hypertensive patients, i.e. elderly patients, those with moderate to severe hypertension and those with target organ manifestation, ought to be the prime candidates for treatment due to more favorable benefit–risk and cost effectiveness ratios.
- Lifestyle modification – primarily weight control and sodium reduction – is an integral part of management of hypertension. Good evidence on efficacy also exists for increased physical activity, moderation of alcohol intake, and ensuring adequate potassium intake.
- Low dose diuretics should be the first line drugs due to proven efficacy and safety; beta-blockers are an attractive alternative. The use of ACE inhibitors, calcium antagonists, angiotensin II blockers, and alpha-blockers ought to be restricted to patients who do not respond to low dose diuretics and beta-blockers or who cannot tolerate them.
- Forty-fold differences in direct drug cost between low dose diuretics and the newer and heavily promoted agents ought to be a strong incentive to enhance use of the former and reduce use of the latter.

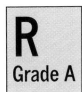

R
Grade A

REFERENCES

1 Joint National Committee on Detection, Evaluation, and Treatment of High Blood Pressure. The Fifth Report of the Joint National Committee on Detection, Evaluation, and Treatment of High Blood Pressure (JNC V). *Arch Intern Med* 1993;**153**:154–83.

2 Joint National Committee on Detection, Evaluation, and Treatment of High Blood Pressure. The Sixth Report of the Joint National Committee on Prevention, Detection, Evaluation, and Treatment of High Blood Pressure (JNC VI). *Arch Intern Med* 1997;**157**:2413–46.

3 Franklin SS, Gustin IVW, Wong ND *et al.* Hemodynamic patterns of age-related changes in blood pressure. The Framingham Heart Study. *Circulation* 1997;**96**:308–15.

4 Burt VL, Whelton P, Roccella EJ *et al.* Prevalence of hypertension in the US adult population. Results from the Third National Health and Nutrition Examination Survey, 1988–1991. *Hypertension* 1995;**25**:305–13.

5 Alderman MH. Blood pressure management: individualized treatment based on absolute risk and the potential for benefit. *Arch Intern Med* 1993;**119**:329–35.

6 Burt VL, Cutler JA, Higgins M *et al.* Trends in the prevalence, awareness, treatment, and control of hypertension in the adult US population. Data from the Health Examination Surveys, 1960 to 1991. *Hypertension* 1995;**26**:60–9.

7 Manolio TA, Cutler JA, Furberg CD *et al.* Trends in pharmacologic management of hypertension in the United States. *Arch Intern Med* 1995;**155**:829–37.

8 Stamler J, Stamler R, Neaton J. Blood pressure, systolic and diastolic, and cardiovascular risks: US population data. *Arch Intern Med* 1993;**153**:598–615.

9 Cutler JA, Psaty BM, MacMahon S, Furberg CD. Public health issues in hypertension control: what has been learned from clinical trials. In: Laragh JH, Brenner BM. eds. New York: Raven Press, 1995, pp 253–70.

10 Cutler JA, Follmann D, Allender PS. Randomized trials of sodium reduction: an overview. *Am J Clin Nutr* 1997;**65**:643S–51S.

11 Whelton PK, He J, Cutler JA *et al.* Effects of oral potassium on blood pressure. Meta-analysis of randomized controlled clinical trials. *JAMA* 1997;**277**:1624–32.

12 Fagard RH. Prescription and results of physical activity. *J Cardiovasc Pharm* 1995;**25**(Suppl 1):S20–S27.

13 Puddey IB, Beilin LJ, Vandongen R, Rouse IL, Rogers P. Evidence for a direct effect of alcohol consumption on blood pressure in normotensive men: a randomized controlled trial. *Hypertension* 1985;**7**:707–13.

14 The Trials of Hypertension Prevention Collaborative Research Group. Effects of weight loss and sodium reduction intervention on blood pressure and hypertension incidence in overweight people with high-normal blood pressure. *Arch Intern Med* 1997;**157**:657–67.

15 Appel LJ, Moore TJ, Obarzanek E *et al.*, for the DASH Collaborative Research Group. A clinical trial of the effects of dietary patterns on blood pressure. *N Engl J Med* 1997;**336**:1117–24.

16 Stamler R, Stamler J, Gosch FC *et al.* Primary prevention of hypertension by nutritional-hygienic means: final report of a randomized, controlled trial. *JAMA* 1989;**262**:1801–7.

17 SHEP Cooperative Research Group. Prevention of stroke by antihypertensive drug treatment in older persons with isolated systolic hypertension: final results of the Systolic Hypertension in the Elderly Program (SHEP). *JAMA* 1991;**265**: 3255–64.

18 Psaty BM, Smith NS, Siscovick DS *et al.* Health outcomes associated with antihypertensive therapies used as first-line agents: a systematic review and meta-analysis. *JAMA* 1997;**277**: 739–45.

19 Siscovick DS, Raghunathan TE, Psaty BM *et al.* Diuretic therapy for hypertension and the risk of primary cardiac arrest. *N Engl J Med* 1994;**330**: 1852–7.

20 Psaty BM, Koepsell TD, Wagner EH, LoGerfo JP, Inui TS. The relative risk of incident coronary heart disease associated with recently stopping the use of beta-blockers. *JAMA* 1990;**263**: 1653–7.

21 Topol EJ, Califf RM, van de Werf F *et al.* Perspectives on large-scale cardiovascular clinical trials for the new millenium. *Circulation* 1997;**95**:1072–82.

22 Staessen JA, Fagard R, Thijs L *et al*, for the Systolic Hypertension – Europe (Syst-Eur) Trial Investigators. Randomised double-blind comparison of placebo and active treatment for older patients with systolic hypertension. *Lancet* 1997; **350**:757–64.

23 Psaty BM, Heckbert SR, Koepsell TD *et al.* The risk of myocardial infarction associated with antihypertensive drug therapies. *JAMA* 1995;**274**: 620–5.

24 Pahor M, Guralnik JM, Corti MC *et al.* Long-term survival and use of antihypertensive medication in older persons. *J Am Geriatr Soc* 1995;**43**: 1191–7.

25 Pahor M, Guralnik JM, Furberg CD, Carbonin P, Havlik RJ. Risk of gastrointestinal haemorrhage with calcium antagonists in hypertensive persons over 67 years old. *Lancet* 1996;**347**:1061–5.

26 Zuccalá G, Pahor M, Landi F *et al.* Use of calcium antagonists and need for perioperative transfusion in older patients with hip fracture: observational study. *Br Med J* 1997;**314**:643–4.

27 Pahor M, Guralnik JM, Salive ME *et al.* Do calcium channel blockers increase the risk of cancer? *Am J Hypertens* 1996;**9**:695–9.

28 Pahor M, Guralnik JM, Ferrucci L *et al.* Calcium channel blockers and incidence of cancer in aged populations. *Lancet* 1996;**348**:493–7.

29 Furberg CD, Psaty BM, Myers JV. Nifedipine: dose-related increase in mortality in patients with coronary heart disease. *Circulation* 1995;**92**: 1326–31 [correction: *Circulation* 1996;**93**: 1475–6].

30 Borhani NO, Mercuri M, Borhani PA *et al.* Final outcome results of the Multicenter Isradipine Diuretic Atherosclerosis Study (MIDAS): a randomized controlled trial. *JAMA* 1996;**276**: 785–91.

31 Alderman MH, Cohen H, Roqué R, Madhavan S. Effect of long-acting and short-acting calcium antagonists on cardiovascular outcomes in hypertensive patients. *Lancet* 1997;**349**:594–8.

32 Curb JD, Pressel SL, Cutler JA *et al*, for the Systolic Hypertension in the Elderly Program Cooperative Research Group. Effect of diuretic-based antihypertensive treatment on cardiovascular disease risk in older diabetic patients with isolated systolic hypertension. *JAMA* 1996;**276**:1886–92.

33 Norwegian Multicenter Study Group. Timolol-induced reduction in mortality and reinfarction in patients surviving acute myocardial infarction. *N Engl J Med* 1981;**304**:801–7.

34 Beta-Blocker Heart Attack Trial Research Group. A randomized trial of propranolol in patients with acute myocardial infarction: I. Mortality results. *JAMA* 1982;**247**:1707–14.

35 Yusuf S, Held P, Furberg C. Update of effects of calcium antagonists in myocardial infarction or angina in light of the second Danish Verapamil Infarction Trial (DAVIT-II) and other recent studies. *Am J Cardiol* 1991;**67**:1295–7.

36 Report of the American College of Cardiology/ American Heart Association Task Force on Practice Guidelines (Committee on Management of Acute Myocardial Infarction). ACC/AHA Guidelines for the management of patients with acute myocardial infarction. *J Am Coll Cardiol* 1996;**28**:1328–428.

37 Pearce KA, Furberg CD, Psaty BM, Kirk J. Comparative cost-effectiveness of first-line drugs for uncomplicated hypertension. *Am J Hypertens* 1998 (in press).

38 Davis BR, Cutler JA, Gordon DJ *et al.* Rationale and design for the Antihypertensive and Lipid Lowering Treatment to Prevent Heart Attack Trial (ALLHAT). *Am J Hypertens* 1996;**9**:342–60.

Glucose abnormalities and cardiovascular disease: "dysglycemia" as an emerging cardiovascular risk factor

16

HERTZEL C. GERSTEIN

INTRODUCTION

Large epidemiologic studies have consistently shown that patients with diabetes mellitus have a 2–4-fold increased risk of cardiovascular disease relative to non-diabetic patients.[1–3] Patients with both type 1 and type 2 diabetes are at increased risk. For patients with type 1 diabetes who present soon after the disease develops, this increased risk is not apparent until 20–30 years after the diagnosis is made. For patients with type 2 diabetes, who represent more than 90% of all patients with diabetes, this increased risk is apparent right at the time of diagnosis and is independent of the duration of diagnosed diabetes.[4–6] For these patients, this observation may be due to a 5–10-year antecedent history of undiagnosed diabetes, preceded by an indeterminate period of elevated glucose levels that are below the diabetic cutoff.[7]

Recent studies suggest that in patients with diabetes, the degree of glucose elevation is directly related to the risk of cardiovascular disease. For non-diabetic patients, a critical overview of the available epidemiologic studies suggests that this continuous relationship extends below the diabetic threshold and includes mildly elevated glucose levels that are generally considered to be normal. There may or may not be a lower glucose threshold to this risk. Thus, like total cholesterol or diastolic hypertension, glucose appears to be a continuous cardiovascular risk factor. Whether or not modification of this risk factor by interventions that lower glucose levels will also prevent cardiovascular disease remains an important and unanswered question.

Table 16.1 Classification of diabetes mellitus[a]

Name	Subtypes	Characteristics	Etiology	Epidemiology
Type 1	A: immune mediated B: idiopathic	Peak onset in teenage years, absent insulin secretion due to β cell damage	Autoimmune, genetics plays a role	∼10% of patients with diabetes; 0.2% of the general population
Type 2	None	Onset usually after age 40; greater than 50% are obese	Genetics plays a key role, many patients are insulin resistant	∼90% of patients with diabetes; ∼10% of the adult population
Gestational	None	Onset during a current pregnancy	Closely related to type 2 diabetes	2–5% of all pregnancies
Other specific types	A to H[b]	Related to a genetic, congenital, acquired pancreatic endocrine or infectious disease or a drug that is associated with β cell dysfunction and/or insulin resistance†	Examples include hemochromatosis, pancreatitis, hypercortisolemia, genetic lesions	∼2% of all patients with diabetes

[a] Adapted from Harris[8] and Expert Committee on the Diagnosis and Classification of Diabetes Mellitus.[8a]
[b] Complete list published in reference 8a.

DEFINITION AND EPIDEMIOLOGY OF DIABETES AND IMPAIRED GLUCOSE TOLERANCE

The diagnosis of diabetes mellitus applies to a heterogeneous group of disorders that are all characterized by high levels of glucose in the blood.[8,8a] This hyperglycemia is due either to absent or minimal insulin secretion from insulin-producing beta cells of the pancreas or to insufficient insulin secretion to overcome a variable degree of "insulin resistance" that is present in a large proportion of the general population. As insulin is the primary hormone that prevents hyperglycemia, by both inhibiting hepatic glucose production and facilitating glucose clearance by muscle, insufficient insulin quickly results in an elevated glucose level. The clinical classification of diabetes and the associated characteristics and suspected causes of each type are listed in Table 16.1.

For many years it was apparent that patients with diabetes had a high risk of developing eye disease, kidney disease, peripheral nerve disease, and cardiovascular disease (i.e. coronary heart disease, cerebrovascular disease, and peripheral vascular disease). In 1979 and 1980 it was also recognized that these complications were occurring in patients with both diagnosed diabetes and asymptomatic, undiagnosed diabetes.[8,9] On the basis of these observations and epidemiologic studies of the risk of diabetic complications according to the fasting and 2-hour glucose level (during a 75 g oral glucose tolerance test) in populations at high risk for diabetes, specific glucose thresholds were defined for the diagnosis of diabetes (Table 16.2). These

Table 16.2 Diagnostic thresholds for diabetes and impaired glucose tolerance. 1997 American Diabetes Association Criteria[8a]

Classification	Casual[b] plasma glucose	Fasting[c] plasma glucose	2-hour postload (75 g glucose) plasma glucose
Diabetes mellitus[a]	≥11.1 mmol/l AND classical signs and symptoms of hyperglycemia	≥7.0 mmol/l	≥11.1 mmol/l
Impaired glucose tolerance	N/A	<7.8 mmol/l	≥7.8 and <11.1 mmol/l
Impaired fasting glucose	N/A	≥6.1 and <7.0 mmol/l	N/A

[a] To confirm a diagnosis of diabetes any of the three criteria needs to be confirmed by one of the three criteria on a subsequent day.
[b] Done at any time of day regardless of time since the last meal.
[c] No caloric intake for ≥8 hours.

specific levels were those above which patients were at high risk of diabetic retinopathy and nephropathy; patients with levels below this threshold had a very low risk for these diabetic complications.[7,8,10] The fact that these thresholds were not chosen to reflect the risk of cardiovascular disease is apparent from many studies demonstrating a high risk of cardiovascular disease in patients with lower glucose levels (see below).

At the time that these thresholds were established, it was clear that a large number of people had glucose levels that fell below the diabetic threshold but that were nevertheless still elevated. This led to the classification of impaired glucose tolerance (IGT), which was defined on the basis of the glucose level (Table 16.2) and not on the basis of any particular clinical characteristics.[8,8a,9] Although people with IGT were at low risk for diabetic retinopathy and nephropathy, they had a higher risk for developing diabetes than people with normal glucose tolerance (defined by a fasting and 2-hour plasma glucose less than 6.1 and 7.8 mmol/l respectively[8a]).

Prevalence estimates

Data from both Canada[11,12] and the United States[13] suggest that approximately 3–5% of all adults have a known diagnosis of diabetes. Large surveys completed in the early 1980s in the United States also showed that the prevalence of undiagnosed diabetes was equal to the prevalence of diagnosed diabetes.[13] Thus, up to 10% of all adults in North America have diabetes. This prevalence varies with age, approaching 15–20% of all people over the age of 64 in the United States.[13] It also varies with race and ethnicity and is higher in aboriginal populations throughout the world, in East Indians, American blacks and Hispanics and in Chinese and Indian migrant communities.[14] The prevalence of IGT varies in a similar pattern; in most populations it is approximately equal to the prevalence of diabetes (both diagnosed and undiagnosed);[14] thus, in the United States the prevalence of IGT and diabetes exceeds 28% of people aged 45–74.[13]

RELATIONSHIP BETWEEN THE GLUCOSE LEVEL AND RETINOPATHY, NEPHROPATHY, AND PERIPHERAL NEUROPATHY

In patients with diabetes, the risk of retinopathy, nephropathy, and neuropathy is highly correlated with various measures of glycemia including fasting plasma glucose, 2-hour postprandial plasma glucose (after a 75 g oral glucose load), and glycated hemoglobin level.[10,15–17] For example, the risk of retinal and renal disease is very low below a fasting glucose of 7.2 mmol/l or a glycated hemoglobin level of 7.0%[10] and increases as these measures increase within the diabetic range.

Therefore, glucose is a continuous risk factor for these complications in patients with diabetes. It is also a modifiable risk factor. The Diabetes Control and Complications Trial[15] clearly showed that for patients with type 1 diabetes, dramatic reductions of the risk of retinopathy (63% risk reduction), laser therapy (51% RR), microalbuminuria (39% RR), clinical proteinuria (54% RR), and neuropathy (60% RR) can be achieved by "tight" glucose control. Similar findings from a small study of thin Japanese patients with type 2 diabetes[17] suggest that the benefits of achieving and maintaining normoglycemia in patients with diabetes is independent of the etiology of the diabetes. This awaits confirmation from the United Kingdom Prospective Diabetes Study (UKPDS).[18]

RELATIONSHIP BETWEEN THE GLUCOSE LEVEL AND THE RISK OF CARDIOVASCULAR DISEASE

The risk of cardiovascular disease in patients with diabetes

As noted above, diabetes is an independent risk factor for cardiovascular disease.[2] People with diabetes have a 2–4-fold higher risk of coronary, cerebrovascular, and peripheral vascular disease than non-diabetic people.[1] The relative risk is greater for women than for men.[1,19] Diabetes is also a poor prognostic factor post myocardial infarction; diabetic patients have a higher inhospital mortality and postdischarge mortality than non-diabetic patients and a higher risk of infarct-related complications.[20,21]

Just as the risk of eye, kidney, and nerve disease increases with the degree of glycemia, a growing number of studies of diabetic patients suggest that the risk of cardiovascular disease also rises with the degree of glycemia. For example, the Wisconsin Epidemiologic Study of Diabetic Retinopathy followed a population based sample of 1210 patients with diabetes presenting before age 30 and 1780 patients with diabetes presenting at or after age 30.[22] In both groups of subjects, 10-year mortality increased with the baseline glycated hemoglobin quartile. After controlling for other risk factors, a 1% increase in glycated hemoglobin was associated with a 10% (older onset subjects) to 18% (younger onset subjects) increase in the hazard of dying from ischemic heart disease.[22] In addition, at least two other smaller population based epidemiologic studies noted a higher rate of CHD[23] or total mortality[24] in subjects with higher glucose levels than in those with better glucose control.

Glucose levels and the risk of cardiovascular disease in non-diabetic patients

Many prospective studies have consistently shown that the relationship between glucose levels and the subsequent risk of cardiovascular disease extends well below the diabetic threshold. For example, after 10 years of follow-up in the Whitehall Study of 18 050 non-diabetic male civil servants, there was an up to two-fold increase in coronary heart disease and stroke mortality in subjects whose 2-hour postload capillary glucose value was greater than 5.4 mmol/l. This increase was independent of age, smoking, blood pressure, cholesterol, and occupation.[25,26] The relationship of non-diabetic range hyperglycemia and cardiovascular disease was also clearly noted after 14 years in the Rancho Bernardo study.[27] In this prospective study of 3458 non-diabetic men and women aged 40–70 with a fasting plasma glucose <7.8 mmol/l, the age-adjusted ischemic heart disease mortality rates approximately doubled in men as the fasting glucose rose from 5 to 7 mmol/l and tripled in women as the fasting glucose rose from 6 to 7.2 mmol/l.

Despite these and other large cohort and cross-sectional studies[28–31] that showed a graded relationship between non-diabetic and even non-impaired glucose tolerance levels of hyperglycemia and cardiovascular disease, some studies did not support such a relationship, especially with only moderate degrees of glucose elevation.[32–34] A systematic overview and meta-analysis of all published cohort studies of mainly non-diabetic populations was therefore done to resolve these discrepancies and to characterize the relationship between glucose levels and cardiovascular disease.[35] This analysis of

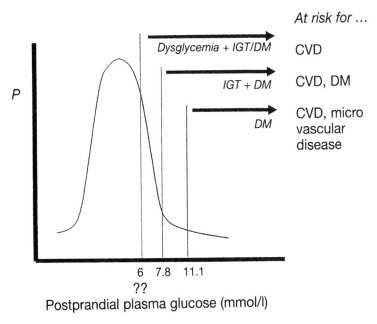

Figure 16.1 Representation of the frequency distribution of glucose levels in the general population, illustrating the point that the significance of glucose as a risk factor for chronic disease depends on the level. Glucose levels above the diabetic threshold are associated with an increasing risk of cardiovascular and microvascular disease, levels above the IGT threshold are associated with an increasing risk of diabetes, and elevated levels above some as yet undefined "dysglycemic" threshold are associated with an increasing risk of cardiovascular disease.

studies describing more than one million person-years of follow-up found that the risk of cardiovascular disease increased continuously with glucose levels above 4.2 mmol/l (75 mg/dl).

Further evidence of the relationship of non-diabetic levels of hyperglycemia to cardiovascular disease was reported in a study of 200 patients with myocardial infarction (36 with diabetes) and 200 matched controls (18 with diabetes).[36] Even after cases and controls with a history of diabetes or whose 2-hour postload glucose values were 7.8 mmol/l or greater (i.e. who had impaired glucose tolerance or diabetes) were excluded from the analysis, fasting glucose levels were significantly higher in cases (6.05 mmol/l) than controls (4.83 mmol/l). Of note, there was no difference in the distribution of fasting insulin.

Therefore, glucose appears to be a continuous cardiovascular risk factor, similar to cholesterol or blood pressure in its dose–response relationship.[37] We have suggested that the term "*dysglycemia*"[38] may be useful for describing this continuous relationship between glucose and cardiovascular disease. Thus, people with dysglycemia alone are at risk for cardiovascular disease, people with dysglycemia and IGT are at higher risk for cardiovascular disease as well as diabetes mellitus, and people with diabetes mellitus are at even higher risk for cardiovascular disease as well as eye, kidney, and nerve disease (Figure 16.1).

MECHANISMS RELATING HYPERGLYCEMIA TO CARDIOVASCULAR DISEASE

Possible explanations for a glucose–cardiovascular disease relationship include:

- direct toxic effects of glucose on cell function and structure;
- indirect effects due to insufficient insulin secretion to maintain normoglycemia;
- a long history of insulin resistance and hyperinsulinemia prior to glucose elevations;
- an association of dysglycemia with other recognized and unrecognized risk factors for cardiovascular disease, including dyslipidemia, hypertension, abdominal obesity, renal damage, and coagulation abnormalities.

Direct toxic effects of glucose

Glycation of a variety of proteins may directly promote cardiovascular disease.[39–42] Glycated albumin promotes albuminuria and endothelial cell dysfunction, glycated red cell membranes are less deformable, glycated LDL apoproteins are more susceptible than non-glycated LDL to uptake by scavenger cells (which would increase foam cell formation), oxidation, and increased platelet aggregation, glycated HDL is less able to transport cholesterol, and glycated fibrin and platelet membranes adversely affect vascular homeostasis. Advanced glycation end product (AGE) proteins also accumulate on vessel walls and in the vessel matrix and may adversely affect endothelial cell function and promote atherosclerosis.[41–43]

Glucose metabolism also results in the formation of reactive oxygen species directly[44] and indirectly through activation of the polyol pathway and AGE formation.[45] Any increased glucose metabolism due to higher ambient glucose levels therefore presents an oxidative stress.[45] Finally, increased glucose metabolism to diacylglycerol may promote vascular cell growth, altered vascular permeability, smooth muscle contraction, and synthesis of various prostaglandins through protein kinase C activation.[46]

Insufficient insulin production

Glucose is the major stimulus for insulin secretion, which in turn prevents rises in glucose levels. Therefore, an elevated glucose level implies a lack of sufficient insulin to maintain normoglycemia. Such a lack of *sufficient* insulin may occur in the presence of both low and high absolute levels of insulin, depending on the degree of insulin resistance.

A number of observations support the possibility that insufficient insulin secretion may be related to cardiovascular disease. First, patients with both type 1 (with no endogenous insulin secretion) and type 2 diabetes (who are not able to make sufficient insulin to prevent hyperglycemia) are at high risk for cardiovascular disease. Intensified insulin therapy may decrease this risk and certainly does not seem to worsen it. Second, patients with hypertension and other cardiovascular risk factors are resistant to the antilipolytic effects of insulin;[47] any decrease in the secretory capacity of insulin would accentuate this and promote free fatty acid transport to the liver. The ensuing hypertriglyceridemia may promote atherosclerosis.[48] Third, patients with cardiovascular disease have increased levels of proinsulin and split products[49,50] – a possible biochemical marker of a failing beta cell.[51] Fourth, many patients with atherosclerosis and/or cardiovascular disease are insulin resistant[52] and require high insulin levels to prevent hyperglycemia. Such a prolonged demand may increase the risk of subsequent beta cell failure and diabetes.[53,54]

Hyperinsulinemia

In non-diabetic people, fasting and 2-hour postload insulin levels rise with fasting and 2-hour glucose levels.[55,56] Thus, even mildly hyperglycemic patients have higher levels of insulin than normoglycemic controls. Moreover, hyperinsulinemia is associated with coronary heart disease[57,58] and many other cardiovascular risk factors including hypertension,[59] left ventricular hypertrophy,[60] elevated levels of triglyceride,[61–63] fibrinogen, von Willebrand factor-related antigen, factor 8 activity, plasminogen activator inhibitor-1 (PAI-1) antigen, and PAI-1 activity,[61] and depressed levels of HDL,[62,63] and tissue plasminogen activator (tPA).[61,64] Insulin may promote hypertension and atherosclerosis by stimulating renal sodium and water retention,[62] stimulating smooth muscle proliferation and vascular growth factor production,[62] sensitizing smooth muscle to the pressor effects of angiotensin II,[65] and increasing noradrenaline release through activation of the sympathetic nervous system.[66]

Despite these associations, the role of hyperinsulinemia in cardiovascular disease remains unclear. First, hyperinsulinemia is not a consistent risk factor in large epidemiologic studies of non-diabetic patients with cardiovascular disease.[67] Second, patients with insulinomas who are insulin resistant, hyperinsulinemic, and *hypoglycemic* have normal lipid profiles and blood pressure and no clinical evidence of cardiovascular disease.[68] Third, studies of intensified insulin therapy in patients with type 1 diabetes taking multiple daily doses of insulin suggest a reduced, not an increased risk for the biochemical changes associated with atherosclerosis.[69] Fourth, the fact that non-diabetic insulin levels are correlated with glucose levels suggests that the association of cardiovascular disease with insulin levels may reflect an association with glucose. The independent contribution of insulin and glucose, and any interaction of the two, to the risk of cardiovascular disease remains unclear despite multivariate analyses.

Association with other risk factors

Hyperglycemia commonly clusters with hypertension, insulin resistance, increased visceral fat, hypertriglyceridemia, and microalbuminuria.[63] It is also associated with obesity, poor socioeconomic status, and low birth weight. As such, the association between glucose and cardiovascular disease may either be due to one of these risk factors or to a common antecedent and not to any direct causal connection.[70,71]

IS GLUCOSE A MODIFIABLE CARDIOVASCULAR DISEASE RISK FACTOR?

A number of randomized controlled trials of intensive versus conventional insulin therapy of patients with both type 1 and type 2 diabetes suggested a non-significant trend in favor of a beneficial cardiovascular effect. These include the Diabetes Control and Complications Trial (DCCT)[15] in patients with type 1 diabetes, the controversial University Group Diabetes Program (UGDP)[72] in patients with type 2 diabetes, and a 6-year Japanese study of intensified versus conventional insulin therapy in patients with type 2 diabetes.[17] The strongest clinical evidence that insulin mediated glycemic control decreases the risk of cardiovascular disease was reported in a Swedish study of myocardial infarction patients randomized to conventional coronary care unit therapy versus an insulin infusion followed by intensified insulin therapy for at least 3 months.[73] Total mortality in the treatment group was reduced by 31% (95% CI 4–51%, $P=0.028$) at 1 year.

Only one small pilot study of 153 men with type 2 diabetes showed a trend towards an increased cardiovascular disease risk with intensified insulin therapy. Despite initial reports to the contrary, there was no significant difference in major or total event rates between the conventional and intensified insulin therapy groups.[74,75]

These data suggest, but do not prove, that insulin mediated tight glycemic control may lower the risk of cardiovascular disease in patients with diabetes mellitus. No intervention studies of the impact of reducing glucose levels in patients with elevated glucose levels that are below the diabetic cutoff have been reported.

CONCLUSION

There are a number of direct and indirect biologic pathways linking dysglycemia to cardiovascular disease. Similar to dyslipidemia, in which ongoing studies are continuing to show the therapeutic value of reducing even minimally elevated lipid levels,[76] dysglycemia may be a continuous modifiable cardiovascular disease risk factor: therapies that reduce elevated glucose levels may reduce the risk of cardiovascular disease.

A number of ongoing studies will address this issue. For patients with newly diagnosed type 2 diabetes, the UKPDS will determine if improved glycemic control prevents cardiovascular disease as well as eye, kidney, and nerve disease. It will end in 1997 after a median follow-up of 4902 randomized subjects for 11 years.[18,77] For patients with impaired glucose tolerance clinical trials of strategies to prevent diabetes, in which cardiovascular disease is a documented secondary outcome, include metformin, the insulin sensitizer troglitazone, diet and exercise (all being tested in the Diabetes Prevention Program), and acarbose (being tested in the Study to Prevent Diabetes). These studies are likely to shed new light on the relationship between glucose and cardiovascular disease and may provide ways of preventing cardiovascular disease in many individuals.

REFERENCES

1 Kannel WB, McGee DL. Diabetes and cardiovascular disease. The Framingham study. *JAMA* 1979;**241**:2035–8.

2 Stamler J, Vaccaro O, Neaton JD, Wentworth D. Diabetes, other risk factors, and 12-yr cardiovascular mortality for men screened in the Multiple Risk Factor Intervention Trial. *Diabetes Care* 1993;**16**:434.

3 Goldbourt U, Yaari S, Medalie JH. Factors predictive of long-term coronary heart disease mortality among 10059 male Israeli civil servants and municipal employees. A 23 year mortality follow-up in the Israeli Ischemic Heart Disease Study. *Cardiology* 1993;**82**:100–21.

4 Jarrett RJ, Shipley MJ. Type 2 (non-insulin-dependent) diabetes mellitus and cardiovascular disease – putative association via common antecedents; further evidence from the Whitehall study. *Diabetologia* 1988;**31**:737–40.

5 Herman JB, Medalie JH, Goldbourt U. Differences in cardiovascular morbidity and mortality between previously known and newly diagnosed adult diabetics. *Diabetologia* 1977;**13**:229–34.

6 Jarrett RJ. Type 2 (non-insulin-dependent) diabetes mellitus and coronary heart disease – chicken, egg or neither? *Diabetologia* 1984;**26**:99–102.

7 Harris MI. Undiagnosed NIDDM: clinical and public health issues. *Diabetes Care* 1993;**16**:642–52.

8 Harris MI. Classification, diagnostic criteria and screening for diabetes. In: Harris MI, Cowie CC, Stern MS *et al.* Eds. *Diabetes in America.* Bethesda: National Institutes of Health, 1995.

8a Expert Committee on the Diagnosis and Classification of Diabetes Mellitus. Report of the Expert Committee on the Diagnosis and Classification of Diabetes Mellitus. *Diabetes Care* 1997;**20**:1183–97.

9 National Diabetes Data Group. Classification and diagnosis of diabetes mellitus and other categories of glucose intolerance. *Diabetes* 1979;**28**:1039–57.

10 McCance DR, Hanson RL, Charles M, *et al.* Comparison of tests for glycated haemoglobin and fasting and two hour plasma glucose concentrations as diagnostic methods for diabetes. *Br Med J* 1994;**308**:1323–8.

11 Young TK, Roos NP, Hammerstrand KM. Estimated burden of diabetes mellitus in Manitoba according to health insurance claims: a pilot study. *Can Med Assoc J* 1991;**144**:318–24.

12 Tan MH, MacLean DR. Epidemiology of diabetes mellitus in Canada. *Clin Invest Med* 1995;**18**:240–6.

13 Kenny SJ, Aubert RE, Geiss LS. Prevalence and incidence of non-insulin-dependent diabetes. In: Harris MI, Cowie CC, Stern MS *et al.* Eds. *Diabetes in America.* Bethesda: National Institutes of Health 1995.

14 King H, Rewers M, WHO Ad Hoc Diabetes Reporting Group. Global estimates for prevalence of diabetes mellitus and impaired glucose tolerance in adults. *Diabetes Care* 1993;**16**:157–77.

15 Diabetes Control and Complications Trial Research Group. The effect of intensive treatment of diabetes on the development and progression of long-term complications in insulin-dependent diabetes mellitus. *N Engl J Med* 1993;**329**:977–86.

16 Krolewski AS, Laffel LMB, Krolewski M, Quinn M, Warram JH. Glycosylated hemoglobin and the risk of microalbuminuria in patients with insulin-dependent diabetes mellitus. *N Engl J Med* 1995;**332**:1251–5.

17 Ohkubo Y, Kishikawa H, Araki E *et al.* Intensive insulin therapy prevents the progression of diabetic microvascular complications in Japanese patients with non-insulin-dependent diabetes

mellitus: a randomized prospective 6-year study. *Diab Res Clin Pract* 1995;**28**:103–17.

18 Turner R, Cull C, Holman R, United Kingdom Prospective Diabetes Study Group. United Kingdom Prospective Diabetes Study 17: a 9 year update of a randomized controlled trial on the effect of improved metabolic control on complications in non-insulin-dependent diabetes mellitus. *Ann Intern Med* 1996;**124**:136–45.

19 Barrett-Connor E, Cohn BA, Wingard DL, Edelstein SL. Why is diabetes mellitus a stronger risk factor for fatal ischemic heart disease in women than in men? The Rancho Bernardo Study. *JAMA* 1991;**265**:627–31.

20 Zuanetti G, Latini R, Maggioni AP, Santoro L, Franzosi MG. Influence of diabetes on mortality in acute myocardial infarction: data from the GISSI-2 study. *J Am Coll Cardiol* 1993;**22**:1788–94.

21 Granger CB, Califf RM, Young S *et al.* Outcome of patients with diabetes mellitus and acute myocardial infarction treated with thrombolytic agents. The Thrombolysis and Angioplasty in Myocardial Infarction (TAMI) Study Group. *J Am Coll Cardiol* 1993;**21**:920–5.

22 Moss SE, Klein R, Klein BEK, Meuer SM. The association of glycemia and cause-specific mortality in a diabetic population. *Arch Intern Med* 1994;**154**:2473–9.

23 Kuusisto J, Mykkanen L, Pyorala K, Laakso M. NIDDM and its metabolic control predict coronary heart disease in elderly subjects. *Diabetes* 1994;**43**:960–7.

24 Andersson DKG, Svardsudd K. Long-term glycemic control relates to mortality in type II diabetes. *Diabetes Care* 1995;**18**:1534–43.

25 Fuller JH, Shipley MJ, Rose G, Jarrett RJ, Keen H. Mortality from coronary heart disease and stroke in relation to degree of glycemia: the Whitehall study. *Br Med J Clin Res Ed* 1983;**287**:867–70.

26 Fuller JH, Shipley MJ, Rose G, Jarrett RJ, Keen H. Coronary-heart-disease risk and impaired glucose tolerance. The Whitehall study. *Lancet* 1980;**8183**:1373–6.

27 Scheidt-Nave C, Barrett-Connor E, Wingard DL, Cohn BA, Edelstein SL. Sex differences in fasting glycemia as a risk factor for ischemic heart disease death. *Am J Epidemiol* 1991;**133**:565–76.

28 Singer DE, Nathan DM, Anderson KM, Wilson PWF, Evans JC. Association of HbA1c with prevalent cardiovascular disease in the original cohort of the Framingham heart study. *Diabetes* 1992;**41**:202–8.

29 Wilson PWF, Cupples A, Kannel WB. Is hyperglycemia associated with cardiovascular disease? The Framingham study. *Am Heart J* 1991;**121**:586–90.

30 Donahue RP, Abbott RD, Reed DM, Yano K. Postchallenge glucose concentration and coronary heart disease in men of Japanese ancestry. Honolulu heart program. *Diabetes* 1987;**36**:689–92.

31 Jackson CA, Yudkin JS, Forrest RD. A comparison of the relationship of the glucose tolerance test and the glycated hemoglobin assay with diabetic vascular disease in the community. The Islington Diabetes Survey. *Diab Res Clin Pract* 1992;**17**:111–23.

32 Pyorala K, Savolainen E, Lehtovirta E, Punsar S, Siltanen P. Glucose tolerance and coronary heart disease: Helsinki Policemen Study. *J Chron Dis* 1979;**32**:729–45.

33 Ohlson LO, Svardsudd K, Welin L *et al.* Fasting blood glucose and risk of coronary heart disease, stroke, and all-cause mortality: a 17-year follow-up study of men born in 1913. *Diabetic Med* 1986;**3**:33–7.

34 Stamler R, Stamler J, Lindberg HA *et al.* Asymptomatic hyperglycemia and coronary heart disease in middle-aged men in two employed populations in Chicago. *J Chron Dis* 1979;**32**:805–15.

35 Coutinho M, Wang Y, Gerstein HC, Yusuf S. Continuous relationship of glucose with cardiovascular events in non-diabetic subjects: a meta regression analysis of 18 studies in 88 000 individuals (American Heart Association 69th Meeting). *Circulation* 1996;**94**:I–214(Abstract).

36 Pais P, Pogue J, Gerstein H *et al.* Risk factors for acute myocardial infarction in Indians: a case-control study. *Lancet* 1996;**348**:358–63.

37 Neaton JD, Wentworth D, MRFIT Research Group. Serum cholesterol, blood pressure, cigarette smoking, and death from coronary heart disease. Overall findings and differences by age for 316, 099 white men. *Arch Intern Med* 1992;**152**:56–64.

38 Gerstein HC, Yusuf S. Dysglycaemia and risk of cardiovascular disease. *Lancet* 1996;**347**:949–50.

39 Lyons TJ. Glycation and oxidation: a role in the pathogenesis of atherosclerosis. *Am J Cardiol* 1993;**71**:26B–31B.

40 Lyons TJ. Lipoprotein glycation and its metabolic consequences. *Diabetes* 1992;**41**:67–73.

41 Vlassara H, Bucala R, Striker L. Pathogenic effects of advanced glycosylation: biochemical, biologic, and clinical implications for diabetes and aging. *Lab Invest* 1994;**70**:138–51.

42 Brownlee M. Glycation and diabetic complications. *Diabetes* 1994;**43**:836–41.

43 Hogan M, Cerami A, Bucala R. Advanced glycosylation endproducts block the antiproliferative effect of nitric oxide. *J Clin Invest* 1992;**90**:1110–15.

44 Baynes JW. Role of oxidative stress in development of complications of diabetes. *Diabetes* 1991;**40**:405–12.

45 Giugliano D, Ceriello A, Paolisso G. Diabetes mellitus, hypertension and cardiovascular disease: which role for oxidative stress? *Metabolism* 1995;**44**:363–8.

46 Kreisberg JI. Hyperglycemia and microangiopathy. Direct regulation by glucose of microvascular cells. *Lab Invest* 1992;**67**:416–26.

47 Hennes MM, O'Shaughnessy IM, Kelly TM *et al.* Insulin-resistant lipolysis in abdominally obese hypertensive individuals. Role of the renin-angiotensin system. *Hypertension* 1996;**28**:120–6.

48 Austin MA, Hokanson JE. Epidemiology of triglycerides, small dense low-density lipoprotein, and lipoprotein(a) as risk factors for coronary heart disease. [Review]. *Med Clin N Am* 1994;**78**:99–115.

49 Bavenholm P, Proudler A, Tornvall P *et al.* Insulin, intact and split proinsulin, and coronary artery disease in young men. *Circulation* 1995;**92**:1422–9.

50 Nordt TK, Schneider DJ, Sobel BE. Augmentation of the synthesis of plasminogen activator inhibitor type-1 by precursors of insulin. A potential risk factor for vascular disease. *Circulation* 1994;**89**:321–30.

51 Haffner SM, Mykkanen L, Valdez RA *et al.* Disproportionately increased proinsulin levels are associated with the insulin resistance syndrome. *J Clin Endocrinol Metabol* 1994;**79**:1806–10.

52 Stern MP. Do non-insulin dependent diabetes mellitus and cardiovascular disease share common antecedents? *Ann Intern Med* 1996;**124**:110–16.

53 Bogardus C. Agonist: the case for insulin resistance as a necessary and sufficient cause of type II diabetes mellitus. *J Lab Clin Med* 1995;**125**:556–8.

54 Taylor SI, Accili A, Imai Y. Insulin resistance or insulin deficiency. Which is the primary cause of NIDDM? *Diabetes* 1994;**43**:735–40.

55 Welborn TA, Wearne K. Coronary heart disease incidence and cardiovascular mortality in Busselton with reference to glucose and insulin concentrations. *Diabetes Care* 1979;**2**:154–60.

56 Barrett-Connor E, Schrott HG, Greendale G *et al.* Factors associated with glucose and insulin levels in healthy postmenopausal women. *Diabetes Care* 1996;**19**:333–40.

57 Fontbonne A, Charles MA, Thibult N *et al.* Hyperinsulinemia as a predictor of coronary heart disease mortality in a healthy population: the Paris Prospective Study, 15 year follow-up. *Diabetologia* 1991;**34**:356–61.

58 Pyorala K. Hyperinsulinemia as predictor of atherosclerotic vascular disease: epidemiologic evidence. *Diabetic Metabol* 1991;**17**:87–92.

59 Denker PS, Pollock VE. Fasting serum insulin levels in essential hypertension. A meta-analysis. *Arch Intern Med* 1992;**152**:1649–51.

60 Sasson Z, Rasooly Y, Bhesania T, Rasooly I. Insulin resistance is an important determinant of left ventricular mass in the obese. *Circulation* 1993;**88**:1431–6.

61 Juhan-Vague I, Thompson SG, Jespersen J. Involvement of the hemostatic system in the insulin resistance syndrome. A study of 1500 patients with angina pectoris. The ECAT Angina Pectoris Study Group. *Arterioscler Thromb* 1993;**13**:1865–73.

62 Elliott TG, Viberti G. Relationship between insulin resistance and coronary heart disease in diabetes mellitus and the general population. *Baillière's Clin Endocrinol Metabol* 1993;**7**:1079–103.

63 Laws A, Reaven GM. Insulin resistance and risk factors for coronary heart disease. *Baillière's Clin Endocrinol Metabol* 1993;**7**:1063–78.

64 Eliasson M, Asplund K, Evrin PE, Lindahl B, Lundblad D. Hyperinsulinemia predicts low tissue plasminogen activator activity in a healthy population: the northern Sweden MONICA study. *Metabol Clin Exp* 1994;**43**:1579–86.

65 Gaboury CL, Simonson DC, Seely EW, Hollenberg NK, Williams GH. Relation of pressor responsiveness to angiotensin II and insulin resistance in hypertension. *J Clin Invest* 1994;**94**:2295–300.

66 Anderson EA, Hoffman RP, Balon TW, Sinkey CA, Mark AL. Hyperinsulinemia produces both sympathetic neural activation and vasodilation in normal humans. *J Clin Invest* 1991;**87**:2246–52.

67 Wingard DL, Barrett-Connor E, Ferrara A. Is insulin really a heart disease risk factor? *Diabetes Care* 1995;**18**:1299–304.

68 Leonetti F, Iozzo P, Giaccari A *et al.* Absence of clinically overt atherosclerotic vascular disease and adverse changes in cardiovascular risk factors in 70 patients with insulinoma. *J Endocrinol Invest* 1993;**16**:875–80.

69 Diabetes Control and Complications Trial (DCCT) Research Group. Effect of intensive diabetes management on macrovascular events and risk factors in the diabetes control and complications trial. *Am J Cardiol* 1995;**75**:894–903.

70 Stern MP. Diabetes and cardiovascular disease: The "common soil" hypothesis. *Diabetes* 1995;**44**:369–74.

71 Jarrett RJ. The cardiovascular risk associated with impaired glucose tolerance. *Diabetic Med* 1996;**13**(3 Suppl 2):S15–S19.

72 Genuth S. Exogenous insulin administration and cardiovascular risk in NIDDM and IDDM. *Ann Intern Med* 1996;**124**:104–9.

73 Malmberg K, Ryden L, Efendic S *et al.* Randomized trial of insulin-glucose infusion followed by

subcutaneous insulin treatment in diabetic patients with acute myocardial infarction (DIGAMI study): effects on mortality at 1 year. *J Am Coll Cardiol* 1995;**26**:57–65.

74 Colwell JA. The feasibility of intensive insulin management in non-insulin-dependent diabetes mellitus. Implications of the Veterans Affairs Cooperative Study on glycemic control and complications in NIDDM. *Ann Intern Med* 1996; **124**:131–5.

75 Abraira C, Johnson N, Colwell JA, VACSDM Group. VA Cooperative Study on glycemic control and complications in type II diabetes (VACSDM): results of the completed feasibility trial. *Diabetes* 1994;**43**(Suppl):59A(abstract).

76 Sacks FM, Pfeffer MA, Moye LA *et al.* The effect of pravastatin on coronary events after myocardial infarction in patients with average cholesterol levels. *N Engl J Med* 1996;**335**: 1001–9.

77 United Kingdom Prospective Diabetes Study Group. UK Prospective Diabetes Study (UKPDS). VIII. Study design, progress and performance. *Diabetologia* 1991;**34**:877–90.

Physical activity and exercise in cardiovascular disease prevention and rehabilitation

17

ERIKA S. FROELICHER,
ROBERTA K. OKA,
GERALD F. FLETCHER

INTRODUCTION

The goal of this chapter is to review the scientific evidence regarding the benefits and safety of physical activity and exercise with respect to a series of health outcomes. A brief coverage of this review is aimed at the adult American population in order to acquaint the physician with the latest recommendations for primary prevention. The major focus, however, is on the coronary population with a minor focus on the elderly, women, and the physically disabled. Existing evidence based reviews and consensus documents are used to support the evidence. The recommendations are deliberately kept very brief, but the necessary references are cited to assist the primary care physician, internist or cardiologist in obtaining such documents.

EVIDENCE FOR BENEFITS OF REGULAR EXERCISE IN ADULTS

An accumulation of scientific evidence provides consistent evidence that light to moderate physical activity in healthy adults reduces the risk for all-cause mortality and cardiovascular disease (CVD) in men and women.[1-3] However, approximately 60% of US adults are not regularly physically active and 25% are inactive.[4] Physical inactivity is a serious, nationwide problem. It poses a major public health challenge with a national burden of unnecessary illnesses and premature death. Physical activity and exercise are pivotal in health promotion and disease prevention, especially now that the evidence for the hazards of being physically inactive are clear.[5] These statistics, representing low levels of exercise in the US population, call for urgent action by health professionals.

Primary care physicians, internists, and cardiologists in particular need to provide evidence based physical activity recommendations to their patients.

Grade A/B

> ### Benefits and adverse effects in adults[5]
>
> Physical activity improves health in the following ways:
> - reduces risk of dying prematurely;
> - reduces risk of dying from heart disease;
> - reduces risk of developing diabetes;
> - reduces risk of developing high blood pressure;
> - helps reduce blood pressure in people who already have high blood pressure.
>
> Other documented health benefits include:
> - reduces the risk of developing colon cancer;
> - reduces feelings of depression and anxiety;
> - helps control weight;
> - helps build healthy bones, muscles, and joints;
> - helps older adults become stronger and better able to move about without falling;
> - promotes psychological well-being.
>
> ### Adverse effects of physical activity
>
> Types of adverse effects:
> - musculoskeletal injuries
> - metabolic abnormalities
> - hematologic and body organ abnormalities
> - hazards
> - infection, allergic, and inflammatory conditions
> - precipitation of cardiac events.
>   1. Most skeletal muscular events are preventable by gradually working up to desirable level, avoiding excessive amounts of activity.
>   2. Serious cardiovascular events can occur with physical exertion. Net effect is lower risk of mortality from cardiovascular disease.

Additionally, the Surgeon General's Report[5] urges health care providers to counsel their patients to do the following.

Recommendations for adults

Recent recommendations for physical activity from the Centers for Disease Control (CDC) and National Institutes of Health (NIH) suggest that American adults should engage in physical activity at a level appropriate to their capacity, needs, and interests. Regular exercise is recommended, preferably daily, of at least 30–45 minutes of brisk walking (3 mph), bicycling or working around the house or yard. Activities may include formal exercise such as walking or jogging or intermittent types of activity that include stair climbing, gardening or housework.[5]

A well rounded exercise program should include both muscular strength training and joint flexibility exercises in order to improve one's ability to perform tasks and to reduce the potential for injury.[3,5] Upper extremity and resistance (strength) training can improve muscle function and evidence suggests that there may be cardiovascular benefit in older patients and those with underlying CVD. This area, however, is rather new and further evidence is needed before recommendations can be made to the public. While these recommendations are especially important for the elderly, persons who have been deconditioned due to recent inactivity or illness may benefit as well. People who are already physically active will benefit even more by increasing intensity or duration of their activity. These recommendations are intended primarily for the healthy sedentary population.[5]

Essentials of physical activity counseling

1. All subjects should be asked about their physical activity status. Questions should address leisure and recreational activities (i.e. sports and exercise), as well as intermittent activity (walking, stair climbing, household and yard work).
2. Assess whether activities meet the current activity recommendation guidelines (i.e. activity should be at least of moderate intensity or equivalent intensity to a brisk walk 3 mph on most or all days).
3. Patients should be assisted in planning an appropriate program of physical activity.

EVIDENCE FOR BENEFITS FROM REGULAR EXERCISE IN THE CORONARY POPULATION

A recent comprehensive evidence based review has been completed on the benefits of exercise in the coronary population.[6] For brevity, this consensus document will be used as a source of evidence along with other consensus documents. The major focus of this review was on coronary patients (including myocardial infarction (MI), coronary artery bypass surgery (CABG), and percutaneous transluminal coronary angioplasty (PTCA)), with a lesser focus on heart failure and cardiac transplantation literature and special populations such as the elderly, women, and physically disabled (see Figure 17.1 for the criteria guiding this review).

Throughout this chapter the following rating system will be applied for the strength of the scientific evidence of the review:

- A – Scientific evidence from well designed and well conducted controlled trials (randomized and non-randomized) provides statistically significant results that consistently support the guideline statement.
- B – Scientific evidence is provided by observational studies or by controlled trials with less consistent results.
- C – Guideline statement supported by expert opinion; the available scientific evidence did not present consistent results or controlled trials were lacking.

CLINICAL AND PHYSIOLOGICAL OUTCOMES IN THE CORONARY POPULATION

A comprehensive review by the Agency for Health Care Policy and Research[6] provides consistent scientific evidence of the benefits of exercise training on a number of outcomes that include morbidity, mortality, exercise tolerance and symptoms (see summary in

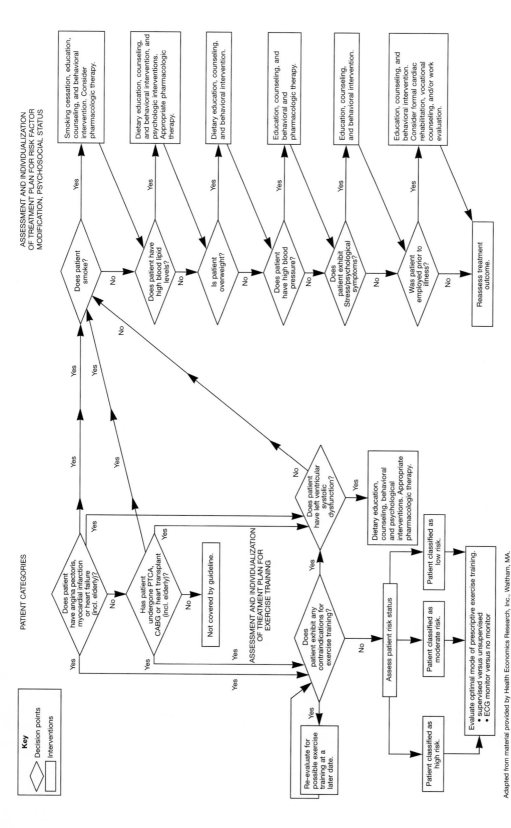

Figure 17.1 Decision tree for cardiac rehabilitation services. (From Wenger *et al*[6])

Adapted from material provided by Health Economics Research, Inc., Waltham, MA.

254

Table 17.1). The evidence is less consistent for the benefit of reduced blood lipids, smoking cessation, psychological well-being, social adjustment and functioning, reduction in excess body weight, and a series of physiologic measures.

Morbidity and safety issues Grade A

Forty-two studies – 15 randomized controlled trials (RCTs), 14 non-randomized studies, and 13 observational studies – provide evidence that exercise training does not change the rate of non-fatal reinfarction. The safety of exercise rehabilitation is well established; rates of infarction and cardiovascular complications are very low.[6] No study documented increased morbidity when comparing patients in the intervention group to the control group, with 4578 patients included in the controlled trials (randomized and non-randomized reviewed).[6]

Reduced mortality Grade B

Thirty-one studies – 17 RCTs, eight non-randomized studies, and six observational studies – provide evidence that exercise training programs significantly reduce total and cardiovascular mortality in patients following MI.[6]

Exercise tolerance Grade A

A total of 114 studies – 46 RCTs, 25 non-randomized studies, and 43 observational studies – demonstrated that exercise training consistently improved objective measures of exercise tolerance, without significant cardiovascular complications or other adverse outcomes. Therefore, appropriately prescribed exercise training is recommended as an integral component of cardiac services, particularly for patients with decreased exercise tolerance. Maintenance of continued exercise training is required to sustain improved exercise tolerance.[6] A minimum duration and frequency of exercise has not been definitively determined and more study is needed in this area.

Strength training (resistance-training) (B)

Seven studies – four RCTs and three non-randomized studies – have shown that strength training improves skeletal muscle strength and endurance in clinically stable coronary patients.[6] In the majority of these studies, weight training was added as a strength training component to the exercise regimens of coronary patients, who had already participated in aerobic exercise training for 3 or more months. Documented benefits occurred with both low and high resistance training. Weight carrying tolerance (time) or increases in skeletal muscle strength after completion of resistance training was reported by all studies. Five of the seven strength training studies demonstrated that submaximal and peak resistance exercise, using a variety of resistance training devices, resulted in significantly lower peak heart rate, pressure rate products, and oxygen

Table 17.1 Summary of evidence for cardiac rehabilitation outcomes: effects of exercise training

Outcome	Evidence base[a]				Strength of evidence[b]
	Total number of studies	Randomized studies	Non-randomized studies	Observational studies	
Exercise tolerance	114	46	25	43	A
Exercise tolerance (strength training)	7	4	3	0	B
Exercise habits	15	10	2	3	B
Symptoms	26	12	7	7	B
Smoking	24	12	8	4	B
Lipids	37	18	6	13	B
Body weight	34	11	7	16	C
Blood pressure	18	9	6	3	B
Psychological well-being	20	9	8	3	B
Social adjustment and functioning	6	2	2	2	B
Return to work	28	10	9	9	A
Morbidity	42 (+2 survey reports)	15	14	13	A
Mortality	31 (+2 survey reports)	17	8	6	B
Pathophysiologic measures: Changes in atherosclerosis	9	5	1	3	A/B
Changes in hemodynamic measurements	5	0	0	5	B
Changes in myocardial perfusion/myocardial ischemia	11	6	2	3	B
Changes in myocardial contractility, ventricular wall motion abnormalities, and/or ventricular ejection fraction	22	9	5	8	B
Changes in cardiac arrhythmias	5	4	0	1	B
Heart failure patients	12	5	3	4	A
Cardiac transplantation patients	5	0	1	4	B
Elderly patients	7	0	1	6	B

[a] Number of studies from scientific literature by type of study design.

[b] Rating for strength of evidence:

A Scientific evidence from well designed and well conducted controlled trials (randomized and non-randomized) provides statistically significant results that consistently support the guideline statement.

B Scientific evidence is provided by observational studies or by controlled trials with less consistent results.

C Guideline statement supported by expert opinion: the available scientific evidence did not present consistent results or controlled trials were lacking.

consumption responses than did maximal treadmill exercise testing.[6] Moreover, angina, ventricular arrhythmias, and ischemic ST segment depression occurred less frequently during resistance testing than during aerobic exercise testing to the point of fatigue.[7-9] These studies therefore provide indirect evidence of the effectiveness of resistance exercise training in selected patients with coronary disease.

A meta-analytic review by Buchner[10] concluded that high intensity exercise programs reported much more gain in strength than did low intensity training. High intensity training was well tolerated by older adults, even those who were frail. Improvements in muscle strength can improve patients' performance of activities of daily living.[11] However, most of the studies involved small numbers of "low risk" male patients, aged 70 years and younger, with good left ventricular function; also, training was of relatively short duration (less than or equal to 12 weeks). Hence the application of this intervention to women coronary patients is at this time based on an extrapolation.

RECOMMENDATION FOR STRENGTH TRAINING EXERCISES

The strength training exercise sessions were typically started 4–6 weeks after MI or CABG and carried out each week. The intensity ranged from 25% to 80% of the one repetition maximal; the most typical format consisted of three 30–60-minute strength training exercise sessions per week for 6–26 weeks.

SAFETY OF STRENGTH TRAINING EXERCISES IN CORONARY PATIENTS

The lack of cardiovascular and orthopedic complications in the 3-year follow-up of strength training was largely attributed to strict preliminary screening and careful supervision.[12] It is unclear if safety can be extrapolated to other populations of coronary or cardiac patients (e.g. women, older men and women patients with low aerobic conditioning, patients at moderate to high cardiovascular risk) and this requires study. However, regimens designed to increase skeletal muscle strength can safely be included in exercise programs of clinically stable coronary patients when appropriate instruction and surveillance are provided.

Symptoms Grade B

Twenty-six studies – 12 RCTs, seven non-randomized studies, and seven observational studies – showed that exercise training decreases both angina pectoris in patients with coronary heart disease (CHD) and symptoms of heart failure in patients with left ventricular (LV) systolic dysfunction. Therefore, exercise training is recommended as an integral component of symptom management for these patients.[6]

Return to work Grade A

Twenty-eight studies – 10 RCTs, nine non-randomized studies, and nine observational studies – provide evidence that do not support an improved rate of return to work as a result of exercise training *alone*. A likely explanation may be that exercise training exerts less influence on return to work than many non-exercise variables including employer attitudes, prior employment status, economic incentives, and the like.[6]

Blood lipid levels Grade B

Thirty-seven studies – 18 RCTs, six non-randomized studies, and 13 observational studies – suggest that exercise training is not recommended as a sole intervention for lipid modification because of inconsistent effects on lipid and lipoprotein levels. Optimal lipid management requires specific dietary and medically indicated pharmacologic management in addition to exercise training.[6]

Smoking cessation Grade A

Twenty-four studies –12 RCTs, eight non-randomized studies, and four observational studies – conclude that exercise training has little or no effect on smoking cessation. Smoking cessation is achieved primarily by targeted smoking cessation strategies.[6] The smoking cessation guidelines developed by an AHCPR evidence guideline panel provide detailed guidance on the optimum strategies for smoking cessation.[13]

Psychological well-being Grade B

Twenty studies – nine RCTs, eight non-randomized studies, and three observational studies – found that exercise training – with or without other cardiac rehabilitation services – generally results in decrease in anxiety and depression and improved physical function.[6] Exercise is therefore recommended to enhance psychological well-being, particularly when it is one component of a multifactorial rehabilitation program. Studies of exercise training in a supervised group setting as a sole intervention do not show consistent improvement in anxiety and depression. Studies of exercise training as a sole intervention are confounded by the consequences of group interactions, formation of social support networks, peer and professional support, and counseling and guidance, all of which may affect depression, anxiety, and self-confidence.

Blood pressure Grade B

Eighteen studies – nine RCTs, six non-randomized studies, and three observational studies – allow the conclusion that exercise training as a sole intervention had no demonstrable effect in lowering blood pressure levels. A multifactorial education, counseling, behavioral, and pharmacologic approach is the recommended strategy for the management of hypertension according to the fifth report of the Joint National Committee on Detection, Evaluation, and Treatment of High Blood Pressure (1993).[14]

Social adjustment and functioning Grade B

Six studies – two RCTs, two non-randomized studies, and two observational studies – provide evidence that exercise training improves social adjustment and functioning and is therefore recommended in the care of cardiac patients. The social benefits from participation in exercise and cardiac rehabilitation are a favorable result. More research is needed to evaluate the impact of cardiac rehabilitation on social adjustment and functioning.[6]

Body weight Grade C

Thirty-four studies – 11 RCTs, seven non-randomized studies, and 16 observational studies – provide evidence that exercise training alone has inconsistent effects on controlling excess body weight and is not recommended as a sole intervention for this risk factor. Optimal management of overweight patients requires multifactorial intervention including intensive nutritional education, counseling and behavioral modification as an adjunct to exercise training. The panel[6] concluded that after a review of behavioral therapy literature involving obese patients, state of the art weight loss programs were shown to be successful. Results of a meta-analysis of 70 studies indicated that weight reduction through dieting can also help normalize plasma lipids and lipoprotein levels in overweight individuals.[15] It is essential to note that the comprehensive use of exercise, education, counseling, and behavioral interventions as a multifactorial approach has consistently yielded much stronger evidence, in terms of health outcomes, than exercise programs alone.

Pathophysiologic measures

ATHEROSCLEROSIS Grade A/B

Nine studies – five RCTs, one non-randomized study, and three observational studies – provide convincing evidence that exercise training as a sole intervention does not result in regression, limitation or progression of angiographically documented coronary atherosclerosis. But regression or limitation in progression of atherosclerosis may occur when exercise training is combined with intense dietary intervention, with or without lipid lowering drugs.[6]

HEMODYNAMIC MEASUREMENT Grade B

Five observational studies provide evidence that exercise training has no effect on development of coronary collateral circulation and produces no consistent changes in cardiac hemodynamic measurements during cardiac catheterization. Exercise training in patients with heart failure and depressed ventricular ejection fraction produces favorable hemodynamic changes in the skeletal musculature. Therefore, cardiac rehabilitation exercise training is recommended to improve skeletal muscle function; however, it does not enhance cardiac hemodynamic function or promote development of collateral coronary circulation.[6]

MYOCARDIAL PERFUSION/MYOCARDIAL ISCHEMIA Grade B

Eleven studies – six RCTs, two non-randomized studies, and three observational studies – provide evidence that exercise training decreases myocardial ischemia as measured by exercise ECG testing, ambulatory ECG recording, and radionuclide perfusion imaging. Exercise training is recommended to improve the measures of myocardial ischemia.[6]

MYOCARDIAL CONTRACTILITY, VENTRICULAR WALL MOTION ABNORMALITIES, AND/OR VENTRICULAR EJECTION FRACTION Grade B

Twenty-two studies – nine RCTs, five non-randomized studies, and eight observational studies – document that exercise training has little effect on ventricular ejection fraction and regional wall motion abnormalities. The effect of exercise training on left ventricular function in patients after anterior wall Q-wave MI with LV dysfunction is inconsistent. Exercise training is not recommended to improve measures of ventricular systolic function.[6]

OTHER CLINICAL POPULATIONS

Heart failure and cardiac transplantation

HEART FAILURE PATIENTS Grade B

Twelve studies – five RCTs, three non-randomized, and four observational studies – provide evidence for the benefit of exercise training in the heart failure population. Exercise training in patients with heart failure and moderate to severe LV dysfunction improves functional capacity and symptoms, without changes in LV function. Exercise training is recommended in these patients to attain functional and symptomatic improvement but there is a potentially higher likelihood of adverse events. In summary, although these studies had small numbers and young populations of patients, predominantly male, and CAD was the major etiology of heart failure, exercise training in patients with heart failure and diminished ventricular systolic dysfunction resulted in documented improvement in functional capacity. The benefits are thought to be due predominantly to adaptation in peripheral circulation and skeletal musculature.[6]

CARDIAC TRANSPLANTATION PATIENTS Grade B

Seven studies – one non-randomized study and six observational studies – suggest that exercise training following cardiac transplantation improves exercise tolerance and is recommended for this purpose. These trials demonstrated that participation in an exercise program produced physiological training responses that included: increased peak oxygen uptake, resting heart rate, decreased peak exercise heart rate, increased resting blood pressure, and decreased peak systolic blood pressure compared with normal controls. No change was observed in peak systolic blood pressure or pressure rate product. However, these studies were uncontrolled and therefore these changes could be either the result of spontaneous improvement or a treatment effect. While there are few studies in this area and no RCTs, initial observations demonstrate efficacy of this intervention.

In addition, it is believed that strength training before the transplantation may help enhance recovery after the operation. However, more research is needed in this area to identify the extent of spontaneous recovery versus the added benefit from exercise intervention.[6,16]

Changes in cardiac arrhythmias Grade B/C

Five studies – four RCTs and one observational study – provide evidence for the role of exercise in patients with arrhythmias. Two of the four RCTs showed that exercising patients, but not the controls, had a reduction in ventricular arrhythmias.[17,18] One demonstrated no statistically significant difference between exercise patients and controls when monitoring ventricular arrhythmia frequency or severity with 24-hour ambulatory ECG.[19] One RCT reported more malignant premature ventricular contractions (PVCs) on 24-hour ambulatory ECG monitoring during exercise training days in exercise patients compared to control patients.[20] The one observational study showed no difference in PVCs at baseline versus after exercise training. Exercise training has inconsistent effects on ventricular arrhythmias.

SPECIAL POPULATIONS

Elderly Grade B

Elderly patients constitute a high percentage of those with MI, CABG, and PTCA and are also at high risk of disability following a coronary event. Seven studies – one non-randomized study and six observational studies – provide the evidence for this review.[6] Also, the Surgeon General's report[5] concludes that physical activity, including strength training (resistance) exercise, appears to be protective against falling and fractures among the elderly, probably by increasing muscle strength and balance. Elderly coronary patients have exercise trainability comparable to younger patients participating in similar exercise rehabilitation. Elderly female and male patients show comparable improvement, but referral to and participation in exercise rehabilitation is less frequent for elderly patients,[5] especially females. Physical activity need *not* be strenuous to achieve health benefits.[11] No complications or adverse outcomes of exercise training in the elderly were described in any study. Although few studies and no randomized controlled trials specifically addressed the efficacy and safety of exercise training and multifactorial rehabilitation in the elderly, the available studies provide important new information of beneficial functional improvement from exercise training for current clinical practice. Elderly patients of both genders should be strongly encouraged to participate in exercise based cardiac rehabilitation and special effort should be taken to overcome the obstacles to entry and participation in cardiac rehabilitation services for elderly patients.

Women Grade B/C

The scientific evidence was either lacking altogether or small numbers of women were included in RCTs, making separate analyses for benefit impossible. This practice resulted in lack of information at best and confusion at worst. If indeed women do experience differing responses than men in exercise training then the effects are likely to be diluted for men and non-informative for women. The consensus of the expert panel[6] was that in most instances women can benefit from exercise training. However, women have unique considerations that require special attention. In studies of CAD patients women tend to be older, live alone more often (they are widowed or divorced), and have fewer economic and social resources. These circumstances require that women be given special attention to minimize the barriers to enrollment in exercise programs and to continuation with the program.

The Center for Women's Health at the National Institutes of Health has as its primary goal compensation for this scientific deficit regarding women's health. Until these new initiatives have been completed and reported in the literature, only scant scientific evidence exists to guide the physician regarding specific recommendations for women.[21] Many studies are now in progress or have already been completed since the formulation of the Center for Women's Health in 1980.

Physically disabled Grade B/C

With the passing of the Americans with Disabilities Act (1990), physicians are now required to address the special exercise training needs of patients with a variety of physical disabilities. People with physical disabilities are advised to see a physician before starting a program of physical activity that is new them.[11] In particular, physically disabled patients with CVD should be referred to the cardiologist for physical therapy or exercise prescription. A recent comprehensive review is available for the reader who requires greater detail than is possible here.[22,23]

GENERAL SAFETY ISSUES

Patients with chronic health problems (i.e. heart disease or diabetes) should first obtain medical clearance before beginning a new exercise program. Skeletal muscle and other injury can be avoided by beginning exercises slowly and gradually building up to the desired amount of exercise (duration, frequency, and intensity) to give skeletal muscles and the cardiovascular system time to adapt. It is recommended that men over 40 and women over 50 consult a physician prior to beginning a vigorous physical activity program. This is to ensure that the patient does not have undiagnosed heart disease or other health problems that may place them at increased risk and that may require special modification in the exercise prescription or the monitoring of their response to the exercise.[5] The ACSM,[24] AHA,[25] and AACVPR[26] have issued guidelines for assessment of an exercise facility prior to beginning an exercise program. A medical evaluation, including an exercise test, is recommended for individuals with known coronary risk factors or a strong family history of CVD. Exercise testing is recommended for persons over 40 years of age, especially if they have two or more risk factors for CVD. But it is not recommended for apparently healthy individuals less than 40 years due to the relatively low predictive value of a positive test.[25]

OTHER ORGANIZATIONAL AND CLINICAL ISSUES

Adherence to exercise (C)

The evidence for exercise interventions for cardiovascular risk reduction has been provided in the preceding pages. However, the extent to which exercise is effective may depend in large part on adherence.[27] Burke and colleagues,[27] in their comprehensive review on adherence, further concluded that non-adherence, whether it occurs early or late in the treatment course, is one mediator of clinical outcomes. Hence, specific attention is given to adherence in this chapter. Barriers to exercise are two-fold: the lack of physicians' exercise prescription and patient non-adherence. Since physicians have had limited clear evidence on reduction of "hard events" until recently, coronary patients have not consistently received physician recommendations regarding exercise or have received suggestions that were too general to be beneficial. Cardiac rehabilitation programs are available for referral by the physician in virtually every major city throughout the U S.

Much of the information on adherence is derived from multifactorial cardiac rehabilitation studies that were designed *not* to evaluate or enhance adherence but to determine the effects of rehabilitation services on other outcomes. These studies demonstrate a progressive decline with longer treatment duration with 20–25% of patients dropping out within the first 3 months, 40–50% between 6 and 12 months, and little further change occurring during the next 3–4 years.[28] Although not confirmed, this trend for high early dropout rates may relate to several factors: cost of the exercise program, insurance reimbursement, convenience associated with program scheduling and facility location, return to work or family demands or simply poor motivation. Alternatively, patients may have mastered their skills and dropped out because of adequate self-care. There are differences in adherence with different modes of delivery of exercise services; what is known about adherence to cardiac rehabilitation is based largely on studies conducted when cardiac rehabilitation content, duration, delivery, and goals were considerably different from what they are at present.

RECOMMENDATIONS TO IMPROVE ADHERENCE

Adherence may be enhanced if the physician understands the factors that affect exercise behavior and accordingly devises an exercise program that is tailored to the needs, preferences, and health status of a given person.[29] Patients, in general, wish to be partners in health care decisions that affect them or their families and improving communication may be a potent adherence enhancing strategy. Attention to the interpersonal relationships between patient and provider can result in greater cooperation and greater patient and provider satisfaction, as well as improved adherence.[30] For example, increased involvement by the patient in clinical decision making has been shown to improve patient satisfaction,[27,28,31,32] patient adherence, and patient outcomes.[28,33,34] In addition, limited evidence supports the importance of involving family members in promoting adherence to cardiac rehabilitation services.[35] If the objective of patient counseling is to permit the patient to make informed decisions about treatments, then a patient may decide to disregard some or all professional advice. This suggests that what is inappropriate behavior from the clinician's perspective (i.e. not following recommendations) may in fact be rational decision making from the patient's perspective.

Many patients make the best decisions they can without considering the importance or even the implications of adherence and carry out their own risk–benefit analysis for each treatment they are offered.[36]

Other factors that may influence patient adherence include emotional support; understanding the patient's (and family's) values, viewpoints, and preferences; and integration of the intervention into the patient's lifestyle, as well as patient characteristics and demographic characteristics; aspects of treatment regimens including complexity, duration, and convenience (e.g. cost, facility location, time of day); and disease factors such as severity of symptoms, among others. Patient perceptions, as well as personal and social circumstances, determine patient decisions about following recommendations.

Adherence to exercise is in general lower than that for pharmacologic interventions; Burke *et al.*[27] suggest that the increased behavioral requirements for maintaining an exercise program may account for this. In general, adherence to the exercise program was better in the home exercise programs than the community based rehabilitation programs.[27] Most likely, the convenience factor can account for these improved rates of adherence.[27]

Strategies to improve adherence

Improving patient–provider communication with more information about CVD and its treatments would likely result in more informed decision making by the patient; providing culturally sensitive care may also improve adherence and perhaps patient outcomes and is likely to improve patient and clinician satisfaction.[37,38] Successful strategies for adherence include:

1. clear communication between patient (family) and provider;
2. emotional support and alleviation of fears and anxieties;
3. understandable and practical explanations about regimens that are compatible with the patient's values, preferences, and expressed needs, acknowledging the patient's social and cultural needs;
4. integration and coordination of patient care to provide continuity of care between transitions.[6]

Alternatives to monitored exercise training (A)

Eleven studies – seven RCTs and four non-randomized studies – informed this question. The evidence suggests that alternative approaches to the delivery of cardiac rehabilitative services, other than traditional supervised group interventions, can be implemented effectively and safely for carefully selected clinically stable patients. Transtelephonic and other means of monitoring and surveillance of patients can extend cardiac rehabilitative services beyond the setting of supervised, structured, group based rehabilitation (see box on page 265 for guide to ECG monitoring). These alternative approaches have the potential to provide cardiac rehabilitation services to low and moderate risk patients who comprise the majority of patients with stable coronary disease, most of whom do not currently participate in supervised, structured rehabilitation.

Recent studies have explored new approaches to deliver cardiac rehabilitation services, with the goals of increasing availability and decreasing costs, while preserving efficacy and safety. Case management approaches to exercise training, smoking cessation, and diet drug management of hyperlipidemia that rely on telephone contact can be provided to appropriately selected patients with coronary disease.

Criteria for electrocardiographic monitoring[39]

1. Two or more MIs.
2. New York Heart Association class 3 or greater.
3. Exercise capacity less than 6 METs.
4. Ischemic horizontal or downsloping ST depression of 4 mm or more or angina during exercise.
5. Fall in systolic blood pressure with exercise.
6. A medical problem that the physician believes may be life-threatening.
7. Previous episode of primary cardiac arrest.
8. Ventricular tachycardia at a workload of less than 6 METs.

Guidelines for participation in supervised and unsupervised exercise training programs are published by the American College of Sports Medicine.[24] In brief, supervision is recommended for patients with two or more major CAD risk factors and patients with known CAD with less than 8 MET functional capacity. Supervision is not suggested in apparently healthy individuals or persons who have equal or more than 8 MET functional capacity. The generalizability of these case management systems to other treatment settings – including university centers, public and community hospitals, and clinics – will depend largely on formulas for reimbursement for services and the extent of

Minimal guidelines for risk stratification

Risk level	Characteristics
Low	No significant left ventricular dysfunction (i.e. ejection fraction $\geq 50\%$)
	No resting or exercise induced myocardial ischemia manifested as angina and/or ST segment displacement
	No resting or exercise induced complex arrhythmias
	Uncomplicated myocardial infarction, coronary artery bypass surgery, angioplasty or atherectomy
	Functional capacity ≥ 6 METs on graded exercise test 3 or more weeks after clinical event
Intermediate	Mild to moderately depressed left ventricular function (ejection fraction 31–49%)
	Functional capacity <5–6 METs on graded exercise test 3 or more weeks after clinical event
	Patients who consistently exceed the intensity of their exercise prescription
	Exercise induced myocardial ischemia (1–2 mm ST segment depression) or reversible ischemic defects (echocardiographic or nuclear radiography)
High	Severely depressed left ventricular function (ejection fraction $\leq 30\%$)
	Complex ventricular arrhythmias at rest or appearing or increasing with exercise
	Decrease in systolic blood pressure of >15 mmHg during exercise or failure to rise with increasing exercise workloads
	Survivor of sudden cardiac death
	Myocardial infarction complicated by congestive heart failure, cardiogenic shock, and/or complex ventricular arrhythmias
	Severe coronary artery disease and marked exercise induced myocardial ischemia (>2 mm ST segment depression)

Note: MET = metabolic equivalent units. From *Guidelines for Rehabilitation Programs* (p. 14) by the American Association of Cardiovascular and Pulmonary Rehabilitation, Champaign, IL: Human Kinetics Books. Copyright 1995 by American Association of Cardiovascular and Pulmonary Rehabilitation. Reprinted by permission.

physician support for this approach, as well as the state regulations regarding medical and health practices. Within each of these settings, managed care programs seeking optimal methods for coronary risk factor reduction and exercise rehabilitation may favor case management systems that provide convenient, individualized health care at low cost.

Risk stratification

Appropriate risk stratification is recommended to minimize any adverse effects that patients might experience (see box on page 265 for risk stratification). This practice is also valuable in aiding the health care provider in deciding the type and intensity at which an exercise regimen will be started and the degree of monitoring and supervision. Furthermore, careful risk stratification also identifies the frequency of surveillance needed for a given patient, alerts the practitioner to promptly respond to changes in patient status, and promotes the safety of exercise training in any delivery system.[6]

FOCUS OF FURTHER SCIENTIFIC STUDY

Scientific studies should address the following areas.[6]

- Evaluate exercise training in special populations, including the elderly, women, different ethnic groups, and low educational and socioeconomic levels.
- Evaluate exercise therapy following contemporary therapies including thrombolysis and acute angioplasty.
- Evaluate effects of exercise training using return to work as a primary outcome.
- Identify factors that promote adherence.
- Identify the optimum degree of supervision and monitoring for high risk groups, such as heart failure, elderly, and those with complex medical problems.
- Evaluate the safety and benefit of exercise training in patients with compensated heart failure and impaired ventricular systolic function.
- Evaluate a variety of different delivery models of exercise therapy.
- Evaluate the safety and specific added benefits of resistance training on cardiac patient outcomes.

SUMMARY

Clear evidence exists for the recommendation of exercise in all individuals for primary preventive purposes. The evidence for patients with CAD is also well substantiated. Further research is indicated to verify how exercise recommendations are best recommended and delivered given the rapidly changing health care practice.

REFERENCES

1 Blair SN, Kohl HW, Paffenbarger RS *et al*. Physical fitness and all cause mortality. A prospective study of healthy men and women. *JAMA* 1989;**262**: 2395–401.

2 Blair SN, Kampert JB, Kohl HW *et al*. Influences of cardiovascular fitness and other precursors on cardiovascular disease and all cause mortality in men and women. *JAMA* 1996;**276**:205–10.

3 National Institutes of Health. Consensus Development Panel on Physical Activity and Cardiovascular Health. Physical Activity and Cardiovascular Health. *JAMA* 1996;**276**:241–6.

4 Powell KE, Thompson PD, Caspers CJ, Kendricks JS. Physical activity and the incidence of coronary heart disease. *Annu Rev Public Health* 1987;**8**: 253–87.

5 US Department of Health and Human Services. *Physical activity and health: a report of the Surgeon General*. Atlanta GA: US Department of Health and Human Services, Centers for Disease Control and Prevention, National Centers for Chronic Disease Prevention and Health Promotion, 1996.

6 Wenger MK, Froelicher ES, Smith LK *et al*. *Cardiac rehabilitation*. Clinical Practice Guideline No. 17. Rockville MD: US Department of Health and Human Services, Public Health Service, Agency for Health Care Policy and Research and the National Heart, Lung & Blood Institute, 1995.

7 Faigenbaum AD, Skrinar GS, Cesare WF, Kraemer WJ, Thomas HE. Physiologic and symptomatic responses of cardiac patients to resistance exercise. *Arch Phys Med Rehabil* 1990;**71**:395–8.

8 Featherstone JF, Holly RG, Amsterdam EA. Physiologic response to weight lifting in coronary artery disease. *Am J Cardiol* 1993;**71**:287–92.

9 Sheldahl M, Wilke NA, Tristani FE, Kalbfleisch JH. Responses of patients after myocardial infarction to carrying a graded series of weight loads. *Am J Cardiol* 1983;**52**:689–703.

10 Buchner DM. Understanding variability in studies of strength training in older adults: meta-analytic perspective. *Top Geriatric Rehabil* 1993;**8**:1–21.

11 Leon AS. ed. *Physical activity and cardiovascular health. A national consensus*. Champaign, IL: Human Kinetics, 1997.

12 Stewart AL, Greenfield S, Hays RD *et al*. Functional status and well-being of patients with chronic conditions: results from the medical outcomes study. *JAMA* 1989;**262**:907–13.

13 Fiori MC, Bailey WC, Cohen SJ *et al*. *Smoking cessation*. Clinical Practice Guideline No. 18. Rockville MD: US Department of Health and Human Services, Public Health Service, Agency for Health Care Policy and Research, 1996.

14 National High Blood Pressure Education Program. *The fifth report of the Joint National Committee on Detection, Evaluation and treatment of high blood pressure*. NIH publication no. 93–1088. Bethesda MD: National Institutes of Health, National Heart, Lung & Blood Institute, 1993.

15 Dattilo AM, Kris-Etherton PM. Effects of weight reduction on blood lipids and lipoprotein: a meta-analysis. *Am J Clin Nutr* 1992;**56**:320–8.

16 Shephard JR. Responses of the cardiac transplant patient to exercise and training. *Exerc Sports Sci Rev* 1992;**20**:297–320.

17 DeBusk RF, Houston N, Haskell W, Fry F, Parker M. Exercise training soon after myocardial infarction. *Am J Cardiol* 1979;**44**:1223–9.

18 Hamalainen H, Luurila OJ, Kallio V, Astrila M, Hakkila J. Long-term reduction in sudden deaths after a multifactorial intervention programme in patients with myocardial infarction: 10-year results of a controlled follow-up study. *Eur Heart J* 1989;**10**:55–62.

19 Todd IC, Ballantyne D. Effects of exercise training on the total ischaemic burden: an assessment by 24 hour ambulatory electrocardiographic monitoring. *Br Heart J* 1992;**68**:560–6.

20 Hogberg E, Schuler G, Kunze B *et al*. Silent myocardial ischemia as a potential link between lack of premonitoring symptoms and increased risk of cardiac arrest during physical strain. *Am J Cardiol* 1990;**65**:853–9.

21 Healy B. Narrowing the gender gaps in biomedical research. *J Myocardial Ischemia* 1992;**4**(1):14–24.

22 Fletcher BJ, Dunbar SB, Felner JM *et al*. Exercise testing and training in physically disabled men with clinical evidence of coronary artery disease. *Am J Cardiol* 1994;**73**:170–4.

23 Heath GW, Fentem PH. *Exerc Sports Sci Rev* 1997; **25**:195–234.

24 American College of Sports Medicine (ACSM). *ACSM's guidelines for exercise testing and prescription*. Baltimore MD: Williams & Wilkins, 1995.

25 American Heart Association. *Strategic plan for promoting physical activity*. Dallas: American Heart Association, 1995.

26 American Association of Cardiovascular and Pulmonary Rehabilitation. *Guidelines for cardiac rehabilitation programs*, 2nd edition. Champaign IL: Human Kinetics, 1995.

27 Burke LE, Dunbar-Jacob JM, Hill MN. Compliance with cardiovascular disease prevention strategies: a review of the research. *Ann Behav Med* 1997; **19**(3): in press.

28 Oldridge NB. Compliance and dropout in cardiac rehabilitation. *J Cardiac Rehab* 1984;**4**:166–77.

29 Blumenthal JA, Gullette ED, Napolitano M, Szczepanski R. Behavioral and psychological issues of cardiac rehabilitation. In Leon AS. ed.

Physical activity and cardiovascular health. A national consensus. Champaign IL: Human Kinetics, 1997.

30 Ewart CK, Stewart KL, Gillilan RE, Kelemen MH. Self-efficacy mediates strength gains during circuit weight training in men with coronary artery disease. *Med Sci Sports Exerc* 1986;**18**: 531–640.

31 Gould KL. Reversal of coronary atherosclerosis: clinical promise as a basis of noninvasive management of coronary artery disease. *Circulation* 1994;**90**:1558–71.

32 Andrew GM, Oldridge NB, Parker JO *et al.* Reasons for dropout from exercise programs in post-coronary patients. *Med Sci Sports Exerc* 1981; **13**: 164–8.

33 Roter DL. Patient participation in patient–provider interaction: the effects of patient questions asking on the quality of interaction, satisfaction, and compliance. *Health Educ Monogr* 1977;**5**: 281–315.

34 Kaplan FH, Greenfield S, Ware JE Jr. Assessing the effect of physician–patient interaction on the outcome of chronic disease. *Med Care* 1989;**27**(3): S110–S127.

35 Sotile WM, Sotile MO, Ewen GS, Sotile LJ. Marriage and family factors relevant to effective cardiac rehabilitation: a review of risk factor literature. *Sports Med Training Rehabil* 1993;**4**:115–28.

36 Donavan JL, Blake DR. Patient non-compliance: deviance or reasoned decision-making? *Soc Sci Med* 1992;**34**:507–13.

37 Epstein LH, Cluss PA. A behavioral medicine perspective on adherence to long-term medical regimens. *J Consult Clin Psychol* 1982;**50**:950–71.

38 Morris LS, Schulz RM. Patient compliance – an overview. *J Clin Pharm Ther* 1992;**17**:283–95.

39 Fletcher GF, Balady G, Froelicher VF, Hartley LH, Haskell WL, Pollock ML. Exercise standards. A statement for healthcare professionals from the American Heart Association. *Circulation* 1996; **86**:340–4.

Psychosocial factors in the primary and secondary prevention of coronary heart disease: a systematic review

18

HARRY HEMINGWAY,
MICHAEL MARMOT

INTRODUCTION

In the past, surveys of the general public have revealed that they believe stress to be a major cause of coronary heart disease (CHD).[1] This tends to upset scientific investigators who despair of trying to educate an irrational public as to the true scientifically established causes. Clinicians too, at times, seem to suffer the same irrational prejudices of the general public in believing a patient's psychological state to be crucial in affecting the course and prognosis of the disease.

Some of the great figures of medical history have considered that coronary disease was importantly related to psychological factors. As is now well known, John Hunter believed his own angina to be brought on by stress. He said that "his life was in the hands of any rascal who chose to annoy or tease him" and on October 16th 1793 "he went to St George's Hospital, and meeting with some things which irritated his mind, and not being perfect master of the circumstances, he withheld his sentiments and . . . dropt down dead".[2] Corvisart drew attention to the "social state: all functions disordered by ever-agitating and ever-renewing causes", thereby emphasizing the importance of prolonged rather than acute stressors.[3] Osler described "arterial degeneration in the worry and strain of modern life" and he talked of the typical coronary patient as one "the indicator of whose engines is always at full steam ahead".[4]

It may not be a general rule but in this case at least, the public, caring clinicians, and great physicians of the past may not all have been wrong. This chapter reviews systematically the prospective studies which have tested specific psychosocial hypotheses and finds evidence for the importance of psychosocial factors in both the etiology and prognosis of CHD. The comparatively limited randomized controlled trial (RCT) evidence is discussed; it has been systematically reviewed elsewhere.[5]

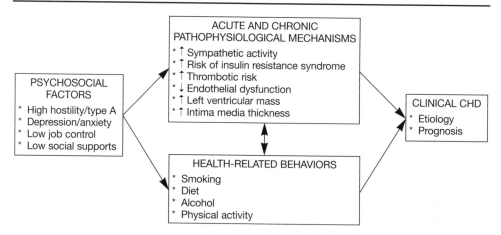

Figure 18.1 Potential pathways by which psychosocial factors may influence CHD etiology and prognosis.

PSYCHOSOCIAL FACTORS

Definition

A major reason for scientific scepticism in this field, apart from an implicit dualism that functions as if the mind and body are not connected, relates to definition and measurement. A psychosocial factor may be defined as a questionnaire based measurement (self-report or external assessment) which potentially relates psychological phenomena to the social environment and to pathophysiological changes. Using psychometric techniques, the validity and reliability (precision) of the instruments used to measure psychosocial factors have been enhanced. By avoiding the unhelpful general term of "stress", recent work has developed theoretical models – for example, the job control–demands–support model of psychosocial work characteristics – which generate specific hypotheses for testing.

How might psychosocial factors be linked to CHD?

Figure 18.1 distinguishes two main putative pathways by which psychosocial factors may affect the risk of CHD: psychosocial factors may act via health-related behaviors and/or via direct pathophysiological effects. Evidence of these mechanisms (reviewed elsewhere[6,7]) is important in making causal inferences and therefore in designing preventive interventions.

First, psychosocial factors may affect behaviors such as smoking, diet, alcohol or physical activity which in turn may influence CHD risk.[8] If such health-related behaviors do lie on the causal pathway between psychosocial factors and CHD, then the approach of many studies to adjust for these factors as confounders may be questioned. Strategies used to change health behaviors and hence alter risk may themselves have an important psychosocial component, although this is not reviewed here.

Second, psychosocial factors may cause direct pathophysiological changes. An extensive literature has demonstrated relationships between acute, shortlived stressors and a wide range of cardiovascular pathophysiology, including endothelial dysfunction[9] and platelet adhesiveness.[10] This raises the important question of the extent to which psychosocial factors act as triggers of an acute event and/or exert chronic cumulative effects on atherosclerotic disease initiation and progression. This review emphasizes prospective cohort studies, often with prolonged follow-up, which, virtually by definition, are unsuited to examining the role of acute psychosocial precipitants of an acute CHD event. Cohort studies are, however, well suited to examination of Corvisart's "ever-agitating" causes and such a chronic role may be argued for each of the psychosocial factors examined.

The pathophysiological effects of psychosocial factors are not confined to acute responses. Monkey models of atherosclerosis demonstrate metabolic, anatomical, and functional disturbances in relation to psychosocial factors (dominance, social support) which may be prevented by beta-blockers.[11] In humans, a growing number of relationships have been demonstrated between psychosocial and pathophysiological factors. Psychosocial work characteristics are associated with elevated plasma fibrinogen,[12] raised left ventricular mass,[13] and the progression of carotid atherosclerosis;[14] type A behavior may be associated with adrenoreceptor density;[15] and depression with low heart rate variability.[16] Studies of psychosocial factors in relation to the quantitative severity of angiographic coronary artery disease may offer potential insights into mechanisms, despite the potential for the selection of such patients to bias results. These studies do not support a relationship between job strain and presence of coronary artery disease[17] and type A behaviour assessed by the structured interview is associated with severity of coronary artery disease only among those under 45 years.[18] Functional aspects of social network ties, rather than size of network, are associated with angiographic severity.[19] Finally, it is plausible that, for example, social supports might influence the access to and outcome of medical care, although there is little direct evidence that this offers an explanation of the effect of social support on coronary risk.

There is a substantial body of evidence for the inverse association between socioeconomic position and CHD.[20] Among the mechanisms linking socioeconomic status with cardiovascular disease may be psychosocial pathways.[20a] Although we do not address the interesting question of whether psychosocial factors might account for the higher rate of CHD in people of lower socioeconomic status, the extent to which socioeconomic status might confound or lie on the causal pathway between psychosocial factors and CHD should not be forgotten.

Method of systematic review

A quality filter was used to select studies for inclusion in the systematic review. Studies were included which had: a prospective, population based design; at least 500 participants (etiological studies in healthy populations) or 100 participants (prognostic studies in CHD patient populations); instruments for exposure measurement used in two or more study populations; fatal or validated non-fatal CHD as outcomes. The purpose of this quality filter was to identify the best available evidence. While cross-sectional studies do not allow inferences about temporal sequence between cause and effect and case-control studies of psychosocial factors are prone to recall bias, it is acknowledged that these (and other studies not reviewed here) have made important contributions to our understanding of psychosocial factors.

Articles were identified by MEDLINE search (1966–1996), manual searching of the bibliographies of retrieved articles and previous review articles and an inhouse bibliographic database. Since no register of published and unpublished studies with psychosocial exposures exists and meticulous hand searching of journals has not been performed, there is a serious potential for publication bias. For this reason a narrative rather than quantitative systematic review is presented. Unbiased estimates of the contribution which psychosocial factors make to CHD causation are particularly important given that randomized controlled trials, at least for primary prevention, are scarcely feasible. Observational studies are therefore likely to remain the main type of evidence on which to base preventive action.

EVIDENCE FOR SPECIFIC PSYCHOSOCIAL FACTORS IN THE ETIOLOGY AND PROGNOSIS OF CHD

Four groups of psychosocial factors were identified using the predefined quality filter: psychological traits (type A behavior, hostility), psychological states (depression, anxiety), psychological interaction with the organization of work (job control–demands–support), and the quantity and quality of social supports. In simple terms this corresponds to a spectrum with mainly psychological components at one end and a stronger social component at the other. Tables 18.1–18.4 detail the prospective etiological and prognostic studies relating to the four groups of psychosocial factors and the box below summarizes the key results. Most published reports emphasize one particular psychosocial factor (even though data may have been collected on a range of factors) and this determined the table in which they were included.

In healthy populations, prospective cohort studies suggest a possible etiological role for:
- depression and anxiety (**Grade B**: 9/10)
- social support (**Grade B**: 5/6)
- low control at work (**Grade B**: 5/8)
- type A/hostility (**Grade B**: 3/8).

In CHD patient populations, prospective studies suggest a prognostic role for:
- depression (**Grade B**: 5/5)
- social support (**Grade B**: 7/7).

Numbers in brackets refer to the (n) unequivocally positive studies / (n) all studies.

Hostility and type A behavior

Type A behavior pattern – the only personality trait which met our review criteria – is characterized by hard driving and competitive behavior, a potential for hostility, pronounced impatience, and vigorous speech stylistics. The instruments for measurement of type A and hostility – the Jenkins Activity Scale, the structured interview, the MMPI, the Bortner Hostility Scale – have been subjected to psychometric testing and incorporated into many cardiovascular cohort studies, more than have reported results. Unlike other psychosocial factors, type A is distinguished by being the subject of numerous intervention trials.[21] Based on early positive findings in Framingham[22] and the Western Collaborative Group 8-year follow-up,[23] among other evidence, the NIH declared type A an independent

Table 18.1 Type A behavior, hostility and CHD

Participants	Exposure	Outcome (n events)	Adjustments	Results
Prospective etiological studies				
Rosenman 1976[23]: 3154 men aged 39–59 years followed for 8.5 years in Western Collaborative Study	Type A	Non-fatal and fatal CHD (257)	Cholesterol, smoking	+ Strong predictor
Haynes 1983[22]: 1674 men and women followed for 8 years in Framingham Study	Type A (Framingham)	Non-fatal MI, coronary insufficiency, angina, CHD death (170)	Age, SBP, cholesterol, smoking, glucose intolerance and other psychosocial factors	+ RR = 2 for men and women
Shekelle 1983[37]: 1877 men aged 40–55 years followed for 20 years in Western Electric	Hostility (MMPI)	Fatal CHD (220)	Age, SBP, cholesterol, smoking, alcohol	+ Strong association
Shekelle 1985[24]: 3110 men followed for 7.1 years in MRFIT	Type A (JAS)	Fatal and non-fatal MI (554)	Age, BP, smoking, cholesterol, alcohol, education	− No association
Johnston 1987[25]: 5936 men aged 40–59 followed for 6.2 years in British Regional Heart Study	Type A (Bortner)	Fatal and non-fatal CHD	Age, social class	− No association
Ragland 1988[38]: 3154 men aged 39–59 years followed for 22 years in Western Collaborative Study	Type A (SI)	Fatal CHD (214)	Age, SBP, cholesterol, smoking	− No association
Hearn 1989[26]: 1399 19-year-old Minnesota students followed for 33 years	Hostility (MMPI)	Non-fatal and fatal CHD and all-cause mortality		− No association
Barefoot 1995[39]: 730 men and women aged 50 years, followed for 27 years	Hostility (Cook-Medley)	Non-fatal MI and all-cause mortality	Age, sex, traditional risk factors	± No association in age, sex-adjusted models with acute MI. Positive association when adjusted for traditional risk factors
Prognostic studies				
Case 1985[40]: 516 patients within 2 weeks of acute MI, followed for 1–3 years	Type A (JAS)	CHD and all-cause mortality (53)	Age, sex, education, rales, ejection fraction, NYHA class, VPD	− No adjusted or unadjusted association
Ragland 1988[41]: 257 men with CHD followed for 11.5 years in Western Collaborative Group	Type A (SI)	Fatal CHD (91)	Follow-up time, type of initial coronary event, and traditional risk factors	− RR 0.58 (0.35–0.96) (type A was protective)
Barefoot 1989[42]: 1467 patients with angiographic disease followed for 5 years	Type A (SI)	Fatal CVD (168) and non-fatal MI (147)		− No association with non-fatal MI
Maruta 1993[43]: 620 general medical patients followed for 20 years	Hostility (MMPI)	Fatal and non-fatal CHD	Age, sex	− No association

JAS, Jenkins Activity Survey; MMPI, Minnesota Multiphasic Personality Inventory; MRFIT, Multiple Risk Factor Intervention Trial; NYHA, New York Heart Association; RR, relative risk; SBP, systolic blood pressure; SI, structured interview; VPD, ventricular premature beats; −, negative study; †, positive study.

273

Table 18.2 Depression and anxiety and CHD

	Participants	Exposure	Outcome (n events)	Adjustments	Results
Prospective etiological studies					
Hallstrom 1986[44]	795 women in Sweden, followed for 12 years	Depression (Hamilton Rating Scale and psychiatric interview)	Angina (25), ischemia ECG changes (39), non-fatal MI (11) and mortality (33)	Age, social class, marital status, conventional risk factors	+ Severity of depression predicted angina but not other outcomes
Hagman 1987[45]	5735 men in Goteburg, Sweden, followed for 2–7 years	Anxiety	Angina without MI (n = 128); physician assessment, Rose screening	Age, cholesterol, BP, smoking, relative weight	+ Strong predictor, particularly for uncomplicated angina
Haynes 1987[46]	1457 men aged 40–64 followed for 10 years in Northwick Park Heart Study	Phobic anxiety (Crown-Crisp)	Fatal (56) and non-fatal (57) CHD	Fibrinogen, cholesterol, factor VII, SBP	+ RR = 3.77 (1.64–8.64) for fatal CHD
Appels 1988[47]	3877 male civil servants, followed for 4.2 years	Depression	Angina, unstable angina, MI (59)	Age, smoking SBP, antihypertensives, cholesterol	+ Combination of low mood, low energy, hopelessness, poor sleep (termed "vital exhaustion"); RR 1.86 for unstable angina and 2.28 for MI for vital exhaustion. No association with negative self-concept and guilt
Anda 1993[48]	2832 US adults aged 45–77 years followed for 12 years in NHANES	Depression (General Well being Schedule)	Fatal and non-fatal CHD (n = 189)	Demographic and risk factors	+ Depressed affect 1.5 (1.0–2.3)
Aromaa 1994[49]	Mini-Finland Health Survey n = 8000 followed for 6.6 years	Depression (GHQ and PSE)	Fatal CHD (91)	Age	+ Risk of CHD death in depressed people 3.36 without pre-existing CVD and 5.52 in those with pre-existing CVD
Kawachi 1994[50]	33 999 US male health professionals aged 42–77 followed for 2 years	Phobic anxiety (Crown-Crisp)	Fatal (40) and non-fatal (128) CHD	Age, BMI, smoking, hypertension, parental history of MI, alcohol, exercise	+ RR = 3.01 (6.08 when sudden cardiac death examined)
Simonsick 1995[51]	1319 (East Boston), 1032 (New Haven), 1110 (Iowa) men and women aged 65, with diagnosed hypertension followed for 6 years (EPESE)	Depression (CES-D)	Cardiovascular mortality	Age	± Inconsistent effect across the three populations

continued

274

Table 18.2 *continued*

	Participants	Exposure	Outcome (n events)	Adjustments	Results
Wassertheil-Smoller 1996[27]	4367 healthy men and women aged over 60, follow-up 4.5 years in SHEP trial	Depression (CES-D)	Non-fatal MI and non-fatal strokes (321)	Baseline depression, age, sex, race, randomization group, education, history of stroke, MI, DM, smoking and baseline ADL	+ An increase in depressive symptoms (but not the baseline scores) predicted 1.18 (1.08–1.30) per 5-unit increase in score
Barefoot 1996[52]	409 men and 321 women born in Glostrup, Denmark, followed for 27 years	Depression (MMPI-OBD scale)	Non-fatal MI (122) and all-cause mortality (290)	Age, conventional CHD risk factors, baseline CHD	+ RR = 1.7 for 2SD difference in depression score
Prognostic studies					
Ahern 1990[53]	353 patients in the Cardiac Arrhythmia Pilot Study, followed for 12 months	8 psychosocial factors including anxiety (Spielberger), depression (Beck Depression Inventory)	Cardiac deaths	Age, left ventricular dysfunction, and previous MI	+ Depression predicted RR 1.3 (type A protective)
Kop 1994[54]	127 patients undergoing successful PTCA, questionnaire administered 2 weeks after discharge	Maastricht Questionnaire for vital exhaustion	Cardiac death MI, subsequent revascularization, increase in coronary atherosclerosis, new angina fatal or non-fatal CHD (29 events)	Severity of coronary artery disease, cholesterol	+ Vital exhaustion predicted events RR 2.7 (1.1–6.3) but P = 0.06 in adjusted models
Ladwig 1994[55]	552 mean 17–21 days post acute MI, followed for 6 months	Depression (interview)	Angina, not returning to work, continuing to smoke	Age, social class, recurrent infarction, rehabilitation, cardiac events and helplessness	+ Depression predicted all outcomes
Frasure-Smith 1995[56]	222 patients aged 24–88 years 5–15 days post acute MI followed for 18 months	Depression (diagnostic interview schedule)	Mortality (21 deaths, 19 cardiac)	Age, left ventricular dysfunction, and previous MI	+ Odds ratio 6.64 (1.8–25.1)
Denollet 1996[57]	268 men, 35 women with angiographically documented CAD participating in rehabilitation program, followed for 7.9 years	Type D personality (tendency to suppress emotional distress), depression, social alienation	All-cause mortality (38, 24 cardiac)	Left ventricular function, number of diseased vessels, low exercise tolerance, lack of thrombocytic therapy	+ Odds ratio of 4.1 (1.9–8.8) for type D and 2.7 for depression

ADL, activities of daily living; CAD, coronary artery disease; CES-D, Center for Epidemiological Studies – Depression; DM, diabetes mellitus; GHQ, General Health Questionnaire; PSE, Present State Examination; MMPI–OBD, Minnesota Multiphasic Personality Inventory – Obvious Depression; PTCA, percutaneous transcutaneous coronary angioplasty.

risk factor for CHD. However, with the publication of negative findings[24-26] it was proposed that a more specific component of type A, namely hostility, might be etiological, although there are conflicting studies. None of the five studies examining type A or hostility in relation to prognosis among patients with CHD has demonstrated an increased risk; indeed, one suggested a protective effect.

Depression and anxiety

There are several reasons why investigations of the relationship between depression and anxiety and CHD differ from those of other psychosocial factors. First, unlike other psychosocial factors, depression and anxiety represent well defined psychiatric disorders, with standardized instruments for measurement. Second, depression and anxiety are commonly the consequence of CHD and the extent to which they are also the cause poses important methodological issues. Third, the ability to diagnose and treat such disorders makes them attractive points for intervention. Finally, depression and CHD could share common antecedents – for example, environmental stressors and social supports.

Table 18.2 shows the results from the seven studies which investigated depression. Six of the seven prospective studies examining the effect of depression in the etiology of CHD were positive. All three of the prospective studies examining the effect of anxiety in the etiology of CHD were positive. Intriguingly, there is some evidence that this effect is strongest specifically for phobic anxiety and sudden cardiac death. Wassertheil-Smoller[27] reported the effect of depression assessed by the Center for Epidemiological Studies – Depression Scale in relation to CVD events among 4367 healthy older people in the SHEP trial. Over a 4.5-year follow-up there were 321 events and an increase in depression symptoms (but not the baseline scores) predicted events, even when controlled for multiple covariates. Such findings are compatible with the hypothesis that premonitory signs of CHD such as angina or breathlessness may have led to the increase in depression. Studies with longer periods of follow-up are less likely to be confounded by the possibility of early disease causing depression, but raise further questions about the time course of exposure. For example, it is possible that there is a common trigger (e.g. viral illness) that precipitates both symptoms of depression and atherothrombotic processes. By examination of subclinical manifestations of CHD (for example, using non-invasive measures of arterial structure and function) before the onset of symptoms, the temporal sequence of the depression–CHD relation might be better understood.

Depression in the postmyocardial infarction (post-MI) patient appears to be of prognostic significance beyond the severity of coronary artery disease. Although discrete major depressive episodes are not uncommon post-MI, depressive symptoms (low mood, poor sleep, low appetite, low motivation, loss of self-esteem, anergia) are more prevalent and it has been proposed that the graded relationship between depression scores and risk, the longlasting nature of the effect, and the stability of the depression measured across time suggest a continuously distributed chronic psychological characteristic.

Job control–demands–support model

The longstanding observation that rates of CHD vary markedly among occupations – more so than can be accounted for by conventional CHD risk factors – generated a

Table 18.3 Job strain (low control and high demands) and CHD

	Participants	Exposure	Outcome (n events)	Adjustments	Results
Prospective etiological studies					
LaCroix 1984[58]	548 men 328 women aged 45–64 followed for 10 years in Framingham Study	Job control/demands (individual and ecological)	Fatal and non-fatal CHD	Age, SBP, cholesterol, smoking	+ Individual measures; all women RR = 2.9, clerical women RR = 5.2, no association in men. Ecological exposure was associated with risk in men and women
Alfredsson 1985[59]	958 096 men and women aged 20–64 years, followed for 1 year	Hectic work and few possibilities for learning (ecological)	Hospitalization for MI (1201)	Age, 10 sociodemographic factors, smoking, heavy lifting	+ RR = 1.5 for hospitalization
Haan 1988[60]	603 male and 299 female Finnish factory workers followed for 10 years	Job control, physical strain, variety (individual)	Fatal and non-fatal CHD (60)	Age, smoking, cholesterol, SBP, alcohol, relative weight	+ OR = 4.95 for low control, low variety, high physical strain vs other
Johnson 1989[61]	7219 employed Swedish men followed for 9 years	Job control, demands, and social support (individual)	CVD mortality (193)	Age	+ Top quality of strain RR = 1.9 overall, 2.6 for clerical men
Read 1989[62]	4737 Hawaiian men aged 45–65 for whom usual and present occupations were the same followed for 18 years	Job control, demands, and their interaction (ecological)	Fatal CHD and non-fatal MI (359)		− No effect of control, demands or their interaction (NS trend for lower strain men to higher CHD)
Alterman 1994[63]	1683 men aged 38–56 years followed for 25 years in Chicago Western Electric Study	Job control, demands, and their interaction (ecological)	CHD mortality (283)	Major coronary risk factors	± Job strain associated with 1.4 (0.92–2.14)
Suadicani 1993[64]	1752 employed men, followed for 3 years	Job influence, monotony, pace, satisfaction, ability to relax	Fatal and non-fatal CHD events (46)		− Inability to relax after work associated with 3-fold increased risk of CHD but none of the other factors
Bosma 1997[28]	6895 men and 3413 women civil servants followed for 5 years in Whitehall II study	Job control, demands (individual, assessed twice 3 years apart, and ecological)	Rose angina (328), doctor diagnosed ischemia (166)	Age, employment grade, smoking, cholesterol, BP, BMI	+ Self-reported or externally assessed low job control predicted CHD
Prognostic studies					
Hlatky 1995[17]	1489 employed patients undergoing coronary angiography, followed for 5 years	Job control, demands (individual)	Prevalence of coronary artery disease, fatal and non-fatal MI (112)	Ejection fraction, extent of coronary atherosclerosis, myocardial ischemia	− Job strain associated with normal coronary arteries; no association with fatal or non-fatal cardiac events

NS, not significant; OR, odds ratio.

Table 18.4 Social supports and CHD

	Participants	Exposure	Outcome (n events)	Adjustments	Results
Prospective etiological studies					
Medalie 1976[65]	10 000 men aged >40 in Israel followed for 5 years	Perceived love and support from spouses	Angina (300)	Age BP, cholesterol, diabetes, ECG abnormalities	+ RR 1.8
Reed 1983[66]	4653 Japanese men in Hawaii followed for 6 years	(1) 9-item network score and (2) factor derived network score	Fatal and non-fatal CHD (218)	Age, SBP, cholesterol, glucose, uric acid, FVC, BMI, physical activity index, alcohol, complex carbohydrates	− Social network associated with CHD prevalence, but not incidence
Orth-Gomer 1987[67] 88	17 433 age 29–74 followed for 6 years	Social network interaction index	All-cause mortality (841) and CVD mortality (414)	Age, education, employment, initial health status, smoking, exercise	+ RR1.5 for ACM and 1.4 for CVD mortality
Kaplan 1988[68]	13 301 men and women aged 39–59 years, followed for 5 years in North Karelia	Social network index	All-cause mortality (598), CVD mortality (297), CHD mortality (223)	Age, education, urban/rural residence	+ Lack of social ties related to CVD mortality (1.5 (1.1–2.1)) and CHD (OR 1.34 (0.9–1.9) for men but not women
Vogt 1992[69]	2603 members of health maintenance organization followed for 15 years	Network scope, network frequency, and network size	All-cause mortality (502) and non-fatal CHD	Age, sex, SES, smoking and subjective health status at baseline	+ Only network scope associated with CHD incidence 1.5 (1.0–2.3) but strong effects on survival in those with CHD
Orth-Gomer 1993[70]	736 middle aged Swedish men followed for 6 years	Emotional support from close persons and support from extended network (social integration)	Non-fatal CHD or CHD death (25)	Age, cholesterol treatment of hypertension, diabetes, BMI, smoking, physical activity	+ Emotional support OR of 3.1 ($P = 0.07$) and 3.8 social integration ($P = 0.04$)

continued

Table 18.4 *continued*

	Participants	Exposure	Outcome (n events)	Adjustments	Results
Prognostic studies					
Ruberman 1984[71]	2320 males 30–69, post-MI followed for 3 years	Social support, life stress	All-cause mortality (128) and sudden cardiac death (68)	Age, myocardial function, ventricular arrhythmia, smoking	+ Combination of social isolation and high life stress associated with RR = 4.5 for all-cause mortality and 5.62 for sudden cardiac death
Wiklund 1988[72]	201 patients with first MI followed for 8.3 years	Social support, depression, and other psychosocial factors	All-cause mortality (48) and non-fatal MI (37)	Hypertension, smoking, angina	+ Being single increased risk of death ($P<0.001$)
Case 1992[73]	1234 participants age 25–75 in diltiazem post-MI trial; followed for 2 years	Living alone, disrupted marriage	Recurrent non-fatal MI or cardiac death (226)	NYHA class, LVEF, education, no beta-blockers, ventricular premature complexes, prior infarction	+ Living alone RR 1.54 (1.04–2.29). No effect of marital disruption
Hedblad 1991[74]	394 68-year-old men, population based study of 24h ECG in Sweden, followed for 5 years	Social support and social network	Fatal CHD, non-fatal MI (17)	Conventional risk factors	+ RR = 4 for low informational support and low emotional support
Williams 1992[75]	1965 patients with angiographically proven CAD, followed for median 9 years	Structural social support (marital status) and functional social support	CVD mortality (237)	LVEF, non-invasive myocardial damage index, conduction disturbances, pain/ischemic index, mitral regurgitation, number of diseased vessels, % stenosis of LMS and LAD coronary arteries, age	+ Unmarried patients without confidant had RR of 3.34 (1.84–6.20)
Berkman 1992[76]	100 men and 94 women aged 65 or more hospitalized with acute MI followed for 6 months	Emotional support	All-cause mortality (76)	Severity of MI, comorbidity, smoking, BP, sociodemographic factors	+ Lack of emotional support RR 2.9 (1.2–6.9)
Jenkinson 1993[77]	1376 patients with suspected acute MI alive at 7 days, follow-up 3 years	Social isolation, life stress, depression, type A	All-cause mortality (247)	Age, previous MI, hospital complications, diabetes, hypertension, car ownership, sex	+ Hazard ratio of 1.49 (1.01–2.18) reduced to 1.33 (0.89–1.98) on adjustment: no effect of type A or depression

BMI, body mass index; CAD, coronary artery disease; CHD, coronary heart disease; CVD, coronary vascular disease; FVC, forced vital capacity; LAD, left anterior descending; LMS, left main stem; LVEF, left ventricular ejection fraction; RR, relative risk; SES, socioeconomic status.

quest for specific components of work which might be of etiological importance. Whilst aspects of the physical work environment may play some role, attention has mainly concentrated on the psychosocial work environment. The dominant "job strain" model of psychosocial work characteristics, as proposed by Karasek and later modified by Hall, grew out of secondary analyses of existing labor force survey data. This model proposes that jobs characterized by low control over work and high conflicting demands might be high strain. A subsequent addition to the model was that social support might buffer this effect. The advantage of the model is that it generates hypotheses for testing.

Table 18.3 shows prospective cohort studies which have examined the relationship between job strain and CHD. Both individual self-report and ecological (assigning a score on the basis of job title) measurements of job strain have been made. The former may be biased by early manifestations of disease, whilst the latter may lack precision. The finding that both methods tend to give reasonably consistent results suggests that they are complementary. Five of the eight studies were positive. There is growing emphasis on the importance of low job control rather than on conflicting demands[28] and it seems likely that these empirical results will necessitate a reformulation of the model. Alternative models of psychosocial work characteristics have been proposed involving an imbalance between the effort at work and rewards received.[29,30]

Quantity and quality of social supports: the buffer theory

Social supports and networks relate to both the number of an individual's social contacts and their quality (including emotional support and confiding support). Marital status – information routinely sought in clinical practice – is a simple measure of social support and the ability of low social support to predict all-cause mortality has long been recognized. It has been proposed that social supports may act to buffer the effect of various environmental stressors and hence increased susceptibility to disease,[31] but until recently there has been little evidence of an etiological link with CHD.

Five of the six prospective cohort studies which investigated aspects of social support in relation to the incidence of CHD were positive. Social supports are the most extensively investigated prognostic psychosocial factor post-MI. All seven of the studies investigating social support in relation to prognosis were positive and the relative risks for two of these studies exceeded 4. However, despite the strength and consistency of these findings, important questions remain unanswered. There is a lack of standardized measurement instruments and, partly for this reason, the relative effect of structural and functional aspects of social supports has yet to be delineated.

MODIFICATION OF PSYCHOSOCIAL FACTORS TO PREVENT CHD ONSET OR RECURRENCE

What are the implications of these findings for cardiological practice? The box below summarizes the main points. When judged on the criteria used for drug interventions, the evidence for psychosocial intervention supports "options to be considered" rather than firm recommendations. There are three ways in which such criteria may not be entirely appropriate when considering psychosocial factors. First, psychosocial interventions – unlike drug and invasive interventions – have few if any adverse effects

---

Implications for cardiological practice: options to consider
- Psychosocial components of cardiac rehabilitation (Grade B)
- Detect and treat depression in CHD patients (Grade B)
- Mobilize social support (Grade B)
- Use socioeconomic status and psychosocial factors to risk-stratify patients (Grade B)

A, strong evidence (at least one well designed RCT or effects strong and consistent across observational studies)
B, moderate evidence (RCT(s) suggest effect despite methodological concerns or observational studies suggest an effect but conflicting data or observational studies alone)
C, limited evidence (published research evidence available but not B or C)

(and may be less costly). Second, psychosocial factors may be interrelated and the quest for a single "toxic component" on which to intervene may not be as fruitful as in the case of, say, serum cholesterol. Few studies have investigated this interrelatedness; instead, researchers have tended to emphasize one factor over others.

A recent meta-analysis of RCTs by Linden et al.[5] has suggested that psychosocial interventions are associated with a 41% reduction in mortality and a 46% reduction in non-fatal events in the first 2 years of follow-up after MI. These RCTs – overwhelmingly in secondary prevention – have tended to be small, without prolonged follow-up; they have involved a diverse range of interventions (relaxation, stress management, counseling), differing in duration and professional setting. Separate analyses, including the larger but *non*-randomized Recurrent Coronary Prevention Project,[32] should be viewed with caution.

With the exception of type A,[21] few of the trials have aimed to modify a single specific psychosocial factor with measurements of the extent to which this was achieved and "hard" CHD endpoints averted. Indeed, one large RCT of psychological rehabilitation found no difference in anxiety and depression and this may in part explain the lack of effect on mortality.[33] The Montreal Heart Attack Readjustment Trial[33a] randomized 903 men and 473 women to psychosocial support or usual care. Among men there was no difference in cardiac or all cause mortality between the intervention and control groups. By contrast, among women there was an excess of cardiac deaths among the intervention group (24/234) compared with the control group (13/239) ($P = 0.051$). The reason for this finding – in the opposite direction to that hypothesized – awaits elucidation.

Most of the trials investigate the contribution of psychosocial intervention in addition to conventional rehabilitation or other lifestyle advice post-MI. Thus, for example, Ornish et al.[34] randomized 53 patients with coronary artery disease to stress management, low fat diet, smoking cessation, and moderate exercise and 43 patients to usual care. However, only 28 patients in the experimental group and 20 patients in the control group agreed to take part – a potential source of selection bias. Although quantitative coronary angiography demonstrated regression of coronary artery disease in 82% of the experimental group at 12-month follow-up, it is not possible to attribute this to the stress management or any other component of the intervention.

The prognostic effect of low social support and depression in those with CHD is strong and consistent. It is therefore reasonable to suggest that improved detection and treatment of depression among CHD patients might improve outcome. Frasure-Smith & Prince[35] randomized 453 male post-MI survivors to monthly monitoring of minor psychiatric morbidity (general health questionnaire) or usual care. The stress management intervention was given to participants whose psychiatric morbidity rose above a critical level; at 1 year the mortality was 4.4% in the intervention group and

8.9% in the control group ($P=0.05$). Two randomized controlled trials[36] modifying social supports post-MI have shown a decrease in cardiac death or reinfarction rates. Since information on patients' families, friends, and colleagues is commonly available to clinicians, this may help to risk-stratify the patient. Clinicians may have a role in mobilizing inactive supports or helping to initiate new supports but the effectiveness awaits demonstration.

The potential for primary prevention in relation to psychosocial factors clearly lies outside the remit of cardiologists. Psychosocial factors themselves are determined largely by social, political, and economic factors and it is therefore policy makers who influence the structure and function of communities – in the public and private domains – who may have scope for primary prevention.

CONCLUSION

Large prospective studies examining specific psychosocial hypotheses suggest the importance of psychosocial factors in relation to CHD etiology and prognosis. Further evidence of a causal role is provided by human and other primate evidence of biological and behavioral pathways mediating these effects. Whilst this review cannot discount the possibility of publication bias, the observational studies suggest etiological roles for social supports, depression and anxiety, and work characteristics and prognostic roles for social supports and depression. However the data that psychosocial interventions reduce mortality post MI are conflicting. In this expanding area of research, future studies might investigate:

- the interrelationship between different psychosocial factors;
- the extent to which effects on CHD are cumulative over the lifecourse or shortlived at different ages;
- the behavioral and biological mechanisms involved;
- the effect of psychosocial factors on different clinical and subclinical outcomes;
- appropriate primary and secondary preventive measures.

REFERENCES

1 Davison C, Davey Smith G, Frankel S. Lay epidemiology and the prevention paradox: the implications of coronary candidacy for health education. *Sociol Health Illness* 1991;**13**:1–19.

2 Acierno LJ. *The history of cardiology.* London: Parthenon, 1994.

3 Corvisart JN. *Essai sur les Maladies et les lesions organiques du Coer et des Gros Vaisseaux.* Paris: Migneret, 1806.

4 Osler W. The Lumleian Lectures on angina pectoris. *Lancet* 1910;i:839–44.

5 Linden W, Stossel C, Maurice J. Psychosocial interventions in patients with coronary artery disease: a meta-analysis. *Arch Intern Med* 1996; **156**:745–52.

6 Schneiderman N, Skyler JS. Insulin metabolism, sympathetic nervous system regulation, and coronary heart disease prevention. In: Orth-Gomer K, Schneiderman N. eds. *Behavioral medicine approaches to cardiovascular disease prevention.* Mawah, New Jersey: Lawrence Erlbaum Associates, 1996.

7 Brunner E. Stress and the biology of inequality. *Br Med J* 1997;**314**:1472–6.

8 Pieper C, Lacroix AZ, Karasek RA. The relation of psychosocial dimensions of work with coronary heart disease risk factors: a meta-analysis of five United States data bases. *Am J Epidemiol* 1989; **129**:483–94.

9 Yeung AC, Vekshtein VI, Krantz DS *et al.* The effect of atherosclerosis on the vasomotor response of coronary arteries to mental stress. *N Engl J Med* 1991;**325**:1551–6.

10 Grignani G, Soffiantino F, Zucchella M *et al.* Platelet activation by emotional stress in patients with coronary artery disease. *Circulation* 1991; **83**:II-128–II-136.

11 Kaplan JR, Manuck SB, Clarkson TB *et al.* Social stress and atherosclerosis in normo-cholesterolemic monkeys. *Science* 1983;**220**:733–5.

12 Brunner EJ, Davey Smith G, Marmot M *et al.* Childhood social circumstances and psychosocial and behavioural factors as determinants of plasma fibrinogen. *Lancet* 1996;**347**:1008–13.

13 Schnall PL, Pieper C, Schwartz JE *et al.* The relationship between 'job strain', workplace diastolic blood pressure, and left ventricular mass index. *JAMA* 1990;**263**:1929–35.

14 Everson SA, Lynch JW, Chesney MA *et al.* Interaction of workplace demands, and cardiovascular reactivity in progression of carotid atherosclerosis: population based study. *Br Med J* 1997;**314**:553–8.

15 Kahn JP, Gully RJ, Cooper TB *et al.* Correlation of type A behaviour with adrenergic receptor density: implications for coronary artery disease pathogenesis. *Lancet* 1987;**2**:937–9.

16 Carney RM, Saunders RD, Freedland KE *et al.*. Association of depression with reduced heart rate variability in coronary artery disease. *Am J Cardiol* 1996;**76**:562–4.

17 Hlatky MA, Lam LC, Lee KL *et al.* Job strain and the prevalence and outcome of coronary artery disease. *Circulation* 1995;**92**:327–33.

18 Williams RB, Barefoot JC, Haney TL. Type A behavior and angiographically documented coronary atherosclerosis in sample of 2,289 patients. *Psychosom Med* 1988;**50**:139–52.

19 Seeman TE, Syme SL. Social networks and coronary artery disease: a comparison of the structure and function of social relationships as predictors of disease. *Psychosom Med* 1987;**49**:341–54.

20 Kaplan GA, Keil JE. Socioeconomic factors and cardiovascular disease: a review of the literature. *Circulation* 1993;**88**:1973–98.

20a Marmot M, Bosma H, Hemingway H *et al.* Contribution of job control and other risk factors to social variations in coronary heart disease incidence. *Lancet* 1997;**350**:235–9.

21 Nunes EV, Frank KA, Kornfield DS. Psychologic treatment for the type A behaviour pattern and for coronary heart disease: a meta-analysis of the literature. *Psychosom Med* 1987;**48**:159–73.

22 Haynes SG, Feinleib M, Kannel WB. The relationship of psychosocial factors to coronary heart disease in the Framingham study: 3. Eight year incidence of coronary heart disease. *Am J Epidemiol* 1980;**111**:37–58.

23 Rosenman RH, Brand RJ, Sholtz RI, Friedman M. Multivariate prediction of coronary heart disease during 8.5 year follow-up in Western Collaborative Group Study. *Am J Cardiol* 1976;**37**:903–9.

24 Shekelle RB, Hulley SB, Neaton JD *et al.* The MRFIT behavior pattern study. II. Type A behavior and incidence of coronary heart disease. *Am J Epidemiol* 1985;**122**:559–70.

25 Johnston DW, Cook DG, Shaper AG. Type A behaviour and ischaemic heart disease in middle-aged British men. *Br Med J* 1987;**295**:86–9.

26 Hearn M, Murray DM, Luepker RB. Hostility, coronary heart disease and total mortality: a 33 year follow up study of university students. *J Behav Med* 1989;**12**:105–21.

27 Wassertheil-Smoller S, Applegate WB, Berge K *et al.* Change in depression as a precursor of cardiovascular events. *Arch Intern Med* 1996;**156**:553–61.

28 Bosma H, Marmot MG, Hemingway H *et al.* Low job control and risk of coronary heart disease in the Whitehall II (prospective cohort) study. *Br Med J* 1997;**314**:558–65.

29 Siegrist J, Peter R, Junge A, Cremer P, Seidel D. Low status control, high effort at work and ischemic heart disease: prospective evidence from blue-collar men. *Soc Sci Med* 1990;**31**:1127–34.

30 Bosma H, Peter R, Siegrist J, Marmot MG. Alternative job stress models and the risk of coronary heart disease: the effort–reward imbalance model and the job strain model. *Am J Public Health* 1997;(in press).

31 Alloway R. The buffer theory of social support – a review of the literature. *Psychol Med* 1987;**17**:91–108.

32 Friedman M, Thoresen CE, Gill JJ. Alteration of type A behaviour and its effect on cardiac recurrences in post myocardial infarction patients: summary results of the recurrent coronary prevention project. *Am Heart J* 1986;**112**:653–65.

33 Jones DA, West RR. Psychological rehabilitation after myocardial infarction: multicentre randomised controlled trial. *Br Med J* 1996;**313**:1517–21.

33a Frasure Smith N, Lesperance F, Prince RH *et al.* Randomised trial of home-based psychosocial nursing intervention for patients recovering from myocardial infarction. *Lancet* 1997;**350**:473–9.

34 Ornish D, Brown SE, Scherwitz LW *et al.* Can lifestyle changes reverse coronary heart disease? The Lifestyle Heart Trial. *Lancet* 1990;**336**:129–33.

35 Frasure-Smith N, Prince R. Long term follow up of the ischaemic heart disease life stress monitoring program. *Psychosom Med* 1989;**51**:485–513.

36 Bucher HC. Social support and prognosis following first myocardial infarction. *J Gen Intern Med* 1994;**9**:409–17.

37 Shekelle RB, Gale M, Ostfeld AM, Paul O. Hostility, risk of coronary heart disease and mortality. *Psychosom Med* 1983;**45**:109–14.

38 Ragland DR. Coronary heart disease mortality in the Western Collaborative Group Study: follow-up experience of 22 years. *Am J Epidemiol* 1988; **127**:462–75.

39 Barefoot JC, Larsen S, von der Lieth L, Schroll M. Hostility, incidence of acute myocardial infarction and mortality in a sample of older Danish men and women. *Am J Epidemiol* 1995;**142**:477–84.

40 Case RB, Heller SS, Case NB, Moss AJ. Type A behavior and survival after acute myocardial infarction. *N Engl J Med* 1985;**312**:737–41.

41 Ragland DR, Brand RJ. Type A behavior and mortality from coronary heart disease. *N Engl J Med* 1988;**318**:65–9.

42 Barefoot JC, Peterson BL, Harrell FEJ. Type A behavior and survival: a follow-up study of 1,467 patients with coronary artery disease. *Am J Cardiol* 1989;**64**:427–32.

43 Maruta T, Hamburgen ME, Jennings CA *et al*. Keeping hostility in perspective: coronary heart disease and the Hostility scale on the Minnesota Multiphasic Personality Inventory. *Mayo Clin Proc* 1993;**68**:109–14.

44 Hallstrom T, Lapidus L, Bengtsson C, Edstrom K. Psychosocial factors and risk of ischaemic heart disease and death in women: a 12 year follow up of participants in the population study of women in Gothenburg, Sweden. *J Psychosom Res* 1986; **30**:451.

45 Hagman M, Wihelmsen L, Wedel H, Pennert K. Risk factors for angina pectoris in a population study of Swedish men. *J Chronic Dis* 1987;**40**: 265–75.

46 Haines AP, Imeson JD, Meade TW. Phobic anxiety and ischaemic heart disease. *Br Med J* 1987;**295**: 297–9.

47 Appels A, Mulder P. Excess fatigue as a precursor of myocardial infarction. *Eur Heart J* 1990;**9**: 758–64.

48 Anda R, Williamson D, Jones D *et al*. Depressed affect, hopelessness, and the risk of ischaemic heart disease in a cohort of US adults. *Epidemiology* 1993;**4**:285–94.

49 Aromaa A, Raitasalo R, Reunanen A *et al*. Depression and cardiovascular diseases. *Acta Psychiatr Scand Suppl* 1994;**377**:77–82.

50 Kawachi I, Sparrow D, Vokonas PS, Weiss ST. Symptoms of anxiety and risk of coronary heart disease. *Circulation* 1994;**90**:2225–9.

51 Simonsick EM, Wallace RB, Blazer DG, Berkman LF. Depressive symptomatology and hypertension associated morbidity and mortality in older adults. *Psychosom Med* 1995;**57**:427–35.

52 Barefoot JC, Schroll M. Symptoms of depression, acute myocardial infarction and total mortality in a community sample. *Circulation* 1996;**93**: 1976–80.

53 Ahern DK, Gorkin L, Anderson JL *et al*. Biobehavioural variables and mortality/cardiac arrest in the Cardiac Arrhythmia Pilot Study. *Am J Cardiol* 1990;**66**:59–62.

54 Kop WJ, Appels A, de Leon CF *et al*. Vital exhaustion predicts new cardiac events after successful coronary angioplasty. *Psychosom Med* 1994;**56**:281–7.

55 Ladwig KH, Roll G, Breithardt G, Budde T, Borggrefe M. Post infarction depression and incomplete recovery 6 months after acute myocardial infarction. *Lancet* 1994;**343**:20–3.

56 Frasure-Smith N, Lesperance F, Talajic M. Depression and 18 month prognosis after myocardial infarction. *Circulation* 1995;**91**: 999–1005.

57 Denollet J, Sys SU, Stroobant N *et al*. Personality as independent predictor of long term mortality in patients with coronary heart disease. *Lancet* 1996;**347**:417–21.

58 Lacroix A, Haynes S. Occupational exposure to high demand/low control work and coronary heart disease incidence in the Framingham cohort. *Am J Epidemiol* 1984;**120**:481.

59 Alfredsson L, Spetz C-L, Theorell T. Type of occupation and near-future hospitalization for myocardial infarction and some other diagnoses. *Int J Epidemiol* 1985;**14**:378–88.

60 Haan MN. Job strain and ischaemic heart disease: an epidemiologic study of metal workers. *Ann Clin Res* 1988;**20**:143–5.

61 Johnson JV, Hall EM, Theorell T. Combined effects of job strain and social isolation on cardiovascular disease morbidity and mortality in a random sample of Swedish male working population. *Scand J Work Environ Health* 1989;**15**:271–9.

62 Reed DM, Lacroix AZ, Karasek RA, Miller D, MacLean CA. Occupational strain and the incidence of coronary heart disease. *Am J Epidemiol* 1989;**129**:495–502.

63 Alterman T, Shekelle RB, Vernon SW, Burau KD. Decision latitude, psychologic demand, job strain, and coronary heart disease in the Western Electric study. *Am J Epidemiol* 1994;**139**:620–7.

64 Suadicani P, Hein HO, Gynetelberg F. Are social inequalities as associated with the risk of ischaemic heart disease a result of psychosocial working conditions? *Atherosclerosis* 1993;**101**: 165–75.

65 Medalie JH, Goldbourt U. Angina Pectoris among 10 000 men. II Psychosocial and other risk factors as evidenced by a multivariate analysis of a five year incidence study. *Am J Med* 1976;**60**:910–21.

66 Reed D, McGee D, Yano K, Feinleib M. Social networks and coronary heart disease among Japanese men in Hawaii. *Am J Epidemiol* 1983; **117**:384–96.

67 Orth-Gomer K, Johnson JV. Social network interaction and mortality. A six year follow up study of a random sample of the Swedish population. *J Chronic Dis* 1987;**40**:949–57.

68 Kaplan GA, Salonen JT, Cohen RD. Social connections and mortality from all causes and from cardiovascular disease: prospective evidence from Eastern Finland. *Am J Epidemiol* 1988;**128**:370–80.

69 Vogt T, Mullooly J, Ernst D, Pope C, Hollis J. Social networks as predictors of ischemic heart disease, cancer, stroke and hypertension: incidence, survival and mortality. *J Clin Epidemiol* 1992;**45**:659–66.

70 Orth-Gomer K, Rosengren A, Wilhelmsen L. Lack of social support and incidence of coronary heart disease in middle-aged Swedish men. *Psychosom Med* 1993;**55**:37–43.

71 Ruberman W, Weinblatt E, Goldberg JD, Chaudhary BS. Psychosocial influences on mortality after myocardial infarction. *N Engl J Med* 1984;**311**:552–9.

72 Wicklund I, Oden A, Sanne H *et al.* Prognostic importance of somatic and psychosocial variables after first myocardial infarction. *Am J Epidemiol* 1988;**128**:787–95.

73 Case RB, Moss AJ, Case N, McDermott M, Eberly S. Living alone after myocardial infarction: impact on prognosis. *JAMA* 1992;**267**:515–19.

74 Hedblad B, Ostergren PO, Hanson BS, Janzon L. Influence of social support on cardiac event rate in men with ischemic type ST-segment depression during ambulatory 24-h long-term ECG recording. The prospective population study "Men born in 1914", Malmo, Sweden. *Eur Heart J* 1992;**13**:433–9.

75 Williams RB, Barefoot JC, Califf RM *et al.* Prognostic importance of social and economic resources among medically treated patients with angiographically documented coronary artery disease. *JAMA* 1992;**267**:520–4.

76 Berkman LF, Leo-Summers L, Horwitz RI. Emotional support and survival after myocardial infarction. A prospective, population-based study of the elderly. *Ann Intern Med* 1992;**117**:1003–9.

77 Jenkinson CM. The influence of psychosocial factors on survival after myocardial infarction. *Public Health* 1993;**107**:305–17.

19 Emerging approaches in cardiovascular prevention

Eva M. Lonn,
Salim Yusuf

INTRODUCTION

Reductions in cholesterol and blood pressure and smoking cessation have been shown to be effective strategies in the prevention of cardiovascular diseases (CVD).[1] However, these "classic" risk factors, along with known non-modifiable risk factors, such as age, gender, and family history, cannot fully explain why certain individuals develop myocardial infarction and stroke, while others do not.[2-4]

These observations suggest that factors other than known risk factors for CHD play an important role in the pathogenesis of coronary artery disease (CAD) and that new preventive therapies aimed at modifying these new risk factors may be additionally useful. In this chapter, we will review a number of emerging risk factors and potential new preventive strategies in cardiovascular medicine. In particular, we will review the evidence for a possible role in CV prevention for oxidation of low density lipoprotein (LDL) and its modification by antioxidants, for the activation of neurohormonal pathways, particularly the renin–angiotensin axis and its modification by angiotensin converting enzyme (ACE) inhibitors in high risk groups, and for hyperhomocysteinemia and its modification by folic acid. Elsewhere in this book, other chapters deal extensively with other emerging risk factors or preventive strategies such as glucose intolerance and use of estrogens.

In addition to identifying and modifying new risk factors, the graded continuous relationship between elevations of traditional risk factors and the risk of disease is being increasingly recognized. For example, there appears to be no threshold at which the relationship between cholesterol and CHD ceases to exist (at least within the range in most Western populations). Similarly, the relationship between blood pressure and the risk of stroke or myocardial infarction is linear (using a doubling scale). These considerations suggest that in individuals at high risk of an event, reductions of cholesterol or blood pressure below "usual" levels may be of substantial benefit. For example, in patients who have already suffered a stroke, lowering blood pressure from a systolic pressure of 140 mmHg to 130 mmHg may be beneficial.[5]

OXIDATIVE STRESS AND USE OF ANTIOXIDANTS IN CARDIOVASCULAR PREVENTION

Pathophysiology and biologic rationale

Extensive laboratory data suggest that oxidative modification of low density lipoprotein (LDL) cholesterol is an important step in the pathogenesis of the atherogenic process.[6,7] Oxidized LDL is potentially more atherogenic than native LDL in many different ways: it is recognized and rapidly taken up by "scavenger" macrophage receptors, giving rise to foam cells; it is directly cytotoxic for endothelial cells and attracts further macrophages to the subintima; it stimulates vascular smooth muscle proliferation in atherosclerotic lesions and autoantibody formation; and contributes to increased vascular tone and coagulability. Experimental studies *in vitro* as well as *in vivo* in different animal models of atherosclerosis suggest that antioxidants could decrease or prevent LDL oxidation and inhibit the atherosclerotic process.[6]

Epidemiology

Epidemiologic studies have generally reported associations between increased intake of various antioxidants and lower CAD risk. Most attention thus far has been directed to the study of naturally occurring antioxidants, particularly the antioxidant vitamins, vitamin E, vitamin C, and beta-carotene, although other antioxidants such as other carotenoids, flavonoids, selenium, magnesium, and monounsaturated fatty acids are also found in natural food products and may reduce LDL oxidation. The major lipid soluble antioxidant vitamins are vitamin E (alpha-tocopherol), the predominant antioxidant present in plasma membranes, tissues and LDL cholesterol and beta-carotene, a precursor of vitamin A. The major water soluble antioxidant vitamin is vitamin C (ascorbic acid), which can regenerate alpha-tocopherol from the tocopheroxyl radical form, thus preserving lipophilic antioxidant within the LDL particles. In addition to food products rich in antioxidant vitamins, antioxidants are available as vitamin supplements, generally at doses much higher than those provided by balanced diets.

A number of epidemiologic studies suggest an inverse association between dietary intake of vegetables and fruits, which are generally rich in antioxidants, and CV risk.[4,8,9] It is unclear, however, which particular components of these dietary products (antioxidants, fiber, low fat, or other factors yet to be identified) might be cardioprotective. In addition, a number of cross-sectional geographic correlation studies suggest a strong inverse association between CHD prevalence and the use of diets rich in antioxidants.[10] Below, we briefly review the information from prospective cohort studies.

VITAMIN E

Several studies including a large number of subjects followed for relatively long periods of time suggest a lower risk for cardiovascular events in vitamin E users after adjustments for other known risk factors as well as for the intake of other antioxidant vitamins[11–15] (Table 19.1). There are, however, several inconsistencies in the available data. Thus, the US Nurses' Health Study and the US Male Health Professionals' Study identified the

Table 19.1 Prospective observational studies of vitamin E and cardiovascular disease

Study participants and location (reference)	Age (yr)	Follow-up (yr)	Comparison groups	Outcomes	Results RR (95% CI)
87 245 female nurses; United States[12]	34–59	8	Upper vs lower quintiles of dietary and supplemental vitamin E intake	437 non-fatal MIs, 115 deaths from CHD	RR = 0.66[a] (0.50–0.87)
34 486 postmenopausal women; United States[13]	56–69	7	Upper vs lower quintiles of vitamin E intake	242 deaths from CHD	Antioxidants from food and vitamin supplements RR = 0.96 (0.62–1.51) Antioxidants from food *without* vitamin supplements RR = 0.38 (0.18–0.80)
39 910 male health professionals; United States[14]	40–75	4	Upper vs lower quintiles of dietary and supplemental vitamin E intake	360 CABGs or PTCAs, 201 non-fatal MIs, 106 deaths from CHD	RR = 0.60 (0.44–0.81)[a]
2748 men; Finland[15]	30–69	14	Upper vs lower tertiles of dietary and supplemental vitamin E intake	186 deaths from CHD	RR = 0.66 (0.42–1.11)[b]
2385 women; Finland[15]	30–69	14	Upper vs lower tertiles of dietary and supplemental vitamin E intake	58 deaths from CHD	RR = 0.35 (0.14–0.88)[b]

CABG, coronary artery bypass grafting; CHD, coronary heart disease; MI, myocardial infarction; PTCA, percutaneous transluminal coronary angioplasty; RR, relative risk; 95% CI, 95% confidence intervals.
[a] Benefits observed for higher vitamin E intake than provided by diet alone, derived largely from prolonged use of supplements.
[b] Benefits derived largely from dietary vitamin E intake (only 3% of the study population took vitamin supplements).

use of high doses of vitamin E in the form of *supplements* for prolonged periods of time as being cardioprotective. These studies suggest that the minimum intake of vitamin E supplements of 100 IU for at least 2 years was associated with a lower cardiovascular risk. Other studies, such as the study in postmenopausal women in the United States and the study of men and women in Finland, identified vitamin E from *food sources* (but not from supplements) to be potentially cardioprotective. In the US Postmenopausal Women's Study, analyses of vitamin E intake from supplements vs diet was specifically examined and in contrast to the US Nurses' Health Study, women taking vitamin E supplements were not found to be at lower risk for developing CVD.

BETA-CAROTENE

The major prospective epidemiologic cohort studies of beta-carotene in cardiovascular disease are summarized in Table 19.2. Significant inconsistencies are noted. In general, however, these studies suggest the possibility of lower risk for adverse cardiovascular outcomes, particularly in men who are current or former smokers, when using larger amounts of dietary beta-carotene provided through nutritional sources or vitamin

Table 19.2 Prospective observational studies of beta-carotene, carotenoids, and cardiovascular disease

Study participants and location (reference)	Age (yr)	Follow-up (yr)	Comparison groups	Outcomes	Results RR (95% CI)
87 245 female nurses; United States[12]	34–59	8	Upper vs lower quintiles of dietary and supplemental carotene intake	437 non-fatal MIs, 115 CHD deaths	P=NS (precise effect not reported)
34 486 postmenopausal women; United States[13]	56–69	7	Upper vs lower quintiles of vitamin A, retinol and carotenoids from food and vitamin supplements	242 CHD deaths	No benefit for vitamin A, retinol or carotenoids from food or from food and vitamin supplements
39 910 male health professionals; United States[14]	40–75	4	Upper vs lower quintiles of dietary and supplemental carotene intake	360 CABGs or PTCAs, 201 non-fatal MIs, 106 CHD deaths	RR=0.71 (0.53–0.86)
2748 men; Finland[15]	30–69	14	Upper vs lower tertiles of dietary and supplemental carotene intake	186 CHD deaths	RR=1.02 (0.70–1.48)
2385 women; Finland[15]	30–69	14	Upper vs lower tertiles of dietary and supplemental carotene intake	58 CHD deaths	RR=0.62 (0.30–1.79)
2974 male pharmaceutical employees; Switzerland[16]	Middle aged	12	Upper vs lower quartiles of serum beta-carotene levels	132 CHD deaths	RR=1.53 (1.07–2.20)
1883 hyperlipidemic men in the placebo group of the LRC-CPPT; United States[17]	47.6	13	Upper vs lower quartiles of serum carotenoid levels	282 CHD deaths and non-fatal MIs	RR=0.64 (0.44–0.92)
1188 men and 532 women; United States[18]	Mean 63.2	8.2	Upper vs lower quartiles of plasma beta-carotene levels	127 CHD deaths	RR=0.57 (0.34–0.95)

CABG, coronary artery bypass grafting; CHD, coronary heart disease; MI, myocardial infarction; NS, not significant; PTCA, percutaneous transluminal coronary angioplasty; RR, relative risk; 95% confidence intervals; LRC-CPPT, Lipid Research Clinics Coronary Primary Prevention Trial.

supplements. A number of epidemiologic studies have also suggested an association between high beta-carotene intake and lower risk of cancer, particularly lung cancer, and these associations are also stronger in current and former smokers. While most epidemiologic studies evaluated beta-carotene intake on levels alone, the Lipid Research Clinic's Coronary Primary Prevention Trial and Followup Study indicated that total serum carotenoid level was more closely related to a lower risk of coronary heart disease in a population of hyperlipidemic men.[17] This suggests that the focus on beta-carotene alone in intervention trials might explain the disappointing results thus far.

VITAMIN C

The National Health and Nutrition Examination Survey (NHANES) prospectively evaluated 11 348 US adults and found a 34% lower standardized mortality ratio (95% CI, 18.1–47.1) among subjects who received 50 mg of vitamin C per day by diet or vitamin supplements compared with those who received less vitamin C.[19] Most other prospective data have not clearly identified vitamin C as a significant cardioprotective agent. Overall, the epidemiologic data evaluating vitamin C and CVD have significant inconsistencies and a number of large prospective epidemiologic studies, after adjusting for other risk factors and for use of other antioxidant vitamins, failed to identify vitamin C as an independent association with lower cardiovascular risk.[14]

These data from epidemiologic studies have several methodological limitations. While most studies have attempted to adjust for different CV risk factors, such adjustments are difficult and may be inadequate. It is possible that lifestyle and dietary patterns not accounted for could contribute to some of the observed apparent lower CV risk in vitamin supplement users compared to non-users. Furthermore, studies which have primarily concentrated on dietary intake of antioxidant vitamins cannot clearly distinguish between the effects of the vitamin itself under investigation, as opposed to other dietary factors (such as high fiber, low fat, other antioxidant substances) which might be prevalent in similar diets.

Randomized clinical trials

In order to address some of the inherent methodologic limitations of observational studies, a number of large, randomized clinical trials of antioxidant vitamins have been conducted and several trials are still ongoing.

TRIALS OF VITAMIN E

Several older studies have evaluated vitamin E in patients with intermittent claudication and angina. These studies were generally small, not always randomized and blinded, and their results are therefore difficult to assess. Some of these studies suggested benefit from vitamin E, particularly in patients with intermittent claudication.[11] More recently, retarded angiographic progression of native coronary atherosclerosis in individuals with a high vitamin E intake has been reported and a small trial of 100 patients following coronary angioplasty found a 46% relative risk reduction ($P=0.06$) for restenosis in patients treated with vitamin E 1200 IU/day.[20,21] Three large randomized trials of vitamin E have been completed (Table 19.3).

The Alpha-Tocopherol Beta-Carotene Cancer Prevention Study (ATBC) is a randomized, double-blind, placebo-controlled primary prevention trial designed primarily to assess the effects of daily supplementation with alpha-tocopherol and beta-carotene on lung and other cancers.[22] A total of 29 133 male smokers from south western Finland were randomly assigned to alpha-tocopherol 50 mg daily or placebo and beta-carotene 20 mg daily or placebo for 5–7 years. Vitamin E did not have any significant effect on CV deaths. However, there was a lower relative risk of angina pectoris incidence (RR = 0.91; 95% CI 0.83–0.99; $P=0.04$).[22,23] A small, unexpected but statistically significant increase in deaths from hemorrhagic stroke and a non-significant reduction in mortality from ischemic stroke were noted in vitamin E recipients. There was no effect on cancer

Table 19.3 Large (>1000 subjects) randomized trials of vitamin E

Trial (reference)	Study participants	Follow-up (yr)	Daily vitamin E dose	Outcomes	Relative risk reduction (%) (95% CI)	
ATBC[22,23]	29 133 male smokers in Finland	6.1	50 mg	Total mortality	−2[b]	(−9 to 5)
				Death from CVD	2	(−8 to 11)
				Angina	9	(1 to 17)
Chinese Study[24]	29 584 adults in Linxian province	5.2	30 mg[a]	Total mortality	9	(0 to 17)
				Death from cerebrovascular disease	9	(−8 to 24)
CHAOS[25]	2002 patients with CAD in the UK	1.4	800 IU/400 IU	Total mortality	−29	(−119 to 24)
				Death from CVD	−10	(−96 to 39)
				Non-fatal MI	77	(53 to 89)

ATBC, Alpha-tocopherol, Beta-carotene Cancer Prevention Study; CHAOS, Cambridge Heart AntiOxidant Study.
[a] In addition to vitamin E, selenium and beta-carotene supplements were used.
[b] Minus sign indicates an increased risk.

deaths. The major limitation of this trial was the low dose used (50 mg daily), which is smaller than the doses suggested by most of the epidemiologic data as being cardioprotective (>100 mg/day). Second, the vitamin E used was synthetic and is less well absorbed compared with the natural forms. Third, it is also unclear whether results from this well defined population of middle aged male smokers from Finland targeted for primary prevention can be generalized to other patient groups.

A second large primary prevention trial conducted in China reported a marginally significant reduction in total mortality (RR = 9%; 95% CI 0–70%) for a combination of vitamin E, beta-carotene, and selenium, with a trend towards reduced CV mortality (RR = 9%; 95% CI −8–24%).[24] The vitamin E dose was also small (30 mg daily), the population studied was very different from a Western population and could have lower baseline antioxidant levels through poor dietary intake, and the study design does not allow the identification of which particular antioxidant contributed to the overall small reduction in mortality.

The Cambridge Heart Antioxidant Study (CHAOS) is a double-blind, placebo-controlled secondary prevention study of 2002 patients with angiographically proven coronary atherosclerosis randomized to vitamin E 800 IU daily or 400 IU daily vs placebo.[25] A highly statistically significant reduction in non-fatal myocardial infarction of 77% and in the combined endpoint of any major CV event of 53% was reported. Although encouraging, this study has many methodological problems and remains inconclusive:

- The baseline characteristics of the study groups were not balanced and completeness of follow-up is uncertain.
- There was a non-significant excess in CV deaths in vitamin E recipients.
- The duration of the study was quite short (median 510 days). The apparent large benefit of vitamin E on non-fatal CV events in this relatively short period of time appears to exceed the size of effects that might be considered plausible from the expected mechanism of action (impact on atherosclerosis) and the epidemiologic data.

Table 19.4 Large randomized trials of beta-carotene

Trial (reference)	Study participants	Follow-up (yr)	Beta-carotene dose	Outcome	Relative risk reduction (%) (95% CI)
ATBC[22,23]	29 133 male smokers in Finland	6.1	20 mg/day	Total mortality	-9^b (-17 to -2)
				Death from CVD	-11 (-23 to 1)
				Death from cancer	-9 (-23 to 3)
				New lung cancer	-18 (-36 to -31)
				Angina	-13 (-27 to 0)
CARET[26]	18 314 male smokers, former smokers and workers exposed to asbestos in the United States	4.0	30 mg/day[a]	Total mortality	-17 (-33 to 3)
				Death from CVD	-26 (-61 to 1)
				Death from cancer	-46 (-100 to -7)
				New lung cancer	-28 (-57 to -4)
PHS[27]	22 071 male physicians in the United States	12.0	50 mg/alternate days	Total mortality	-2 (-11 to 7)
				Death from CVD	-9 (-27 to 7)
				Death from cancer	-2 (-18 to 11)
				New lung cancer	7 (-27 to 32)
				Myocardial infarction	4 (-9 to 16)
				Stroke	4 (-11 to 17)
SCPS[18]	1188 men and 532 women in the United States	8.2	50 mg/day	Total mortality	-3 (-30 to 18)
				Death from CVD	-16 (-64 to 18)
				Death from cancer	17 (-29 to 56)

ATBC, Alpha-tocopherol, Beta-carotene Cancer Prevention Study; CARET, β-Carotene and Retinol Efficacy Trial; PHS, Physicians' Health Study; SCPS, Skin Cancer Prevention Study.

[a] Patients randomized to beta-carotene also received 25 000 U/day of retinol (vitamin A).
[b] Minus sign indicates an increased risk.

- The overall number of events was relatively small, that is, 14 non-fatal myocardial infarcts and 27 CV deaths in the vitamin E group and 41 and 23 events respectively in placebo-treated patients. Therefore, it would be premature to conclude at present that vitamin E use reduces the risk of CV events.

A number of large randomized clinical trials of vitamin E are currently ongoing and widespread use of vitamin E in CV prevention should await their results.

TRIALS OF BETA-CAROTENE

A number of large, long-term, well-designed randomized trials of beta-carotene in primary prevention have recently been reported (Table 19.4). These studies have consistently failed to show benefit from beta-carotene, in the prevention of both CVD and cancer. Furthermore, concern about an increased risk of cancer was present in some investigations.

In the ATBC trial, the total mortality was 8% higher (95% CI 1–16%; $P=0.02$) among participants who received 20 mg of beta-carotene daily[22] and there were trends towards increased deaths from lung cancer as well as ischemic heart disease, although this did not reach statistical significance.

The Beta-Carotene and Retinol Efficacy Trial (CARET) randomized 18 314 current or former smokers and workers exposed to asbestos to a combination of 30 mg of beta-carotene per day and 25 000 IU of retinol (vitamin A) or placebo.[26] The primary study endpoint was lung cancer. After an average follow-up of 4 years, this study was terminated earlier than planned due to an increase in lung cancer incidence in individuals randomized to beta-carotene and vitamin A (RR for cancer = 1.28; 95% CI 1.04–1.57; $P=0.02$). Also, the total mortality was 17% higher in the active treatment group ($P = 0.02$), with increased deaths from lung cancer and CV causes.

The Physicians' Health Study (PHS) enroled 22 071 male physicians, 42–84 years of age, in the United States.[27] These were randomized to receive beta-carotene 50 mg on alternate days or placebo and were followed for an average of 12 years. There were no significant differences in the incidence of CVD, cancers or in overall mortality. The possibility of late vs early differences was investigated and no differences in early or late overall incidence of these events was noted.

Smaller randomized clinical trials of beta-carotene, designed primarily to assess effects on skin cancer, also failed to demonstrate any reduction in mortality from CVD or other causes.[18] A study by Greenberg *et al.* outlines the apparent discrepancy between epidemiologic investigations and clinical trial results.[18] Beta-carotene plasma levels were measured at baseline and individuals in the highest quartile of plasma beta-carotene levels had a lower risk of death from all causes, compared with the lowest quartile. However, results of the randomized trial did not reveal any effects on total or CV mortality associated with beta-carotene supplementation for a median of 8.2 years. These data suggest that beta-carotene levels may have been a marker associated with other factors that may have been related to CVD.

TRIALS OF VITAMIN C

There have been no large trials of vitamin C supplementation. In a trial of 578 patients admitted to a geriatric hospital, supplementation with 200 mg of vitamin C daily did not reduce mortality at 6 months.[28] The Chinese trial discussed in the section on vitamin E reported no reduction in total mortality in individuals randomized to a combination of vitamin C and molybdenum.[24] There was also no effect on mortality from cerebrovascular disease.

CLINICAL TRIALS USING OTHER ANTIOXIDANTS

Probucol is a lipid lowering agent which reduces low density lipoprotein (LDL) but also lowers high density lipoprotein (HDL) and has been shown to be a potent antioxidant in a number of experimental studies. The Probucol Quantitative Regression Swedish Trial (PQRST) in 274 hypercholesterolemic subjects failed, however, to reveal any benefit in the progression of femoral atherosclerosis.[29] This lack of benefit from probucol may be related to the significant reduction in HDL cholesterol (by 24%) in patients treated with probucol, compared with those in the placebo group.

Antioxidants – conclusions and recommendations

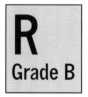

R

Grade B

Vitamin E

While attractive, the antioxidant hypothesis remains at present unproven. The most promising data relate to vitamin E, but these are inconclusive and do not warrant its widespread use at present. The strong biologic rationale and epidemiologic data relating antioxidants to lower CV risk justify ongoing trials of vitamin E and new antioxidant agents in further evaluating this hypothesis.

RENIN–ANGIOTENSIN AXIS AND IMPACT OF ANGIOTENSIN CONVERTING ENZYME (ACE) INHIBITORS

Pathophysiology and biologic rationale

Experimental and human studies suggest that ACE inhibitors may reduce CV risk through both cardioprotective and vasculoprotective effects mediated by blocking both circulating and tissue renin–angiotensin systems, as well as by bradykinin potentiation.[30] ACE inhibitors are antiproliferative, have antimigratory effects on smooth muscle cells, restore endothelial-mediated vascular reactivity, and have antithrombotic action by decreasing platelet aggregation and enhancing endogenous fibrinolysis.[31,32]

Epidemiologic and genetic studies: link between the renin–angiotensin system and the risk for myocardial infarction

The prospective cohort study of Alderman *et al.* in 1717 subjects with mild to moderate hypertension followed for a mean of 8.3 years reported a 5.3-fold increased and independent risk of myocardial infarction among subjects with high vs those with low renin profiles.[33] However, Meade *et al.*[34] failed to demonstrate associations between plasma renin levels and risk for myocardial infarction in normotensive individuals and it remains uncertain whether correlations between plasma renin levels and CV risk may be restricted to certain specific groups such as hypertensive individuals.

A number of recent investigations report significant associations between the ACE-DD genotype, which identifies individuals with higher levels of circulating ACE and risk for CVD, although other studies failed to confirm these findings.[35] Overall, as summarized in a recent meta-analysis, it appears that the ACE-DD genotype is associated with a moderately increased CV risk, particularly in certain ethnic groups such as the Japanese, and in individuals developing CHD in the absence of hyperlipidemia and other classic risk factors for atherosclerosis.[36] The ACE-DD genotype is quite prevalent and is observed in about a quarter of the population. Therefore, this hypothesis, if proven, has substantial therapeutic and public health implications. The obvious question which requires further investigation is the role of intervention with ACE inhibitors (or angiotensin II blockers) in individuals with the ACE-DD genotype and higher levels of circulating ACE and angiotensin II.

Randomized clinical trials

The potential for ACE inhibitors to prevent major ischemic events and to therefore alter the natural history of atherosclerotic disease has been brought into focus by the results of the Studies of Left Ventricular Dysfunction (SOLVD)[37] and the Survival and Ventricular Enlargement (SAVE) trials,[38] which separately demonstrated a significant reduction in the risk for acute myocardial infarction in patients with documented CVD and low ejection fraction treated with ACE inhibitors for approximately 40 months. Pooled results of the SOLVD Treatment trial, SOLVD Prevention trial, the SAVE study, the Acute Infarction Ramipril Efficacy Study (AIRE),[39] and the Trandolapril Cardiac Evaluation studies (TRACE)[40] indicate a 21% (95% CI 11–29%; $P = <0.002$) relative risk reduction for myocardial infarction associated with ACE inhibitor therapy. In addition, other related ischemic endpoints, mainly hospitalizations for unstable angina in the combined SOLVD trials (RR = 20%; 95% CI 9–29%; $P = 0.001$) and revascularization procedures in the SAVE trial (RR = 24%; 95% CI 6–39%, $P = 0.014$) were also significantly reduced in patients treated with enalapril and captopril respectively. These trials included patients with low left ventricular ejection fraction or heart failure. These patients were likely to have elevations of renin and angiotensin levels; therefore, the data from these trials cannot be extrapolated to other high risk populations who may not have left ventricular dysfunction. The benefit was seen, however, in a number of different subgroups and the relationship between the degree of LV dysfunction and reduction in myocardial infarction was weak ($P = 0.04$), so that the role of ACE inhibitors in preventing myocardial infarction in high risk patients without LV dysfunction deserves further exploration.

The effects of ACE inhibitors on myocardial infarction risk in major clinical trials are summarized in Table 19.5, which emphasizes the importance of prolonged therapy in attaining benefits. The observed time course in the reduction of acute ischemic events (with a 6- to 12-month lag) resembles the results of trials of cholesterol lowering and suggests that the mechanism for the observed anti-ischemic action of ACE inhibitors is unlikely to be related solely to the beneficial hemodynamic effect of these drugs, which is generally noted immediately and is not expected to increase with time (Figure 19.1). These observations suggest that ACE inhibitors decrease the incidence of ischemic events by multiple mechanisms, including the prevention of coronary atherosclerosis progression and/or stabilization of atherosclerotic plaques.

Direct proof of potential benefits of ACE inhibitors in patients without left ventricular dysfunction is currently not available and is under investigation in several large ongoing clinical trials.

ACE INHIBITORS – CONCLUSIONS AND RECOMMENDATIONS

ACE inhibitors are currently indicated in all patients with clinical manifestations of congestive heart failure and in individuals with asymptomatic left ventricular dysfunction. They are also effective antihypertensive agents and have been demonstrated to reduce the progression of renal disease in diabetic patients. Recent studies also suggest an important role for ACE inhibitors in the management of acute myocardial infarction. The preventive use of ACE inhibitors in high risk individuals with preserved left

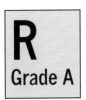

R

Grade A

For high risk
patients

Table 19.5 Effects of ACE inhibitors on MI — impact of duration of treatment

Mean duration of treatment trial(s)	Patient characteristics	Number of MI (% of patients)		Relative risk reduction (%) (95% CI)	P
		ACE inhibitors	Placebo		
≤6 months					
CONSENSUS II	Unselected patients with acute MI	271 (8.9)	268 (8.8)	−1 (−21,15)	NS
GISSI-3	Unselected patients with acute MI	303 (3.2)	292 (3.1)	−4 (−23,12)	NS
ISIS-4	Unselected patients with acute MI	1162 (4.0)	1101 (3.8)	−6 (−15,3)	NS
CCS-1	Unselected patients with acute MI	Not reported			
SMILE	Acute anterior MI; not eligible for thrombolysis	8 (1.0)	5 (0.6)	37 (−20,80)	NS
Overall				*−5 (−10,2)*	
15 months					
AIRE[a]	Clinical evidence of HF early post-MI	81 (8.0)	88 (8.9)	9 (−22,35)[a]	NS
26.5 months					
TRACE	EF ≤35% early post-MI	97 (11.1)	111 (12.7)	14 (−10,31)	NS
38–42 months[a]					
SOLVD Prevention	EF ≤35% without HF	161 (7.6)	204 (9.1)	24 (6,38)	0.01
SOLVD Treatment	EF ≤35% with HF	127 (9.9)	156 (12.3)	23 (2,39)	0.02
SAVE	EF ≤40% early post-MI	133 (11.9)	170 (15.2)	25 (5,40)	0.05
Overall				*23 (11,32)*	0.001

MI, myocardial infarction, EF, left ventricular ejection fraction; HF, heart failure; CI, confidence intervals; CONSENSUS II, Cooperative New Scandinavian Enalapril Survival Study II; GISSI-3, Gruppo Italiano per lo Studio della Soppravivenza nell'Infarcto miocardico-3; ISIS-4, Fourth International Study of Infarct Survival; CCS-1, Chinese Captopril Study-1; SMILE, Survival of Myocardial Infarction Long-term Evaluation; AIRE, Acute Infarction Ramipril Efficacy; TRACE, Trandolapril Cardiac Evaluation study group; SOLVD, Studies of Left Ventricular Dysfunction; SAVE, Survival And Ventricular Enlargement trial.
[a] Long-term follow-up of the UK component of AIRE (AIREX) demonstrates a significant reduction in fatal MI.

ventricular function remains at present speculative and should await results of ongoing large clinical trials.

HOMOCYSTEINE AND VASCULAR DISEASE

Pathophysiology and biologic rationale

Homocysteine is a sulfur-containing amino acid produced during catabolism of the essential amino acid methionine. It can be irreversibly degraded by cystathionine-beta-

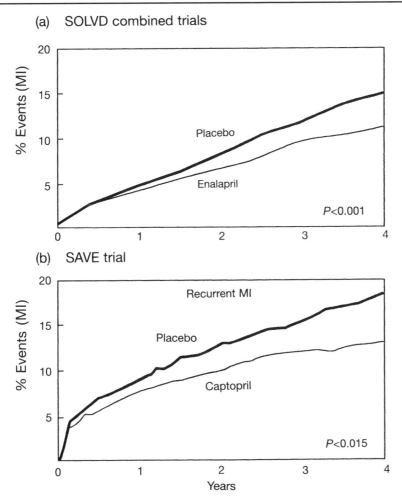

(a) SOLVD combined trials

(b) SAVE trial

Figure 19.1 (a) Cumulative incidence of myocardial infarction (MI) in the combined Studies of Left Ventricular Dysfunction (SOLVD). (b) Incidence of recurrent MI in the Survival and Ventricular Enlargement (SAVE) trial. In both studies, differences in the incidence of MI between ACE inhibitor and placebo-treated patients started to become apparent after 6–12 months of therapy and continued to widen thereafter. (Adapted with permission from *The Lancet* and *New England Journal of Medicine*.)

synthase, a process requiring vitamin B_6 as a cofactor. Alternatively, homocysteine can be remethylated to conserve methionine in a process requiring methionine synthase and methylcobalamin (vitamin B_{12}) as a cofactor and methyl-tetrahydrofolate reductase (MTHFR) as a cosubstrate. This metabolic pathway requires an adequate supply of folate and the enzyme MTHFR. Genetic and acquired abnormalities in the function of these enzymes or deficiencies in folate or vitamin B_6 or B_{12} cofactors can therefore lead to elevated concentrations of intracellular homocysteine, which is then released to the plasma. Very high levels of plasma homocysteine lead to homocystinuria, which is caused by the rare homozygous deficiency of cystathionine-beta-synthase or the even more infrequent homozygous deficiency in MTHFR or defects in cobalamin metabolism. These distinct genetic abnormalities, which share very high levels of plasma homocysteine, have typical clinical manifestations, including severe premature atherosclerotic and thromboembolic disease. Histopathologically, this vascular disease is characterized by vascular endothelial injury, vascular smooth muscle cell proliferation, progressive arterial stenosis, and hemostatic changes consistent with a prothrombotic state. These findings have led McCully to formulate the homocysteine theory of atherosclerosis.[41]

More recently, the role of modest elevations in homocysteine without associated homocystinuria in the causation of atherosclerotic and thromboembolic vascular disease has been investigated. Such "modest" elevations in plasma homocysteine can be related to genetic, physiologic, pathologic, and nutritional factors. Thus, heterozygous MTHFR mutations (e.g. thermolabile MTHFR), age, gender, postmenopausal status in women, smoking, sedentary lifestyle, dietary factors including increased intake of animal proteins which have a higher methionine content and low intake of folate, vitamins B_6 and B_{12}, renal failure, transplantation, and medications such as corticosteroids and cyclosporin have been associated with hyperhomocysteinemia.[42]

Potential mechanisms of athero- and thrombogenicity associated with elevated homocysteine levels include:

- endothelial dysfunction related to direct endothelial cell damage and impaired production of nitric oxide;[43]
- stimulation of smooth muscle cell proliferation;[44]
- lipid abnormalities, including increased plasma triglycerides and increased susceptibility to oxidation of LDL;[45]
- increased thrombogenicity mediated by promoting the adherence of platelets and release of platelet-derived growth factors due to homocysteine-induced endothelial damage, activation of factor V, factor Xa, inhibition of protein C activation, inhibition of cell surface expression of thrombomodulin, and decreased tissue plasminogen activator (tPA) activity.[46]

Epidemiology

Elevated plasma homocysteine levels have been associated with other risk factors for cardiovascular disease, such as male gender, old age, smoking, high blood pressure, elevated cholesterol levels, and lack of exercise in population based cross-sectional studies.[47] Several studies have also demonstrated associations between the anatomic extent of coronary or carotid atherosclerosis and plasma homocysteine levels. Thus, in a cross-sectional investigation of the Framingham Heart Study, the odds ratio for carotid artery stenosis of $\geq 25\%$ was 2.0 (95% CI 1.4–2.9) for subjects with the highest plasma homocysteine concentrations as compared with those with the lowest concentrations.[48] A case-control study from the Atherosclerosis Risk in Communities Study (ARIC) found that the odds ratio for having a thickened carotid artery wall was 3.15 for subjects in the top quintile of plasma homocysteine levels, compared with those in the bottom quintile.[49] A number of cross-sectional epidemiologic studies, as well as prospective and retrospective case-control studies, have generally also confirmed strong associations between high plasma homocysteine levels and risk for coronary artery disease, stroke or peripheral vascular disease.

Boushey *et al.* reviewed the major epidemiologic investigations of homocysteine and CVD up to 1995 and pooled their results in a meta-analysis which quantifies the magnitude of risk associated with elevated homocysteine levels.[50] In this analysis, a linear, independent risk for increment in homocysteine and cardiovascular risk was found. Every 5 µmol/l increment in homocysteine was found to be associated with an increased odds ratio for coronary artery disease of 1.6 for men (95% CI 1.4–1.7) and 1.8 for women (95% CI 1.3–1.9). The risk was also increased for other common vascular disorders: 1.5 for cerebrovascular disease and 6.8 for peripheral vascular disease. Similar data were reported for venous thromboembolic disorders.[51]

While overall positive associations between increased plasma homocysteine without provocation or increased levels following methionine loading have been reported in epidemiologic investigations, the number of well conducted, large prospective studies is small and there are some inconsistencies in the available data. In the Physicians' Health Study with a 5 year follow-up, plasma homocysteine levels above the 95th percentile of the control distribution were associated with a 3.4-fold increased risk of myocardial infarction[52] at 5 years; however, the relative risk was substantially reduced to 1.7 by 7.5 years of follow-up, which was no longer statistically significant.[53] Also within the Physicians' Health Study, moderately elevated plasma total homocysteine levels were not found to be a major risk factor for angina requiring bypass graft surgery.[54] This suggests that elevated homocysteine may either be a response to atherosclerosis or a thrombogenic factor.

Randomized clinical trials

Homocysteine levels can be easily reduced by supplementation with folic acid and possibly vitamins B_6 and B_{12} or a combination of these. While these represent very simple, inexpensive and likely risk-free interventions, trials evaluating these supplements have not been conducted thus far. In the United States, Canada and other countries, fortification of grains with folic acid is planned primarily for the prevention of neural tube defects. While this is a positive health policy initiative, it is expected that the amounts of folic acid used will be insufficient to effectively reduce homocysteine levels in a large proportion of individuals. Therefore, it is timely to evaluate the impact of folate alone or combined with vitamin B_6 and B_{12} in reducing major clinical cardiovascular events and on atherosclerosis progression.

Homocysteine – conclusions and recommendations

Overall, the current experimental and epidemiologic data suggest that reducing homocysteine could represent an effective, simple intervention. Confirmation from clinical trials is, however, not available. In the meantime, it appears prudent to ensure adequate dietary intake of folate and vitamins B_6 and B_{12}.

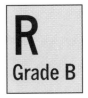

R

Grade B

In the presence of hyperhomocysteinemia

CONCLUSIONS

This chapter summarizes the evidence on antioxidants, reductions in homocysteine levels, and modulating the renin–angiotensin axis. These areas are promising, but definite conclusions must await the results of ongoing, large randomized trials. Additional areas not covered include lowering Lp(a), hormone replacement, use of selective estrogen receptor modulation, modifying coagulation parameters, enhancing fibrinolysis, and modifying psychosocial factors. Some of these are covered in other chapters.

REFERENCES

1 Goldman L, Cook EF. The decline in ischemic heart disease mortality rates. An analysis of the comparative effects of medical interventions and changes in lifestyle. *Ann Intern Med* 1984;**101**: 825–36.

2 Gordon T, Garcia-Palmieri MR, Kagan A, Kannel WB, Schiffman J. Differences in coronary heart disease in Framingham, Honolulu and Puerto Rico. *J Chron Dis* 1974;**27**:329–44.

3 Verschuren WMM, Jacobs DR, Bloemberg BPM *et al.* Serum total cholesterol and long-term coronary heart disease mortality in different cultures. Twenty-five-year follow-up of the Seven Countries Study. *JAMA* 1995;**274**:131–6.

4 Kannel WB, Castelli WP, Gordon T. Cholesterol in the prediction of atherosclerotic disease. New perspectives based on the Framingham Study. *Ann Intern Med* 1979;**90**:85–91.

5 Rogers A, MacMahon S, Gamble G *et al.* Blood pressure and risk of stroke in patients with cerebrovascular disease. *Br Med J* 1996;**313**:147.

6 Steinberg D. Antioxidants in the prevention of human atherosclerosis. Summary of the proceedings of a National Heart, Lung and Blood Institute workshop: September 5–6, 1991, Bethesda, Maryland. *Circulation* 1992;**85**: 2338–43.

7 Berliner JA, Navab M, Fogelman AM *et al.* Atherosclerosis: basic mechanisms. Oxidation, inflammation and genetics. *Circulation* 1995;**91**: 2488–96.

8 Rimm EB, Ascherio A, Giovannucci E *et al.* Vegetable, fruit, and cereal fiber intake and risk of coronary heart disease among men. *JAMA* 1996;**275**:447–51.

9 Hertog MG, Feskens EJ, Holman PC, Katan MB, Kromhout D. Dietary antioxidant flavonoids and risk of coronary heart disease: the Zutphen Elderly Study. *Lancet* 1993;**342**:1007–11.

10 Gey KF, Puska P, Jordan P, Moser UK. Inverse correlation between plasma vitamin E and mortality from ischemic heart disease in cross-cultural epidemiology. *Am J Clin Nutr* 1991;**53**: 326S–34S.

11 Jha P, Flather M, Lonn E, Farkouh M, Yusuf S. The antioxidant vitamins (E,C and beta-carotene) and cardiovascular disease: a critical summary of epidemiological and clinical trial data. *Ann Intern Med* 1995;**123**:860–72.

12 Stampfer MJ, Hennekens CH, Manson JE *et al.* Vitamin E consumption and the risk of coronary disease in women. *N Engl J Med* 1993; **328**: 1444–9.

13 Kushi LH, Fulsom AR, Prineas RJ *et al.* Dietary antioxidant vitamins and death from coronary heart disease in postmenopausal women. *N Engl J Med* 1996;**334**:1156–62.

14 Rimm EB, Stampfer MJ, Ascherio A *et al.* Vitamin E consumption and the risk of coronary heart disease in men. *N Engl J Med* 1993;**328**:1450–6.

15 Knekt P, Reunanen A, Jarvinen R *et al.* Antioxidant vitamin intake and coronary mortality in a longitudinal population study. *Am J Epidemiol* 1994;**139**:1180–90.

16 Gey KF, Moser UK, Jordan P *et al.* Increased risk of cardiovascular disease at suboptimal plasma concentrations of essential antioxidants: an epidemiological update with special attention to carotene and vitamin C. *Am J Clin Nutr* 1993; **57**(5 Suppl):787S–97S.

17 Morris DI, Kritchevsky SB, Davis CE. Serum carotenoids and coronary heart disease. The Lipid Research Clinics Coronary Primary Prevention Trial and Follow-up Study. *JAMA* 1994;**272**: 1439–41.

18 Greenberg ER, Baron JA, Karagas MR *et al.* Mortality associated with low plasma concentration of beta-carotene and the effect of oral supplementation. *JAMA* 1996;**275**:699–703.

19 Enstrom JE, Kanim LE, Klein MA. Vitamin C intake and mortality among a sample of the United States population. *Epidemiology* 1992;**3**: 194–202.

20 Hodis HN, Mack WJ, Labree JL *et al.* Serial coronary angiographic evidence that antioxidant vitamin intake reduces progression of coronary artery atherosclerosis. *JAMA* 1995;**273**: 1849–54.

21 DeMaio SJ, King SB III, Lembo NJ *et al.* Vitamin E supplementation, plasma lipids and incidence of restenosis after percutaneous transluminal coronary angioplasty (PTCA). *J Am Coll Nutr* 1992;**11**:68–73.

22 The Alpha-Tocopherol, Beta Carotene Cancer Prevention Study Group. The effect of vitamin E and beta carotene on the incidence of lung cancer and other cancers in male smokers. *N Engl J Med* 1994;**330**:1029–35.

23 Rapola JM, Virtamo J, Haukka JK *et al.* Effect of vitamin E and beta carotene on the incidence

of angina pectoris: a randomized, double-blind, controlled trial. *JAMA* 1996;**275**:693–8.

24 Blot WJ, Li JY, Taylor PR *et al.* Nutrition intervention trials in Linxian, China: supplementation with specific vitamin/mineral combinations, cancer incidence, and disease-specific mortality in the general population. *J Natl Cancer Inst* 1993;**85**:1483–92.

25 Stephens NG, Parsons A, Schofield PM *et al.* Randomized controlled trial of vitamin E in patients with coronary disease: Cambridge Heart Antioxidant Study (CHAOS). *Lancet* 1996;**347**:781–6.

26 Omenn GS, Goodman GE, Thornquist MD *et al.* Effects of a combination of beta carotene and vitamin A on lung cancer and cardiovascular disease. *N Engl J Med* 1996;**334**:1150–5.

27 Hennekens CH, Burning JE, Manson JE *et al.* Lack of effect of long-term supplementation with beta carotene on the incidence of malignant neoplasms and cardiovascular disease. *N Engl J Med* 1996;**334**:1145–49.

28 Wilson TS, Datta SB, Murrell JS, Andrews CT. Relation of vitamin C levels to mortality in a geriatric hospital: a study of the effect of vitamin C administration. *Age Aging* 1973;**2**:163–71.

29 Walldius G, Erikson U, Olsson AG *et al.* The effect of probucol on femoral atherosclerosis: the Probucol Quantitative Regression Swedish Trial (PQRST). *Am J Cardiol.* 1994;**74**:875–83.

30 Lonn EM, Yusuf S, Prabhat J *et al.* Emerging role of angiotensin-converting enzyme inhibitors in cardiac and vascular protection. *Circulation* 1994;**90**:2056–69.

31 Mancini GBJ, Henry GC, Macaya C *et al.* Angiotensin-converting enzyme inhibition with quinapril improves endothelial vasomotor dysfunction in patients with coronary artery disease. The TREND (Trial on Reversing ENdothelial Dysfunction) study. *Circulation* 1996;**94**:258–65.

32 Wright RA, Flapan AD, Alberti KG *et al.* Effects of captopril therapy on endogenous fibrinolysis in men with recent, uncomplicated myocardial infarction. *J Am Coll Cardiol* 1994;**24**:67–73.

33 Alderman MH, Madhavan SH, OOi WL *et al.* Association of the renin-sodium profile with the risk of myocardial infarction in patients with hypertension. *N Engl J Med.* 1991;**324**:1098–104.

34 Meade TW, Cooper JA, Peart WS. Plasma renin activity and ischemic heart disease. *N Engl J Med* 1993;**329**:616–19.

35 Cambien F, Poirier O, Lecerf L *et al.* Deletion polymorphism in angiotensin-converting enzyme gene associated with parental history of myocardial infarction. *Nature* 1992;**359**:641–4.

36 Samani NJ, Thompson JR, O'Toole L, Channer K, Woods KL. A meta-analysis of the association of the deletion allele of the angiotensin-converting enzyme gene with myocardial infarction. *Circulation* 1996;**94**:708–12.

37 Yusuf S, Pepine CJ, Garces C *et al.* Effect of enalapril on myocardial infarction and unstable angina in patients with low ejection fractions. *Lancet* 1992;**340**:1173–8.

38 Rutherford JD, Pfeffer MA, Moye LA *et al*, on behalf of the SAVE Investigators. Effects of captopril on ischemic events after myocardial infarction. Results of the Survival and Ventricular Enlargement trial. *Circulation* 1994;**90**:1731–8.

39 The Acute Infarction Ramipril Efficacy (AIRE) Study Investigators. Effect of ramipril on mortality and morbidity of survivors of acute myocardial infarction with clinical evidence of heart failure. *Lancet* 1993;**342**:821–8.

40 Kober L, Torp-Pederson C, Carlsen JE *et al.* for the Trandolapril Cardiac Evaluation (TRACE) Study Group. A clinical trial of the angiotensin-converting-enzyme inhibitor trandolapril in patients with left ventricular dysfunction after myocardial infarction. *N Engl J Med* 1995;**333**:1670–6.

41 McCully KS, Wilson RB. Homocysteine theory of arteriosclerosis. *Atherosclerosis* 1975;**22**:215–27.

42 Ueland PM, Refsum H, Brattstrom L. Plasma homocysteine and cardiovascular disease. In: Francis RB. Ed. *Atherosclerotic cardiovascular disease, hemostasis and endothelial function.* New York: Marcel Dekker, 1992.

43 Tawakol A, Omland T, Gerhard M, Wu JT, Creager MA. Hyperhomocyst(e)inemia is associated with impaired endothelium-dependent vasodilation in humans. *Circulation* 1997;**95**:1119–21.

44 Tsai JC, Perella MA, Yoshizumi M *et al.* Promotion of vascular smooth muscle growth by homocysteine: a link to atherosclerosis. *Proc Natl Acad Sci USA* 1994;**91**:6369–73.

45 Frascher G, Karnaukhova E, Muehl A, Hoeger H, Lubec B. Oral administration of homocysteine leads to increased plasma triglycerides and homocysteic acid-additional mechanisms in homocysteine induced endothelial damage? *Life Sci* 1995;**57**:813–17.

46 Mayer EL, Jacobson DW, Robinson K. Homocysteine and coronary atherosclerosis. *J Am Coll Cardiol* 1996;**27**:517–27.

47 Nygard O, Vollset SE, Refsum H *et al.* Total plasma homocysteine and cardiovascular risk profile. *JAMA* 1995;**274**:1526–33.

48 Selhub J, Jacques PF, Bostom AG *et al.* Association between plasma homocysteine concentrations and extracranial carotid-artery stenosis. *N Engl J Med* 1995;**332**:286–91.

49 Malinow MR, Nieto FJ, Szklo M, Chambless LE. Carotid artery intimal-medial wall thickening and

plasma homocyst(e)ine in asymptomatic adults. The Atherosclerosis Risk in Communities Study. *Circulation* 1993;**87**:1107–13.

50 Boushey CJ, Beresford SAA, Omenn GS, Motulsky AG. A quantitative assessment of plasma homocysteine as a risk factor for vascular disease. Probable benefits of increasing folic acid intakes. *JAMA* 1995;**274**:1049–57.

51 Den Heijer M, Koster T, Blom HJ *et al.* Hyperhomocysteinemia as a risk factor for deep-vein thrombosis. *N Engl J Med.* 1996;**334**: 759–62.

52 Stampfer MJ, Malinow MR, Willett WC *et al.* A prospective study of plasma homocyst(e)ine and risk of myocardial infarction in US physicians. *JAMA* 1992;**268**:877–81.

53 Chasan-Taber L, Selhub J, Rosenberg IH *et al.* A prospective study of folate and vitamin B$_6$ and risk of myocardial infarction in US physicians. *J Am Coll Nutr* 1996;**15**:136–43.

54 Verhoef P, Hennekens CH, Allen RH *et al.* Plasma total homocysteine and risk of angina pectoris with subsequent coronary artery bypass surgery. *Am J Cardiol* 1997;**79**:799–801.

Cost-effectiveness of prevention of cardiovascular disease

20

CHEN Y. TUNG,
DANIEL B. MARK

INTRODUCTION

Medical care for cardiovascular disease is expensive. In the US, the total annual direct cost of caring for coronary heart disease, stroke, hypertension, and heart failure patients is estimated to be $159 billion with another $25 billion lost due to the effects of these diseases on employment and productivity.[1] Although Canada, Western Europe and many other industrialized countries spend less on medical care than the US, their incidence and prevalence of cardiovascular diseases are similar and their spending on this segment of the medical population as a proportion of all medical spending is comparable to the US. Since cardiovascular diseases are chronic diseases, therapies are largely palliative rather than curative. Patients may live 20 or 30 years with these disorders during which period of time they can experience numerous cardiovascular complications, often necessitating expensive hospitalizations and interventions.

In this context, it is easy to see why preventive medical care is appealing. By pre-empting the first manifestation of disease, the entire set of downstream consequences (with their attendant morbidity and cost) are also prevented. However, because it is rarely (if ever) possible to know precisely which at-risk subject will develop clinically manifest disease, preventive therapies must be given to many in order to protect a few. Consequently, the number needed to treat to prevent one new case of cardiovascular disease is often quite large. And since preventive therapies must generally be used indefinitely, the associated lifetime treatment costs are often substantial. For this reason, the economic attractiveness (assessed as the cost per additional unit of medical benefit produced) of preventive therapies has been controversial.[2]

In an earlier chapter, Hlatky reviewed the basic principles of cost-effectiveness analysis (see Chapter 6). As he pointed out, cost-effectiveness is a type of economic analysis that relates the extra benefits of a new strategy or therapy to the extra costs required to produce these benefits. Most commonly, such cost-effectiveness ratios are expressed as dollars (or other currency) required to add an extra life-year (or a quality-adjusted life-year) with the new therapy. In this context, an economically attractive ("cost-effective") therapy is one that yields an extra life-year for ≤ $50 000 while an economically unattractive ("not cost-effective") therapy is one that requires ≥ $100 000 for every extra life-year produced. (These benchmarks should not be interpreted dogmatically.[3]) For reasons reviewed in detail by Hlatky, the incremental effectiveness of a new therapy often has a much greater impact on its cost-effectiveness ratio than its incremental cost. Consequently, therapies where the number needed to treat to produce one extra unit of benefit (e.g. one extra survivor, one extra CAD-free subject) is large may not be economically attractive at even a modest price per subject treated, whereas therapies that are very effective or are applied to high risk populations may be economically attractive at a substantially greater cost per subject.

Preventive therapies are now typically divided into those used in disease-free subjects to prevent the initial manifestation of disease (i.e. primary prevention) and those used to prevent complications or disease progression in patients with established disease (i.e. secondary prevention). In this chapter, we will review what is known about the economics of both types of prevention for atherosclerotic coronary artery disease.

LIPIDS

Primary prevention

Many observational studies (reviewed in Chapter 13) have established a strong dose–response relationship between cholesterol level and risk of coronary artery disease (CAD). These data suggest that therapies that reduce cholesterol the most should prevent the greatest number of coronary events. Trials evaluating the first generation of lipid lowering agents (e.g. Helsinki [gemfibrozil], LRC-CPPT [cholestyramine], and WHO [clofibrate]) yielded modest reductions in cholesterol (~10%) and produced equivocal clinical results. Given the limited clinical effectiveness of these agents, cost-effectiveness analyses indicated that cholesterol reduction using them in primary prevention was economically unattractive, although therapy targeted at high risk subjects with multiple risk factors had a more favorable economic profile.[4] With HMG-CoA reductase inhibitors (statins), cholesterol reductions of 20–30% or more can be achieved and the cost-effectiveness of preventive therapy with these agents appears more favorable.

The most important study of primary prevention with statin therapy is the West of Scotland Coronary Prevention Study (WOSCOPS). WOSCOPS randomized 4159 men between the ages of 45 and 65 without overt coronary disease who had LDL cholesterol levels ≥ 155 mg/dl to either pravastatin (40 mg/d) or placebo.[5] During the mean follow-up of 4.9 years, pravastatin reduced the total cholesterol by 20% and decreased all-cause mortality by 22% (P=0.051). In absolute terms, at the end of 5 years the pravastatin arm had five per 1000 fewer deaths (P=0.13), 19 per 1000 fewer myocardial infarctions (MIs) (P<0.0001), 14 per 1000 fewer diagnostic catheterizations (P=0.007) and eight per 1000 fewer revascularization procedures (P=0.009) compared with usual care.

To evaluate the economic profile of statin therapy in primary prevention, Caro and colleagues used the WOSCOPS database along with long term survival of Scottish subjects (matched to the WOSCOPS subjects on age, gender, and cardiac event profile) obtained from the Scottish Record Linkage system.[6] This allowed the creation of a full survival curve for each treatment arm (empirical data for 5 years, Scottish survival data after 5 years based on subject event profile). Cost data were derived from Scottish 1996 medical prices and are cited below in their US dollar equivalents. Caro and coworkers estimated that to prevent one extra subject from moving from an asymptomatic state to clinical disease (indicated in the WOSCOPS database by death, MI, stroke, revascularization or angina), 31.4 men would need to be started on statin therapy. Pravastatin therapy (the average daily dose in the trial was 40 mg) was assigned a cost of $934 per year. The investigators estimated a drug treatment cost (over 5 years) of $3735 per subject with a cost offset of $85 per subject due to adverse events prevented by treatment, leaving a net undiscounted 5-year incremental cost per subject of $3650 ($3196 discounted at 6%). On the medical benefit side, the investigators projected an average (undiscounted) increase in life expectancy per subject of 0.25 years (approximately 0.10 years discounted). The resulting base-case cost-effectiveness ratio indicated that statin therapy as primary prevention in the WOSCOPS population added an additional life year at a cost of $32 600. Using the benchmarks cited earlier, this would be an economically attractive therapy (i.e. <$50 000 per life year added).

In contrast with these results, Goldman and colleagues found that primary prevention with lovastatin was not economically attractive except in the highest risk subgroups (e.g. middle aged men with cholesterol levels >300 mg/dl and several other risk factors).[7] Their analysis was based on pooled literature data regarding the efficacy of statin therapy and on the coronary heart disease (CHD) policy model, a computer simulation model that estimated the annual incidence of coronary disease in subjects aged 35–84 based on their risk factor profile.[8]

There are several possible reasons why the WOSCOPS analysis and the Goldman analysis reached different conclusions about the use of statin therapy as primary prevention. The most important is probably the different comparison (standard care) strategies used in the two analyses. Goldman and colleagues assumed that the new strategy being evaluated was a primary prevention program (added to a pre-existing secondary prevention program) and the comparison strategy was secondary prevention alone. By making secondary prevention with statin therapy part of standard care, the CHD policy model diminished the incremental benefits attributable to the primary prevention statin program without diminishing its costs (thereby increasing the cost per unit of benefit). From a policy point of view this is appropriate; because (as will be discussed below) the secondary prevention program is more economically attractive, it would logically be instituted first. Having put this program in place, the Goldman analysis asked whether now adding a primary prevention program to it was economically attractive (and concluded it was generally not). In contrast, Caro and colleagues made no explicit assumptions about the existence of a secondary prevention program in their subjects who developed clinical disease. While some of the Scottish subjects used in the WOSCOPS analysis to estimate life expectancy may have received statin therapy for secondary prevention, the prevalence of this would likely be quite low (given that many of the follow-up data used in the analysis were accrued between 1981 and 1994). Thus, the WOSCOPS model compared combined primary prevention against no use of statin therapy (i.e. no explicit use of secondary prevention statin therapy).

It is also possible that since coronary disease death rates are higher in Scotland than in the US, the middle aged asymptomatic Scottish males enroled in WOSCOPS were relatively high risk subjects by US criteria.[1] As discussed earlier, the higher risk the subject, the smaller the number needed to treat to prevent one new event and the more cost-effective a therapy will be.

R

Grade B

To the extent that secondary prevention with statin therapy is widely used and represents an accepted standard of care in a particular health care system, the results of the Goldman analysis would be more relevant. If such therapy is not widely used, the WOSCOPS analysis would be more germane for decision makers. The differences between the WOSCOPS analysis and the Goldman analysis highlight the importance of carefully defining the comparison strategy in any cost-effectiveness study. Cost-effectiveness analyses do not define invariant medical (or economic) truths. A therapy or strategy is economically attractive relative to a specifically defined alternative in a particular population at a given time. If the circumstances assumed in the analysis change materially, cost-effectiveness will need to be reassessed.

Secondary prevention

For patients with known CAD, several recently completed clinical trials have demonstrated significant clinical benefit for statin therapy. The Scandinavian Simvastatin Survival Study (4S) was a double-blind, placebo-controlled trial of adjusted dose simvastatin in 4444 men and women between the ages of 35 and 60 with a history of angina or prior MI and total cholesterol levels between 210 and 310 mg/dl despite dietary interventions.[9] Median follow-up was 5.4 years. The majority of patients received 20 mg/day of simvastatin but more than one-third required 40 mg/day. Simvastatin reduced total cholesterol by 25%, LDL-C by 35%, and decreased all-cause mortality by 30% ($P=0.003$). In absolute terms, over the 5-year study period the simvastatin arm had 32 per 1000 fewer deaths, 47 per 1000 fewer non-fatal MIs, and 59 per 1000 fewer revascularization procedures.

Pedersen and colleagues evaluated the incremental cost of simvastatin therapy in the 4S trial.[10] During the 5.4 years of trial follow-up, simvastatin therapy reduced hospitalizations for acute cardiovascular disease by 26% ($P<0.0001$) and total hospital days by 5138 ($P<0.0001$). The beneficial effect of simvastatin on hospitalization first became evident after 10 months of therapy, became statistically significant after 22 months, and appeared to increase over time. The use of antianginal and other cardiovascular drugs was not altered by statin therapy. Using US DRG based reimbursement rates as cost weights, Pedersen and coworkers estimated that simvastatin therapy would save an average of $3872 per patient due to a reduced need for hospitalization. The cost of the drug itself over the 5-year trial period averaged $4400 (discounted) per patient. Added to this was the cost of laboratory monitoring of the statin therapy (3–4 lipid and transaminase measurements in the first year, annually thereafter), which amounted to $250 (discounted) per patient. Thus, the net cost of the statin arm in the 4S trial over a mean of 1915 days of follow-up was $778 per patient, which equates to approximately $148 per patient per year.[10]

Several cost-effectiveness analyses of the 4S data have been presented. Two have attempted to provide a US perspective on the results of this Swedish trial. Schwartz and colleagues calculated a cost per life-year added with statin therapy of $18 100, with a cost per quality adjusted life-year added of $15 100.[11] These investigators made the conservative assumption that the costs and benefits of statin therapy would accrue only for the 5-year duration of the trial. Extrapolating the data to a lifetime perspective improved the cost per life-year saved to $5800.

In a separate analysis of the same data, Johanesson and colleagues constructed a modified Markov model to estimate the cost-effectiveness of using statin therapy for 5 years as secondary prevention for subgroups defined by age, sex, and cholesterol level.[12] The increased life expectancy produced by statin therapy was estimated from the 4S trial data. For a 59-year-old male with a pretreatment cholesterol level of 261 mg/dl, life expectancy was prolonged by 0.28 years; for a 59-year-old woman, the corresponding figure was 0.16 years. Cost figures were derived from four Swedish hospitals and converted to US dollars. For the prototypical 59-year-old man cited above, treatment costs averaged $2242 with a cost offset of $718 due to reduced morbidity, leaving a net incremental cost of $1524 per patient. The cost per year of life added with statin therapy for this patient was $5400.[12] For the corresponding 59-year-old woman, the net incremental cost was $1685 and the cost per life-year added with statin therapy was $10 500. The cost-effectiveness of 5 years of simvastatin ranged from $3800 per life-year added for a 70-year-old man with a cholesterol of 309 mg/dl to $27 400 for a 35-year-old woman with a cholesterol of 213 mg/dl. Extensive sensitivity analyses showed that statin therapy as secondary prevention was economically attractive under a wide range of assumptions.

Differences between cardiovascular care in Sweden and North America raise the question of how generalizable an economic analysis of the 4S trial is. For example, Swedish use of coronary revascularization procedures was far lower than in both the US and many European countries. In the 4S trial, the 5-year rate of revascularization was 17.2% in the placebo arm and 81% of those procedures were coronary bypass surgeries. With the higher procedure rates in the US, even a modest relative reduction in the need for revascularization could generate greater cost savings than were seen in 4S. In addition, important benefits of therapy may be seen in patients who have undergone revascularization. For example, in the Post Coronary Artery Bypass Graft Trial, aggressive lipid lowering with lovastatin to an LDL cholesterol <100 mg/dl reduced the need for repeat revascularization over a 4-year follow-up by 29% relative to moderate lipid lowering therapy.[13]

The CARE (Cholesterol and Recurrent Events) trial randomized 4159 post-MI patients with an average total cholesterol of 209 mg/dl to either pravastatin 40 mg/d or placebo.[14] After 5 years of follow-up, death and non-fatal MI were reduced by 24% ($P=0.003$). On an absolute basis, pravastatin therapy reduced coronary deaths by 11 per 1000 ($P=0.10$), non-fatal MIs by 18 per 1000 ($P=0.02$), and revascularization procedures by 47 per 1000 ($P<0.001$). Although an economic analysis of this trial has not yet been reported, evaluation of the absolute reduction in event rates suggests the cost-effectiveness ratio for statin therapy in this population will be less favorable than 4S but more favorable than the West of Scotland Study.

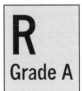

R
Grade A

TOBACCO

Cigarette smoking has many adverse health effects, among which is a significant risk of coronary disease. Given the addictive nature of smoking, most smoking cessation programs have limited success (~6% more patients stop smoking in 12 months than controls).[15] As reviewed in previous chapters, observational data suggest that those who succeed in quitting experience a sharp decline in the high cardiovascular risk associated with smoking in the first 6 months and their risk reaches the level of non-smokers after 1–2 years. This decrease in cardiovascular risk from smoking cessation has been estimated to increase life expectancy for each quitter by between 2 and 5 years.[16]

In a primary prevention study, Cummings and colleagues created a model to examine the cost-effectiveness of physician counseling (versus no counseling) on smoking cessation.[17] In their model, the authors assumed physician counseling led to a 2.7% decrease in smoking at 1 year with a subsequent 10% relapse rate. They assumed that the cost of this brief advice would be $12. These data yielded cost-effectiveness ratios from about $1000 to $1400 per year of life saved for men and from about $1700 to $3000 per year of life saved for women. Sensitivity analysis of a worst-case scenario (cost increased to $45, cessation rate decreased to 1%, 50% relapse after the first year) still indicated that brief physician advice to quit smoking was economically attractive. Although physician counseling is only very modestly effective, it remains an important prevention strategy because it is so inexpensive.

A similar analysis was performed by Oster and coworkers comparing nicotine gum as an adjunct to physician advice versus physician advice alone.[18] Based on randomized clinical trials, the authors assumed that nicotine gum for 4 months resulted in a cessation rate of 6.1% versus 4.5% for physician counseling. The cost of 4 months of nicotine gum was $161 (1984 figures). The cost-effectiveness ratios for this form of smoking cessation intervention ranged from about $6000 to $9000 per life-year added for men and about $9500 to $13 000 for women.

In the arena of secondary prevention, Krumholz and colleagues evaluated the effect of a nurse counseling smoking cessation program for post-MI patients.[19] Data from a previously published randomized trial were used in a decision model to define the 1-year quit rate and postcessation mortality.[20] The model assumed an incremental life expectancy of 1.7 years per quitter. The estimated cost of the program was $100 per patient. With an incremental smoking cessation rate of 26%, the program's cost-effectiveness ratio was highly favorable at $265 per life-year added. Sensitivity analyses showed that the cost-effectiveness ratio remained attractive at below $10 000 per life-year added if only 1% of smokers quit (instead of 26%) or if quitters gained only 0.1 year of life expectancy (instead of 1.7 years).

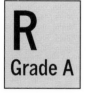

R
Grade A

For those who are able to stop smoking, observational data suggest significant gains in life expectancy. When these favorable estimates are combined with the relatively modest cost of smoking cessation interventions, these programs appear very economically attractive.

HYPERTENSION

Hypertension is an ideal disease for preventive therapy. It is a highly prevalent disorder with more than 60 million Americans (one in four adults) estimated to have the disease.[1] If untreated, hypertension leads to significant morbidity and mortality with coronary disease, heart failure, and strokes as the main cardiovascular complications. Finally, numerous interventions capable of lowering the blood pressure are available, including a wide spectrum of antihypertensive pharmacologic agents.

Using data from the Framingham study, Stason and Weinstein evaluated the cost-effectiveness of treatment of hypertension as primary prevention by modeling stepped care from screening for hypertension to drug compliance.[21] When stratified by initial blood pressure, age, gender, and race, most subgroups had cost-effectiveness ratios of less than $50 000 per quality-adjusted life-year. Not surprisingly, the cost-effectiveness was more favorable for those with higher initial blood pressures. Other determinants of cost-effectiveness were gender, age, and compliance.

Because hypertension usually requires lifetime therapy and as most antihypertensive agents are equally efficacious at reducing blood pressure, an important determinant of the economic profile of this form of prevention is the cost of the antihypertensive regimen. Edelson evaluated the cost-effectiveness of five specific monotherapies in persons without coronary disease aged 35–64.[22] The study involved simulation of 20 years of therapy (1990–2010) based on the coronary heart disease policy model. Effectiveness data were based on a meta-analysis of 153 studies in the literature. A key assumption was that if different agents produce the same reduction in diastolic blood pressure then the clinical benefit would be the same. Of the five agents studied, propranolol and hydrochlorothiazide had the most favorable cost-effectiveness ratios at $10 900 and $16 400 per year of life saved, respectively (expressed in 1987 dollars). Captopril had a higher cost and a lower estimated reduction in diastolic blood pressure, yielding a cost-effectiveness ratio of $72 100 per life-year saved. A limitation of the study was that estimates of 20-year outcomes were based on trials often lasting only several months. More recently, Littenberg modeled the cost-effectiveness of treating mild hypertension (diastolic pressure from 90 to 105) and also found the cost-effectiveness ratio was more attractive when the least costly antihypertensive agent was used.[23]

Even though the various antihypertensive agents are all capable of lowering blood pressure, only diuretics and beta-blockers have been shown to reduce cardiovascular morbidity and mortality in randomized clinical trials.[24] Data regarding the long term improvements in survival and reduction in cardiovascular disease for the other agents are inconclusive or absent. The recent controversy regarding calcium-channel blockers and potential increase in mortality serves as a reminder that we cannot assume that lower blood pressure means reduced cardiovascular disease and improved survival.[24]

Although no recent economic models have evaluated treatment of hypertension in the elderly, an overview of the available randomized trial data showed that 2–4 times as many younger subjects needed to be treated for 5 years to equal the benefits of therapy in preventing morbid and fatal events in the older population.[25] Thus, the economic profile of treatment in the elderly would be expected to be correspondingly favorable.

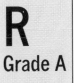

No large randomized clinical trials have evaluated hypertension control as secondary prevention and no cost-effectiveness models addressing this issue have been published.

EXERCISE

Many epidemiologic data support the idea that exercise on a regular basis is associated with less coronary heart disease and improved longevity. The improved outcomes are attributed, at least in part, to improvements in blood pressure, weight, and cholesterol levels. Analysis of the economic benefits of regular exercise in the primary prevention of cardiovascular disease has been limited to model simulations of clinical outcomes based on epidemiologic data. In 1000 hypothetical 35-year-old males, a 2000 Kcal/week jogging program (~20 miles) was assumed to reduce CHD risk by 50% compared with no exercise.[26] Direct costs attributed to the program included exercise equipment and a portion of an annual physician visit ($100 per year). The model also used a sliding scale of indirect costs due to lost productivity for time spent in jogging based on how much the individual disliked exercise ($9.00 per hour for subjects who disliked exercise, $4.50 per hour for neutral subjects, and $0 for subjects who enjoyed exercise).

The cost-effectiveness ratio using direct costs was $1395 per quality-adjusted life-year added; with the indirect costs, the ratio increased to $11 313 for regular exercise versus no exercise. The model assumed that compliance was 100% even for those who disliked exercise.

Most studies of exercise as secondary prevention in coronary disease involve structured programs of cardiac rehabilitation in post-MI patients. Because of limited sample size, no single randomized trial has definitely shown that cardiac rehabilitation reduces cardiac events. Two meta-analyses pooled data from the available trials and estimated a 20–25% reduction in death and non-fatal MI with cardiac rehabilitation in post-MI patients.[27,28] In 1993, Oldridge published an economic evaluation of an 8-week cardiac rehabilitation program in post-MI patients with mild to moderate depression and/or anxiety.[29] There were no differences in mortality or non-fatal MI, but quality of life, as measured by the time trade-off method, did improve, leading to 0.052 quality-adjusted life-years gained during the 1 year of follow-up. The corresponding cost-effectiveness ratio in this analysis was around $10 000 per quality-adjusted life-year added. Overall, the utility of structured cardiac rehabilitation programs is restricted due to limited availability and low rates of participation by eligible patients.

R Grade A/B

PHARMACOLOGIC SECONDARY PREVENTION

R Grade A

R Grade A

For those with coronary disease, aspirin therapy leads to a substantial reduction in death and non-fatal MI, while its costs and long term side effects are minimal.[30] Even though there are no formal cost-effectiveness analyses of aspirin therapy, its efficacy and low price make aspirin a "best buy" for secondary prevention therapy.

For post-MI patients, several trials have shown that beta-blockers prevent death and cardiac events. Goldman and coworkers performed a cost-effectiveness analysis of beta-blocker therapy after an acute MI in men.[31] The model assumed a mortality reduction of 25% per year for the first 3 years of therapy and 7% per year for years 4–6 with gradual attenuation over a subsequent 9-year period, based on an overview of the available literature. After 6 years of therapy, the model assumed beta-blockers were discontinued. The average cost of propranolol therapy used in this study was $208 per patient per year (1987 dollars). The cost-effectiveness ratios ranged from $2300 per life-year added in high risk patients up to $13 600 per life-year saved for low risk patients. The beta-blocker trials upon which this model was based were all completed in the prethrombolytic era and the cost-effectiveness of this form of secondary prevention has not been re-examined in patients undergoing reperfusion therapy. Furthermore, recent analyses of the Beta Blocker in Heart Attack Trial (BHAT) showed that MI patients who survived the first year with low to moderate risk courses (the typical profile of a postreperfusion therapy patient) did not evidence any long term benefit from beta-blockers.[32]

Angiotensin converting enzyme (ACE) inhibitor efficacy in secondary prevention was demonstrated in the SAVE (Survival And Ventricular Enlargement) trial, a double-blinded, placebo-controlled trial of captopril in 2231 acute MI survivors with an ejection fraction (EF) ≤40%. SAVE showed a 19% reduction in mortality during the average follow-up of 3.5 years. Based on SAVE results, Tsevat and colleagues created a decision model to determine the cost-effectiveness of ACE inhibitors in 50–80-year-old acute MI survivors with an EF of ≤40%.[33] Assuming that the survival benefits of captopril extended beyond 4 years, the cost-effectiveness ratios averaged $10 400 per quality-adjusted life-year or less (1991 dollars), depending on age. The use of 6 weeks of lisinopril therapy in acute MI patients was recently reported to be economically attractive ($2300 per extra death avoided at 6 weeks), based on the GISSI-3 trial data.[34]

PREVENTIVE STRATEGIES RIPE FOR COST-EFFECTIVENESS ANALYSIS

Multiple risk factor interventions

The studies reviewed thus far have focused on the cost-effectiveness of single risk factor interventions independent of other risk factors. In clinical practice, patients have multiple risk factors that require multiple concurrent interventions. The Stanford Coronary Risk Intervention Program (SCRIP) evaluated the effect of multifactor risk modification on the progression of angiographic CAD in 300 patients.[35] The intervention program consisted of exercise, dietary modifications, weight loss, lipid lowering pharmacotherapy, and smoking cessation. After 4 years, patients in the intervention arm had on average a 20% increase in exercise capacity, a 4% decrease in weight, and a 22% reduction in LDL cholesterol compared with those receiving usual care. Angiographically, those in the risk intervention arm had significant attenuation of coronary disease progression. In addition, there was a decrease in the composite endpoint of death, non-fatal MI, percutaneous transluminal coronary angioplasty (PTCA) and coronary artery bypass graft (CABG) ($P = 0.05$). Based on these results and the reduction in cardiac hospitalizations, Superko estimated the net cost of the program at $630 per patient per year.[36]

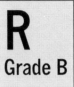

Diabetes

Diabetes leads to many long term complications including retinopathy, neuropathy, nephropathy, and atherosclerosis. However, only recently has control of glucose level been shown to reduce these complications. The DCCT (Diabetes Control and Complications Trial) randomized 1441 insulin-dependent diabetic patients to intensive insulin therapy versus conventional therapy with a mean follow-up of 6.5 years.[37] The intensive therapy arm showed significant reductions in retinopathy, neuropathy, and nephropathy. However, since there were few cardiovascular events in this primary prevention study, the lower rate of cardiovascular events in the intensive therapy arm was not significant ($P = 0.08$). A Monte Carlo simulation model based on the reduction of renal, neurological, and retinal complications estimated that the cost-effectiveness of lifetime intensive insulin therapy compared with conventional therapy was $28 661 per life-year added.[38]

Hormone replacement therapy

Compared to men, women's risk of coronary disease is low until the menopause, when the risk increases progressively. Numerous observational studies of estrogen replacement therapy in postmenopausal women have demonstrated a marked reduction in cardiac events (see Chapter 1). However, these findings are confounded by the generally healthier lifestyles and higher socioeconomic status of women who take estrogen replacement therapy. Estrogen also produces other important effects including a lower risk of osteoporosis, an increased risk of endometrial cancer (prevented by concurrent progesterone therapy), and a possibly increased risk of breast cancer. The benefits and risks of estrogen replacement therapy are currently under study in several ongoing randomized clinical trials (Heart Estrogen-Progestin Replacement Study and Women's Health Initiative). A preliminary cost-effectiveness analysis based on the earlier epidemiologic effectiveness literature (50% decrease in coronary heart disease deaths, 36% increase in breast cancer) yielded a cost of $12 620 per life-year added for a 10-year course of estrogen therapy (1990 dollars).[39]

Antioxidants

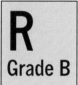

Antioxidants are thought to have a role in the prevention of atherosclerosis through the inhibition of LDL cholesterol oxidation (see Chapter 19). Some observational studies have shown a higher intake of vitamin E to be associated with lower rates of coronary disease. CHAOS (Cambridge Heart Anti-Oxidant Study) was a double-blinded, placebo-controlled trial of vitamin E in 2002 patients with angiographically proven CAD.[40] After 1.4 years, vitamin E was associated with a 23% reduction in non-fatal MI ($P=0.005$); however, this therapy was also associated with a non-significant increase in total mortality. A cost-effectiveness analysis of vitamin E prevention therapy will need to await the results of ongoing, large scale mortality trials.

CONCLUSIONS

Based on the cost-effectiveness data available, the following preventive strategies are considered economically attractive:

- secondary prevention with statins in hyperlipidemia;
- smoking cessation programs for both primary and secondary prevention;
- treatment of hypertension for primary prevention, especially with beta-blockers and thiazide diuretics;
- primary prevention with a regular exercise program;
- secondary prevention with cardiac rehabilitation;
- for post-MI patients, the use of beta-blockers and ACE inhibitors.

Even though no formal cost-effectiveness analysis has been done for aspirin (in secondary prevention), given its low cost and substantial clinical benefits, it should be considered in the "best buy" category. The cost-effectiveness of primary prevention with statins in hyperlipidemia remains unsettled. For the following preventive strategies we await more clinical effectiveness data prior to the consideration of cost-effectiveness analysis: hormone replacement therapy as primary prevention in postmenopausal women, antioxidants in secondary prevention and achieving euglycemia in diabetics for both primary and secondary prevention. Finally, it is important to keep in mind that as therapeutic options and their associated costs change, cost-effectiveness will need to be reassessed.

Acknowledgment

We are indebted to Tracey Simons MA for her assistance in the preparation of this chapter.

REFERENCES

1 American Heart Association. 1997 *heart and stroke statistical update*.

2 Weinstein MC. Economics of prevention. The costs of prevention. *J Gen Intern Med* 1990;**5**(Suppl): S89–S92.

3 Mason J, Drummond M, Torrance G. Some guidelines on the use of cost effectiveness league tables. *Br Med J* 1993;**306**:570–2.

4 Goldman L, Gordon DJ, Rifkind BM *et al.* Cost and health implications of cholesterol lowering. *Circulation* 1992;**85**:1960–8.

5 Shepherd J, Cobbe SM, Ford I *et al.* for the West of Scotland Coronary Prevention Study Group. Prevention of coronary heart disease with pravastatin in men with hypercholesterolemia. *N Engl J Med* 1995;**333**:1301–7.

6 Caro J, Klittich W, McGuire A *et al.* for the West of Scotland Coronary Prevention Study Group. The West of Scotland Coronary Prevention Study: weighing the costs and benefits of primary prevention with pravastatin. *Br Med J* 1997;(in press).

7 Goldman L, Weinstein MC, Goldman PA, Williams L. Cost effectiveness of HMG-CoA reductase inhibition for primary and secondary prevention of coronary heart disease. *JAMA* 1991;**265**: 1145–51.

8 Weinstein MC, Coxson PG, Williams LW *et al.* Forecasting coronary heart disease incidence, mortality, and cost: the coronary heart disease policy model. *Am J Public Health* 1987;**77**: 1417–26.

9 Scandinavian Simvastatin Survival Study Group. Randomised trial of cholesterol lowering in 4444 patients with coronary heart disease: the Scandinavian Simvastatin Survival Study (4S). *Lancet* 1994;**344**:1383–9.

10 Pedersen TR, Kjekshus J, Berg K *et al.* for the Scandinavian Simvastatin Survival Group. Cholesterol lowering and the use of healthcare resources: results of the Scandinavian Simvastatin Survival Group. *Circulation* 1996;**93**: 1796–802.

11 Schwartz JS, Kjekshus J, Pedersen TR. Impact of cholesterol lowering on resource use and cost among patients with coronary heart disease (CHD): results from the 4S. *Circulation* 1995;**92**: 510A.

12 Johannesson M, Jonsson B, Kjekshus J *et al.*, for the Scandinavian Simvastatin Survival Group. Cost effectiveness of simvastatin treatment to lower cholesterol levels in patients with coronary heart disease. *N Engl J Med* 1997;**336**:332–6.

13 The Post Coronary Artery Bypass Graft Trial Investigators. The effect of aggressive lowering of low-density lipoprotein cholesterol levels and low-dose anticoagulation on obstructive changes in saphenous vein coronary artery bypass grafts. *N Engl J Med* 1997;**336**:153–62.

14 Sacks FM, Pfeffer MA, Moye LA *et al.* for the CARE Investigators. Cholesterol And Recurrent Events (CARE). *N Engl J Med* 1996;**335**:1001–9.

15 Ockene JK. Smoking intervention: a behavioral, educational, and pharmacologic perspective. In: Ockene IS, Ockene JK. eds. *Prevention of coronary heart disease*. Boston: Little, Brown, 1992, pp 201–30.

16 Tsevat J, Weinstein MC, Williams LW, Tosteson ANA, Goldman L. Expected gains in life expectancy from various coronary heart disease risk factor modifications. *Circulation* 1991;**83**: 1194–201.

17 Cummings SR, Rubin SM, Oster G. The cost-effectiveness of counseling smokers to quit. *JAMA* 1989;**261**:75–9.

18 Oster G, Huse DM, Delea TE, Colditz GA. Cost-effectiveness of nicotine gum as an adjunct to physician's advice against cigarette smoking. *JAMA* 1986;**256**:1315–18.

19 Krumholz HM, Cohen BJ, Tsevat J, Pasternak RC, Weinstein MC. Cost-effectiveness of a smoking cessation program after myocardial infarction. *J Am Coll Cardiol* 1993;**22**:1697–702.

20 Taylor CB, Houston-Miller N, Killen JD, DeBusk RF. Smoking cessation after acute myocardial infarction: effects of a nurse-managed intervention. *Ann Intern Med* 1990;**113**:118–23.

21 Weinstein MC, Stason WB. *Hypertension: a policy perspective*. Cambridge: Harvard University Press, 1976.

22 Edelson JT, Weinstein MC, Tosteson AN *et al.* Long-term cost-effectiveness of various initial monotherapies for mild to moderate hypertension. *JAMA* 1990;**263**:407–13.

23 Littenberg B. A practice guideline revisited: screening for hypertension. *Ann Intern Med* 1995; **122**:937–9.

24 Psaty BM, Smith NL, Siscovick DS *et al.* Health outcomes associated with antihypertensive therapies used as first-line agents: a systematic review and meta-analysis. *JAMA* 1997;**277**: 739–45.

25 Mulrow CD, Cornell JA, Herrera CR *et al.* Hypertension in the elderly: implications and generalizability of randomized trials. *JAMA* 1994; **272**:1932–8.

26 Hatziandreu EI, Koplan JP, Weinstein MC, Caspersen CJ, Warner KE. A cost-effectiveness analysis of exercise as a health promotion activity. *Am J Public Health* 1988;**78**:1417–21.

27 Oldridge NB, Guyatt GH, Fischer ME, Rimm AA. Cardiac rehabilitation after myocardial infarction: combined experience of randomized clinical trials. *JAMA* 1988;**260**:945–50.

28 O'Connor GT, Buring JE, Yusuf S *et al.* An overview of randomized trials of rehabilitation with exercise after myocardial infarction. *Circulation* 1989;**80**: 234–44.

29 Oldridge N, Furlong W, Feeny D *et al.* Economic evaluation of cardiac rehabilitation soon after acute myocardial infarction. *Am J Cardiol* 1993; **72**:154–61.

30 Antiplatelet Trialists' Collaboration. Collaborative overview of randomized trials of antiplatelet therapy. I. Prevention of death, myocardial infarction, and stroke by prolonged antiplatelet therapy in various categories of patients. *Br Med J* 1994;**308**:81–106.

31 Goldman L, Sia STB, Cook EF, Rutherford JD, Weinstein MC. Costs and effectiveness of routine therapy with long-term beta-adrenergic antagonists after acute myocardial infarction. *N Engl J Med* 1988;**319**:152–7.

32 Viscoli CM, Horwitz RI, Singer BH. Beta-blockers after myocardial infarction: influence of first-year clinical course on long-term effectiveness. *Ann Intern Med* 1993;**118**:99–105.

33 Tsevat J, Duke D, Goldman L *et al.* Cost-effectiveness of captopril therapy after myocardial infarction. *J Am Coll Cardiol* 1995;**26**:914–19.

34 Franzosi MG, Maggioni AP, Santoro E, Tognoni G, for the GISSI-3 Trial. Cost-effectiveness analysis of an early lisinopril use in patients with acute myocardial infarction: results from GISSI-3 Trial. *J Am Coll Cardiol* 1997;**29**:49A.

35 Haskell WL, Alderman EL, Fair JM *et al.* Effects of intensive multiple risk factor reduction on coronary atherosclerosis and clinical cardiac events in men and women with coronary artery disease: the Stanford Coronary Risk Intervention Project (SCRIP). *Circulation* 1994;**89**:975–90.

36 Superko HR. Sophisticated primary and secondary atherosclerosis prevention is cost effective. *Can J Cardiol* 1995;**11**:35–40.

37 The Diabetes Control and Complications Trial Research Group. The effect of intensive treatment of diabetes on the development and progression of long-term complications in insulin-dependent diabetes mellitus. *N Engl J Med* 1993;**329**: 977–86.

38 The Diabetes Control and Complications Trial Research Group. Lifetime benefits and costs of intensive therapy as practiced in the Diabetes Control and Complications Trial. *JAMA* 1996; **276**:1409–15.

39 Tosteson ANA, Weinstein MC. Cost effectiveness of hormone replacement therapy after the menopause. *Baillière's Clin Obstet Gynaecol* 1991; **5**:943–59.

40 Stephens NG, Parsons A, Schofield PM *et al.* Randomised controlled trial of vitamin E in patients with coronary disease: Cambridge Heart Antioxidant Study (CHAOS). *Lancet* 1996;**347**: 781–6.

Estrogens and cardiovascular disease

21

JACQUES E. ROSSOUW

In the United States the number of women who die annually from cardiovascular disease is higher than that of men. In 1992, major cardiovascular diseases accounted for 474 601 deaths in women and 439 307 deaths in men.[1] The number of deaths from coronary heart disease (CHD) was slightly lower in women (233 136) compared to men (246 913), but the number of deaths from stroke was higher in women (67 124) than in men (56 645), as were the number of deaths from pulmonary embolism (5097 in women compared to 4149 in men). In summary, cardiovascular disease is at least as large a health problem in women as in men and for some conditions, the disease burden is greater in women than in men.

However, CHD in particular occurs at a later age in women than in men and this is part of the reason why early trials (including estrogen trials) attempting to prevent "premature" CHD focused on middle aged men. On average, CHD death occurs about 10 years later in women (Figure 21.1). The incidence rate of CHD mortality rises after age 65 and rises particularly steeply after age 75. Though their rates are lower at any age, the fact that there are more older women explains why the absolute numbers of CHD events are similar. The great majority of CHD events in women occur after age 75. Deaths from strokes and pulmonary embolism also rise markedly with age. Since CHD and strokes are the major contributors to overall cardiovascular disease rates, estrogen effects on these conditions will dominate the overall cardiovascular outcome.

The sex differential in the age of onset of CHD is one of the reasons why estrogen is of interest as a potential preventive treatment for CHD. Lipid levels in children of both sexes are similar until puberty, when HDL cholesterol levels fall by about 10 mg/dl in boys only, while LDL cholesterol levels decrease by about 5 mg/dl in girls.[2] These changes may be attributable to rising androgen and estrogen levels in boys and girls respectively. The sex differential for HDL cholesterol persists through most of adult life, but is less marked in older persons. LDL cholesterol levels rise during adulthood and in older women LDL cholesterol levels eventually catch up with those in men. Estrogen levels in women gradually decline starting some years before the menopause, during which time LDL cholesterol levels rise and HDL cholesterol levels decrease.[3] These lipid changes may underlie the lower CHD risk in premenopausal women and the gradual increase in postmenopausal women. Women who have a premature menopause, especially a

315

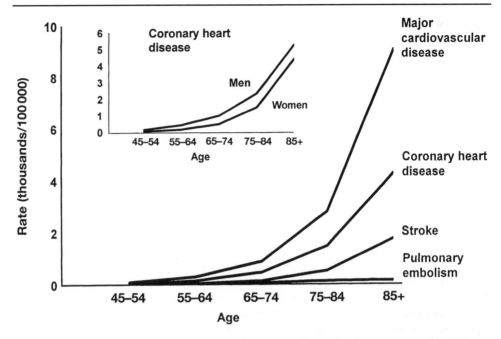

Figure 21.1 Mortality rates by 10-year age groups for major cardiovascular disease, coronary heart disease, stroke, and pulmonary embolism in US women, 1992.[1] Inset: Comparison of coronary heart disease mortality rates by age for men and women.

surgical menopause with removal of the ovaries, have a higher CHD risk which can be abolished by the administration of estrogen.[4] When exogenous estrogen is administered to postmenopausal women, LDL cholesterol levels decrease, HDL cholesterol levels increase, and triglyceride levels increase.[5–8] However, exogenous estrogen also has multiple other effects. Some changes in coagulation factors are potentially favorable (e.g. a decrease in fibrinogen level[6–8]) while others are potentially unfavorable (e.g. an increase in factor VII[7,8]), and the net effect of estrogen on coagulation is uncertain. Other potential influences of estrogen on vascular biology include direct effects on the vessel wall, which improve blood flow,[9,10] and antioxidant properties that may slow the early stages of atherosclerosis. It should be noted that many, but not all, of the biologic effects of estrogen are counteracted by progestin which is now commonly prescribed in combination with estrogen in women with an intact uterus.[6–8]

Thus, there is a plethora of potential mechanisms by which estrogen may reduce the risk of CHD. Unfortunately, the existence of mechanisms does not necessarily translate into clinical benefit. A treatment that has a favorable effect on an intermediate mechanism may decrease the incidence of the clinical event of interest, may have no effect or may actually increase the event. It may also have unanticipated adverse effects on other clinical events.[11] For example, a number of early lipid lowering drugs such as thyroxin and estrogen were abandoned after it was found that though they decreased cholesterol levels they also increased the cardiovascular morbidity and mortality in men.[12] Similarly, some calcium-channel blockers are effective at lowering blood pressure, but increase total mortality.[13]

OBSERVATIONAL STUDIES

Coronary heart disease

More than 30 observational studies have consistently suggested that women who are taking estrogen appear to have a lower risk of heart disease[14–19] and a few studies have also shown similar apparent risk reductions for estrogen when used in combination with progestin.[17–19] Only a few key studies will be reviewed in detail, because they sufficiently illustrate the findings from observational studies and their limitations.

THE NURSES' HEALTH STUDY

The women in this study comprise one of the largest and best studied cohorts in the US.[17] The 1976 baseline examination included 121 700 nurses aged 30–55 years, of whom 21 726 were postmenopausal. With the passage of time a progressively larger proportion entered the menopause and have contributed data to a series of papers on the associations between menopause, hormone replacement therapy, and cardiovascular disease. Data on hormone use and health status were updated biennially by questionnaire. The most recent analysis included 59 337 women with up to 16 years average follow-up for a total experience of 662 891 person-years. Women who had never used hormones accounted for half the data, while current users and past users accounted for about one-quarter each. Conjugated equine estrogen accounted for about two-thirds of the estrogen used. Proportional hazards models were used to calculate relative risks for the incidence of clinical outcomes, using women who had never used hormones as the reference group. Multivariate adjustment for age, age at menopause, body mass index, cigarette smoking, hypertension, elevated cholesterol levels, diabetes, family history of myocardial infarction, prior use of oral contraceptives, type of menopause (natural or surgical), and 2-year time interval was performed.

The analyses included 584 non-fatal myocardial infarctions, 186 deaths due to coronary disease, 572 strokes, and 553 instances of coronary revascularization procedures (angioplasty or bypass surgery). The adjusted relative risk of major coronary disease in current users compared to never-users was 0.60 (95% CI 0.47–0.76), and in past users it was 0.85 (0.71–1.01). The relative risk increased towards unity with time since last use, even last use as recently as 3 years ago (Figure 21.2). Among current users, longer duration of use was associated with a (non-significant) trend towards a higher relative risk, as was increasing dose of estrogen, though the risk remained below unity. Current users of estrogen alone had a relative risk of 0.60 (0.43–0.83) and current users of estrogen with progestin had a relative risk of 0.39 (0.19–0.78). The relative risk was lower in younger than in older women. In contrast to the findings for major coronary disease, coronary revascularization procedures were equally common in current users compared to never-users (relative risk 0.99; 95% CI 0.78–1.26).

Taken at face value, the data from the Nurses' Health Study indicate that current estrogen use is associated with a lower relative risk of major coronary disease irrespective of whether progestin was added or not. The progestin use data are scanty in that there were only eight cases of major coronary disease in 27 161 person-years of follow-up compared to 47 cases in 82 626 person-years of follow-up for estrogen alone. Nonetheless, the progestin data are consistent with those of other studies.[8,19]

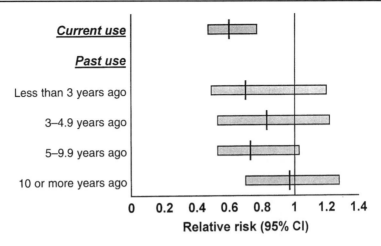

Figure 21.2 Relative risks and 95% confidence intervals for coronary heart disease in the Nurses' Health Study, comparing current users and past users of estrogen with never-users.[17]

The design feature of updating the hormone and health status data every 2 years provides specific insights into some of the biases that may be operating. The finding that current users, but not past users, exhibit a lower risk of major coronary disease may be explained by immediate and direct effects on the vessel wall or on coagulation factors which rapidly disappear when the estrogen is withdrawn. However, an immediate beneficial effect on the vessel wall is made unlikely by the finding that there was no reduction in relative risk of coronary revascularization in current estrogen users. Most patients undergo revascularization for symptoms and if estrogens had a direct effect symptoms would have been less likely in users and when they occurred might well have led to the discontinuation of estrogen. In both cases the result would be a lower rate of revascularization in estrogen users and it is worrisome that this was not observed. At a minimum, the unchanged relative risk for revascularization questions the idea that estrogen has an immediately beneficial effect in women with existing CHD, and keeping in mind the greater likelihood of discontinuation in users who develop symptoms, estrogen may even have a deleterious effect. Another possible explanation, that estrogen users may have been under closer medical surveillance and would therefore be more likely to receive surgical intervention, is untenable in a population of nurses. The data in regard to revascularization have implications for the interpretation of the data for CHD events: if estrogens confer no immediate benefit, the finding of lower CHD rates in current users (but not past users) may be due to the placebo effect known to operate in subjects who are regularly taking medications or to selection bias as to who goes onto estrogen and who is removed from therapy. It is likely that many women with symptoms of heart disease are selectively disbarred or removed from therapy, which would decrease the relative risk for women who remain on therapy and increase that for women who go off therapy.

On the other hand, the study also provides little evidence of long term beneficial effects of estrogen, as might have been expected if it operated through a lipid mechanism. Past users, even those who stopped less than 3 years ago, did not show significant benefit and among current users there were non-significant trends towards higher risk with longer duration of use and higher doses – the opposite of what might have been expected from an antilipemic agent. Aside from the generic issue of how much weight

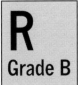

to accord observational studies (see below), these observations suggest that the findings of the Nurses' Health Study should not be taken as strong evidence for a cardioprotective effect of estrogen.

UPPSALA STUDY

The most extensive report of the European experience comes from Sweden.[18] This was a prospective cohort study linking hormone prescriptions over a 3-year period (1977–1980) to the central health records (1977–1983) of the entire female population of the Uppsala health care region (1.4 million). Pharmacy records identified 23 174 women aged 35 years and older who were prescribed hormones and their incidence of myocardial infarction was compared to that of the background population. Average follow-up time for the hormone cohort was 5.8 years for a total of 133 372 person-years, during which time 227 myocardial infarctions were recorded. There were 8162 myocardial infarctions during 2.1 million person-years in the background population. Because this was a record linkage study, it was not possible to characterize the study population in any detail beyond age, date of prescription, and type of hormone prescribed. Questionnaire interviews with a subsample indicated that the women prescribed hormones were more likely to have had an oophorectomy or hysterectomy, to exercise, to be leaner, to be current smokers, and to have a higher level of education. It was not possible to make direct adjustments for these factors in the analysis. The subsample findings also indicated that about half the women who entered the cohort in the first 15 months were current users filling repeat prescriptions, while those who entered later were new users. By the end of the observation period almost four-fifths of the cohort were no longer taking hormones. Therefore, women who entered early had a longer estimated average exposure to hormones (about 5 years) than those who entered later (about 3 years). Since information on prescriptions during the years 1981–1983 was not available for the entire cohort, it is not possible to make a clear distinction between current users and past users. This complicates the interpretation of the data on relative risk for myocardial infarction.

The types of hormones used in the Uppsala Study differed from those in the Nurses' Health Study. About one-quarter received a specific combined estradiol-levonorgestrel pill, one-half received either estradiol or conjugated equine estrogen (sometimes with a progestin), and one-quarter received other estrogens (chiefly estriol compounds of weak potency). The main findings were that the age-adjusted relative risk of myocardial infarction in hormone users was 0.81 (0.71–0.92), in users of the more potent estradiol or conjugated equine estrogen compounds it was 0.74 (0.61–0.88), and in users of the weaker other estrogens it was 0.90 (0.74–1.08). Further subgroup analyses indicated a relative risk for users of the combined pill of 0.50 (0.28–0.80), and for users of estradiol or conjugated equine estrogen of 0.80 (0.65–0.97) (Figure 21.3). Thus, the addition of the progestin levonorgestrel to estradiol did not abolish the apparent cardioprotective effect of estradiol. In this respect the findings are similar to those of the Nurses' Health Study. Younger women appeared to benefit more than older women. In the Uppsala Study it was not possible to examine whether current use of hormones had a different impact from past use, though it is worth noting that the relative risks for myocardial infarction in the hormone users were highest in the first few years, when more of the women would have been current users and would have used the hormones for a longer period of time. These women should have benefited most if the hormones

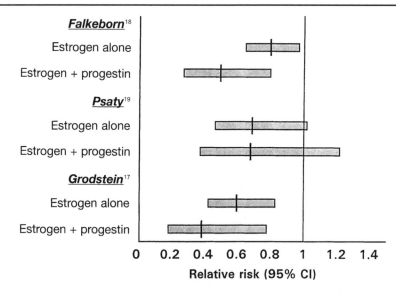

Figure 21.3   Relative risks and 95% confidence intervals for coronary heart disease comparing users of estrogen alone, and of estrogen with progestin, with non-users in three studies.

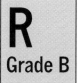

were protective, but they did not. Conversely, the lowest relative risks were recorded at the end of the observation period, when only about one-fifth of the women were still taking hormones. These internal inconsistencies raise some doubt about the validity of the investigators' conclusion that the hormones were indeed cardioprotective.

Cerebrovascular disease

The data for stroke are less consistent than those for coronary heart disease.[14,17,20–28] Among the 11 published observational studies, seven had a nominal decrease in relative risk for stroke in hormone users (three statistically significant)[14,20,23] and four had a nominal increase (one statistically significant)[27] (Figure 21.4). A recent meta-analysis of stroke studies suggested that in aggregate, estrogen users had the same risk for all strokes as non-users.[16] However, an examination of data from the Nurses' Health Study looking at subtypes of strokes is not reassuring.[17] Even though the relative risk for all strokes (121 cases) in current hormone users was 1.03 (0.82–1.31), for ischemic strokes (73 cases) there was a significant 40% excess, relative risk 1.40 (1.02–1.92). Furthermore, for all strokes there was a significant increase in relative risk with increasing dose of current estrogen (P for trend = 0.047), with a point estimate as high as 1.86 (0.59–5.90) at the highest dose of more than 1.25 mg conjugated equine estrogen. Users of estrogen alone tended to have a higher risk than users of estrogen in combination with progestin. There was no excess of strokes in past users. The results of the Uppsala Study were different: the relative risk for all strokes in hormone users was 0.90 (0.81–0.99) and there was no excess risk in any hormone subgroup or by type of stroke.[20] However, as noted above, the studies are not readily compared because of methodologic differences.

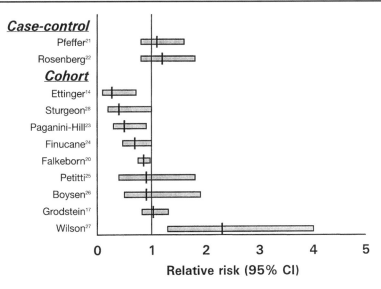

Figure 21.4 Relative risks and 95% confidence intervals for all strokes comparing users of estrogen with non-users in 11 studies.

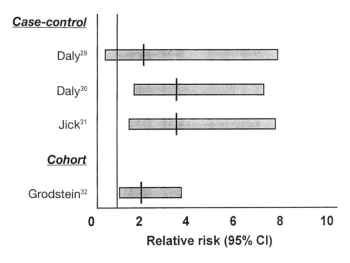

Figure 21.5 Relative risks and 95% confidence intervals for venous thromboembolism comparing users of estrogen with non-users in four studies.

Venous thromboembolism

One recent cohort study and three case-control studies have provided the first indication that hormone replacement therapy carries an increased risk of venous thromboembolism (deep vein thrombosis and pulmonary embolism).[29-32] The studies are consistent in showing an increased relative risk for current use of hormones (Figure 21.5). The small case-control study of Daly *et al.* (18 cases)[29] reported a non-significant relative risk of 2.3 (0.6–8.1), while two larger case-control studies reported significantly elevated relative risks of 3.6 (1.8–7.3; 44 cases) and 3.6 (1.6–7.8; 42 cases)[30,31] and in the Nurses' Health Study cohort a relative risk of 2.1 (1.2–3.8; 123 cases) was reported.[32]

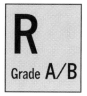

Grade A/B

The two studies that had separate data on past and current use reported significantly elevated relative risks for current use only. In all three studies with data, recent onset of current use conferred higher risk than long duration of use, consistent with an immediate effect on coagulation factors.[30–32] Two out of three studies had evidence of a dose–response relationship.[31,32] Estrogen alone, as well as estrogen with progestin, appeared to be associated with a higher risk.

General critique of observational studies of estrogen and cardiovascular disease

The findings from observational studies need to be treated with a great deal of caution. In general, women who take estrogen are healthier than women who do not.[33] Estrogen users have a lower risk of death from almost all causes, including cancers and other diseases with no plausible biological relationship to estrogens.[28,33] The studies with the lowest relative risks for CHD death also have the lowest risk for cancer death.[34] Unintended selection of healthy women may explain these findings and may also contribute to an exaggerated estimate of a cardioprotective effect and an underestimation of adverse effects. Importantly, a better health profile has been shown to be present even before women are prescribed estrogens.[35] Women who have recently stopped HRT have higher relative risks for all causes of death, indicating cessation of treatment when risk factors or early disease become manifest.[28] The selection of who is placed on treatment and who is taken off treatment, rather than the treatment itself, may account for much of the lower subsequent risk of disease, including heart disease, in women who are currently on hormone replacement therapy (HRT).

It is impossible to correct for all the potential biases in analysing observational data. Measurement of potential confounding factors may be inadequate and confounders that have not been measured cannot be corrected for. Furthermore, combining the results of the observational studies in meta-analyses is not helpful and may even be misleading. If there is a systematic bias in study data, then combining the data of all studies ascribes a significance level to the bias, but does not illuminate the basic question.[36] In spite of their consistency in the case of CHD, it is impossible to tell from the observational studies whether estrogen use confers real benefit for CHD or what the size of any effect might be. In the case of stroke, the observational studies are not consistent and thus are even less helpful. For venous thromboembolism, the findings are consistently in an adverse direction. Given the healthy user selection biases towards showing benefit, the adverse findings for venous thromboembolism have a high degree of credibility.

Reliable information can be obtained from randomized controlled clinical trials which, if large enough, will eliminate the possibility that differences between study groups account for the results. Even though insufficient for public health recommendations, the observational data are certainly strong enough to justify the need for trials directly measuring effects on all these clinical outcomes. The fallacy of relying on observational data has been illustrated by recent experience with beta-carotene. Even though a substantial body of epidemiologic data, buttressed by plausible biological mechanisms, suggested that beta-carotene is associated with lower risk of CHD and cancer,[37,38] when the hypothesis was put to the test in three separate clinical trials no benefit for CHD could be shown.[39–41] Rather, in two of the trials there was an excess of deaths, particularly deaths due to cardiovascular disease and lung cancer.[39,40]

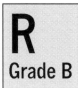

Estrogen and cardiovascular disease

- Cardiovascular disease is a major health problem in postmenopausal women.
- Observational studies suggest that estrogen replacement might lower CHD risk, have no effect on stroke, and increase risk of thromboembolism and breast cancer.
- Because of healthy user biases the observational studies are likely to overestimate the benefits and underestimate the risks of long term estrogen use
- Current clinical trials will quantify the real effects of estrogen on clinical disease outcomes.

CLINICAL TRIALS

Clinical trials measuring the effects of estrogen on potential mediators of a clinical effect on CHD have confirmed that estrogen has multiple effects on blood lipids, coagulation factors, and other potential mediators of CHD.[5–8] The effects of estrogen on blood lipids (lowering LDL cholesterol, raising HDL cholesterol) are regarded as being favorable in spite of a propensity to raise triglycerides. Similarly, the effects on vascular reactivity and blood flow are promising even though these physiologic findings have not been related to clinical disease outcomes.[9,10] The data on coagulation factors are mixed and it is not at all clear whether the net effect is favorable or unfavorable.[6–8]

Currently, there are data from only one trial of estrogen to prevent clinical CHD in women.[42] Published in 1979, the study was too small to provide meaningful results. Eighty-four matched pairs of postmenopausal women were randomly assigned to conjugated equine estrogen 2.5 mg daily with cyclic medroxyprogesterone acetate 10 mg on 7 days of the month. During 10 years of follow-up there were three myocardial infarctions in the placebo group and one in the hormone group. Larger trials were done in men in the 1960s and 1970s using relatively high doses of estrogen as a lipid lowering agent to prevent CHD. The largest trial was nested in the Coronary Drug Project, where conjugated equine estrogen in doses of 2.5 mg and 5 mg daily or placebo was administered to men aged 30–64 years who had previously suffered a myocardial infarction. The trial of estrogen 5 mg daily in 3907 men was stopped after 2 years because of an excess of CHD in the estrogen (11%) compared to the placebo (7%) group and also an excess of venous thromboembolism and an adverse trend in total mortality.[43] The trial using the lower dose of 2.5 mg estrogen in 3890 men was also stopped ahead of time at 4.7 years because of excess cancer and thromboembolism, together with an adverse trend for total mortality.[44] At the time of stopping the trial, the rates of CHD in the estrogen and placebo groups were identical at 23%. Three small secondary prevention trials in men provided mixed results with no real indication of benefit for preventing reinfarction (Table 21.1).[45–47] Thus, even though estrogen has the same lipid lowering effect in men as in women, a substantial body of clinical trial data has failed to show benefit and in the largest study there was sufficient evidence of harm to mandate the early stopping of the trial.

The state of uncertainty about the risks and benefits of long term estrogen (and progestin) use has prompted the initiation of three large clinical trials in women. The Heart and Estrogen/Progestin Study (HERS) of over 2700 women is a secondary prevention trial of estrogen and progestin in women with a uterus who have had a documented previous myocardial infarction and will report around the year 2000. The

Table 21.1 Results of randomized trials of estrogen to prevent coronary heart disease

	Drug, daily dose	Duration in years	Number of participants	Rate of CHD (%)	
				Placebo	Estrogen
Women					
Nachtigall[42]	CEE 2.5 mg + cyclic MPA 10 mg	10	168	3.6	1.2
Men					
Marmorston[47]	CEE 1.25–2.5 mg	2	185	23.6	8.1
Oliver[45]	Ethinyl estradiol 200 µg	5	100	48.0	44.0
Schoch[46]	CEE 1.25 mg	3	284	29.3	36.2
CDP[43]	CEE 5 mg	2 (stopped early)	3907	7.5	11.0
CDP[44]	CEE 2.5 mg	4.7 (stopped early)	3890	23.4	23.3

CEE, conjugated equine estrogens; MPA, medroxyprogesterone acetate.

Women's Health Initiative (WHI), which includes a large clinical trial of 27 500 women with and without a uterus and with and without previous heart disease, will test both estrogen alone and estrogen with progestin depending on uterus status. The results will be available after 2005. In the United Kingdom, the Medical Research Council has launched a trial very similar to WHI, except that one treatment arm includes estrogen and progestin in women who do not have a uterus. In aggregate, these trials have the ability to answer all the major questions about the risks and benefits of long term HRT.

RISKS AND BENEFITS OF ESTROGENS

In the virtual absence of trial data using clinical outcomes in women, any discussion of cardiovascular risks and benefits is highly speculative. The observational data suggest that estrogen use is associated with a potential reduction in CHD, no effect on stroke overall (but a possible increase in ischemic stroke), and an increase in venous thromboembolism. As indicated above, there is good reason to think that the observational data overstate the benefits and understate the risks. The final answer will not be found within the observational studies because of their potential for bias. Clinical trials will provide an unbiased estimate of the true effect of estrogen and these effects may then be contrasted with those suggested by observational studies. At one extreme, it is possible that estrogen is indeed cardioprotective and there is no healthy user bias, in which case the trials will confirm the observational data and the overall effect on cardiovascular disease would be beneficial, given that CHD is more common than either stroke or pulmonary embolism. At the other extreme, it is possible that estrogen is not cardioprotective and the bias in observational studies is strong, in which case the real overall effect on cardiovascular disease would be adverse. All kinds of intermediate outcomes are possible, ranging from modest benefit to no effect to a modestly adverse outcome.

It is possible to construct a unifying hypothesis for the findings from observational studies and clinical trials in men. The cardiovascular effects of estrogen might depend on the balance between favorable lipid changes and unfavorable coagulation changes[48]

and on the relative importance of these changes in different parts of the vascular system. For example, for CHD the effects of favorable lipid changes might predominate, for stroke the lipid and coagulation changes might be in balance, and for venous thromboembolism unfavorable coagulation changes might predominate. There could also be a dose-dependent effect, in that the coagulation changes may predominate at higher doses.[48] This would explain the higher CHD incidence found in some trials using high doses of estrogen in men and the trend towards less apparent benefit for CHD (and increased risk for stroke) at doses of 1.25 mg and higher in the Nurses' Health Study. Tension between the lipid and coagulation changes would also fit with the observational study findings that the combination of estrogen with progestin is associated with a risk reduction for CHD similar to that of estrogen alone. Progestins blunt both the increases in HDL cholesterol and the increases in factor VII caused by estrogen and thus their net effect on CHD might be neutral.

Aside from the cardiovascular risks and benefits, estrogen also has a potential for affecting many other diseases. The most pertinent risk is that of cancer, especially cancers of the breast and endometrium. It appears that cancer of the endometrium can be avoided by adding progestin in women with a uterus (though long term data on this point are not available). The effect of estrogen on cancer of the breast is uncertain, because only observational data exists at this point. These data suggest little risk for short term use (less than 5 years), but increased risk for current use over longer periods of time.[16,49] For reasons previously discussed, the observational data may underestimate the risk of breast cancer. Other potential risks include pancreatitis (resulting from the aggravation of pre-existing hypertriglyceridemia) and cholecystitis. Disease conditions that may benefit from estrogen use include osteoporotic fractures and Alzheimer's disease. Further, any consideration of the risks and benefits of estrogen use has to include the balance of effects on overall quality of life. The avoidance of disease is the most important determinant of good quality of life, but symptoms caused by hormones (e.g. breast tenderness, bleeding, mood changes) or alleviated by hormones (e.g. urinary symptoms, vaginal atrophy) enter into consideration as well.

R
Grade B

TREATMENT RECOMMENDATIONS

Based on current evidence estrogen should not be considered for prevention or treatment of CHD. Neither primary prevention of CHD nor prevention of reinfarction has been demonstrated in clinical trials in women and there are questions about the long term safety of estrogen. Breast cancer is the most prominent safety concern, but an increased rate of thromboembolism also raises concerns about the effects of estrogen on blood coagulation. There are a number of effective and safe prevention treatments for CHD, backed by rigorous evidence including clinical trials. The existence of these alternative treatments means that there are no pressing reasons to consider using the unproven and potentially unsafe estrogen. The better proven treatments include those that ameliorate the traditional risk factors (high blood pressure, high blood cholesterol, smoking cessation) or have effects on platelet function (low dose aspirin) or myocardial oxygen demand (beta-blockers). Each of these treatments works in women as well as in men, and they have been shown to reduce CHD events without increasing non-cardiac mortality, so that the net effect tends towards a lower total mortality.

Similarly, estrogen is not a first line treatment for lipid disorders. Estrogen undoubtedly lowers LDL cholesterol and raises HDL cholesterol, but the same questions about long term safety militate against its use for this purpose. In women with a uterus, the concomitant administration of a progestin will reduce the HDL raising effect of estrogen and the regimen will cause the resumption of vaginal bleeding in the majority of women. The triglyceride raising effects of estrogen may precipitate pancreatitis in those with pre-existing hypertriglyceridemia. With the advent of the HMG-CoA reductase inhibitors, there is now a very effective and safe treatment for high LDL cholesterol which lowers CHD mortality. These drugs also have potentially clinically important HDL raising and triglyceride lowering effects and are remarkably free of side effects. The use of these drugs for the treatment of most lipid disorders appears to be a far more rational choice than the use of estrogen.

Treatment guidelines

- Estrogen should not be used for the prevention or treatment of CHD.
- Alternative proven effective and safe treatments are available for the prevention and treatment of CHD.
- Estrogen is not a first line treatment for high LDL cholesterol levels
- Estrogen may occasionally be used as a second line treatment for high LDL cholesterol levels if other lipid lowering drugs cannot be used.
- Estrogen prescribed for another condition (e.g. osteoporosis) in a woman with high LDL cholesterol levels may obviate the need for another lipid lowering therapy.
- Contraindications to estrogen include raised triglyceride levels or a history of thromboembolism or breast cancer.

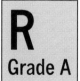

However, there may be a place for estrogen as a second line treatment for lipid disorders in the rare situation where the standard lipid lowering therapies cannot be used or have been ineffective. There may also be a place for estrogen as lipid lowering therapy when the estrogen is prescribed for other reasons. For example, in a woman with menopausal symptoms or with osteoporosis who also has a high LDL cholesterol, the prescription of estrogen may avoid the use of a second drug. Because of the safety concerns, the estrogen dose should be the lowest consistent with a therapeutic effect, and in a woman with a uterus, the estrogen should be coadministered with a progestin to protect the uterus. Estrogen should not be used in women with blood triglyceride levels above 400 mg/dl or in those with a history of active or recent thromboembolism or who have ever had breast cancer. If estrogen is used, regular monitoring for breast cancer is mandatory.

These treatment guidelines are subject to modification once the results from clinical trials become available. If the trials show substantial benefit for CHD prevention and minimal risk, estrogen may become a first line treatment for CHD and lipid disorders in women, either alone or in combination with other treatments. It should be noted that several recent treatment guidelines allow for more liberal use of estrogen than those discussed above.[50-52] However, all these bodies also stress that clinical trials are needed. This puts the authors of the guidelines in the uncomfortable position of making a recommendation without having the requisite evidence. A more responsible position is not to recommend estrogens until the evidence is available. In the meantime, there is no shortage of alternatives proven to be effective and safe.

REFERENCES

1 National Center for Health Statistics. *Vital statistics of the United States, 1992, vol II, mortality, part A.* Washington: Public Health Service, 1996.

2 National Heart, Lung, and Blood Institute. *The Lipid Research Clinics population studies data book: volume I – the prevalence study.* Bethesda: US Department of Health and Human Services, NIH Pub. No. 80–1527, 1980.

3 Matthews KA, Meilahn E, Kuller LH *et al.* Menopause and risk factors for coronary heart disease. *N Engl J Med* 1989;**321**:641–6.

4 Colditz GA, Willett WC, Stampfer MJ *et al.* Menopause and the risk of coronary heart disease in women. *N Engl J Med* 1987;**316**:1105–10.

5 Walsh BW, Schiff I, Rosner B *et al.* Effects of postmenopausal estrogen replacement on the concentrations and metabolism of plasma lipoproteins. *N Engl J Med* 1991;**325**:1196–204.

6 Writing Group. Effects of estrogen or estrogen/progestin regimens on heart disease risk factors in postmenopausal women. The Postmenopausal Estrogen/Progestin Interventions (PEPI) Trial. *JAMA* 1995;**273**:199–208.

7 Lobo RA, Pickar JH, Wild RA, Walsh B, Hirvonen E. Metabolic impact of adding medroxy-progesterone acetate to conjugated estrogen therapy in postmenopausal women. *Obstet Gynecol* 1994;**84**:987–95.

8 Medical Research Council's General Practice Research Framework. Randomized comparison of estrogen versus estrogen plus progestogen hormone replacement therapy in women with a hysterectomy. *Br Med J* 1996;**312**:473–8.

9 Leiberman EH, Gerhard MD, Uehata A *et al.* Estrogen improves endothelium-dependent, flow-mediated vasodilatation in postmenopausal women. *Ann Intern Med* 1994;**121**:936–41.

10 Rosano GMC, Sarrel PM, Poole-Wilson PA, Collins P. Beneficial effect of estrogen on exercise-induced myocardial ischaemia in women with coronary artery disease. *Lancet* 1993;**342**:133–6.

11 Fleming TR, DeMets DL. Surrogate end points in clinical trials: are we being misled? *Ann Intern Med* 1996;**125**:605–13.

12 Gould AL, Rossouw JE, Santanello NC, Heyse JF, Furberg CF. Cholesterol reduction yields clinical benefit: a new look at old data. *Circulation* 1995; **91**:2274–82.

13 Furberg CD, Psaty BM, Meyer JV. Nifedipine. Dose-related increase in mortality in patients with coronary heart disease. *Circulation* 1995;**92**: 1326–31

14 Ettinger B, Friedman GD, Bush T, Quesenberry CP. Reduced mortality associated with longterm postmenopausal estrogen therapy. *Obstet Gynecol* 1996;**87**:6–12.

15 Stampfer MJ, Colditz GA. Estrogen replacement therapy and coronary heart disease: a quantitative assessment of the epidemiologic evidence. *Prev Med* 1991;**20**:47–63.

16 Grady D, Rubin SM, Petitti DB *et al.* Hormone therapy to prevent disease and prolong life in postmenopausal women. *Ann Intern Med* 1992; **117**:1016–37.

17 Grodstein F, Stampfer MJ, Manson JE *et al.* Postmenopausal estrogen and progestin use and the risk of cardiovascular disease. *N Engl J Med* 1996;**335**:453–61.

18 Falkeborn M, Persson I, Adami HO *et al.* The risk of acute myocardial infarction after estrogen and estrogen-progestogen replacement. *Br J Obstet Gynaecol* 1992;**99**:821–8.

19 Psaty BM, Heckbert SR, Atkins D *et al.* The risk of myocardial infarction associated with the combined use of estrogens and progestins in postmenopausal women. *Arch Intern Med* 1994; **154**:1333–9.

20 Falkeborn M, Persson I, Terent A *et al.* Hormone replacement therapy and stroke. *Arch Intern Med* 1993;**153**:1201–9.

21 Pfeffer RI, van den Noort S. Estrogen use and stroke risk in postmenopausal women. *Am J Epidemiol* 1976;**103**:445–56.

22 Rosenberg SH, Fausone V, Clark R. The role of estrogens as a risk factor for stroke in postmenopausal women. *West J Med* 1980;**133**: 292–6.

23 Paganini-Hill A, Ross RK, Henderson BE. Postmenopausal oestrogen treatment and stroke: a prospective study. *Br Med J* 1988;**297**:519–22.

24 Finucane FF, Madans JH, Bush TL, Wolf PH, Kleinman JC. Decreased risk of stroke among postmenopausal hormone users. *Arch Intern Med* 1993;**153**:73–9.

25 Petitti DB, Wingerd J, Pellegrin F, Ramcharan S. Risk of vascular disease in women: smoking, oral contraceptives, noncontraceptive estrogens, and other factors. *JAMA* 1979;**242**:1150–4.

26 Boysen G, Nyboe J, Appleyard M *et al.* Stroke incidence and risk factors for stroke in Copenhagen, Denmark. *Stroke* 1988;**19**: 1345–53.

27 Wilson PWF, Garrison RJ, Castelli WP. Postmenopausal estrogen use, cigarette smoking, and cardiovascular morbidity in women over 50: the Framingham Study. *N Engl J Med* 1985;**313**: 1038–43.

28 Sturgeon SR, Schairer C, Brinton LA, Pearson T, Hoover RN. Evidence of a healthy estrogen user survivor effect. *Epidemiology* 1995;**6**:227–31.

29 Daly E, Vessey MP, Painter R, Hawkins MM. Case-control study of venous thromboembolism risk in users of hormone replacement therapy (letter). *Lancet* 1996;**348**:1027.

30 Daly E, Vessey MP, Hawkins MM *et al*. Risk of venous thromboembolism in users of hormone replacement therapy. *Lancet* 1996;**348**:977–80.

31 Jick, H, Derby LE, Meyers MM, Vasilakis C, Newton KM. Risk of hospital admission for idiopathic venous thromboembolism among users of postmenopausal estrogens. *Lancet* 1996;**348**:891–983.

32 Grodstein F, Stampfer MJ, Goldhaber SZ *et al*. Prospective study of exogenous hormones and risk of pulmonary embolism in women. *Lancet* 1996;**348**:983–7.

33 Barrett-Connor E, Wingard DL, Criqui MH. Postmenopausal estrogen use and heart disease risk factors in the 1980s. *JAMA* 1989;**261**:2095–100.

34 Postuma WFM, Westendorp RG, Vanderbrouke JP. Cardioprotective effect of hormone replacement therapy in postmenopausal women: is the evidence biased? *Br Med J* 1994;**308**:1268–9.

35 Matthews KA, Kuller LH, Wing RR, Meilahn EN, Plantinga P. Prior to use of estrogen replacement therapy, are users healthier than nonusers? *Am J Epidemiol* 1996;**143**:971–8.

36 Shapiro S. Meta-analysis/Shmeta-analysis. *Am J Epidemiol* 1994;**140**:771–7.

37 Gaziano JM, Manson JE, Buring JE, Hennekens CH. Dietary antioxidants and cardiovascular disease. *Ann NY Acad Sci* 1992;**669**:249–59.

38 Menkes MS, Comstock GW, Vuilleumier JP *et al*. Serum beta-carotene, vitamins A and E, selenium, and the risk of lung cancer. *N Engl J Med* 1986;**315**:1250–4.

39 Alpha-Tocopherol, Beta Carotene Cancer Prevention Study Group. The effect of vitamin E and beta carotene on the incidence of lung cancer and other cancers in male smokers. *N Engl J Med* 1994;**330**:1029–35.

40 Omenn GS, Goodman GE, Thornquist MD *et al*. Effects of a combination of beta carotene and vitamin A on lung cancer and cardiovascular disease. *N Engl J Med* 1996;**334**:1150–5.

41 Hennekens CH, Buring JE, Manson JE *et al*. Lack of effect of long-term supplementation with beta carotene on the incidence of malignant neoplasms and cardiovascular disease. *N Engl J Med* 1996;**334**:1145–9.

42 Nachtigall LE, Nachtigall RH, Nachtigall RD, Beckman EM. Estrogen replacement therapy II: a prospective study in the relationship to carcinoma and cardiovascular and metabolic problems. *Obstet Gynecol* 1979;**54**:74–9.

43 Coronary Drug Project Research Group. The Coronary Drug Project: initial findings leading to modifications of its research protocol. *JAMA* 1970;**214**:1303–13.

44 Coronary Drug Project Research Group. The Coronary Drug Project: findings leading to discontinuation of the 2.5 mg/day estrogen group. *JAMA* 1973;**226**:652–7.

45 Oliver MF, Boyd GS. Influence of reduction in serum lipids on prognosis of coronary heart disease. *Lancet* 1961;**ii**:499–505.

46 Schoch HK. The U.S. Veterans Administration Cardiology Drug-Lipid Study: an interim report. In: Holmes WL, Carlson LA, Paoletti R. eds. *Drugs affecting lipid metabolism*. New York: Plenum Press, 1969, pp 405–20.

47 Marmorston J, Moore FJ, Kuzma TO, Magidson O, Weiner J. Effect of Premarin on survival in men with myocardial infarction. *Proc Soc Exp Biol Med* 1960;**105**:618–20.

48 Psaty BM, Heckbert SR, Atkins D *et al*. A review of the association of estrogens and progestins with cardiovascular disease in postmenopausal women. *Arch Intern Med* 1993;**153**:1421–7.

49 Colditz GA, Hankinson SE, Hunter DJ *et al*. The use of estrogens and progestins and the risk of breast cancer in postmenopausal women. *N Engl J Med* 1995;**332**:1589–93.

50 American College of Physicians. Guidelines for counseling post-menopausal women about preventive hormone therapy. *Ann Intern Med* 1992;**117**:1038–41.

51 Expert Panel. Summary of the Second Report of the National Cholesterol Education Program (NCEP) Expert Panel on Detection, Evaluation, and Treatment of High Blood Cholesterol in Adults (ATP-II). *JAMA* 1993;**269**:3015–23.

52 American College of Obstetricians and Gynecologists. *Hormone replacement therapy*. Technical bulletin number 166. Washington: ACOG, 1992.

Ethnicity and cardiovascular disease

22

SONIA S. ANAND,
SALIM YUSUF

INTRODUCTION

The major risk factors for cardiovascular disease (CVD), which include elevated blood pressure, elevated cholesterol, cigarette smoking, and diabetes, have been derived from epidemiologic studies conducted primarily in white populations.[1] Globally, non-white populations constitute the majority of the world's population although the most influential risk factors for CVD in these populations remain unconfirmed. Ethnicity-related research is important as it documents the rates of known risk factors for a disease, identifies new risk factors, provides us with clues regarding similarities and differences in disease causation, and allows us to define high risk populations for specific diseases. Furthermore, it helps us to understand variations in responses to preventive strategies, medical therapies and health care utilization patterns, and, most importantly, it leads to specific prevention strategies that are appropriately tailored to the major ethnic groups. Therefore, studies that explore reasons for the differences in CVD rates among ethnic populations are of major public health importance.

GENERAL ISSUES

Defining ethnic groups

A *racial* group refers to a population who share a common gene pool and assumes that important genetic differences exist between racial groups.[2] On the other hand, an *ethnic* group refers to a population who share common cultural characteristics such as language, religion, and diet. Therefore the concept of ethnicity relies more on a shared cultural definition of identity than solely on biological similarity. Given that variations in disease rates between populations may be explained by socioeconomic, sociocultural, biological, and genetic factors, classification by ethnic origin rather than race is desirable.[2]

Table 22.1 Disability-adjusted life-year lost (hundreds of thousands) from ischemic heart disease in 1990 (projected data from the World Bank)[4]

Region	Male	Female
Sub-Saharan Africa	6.7	5.4
China	24.8	17.6
India	49.5	31.9
Other Asia/Islands	35.4	26.7
Latin America/Caribbean	16	11.3
Middle East	15.5	10.6
Formerly Socialist Economies of Europe	45.2	34.3
Market Economies	56.4	37.2
Total World	249.6	175.0

Note that disability-adjusted life-years lost from CHD in India are only slightly lower than all the market economies combined.

INTERPRETATION OF STUDIES IN ETHNIC POPULATIONS

The methodologic limitations of studies of ethnic populations must be recognized.[3] Mortality statistics often provide the first clues that differences in CVD rates exist among ethnic groups. Although most developed countries have established mortality statistics, division of these rates by ethnic groups is not uniform. These variations in the manner in which mortality rates between countries are reported make it difficult to ascribe observed differences in disease rates to ethnic differences as many potential confounders exist, including differences in disease definitions, socioeconomic status, age, degree of acculturation, and other demographic variables. Unfortunately, mortality statistics in developing countries are often not available and conclusions about disease rates are usually based upon data from sample registration systems, community surveys and hospital admissions. The disability-adjusted life-year has been used by international organizations like the World Bank and the World Health Organization to summarize the information on mortality. This measure allows global comparisons of the impact of various diseases between developed and developing countries,[4] based on estimates derived from data of varying methodologic quality (Table 22.1). Nevertheless, these kinds of data are useful approximations of the relative disease burden in various countries.

Worldwide patterns of disease

The major non-communicable diseases are CVD, cancer, and diabetes and they account for 75% of worldwide deaths in industralized countries and 40% of deaths in developing countries.[5] Half of these deaths are due to CVD and total approximately 12 million deaths per year worldwide.[5] In most developed countries CVD rates are declining due to CVD risk factor modification and improved secondary prevention strategies. However, in developing countries an epidemiologic transition from acute infectious diseases to a rise in the major non-communicable diseases is occurring. The reasons for this transition include an increasing life expectancy associated with a decline in childhood and adult deaths from infections, and an increase in the prevalence of CVD risk factors associated with industrialization and urbanization.[5]

Table 22.2 Intercountry CVD mortality rates 1993[73][a]

Country	CHD mortality rates (men)	CBVD mortality rates (men)	CHD mortality rates (women)	CBVD mortality rates (women)
Russian Federation	556	288	278	225
Finland	326	107	154	89
US	231	52	124	45
China – urban[b]	112	253	80	181
France	87	35	37	25
China – rural	47	225	34	156
Japan	46	93	25	67

[a] Rates for ages 35–74, per 100 000 of the European population, 1993.
[b] Note the major urban–rural gradient for CHD but not for CBVD in China.

Population differences in the CVD mortality rates are influenced by geographic and environmental factors. Ethnic variations in disease rates are closely tied to geographic patterns of disease.[6] Often the first clue that ethnic variations in disease burden exist comes from observations made between countries. These geographic differences have provided many of the initial hypotheses of the association between lifestyle factors and CVD. One of the first epidemiologic studies to highlight the variation in CHD rates between countries was the Seven Countries Study.[7] In this major longitudinal cohort study, 16 cohorts of men aged 49–59 years were examined and followed for CHD mortality and total mortality. Large differences in CHD mortality between countries were observed, with low CHD rates in Japan and the Mediterranean countries and high CHD rates in Finland and the US. These differences were in large part explained by differences in diet, serum cholesterol, and blood pressure. More recent data from WHO MONICA (MONItoring of trends and determinants in CArdiovascular disease), a CVD surveillance project which includes 117 reporting units in 40 centers from 26 countries,[8] indicate that a greater than 14-fold difference in CHD mortality for men and more than 11-fold differences in CHD mortality for women exists between countries (Table 22.2). These intercountry observations have raised questions as to whether these differences are due to differences in ethnic group susceptibility to CVD, differences in environmental factors or both.

Migrant groups

Observational studies reveal that when members of a given ethnic group change to a new environment (migration) their physical response to a given set of environmental factors differs from those who remain in their native lands. This suggests that environmental influences are very powerful factors in CVD causation. Conversely, despite different environments, similarities in rates within an ethnic group suggest a predominant genetic propensity towards or protection from CVD. Comparing the mortality rates of long-settled migrants to the disease rates in their country of origin helps to establish the relative contribution of genetic and environmental influences to differences in mortality rates. The Ni-Ho-San Study of Japanese migrants to Hawaii and San Francisco revealed that changes in disease rates in this population likely reflected changing environmental influences.[9] The 12-year age-adjusted mortality rates for CHD compared to rates in Japan were higher in Hawaii and highest in California. More than half of the increase in CHD was attributable to different levels of conventional risk factors, as the US cohort had a higher fat diet and higher mean serum cholesterol compared to the Hawaiian or Japanese cohorts.[9] This suggests that the low rates of CHD mortality in Japan may be attained in Japanese migrants by maintaining their risk factors at levels similar to those in Japan.

SPECIFIC ETHNIC GROUPS

In the following sections we will review the CVD profile of seven major ethnic groups. Based on the best available data, we will document their disease burden and changes in disease rates over time and review common/influential CVD risk factors. We then suggest special ethnic group-specific preventive strategies which need to be developed or reinforced.

European origin

People of European origin include those who originate from Northern Europe, such as the Nordic countries and Germany, Western Europe including the UK and France, Southern Europe including Spain and Italy, and Eastern Europe which includes the Slavic countries.

DISEASE BURDEN

Differences in the age standardized mortality rates (ASMR) vary widely between European populations. Data from the WHO indicate that wide variations in disease rates exist between the Eastern European countries and Southern European countries such as Italy and France.[10] In 1994, the ASMR for CHD among males in the Russian Federation was 556 per 100 000 compared to 87 per 100 000 among males in France.[10] The cerebrovascular disease (CBVD) ASMR was 288 per 100 000 among males in the Russian Federation compared to 35 per 100 000 in France.[10] Although in all countries the CVD mortality rates are much lower among women, these impressive between-country differences persist (Table 22.2). Over the past 30 years most European countries have experienced declines in the CVD mortality rates. The Eastern European countries continue to have among the highest rates of CHD and CBVD in the world, with a few showing a decline and several showing an increase.[11]

COMMON RISK FACTORS

Across several European populations the high rates of CVD are mainly attributable to the major risk factors for vascular disease in white populations, namely diets high in saturated fats, elevated serum cholesterol, elevated blood pressure, diabetes, and smoking. The epidemic of CHD in the Eastern European countries is related to high levels of smoking and diets high in saturated fat.[6] Research to explain why the Italian and French populations remain relatively "protected" from CHD has yielded numerous hypotheses. It is likely that dietary variations account for the differences in disease rates.

It is believed that the high consumption of monounsaturated fats such as olive oil and antioxidants is responsible for the low rates of CHD in Italy. In France, despite having similar saturated fat consumption, serum cholesterol, blood pressure, and smoking, the CHD mortality rate remains very low.[12] This immunity to CHD has been attributed to a high consumption of ethanol (wine), which is usually ingested with meals and may offer cardioprotection by increasing HDL cholesterol levels or inhibiting postprandial hyperlipidemia and platelet aggregation.[13] Despite this relative protection from CHD, the total mortality rate in France is no different from other Western countries which suggests an increase in alcohol-related non-CHD deaths such as cirrhosis.[13]

INFLUENTIAL RISK FACTORS

CHD, like other epidemics, relates closely to social conditions and its prevalence appears to be strongly related to the social and cultural conditions of society, more so than to its genetic make-up. This is evidenced by the rapid declines in the rates of CHD in parallel to economic changes in the US and Japan and the increase in CHD rates in the Eastern European countries. These changes have occurred too quickly for changes in gene frequencies to be responsible.[6] Therefore, rather than differences in CHD rates between populations being largely due to genetic differences, broad variations in CHD rates appear to be mostly explained by consideration of three factors: nutrition (high fat diets), smoking, and economic factors.

SPECIAL APPROACHES TO PREVENTION

It is clear that major lifestyle changes and vigilant treatment of risk factors result in declines in CVD rates. In Finland, an impressive 60% reduction in CHD mortality and stroke was observed between 1972 and 1994 and it is estimated that approximately 75% of this decline in CHD mortality can be explained by a substantial lowering of serum cholesterol by 14% (0.93 mmol/l) in men and by 18% (1.19 mmol/l) in women, diastolic blood pressure by 5% (6.6 mmHg) in men and 13% (12.7 mmHg) in women, and a significant reduction in smoking (18% in men).[14] Furthermore, in the US a 34% decline in CHD mortality occurred between 1980 and 1990. One-quarter of this decline is attributable to primary prevention efforts and 29% is explained by secondary prevention efforts such as reduction in serum cholesterol, diastolic blood pressure, and smoking. Furthermore, 43% of this decline is attributed to improved medical and surgical management in patients with established coronary disease.[15] More recently in Poland, during the 1990s, a rapid decrease (about 25%) in CHD deaths in early middle age has been observed. This decline in CHD rates is attributed in large part to marked dietary changes such as the reduced consumption of animal fats.[16] Therefore, decreasing the consumption of animal fat, diastolic blood pressure, and tobacco consumption can lead to large reductions in CHD deaths.

Japanese

DISEASE BURDEN

Mortality rates from CVD are much lower in Japan than Western countries.[10] Initial data from the Seven Countries Study confirmed that the Japanese experience relatively lower rates of CVD compared to Western populations.[17] In Japan, the pattern of CVD differs from Western populations as they tend to experience relatively higher proportions of CBVD (ASMR: men 93, women 67/10 000) and less CHD (ASMR: men 46, women 25/100 000).

TEMPORAL TRENDS

In parallel with a rise in economic prosperity, the CHD rates in Japan have declined more markedly than those in Western countries. Given the low rate of CHD in Japan, the life expectancy in Japan is among the highest in the world.[18] Furthermore, mortality from CBVD has also declined substantially in men and women in Japan since 1950.[18] Dietary changes such as reduction in salt consumption and increased pharmacologic treatment of hypertension are probably responsible for this decline.[18]

COMMON RISK FACTORS

A review of CVD risk factors in the Japanese population reveals that hypertension is the most important CVD risk factor, more so than cholesterol and cigarette smoking.[18] However, low serum cholesterol related to a diet low in saturated fat and cholesterol is likely to be responsible for the low rates of CHD mortality observed in the Japanese. Despite the fact that two-thirds of Japanese men smoke, CHD rates remain unexpectedly low. Furthermore, the prevalence of non-insulin-dependent diabetes mellitus (NIDDM) in Japanese males and females is higher than the rates in most Western countries. In the Hisayama Cohort Study the prevalence of NIDDM was 13% in males and 9% in females and the relative risk of NIDDM for CVD was 3.0 (1.8–5.2).[19] Therefore, NIDDM appears to be an emerging and important risk factor for both stroke and CHD in the general Japanese population.[19]

INFLUENTIAL RISK FACTORS

Over the last 30 years blood pressure levels have declined in Japan due to increased diagnosis and treatment of hypertension.[18] However, during this period a 2–3-fold increase in glucose tolerance and NIDDM, as well as obesity and hypercholesterolemia (the mean cholesterol is only 10% lower than in the US in 1989), has occurred.[18] The increase in diabetes, obesity, and serum cholesterol is likely due to "westernization" of the Japanese lifestyle. It is possible that as cholesterol and glucose levels rise the impact of the high cigarette smoking may become manifest.

MIGRANT PATTERNS

The Ni-Ho-San Study demonstrated that the rates of CHD and CBVD mortality rates in Hawaii are intermediate between rates in Japan and California.[9] The gradients in CVD risk factors paralleled these disease gradients. This indicates that environmental factors contributed significantly to the risk factor profiles and disease rates of this migrant Japanese population.

SPECIAL APPROACHES TO PREVENTION/TREATMENT

With increasing adoption of urban lifestyles in Japan, the rates of CHD risk factors are approaching those of Americans. The differences in CHD rates between Japan and the

US demonstrate consistent relationships between diet, serum cholesterol, and CHD. Recent studies have documented that the average serum cholesterol concentration among the Japanese has increased from 1980 to 1989. The age-adjusted total serum cholesterol levels increased from 4.84 to 5.22 mmol/l in men and from 4.91 to 5.24 mmol/l among women and this, combined with the increased prevalence of cigarette smoking among Japanese males (59%), suggests that Japan may soon experience a significant increase in CHD rates.[18] Therefore, maintenance of a low fat diet, avoidance of obesity through decreased energy intake and regular physical activity will likely prevent the development of the cholesterol and glucose intolerance. Avoidance of cigarette smoking is also critical. This change in the CVD risk factor profile has led to a changing pattern of CVD among Japanese in Japan: a significant decrease in morbidity and mortality from CBVD and no significant changes in the risk of CHD. However, if the change in risk factors continues CHD rates may show an increase in this population.

Chinese

DISEASE BURDEN

Although the overall mortality from CVD is less in China than in Western countries, CVD is the most common cause of death in mainland China and Taiwan. When compared to Western populations, the Chinese experience higher stroke rates and relatively lower rates of CHD, a pattern similar to that observed in Japan. In China, the ASMR for CHD in men aged 35–74 was 112/100 000 and in women 80/100 000.[10] These rates are five-fold lower than the highest rates observed in the MONICA project from Western and Eastern Bloc countries.[10] The ASMR for CBVD from 1994 was 253 in Chinese men aged 35–74 and 181/100 000 in women.[11] Comparison with five stroke registries from the West suggests that intracerebral hemorrhage occurs between two and three times more frequently in the Chinese than in white Caucasians.[20] Only 6–12% of strokes in whites are reported as intracerebral hemorrhages compared to 25–30% of hemorrhagic strokes in Chinese.[11]

TEMPORAL TRENDS

Death rates from major adult CVD (particularly CHD) have been increasing in China in recent decades.[21] Mortality attributable to CVD increased from 86/100 000 (12% of total deaths) in 1957 to 214/100 000 (36%) in a recent analysis of urban Chinese.[21] Although most Western countries report a decline in CVD mortality, the decline in stroke deaths in China has not been as striking. A recent study in Shanghai from 1984 to 1991 reported no changes in the stroke incidence, yet a decline in the case fatality rate from stroke in both rural and urban China.[20]

COMMON RISK FACTORS

A case-control study from Hong Kong of acute myocardial infarction (AMI) sufferers provides evidence that conventional risk factors for CHD in Chinese remain important.[22] The odds ratio for AMI associated with cigarette smoking was 4.3, 3.3 for hypertension, and 2.4 for diabetes. Although the mean serum cholesterol among Chinese would be

Table 22.3 North–South and urban–rural comparisons of CVD risk factors in China[25]

Factor	Beijing – urban	Beijing – rural	Guangzhou – urban	Guangzhou – rural
Hypertension – men (%)	29.6	25.5	9.5	7.6
Hypertension – women (%)	25.1	17.9	12.4	4.1
Cholesterol – men (mmol/l)	4.78	4.42	4.71	4.11´
Cholesterol – women (mmol/l)	4.83	4.34	4.83	4.1
HDL – men (mmol/l)	1.37	1.39	1.29	1.26
HDL – women (mmol/l)	1.52	1.47	1.37	1.24
Smoking – current men (%)	71	78	73	77
Smoking – current women (%)	23	31	3	7
BMI – men	23	22	21	20
BMI – women	24	23	22	20

considered low by Western standards, a prospective observational study of approximately 9000 Chinese in urban Shanghai demonstrated that serum cholesterol was directly related (continuous relationship) to CHD mortality even at these low levels.[23] Cigarette smoking is highly prevalent among Chinese males as approximately 40–60% of men smoke and there is evidence that these rates are increasing.[24]

INFLUENTIAL RISK FACTORS

Although the rates of cigarette smoking are high, hypertension appears to be the most influential risk factor for CVD in this group. However, with increasing urbanization and subsequent increase in serum cholesterol, the interaction between smoking and cholesterol may lead to increased rates of CHD.

GEOGRAPHIC VARIATIONS

Trends in morbidity and mortality from CVD within China indicate that the mortality rate attributable to CVD is higher in North China (Beijing) than in South China (Guangzhou).[25] Furthermore, comparison of urban and rural areas in China indicates that CHD rates increase by two-fold in urban areas compared to rural areas (48 vs 23/100 000).[25] The prevalence of hypertension, mean serum cholesterol, and mean body mass index (BMI) were all lower in the South compared to the North and in rural compared to urban areas (Table 22.3). However, the greatest differences in the prevalence of cigarette smoking exist between men and women (74% vs 20%) and this does not share the same geographic distribution as do the other major CVD risk factors.

MIGRANT PATTERNS

Data from Chinese migrants to Singapore and Mauritius provide evidence that the effects of exposure to urban environments lead to adverse risk factor profiles for CVD.[26,27] In a comparative study of Chinese migrants to Mauritius the prevalence of CHD by ECG was six times greater (24% vs 4%) than in Beijing, China. Also, the prevalence of diabetes and the mean serum cholesterol was higher in Mauritius Chinese (5.5 mmol/l) than in Beijing Chinese (4.4 mmol/l), whereas the prevalence of hypertension and smoking was greater in Beijing.[26] Therefore, although the prevalence of hypertension and smoking may decline with migration, the rates of obesity, late onset diabetes, elevated serum cholesterol, and CHD appear to increase.

SPECIAL APPROACHES TO PREVENTION

Economic modernization in China is resulting in an increased prevalence of conventional CVD risk factors over time in urban populations.[28] This offers a major challenge for prevention efforts among urban Chinese, both in China and abroad, as the Chinese, who have traditionally had a very low prevalence of CHD, will likely not remain protected from developing CHD with their changes in lifestyle. Important prevention strategies in this group include smoking cessation/prevention and maintenance of a "rural diet" (high fiber, low fat consumption) to prevent increases in BMI, diabetes, serum cholesterol, and hypertension.

South Asians

South Asians refer to people who originate from India, Sri Lanka, Bangladesh, and Pakistan.

DISEASE BURDEN

Studies of South Asian migrants demonstrate that they suffer a higher mortality from CHD when compared to other ethnic groups (Table 22.4).

Within India

There are relatively few mortality studies from India as there is no uniform completion of death certificates and no centralized death registry for CVD.[29] However, the WHO and the World Bank data indicate that deaths attributable to CVD disease have increased in parallel with the expanding population in India and it now accounts for a large proportion of disability-adjusted life-years. Of all deaths in 1990, approximately 25% were attributable to CVD, which is greater than the 9% due to diarrheal diseases, the 12% due to respiratory infections, and the 5% due to tuberculosis.[4]

South Asian migrants

Studies of South Asian migrants to countries such as the United Kingdom, South Africa, Singapore, and North America provide evidence that South Asians suffer between 1.11 and 3.19 times higher CHD mortality compared to other ethnic groups (Table 22.4).[30]

TEMPORAL TRENDS

In India the CHD rate is expected to rise in parallel with the increase in life expectancy due to an increase in per capita income and a decline in infant mortality. The average life expectancy has increased from 47 years in 1960 to 58 in 1990. This trend is expected to continue with life expectancy at birth reaching 70 years by 2030, leading

Table 22.4 Standardized mortality ratios (per 100 000) for CHD in South Asians worldwide[a]

Study year	Country	Reference population	Age	SMR
Wyndham[74] 1968–77	South Africa	Whites	15–64	300
Steinberg[75] 1968–85	South Africa	Whites	35–74	502
Baligadoo[76]	Mauritius	Europeans	40–45	260
Toumilehto[77] 1971–80	Fiji	Melanesians	40–60+	350
Beckles[78] 1977–84	Trinidad	Blacks	35–69	260
Hughes[79] 1980–4	Singapore	Chinese	30–69	380
Hughes[79] 1980–4	Singapore	Malays	30–69	190
Adelstein[80] 1970–2	UK	Whites	20+	115
McKeigue[81] 1979–83	UK	Whites	20–64	160
Balarajan[32] 1979–83	UK	Whites	20–69	M136 M146
Sheth[33] 1979–83	Canada	Whites	35–74	M122 F139
Sheth[33] 1979–83	Canada	Chinese	35–74	M329 F344
Sheth[33] 1989–93	Canada	Whites	35–74	M95 F131
Sheth[33] 1989–93	Canada	Chinese	35–74	M275 F369

[a] Standardized mortality to reference indigenous population of 100.

to large increases in CVD prevalence.[31] Although the CHD mortality rate of South Asians compared to other populations remains high, a decline in CHD rates has been observed in most South Asian migrants over the past 10 years, although this decline has been less than that observed in the general population in most countries except Canada.[32,33]

COMMON RISK FACTORS

South Asians, despite having increased rates of CHD, do not display an excess of conventional cardiovascular risk factors such as smoking, hypertension or elevated cholesterol.[34,35] However, these factors remain strongly associated with the development of CHD in South Asians. Data from a case-control study in Bangalore, India,[36] in which 300 cases of AMI were compared to 300 age- and sex-matched controls, revealed an increasing relative risk of MI as the number of conventional risk factors increased. The odds ratio for smoking was 3.6, 2.6 for diabetes, and 2.7 for hypertension. In this study serum cholesterol did not seem to differ between cases and controls and the levels were similar to Western values. Cross-sectional studies of CHD risk factors in South Asians have identified that this group suffers a high prevalence of impaired glucose tolerance, central obesity, elevated triglycerides, and low HDL cholesterol.[35] The prevalence of impaired glucose tolerance and NIDDM is 4–5 times higher in South Asian migrants than in Europeans by the age of 55 (20% vs 4%).[34,35] The prevalence of diabetes in South Asians in the UK was 10–19%, 21% in Trinidad, 25% in Fiji, 22% in South Africa, 25% in Singapore, and 20% in Mauritius.[35] In rural India it is 3% and 11–30% in urban India, which is similar to the rates reported among Indians living abroad.[37] There is preliminary evidence that South Asians have elevated levels of Lp(a), a lipoprotein which is genetically mediated and associated with increased atherosclerosis and thrombogenesis.[38]

INFLUENTIAL RISK FACTORS

Glucose intolerance, abdominal obesity, and its associated dyslipidemia appear to be the dominant factors associated with the development of CHD in South Asians. Increasingly, data support the idea that elevations of glucose in the non-diabetic range, is prevalent in South Asians, and is associated with the development of atherosclerosis.[39]

GEOGRAPHIC VARIATIONS

Epidemiologic data support a striking urban–rural difference in the prevalence of CHD and CHD risk factors in South Asians living in India and abroad.[40] Data from India demonstrate at least a two-fold excess of CHD in urban compared to rural environments. A recent overview of prevalence surveys in India reported a nine-fold increase of CHD in urban centers, compared with a two-fold increase in rural populations over two decades of study.[41] Data from a study by Reddy conducted in 1989–94 in which a population based sample from urban Delhi was compared to a similar sample from rural Haryana revealed the CHD prevalence was 10/1000 in Delhi compared to 2/1000 in Haryana.[42] Associated with this increase in CHD rates in urban areas is an increase in the prevalence of lipid and glucose abnormalities, impaired glucose tolerance (IGT) and NIDDM, lower HDL cholesterol, and higher triglycerides, Increased abdominal obesity, BMI, and hypertension are observed in the urban areas compared to the rural areas (Table 22.5). By contrast, the rates of tobacco smoking are higher within rural environments among both men and women.

MIGRATION PATTERNS

An urban–rural difference in CHD prevalence and risk factors is observed within India and abroad. A recent study which compared the risk profiles of urban South Asians living in the UK with their siblings living in India (Table 22.6) revealed that the UK cohort had a higher BMI (27 vs 23), systolic BP (144 mmHg vs 137 mmHg), total cholesterol (6.35 vs 5.0 mmol/l), lower HDL cholesterol (1.14 vs 1.27 mmol/l), and higher fasting glucose (5.4 vs 4.6 mmol/l) compared to their siblings. Lp(a), which is genetically determined, was similarly high in both groups.[43]

PREVENTION STRATEGIES

Changes in the risk factor profiles of South Asians are attributable to lifestyle changes associated with urbanization such as decreased physical activity and dietary changes (higher fat consumption, decreased vegetarianism, decreased fiber) which lead to obesity

Table 22.5 Urban–rural comparisons of CVD risk factors in India

Factor	Delhi – urban	Haryana – rural
Diabetes mellitus – men (%)	10.9	2.9
Diabetes mellitus – women (%)	11.2	2.6
Hypertension – men (%)	25.5	14
Hypertension – women (%)	29	10.8
Cholesterol – men (mmol/l)	4.96	4.4
Cholesterol – women (mmol/l)	5.01	4.28
HDL – men (mmol/l)	1.01	1.02
HDL – women (mmol/l)	1.12	1.08
Smoking – current men (%)	28.7	54.7
Smoking – current women (%)	2.6	25.3
BMI – men	23.6	19.9
BMI – women	25.1	20.3
W/H ratio – men	0.99	0.95
W/H ratio – women	0.83	0.83

Adapted from Reddy et al.[42]

Table 22.6 Migrant comparison of South Asians from India and the UK

	Indian subcontinent	Sibling migrants UK	Significance
Mean age (years)	45	46	NS
Serum glucose – men (mmol/l)	4.5	5.7	0.001
Serum glucose – women (mmol/l)	4.7	5.1	0.05
Serum cholesterol – men (mmol/l)	4.9	6.5	0.001
Serum cholesterol – women (mmol/l)	5.1	6.2	0.001
HDL cholesterol – men (mmol/l)	1.21	1.12	NS
HDL cholesterol – women (mmol/l)	1.34	1.16	0.05
Serum Lp(a) – men (mg/dl)	17.4	18.8	NS
Serum Lp(a) – women (mg/dl)	18.9	20.4	NS
Systolic/diastolic blood pressure – men (mmHg)	132/87	146/93	0.001/NS
Systolic/diastolic blood pressure – women (mmHg)	142/88	143/86	NS/NS
BMI – men	22.9	26.8	0.001
BMI – women	22.7	27.4	0.001

and its harmful sequelae. Clearly strategies to prevent the development of obesity are required to decrease the number of South Asians who suffer from glucose intolerance, its associated dyslipidemia, and ultimately CHD.

Hispanics

The term "Hispanic" includes Cuban-Americans, Mexican-Americans, and Puerto Rican-Americans. There are approximately 20 million Mexican-Americans living in the US and they comprise approximately 9% of the US population.[44] The majority of information on CVD in Hispanics has been derived from studies in Mexican-Americans.

DISEASE BURDEN

Although death certificate registries report that the age-adjusted mortality rates for major CVD among Mexican-Americans are lower than those of African-Americans and whites in the US,[45] recent data from the Corpus Christi Heart Project (CCHP), Texas, reported a greater incidence of MI in Mexican-Americans compared to non-Hispanic whites over a 4-year period.[46] This population based surveillance project, conducted between 1988 and 1992, reported that age-adjusted incidence ratios comparing Mexican-Americans to non-Hispanic whites were 1.52 (95% CI 1.28–1.80) and 1.25 (95% CI 1.10–1.42) among women and men respectively.[46] Although cross-sectional studies reveal a similar or lower prevalence of MI among Mexican-Americans than non-Hispanic whites, the CCHP has reported a greater case fatality rate following MI among Mexican-Americans than non-Hispanic whites. Therefore, a lower CHD prevalence in Mexican-Americans does not necessarily reflect a lower incidence of CHD.

Under the age of 60 years Hispanics have a significantly elevated CBVD death rate compared to non-Hispanics whites (men 32 vs 19, women 23 vs 18/100 000 respectively). However, in older age categories the CBVD rate in Hispanics is substantially lower than whites (men 589 vs 765, women 535 vs 847 per 100 000).[47] Therefore, overall the CBVD death rate over 45 years of age in Hispanics is lower when compared to whites (men 115 vs 147/100 000 and women 110 vs 209/100 000).[48]

TEMPORAL TRENDS

Although declines in CHD and CBVD mortality have occurred in Mexican-Americans over the past 20 years, this decline has been less than that among non-Hispanic whites.[47,49]

COMMON RISK FACTORS

The Hispanic Health and Nutrition Examination (HHANES) demonstrated that Hispanics suffer a high prevalence of conventional CVD risk factors such as hypertension (17% prevalence), smoking, serum cholesterol (mean 5.35 mmol/l), diabetes (24% prevalence), and obesity (29% men, 39% women), compared to non-Hispanic whites.[50] The San Antonio Heart Study reported that Mexican-Americans had 2.5 times the prevalence of NIDDM compared to the non-Hispanic whites as diagnosed by the oral glucose tolerance test.[51] They also observed that a socioeconomic gradient existed within the Hispanic population, with diabetes being more prevalent in the lower socioeconomic groups.[51] Furthermore, Mexican-Americans have higher blood concentrations of triglycerides and lower HDL cholesterol levels compared to non-Hispanic whites.[44]

INFLUENTIAL RISK FACTORS

Glucose intolerance appears to be the most influential risk factor for CHD among Mexican-Americans.[52] The greater mortality observed among Mexican-Americans following MI in comparison to non-Hispanic whites is attributed in large part to the increased prevalence of diabetes.[52] Furthermore, glucose intolerance also defines which Mexican-Americans are more likely to suffer CHD events within their own population, as diabetic Mexican-Americans are four times more likely to suffer a MI compared to their non-diabetic counterparts.[53]

GEOGRAPHIC VARIATIONS

This population suffers a high prevalence of glucose metabolic derangements upon the adoption of an urban lifestyle.

SPECIAL APPROACHES TO PREVENTION/TREATMENT

Due to the discrepant data concerning the CHD mortality rates of Mexican-Americans, despite their adverse risk factor profile many researchers believe they remain "protected" from CHD.[54] Clearly, the burden of CHD among Mexican-Americans is considerable and risk factor modification of conventional CHD risk factors must be initiated. Furthermore, primary prevention strategies such as prevention of obesity through dietary changes and increased physical activity will reduce the rate of glucose intolerance in this group. Promotion of these strategies is important given that Mexican-Americans are less likely to receive treatment for diabetes, hypercholesterolemia, and hypertension compared to non-Hispanic whites.[46] Therefore it is critical that ethnically sensitive strategies are developed to bring about both primary and secondary prevention in this growing group of Americans.

Aboriginal populations

DISEASE BURDEN

Although mortality rates for CVD among aboriginal populations appear to be lower than whites, CHD is the leading cause of death in North American Indian and Alaskan native males and females.[44] Although research in this ethnic group is limited, the Strong Heart Study,[55] which was initiated in 1988, studied 4549 American natives aged 45–74 years from 13 tribes in the Southern US. The prevalence estimates of definite MI in those aged 45–74 years from 13 tribes in the Southern US. The prevalence estimates of definite MI in those aged 45–74 years were 2.8% in men without diabetes and 5.3% in men with diabetes, 0.4% in women without diabetes, and 1.4% in women with diabetes. Data from other US cohort studies indicate that native Americans may have a lower prevalence of MI than whites (7.9%), African-Americans (6.1%), and Hispanics (5.6%).[55] However, data from Canada indicate that native Canadians suffer higher rates of CHD compared to the general population.[56]

There is little published information concerning the epidemiology of CBVD in native populations. In the US the CBVD mortality rate under the age of 65 years is similar in native Americans and white Americans and substantially lower than rates in African-Americans.[57] Over the age of 65, the CBVD rate in native Americans is substantially lower than whites. The age-adjusted mortality rate for CBVD in native American men in 1988–98 was approximately 80/100 000 compared to 120/100 000 in white American men and 60/100 000 compared to 100/100 000 in native women compared to white American women.[57] In Canada, the ASMR (0–64 years) among natives on Indian reservations is 1.44 for males and 1.93 for females compared to the general population.

TEMPORAL TRENDS

As more native Indians give up their traditional hunter-gatherer lifestyles and adopt "urban" lifestyles, the prevalence of CVD and CVD risk factors increases. Data from Canada, in which the time periods 1979–83 and 1984–85 were compared, revealed that a decline in CHD rates of 22% occurred in native men, whereas the rates of CHD *increased* by 5% among native women.[58] The age-adjusted rates of CBVD mortality declined over the period 1980–90 in native Americans by approximately 20%, which is slightly lower than the 26% decline observed in white Americans.[57]

COMMON RISK FACTORS

The common CHD risk factors in native men and women include diabetes, obesity, and low HDL cholesterol. The prevalence of cigarette smoking is increasing among native Indians yet it varies greatly between reserves.[55] The prevalence of diabetes in the Strong Heart Study was an astounding 48% in the 45–64 year age group compared to approximately 5.5% in the US general population and the prevalence of obesity was between 26 and 41%, with an average BMI of 31 and waist:hip ratio of 0.96 in men. Interestingly, the prevalence of hypertension and elevated serum cholesterol among natives appears to be lower when compared to the general US population. However, the prevalence of low HDL cholesterol is greater in this group as approximately 25% of native men have a HDL cholesterol values less than 0.90 mmol/l.

INFLUENTIAL RISK FACTORS

Clearly glucose intolerance amongst native Indians is the most influential risk factor for future CHD. Native men and women who are diabetic are 2–4 times more likely to suffer CVD than non-diabetics.[59] In the Strong Heart Study other important risk factors for CHD included hypertension, obesity, smoking, and low HDL cholesterol.[55]

GEOGRAPHIC VARIATIONS

Studies in aboriginal populations in North America have revealed that important regional and intertribal differences exist in the prevalence of diabetes, IGT, cigarette smoking, and disease rates.[55,57] Most of the current data on native CVD rates and risk factors have come from studies of natives living on reserves. There is relatively little information regarding these profiles in city-dwelling natives.

SPECIAL APPROACHES TO PREVENTION/TREATMENT

In order to devise preventive strategies for CVD in native populations, more research into the epidemiology of CVD risk factors and CVD must be performed. Specifically, research into the epidemiology of CVD profiles of native Indians who do not live on reservations must be emphasized, as it is very likely that urban natives may have different CVD risk factor profiles and disease rates from reservation populations. This information will be important in developing culturally sensitive risk factor modification and education programs for native populations.

Blacks of African origin

DISEASE BURDEN

CVD mortality data from countries in sub-Saharan Africa are limited, as only 1.1% of all deaths are registered with a central agency.[60] Data from other sources, such as sample registries, and small scale population studies in 1990 indicate that the prevalence of acute MI in males and females of all ages was 3.4/100 000 and the mortality from acute MI in 1990 was 41/100 000.[60] These rates are considerably lower than those of whites and South Asians who live in Africa, as well as rates of most Western countries which are on average five times higher.[60,61] Even so, in sub-Saharan Africa the proportional mortality rate from CHD accounts for 26% of all deaths and in the 60–70-year age group, for over 80% of all deaths.[60] Furthermore, the case fatality rate of CHD is higher in sub-Saharan Africa compared to Western countries, meaning that once an individual develops CHD in sub-Saharan Africa the probability of death is higher than in Western countries. This likely reflects the limited access to acute and chronic treatment strategies.

RISK FACTORS

The prevalence of most conventional risk factors for CHD is lower among blacks compared to other groups within Africa and the world, with the exception of hypertension and perhaps smoking among urban blacks.[61–63] Data from the WHO Inter-Health Program, a substudy of the MONICA project, assessed the risk factor profile of men and women aged 35–64 years from Tanzania.[62] The prevalence of smoking was 37% among men and 3.9% among women, the mean BMI was 21 in men and 22 in women, the mean BP was 126/79 mmHg among men compared to 125/79 mmHg in women, the mean serum cholesterol was 4.1 mmol/l in men and 4.3 mmol/l in women. When compared to the risk factor profile of other developing and developed countries, the Tanzanians' was more favorable, with the exception of smoking among men. Furthermore, the prevalence of multiple risk factors for CHD was low, as 65% of the population had no identifiable risk factors, 30% had a single risk factor, and only 5% had at least two risk factors, compared to 50%, 40%, and 10% in the US.[62]

GEOGRAPHIC VARIATIONS

In most urban and virtually all rural regions of sub-Saharan Africa the prevalence of traditional CVD risk factors among blacks is low. However, with urbanization an increase in conventional cardiovascular risk factors and CVD rates is expected.[64] An example of this is found in South Africa, as the rapid migration of blacks to urban centers has led to increased poverty, obesity, hypertension, and LDL cholesterol and a decrease in HDL cholesterol.

SPECIAL APPROACHES TO DISEASE PREVENTION

Although CHD rates among people of African origin remain relatively low, the data are limited and given the increased migration of blacks to urban centers and a subsequent rise in the number of conventional CHD risk factors, the rates of CHD and CBVD are expected to rise. Primary prevention strategies such as reducing the availability of saturated fats and increasing the availability of monounsaturated fats, control of cigarette smoking by increasing the price of cigarettes, controlling the amount of salt consumption, and promoting regular physical activity are required on a community level, especially among urban populations. Key primary and secondary prevention strategies among blacks include control of hypertension and effective antismoking campaigns.

West Indies

DISEASE BURDEN

In Trinidad, data from 1989 reveal that the age-adjusted incidence of CHD in people of African origin was 7/1000 person-years at risk among men and 5/1000 person-years at risk among women. The rate in men approximated that of males of European descent (6.45/1000), whereas the rates among women were higher in blacks (5 vs 2.9/1000). The rates in both gender groups were substantially lower than males (16/1000) and females (13/1000) of South Asian origin.[65]

RISK FACTORS

The most prevalent and influential risk factor among West Indian blacks is hypertension. In Trinidad the prevalence of hypertension among African blacks was 33%, diabetes 8.1%, and smoking 39%.[65] Furthermore, the mean HDL and LDL cholesterol in men was 1.03 and 4.04 mmol/l, and in women 1.30 and 4.11 mmol/l. The most important predictors of CHD in this cohort were hypertension, high LDL cholesterol, low HDL cholesterol, and diabetes mellitus.

African-Americans

African-Americans are the largest non-white population in the US and represent approximately 12% of the population.

DISEASE BURDEN

CVD is the leading cause of death among African-Americans and the incidence of both CHD and CBVD is higher in African-Americans compared to white Americans. The CHD mortality rate in African-American males is 2.4% higher than in white males (138.1 vs 134.8/100 000) and 33% higher in African-American women compared to white American women (85 vs 64/100 000).[44] Also, sudden cardiac death (defined by ICD codes 410–414) is more common among African-American men (137/100 000) compared to white American men (122/100 000) aged 35–74 years and women (67 vs 41/100 000) respectively.[66] The CBVD mortality rate is 98% higher in African-American males compared to white males (52 vs 26/100 000) and 77% higher in African-American females compared to white females (40 vs 22/100 000).[44]

TEMPORAL TRENDS

Although there has been a decline in mortality rates from CVD in both African-Americans and white Americans over the past 30 years, these declines have been less marked in African-Americans.[44]

COMMON RISK FACTORS

Compared to whites, African-Americans develop high blood pressure at an earlier age and it is more severe.[44] The reason for black–white differences in hypertension prevalence likely involves a complex interaction between environmental response to diet and stress and a potential genetic/physiologic difference such as differences in sodium/potassium excretion, perhaps linked to their origins in Africa.

Serum cholesterol levels are no higher than those in white Americans, as 47% of African-American men have cholesterol values over 5.2 mmol/l compared to 54% of white males and 51% of women have levels greater than 5.2 mmol/l compared to 53% of white females.[44] On average, African-Americans have higher HDL cholesterol levels compared to whites, a difference which is more marked among women.[44]

The prevalence of cigarette smoking is greater among African-American males (33% vs 27%) than in white men, whereas fewer African-American females smoke compared to white American women.[44] Obesity is an emerging problem among African-Americans, especially in women, as approximately 50% of African-American women are reported to be overweight, compared to 33% of white American women.[44] Closely linked to the prevalence of obesity is a low prevalence of self-reported regular physical activity. Approximately 65% of African-Americans lead a sedentary lifestyle compared to about 56% of whites.[44] Furthermore, the prevalence of diabetes in African-Americans is higher than in whites, as demonstrated by NHANES II conducted from 1976 to 1980 in which African-Americans aged 20–74 years had a NIDDM prevalence of 9.9% compared to 6% in white Americans.[44] Furthermore, the rate of NIDDM is increasing faster among African-Americans than among whites, especially in women, as it is closely tied to the development of obesity.[44]

Although elevated levels of Lp(a) are found more often in African-Americans than in whites, it is unclear whether elevated Lp(a) levels are related to an increased CHD risk among African-Americans.[67] However, even after consideration of "biomedical" differences in conventional risk factor prevalence such as hypertension, smoking, and obesity, other factors likely play a role in the slower decline in CVD rates which has been observed among blacks. Differences in socioeconomic status between African-Americans and whites translate into decreased access to medical therapies and hospital services which result in the performance of fewer diagnostic tests and coronary revascularization procedures.[68,69]

INFLUENTIAL RISK FACTORS

Black and white differences in CVD mortality appear to be largely due to differences in hypertension prevalence. However, late onset diabetes is an increasing problem among

African-Americans due to the increase in obesity. Even so, at least 30% of the excess CHD mortality between blacks and whites can be accounted for by differences in socioeconomic status and these socioeconomic differentials lead to less access to health care services and acceptance of preventive strategies.[68]

GEOGRAPHIC VARIATIONS

African-Americans in the south-eastern US have a greater prevalence of hypertension and higher death rates from CBVD than those from other regions of the country.[44] This pattern is also observed among white Americans so it is likely that certain environmental factors are responsible for this difference.

SPECIAL APPROACHES TO PREVENTION/TREATMENT

The rates of CHD among blacks in Africa are relatively low compared to the rates in most Western countries, although with urbanization, both within Africa and among migrant Africans in the West Indies and the US, the rates of CVD are comparable or higher than the rates of most Western countries. As in other populations, conventional CVD risk factors remain important, but the dominant CVD risk factor among people of African origin is hypertension. Special efforts at detection, prevention, and treatment of hypertension, both through lifestyle changes and appropriate pharmacologic therapy, are necessary. In the US, the socioeconomic disparity of this population results in an enhanced disease burden. This black–white differential in disease rates, risk factors and access to medical treatments necessitates specific prevention strategies for this group. Such strategies include primary prevention programs to prevent unhealthy lifestyle behaviors such as poor dietary practices and cigarette smoking. As these risk factors are closely tied to low socioeconomic status, other factors besides "biomedical" ones must be targeted. Health care providers must ensure equal access to health care services, especially among the poorer black population. However, in order to overcome the larger differential in socioeconomic status between African-Americans and whites, overall changes to social policy are required at the national level.

Studies of multiple ethnic groups

Studies of diverse ethnic populations who reside in a single country and hence are exposed to a similar environment indicate that the pattern of CHD mortality within these groups initially resembles that of their home country. However, through the process of acculturation, prolonged exposure to new environmental factors results in similarities in CVD risk factors and trends within a multiethnic population.

A study of multiple ethnic groups in the US revealed that CVD mortality rates were highest among African-Americans, followed by whites and Hispanics.[70] By contrast, Japanese, Chinese, Koreans, and Filipinos had much lower CHD mortality rates. Another study conducted in California between 1985 and 1990 compared CHD and CBVD death rates in six ethnic groups. Once again, African-American men and women in all age groups were found to have the highest CVD death rates. Hispanics, Chinese, and Japanese had much lower CVD rates although the CBVD deaths were proportionally a more important cause of death among the Chinese and Japanese. Furthermore, a study which

347

compared the rates of hospitalization for CHD among Asian-Americans with Americans in Northern California revealed that the risk of hospitalization for CHD was lowest among the Chinese-Americans (0.6) and highest among the South Asians (3.7, P<0.001).[71] Recent data from the UK reveal that although the CHD mortality rates were approximately 43% higher among South Asian men and women compared to the general UK population (ASMR: men 282/100 000, women ASMR 89/100 000), among South Asians a decline in the CHD rates of 26% in men and 18% in women occurred.[72] This is in keeping with a decline in CHD mortality in the UK as a whole over the past decade.

In Canada, an analysis of the Canadian national mortality database of South Asians, Chinese and Canadians of European origin demonstrated that the ASMR per 100 000 for CHD in South Asians (men 320, women 144) was similar compared to European Canadians (men 320, women 110), yet was much higher than Chinese (men 107, women 40). Furthermore, a significant decline in CHD death rates from 1979–83 to 1989–93 was observed in all groups with the greatest declines being apparent among South Asian men and women compared to European Canadians and Chinese respectively (men 22%, 13%, and 5.4% and women 6%, 4%, and 2%)[33] (Table 22.4). Furthermore, in Canada the inverse socioeconomic status–mortality relationship is observed in European Canadians but not in South Asians and Chinese. This raises the issue of whether this relationship is *acquired* within societies and therefore is potentially preventable/modifiable.

CONCLUSIONS

CVD accounts for the largest percentage of deaths worldwide (Table 22.7). To date, recognition and modification of the major CVD risk factors have led to declines in CVD rates in most Western countries, although these declines have lagged behind in most non-white populations. Socioeconomic development, urbanization, and increasing life expectancy have led to a progressive rise in the CVD rates in developing countries such as India and China.

It is clear that elevated serum cholesterol, elevated blood pressure, cigarette smoking, and glucose intolerance are the major risk factors for CHD and CBVD in most populations. However, the prevalence of these factors and the strength of association of these factors with CVD varies between ethnic groups. Furthermore, other risk or protective factors (levels of endogenous fibrinolysis, dietary factors such as flavonoids and antioxidants) likely exist. Identification of these factors is important so that new approaches to prevention of CVD in these populations may be developed. Research into ethnic populations who suffer adverse glucose and lipid changes upon adoption of urban lifestyles (i.e. Hispanics, Aboriginals, and South Asians) should be a priority as a greater proportion of these groups are experiencing increases in CVD rates. Furthermore, in developed countries, research into reasons for social disparity and its impact on the distribution of CVD risk factors among ethnic groups must be continued so specific interventions may be developed to reduce the adoption of unhealthy lifestyle behaviors and remove barriers to health care services. Ultimately all of this information will lead to special strategies for prevention which may be tailored to ethnic populations and generate important areas for future study.

Table 22.7 Summary of disease rates and risk factors among major ethnic groups. Based mainly on studies conducted in North America. (Note that disease rates will vary by study but this table provides a useful but approximate comparison between ethnic groups)

	US whites[44]	Chinese[10]	Japanese[10]	South Asian[33]	African-American[44]	Hispanic[44]	Aboriginal[57]
Disease pattern	Reference population	↓↓CHD ↑↑CBVD	↓↓CHD ↑↑CBVD	↑↑CHD ↑↑CBVD	↑↑CHD ↑↑CBVD	↑↑CHD ↓↓CBVD	↓↓CHD ↓↓CBVD
CHD mortality per 100 000 in North America	M 135 F 64	M 44 F 23	M 79 F 41	M 135 F 84	M 138 F 85	M 205 F 80	M 86 F 48
CBVD mortality per 100 000 in North America	M 26 F 22	M 24 F 27	M 26 F 23	M 25 F 25	M 52 F 26	M 32 F 23	M 23 F 23
CHD prevalence	7.5%	China: 4% Mauritius: 24%	Japan: 5%	Rural India: 2.7% Urban India: 10% Abroad: 17%	6.9%	5.6%	4%
Temporal pattern	↓↓CHD ↓↓CBVD	↑↑CHD ↓↓CBVD	-CHD ↓↓CBVD	↑↑CHD in India ↓↓CHD abroad ↓↓CBVD abroad	↓↓CHD[a] ↓↓CBVD[a]	↓↓CHD ↓↓CBVD[a]	↑↑CHD ↓↓CBVD[a]
Common risk factors[b]	Cholesterol Smoking Hypertension Diabetes Obesity	Hypertension Smoking	Hypertension Smoking	Cigarette smoking Abdominal obesity Hypertension Dysglycemic[d]	Hypertension Obesity Low SES Diabetes/IGT Smoking	Diabetes/IGT Hypertension Smoking Low HDL Obesity	Diabestes Obesity Smoking
Protective factors		Low cholesterol ? Antithrombotic factors	Low cholesterol ? Antithrombotic factors	Rural lifestyle	↑↑HDL cholesterol	Rural lifestyle	Rural lifestyle
Increasing risk factors with urbanization	Obesity Sedentary Lifestyle	↑↑Cholesterol Smoking Diabetes Obesity	↑↑Cholesterol Smoking Diabetes Obesity	Diabetes Obesity Hypertension Cholesterol	Diabetes Obesity	Diabetes Obesity	Diabetes Obesity
Prevention strategy[c]	Low fat diet Exercise Prevent smoking	Control BP Maintenance of traditional diet Prevent smoking	Control BP Maintenance of traditional diet Prevent smoking	Low fat diet Prevent obesity Exercise Blood glucose control	Improved access to care Control BP Prevent obesity	Low fat diet Weight loss Exercise Blood glucose control	Low fat diet Weight loss Exercise Blood glucose control

[a] Decline slower than in US whites.
[b] Ordered by decreasing importance.
[c] All factors matter but special attention paid to.
[d] Fasting blood glucose >4.9 mmol/l.

REFERENCES

1 Lenfant C. Task force on research in epidemiology and prevention of cardiovascular diseases [news]. *Circulation* 1994;**90**:2609–17.

2 Cooper R. A note on the biologic concept of race and its application in epidemiologic research. *Am Heart J* 1984;**108**:715–22.

3 Chaturvedi N, McKeigue PM. Methods for epidemiological surveys of ethnic minority groups [see comments]. [Review]. *J Epidemiol Community Health* 1994;**48**:107–11.

4 Murray CJ. Quantifying the burden of disease: the technical basis for disability-adjusted life years. *Bull WHO* 1994;**72**:429–45.

5 Lopez AD. Assessing the burden of mortality from cardiovascular diseases. *World Health Stat Quart* 1993;**46**:91–6.

6 Marmot M. Coronary heart disease: rise and fall of a modern epdiemic, In:Marmot M, Elliot P. eds. *Coronary heart disease epidemiology.* Oxford: Oxford University Press, 1995, pp 3–19.

7 Menotti A, Keys A, Kromhout D *et al.* Inter-cohort differences in coronary heart disease mortality in the 25-year follow-up of the seven countries study. *Eur J Epidemiol* 1993;**9**:527–36.

8 Siegfried B. WHO MONICA Project: objectives and design. *Int J Epidemiol* 1989;**18**:S29–S37.

9 Benfante R. Studies of cardiovascular disease and cause-specific mortality trends in Japanese-American men living in Hawaii and risk factor comparisons with other Japanese populations in the Pacific region: a review. *Human Biol* 1992; **64**:791–805.

10 *World health statistical annual 1994.* Geneva: WHO, 1994.

11 Thorvaldsen P, Asplund K, Kuulasmaa K, Rajakangas AM, Schroll M. Stroke incidence, case fatality, and mortality in the WHO MONICA project. World Health Organization monitoring trends and determinants in cardiovascular disease [published erratum appears in *Stroke* 1995;**26**(8): 1504]. *Stroke* 1995;**26**:361–7.

12 Artaud-Wild SM, Connor SL, Sexton G, Connor WE. Differences in coronary mortality can be explained by differences in cholesterol and saturated fat intakes in 40 countries but not in France and Finland. A paradox [see comments]. *Circulation* 1993;**88**:2771–9.

13 Criqui MH, Ringel BL. Does diet or alcohol explain the French paradox? *Lancet* 1994;**344**:1719–23.

14 Vartiainen E, Puska P, Pekkanen J, Tuomilehto J, Jousilahti P. Changes in risk factors explain changes in mortality from ischaemic heart disease in Finland. *Br Med J* 1994;**309**:23–7.

15 Hunink MG, Goldman L, Tosteson A *et al.* The recent decline in mortality from coronary heart disease, 1980–1990. *JAMA* 1997;**277**:535–42.

16 Zatonski W. The development of Poland's health situation after 1988. 1996 (personal communication).

17 Vartiainen E, Puska P, Jousilahti P *et al.* Twenty-year trends in coronary risk factors in north Karelia and in other areas of Finland. *Int J Epidemiol* 1994;**23**:495–504.

18 Iso H, Komachi Y, Shimamoto T, Iida M. Trends for cardiovascular risk factors and disease in Japan: implications for primordial prevention. 1996(personal communication).

19 Fujishima M, Kiyohara Y, Kato I *et al.* Diabetes and cardiovascular disease in a prospective population survey in Japan. *Diabetes* 1996;**45**:S14–S16.

20 Hong Y, Bots ML, Pan X *et al.* Stroke incidence and mortality in rural and urban Shanghai from 1984 through 1991. Findings from a community-based registry. *Stroke* 1994;**25**:1165–9.

21 Woo KS, Donnan SP. Epidemiology of coronary arterial disease in the Chinese. [Review]. *Int J Cardiol* 1989;**24**:83–93.

22 Donnan SP, Ho SC, Woo J *et al.* Risk factors for acute myocardial infarction in a southern Chinese population. *Ann Epidemiol* 1994;**4**:46–58.

23 Chen Z, Peto R, Collins R *et al.* Serum cholesterol concentration and coronary heart disease in population with low cholesterol concentrations [see comments]. *Br Med J* 1991;**303**:276–82.

24 Tao SC, Huang ZD, Wu XG *et al.* CHD and its risk factors in the People's Republic of China. *Int J Epidemiol* 1989;**18**:S159–S163.

25 People's Republic of China–United States Cardiovascular and Cardiopulmonary Epidemiology Research Group. An epidemiological study of cardiovascular and cardiopulmonary disease risk factors in four populations in the People's Republic of China. *Circulation* 1992;**85**:1083–96.

26 Li N, Tuomilehto J, Dowse G *et al.* Electrocardiographic abnormalities and associated factors in Chinese living in Beijing and in Mauritius. The Mauritius Non-Communicable Disease Study Group. *Br Med J* 1992;**304**: 1596–601.

27 Hughes K, Yeo PP, Lun KC *et al.* Cardiovascular diseases in Chinese, Malays, and Indians in Singapore. II. Differences in risk factor levels. *J Epidemiol Community Health* 1990;**44**:29–35.

28 Chonhua Y, Zhaosu W, Yingkai W. The changing pattern of cardiovascular diseases in China. *World Health Stat Quart* 1993;**46**:113–18.

29 Reddy KS. Cardiovascular diseases in India. *World Health Stat Quart* 1993;**46**:101–7.

30 Enas EA Yusuf S, Mehta J. Prevalence of coronary artery disease in Asian Indians. *Am J Cardiol* 1992;**70**:945–9.

31 Lowy AGJ, Woods KL, Botha JL. The effects of demographic shift on coronary heart disease mortality in a large migrant population at high risk. *J Public Health Med* 1991;**13**:276–80.

32 Balarajan R. Ethnic differences in mortality from ischemic heart disease and cerebrovascular disease in England and Wales. *Br Med J* 1991; **302**:560–4.

33 Sheth T, Chagani K, Nargundkar M *et al.* Ethnic differences in cause-specific mortality: South Asians, Chinese, whites in Canada. *Eur Heart J* 1996;**17**:234 (Abstract).

34 McKeigue PM, Ferrie JE, Pierpoint T, Marmot MG. Association of early-onset coronary heart disease in South Asian men with glucose intolerance and hyperinsulinemia. *Circulation* 1993;**87**:152–61.

35 McKeigue PM, Shah B, Marmot MG. Relation of central obesity and insulin resistance with high diabetes prevalence and cardiovascular risk in South Asians [see comments]. *Lancet* 1991;**337**: 382–6.

36 Pais P, Pogue J, Gerstein H *et al.* Risk factors for acute myocardial infarction in Indians: a case control study. *Lancet* 1996;**348**:358–63.

37 Ramachandran A, Dharmaraj D, Snehalatha C, Viswanathan M. Prevalence of glucose intolerance in Asian Indians. *Diabetes Care* 1992; **15**:1348–55.

38 Anand S, Enas E, Pogue J *et al.* Elevated lipoprtoein (a), low HDL cholesterol and elevated glucose in South Asians compared to North American Whites. *Eur Heart J* 1996;**17**:398.

39 Gerstein HC, Yusuf S. Dysglycaemia and risk of cardiovascular disease. *Lancet* 1996;**347**: 949–50.

40 Reddy S. Coronary heart disease in different racial groups. In:Yusuf S, Wilhelmsen L. eds. *Advanced issues in prevention and treatment of atherosclerosis.* Surrey: Euromed Communications, 1995, pp 47–62.

41 Gupta R, Gupta VP. Meta-analysis of coronary heart disease prevalence in India. *Indian Heart J* 1996;**48**:241–5.

42 Reddy S. ICMR cross-sectional study of CHD risk factors in urban and rural India. 1997; (Abstract).

43 Bhatnagar D, Anand IS, Durrington PN *et al.* Coronary risk factors in people from the Indian subcontinent living in west London and their siblings in India [see comments]. *Lancet* 1995; **345**:405–9.

44 American Heart Association. *Heart and stroke facts: 1996 statistical supplement.* Dallas, TX: American Heart Association, 1995.

45 Becker T, Wiggins C, Key C, Samet J. Ischemic heart disease mortality in Hispanic American Indians and non-Hispanic whites in New Mexico, 1958–1982. *Circulation* 1988;**78**:302–9.

46 Goff D, Nichaman M, Chan W *et al.* Greater incidence of hospitalized myocardial infarction among Mexican-Americans than non-Hispanic whites: The Corpus Christi Heart Project, 1988–1992. *Circulation* 1997; (in press).

47 Gillum RF. Epidemiology of stroke in Hispanic Americans. *Stroke* 1995;**26**:1707–12.

48 Morgenstern L, Spears W, Goff D, Grotta J, Nichaman M. African Americans and women have the highest stroke mortality in Texas. *Stroke* 1997;**28**:15–18.

49 Stern M, Gaskill S. Secular decline in death rates due to ischemic heart disease in Mexican Americans and non-Hispanic whites, Texas 1970–1980. *Circulation* 1987;**76**:1245–50.

50 Pappas G, Gergen PJ, Carroll M. Hypertension prevalence and the status of awareness, treatment, and control in the Hispanic Health and Nutrition Examination Survey 1982–84. *Am J Public Health* 1990;**80**:1431–6.

51 Haffner SM, Valdez RA, Hazuda HP *et al.* Prospective analysis of the insulin-resistance syndrome (syndrome X). *Diabetes* 1992;**41**: 715–22.

52 Goff DC Jr, Ramsey DJ, Labarthe DR, Nichaman MZ. Greater case-fatality after myocardial infarction among Mexican Americans and women than among non-Hispanic whites and men. The Corpus Christi Heart Project [see comments]. *Am J Epidemiol* 1994; **139**:474–83.

53 Goff DC Jr, Ramsey D, Labarthe DR, Nichaman MZ. Acute myocardial infarction and coronary heart disease mortality among Mexican Americans and non-Hispanic whites in Texas, 1980 through 1989. *Ethnicity Dis* 1993;**3**:64–9.

54 Goff DC Jr, Varas C, Ramsey DJ *et al.* Mortality after hospitalization for myocardial infarction among Mexican Americans and non-Hispanic whites: the Corpus Christi Heart Project. *Ethnicity Dis* 1993; **3**:55–63.

55 Howard BV, Lee ET, Cowan LD *et al.* Coronary heart disease prevalence and its relation to risk factors in American Indians. The Strong Heart Study. *Am J Epidemiol* 1995;**142**:254–68.

56 MacMillan H, MacMillan A, Offord D, Dingle J. Aboriginal health. *Can Med Assoc J* 1996;**155**: 1569–78.

57 Gillum RF. The epidemiology of stroke in Native Americans. *Stroke* 1995;**26**:514–21.

58 Mao Y, Moloughney B, Semenciw R, Morrison H. Indian reserve and registered Indian mortality in Canada. *Can J Public Health* 1992;**83**:350–3.

59 Howard BV, Lee ET, Fabsitz RR *et al.* Diabetes and coronary heart disease in American Indians: The Strong Heart Study. *Diabetes* 1996;**45**(Suppl 3): S6–13.

60 Murray CJ, Lopez AD. Mortality by cause for eight regions of the world: Global Burden of Disease Study. *Lancet* 1997;**349**:1269–76.

61 Murray CJL, Lopez AD. Alternative projections of mortality and disability by cause 1990–2020: Global Burden of Disease Study. *Lancet* 1997;**349**: 1498–504.

62 Berrios X, Koponen T, Huiguang T *et al.* Distribution and prevalence of major risk factors of noncommunicable diseases in selected countries: the WHO Inter-Health Programme. *Bull WHO* 1997;**75**:99–108.

63 Seedat YK. Ethnicity, hypertension, coronary heart disease, and renal diseases in South Africa. *Ethnicity Health* 1996;**1**:349–57.

64 Akinkugbe OO. World epidemiology of hypertension. In: Hall WD, Saunders E, Shulman NB, eds. *Hypertension in blacks: epidemiology, pathophysiology, and treatment.* St Louis: Year Book Publishers, 1985, pp 13–16.

65 Miller GJ, Beckles GL, Maude GH *et al.* Ethnicity and other characteristics predictive of coronary heart disease in a developing community: principal results of the St James Survey, Trinidad. *Int J Epidemiol* 1989;**18**:808–17.

66 Gillum RF. Sudden coronary death in the United States: 1980–1985. *Circulation* 1989;**79**:756–65.

67 Moliterno DJ, Jokinen EV, Miserez AR *et al.* No association between plasma lipoprotein(a) concentrations and the presence or absence of coronary atherosclerosis in African-Americans. *Arterioscler Thromb Vasc Biol* 1995;**15**:850–5.

68 Geronimus AT, Bound J, Waidmann TA, Hillemeier MM, Burns PB. Excess mortality among blacks and whites in the United States [see comments]. *N Engl J Med* 1996;**335**:1552–8.

69 Fang J, Madhavan S, Alderman MH. The association between birthplace and mortality from cardiovascular causes among black and white residents of New York City [see comments]. *N Engl J Med* 1996;**335**:1545–51.

70 Frerichs RR, Chapman JM, Maes EF. Mortality due to all causes and to cardiovascular diseases among seven race-ethnic populations in Los Angeles County, 1980. *Int J Epidemiol* 1984;**13**: 291–8.

71 Klatsky AL, Tekawa I, Armstrong MA, Sidney S. The risk of hospitalization for ischemic heart disease among Asian Americans in northern California. *Am J Public Health* 1994;**84**:1672–5.

72 Balarajan R. Ethnicity and variations in mortality from coronary heart disease. *Health Trends* 1996; **28**:45–51.

73 Tunstall-Pedoe H, Kuulasmaa K, Amouyel P *et al.* Myocardial infarction and coronary deaths in the World Health Organization MONICA Project. Registration procedures, event rates, and case-fatality rates in 38 populations from 21 countries in four continents. *Circulation* 1994;**90**:583–612.

74 Wyndham CH. Trends with time of cardiovascular mortality rates in the populations of the RSA for the period 1968–1977. *South African Med J* 1982; **61**:987–93.

75 Steinberg WJ, Balfe DL, Kustner HG. Decline in the ischaemic heart disease mortality rates of South Africans, 1968–1985. *South African Med J* 1988;**74**:547–50.

76 Baligadoo S, Manraj M, Krishnamoorthy R, Jankee S, Ramaswamy R. Genetic contribution to the high mortality from coronary disease in Indian Diaspora: case study of Mauritius. *Eur Heart J* 1994;**15**:162 (Abstract).

77 Tuomilehto J, Ram P, Eseroma R, Taylor R, Zimmet P. Cardiovascular diseases and diabetes mellitus in Fiji: analysis of mortality, morbidity and risk factors. *Bull WHO* 1984;**62**:133–43.

78 Beckles GL, Miller GJ, Kirkwood BR *et al.* High total and cardiovascular disease mortality in adults of Indian descent in Trinidad, unexplained by major coronary risk factors. *Lancet* 1986;**1**:1298–301.

79 Hughes K, Lun KC, Yeo PP. Cardiovascular diseases in Chinese, Malays, and Indians in Singapore. I. Differences in mortality. *J Epidemiol Community Health* 1990;**44**:24–8.

80 Adelstein AD, Marmot MG, Bulusu L. Migrant studies in Britain. *Br Med Bull* 1984;**40**:315–19.

81 McKeigue PM, Marmot MG. Mortality from coronary heart disease in Asian communities in London. *Br Med J* 1988;**297**:903.

Part III
Specific cardiovascular disorders
i: Stable coronary artery disease

BERNARD J GERSH, Editor

Grading of recommendations and levels of evidence used in *Evidence Based Cardiology*

GRADE A

Level 1a   Evidence from large randomized clinical trials (RCTs) or systematic reviews (including meta-analyses) of multiple randomized trials which collectively has at least as much data as one single well-defined trial.

Level 1b   Evidence from at least one "All or None" high quality cohort study; in which ALL patients died/failed with conventional therapy and some survived/succeeded with the new therapy (eg chemotherapy for tuberculosis, meningitis, or defibrillation for ventricular fibrillation); or in which many died/failed with conventional therapy and NONE died/failed with the new therapy (eg penicillin for pneumococcal infections).

Level 1c   Evidence from at least one moderate sized RCT or a meta-analysis of small trials which collectively only has a moderate number of patients.

Level 1d   Evidence from at least one RCT.

GRADE B

Level 2   Evidence from at least one high quality study of non-randomized cohorts who did and did not receive the new therapy.

Level 3   Evidence from at least one high quality case control study.

Level 4   Evidence from at least one high quality case series.

GRADE C

Level 5   Opinions from experts without reference or access to any of the foregoing (eg argument from physiology, bench research or first principles).

A comprehensive approach would incorporate many different types of evidence (eg RCTs, non-RCTs, epidemiologic studies, and experimental data), and examine the architecture of the information for consistency, coherence and clarity. Occasionally the evidence does not completely fit into neat compartments. For example, there may not be an RCT that demonstrates a reduction in mortality in individuals with stable angina with the use of beta-blockers, but there is overwhelming evidence that mortality is  reduced following MI. In such cases, some may recommend use of beta-blockers in angina patients with the expectation that some extrapolation from post-MI trials is warranted. This could be expressed as Grade A/C. In other instances (e.g. smoking cessation or a pacemaker for complete heart block), the non-randomized data are so overwhelmingly clear and biologically plausible that it would be reasonable to consider these interventions as Grade A.

Recommendation grades appear either in a shaded margin box with an 'R' logo as shown, or within the text, for example Grade A.

Anti-ischemic drugs

23

LIONEL H. OPIE

A major problem . . . is the lack of sufficient data comparing antianginal and placebo treatment.[1]

The major anti-ischemic drugs are, in historical order of appearance, the nitrates, the beta-adrenergic blockers, and the calcium-channel antagonists. In addition, there is increasing evidence that the angiotensin converting enzyme (ACE) inhibitors and the statin lipid lowering drugs have indirect anti-ischemic properties. Preservation of endothelial function may also be an indirect anti-ischemic procedure. The antiplatelet agents including aspirin and the new GPIIb/II receptor blockers, as well as the antithrombotics and thrombolytics, will not be considered here but in the following section of Part III on acute ischemic syndromes. Special attention will be paid to the potential effect of the standard anti-ischemic drugs not just in giving symptomatic relief of angina, but, in keeping with the aim of this book, on hard outcome endpoints such as reinfarction and mortality.

WHAT IS ISCHEMIA?

Ischemia of the myocardium is probably the most important cause of cardiovascular and total mortality and morbidity in Western societies, yet ischemia is difficult to define.[2] Although there are many definitions, in the end they come down to an inadequate blood supply to the myocardium. The Greek *ischo* means "to hold back" and *haima* means "blood". The word ischemia was, it seems, first used by Rudolf Virchow in 1858, to describe a situation in which limitation of blood flow resulted from an increased resistance to blood flow. The "modern" concept of supply–demand imbalance as a cause of ischemia dates back to observations made nearly two hundred years ago on the exercising limb.[3]

If we call into vigorous action a limb around which we . . . applied a ligature, we find then that the member can only support its action for a very short time; for now its supply of energy and its expenditure do not balance each other.

Myocardial ischemia therefore exists when the reduction of coronary flow is so severe that the supply of oxygen is inadequate for the demands of the tissue, which is the

Table 23.1 The clinical spectrum of acute ischemia and the various drugs used

Clinical syndrome	Pathophysiology	Drug therapy	Outcome in RCTs
Effort angina	Imbalance of oxygen supply–demand	Nitrates, beta-blockers, calcium antagonists	None for nitrates, limited for others
Unstable angina	As above, prolonged	As above, antithrombotics	None for anti-ischemic drugs
Threatened MI	As above prior to start of cell necrosis	Beta-blockade	Possible benefit for beta-blockade, harm for nifedipine
Ischemic arrhythmias	Ischemia-induced rise in cell calcium and cyclic AMP; increased Purkinje fibers; lipid changes	Beta-blockade	Indirect evidence strongly favors beta-blockade, but no RCTs have been directed towards ischemic arrhythmias

RCTs, randomized controlled trials

generally accepted situation in acute effort angina. Ischemia is often distinguished from infarction, the latter reflecting prolonged irreversible ischemia with myocardial cell death. Therefore the ischemia is also the underlying situation in unstable angina and the very early phase of the clinical syndrome of acute myocardial infarction (AMI), when reperfusion can still reverse the ischemic myocardial damage. Myocardial ischemia is also thought to contribute, together with the underlying anatomical substrate, to the potentially lethal ventricular arrhythmias found in patients with ischemic heart disease.

Myocardial ischemia may also occur chronically, as proposed for hibernation. In the latter case, the proposal is that the myocardium has undergone a chronic adaption to ischemia by downregulation of contraction. The simplified concept is "little blood, little work".[4]

Therefore, there is a wide spectrum of conditions in which myocardial ischemia is clinically relevant (Table 23.1) and for which anti-ischemic drugs can be used. As will be argued, the hard evidence for their long term benefit is, in general, strikingly absent.

GENERAL ASPECTS OF SAFETY AND EFFICACY

Safety and efficacy are ultimately linked: the more pronounced the beneficial effects of a therapeutic regimen, the greater the degree of side effects that may be tolerated. A drug that significantly prolongs life, such as alteplase or streptokinase in AMI, is recommended for use despite an increased incidence of hemorrhagic stroke, because a consideration of the combined endpoints of mortality plus stroke favor the use of the drug. There exists a hierarchy for the significance of endpoints, the most important primary endpoint being prolongation of life, with secondary endpoints being an improved quality of life either by reduction of morbidity or by relief of symptoms such as anginal pain. Tertiary endpoints are those that neither improve the quantity nor the quality of life, but which are expected to prevent disease by reducing risk factors; examples are treating arterial hypertension or lowering elevated blood lipid levels in otherwise normal individuals.

Evidence for the first of these endpoints is in general scant in relation to the anti-ischemic drugs. Information gathered in one situation is not necessarily directly relevant to another. Thus, for example, the benefits of beta-blockade in postmyocardial infarct (MI) prevention[5] do not necessarily show that these drugs also prolong life in stable effort angina. The present author agrees with Hjemdahl *et al.*[1] that the pathophysiological situation in patients with symptomatic angina is often very different from that in the post-MI setting. In MI, there is a zone of dead tissue, and depending on its size there will be reactive remodeling in the rest of the ventricle, introducing a different pathophysiological situation and predisposing to left ventricular (LV) failure. Also, the presence of viable and non-viable myocardium creates electrical inhomogeneity that predisposes to re-entry with risks of lethal ventricular arrhythmias. Furthermore, the possibility of the coexistence of stunning, hibernation, and preconditioning, collectively called the new ischemic syndromes, all predispose to a highly complex and multifarious spectrum that constitutes ischemic LV dysfunction.[6] Although some of these abnormalities may be found in chronic stable angina, because there may be coexisting previous MI, nonetheless the predominant and basic pathology is in the one case transient myocardial ischemia causing effort angina, and in the other case dead tissue with reactive ventricular remodeling. Nonetheless, a sizable portion of patients in studies on chronic stable angina – up to one-third – have had previous infarcts.[1] Post-MI angina therefore merits specific consideration, but again outcome studies are missing.

HOW IS SAFETY ASSESSED? THE HIERARCHY OF EVIDENCE

Safety is not well defined but could be regarded as the absence of significant adverse effects when the drug is used with due regard for its known contraindications. Safety implies the added assurance that there are no hidden dangers in the legitimate use of the drug. Evidence for safety, like evidence for efficacy, can come from a variety of sources. There is a hierarchy of evidence regarding safety, starting from anecdotal case reports as the least reliable, followed by case series, case control studies, cohort studies, and going through to more coherent information with emphasis on large controlled randomized trials (RCTs) and carefully conducted meta-analyses of these trials, leading to acceptance of the overall evidence as favoring a position where the benefit and the safety of a drug group is well established (which is the most reliable evidence). For example, in the case of calcium antagonists, most of the current evidence on adverse effects comes from case control or cohort studies or small RCTs. Such data are subject to serious intrinsic problems of the methodology which can generate hypotheses without being capable of proof or otherwise. On the other hand, in the case of beta-blockers, there is substantial evidence for benefit in the data on post-MI patients from many large trials,[5] whereas among the calcium antagonists, only for verapamil is there good evidence, which is limited by the small numbers involved.

SAFETY CONCERNS REGARDING CALCIUM ANTAGONISTS

Recently a number of safety concerns have been raised in relation to calcium antagonists, and to some extent also in relation to beta-blockers. Many of these are based on case-control or cohort studies, which are not a reliable source of information.[7] There are major contradictions between the studies. The question of cancer and gastrointestinal hemorrhage as possible side effects is reviewed by the WHO–ISH committee, without a causative association being found.[8] In the case of cancer, one small cohort study is outweighed by two bigger negative studies.[9,10] In the case of hemorrhage, the evidence is incomplete and not supported by prospective studies. In general, it is the short acting calcium antagonists[11] and particularly short acting nifedipine that have been associated with adverse effects.[12]

There is long standing good evidence that short acting instant release (IR) nifedipine in capsule form can increase mortality in acute ischemic syndromes[13,14] so that it is contraindicated in unstable angina or early phase MI unless accompanied by beta-blockade. It follows that: (1) the mechanism of the adverse effects of IR nifedipine is very probably by reflex adrenergic activation, and (2) even in stable effort angina, neither short acting nifedipine nor any other short acting dihydropyridine should be used in the absence of an accompanying beta-blocker. Indirect data from a meta-analysis of effort angina[15] could also suggest that a short acting dihydropyridine should be avoided in effort angina.

Safety concerns have also been raised in relation to beta-blockers. Case control studies have raised the possibility of an increased incidence of sudden cardiac arrest or death in hypertensive patients treated by beta-blockade.[16,17] Again, the potential weakness of case control studies must be emphasized.

R

Grade A

SAFETY vs SAFE USE

Whenever a serious side effect of any given drug becomes known, and acted on, then that safety issue should be obviated so that the drug becomes safer. For example, beta-blockers are no longer given to patients with pre-existing excess bradycardia or sick sinus syndrome or asthma. In that sense, the increased mortality long known in relation to the use of IR nifedipine in acute ischemic syndromes is a safety issue that should already have been overcome by the appropriate warnings.

RCTs OF CALCIUM ANTAGONISTS AND BETA-BLOCKERS IN EFFORT ANGINA

Regarding trials with outcome endpoints, there are only two relatively small RCTs which compare calcium antagonists with beta-blockers in effort angina, neither trial having a placebo arm. In the APSIS[18] study, slow release verapamil was compared with metoprolol, the main prognostic endpoints being a combination of morbidity and mortality (total and cardiovascular), and non-fatal cardiovascular complications including myocardial infarction, revascularization, stroke, and peripheral vascular events, as well as treatment failure. These endpoints did not differ significantly between the treatments, nor were side effects or quality of life indices different between the two drugs. Even though 809 patients were followed for more than 3 years on the average, for a total of almost 1400 patient years per treatment group, the trial was not large enough to exclude the possibility that there could still be significant differences in a single endpoint such as mortality between the agents, because of the very low death rate, which was about 2% per year of follow-up. Regarding mortality, it is impossible to exclude that either drug might be better than the other, or that one or the other drugs might be better or worse than placebo (not tested). Studies to settle the mortality issue are unlikely to be undertaken, so we must evaluate the combined endpoints actually tested. On present evidence there are not enough data to conclude that either the calcium antagonists or the beta-blockers differ one from the other or from placebo. The exception to this statement relates to the adverse effects of IR nifedipine in acute ischemic syndromes, and by extrapolation to the avoidance of such drugs in effort angina unless used with beta-blockade.

TIBET[19] compared slow release nifedipine (twice daily formulation) with atenolol. As there were three treatment arms including the combination of these drugs, and only 682 patients in total to start with, there were only 450 patient years in each group. Outcome was assessed by a combination of endpoints considered either "hard" (cardiac mortality, MI or unstable angina) or "soft" (revascularization or treatment failure). For a mean follow-up of 2 years, there were totals of 47 endpoints in the atenolol group, 46 in the nifedipine group, and 31 in the combination group. Total deaths were not reported, but cardiac deaths were 3, 6 and 4 respectively. There were no differences between the groups in the predetermined endpoints, and the only difference of note was more drop-outs in the nifedipine group (40% vs 27% for atenolol and 29% for the combination, this difference being highly significant with $P=0.001$). Thus the major conclusion of this study is that it is underpowered for hard endpoints and even for combined hard and soft endpoints. The major firm conclusion is the poor tolerance of nifedipine tablets.

The ASIST[20] study is the only one in mild effort angina or silent ischemia that compares a beta-blocker, atenolol, with placebo. Patients with moderate to severe angina were excluded. Over one year, atenolol gave better event-free survival, using a mixed bag of endpoints, including death, resuscitation, non-fatal myocardial infarction, hospitalization for unstable angina, aggravation of angina, and revascularization. There were only a few serious events and the most evident difference was that there was less aggravation of angina with atenolol (9 of 152 vs 26 of 154 with placebo, $P=0.003$). This trial, therefore, tells us that atenolol is antianginal, which is not surprising.

The combined message emerging from APSIS, TIBET, and ASIST is this: the real problem is that the incidence of hard endpoints such as mortality, infarction, or unstable angina is so low in chronic stable effort angina, that vast trials would be needed to show beyond doubt that calcium antagonists or beta-blockers do more than relieve symptoms. Because of the rather low death rate, with cardiac deaths at about 1% per year, these trials could have missed large relative differences of 30–40% in death between the agents, although any differences in the absolute death rate would remain small even in a mega-trial. From the expected effect of trial size on trial results,[5] it can be estimated that, to study 600 total deaths in effort angina, even with a risk reduction of one-quarter, would need about 30 000 patients in a long term trial (60 000 if the endpoint is cardiac mortality) to show any differences between calcium antagonists and beta-blockers. Trials of this size are, in the view of the present author, unlikely ever to be undertaken. Rather, it makes sense to select high risk patients with clusters of risk factors such as age, male gender, hypertension, smoking, and hypercholesterolemia. Alternatively, trials carefully designed to establish whether or not two treatments have an equivalent effect may be considered because fewer numbers are required than in mega-trials.[21] From the point of view of evidence based medicine, the data currently available are insufficient, even though the efficacy and safety of the calcium antagonist under test was in the same range as that of the beta-blocker in both the APSIS and TIBET trials.

RCTs OF NITRATES IN EFFORT ANGINA

There are no such trials reported and none is being planned. Nitrates therefore remain strictly in the realm of agents that provide symptomatic relief, without evidence for outcome benefit. Theoretically, the reflex tachycardia that they invoke might adversely affect the long term outcome in ischemic states.

UNSTABLE ANGINA AS AN EXAMPLE OF PROLONGED ISCHEMIA

This condition has two major components: acute myocardial ischemia, and a disturbance of the thrombotic mechanism. Antianginal drugs therefore constitute only part of the therapy. In contrast to the good data on the benefit of heparin and aspirin, there is again no good evidence for the benefit of nitrates in unstable angina. Compared with intravenous diltiazem, intravenous nitroglycerin was less effective on short term endpoints such as refractory angina and MI.[22] Regarding long term outcome with nitrates in unstable angina, there has been only one trial, which compared transdermal nitroglycerin with placebo therapy over 4 months, each arm receiving in addition conventional medical treatment. Outcome events such as death, MI or refractory angina were similar in the nitrate and placebo arms.[23]

In the case of beta-blockade, there are no good studies, the only one available showing an insignificant trend to short term benefit as measured by the decrease in recurrent ischemia or MI within 48 hours.[24] Neither of two older studies had hard endpoints.[25,26]

There is a difference in the safety profile of the DHPs (dihydropyridines) and the non-DHPs (such as verapamil and diltiazem). Of the DHPs, only IR nifedipine has been well tested, with an adverse outcome in two trials. In the HINT study,[21] IR nifedipine was inferior to placebo with MI within 48 h as an endpoint (odds ratio 2.0, confidence intervals 1.1–3.6) so that the trial was stopped,[24] while in the other study[27] there was an increase in early mortality. The heart rate increasing effect of the IR nifedipine[27] was probably the result of adrenergic activation because a benefit for the addition of IR nifedipine to prior beta-blockade was shown in both these trials and also by Gerstenblith *et al.*[28] By contrast, the non-DHP diltiazem was successfully used in comparison with a nitrate, both agents being given intravenously with a relative risk of 0.49 in favor of diltiazem for short term events, chiefly recurrent pain.[22] Diltiazem decreased the heart rate whereas the nitrate increased it. Although there has been no similar trial with verapamil, several smaller trials suggest efficacy.[29–31] While it is possible that long acting DHPs such as amlodipine that do not increase the heart rate might be safe in unstable angina, no such trials are likely to be done. The conclusion from the safety point of view is that the non-DHP diltiazem is best tested without the trial being large enough to yield outcome data, that verapamil may be similar in its effects though even less well tested, and that the DHPs as a group are relatively contraindicated with short acting nifedipine (and nicardipine) totally contraindicated.

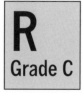

R

Grade C

PRINZMETAL'S VARIANT ANGINA

This type of angina at rest is caused by coronary spasm and is specifically relieved by calcium antagonists. There are no outcome studies with hard endpoints, perhaps because the condition is potentially fatal and therefore placebo-controlled trials would be impossible. Some of the studies with remission of attacks as endpoint are reviewed by Opie and Maseri.[32] Short acting agents are standard. Of these, nifedipine should not be used unless the diagnosis is firm, and it is sure that the patient does not have unstable angina or threatened MI.

THREATENED INFARCTION

In this situation where ischemia is threatening to develop into infarction, IR nifedipine had adverse short term (2-week) effects in a relatively small randomized trial, in which mortality was increased from 0 of 82 placebo patients to 7 of 89 nifedipine patients ($P=0.018$).[13] By contrast, in another relatively small trial with propranolol started intravenously within 4 hours of the onset of symptoms of AMI and then continued orally, there were fewer completed infarcts as shown by a limitation of blood enzyme rise,[26] and the incidence of ventricular fibrillation was less.[33] These small trials do not provide definitive information but are in agreement with the general concept that adrenergic activation is harmful in threatened infarction[26,34] so that beta-blockade is the preferred mode of therapy. This recommendation is, however, not based on good trial data.

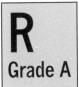

POST-INFARCT EFFORT ANGINA

Two large RCTs suggest that long term post AMI therapy by IR nifedipine in standard doses is not beneficial or possibly harmful.[14,35] Angina was not a specific endpoint. Even though evidence from cohort studies is contradictory,[36,37] this agent is far from ideal for post-MI patients with angina.

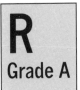

Only one of the post-MI trials with calcium antagonists specifically reported on the incidence of angina pectoris in a subgroup of the postinfarct DAVIT II study,[38] in which verapamil 360 mg per day was started 7–15 days following infarct and continued for up to 18 months. Verapamil was significantly antianginal.[39] Regarding the outcome of the DAVIT II study as a whole, in the verapamil group there was a reduction (RR 0.80, CI 0.64–0.99) in the combined endpoint predetermined as death and/or reinfarction. Although total mortality did not fall, the RR was also 0.80 (CI 0.61–1.05), and the lack of significance could possibly be ascribed to the relatively small numbers involved. Regarding heart failure, analysis of predetermined subgroups, undertaken before the code was broken, showed that in patients without prior heart failure during their stay in the coronary care unit, there was a mortality reduction ($P=0.024$). There was no effect of verapamil, either beneficial or harmful, in those with *prior* (not concurrent) heart failure. However, subgroup analysis even with predetermined endpoints is open to criticism.

Regarding diltiazem, the MDPIT postinfarct study in which diltiazem was given as 240 mg per day for a mean of 25 months, did not report on effort angina.[40] An earlier study in which diltiazem was given for 14 days after non-Q wave infarction found no difference in the incidence of chest pain "recognized as angina pectoris".[41] Outcome evidence that this drug increases cardiac events (cardiac deaths and/or non-fatal infarction) in post-MI patients with congestive heart failure cannot be disputed.[40]

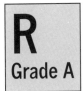

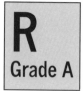

Regarding beta-blockers, there is impressive evidence that these drugs prolong life in postinfarct patients.[5] Therefore, although there appear to be no formal trials on antianginal properties in postinfarct patients, the large number of postinfarct trials and the many patients studied, mean that these drugs have more overall compelling evidence in their favor in the postinfarct situation than does verapamil and much more compelling evidence than for the DHP calcium antagonists. First principles suggest it is likely that they are exerting their benefit at least in part by an anti-ischemic effect, although a beneficial effect on remodeling and postinfarct heart failure is a reasonable alternative.[42,43]

ISCHEMIC ARRHYTHMIAS

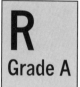

The Cape Town hypothesis is that beta-blockers have a ventricular antiarrhythmic effect in AMI by limiting metabolic changes such as increased levels of cyclic AMP in the ischemic tissue.[34,44] Nonetheless, other modes of action are possible, for example by inhibition of the current I_f that initiates pacemaker activity in injured Purkinje cells. A meta-analysis has shown that beta-blockade is effective when given as prophylactic antiarrhythmic therapy in the context of AMI and that it reduces mortality with an odds ratio of 0.81 in 55 trials.[45] Further evidence for outcome benefit for beta-blockers, as in post-infarct patients, comes from the Cardiac Arrhythmia Suppression Trial (CAST) in which prior beta-blockade therapy was associated with a one-third reduction in arrhythmic death or cardiac arrest.[43] By contrast, calcium antagonists had a slightly increased relative risk, albeit not of statistical significance. Yet these findings do not prove that the beta-blockers were acting as anti-ischemic agents, and only provide indirect evidence that beta-blockers are safe when deliberately chosen as anti-ischemic drugs in other clinical situations.

CALCIUM ANTAGONISTS IN STABLE ANGINA AFTER ANGIOPLASTY

There is no convincing evidence that pharmacological therapy alters the incidence of restenosis. There is some evidence from a meta-analysis that calcium antagonists as a group may help to prevent restenosis,[46] which should mean lessened effort angina – a possibility that was not reported. In one specific study over 6 months, twice daily verapamil reduced restenosis following percutaneous transluminal coronary angioplasty (PTCA), but only in patients with stable angina.[47] Beta-blockers appear to be untested in this situation.

CONGESTIVE HEART FAILURE AND EFFORT ANGINA

There are no studies with this combination as a predetermined endpoint. Indirect evidence suggests a role for ACE inhibitors. Of interest, in the PRAISE study[48] amlodipine (despite increasing pulmonary edema) lessened mortality in the subgroup of patients without a history of angina, but not in those with angina.

ACE INHIBITORS AS POTENTIAL ANTI-ISCHEMIC DRUGS

There are at least four potentially anti-ischemic mechanisms whereby ACE inhibitors may operate. First, angiotensin II is known to facilitate sympathetic adrenergic transmission, also in humans.[49] Second, ACE inhibitors, by formation of bradykinin, indirectly promote the formation of nitric oxide, which in turn inhibits myocardial oxygen consumption.[50] Third, ACE inhibitors are potentially antihypertensive and thereby reduce the afterload. Fourth, in 15 hypertensive patients of whom 11 had effort angina, ACE inhibitors improved coronary flow reserve after long term therapy.[51] The mechanism may be by reversal of endothelial dysfunction.[52] Not surprisingly, these agents have a documented antianginal effect in hypertensive patients with angina[53,54] without, however, any outcome data. In patients with low ejection fractions, below 35%, chronic therapy by enalapril in the Studies of Left Ventricular Dysfunction (SOLVD) trials led to less hospital admissions for unstable angina, and therefore might well have reduced stable effort angina, but the data are not clear on this point.[55] In the SAVE study there was an unexpected reduction in recurrent MI in the group given captopril.[56] The hypothesis that ACE inhibitors can protect against manifestations of ischemic heart disease is under test in several very large trials with mellifluous acronyms such as PEACE and HOPE. In "standard" angina of effort, without hypertension or heart failure, ACE inhibitors have an inconstant effect, as reviewed elsewhere.[57] Any outcome benefit in patients with ischemic heart disease as opposed to heart failure remains controversial and multifactorial in origin.[58] Logically, the expected benefit would be more in patients with more severe ischemia and a greater activation of the adrenergic and renin–angiotensin systems.[59]

STATINS AS POTENTIAL ANTI-ISCHEMIC DRUGS

Statins have made a considerable difference to the mortality of patients with ischemic heart disease in several studies. In the West of Scotland Coronary Prevention Study (WESCOPS), pravastatin was able to reduce hard endpoints in middle aged hypercholesterolemic men without prior MI. In this group, the occurrence of angina pectoris was highly correlated ($P<0.0001$) with the primary endpoint which was definite coronary heart disease death or non-fatal MI.[60] Therefore, in hypercholesterolemic males with angina, statins are able to reduce hard endpoints. That they have a direct anti-ischemic effect is shown by reduction of ST segment deviations on 48-hour Holter traces in patients with stable angina pectoris, documented coronary artery disease and pre-existing antianginal therapy, the latter not being specified.[61] Nonetheless, there is no formal proof that these agents have clinical antianginal efficacy.

DIURETICS AS POTENTIAL ANTI-ISCHEMIC DRUGS

Short term diuretic therapy has an antianginal effect, possibly by reduction of the left ventricular preload.[62] No outcome data are available. Some case-control studies on hypertensive patients have suggested increased mortality on diuretics when given in high doses and without potassium supplementation.[16,17]

CONCLUSIONS

There are few if any satisfactory outcome studies available with the conventional antianginal drugs in effort angina. There are no trials at all on nitrates, and only rather small trials comparing beta-blockers and calcium antagonists. Some indirect evidence suggests that the ACE inhibitors and statins may have antianginal properties. Adequately powered outcome trials in patients with cardiac death and non-fatal MI as endpoints in effort angina would require mega-trials in view of the low incidence of these events. It would be more practicable to select high risk categories or to aim trials at showing drug equivalence. In unstable angina, where ischemia is prolonged, there are no good trials showing that nitrates, beta-blockers or calcium antagonists – all commonly used drugs – have outcome benefit. Although beta-blockers have good evidence favoring their use as prophylactic antiarrhythmic drugs in AMI, with a reduction in mortality shown by meta-analysis, it is not certain that they are acting as anti-ischemic drugs in this situation.

Key points

- Standard anti-ischemic drugs (nitrates, beta-blockers, calcium antagonists) relieve anginal pain but their effect on outcome in effort angina is not known. Two relatively small trials suggest equivalence between calcium antagonists and beta-blockers. It is desirable but unlikely that mega-trials will be conducted to settle this issue.
- Likewise in unstable angina, outcome data for the anti-ischemic agents are lacking.
- An exception is short acting nifedipine, which in two trials in acute ischemic syndromes has increased mortality, probably by reflex adrenergic activation.
- The closer the patient is to AMI, the stronger are the data for the safety of beta-blockers.
- In the postinfarct phase the data for safety and efficacy of beta-blockers are especially strong. The only calcium antagonist with good evidence for safety is verapamil, but without mortality benefit in the relatively small trials conducted.
- In acute ischemic ventricular arrhythmias, there is indirect evidence for the prophylactic effect of beta-blockers on mortality, even though there is no formal trial.
- Indirect evidence in the absence of formal trials also suggests that statins and angiotensin converting enzyme inhibitors have some anti-ischemic properties.

REFERENCES

1 Hjemdahl P, Eriksson SV, Held C, Rehnqvist N. Prognosis of patients with stable angina pectoris on antianginal drug therapy. *Am J Cardiol* 1996; 77:6D–15D.

2 Hearse DJ. Myocardial ischaemia: can we agree on a definition for the 21st century? *Cardiovasc Res* 1994;28:1737–44.

3 Burns A. *Observations on some of the most frequent and important diseases of the heart; on aneurysm of the thoracic aorta; on preternatural pulsation in the epigastric region; and on the unusual origin and distribution of some of the large arteries of the human body.* Edinburgh: Bryce, 1809.

4 Rahimtoola SH. The hibernating myocardium. *Am Heart J* 1989;117:211–21.

5 Yusuf S, Peto R, Lewis J *et al.* Beta blockade during and after myocardial infarction: an overview of the randomized trials. *Prog Cardiovasc Dis* 1985; 27:335–71.

6 Opie LH. The multifarious spectrum of ischemic left ventricular dysfunction: relevance of new ischemic syndromes. *J Mol Cell Cardiol* 1996;28: 2403–14.

7 Yusuf S, Garg R, Zucker D. Analyses by the intention-to-treat principle in randomized trials and databases. *PACE* 1991;14:2078–82.

8 WHO-ISH Study. Ad Hoc Subcommittee of the Liaison Committee of the World Health Organisation and the International Society of

Hypertension. Effects of calcium antagonists on the risks of coronary heart disease, cancer and bleeding. *J Hypertens* 1997;**15**:105–15.

9 Jick H, Jick S, Derby LE *et al*. Calcium-channel blockers and risk of cancer. *Lancet* 1997;**349**: 525–8.

10 Olsen JH, Sorensen HT, Friis S *et al*. Cancer risk in users of calcium channel blockers. *Hypertension* 1997;**29**:1091–4.

11 Alderman MH, Cohen H, Rogue R, Medhaven S. Effect of long-acting and short-acting calcium antagonists on cardiovascular outcomes in hypertensive patients. *Lancet* 1997;**349**:594–8.

12 Pahor M, Guralnik JM, Corti M *et al*. Long term survival and use of antihypertensive medications in older persons. *J Am Geriat Soc* 1995;**43**: 1191–7.

13 Muller J, Morrison J, Stone P *et al*. Nifedipine therapy for patients with threatened and acute myocardial infarction: a randomized, double-blind, placebo-controlled comparison. *Circulation* 1984;**69**:740–7.

14 SPRINT II Study, Goldbourt U, Behar S *et al*. Early administration of nifedipine in suspected acute myocardial infarction. The Secondary Prevention Reinfarction Israel Nifedipine Trial 2 Study. *Arch Intern Med* 1993;**153**:345–53.

15 Glasser SP, Clark PI, Lipicky RJ *et al*. Exposing patients with chronic, stable, exertional angina to placebo periods in drug trials. *JAMA* 1991; **265**:1550–4.

16 Hoes AW, Grobbee DE, Lubsen J *et al*. Diuretics, β-blockers, and the risk for sudden cardiac death in hypertensive patients. *Ann Intern Med* 1995; **123**:481–7.

17 Siscovick DS, Raghunathun TE, Psaty BM. Diuretic therapy for hypertension and the risk of primary cardiac arrest. *N Engl J Med* 1994;**330**: 1852–7.

18 Rehnqvist N, Jjemdahl P, Billing E, Bjokander I, Eriksson SV. Effects of metoprolol vs verapamil in patients with stable angina pectoris. The Angina Prognosis Study in Stockholm (APSIS). *Eur Heart J* 1996;**17**:76–84.

19 Dorgio HJ, Ford I, Fox KM, on behalf of the TIBET study group. Total Ischaemic Burden European Trial (TIBET): effects of ischaemia and treatment with atenolol, nifedipine SR and their combination on outcome in patients with chronic stable angina. *Eur Heart J* 1996;**17**:104–12.

20 Pepine C, Cohn PF *et al*. Effects of treatment on outcome in mildly symptomatic patients with ischemia during daily life. The Atenolol Silent Ischemia Study (ASIST). *Circulation* 1994;**90**: 762–8.

21 Hampton JR. Alternatives to mega-trials in cardiovascular disease. *Cardiovasc Drugs Ther* 1996;**10**:759–65.

22 Gobel E, Hautvast R, van Gilst W *et al*. Randomised double-blind trial of intravenous diltiazem versus glyceryl trinitrate for unstable angina pectoris. *Lancet* 1995;**346**:1653–7.

23 Ardissino D, Merlini PA, Savonitto S *et al*. Effect of transdermal nitroglycerin on N-acetylcysteine, or both, in the long-term treatment of unstable angina pectoris. *J Am Coll Cardiol* 1997;**29**: 941–7.

24 HINT Study. Early treatment of unstable angina in the coronary care unit, a randomised, double-blind placebo controlled comparison of recurrent ischemia in patients treated with nifedipine or metoprolol or both. Holland Inter-university Nifedipine Trial. *Br Heart J* 1986;**56**:400–13.

25 Fischl SJ, Herman MV, Gorlin R. The intermediate coronary syndrome. Clinical, angiographic and therapeutic aspects. *N Engl J Med* 1973;**288**: 1193–8.

26 Norris RM, Sammel NL, Clarke ED, Smith WM. Protective effect of propranolol in threatened myocardial infarction. *Lancet* 1978;**ii**:907–9.

27 Muller J, Turi Z, Pearl D *et al*. Nifedipine and conventional therapy for unstable angina pectoris: a randomized, double-blind comparison. *Circulation* 1984;**69**:728–33.

28 Gerstenblith G, Ouyang P, Achuff SC *et al*. Nifedipine in unstable angina. A double-blind, randomized trial. *N Engl J Med* 1982;**306**: 885–9.

29 Mauritson DR, Johnson SM, Winniford MD *et al*. Verapamil for unstable angina at rest: a short-term randomized, double-blind study. *Am Heart J* 1983;**106**:652.

30 Mauri F, Marfici A, Briaghi M *et al*. Effectiveness of calcium antagonist drugs in patients with unstable angina and proven coronary artery disease. *Eur Heart J* 1988;**9**:158–63.

31 Capucci A, Bassein L, Bracchetti D *et al*. Propranolol v. verapamil in the treatment of unstable angina. A double-blind cross-over study. *Eur Heart J* 1983;**4**:148–54.

32 Opie LH, Maseri A. Vasospastic angina. In: Krebs R, ed. *Treatment of cardiovascular disease by Adalat (nifedipine)*. Stuttgart: Schattauer, 1986.

33 Norris RM, Brown MA, Clarke ED *et al*. Prevention of ventricular fibrillation during acute myocardial infarction by intravenous propranolol. *Lancet* 1984;**ii**:883–6.

34 Opie LH. Myocardial infarct size. 2. Comparison of anti-infarct effects of β-blockade, glucose-insulin-potassium, nitrates and hyaluronidase. *Am Heart J* 1980;**281**:1462–4.

35 SPRINT I Study. Secondary Prevention Reinfarction Israeli Nifedipine Trial. A randomized intervention trail of nifedipine in patients with acute myocardial infarction. *Eur Heart J* 1988;**9**: 354–64.

36 Braun S, Boyko V, Behar S *et al*. Calcium antagonists and mortality in patients with coronary artery disease: a cohort study of 11, 575 patients. *J Am Coll Cardiol* 1996;**28**:7–11.

37 Koenig W, Lowel H, Lewis M, Hormann M. Long-term survival after myocardial infarction: relationship with thrombolysis and discharge medication. Results of the Augsburg myocardial infarction follow-up study. *Eur Heart J* 1996;**17**: 1199–206.

38 Jespersen CM, Hansen JF, Mortensen LS. Danish Study Group on Verapamil in Myocardial Infarction: the prognostic significance of post-infarction angina pectoris and the effect of verapamil on the incidence of angina pectoris and prognosis. *Eur Heart J* 1994;**15**:270–6.

39 DAVIT Study, Jespersen CM, Hansen JF, Mortensen LS. The prognostic significance of post-infarction angina pectoris and the effect of verapamil on the incidence of angina pectoris and prognosis. *Eur Heart J* 1994;**15**:270–6.

40 MDPIT Study. The Multicenter Diltiazem Postinfarction Trial Research Group. The effect of diltiazem on mortality and reinfarction after myocardial infarction. *N Engl J Med* 1988;**319**: 385–92.

41 Gibson RS, Boden WE, Theroux P *et al*. Diltiazem and reinfarction in patients with non-Q-wave myocardial infarction. *N Engl J Med* 1986;**315**: 423–9.

42 Lichstein E, Hager D, Gregory JJ *et al*. Relation between beta-adrenergic blocker use, various correlates of left ventricular function and the chance of developing congestive heart failure. *J Am Coll Cardiol* 1990;**16**:1327–32.

43 Kennedy HL, Brooks MM, Barker AH *et al*. β-blocker therapy in the cardiac arrhythmia suppression trial. *Am J Cardiol* 1994;**74**: 674–80.

44 Lubbe WH, Podzuweit T, Opie LH. Potential arrhythmogenic role of cyclic adenosine monophosphate (AMP) and cytosolic calcium overload: implications for prophylactic effects of beta-blockers in myocardial infarction and proarrhythmic effects of phosphodiesterase inhibitors. *J Am Coll Cardiol* 1992;**19**: 1622–33.

45 Teo KK, Yusuf S, Furberg CD. Effects of prophylactic antiarrhythmic drug therapy in acute myocardial infarction. *JAMA* 1993;**270**: 1589–95.

46 Hillegass WB, Ohman M, Leimberger JD, Califf RM. A meta-analysis of randomized trials of calcium antagonists to reduce restenosis after coronary angioplasty. *Am J Cardiol* 1994;**73**:835–9.

47 Hoberg E, Kubler W. Prevention of restenosis after PTCA: role of calcium antagonists. *J Cardiovasc Pharmacol* 1991;**18**(Suppl 6):S15.

48 Packer M, O'Connor C, *et al*. for the Prospective Randomized Amlodipine Survival Evaluation Study Group. Effect of amlodipine on morbidity and mortality in severe chronic heart failure. *N Engl J Med* 1996;**335**:1107–14.

49 Lyons D, Webster J, Benjamin N. Angiotensin II. Adrenergic sympathetic construction action in humans. *Circulation* 1995;**91**:1457–60.

50 Zhang X, Xie Y-W, Nasjletti A *et al*. ACE inhibitors promote nitric oxide accumulation to modulate myocardial oxygen consumption. *Circulation* 1997;**95**:176–82.

51 Motz W, Strauer BE. Improvement of coronary flow reserve after long-term therapy with enalapril. *Hypertension* 1996;**27**:1031–8.

52 TREND Study, Mancini GB, Henry GC, Macaya C *et al*. Angiotensin-converting enzyme inhibition with quinapril improves endothelial vasomotor dysfunction in patients with coronary artery disease. The TREND (Trial on Reversing Endothelial Dysfunction) Study. *Circulation* 1996; **94**:258–65.

53 Akhras F, Jackson G. The role of captopril as single therapy in hypertension and angina pectoris. *Int J Cardiol* 1991;**33**:259–66.

54 Stumpe KO. Overlack A, on behalf of the Perindopril Therapeutic Safety Study Groups (PLUTS). A new trial of the efficacy, tolerability and safety of angiotensin-converting enzyme inhibition in mild systemic hypertension with concomitant diseases and therapies. *Am J Cardiol* 1993;**71**:32E–7E.

55 Yusuf S, Pepine CJ, Garces C *et al*. Effect of enalapril on myocardial infarction and unstable angina in patients with low ejection fractions. *Lancet* 1992; **340**:1173–8.

56 Pfeffer MA, Braunwald E, Moye LA. Effect of captopril on mortality and morbidity in patients with left ventricular dysfunction after myocardial infarction. Results of the Survival and Ventricular Enlargement trial. *N Engl J Med* 1992;**327**: 669–77.

57 Opie LH. *Angiotensin converting enzyme inhibitors: Scientific basis for clinical use*. New York: Author's Publishing House, 1992.

58 Young JB. Reduction of ischemic events with angiotensin-converting enzyme inhibitors: lessons and controversy emerging from recent clinical trials. *Cardiovasc Drugs Ther* 1995;**9**: 89–102.

59 Remme WJ, Kruyssen DA, Look MP *et al*. Systemic and cardiac neuroendocrine activation and severity of myocardial ischemia in humans. *J Am Coll Cardiol* 1994;**23**:82–91.

60 WESCOPS Study. The West of Scotland Coronary Prevention Study Group. Baseline risk factors and their association with outcome in the West of Scotland Coronary Prevention Study. *Am J Cardiol* 1997;**79**:756–62.

61 van Boven AJ, Jukema W, Zwinderman AH *et al.* Reduction of transient myocardial ischemia with pravastatin in addition to the conventional treatment in patients with angina pectoris. *Circulation* 1996;**94**:1503–5.

62 Parker JD, Parker AB, Farrell B, Parker JO. Effects of diuretic therapy on the development of tolerance to nitroglycerin and exercise capacity in patients with chronic stable angina. *Circulation* 1996;**93**:691–6.

24 Chronic coronary artery disease: coronary artery bypass surgery vs percutaneous transluminal coronary angioplasty vs medical therapy

CHARANJIT S. RIHAL,
BERNARD J. GERSH,
SALIM YUSUF

INTRODUCTION

Coronary artery disease is the leading cause of death in developed countries and is a major determinant of health care resource use and costs, and lost productivity due to illness. It is likely to maintain that status as demographic changes leading to a higher proportion of persons in older age groups continue and patients with previous cardiac procedures return with recurrent symptoms.

Since the original descriptions of surgical[1] and percutaneous[2] revascularization, the past two decades have witnessed technical advances such that the number of revascularization procedures has continued to increase yearly. By 1994 more than 428 000 percutaneous transluminal coronary angioplasty (PTCA) and 501 000 coronary artery bypass graft (CABG) procedures had been performed in the United States.[3] Both these procedures and their variations have significant potential to improve morbidity and mortality among a large number of patients. However, the indiscriminate application of these procedures may increase both costs and morbidity and mortality. We believe that rational application, informed by the evidence, will lead to medically appropriate, yet cost-effective approaches.

Which patients should receive CABG and PTCA for chronic coronary artery disease? Choosing myocardial revascularization techniques requires a thorough knowledge of the pertinent evidence, relative efficacies, estimation of individual risk-to-benefit ratios, and an understanding of the limitations of each procedure. Currently, practicing clinicians are confronted with a wide range of treatment options for chronic coronary artery disease, and treatment modalities continue to evolve rapidly. This chapter reviews the published evidence comparing CABG, PTCA, and medical therapy for chronic coronary artery disease. It attempts to place the evidence from recent trials that compared modes of revascularization in the context of previous data that compared CABG with medical therapy. Limitations of the available data and application to clinical practice are also discussed.

The medical management of patients with chronic coronary artery disease is reviewed in detail elsewhere (Chapters 23 and 31). Patients with chronic coronary artery disease may be those who have recovered after a myocardial infarction or unstable angina or those with chronic stable angina. All patients should be treated routinely with aspirin. If they have previously had a myocardial infarction, they should receive a beta-blocker for secondary prophylaxis to reduce the risk of death or recurrent myocardial infarction. Patients with heart failure or those with markers of left ventricular dysfunction should also receive an angiotensin converting enzyme inhibitor. Patients with angina pectoris should initially be managed with beta-blockers and nitrates. If symptoms continue or side effects develop, calcium-blockers are useful alternatives. It is our preference to use calcium antagonists that lower the heart rate (e.g., diltiazem or verapamil). If medical therapy fails (refractory angina) or patients have objective evidence of significant ischemia, angiography is indicated. In all patients, an assessment of risk factors (increase in lipids, blood pressure, glucose, or overweight) should be performed and appropriately controlled. In addition, every effort to get smokers to give up their habit should be emphasized and, if necessary, smokers should be referred to smoking cessation clinics. A comprehensive approach to the medical management of patients is the underlying foundation of management of all patients with chronic coronary artery disease. In the subsequent sections, we discuss the role of revascularization in appropriately selected patients.

Considered empirically, there are three broad indications for myocardial revascularization: to improve or alleviate symptoms caused by myocardial ischemia, to improve the likelihood of long term survival, and to prevent non-fatal events such as myocardial infarction or progression to congestive heart failure. With respect to these outcomes, the following questions can be asked: how does CABG compare with medical therapy, how does PTCA compare with medical therapy, and how does PTCA compare with CABG when revascularization is required?

CABG vs MEDICAL THERAPY

Three landmark prospective randomized studies provide the bulk of the data on which current practice is based: the European Coronary Surgery Study (ECSS), the Veterans Administration (VA) Coronary Artery Bypass Surgery Cooperative Study Group, and the Coronary Artery Surgery Study (CASS).[4-6] These trials and numerous retrospective studies from associated registries demonstrated that the absolute mortality benefit of CABG was proportional to the long term risk of medical therapy.[5-7] Although both the VA study and CASS failed to demonstrate an overall mortality difference between medical and surgical groups that was statistically significant, subgroups in which CABG was superior to medical therapy were identified early. These subgroups included patients with left main coronary artery disease[8,9] or left main "equivalent" disease[10] and patients with three vessel disease with left ventricular dysfunction.[11] The ECSS trial demonstrated a reduction in mortality overall that was statistically significant. The results appeared most marked in patients with left main coronary artery disease, three vessel disease, or two vessel disease with stenosis of the proximal left anterior descending artery.[4,9]

Interpretation of these results has numerous limitations. The trials were confined to patients age 65 years or younger (whereas more than 50% of CABG procedures are now performed among this group).[3] Only CASS included women, and only 14% of the patients in CASS received an internal thoracic conduit. This conduit was not used in the other trials. At the time, lipid lowering agents were not widely used, HMG-CoA reductase inhibitors were not available, and aspirin was not widely used in either medical or surgical patients. High risk patients such as those with severe angina and left main coronary artery stenosis were underrepresented in these trials. Nonetheless, the results delivered a consistent message, which holds true in the current era, namely, that the benefits of coronary revascularization, in comparison with medical therapy, were proportional to baseline risk, as defined by anatomic and physiologic markers such as the number of diseased vessels, involvement of the proximal left anterior descending artery, degree of myocardial ischemia, and global left ventricular function. Although these studies provided the basis for numerous investigations on the role of myocardial revascularization, each trial was relatively small (350–400 patients per treatment arm) and definitive conclusions cannot be drawn, especially with regard to various subgroups of interest. However, more definitive conclusions can be drawn if the data from all the trials are considered together.

A systematic review (meta-analysis) of seven randomized trials of CABG versus an initial strategy of medical therapy for chronic coronary artery disease has been published.[7] In addition to the three major trials cited above, the report included four small trials (50 patients per treatment arm). In all, 2649 patients randomly allocated to CABG or medical therapy were included. All contributing trials were conducted in the 1970s and early 1980s and primarily included patients with stable angina pectoris. Those with medically refractory or unstable angina generally were not included. For purposes of the meta-analysis, original clinical and angiographic data were collected and analysed with uniform definitions. Abnormal ejection fraction was defined as $\leq 50\%$ and significant coronary stenosis was defined as >50% diameter reduction. Baseline angiographic and clinical characteristics are listed in Table 24.1. Of the patients enrolled, 20% had an abnormal ejection fraction and the majority had three vessel (50.6%) or left main coronary artery disease (6.6%). Most of the patients were between 40 and 60 years old and almost all were male. About one-half of the patients were taking beta-adrenergic blockers, but only 3% were receiving antiplatelet drugs; however, this proportion increased during follow-up.

Cumulative mortality over 12 years of follow-up is shown in Figure 24.1. At 5, 7, and 10 years, 10.2%, 15.8%, and 26.4% of patients, respectively, assigned to CABG had died, whereas 15.8%, 21.7%, and 30.5% of their medically assigned counterparts had died. Risk reductions (RR) were significant at all three time points (RR 0.61, 0.68, 0.83) even though 40% of patients initially assigned to medical treatment underwent CABG by 10 years. Because such crossovers occurred in the highest risk medical patients (left main coronary artery or three vessel disease, unstable angina), these trials would tend to underestimate the real benefits of CABG in comparison with medical therapy alone, and this underestimation would be greatest among high risk subsets. Because of the perioperative mortality associated with CABG, overall mortality was unchanged

R

Grade A

Table 24.1 Clinical and angiographic characteristics of patients enrolled in randomized trials of CABG vs medical therapy

Characteristic	% of patients
Age distribution (yr)	
<40	8.5
41–50	38.2
51–60	46.0
>60	7.3
Ejection fraction ($n=2474$)	
<40	7.2
40–49	12.5
50–59	28.0
≥ 60	52.3
Male	96.8
Severity of angina (CCS)	
None	11.2
Class I or II	53.8
Class III or IV	35.0
History	
Myocardial infarction	59.6
Hypertension	26.0
Heart failure	4.0
Diabetes mellitus	9.6
Smoking ($n=1949$)	83.5
Current smokers ($n=2298$)	45.5
ST segment depression >1 mm	
Resting ($n=2423$)	9.9
Exercise ($n=1985$)	70.5
Drugs at baseline	
Beta-blockers ($n=2308$)	47.4
Antiplatelet agents ($n=1195$)	3.2
Digitalis ($n=2319$)	12.9
Diuretics ($n=1940$)	12.6
No. of vessels diseased	
Left main artery	6.6
One vessel[a]	10.2
Two vessels[a]	32.4
Three vessels[a]	50.6
Location of disease	
Proximal left anterior descending	59.4
Left anterior descending diagonal	60.4
Circumflex	73.8
Right coronary	81.6

Data on some characteristics are not available for all patients: where data are available in less than 90% of the patients, numbers of patients with available data are shown in parentheses.

[a] Without left main artery.

From Yusef S *et al.*,[7] by permission of The Lancet Ltd.

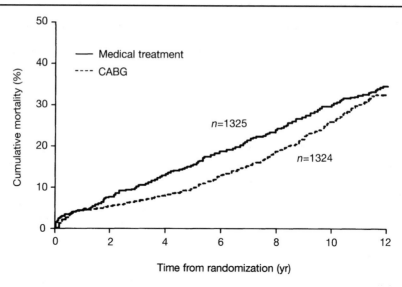

Figure 24.1 Overall survival after random allocation to medical treatment or coronary artery bypass graft. (From Yusuf S *et al.*,[7] by permission of The Lancet Ltd.)

early in the course of the trial. As with any prophylactic surgical treatment, enrolled subjects must survive long enough to accrue a net benefit from treatment. In this case, a significant net benefit was not seen in favor of CABG for 2–3 years (Figure 24.1). During long term follow-up, the advantage in favor of an initial strategy of CABG substantially widened up to 5–7 years, before again narrowing by 10–12 years. This tendency for the relative – but not the absolute – benefit to converge is likely due to a high rate of crossover among highest risk subsets, the development of graft atherosclerosis, and progression of underlying native vessel disease.

Significant heterogeneity of treatment effect was observed among angiographic and clinical subgroups (Table 24.2). In general, the survival advantage of CABG over medical therapy was proportional to the number of diseased coronary arteries (significant for three vessel [RR 0.58; $P<0.001$] and left main coronary artery [RR 0.32; $P=0.004$] disease) and, in particular, to involvement of the left anterior descending (LAD) coronary artery (RR 0.58, even if only one or two vessel disease). Relative benefits were similar regardless of left ventricular function (RR 0.61 [normal]; RR 0.59 [abnormal]). However, *absolute* benefit was greater among patients with an abnormal ejection fraction because the risk of death was twice as high in this group (5-year medical mortality rate of 25.2% with ejection fraction <50% vs 13.3% if >50%). Similarly, absolute and, to some extent, relative mortality benefits were greater among patients with evidence of myocardial ischemia (abnormal exercise test results or severe angina).

To further put the relative and absolute benefits of CABG into perspective, a risk score stratified by clinical and angiographic markers was developed. This indicated that patients at high risk (5-year medical mortality, 23%) experienced a clinically and statistically highly significant improvement in survival (RR 0.50; $P=0.001$). Those at moderate risk (5-year medical mortality, 11.5%) also benefited (RR 0.63; $P=0.05$), but absolute benefits were smaller. In contrast, no evidence was observed of survival benefit among those at low risk (5-year medical mortality, 5.5%; RR 1.18; $P=0.70$).

As mentioned above, among patients in whom a survival benefit cannot be expected, there are two broad potential indications for CABG: to alleviate symptoms of angina

Table 24.2 Outcomes of various subgroups in medical therapy (MT) vs CABG trials at 5 years

Subgroup	Overall numbers		MT mortality rate (%)	Odds ratio (95% CI)	P for CABG vs MT	P for interaction
	Deaths	Patients				
Vessel disease	21	271	9.9	0.54 (0.22–1.33)	0.18	0.19
One vessel						
Two vessels	92	859	11.7	0.84 (0.54–1.32)	0.45	
Three vessels	189	1341	17.6	0.58 (0.42–0.80)	<0.001	
Left main artery	39	150	36.5	0.32 (0.15–0.70)	0.004	
No LAD disease	50	606	8.3	1.05 (0.58–1.90)	0.88	0.06
One or two vessels						
Three vessels	46	410	14.5	0.47 (0.25–0.89)	0.02	
Left main artery	16	51	45.8	0.27 (0.08–0.90)	0.03	
Overall	112	1067	12.3	0.66 (0.44–1.00)	0.05	
LAD disease present	63	524	14.6	0.58 (0.34–1.01)	0.05	0.44
One or two vessels						
Three vessels	143	929	19.1	0.61 (0.42–0.88)	0.009	
Left main artery	22	96	32.7	0.30 (0.11–0.84)	0.02	
Overall	228	1549	18.3	0.58 (0.43–0.77)	0.001	
LV function	228	2095	13.3	0.61 (0.46–0.81)	<0.001	0.90
Normal						
Abnormal	115	549	25.2	0.59 (0.39–0.91)	0.02	
Exercise test status	102	664	17.4	0.69 (0.45–1.07)	0.10	0.37
Missing						
Normal	60	585	11.6	0.78 (0.45–1.35)	0.38	
Abnormal	183	1400	16.8	0.52 (0.37–0.72)	<0.001	
Severity of angina (CCS)						
Class 0, I, II	178	1716	12.5	0.63 (0.46–0.87)	0.005	0.69
Class III, IV	167	924	22.4	0.57 (0.40–0.81)	0.001	

From Yusuf S *et al*,[7] by permission of the Lancet Ltd.

pectoris over and above medical therapy and to reduce the incidence of non-fatal outcomes, such as myocardial infarction, congestive heart failure, and hospitalization. Registry studies have suggested a favorable impact on late myocardial infarction among highest risk subsets, such as patients with three vessel disease and severe angina pectoris.[12] Similarly, CABG generally is considered to improve or to relieve angina pectoris in a much broader group of patients than the subgroups in which it has been found to be superior in extending survival. In the meta-analysis of all CABG vs medical therapy trials, no overall impact of CABG surgery on subsequent infarction could be demonstrated. This was due primarily to an excess of infarction in the perioperative period (10.3% incidence of death or myocardial infarction at 30 days) among those assigned to surgery.[7] Although the risk of subsequent myocardial infarction was lower during extended follow-up, this was not statistically significant (24.4% incidence of death or myocardial infarction at 5 years for the CABG group vs 30.7% for the medical group).[7] It is unfortunate that most trials did not prospectively collect data on rehospitalization for unstable angina, quality of life, or cost.

Few randomized data from the modern era compare CABG with medical therapy. The Asymptomatic Cardiac Ischemia Pilot (ACIP) prospectively assigned 558 patients with asymptomatic but proven ischemia (positive exercise test results or ambulatory

R

Grade **A/B**

373

electrocardiographic monitor) to two medication strategies versus routine revascularization.[13,14] Among the 192 patients assigned to a revascularization strategy, 78 had CABG and 92 had PTCA.[13] The other 37 patients did not undergo the assigned procedure. Despite the relatively small sample size, after 2 years of follow-up, mortality was significantly lower among the patients assigned to routine revascularization (1.1% vs 6.6% and 4.4% for the two medical groups, $P<0.02$).[15] Rates of death or myocardial infarction were 12.1% (angina-guided), 8.8% (ischemia-guided), and 4.7% (revascularization, $P<0.04$). Similarly, rates of non-protocol revascularization (29% of medically assigned patients "crossed over") and hospital admissions were significantly lower among the revascularization group. Although designed as a pilot study, the observed risk reductions in the ACIP were dramatic and suggest that, among patients with evidence of myocardial ischemia, revascularization may be even more superior than previously thought in the context of modern revascularization techniques. They also point to a need for larger, more definitive randomized trials testing modern revascularization techniques, so that reliable estimates of effect size with narrower confidence intervals can be made.

R

Grade A

In summary, CABG improves long term survival in a broad spectrum of patients at moderate to high risk with medical therapy. Although a relative risk reduction of about 40% can be expected overall in comparison with medical therapy, absolute benefits are proportional to the expected risk with medical therapy. As such, absolute benefit is greatest among those at highest risk with medical therapy (5-year mortality >20%). Clinical and angiographic markers of risk, including severity of coronary artery disease, left ventricular dysfunction, and myocardial ischemia, can identify patients in various risk strata. Importantly, about 60% of patients enrolled in these trials had three vessel or left main coronary artery disease and about 20% had left ventricular dysfunction. The data are limited by the relatively small sample sizes of individual trials, the exclusion of women, and by the fact the data are 20 years old.

During the past two decades, advances have occurred in both surgical and medical treatments, and these potentially could alter the results if the trials were performed today. For example, arterial conduits, such as the left internal thoracic artery, are now preferred because of markedly superior long term patency rates, and the benefits of aggressive lipid lowering and chronic antiplatelet therapy have been demonstrated.[16,17] Despite these limitations, the available data are still the basis for current surgical practice in chronic coronary artery disease. Pilot data from ACIP suggest an accentuation of benefits with modern revascularization techniques and point to a need for modern trials.

ROLE OF CORONARY ANGIOPLASTY

Since its introduction in the late 1970s,[2] PTCA has gained wide acceptance by physicians and patients for the treatment of coronary artery stenoses. PTCA was developed primarily as a treatment for single vessel coronary artery disease, and more than 90% of PTCA procedures are still performed for this reason.[18,19] However, its role in multivessel disease is expanding. Rates of procedural success and complications[18,19] have been well described in large observational databases, but relatively few prospective randomized data are available about whether a patient with single vessel disease is best treated with medical therapy, PTCA, or CABG.

PTCA vs MEDICAL THERAPY

Few prospective randomized studies have directly compared PTCA with medical therapy. The first randomized trial of PTCA (A Comparison of Angioplasty with Medical Therapy in the Treatment of Single Vessel Coronary Artery Disease – ACME), was published in 1992,[20] 13 years after Gruentzig's initial report.[2]

In ACME, 212 patients with stable, single vessel coronary artery disease (70–99% stenosis) and exercise-induced myocardial ischemia were randomly assigned to PTCA or medical therapy and followed for 6 months. No patient assigned to PTCA died, and one patient in the medical arm died after a non-protocol PTCA. Even though PTCA was technically successful in only 80% of patients, the proportion of patients free of angina at 6 months was greater in the PTCA arm (64% vs 46%, P<0.01), and the mean number of monthly anginal episodes among those who were still symptomatic decreased. The use of medication among patients who underwent PTCA was significantly reduced but not eliminated. Treadmill exercise duration increased significantly more among the PTCA arm, even though the use of concomitant antianginal medications was discontinued before the test (increase, 2.1 vs 0.5 minutes; P<0.0001). However, the modest subjective (including psychologic wellbeing scores) and objective improvement in anginal symptoms among the PTCA group was at a significant price and included two emergency CABG operations and five myocardial infarctions. By 6 months, seven patients in the PTCA group had undergone CABG, compared with none in the medical arm, and 16 patients had required non-protocol PTCA, compared with 11 in the medical arm. No difference in rates of myocardial infarction was observed (five in the PTCA arm vs three in the medical arm) by 6 months.

These findings are reinforced by an even smaller trial of medical therapy versus PTCA for *asymptomatic* single vessel disease, with 88 patients in total and published in abstract form.[21] After 2 years of follow-up, no important differences emerged with respect to myocardial infarction (1 vs 2, medical vs PTCA, respectively), angina (11 vs 9), death (1 vs 0), or non-protocol revascularization (9 vs 7).

The results of the Randomized Intervention Treatment of Angina (RITA)-2 trial have been published recently.[22] This prospective, randomized trial of 1018 patients with stable coronary artery disease was conducted at 20 sites in the United Kingdom and Ireland and tested the hypothesis that elective PTCA would reduce the combined frequency of all-cause death and definite non-fatal myocardial infarction. Patients with recent unstable symptoms were excluded and 80% of patients had Canadian Cardiovascular Society (CCS) class 0 to II angina (47% class 0 or I and 33% class II) and 78% were taking one or two antianginal drugs at enrollment. Also, 60% of the patients had single vessel coronary artery disease, 33% had two vessel disease, and 7% had three vessel disease; only 6% of the patients had significant left ventricular dysfunction. Results over a median 2.7-year follow-up period are summarized in Figure 24.2. Eighteen deaths occurred (average mortality, 0.7% per year), and the primary endpoint of death or myocardial infarction occurred in 6.3% of PTCA patients and 3.3% of patients assigned to medical therapy (absolute difference, 3.0%; 95% confidence interval, 0.4–5.7%; P = 0.02). The difference was attributable mainly to one death and seven myocardial infarctions among patients undergoing PTCA. The combined rates of death, myocardial infarction, and non-protocol revascularization were about 25% in both groups by 3 years of follow-up and were primarily due to worsening of symptoms among the medical group. Angina pectoris and treadmill exercise time improved significantly in both groups,

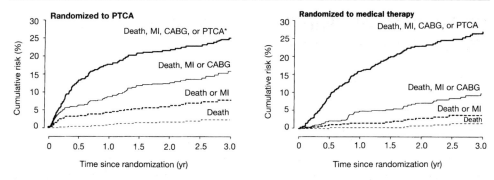

Figure 24.2 Cumulative risk of PTCA, CABG, myocardial infarction or death; * denotes PTCA in addition to randomized PTCA. (Modified from RITA-2 Trial participants,[22] by permission of The Lancet Ltd.)

especially in the PTCA group (absolute 16.5% excess of grade 2 or worse angina in the medical group at 3 months). Because patients with severe symptoms among both groups underwent non-protocol revascularization during 3 years of follow-up, the difference in reported angina decreased (absolute 7.6% difference in grade 2 angina or worse). Patients with grade 2 or worse angina appeared to benefit from PTCA, with a 20% lower incidence of angina and 1 minute longer treadmill exercise times, whereas patients with mild symptoms at enrollment derived no significant improvement in symptoms.

A reasonable conclusion appears to be that among patients with low risk coronary artery disease (average mortality, 0.7% per year in RITA-2), PTCA (plus needed antianginal medications) can improve symptoms short term in comparison with medications alone. However, no apparent reduction can be expected in the need for subsequent PTCA, myocardial infarction, or CABG. These data suggest that PTCA is indicated for single vessel disease if the desired level of anginal relief cannot be achieved with medical therapy. It is also only important to remember that coronary angiography, indispensable in establishing the diagnosis and guiding invasive treatment, cannot predict sites of future coronary occlusion. The majority of so-called culprit lesions are mild (<50% diameter stenosis) before acute infarction, and the site of acute occlusion frequently is not the most severe previous stenosis.[23–26]

On the basis of these data, "prophylactic" PTCA for mild symptoms cannot be recommended; however, because of the extremely small total sample size and short follow-up, the possibility that clinically important differences (or type II error) were missed cannot be excluded. These data do not address whether new interventional and medical therapies, such as stents[27–29] (used in 8% of patients in RITA-2), HMG-CoA reductase inhibitors,[30] and antiplatelet antibodies,[31] may significantly mitigate the observed risks and benefits. Stents, in particular, may significantly enhance observable benefits among patients undergoing percutaneous revascularization. In a report of 120 patients randomly assigned to undergo PTCA or stenting for the treatment of a proximal left anterior descending artery stenosis, both angiographic restenosis (19% vs 40%, $P = 0.02$) and survival free of death, myocardial infarction, or recurrent angina by 1 year (13% vs 30%, $P = 0.04$) were significantly lower among patients undergoing stenting. The long term benefits of stenting were observed even though initial procedural success rates were equivalent (95% stent group, 93% PTCA group).[27]

R

Grade A

THEORETIC CONSIDERATIONS FOR COMPARISON OF CABG, PTCA, AND MEDICAL THERAPY

PTCA emerged approximately 10 years after CABG had become an accepted surgical alternative for patients with severe coronary artery disease. Although PTCA was originally conceived as an alternative to CABG, rates of both PTCA and CABG have increased consistently, and they parallel one another.[3] This, together with the fact that most PTCA procedures have been performed for single vessel disease, suggests that PTCA has been used primarily as an alternative to medical therapy rather than to CABG. More recently, with increased experience, improvements in equipment, and development of new technologic devices, the scope of PTCA has increasingly included subsets of patients previously referred for CABG. Several prospective randomized trials have directly compared multivessel PTCA and CABG. Before reviewing the results of these trials (which compare two active invasive therapies without medical or placebo controls), several general considerations for such a comparison need to be reviewed.

As mentioned above, when comparing PTCA with CABG, several outcomes can be assessed: mortality, symptoms, non-fatal events (such as non-fatal myocardial infarction), costs, and surrogate laboratory endpoints (such as left ventricular function). Because neither PTCA nor CABG has been demonstrated to decrease the incidence of non-fatal myocardial infarction in comparison with medical therapy, myocardial infarction is unlikely to be sensitive to a possible differential impact of the two procedures. Similarly, inclusion of low risk subgroups in which CABG has *not* been shown to improve survival compared with medical therapy, such as single vessel disease, would decrease the ability to demonstrate mortality differences. An exception would occur if PTCA were significantly worse than medical therapy or substantially superior to CABG (both of which can be considered unlikely).

It has been demonstrated that CABG is associated with an approximately 50% risk reduction in moderate and high risk subgroups at 5 years, in comparison with medical therapy. The detection of a relative risk difference of 10–20% between CABG and PTCA would be clinically relevant. If such a comparison indicated superiority of PTCA over CABG, it could reasonably be concluded that PTCA was superior to both medical therapy (indirect extrapolation) and CABG (direct inference). However, if a 20% difference in the relative risk of mortality in favor of CABG existed, surgical revascularization would generally be preferred over PTCA in such patients if the goal is improvement in prognosis. If the available data from such a comparison were large, the confidence interval of any observed difference would be narrow enough (for example, 20% ± 10%) to suggest that PTCA was superior to medical therapy to a clinically worthwhile extent, an indirect extrapolation necessitated by lack of a medical control arm.

If no difference were observed between CABG and PTCA, it could be concluded that PTCA is equivalent to CABG only if trials were large enough to reliably detect or exclude relative differences in mortality of about 20% (with narrow confidence intervals) and included a large number of patients in whom CABG has been shown to improve prognosis. Because approximately 600 deaths would be needed in the "control" group to exclude a relative risk difference of 20% with 90% power, trials with about 4000 moderate to high risk patients per treatment arm would be needed. However, if a 30% risk difference was considered the smallest clinically important difference, trials of about 2000 patients in each group would be required. Moreover, in such a comparison, if the confidence limits of any difference included the possibility that PTCA was worse than

CABG by 50% (relative risk), it could not be inferred that PTCA had any favorable impact on survival in comparison with medical therapy.

These considerations indicate that to reliably compare the relative impact of PTCA vs CABG and to avoid missing clinically important differences (risk reductions on the order of 20%), the following conditions need to be met:

1. inclusion of subgroups in which surgery has been shown to be superior to medical therapy;
2. inclusion of sufficient numbers of patients (that is, adequate statistical power);
3. follow-up of at least 3–4 years to accrue a sufficient number of endpoints and to obtain data well beyond the early period when periprocedural mortality rates have a substantial influence (ideally, follow-up would be extended to 10 years to assess the late effects of both procedures);
4. a high rate of compliance to the original treatment allocation; if a substantial proportion of patients "cross over" (30–40% by 5 years), the ability to detect differences in survival decreases markedly.

Among low risk patients (annual mortality <2% per year) it may be moot to assess mortality differences between PTCA and CABG because CABG has not been shown to decrease mortality. Moreover, conducting a trial to detect clinically important differences in such patients would be extremely difficult because of the large number of patients that would be required. For example, if a 1% annual mortality rate is assumed for the medical group, 8000 patients would need to be followed for 5 years to detect reliably a 30% risk reduction or 16 000 patients followed for the same period to detect a 20% risk reduction. Furthermore, in such low risk patients, any absolute benefit is likely to be too small to justify the costs and risks associated with revascularization. A large difference (for example, a 50% risk reduction that could be demonstrated with about 4000 randomized patients) would be extremely unlikely.

Therefore, among low risk patients, the most relevant comparison is between PTCA and medical therapy. Any such trials are unlikely ever to demonstrate a difference in mortality between PTCA and medical therapy (unless PTCA were harmful). However, effects on a combined clinical variable could be compared, potentially including non-fatal events such as myocardial infarction, severe angina, costs, and need for further revascularization procedures. Non-fatal events in a composite endpoint would need to be chosen carefully. Neither CABG nor PTCA has been shown to reduce the risk of subsequent non-fatal myocardial infarction, and inclusion of such an endpoint would dilute relative differences and decrease the likelihood of detecting differences. Both PTCA and CABG are effective in relieving angina and myocardial ischemia, and a relevant composite end point could include death plus severe angina. Such trials are feasible and could provide clinically relevant answers. It must be borne in mind that invasive procedures may increase rates of myocardial infarction (perioperative risk) while decreasing subsequent angina pectoris.

PTCA vs CABG IN SINGLE VESSEL DISEASE

Although medical therapy generally is indicated first, revascularization may be indicated for symptom relief. Both PTCA and CABG offer a high rate of procedural success in such patients. However, it has not been clear which of these is the optimal mode of revascularization for these patients. Three randomized trials have provided data comparing PTCA and CABG for single vessel disease; the first was published in 1994.[32] It was a single-center Swiss trial in which 134 patients with isolated proximal left anterior descending coronary artery stenosis were randomly assigned to angioplasty or CABG with a left internal thoracic artery conduit. Over 2.5 years of follow-up, only one cardiac death occurred in the CABG group and none in the PTCA group, confirming the general low risk status of these patients. No significant difference was found in cardiac death plus myocardial infarction (4.5% CABG vs 11.7% PTCA, $P=0.21$), and the only significant difference between the two groups was a higher rate of repeat revascularization in the PTCA group (34%) because of restenosis. Relief of angina was achieved in a high proportion of each group (more than 95% CCS class I at 1 year), and no difference in the duration of the exercise test was found.

Similar results were found in the British RITA and Brazilian MASS studies. RITA included 456 patients with single vessel disease.[33] After 2.5 years of follow-up, no significant difference in death plus myocardial infarction was found (16 CABG vs 24 PTCA) among patients with single vessel disease, but patients randomized to PTCA required a significantly greater number of repeat procedures (38% vs 11%, $P=0.01$). MASS was a very small trial of 214 patients with isolated stenosis of the proximal left anterior descending coronary artery and, to date, incorporated the only three-way randomization among PTCA, CABG, and medical therapy. Rates of death (one in each group) or non-fatal myocardial infarction (one CABG, two PTCA) were very low over a mean 3-year follow-up period. Twenty-one PTCA patients (29%) required repeat revascularization. After 3 years, 98% of patients assigned to CABG and 82% assigned to PTCA were free of angina, compared with only 32% of those in the medical group. No patient in any treatment group had severe angina (class III or IV).

In the meta-analysis of Pocock et al.,[34] 732 patients had single vessel disease. Of the 358 patients in the CABG group, 16 (4.5%) experienced cardiac death or myocardial infarction in the first year, versus 27 of 374 PTCA (7.2%) patients. Because no such difference was found for multivessel disease, caution is needed to avoid overinterpretation of these data. When all-cause death over all patient years of follow-up is considered, no significant differences are found (3.7% PTCA vs 3.1% CABG; odds ratio 1.13; 95% CI 0.50–2.6). Rates of all-cause death or myocardial infarction were slightly higher in the PTCA group than the CABG group (10.1% vs 6.1%; odds ratio 1.71; 95% CI 1.01–2.90 $P<0.05$). Rates of angina grade 2 or worse were low at 1 year in both groups (6.5% CABG, 14.6% PTCA, $P<0.01$) and at 3 years (12.5% CABG, 15.4% PTCA, $P=0.11$). Rates of additional revascularization procedures were significantly lower at 1 year in the CABG group (3.6% vs 30.5% in the PTCA group).

In summary, the data available suggest that both PTCA and CABG are highly effective in providing symptom relief for patients with severe single vessel coronary artery disease. Neither procedure is associated with an unequivocal reduction in mortality or myocardial infarction compared with the other. Patients undergoing PTCA have a greater likelihood of repeat procedures, because of the unsolved problem of restenosis. If this is acceptable to patients and their physicians, then PTCA offers a simpler and much less invasive mode of revascularization; however, less invasive means of performing CABG are under development. Of note, the meta-analysis of CABG versus medical therapy trials suggested a mortality benefit for CABG in one or two vessel disease with involvement of the proximal left anterior descending coronary artery (RR 0.58; 95% CI 0.34–1.01).[7] These patients have a large area of myocardium at jeopardy and are at higher risk of death than those with other forms of single vessel disease. For single vessel disease, the current conclusions and recommendations are based on a relatively small number of patients, and the possibility that potentially important differences between therapies were missed cannot be ruled out.

PTCA vs CABG IN MULTIVESSEL DISEASE

For multivessel disease, CABG has remained the mainstay of therapy for moderate and high risk subgroups, such as those with severe two or three vessel disease, especially in the presence of left ventricular dysfunction. Technologic advances in the past 5–7 years have increasingly allowed wider application of PTCA, and a number of prospective, randomized trials have directly compared PTCA with CABG. The group of patients with multivessel disease is a heterogeneous group – heterogeneity in the location and extent of anatomic stenosis, clinical symptoms, ventricular function, and coexistent disease – and, thus, needs to be evaluated carefully when comparing trial results.

There are nine randomized studies comparing PTCA and CABG in the treatment of multivessel disease.[32,33,35–41] Although these studies are heterogeneous in regard to design, methods, and stage of follow-up, they are broadly comparable and it is instructive to consider them together. A systematic review of eight randomized trials of CABG vs PTCA has been published.[34] This collaborative effort encompassed European, North American, and South American trials, although the largest trial, the Bypass Angioplasty Revascularization Investigation (BARI, see below), was not included because the data were not publicly available at the time. There were five single-center trials, two multicenter trials, and one international trial. The main characteristics of these trials are compared in Tables 24.3 and 24.4. No trial individually was powered to detect or to exclude differences in mortality, and various composite clinical endpoints were used. All trials shared certain important features: treatment allocation to PTCA or CABG was randomly assigned, a high degree of compliance with the assigned therapy was achieved (more than 95%), and follow-up data describing vital status, incidence of myocardial infarction, and prevalence of angina pectoris (and/or measures of myocardial ischemia) were collected. Length of follow-up varied, and in some instances, additional follow-up is planned.

The meta-analysis included 3371 patients: 1661 patients randomized to CABG and 1710 to PTCA. The incidence of major endpoints during an aggregate mean follow-up period of 2.7 years was found to be nearly identical: 4.4% of patients randomized to CABG and 4.6% of patients randomized to PTCA had died (RR 1.08; 95% CI 0.79–1.50); death or myocardial infarction occurred in 7.6% of those who had CABG and in 7.9% of those who had PTCA (RR 1.10; 95% CI 0.89–1.37) (Figure 24.3). Repeat revascularization within 1 year was required in 33.7% of PTCA patients (including 18% who underwent CABG), but in only 3.3% of those initially assigned to CABG (P<0.0001). The prevalence of angina pectoris (at least class 2) was significantly higher in the PTCA group at 1 year, but at 3 years this difference had decreased (Figure 24.4) as rates of repeat revascularization increased in the PTCA patients.

The largest of the PTCA vs CABG trials, the Bypass Angioplasty Revascularization Investigation (BARI), was published in 1996.[42] It was designed originally as an "equivalence" trial, and sample size calculations were predicated on an estimated 5-year mortality of about 5%, with the goal that the upper 95% confidence limit for any observed difference would not exceed 2.5% ("the maximum acceptable absolute difference

Table 24.3 Main characteristics of nine prospective randomized trials of PTCA vs CABG

	BARI	CABRI	EAST	ERACI	GABI	MASS	RITA	Swiss	Toulouse
Location	North America, multicenter	Europe, multicenter	Emory University (Atlanta, GA), single-center	Argentina, single-center	Germany, multicenter	Brazil, single-center	Britain, multicenter	Switzerland, single-center	France, single-center
Patients screened (*n*)	25 200	?	5118	1409	8981	?	17 237	?	?
Randomized (%)	1829 (7.3)	1054	392 (7.7)	127 (9.0)	359 (4.0)	214	1011 (4.8)	142	152
Equivalent revascularization required	No	No	No	No	Yes	Yes	Yes	Yes	Yes
Follow-up									
Planned duration (yr)	10	5–10	3	3	1	3.5	5	2.5	3
Completed	No	No	Yes	Yes	Yes	Yes	No	Yes	Yes
Primary endpoint	Mortality, MI	Mortality, non-fatal MI, angina, functional capacity	Combined death, MI, and large thallium defect	Combined death, MI, and angina	Freedom from angina at 1 year (>CCS 2)	Combined cardiac death, MI, refractory angina	Combined death and MI	Death, MI, repeat revascularization	?

Adapted from Raco D, Rihal CS, Yusuf S. Ramdomized trials of PTCA: comparison of medical and surgical therapy. In: Grech ED, Ramsdale DR, eds. *Practical interventional cardiology.* St Louis: Mosby, 1997, pp 317–26.

Table 24.4 Patient profiles in nine randomized trials of PTCA vs CABG

	BARI	CABRI	EAST	ERACI	GABI	MASS	RITA	Swiss	Toulouse
No. of stenotic vessels (%)									
One	0	0	0	0	0	100	45	100	—
Two	56	58	60	55	81	—	43	—	49
Three	43	40	40	45	19	—	12	—	14
Mean ejection fraction (%)	58	63	61	61	?	75	?	?	?
Average age (yr)	61	61	62	57	59	56	57	56	?
CCS class 3 or 4 angina (%)	?	65	80	?	65	?	60	89	?
Mammary artery used (% of CABG procedures)	82	?	90	77	37	100	74	100	?
Male/female	74:26	63:37	74:26	54:46	80:20	58:42	81:19	80:20	?
Previous MI (%)	?	41	41	32	47	?	43	0	?

Adapted from Raco D, Rihal CS, Yusuf S. Randomized trials of PTCA: comparison of medical and surgical therapy. In: Grech ED, Ramsdale DR, eds. *Practical interventional cardiology.* St Louis: Mosby, 1997, pp 317–26.

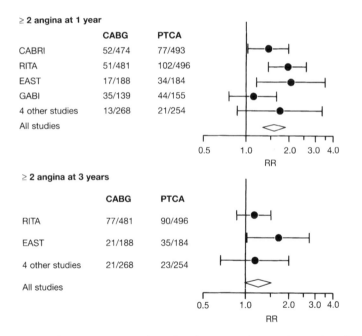

Trial	CABG		PTCA	
	(n)	(%)	(n)	(%)
CABRI	29	(5.7)	43	(7.9)
RITA	31	(6.2)	34	(6.7)
EAST	33	(18.4)	24	(13.7)
GABI	18	(10.2)	10	(5.5)
Toulouse	6	(7.9)	6	(7.9)
MASS	1	(1.4)	5	(6.9)
Swiss	2	(3.0)	6	(8.8)
ERACI	7	(10.9)	8	(12.7)
All trials	127		135	

Figure 24.3 Cardiac death and myocardial infarction for PTCA group compared with CABG group in the first year after randomization. (From Pocock SJ et al.,[34] by permission of The Lancet Ltd.)

≥ 2 angina at 1 year

	CABG	PTCA
CABRI	52/474	77/493
RITA	51/481	102/496
EAST	17/188	34/184
GABI	35/139	44/155
4 other studies	13/268	21/254
All studies		

≥ 2 angina at 3 years

	CABG	PTCA
RITA	77/481	90/496
EAST	21/188	35/184
4 other studies	21/268	23/254
All studies		

Figure 24.4 Prevalence of angina pectoris (at least class 2) at 1 and 3 years after random allocation to PTCA or CABG. (From Pocock SJ et al.,[34] by permission of The Lancet Ltd.)

between the CABG and PTCA event rates").[39] Approximately 30% of screened angiograms of patients with multivessel disease were considered eligible and 1829 patients were enrolled. About 40% of these patients had three vessel disease, and 22% had an ejection fraction <50%. Assignment to PTCA or CABG was randomly allocated, and follow-up was for 5 years before the first results were presented.

In BARI, the 5-year mortality among patients assigned to CABG was 10.7%, and 13.7% among those assigned to PTCA (absolute difference, 3.0%; 95% CI −0.2 to 6.0%;

Table 24.5 All-cause mortality after randomized assignment to PTCA or CABG

Trial	PTCA Obs/Tot	CABG Obs/Tot	Odds ratio	95% CI
BARI	125/915	111/914	1.14	0.87–1.50
CABRI	21/541	14/513	1.43	0.73–2.81
EAST	14/198	12/194	1.15	0.52–2.55
ERACI	3/63	3/64	1.02	0.20–5.20
GABI	4/182	9/177	0.44	0.15–1.32
MASS	1/72	1/70	0.97	0.06–15.70
RITA	16/510	18/501	0.87	0.44–1.72
Swiss	3/68	1/66	2.70	0.37–19.60
Toulouse	5/76	7/76	0.70	0.22–2.26
Total	192/2625	176/2575	1.09	0.88–1.35

Obs, observed; Tot, total.
Between-trial test for heterogeneity, χ^2 (df = 8) = 5.17.
Fixed effects model.

$P = 0.19$). The near 22% relative risk reduction in favor of CABG did not reach statistical significance, but the study had less than 40% power to reliably detect such a difference. The incidence of death or Q wave myocardial infarction by 5 years was 19.4% and 21.3% for the CABG and PTCA groups, respectively. Although 54% of the PTCA group required additional revascularization procedures, compared with 8% of the CABG group, 69% of those assigned to PTCA did not require subsequent CABG. Among treated diabetics (which was not one of the four subgroup analyses designated *a priori*), a significant mortality difference in favor of CABG was found (5-year mortality, 19.4% CABG vs 34.5% PTCA; $P = 0.003$). The authors concluded that multivessel PTCA did not compromise 5-year survival, with the exception of treated diabetics, although subsequent revascularization is required more frequently.

UPDATED META-ANALYSIS

BARI was published after the Pocock meta-analysis. Results of systematic reviews of all-cause mortality (death or myocardial infarction) and non-protocol revascularization after the initial randomly assigned treatment are presented in Tables 24.5–24.7. The data are from the original publications or, if lacking, from the meta-analysis of Pocock et al.[34] Total mortality did not differ between the PTCA and CABG groups (7.3% vs 6.8%; odds ratio 1.09; 95% CI 0.88–1.35). Currently, a separate analysis cannot be performed for diabetic or other subgroups. Similarly, the combined endpoint of death or myocardial infarction did not differ between the groups (13.8% PTCA vs 13.4% CABG; odds ratio 1.05; 95% CI 0.89–1.23).

Substudies have demonstrated that PTCA and CABG produce similar benefits on quality of life measures and return to employment and are roughly equivalent in cost over 3–5 years of follow-up.[43–46] CABG is associated with more complete revascularization, but differences in degree of revascularization of major lesions are less pronounced.[45]

In summary, nine trials have randomized 5200 patients with multivessel coronary artery disease to PTCA or CABG. No clear superiority of one procedure over the other

Table 24.6 Death or myocardial infarction after randomized assignment to PTCA or CABG

Trial	PTCA Obs/Tot	CABG Obs/Tot	Odds ratio	95% CI
BARI	195/915	179/914	1.11	0.89–1.40
CABRI	35/541	32/513	1.04	0.63–1.71
EAST	43/198	50/194	0.80	0.50–1.27
ERACI	9/63	8/64	1.17	0.42–3.22
GABI	11/182	22/177	0.47	0.23–0.95
MASS	3/72	2/70	1.47	0.25–8.68
RITA	50/510	43/501	1.16	0.76–1.77
Swiss	11/68	3/66	3.43	1.14–10.35
Toulouse	6/76	6/76	1.00	0.31–3.24
Total	363/2625	345/2575	1.05	0.89–1.23

Obs, observed; Tot, total.
Between-trial test for heterogeneity, χ^2 (df = 8) = 11.33.
Fixed effects model.

Table 24.7 Non-protocol revascularization after randomized assignment to PTCA or CABG

Trial	PTCA Obs/Tot	CABG Obs/Tot	Odds ratio	95% CI
BARI	494/915	73/914	8.58	7.04–10.46
CABRI	163/541	18/513	6.49	4.71–8.93
EAST	107/198	25/194	6.28	4.13–9.55
ERACI	20/63	2/64	7.26	2.91–18.14
GABI	91/182	9/177	9.29	5.86–14.73
MASS	29/72	0/70	11.72	5.20–26.42
RITA	189/510	20/501	7.50	5.53–10.16
Swiss	29/68	2/66	9.13	4.10–20.32
Total	1122/2549	149/2499	7.87	6.92–8.95

Obs, observed; Tot, total.
Between-trial test for heterogeneity, χ^2 (df = 7) = 4.92.
Fixed effects model.

has been demonstrated, with the possible exception of treated diabetics, an observation that needs to be confirmed. Whereas patients who initially undergo multivessel PTCA require more repeat procedures, initial morbidity is less and overall anginal relief is nearly equivalent by 3 years. Clearly, restenosis is the major limitation of PTCA, but most patients can be managed successfully with a strategy of one or more PTCA procedures, as needed, avoiding CABG (or perhaps keeping it in reserve) in about two-thirds of patients over 5 years.

Can it be concluded, then, that PTCA and CABG are equivalent modes of revascularization for multivessel disease among angiographically eligible patients, except for the unsolved problem of restenosis? To answer this question, it is necessary to consider the marked heterogeneity of what is termed "multivessel disease". A patient with discrete lesions of the right coronary and circumflex arteries who has a normal left ventricle or a patient with diffuse three vessel disease and an ejection fraction of

30% can be rightly classified under the term "multivessel disease"; yet, the prognoses, risks, and potential benefits of revascularization vary considerably.

In the recent PTCA vs CABG trials, enrolled patients were relatively low risk: fewer than 20% had left ventricular dysfunction and almost 70% had one or two vessel disease. In the meta-analysis of Pocock et al.,[34] the observed first-year mortality of 2.6% and 1.1% per year thereafter confirm the relatively low risk status of these patients (however, no medical control arms were present). Patients enrolled in BARI had higher observed mortality rates and more closely approximated moderate risk patients, but this was due primarily to the higher proportion of patients with diabetes mellitus. Overall, in BARI, nearly 60% of patients had two vessel coronary artery disease. In contrast, patients enrolled in the earlier trials of CABG vs medical therapy had a 20% prevalence of significant left ventricular dysfunction and 60% had three vessel or left main coronary artery disease.[7] Thus, the current PTCA vs CABG trials include a high proportion of patients in whom CABG has *not* been shown to be superior to medical therapy. Moreover, the total enrollment of 5200 patients falls short of what would be needed to demonstrate clinically important differences in mortality of 20–30% among low and moderate risk patients. It is reasonable to surmise that if CABG were superior to PTCA in moderate and high risk patients, the current PTCA vs CABG trials would have low power to reliably detect significant differences and that such a difference cannot be ruled out. Large mortality differences of the order of 40–50%, however, are unlikely, given the current data.

LIMITATIONS OF CURRENT RANDOMIZED DATA

In a rapidly evolving field, all trials designed to address specific clinical questions begin to become obsolete with publication. This is especially notable for the CABG versus medical therapy trials performed 20–25 years ago. The wide application of antiplatelet and antihyperlipidemic therapy in current practice may significantly mitigate the published results. Temporal changes in angioplasty and surgical techniques are continuing and, in some cases, accelerating. The development of new interventional devices designed to deal with procedural complications, specific high risk lesions, or previously unapproachable lesions has broadened the scope of percutaneous procedures. Coronary stents have decreased the incidence of both emergency and late CABG and likely have a mitigating effect on the recalcitrant problem of restenosis. New adjunctive medical therapies such as ticlopidine and platelet IIb/IIIa receptor antibodies are having a major impact on interventional procedures. CABG, too, has undergone significant technologic advances. Internal thoracic arterial conduits are in widespread use, with excellent long-term patency, improved myocardial preservation techniques, and adjunctive medical therapies, and less invasive surgical approaches have been developed.

Specific methodologic concerns also exist about the available data. Trials of surgical procedures inherently are logistically complex; as a result, all trials reviewed above are small and the possibility of missing potentially important differences cannot be ruled out. Although systematic reviews, preferably based on individual patient data, can provide some redress, larger definitive trials are preferable. Follow-up in many trials has been short, and more definitive conclusions await collection of additional data and endpoints. Commonly, in trials of invasive treatments, "crossover" to the other therapy occurs with increasing frequency during the course of follow-up, necessitating

GR	VD	95%	LAD	CABG better Medicine better
1	1	No		
2	1	Yes		
3	2	No		
4	2	Yes		
5	1	Yes	95% Prox	
	2	Yes	95%	
6	2	Yes	95% Prox	
	3	No	Yes	
7	3	Yes	Yes	
8	3	Yes	Prox	
9	3	Yes	95% Prox	

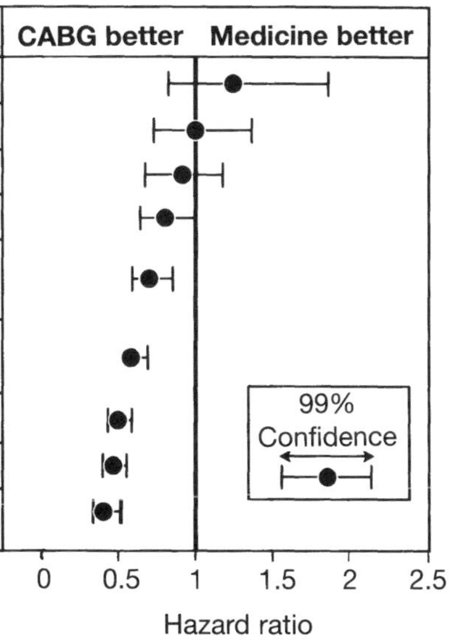

Hazard ratio

Figure 24.5 Adjusted hazard ratios comparing CABG and medical therapy (MT) for the nine coronary anatomy groups. GR, group; VD, number of diseased vessels; LAD, left anterior descending coronary artery; Prox, proximal; 95%, ≥95% coronary artery stenosis. (From Jones RH *et al.*,[51] by permission of Mosby–Year Book, Inc.)

consideration of therapeutic strategies rather than specific treatments. As with many large surgical trials, the generalizability of results to medical centers with a lower volume and different levels of experience remains unproven.[47–49] The greatest limitation of the currently available data is the lack of large trials incorporating all three major approaches to patients with coronary artery disease: medical, interventional, and surgical. Until such trials are performed, comparative data are likely to remain limited to observational databases.[50]

DATABASE STUDIES

Prospective randomized trials provide the highest level of evidence for clinical decision making; nonetheless, information from trials frequently must be supplemented and enhanced by observational studies. Long term survival for 9263 patients with angiographically documented coronary artery disease has been reported recently by Duke University Medical Center.[50,51] Although treatment assignment was non-random, the prospective 97% complete follow-up of this consecutive series provided unique insight into the relative efficacies of various treatments with concurrent controls (2449 patients, medical only; 2924, PTCA; 3890, CABG). Nine risk strata based on number and extent of coronary artery disease were identified (left main coronary artery disease and <75% stenoses were excluded). Long term survival comparisons between treatments were assessed by Cox proportional hazards models and Kaplan–Meier survival analysis. CABG was significantly associated with improved long term outcomes in comparison with medical therapy among patients in moderate and high risk strata: for three vessel disease ($n = 2771$), odds ratio 0.44; 95% CI 0.42–0.80 (Figure 24.5). PTCA, however, was superior to medical therapy only among low risk strata.[51]

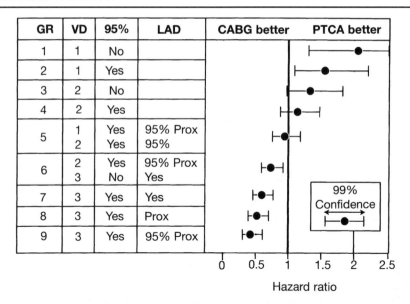

GR	VD	95%	LAD	CABG better PTCA better
1	1	No		
2	1	Yes		
3	2	No		
4	2	Yes		
5	1	Yes	95% Prox	
	2	Yes	95%	
6	2	Yes	95% Prox	
	3	No	Yes	
7	3	Yes	Yes	
8	3	Yes	Prox	
9	3	Yes	95% Prox	

Hazard ratio

Figure 24.6 Adjusted hazard ratios comparing CABG and PTCA for the nine coronary anatomy groups. GR, group; VD, number of diseased vessels; LAD, left anterior descending coronary artery; Prox, proximal; 95%, ≥ 95% coronary artery stenosis. (From Jones RH *et al.*,[51] by permission of Mosby–Year Book, Inc.)

In comparison with PTCA, CABG was associated with improved outcomes among high risk strata, namely, all patients with three vessel disease and two vessel disease with 95% involvement of the proximal left anterior descending coronary artery. Conversely, adjusted hazard ratios demonstrated the clear superiority of PTCA over CABG among low risk patients (Figure 24.6) and a trend toward superiority among moderate risk patients. In summary, these prospective observational data indicate equivalence or superiority of revascularization over medical therapy among *all* subgroups, with CABG favored for high risk strata and PTCA for low risk strata. In no subgroup was medical therapy clearly superior to revascularization. These data must, however, be interpreted extremely cautiously and considered tentative until confirmed by prospective randomized trials.

These prospective observational data are broadly consistent with the previously presented framework placing PTCA vs CABG trials in the context of CABG vs medical therapy trials. Although a definite benefit of CABG over medical therapy for one and two vessel disease could not be demonstrated in the randomized trials (with the possible exception of proximal left anterior descending coronary artery disease), non-significant trends favoring CABG were found. The relatively low number of observed events (113 deaths over 5 years) in these trials may have precluded detection of a benefit (type II error). The Duke observational data extend the randomized trials and, by virtue of the much larger number of events (in turn, related to the larger number of patients and longer duration of follow-up), allow further characterization of possible treatment differences. As with any non-randomized study, significant limitations to the data remain and definitive conclusions await performance of larger randomized trials. Because treatment selection was non-random, bias cannot be excluded. Moreover, determination of time zero was arbitrary and deaths occurring while awaiting revascularization were assigned to medical therapy, which would tend to inflate event rates among medical patients. This misclassification problem is mitigated to some extent by revascularization deaths that occurred after a period of deterioration while the subjects were receiving medical therapy.

CURRENT RECOMMENDATIONS FOR MYOCARDIAL REVASCULARIZATION IN PATIENTS WITH CHRONIC STABLE ANGINA

CABG vs medical therapy

1. Among patients with medically refractory angina pectoris, CABG is indicated for symptom improvement. ⬚Grade A⬚
2. Among patients with medically stable angina pectoris, CABG is indicated for left main coronary artery or three vessel disease (regardless of left ventricular function) for prolongation of life. This is a class A recommendation based on level la evidence. ⬚Grade A⬚
3. CABG may be indicated for prolongation of life if the proximal left anterior descending coronary artery is involved (regardless of the number of diseased vessels). This is a class A recommendation based on level la evidence. ⬚Grade A⬚

PTCA vs medical therapy

1. Among patients with medically refractory angina pectoris, PTCA is indicated for symptom improvement. ⬚Grade A⬚
2. PTCA may be indicated in the presence of severe myocardial ischemia, regardless of symptoms. It is unclear whether PTCA improves survival in comparison with medical treatment among patients with one or two vessel disease. This is a class B recommendation based on level 2 evidence. ⬚Grade B⬚
3. In the absence of symptoms or myocardial ischemia, PTCA is not indicated (merely for the presence of an anatomic stenosis). ⬚Grade A⬚

PTCA vs CABG

1. For single vessel disease, both PTCA and CABG provide excellent symptom relief but repeat revascularization procedures are required more frequently after PTCA. This is a class A recommendation based on level 1c evidence. Intracoronary stenting may be the preferred option (class A, level 1c), but direct comparison with CABG is lacking. ⬚Grade A⬚
2. For treated diabetics with two or three vessel disease, CABG may be the treatment of choice. Additional data are needed. This is a class A recommendation based on level 1a evidence. ⬚Grade A⬚
3. For non-diabetics, both multivessel PTCA and CABG are acceptable alternatives. The choice of PTCA or CABG for initial treatment will depend primarily on local expertise and patient and physician preference. This is a class A recommendation based on level 1a evidence. The following caveats should be considered: ⬚Grade A⬚

- In general, PTCA will be preferred for patients at low risk and CABG for patients at high risk.
- Large differences in mortality (40–50%) are unlikely, but smaller, potentially important differences in mortality (20–30%) cannot be ruled out, given the available data.
- CABG is associated with more complete revascularization and superior early relief of angina, but these differences are lessened after 3–5 years.
- No significant differences in rates of myocardial infarction have been demonstrated.
- Repeat revascularization procedures are required significantly more often after PTCA.
- Initial costs, quality of life, and return to work are initially more favorable with PTCA than CABG, but these variables roughly equalize over 3–5 years.

REFERENCES

1 Favaloro RG. Saphenous vein autograft replacement of severe segmental coronary artery occlusion: operative technique. *Ann Thorac Surg* 1968;**5**:334–9.

2 Gruntzig AR, Senning A, Siegenthaler WE. Nonoperative dilatation of coronary-artery stenosis: percutaneous transluminal coronary angioplasty. *N Engl J Med* 1979;**301**:61–8.

3 Greaves EJ, Gillum BS. *1994 Summary: National Hospital Discharge Survey. Advance data from Vital and Health Statistics*, no. 278. Hyattsville, Maryland: National Center for Health Statistics, 1996.

4 European Coronary Surgery Study Group. Long-term results of prospective randomised study of coronary artery bypass surgery in stable angina pectoris. *Lancet* 1982;**ii**:1173–80.

5 The VA Coronary Artery Bypass Surgery Cooperative Study Group. Eighteen-year follow-up in the Veterans Affairs Cooperative Study of Coronary Artery Bypass Surgery for stable angina. *Circulation* 1992;**86**:121–30.

6 Alderman EL, Bourassa MG, Cohen LS *et al.* Ten-year follow-up of survival and myocardial infarction in the randomized Coronary Artery Surgery Study. *Circulation* 1990;**82**:1629–46.

7 Yusuf S, Zucker D, Peduzzi P *et al.* Effect of coronary artery bypass graft surgery on survival: overview of 10-year results from randomised trials by the Coronary Artery Bypass Graft Surgery Trialists Collaboration. *Lancet* 1994;**344**:563–70.

8 Caracciolo EA, Davis KB, Sopko G *et al.* Comparison of surgical and medical group survival in patients with left main coronary artery disease. Long-term CASS experience. *Circulation* 1995;**91**:2325–34.

9 Prospective randomised study of coronary artery bypass surgery in stable angina pectoris. Second interim report by the European Coronary Surgery Study Group. *Lancet* 1980;**ii**:491–5.

10 Caracciolo EA, Davis KB, Sopko G *et al.* Comparison of surgical and medical group survival in patients with left main equivalent coronary artery disease. Long-term CASS experience. *Circulation* 1995;**91**:2335–44.

11 Passamani E, Davis KB, Gillespie MJ, Killip T. A randomized trial of coronary artery bypass surgery. Survival of patients with a low ejection fraction. *N Engl J Med* 1985;**312**:1665–71.

12 Myers WO, Schaff HV, Fisher LD *et al.* Time to first new myocardial infarction in patients with severe angina and three-vessel disease comparing medical and early surgical therapy: a CASS registry study of survival. *J Thorac Cardiovasc Surg* 1988;**95**:382–9.

13 Chaitman BR, Stone PH, Knatterud GL *et al.* Asymptomatic Cardiac Ischemia Pilot (ACIP) study: impact of anti-ischemia therapy on 12-week rest electrocardiogram and exercise test outcomes. The ACIP Investigators. *J Am Coll Cardiol* 1995;**26**:585–93.

14 Rogers WJ, Bourassa MG, Andrews TC *et al.* Asymptomatic Cardiac Ischemia Pilot (ACIP) study: outcome at 1 year for patients with asymptomatic cardiac ischemia randomized to medical therapy or revascularization. The ACIP Investigators. *J Am Coll Cardiol* 1995;**26**: 594–605.

15 Davies RF, Goldberg AD, Forman S *et al.* Asymptomatic Cardiac Ischemia Pilot (ACIP) study two-year follow-up: outcomes of patients randomized to initial strategies of medical therapy versus revascularization. *Circulation* 1997;**95**: 2037–43.

16 Randomised trial of cholesterol lowering in 4444 patients with coronary heart disease: the Scandinavian Simvastatin Survival Study (4S). *Lancet* 1994;**344**:1383–9.

17 West of Scotland Coronary Prevention Study: identification of high-risk groups and comparison with other cardiovascular intervention trials. *Lancet* 1996;**348**:1339–42.

18 Detre K, Holubkov R, Kelsey S *et al*. One-year follow-up results of the 1985–1986 National Heart, Lung, and Blood Institute's Percutaneous Transluminal Coronary Angioplasty Registry. *Circulation* 1989;**80**:421–8.

19 Detre K, Holubkov R, Kelsey S *et al*. Percutaneous transluminal coronary angioplasty in 1985–1986 and 1977–1981. The National Heart, Lung, and Blood Institute Registry. *N Engl J Med* 1988;**318**:265–70.

20 Parisi AF, Folland ED, Hartigan P. A comparison of angioplasty with medical therapy in the treatment of single-vessel coronary artery disease. Veterans Affairs ACME Investigators. *N Engl J Med* 1992;**326**:10–16.

21 Sievers B, Hamm CW, Herzner A, Kuck KH. Medical therapy versus PTCA: a prospective, randomized trial in patients with asymptomatic coronary single vessel disease (Abstract). *Circulation* 1993;**88**:I-297.

22 RITA-2 Trial Participants. Coronary angioplasty versus medical therapy for angina: the second Randomised Intervention Treatment of Angina (RITA-2) trial. *Lancet* 1997;**350**:461–8.

23 Little WC, Constantinescu M, Applegate RJ *et al*. Can coronary angiography predict the site of a subsequent myocardial infarction in patients with mild-to-moderate coronary artery disease? *Circulation* 1988;**78**:1157–66.

24 Ambrose JA, Tannenbaum MA, Alexopoulos D *et al*. Angiographic progression of coronary artery disease and the development of myocardial infarction. *J Am Coll Cardiol* 1988;**12**:56–62.

25 Giroud D, Li JM, Urban P, Meier B, Rutishauser W. Relation of the site of acute myocardial infarction to the most severe coronary arterial stenosis at prior angiography. *Am J Cardiol* 1992;**69**:729–32.

26 Hackett D, Verwilghen J, Davies G, Maseri A. Coronary stenoses before and after acute myocardial infarction. *Am J Cardiol* 1989;**63**:1517–18.

27 Versaci F, Gaspardone A, Tomai F *et al*. A comparison of coronary-artery stenting with angioplasty for isolated stenosis of the proximal left anterior descending coronary artery. *N Engl J Med* 1997;**336**:817–22.

28 Serruys PW, de Jaegere P, Kiemeneij F *et al*. A comparison of balloon-expandable-stent implantation with balloon angioplasty in patients with coronary artery disease. Benestent Study Group. *N Engl J Med* 1994;**331**:489–95.

29 Fischman DL, Leon MB, Baim DS *et al*. A randomized comparison of coronary-stent placement and balloon angioplasty in the treatment of coronary artery disease. Stent Restenosis Study Investigators. *N Engl J Med* 1994;**331**:496–501.

30 Schafer AI. Hypercoagulable states: molecular genetics to clinical practice. *Lancet* 1994;**344**:1739–42.

31 Harker LA. Platelets and vascular thrombosis. *N Engl J Med* 1994;**330**:1006–7.

32 Goy JJ, Eeckhout E, Burnand B *et al*. Coronary angioplasty versus left internal mammary artery grafting for isolated proximal left anterior descending artery stenosis. *Lancet* 1994;**343**:1449–53.

33 Coronary angioplasty versus coronary artery bypass surgery: the Randomised Intervention Treatment of Angina (RITA) trial. *Lancet* 1993;**341**:573–80.

34 Pocock SJ, Henderson RA, Rickards AF *et al*. Meta-analysis of randomised trials comparing coronary angioplasty with bypass surgery. *Lancet* 1995;**346**:1184–9.

35 King SB III, Lembo NJ, Weintraub WS *et al*. A randomized trial comparing coronary angioplasty with coronary bypass surgery. Emory Angioplasty versus Surgery Trial (EAST). *N Engl J Med* 1994;**331**:1044–50.

36 Hamm CW, Reimers J, Ischinger T *et al*. A randomized study of coronary angioplasty compared with bypass surgery in patients with symptomatic multivessel coronary disease. German Angioplasty Bypass Surgery Investigation (GABI). *N Engl J Med* 1994;**331**:1037–43.

37 First-year results of CABRI (Coronary Angioplasty versus Bypass Revascularization Investigation). CABRI Trial Participants. *Lancet* 1995;**346**:1179–84.

38 Rodriguez A, Boullon F, Perez-Baliño N *et al*. Argentine Randomized Trial of Percutaneous Transluminal Coronary Angioplasty Versus Coronary Artery Bypass Surgery in Multivessel Disease (ERACI): in-hospital results and 1-year follow-up. ERACI Group. *J Am Coll Cardiol* 1993;**22**:1060–7.

39 Williams DO, Baim DS, Bates E *et al*. Coronary anatomic and procedural characteristics of patients randomized to coronary angioplasty in the Bypass Angioplasty Revascularization Investigation (BARI). *Am J Cardiol* 1995;**75**:27C–33C.

40 Puel J, Karouny E, Marco F *et al*. Angioplasty versus surgery in multivessel disease: immediate results and in-hospital outcome in a randomized prospective study (Abstract). *Circulation* 1992;**86**:I-372.

41 Hueb WA, Bellotti G, de Oliveira SA *et al*. The Medicine, Angioplasty or Surgery Study (MASS):

a prospective, randomized trial of medical therapy, balloon angioplasty or bypass surgery for single proximal left anterior descending artery stenoses. *J Am Coll Cardiol* 1995;**26**:1600–5.

42 Comparison of coronary bypass surgery with angioplasty in patients with multivessel disease. The Bypass Angioplasty Revascularization Investigation (BARI) Investigators. *N Engl J Med* 1996;**335**:217–25.

43 Pocock SJ, Henderson RA, Seed P, Treasure T, Hampton JR. Quality of life, employment status, and anginal symptoms after coronary angioplasty or bypass surgery. 3-year follow-up in the Randomized Intervention Treatment of Angina (RITA) Trial. *Circulation* 1996;**94**:135–42.

44 Zhao XQ, Brown BG, Stewart DK *et al*. Effectiveness of revascularization in the Emory Angioplasty versus Surgery Trial. A randomized comparison of coronary angioplasty with bypass surgery. *Circulation* 1996;**93**:1954–62.

45 Weintraub WS, Mauldin PD, Becker E, Kosinski AS, King SB III. A comparison of the costs of and quality of life after coronary angioplasty or coronary surgery for multivessel coronary artery disease. Results from the Emory Angioplasty versus Surgery Trial (EAST). *Circulation* 1995;**92**:2831–40.

46 Rodriguez A, Ahualli P, Perez-Baliño N *et al*. Argentine Randomized Trial of Percutaneous Transluminal Coronary Angioplasty versus Coronary Artery Bypass Surgery in Multivessel Disease (ERACI): late cost and three years follow up results (Abstract). *J Am Coll Cardiol* 1994;**23**:469A.

47 Ellis SG, Nowamagbe O, Bittl JA *et al*. Analysis and comparison of operator-specific outcomes in interventional cardiology. From a multicenter database of 4860 quality-controlled procedures. *Circulation* 1996;**93**:431–9.

48 Ellis SG, Weintraub W, Holmes D *et al*. Relation of operator volume and experience to procedural outcome of percutaneous coronary revascularization at hospitals with high interventional volumes. *Circulation* 1997;**95**:2479–84.

49 Jollis JG, Peterson ED, Nelson CL *et al*. Relationship between physician and hospital coronary angioplasty volume and outcome in elderly patients. *Circulation* 1997;**95**:2485–91.

50 Mark DB, Nelson CL, Califf RM *et al*. Continuing evolution of therapy for coronary artery disease. Initial results from the era of coronary angioplasty. *Circulation* 1994;**89**:2015–25.

51 Jones RH, Kesler K, Phillips HR III *et al*. Long-term survival benefits of coronary artery bypass grafting and percutaneous transluminal angioplasty in patients with coronary artery disease. *J Thorac Cardiovasc Surg* 1996;**111**:1013–25.

Part III
Specific cardiovascular disorders
ii: Acute ischemic syndromes

JOHN A CAIRNS and BERNARD J GERSH, Editors

Grading of recommendations and levels of evidence used in *Evidence Based Cardiology*

GRADE A

Level 1a   Evidence from large randomized clinical trials (RCTs) or systematic reviews (including meta-analyses) of multiple randomized trials which collectively has at least as much data as one single well-defined trial.

Level 1b   Evidence from at least one "All or None" high quality cohort study; in which ALL patients died/failed with conventional therapy and some survived/succeeded with the new therapy (eg chemotherapy for tuberculosis, meningitis, or defibrillation for ventricular fibrillation); or in which many died/failed with conventional therapy and NONE died/failed with the new therapy (eg penicillin for pneumococcal infections).

Level 1c   Evidence from at least one moderate sized RCT or a meta-analysis of small trials which collectively only has a moderate number of patients.

Level 1d   Evidence from at least one RCT.

GRADE B

Level 2   Evidence from at least one high quality study of non-randomized cohorts who did and did not receive the new therapy.

Level 3   Evidence from at least one high quality case control study.

Level 4   Evidence from at least one high quality case series.

GRADE C

Level 5   Opinions from experts without reference or access to any of the foregoing (eg argument from physiology, bench research or first principles).

A comprehensive approach would incorporate many different types of evidence (eg RCTs, non-RCTs, epidemiologic studies, and experimental data), and examine the architecture of the information for consistency, coherence and clarity. Occasionally the evidence does not completely fit into neat compartments. For example, there may not be an RCT that demonstrates a reduction in mortality in individuals with stable angina with the use of beta-blockers, but there is overwhelming evidence that mortality is  reduced following MI. In such cases, some may recommend use of beta-blockers in angina patients with the expectation that some extrapolation from post-MI trials is warranted. This could be expressed as Grade A/C. In other instances (e.g. smoking cessation or a pacemaker for complete heart block), the non-randomized data are so overwhelmingly clear and biologically plausible that it would be reasonable to consider these interventions as Grade A.

Recommendation grades appear either in a shaded margin box with an 'R' logo as shown, or within the text, for example Grade A.

Unstable angina

25

PIERRE THÉROUX,
JOHN A CAIRNS

DEFINITION AND INCIDENCE

Ustable angina encompasses a spectrum of symptomatic manifestations of ischemic heart disease, intermediate between stable angina and acute myocardial infarction.[1-3] Early publications identified a variety of premonitory symptoms in people who eventually went on to develop myocardial infarction (MI) or sudden coronary death. The concept of impending acute coronary artery occlusion due to thrombosis evolved in the 1930s,[4,5] and eventually there were prospective trials among patients with syndromes which may in retrospect be called unstable angina, documenting high rates of MI and death. In 1971, Fowler[6] used the term "unstable angina" which was subsequently popularized by Conti and has come to be widely used.

Three general chest pain patterns characterize unstable angina. First is that of the recent onset (within the past 4–8 weeks) of angina of at least Canadian Cardiovascular Society (CCS) Class III in severity. A second pattern is that of progressive or crescendo pain that has distinctly changed, having become more frequent, easily induced, severe or prolonged, or less responsive to nitroglycerin. Thirdly, there may be pain at rest and emotional ease lasting longer than 15–20 minutes. Variant or Prinzmetal's angina, characterized by episodic ischemic pain, often severe in degree, usually occurring at

Clinical presentation of unstable angina		
I	New onset angina	Onset within post 4–8 weeks, at least CCS grade III
II	Crescendo angina	Previously stable angina which has become distinctly more frequent, easily induced, severe, or prolonged, or less responsive to nitroglycerin
III	Rest angina	Angina occurring at rest and lasting longer than 15–20 minutes

- Encompassed within this spectrum of symptomatic manifestations of ischemic heart disease are variant or Prinzmetal's angina and angina in the early post-MI period (>24 hours). Non-Q wave MI generally cannot be differentiated from unstable angina on initial clinical presentation and the initial management is not different. ST and T wave abnormalities are common.
- The development of new Q waves or the elevation of cardiac enzymes to more than twice normal defines the occurrence of MI.

rest, accompanied by predominant ST segment elevation, and often by ventricular arrhythmias, is generally included with the other syndromes of unstable angina.[7] The full syndrome of variant angina is rare, but lesser degrees of ST segment elevation without marked accompanying symptoms are relatively common. It has been recognized for many years that angina in the first few weeks following MI has a serious prognosis,[8] and including such patients within the definition of unstable angina has aided management.

Perceptions of a gradient of risk from new onset, to crescendo, to prolonged rest angina,[1] have been augmented by a recent well documented case series.[9] Braunwald has suggested a classification which attempts to incorporate features of the pain pattern, history of coronary artery disease, ECG abnormalities, and response to treatment.[10] Some attempts have been undertaken to assess the clinical value of this classifications scheme.[11,12] More exhaustive classifications, including angina equivalence, medication used, severity, clinical background, provocative factors, extent of atherosclerosis, dynamics of coronary obstructions and left ventricular function might be useful for the development of algorithms for risk evaluation and treatment.

When patients present with a severe rest pain pattern, often accompanied by electrocardiographic (ECG) abnormalities, it may be quite unclear whether the diagnosis is unstable angina or non-Q wave infarction in evolution until enzyme levels become available. In general, elevation of standard cardiac enzymes beyond twice the upper limit of normal defines the syndrome as MI and not unstable angina. With the advent of new and very sensitive and specific parameters of myocardial necrosis such as troponin T and I,[13] differentiation between unstable angina and MI may be sharpened. Small elevations of troponin T or troponin I, with or without CK elevations, are associated with a worsened prognosis.[13,14] When there is initial uncertainty as to whether the diagnosis is unstable angina or non-Q wave infarction, the acute management does not depend upon differentiating the two. Accordingly, the inclusion criteria in current clinical trials encompass those patients presenting with either unstable angina or non-Q wave infarction in evolution.[15] The diagnosis of unstable angina does not require the presence of an abnormal ECG, although often there are ST segment and T wave abnormalities and their presence increases the specificity of the diagnosis of acute myocardial ischemia and indicates a worse prognosis.[16–18] Current information on the prevalence of ECG abnormalities is difficult to obtain, in part because ECG criteria are often used to define eligibility for clinical studies. Langer et al.[18] reported 196 patients hospitalized with unstable angina diagnosed as rapid acceleration of previous anginal symptoms to include rest pain or prolonged ischemic chest pain of more than 20 minutes duration without evidence of acute MI. After various exclusions, 135 patients remained and of these, the admitting ECG showed ST segment depression in 25%, ST segment elevation in 16%, both in 4%, and none in 55%.

The clinical diagnosis of unstable angina is in most settings based upon (1) the presence of an unstable ischemic pain pattern of at least CCS grade III and (2) accompanying evidence of significant underlying coronary artery disease. The evidence may be historical, based on previous MI, percutaneous transluminal coronary angioplasty (PTCA), coronary artery bypass graft (CABG), exercise testing or coronary angiography, or it may arise from ECG patterns of previous infarction or present ST and T wave abnormalities in association with the pain. Acute MI must be ruled out.

In clinical trials of unstable angina, there is a reasonably consistent attempt to define an unstable pain pattern, and to require objective parameters of underlying coronary artery disease. Rest pain is always included, but the inclusion of non rest pain patterns varies from trial to trial as does the requirement for transient ECG abnormalities. Those studies including patients with a crescendo pattern but without rest pain, will have fewer ischemic outcome events than those focusing on rest pain patients.[14] Even with rigorous diagnostic criteria, some patients without coronary artery disease continue to be entered into these trials.[19]

In the United States in the 1990s, hospital discharges for unstable angina (UA) exceed 700 000 annually, about equal to those for MI, one-third of which are of the non-Q wave type.[20,21] Admission rates for MI and UA are increasing,[20,22] likely as a result of changes in patterns of practice and referral in accordance with the emphasis on primary and secondary prevention and earlier intervention. Public education programs may also favor early diagnosis, referral, and treatment.

The validity of the figures for the incidence of UA is uncertain. The syndrome is heterogeneous, with a wide spectrum of clinical presentations and severity. In its broadest definition, the term unstable angina could include all patients with the initial occurrence or increasing severity of angina. Using a more restricted definition of unstable angina, the Framingham study showed that UA was the first manifestation of coronary artery disease in only about 10% of patients when patients with evolving MI were retrospectively excluded.[23] Although the more unstable patients are likely to be hospitalized in coronary care units (CCUs), the disposition of the majority of patients with milder presentations is governed by factors such as the availability of monitored beds and local practice patterns, and there is much variability among hospitals, regions, and countries. A relative lack of standardization of diagnostic criteria and terminology in the recording of final hospital diagnoses influences the validity of national incidence statistics. More valid and precise data can be derived from more rigorous CCU registries, but the generalizability of such data is limited.

NATURAL HISTORY

The natural history of unstable angina is determined by the severity and extent of coronary artery disease, the presence of comorbid conditions, age, and the ischemic pain pattern which may range from the simple onset of new angina, to profound and prolonged episodes of angina at rest, accompanied by LV dysfunction and resistance to medical therapy.[3] Outcomes have improved dramatically as therapeutic advances have been made. Prior to routine prescription of bedrest, nitrates, and beta-blockers for UA, by 1 month the rate of MI was about 40% and of death about 25%.[1,2] By the 1970s these rates had fallen to about 10% and 2%.[1,2] In 1979–80, a study of all patients hospitalized with UA in Hamilton, Canada over a 1-year period noted inhospital and 1-year mortalities of 1.5% and 9.2% respectively.[24] By the time of the re-evaluation of heparin in the late 1980s, study inclusion criteria had shifted toward patients at somewhat higher risk and some trials included patients with non-Q wave MI. In these trials, by about 5 days, the rate of the composite outcome of death or non-fatal MI was about 10%.[25,26] This rate was reduced to about 4% with the use of heparin and aspirin. A recent large trial among patients with UA or non-Q wave MI, reported that among those patients with UA, by 6 weeks the rate of non-fatal MI was 6.5% and of death was 1.2%.[15]

PATHOPHYSIOLOGY

Unstable angina is a clinical manifestation of acute myocardial ischemia; it is the consequence of a build-up of pathophysiologic events occurring at the site of an active coronary artery plaque. The understanding of these events has progressed from the simple description of plaques as visualized by coronary angiography, to investigation of cell biology. The exponential growth of knowledge has stimulated parallel development of evidence based therapy.

The presence of obstructive atherosclerosis was almost invariably described in the early angiography studies of UA, providing a rationale to attempt coronary revascularization procedures. Angiographic description of lesions in terms of severity and of number of diseased vessels did not, however, allow differentiation of UA from other manifestations of coronary artery disease, including stable angina and MI.[27] Disease severity was also found to be highly variable between patients, from absence of significant stenoses to presence of left main disease in 5–10% of patients, and single-, two- or three-vessel disease in respectively 20%, 30%, and 40%. Patients with no significant stenoses were considered to be experiencing atypical UA, with a favorable prognosis.

The concept of a fixed obstruction to blood flow was challenged as transient, dynamic, and often complete obstruction was observed in patients with vasospastic disease.[28] It rapidly became clear that UA was associated with a rapid progression of the severity of obstruction in one active coronary lesion.[29] Careful analyses of the morphology of these culprit stenoses revealed features suggestive of plaque disruption and of presence of intraluminal thrombi.[19,30] These findings were confirmed in a few angioscopic studies. Meticulous pathologic description of plaque morphology and structure was then carried out, introducing a new era of understanding and progress.[31,32]

Falk showed the presence of occlusive thrombi in patients dying suddenly after repetitive episodes of UA; these thrombi were of various ages, coinciding with the previous episodes of ischemia.[31] Davies and Thomas described coronary thrombosis on a ruptured plaque in 95% of sudden death victims.[32] These plaques were of only moderate severity, with an inner core rich in cholesterol and cholesterol esters, and a thin fibrous cap, poor in connective tissue and smooth muscle cells, rendering them friable and prone to rupture under a local rheologic stress.[33] At microscopy, these plaques have a high density of monocytes–macrophages, mast cells, lymphocytes and neutrophils.[34] This active plaque is the site of intense inflammatory reaction involving interaction of multiple cells, secretion of matrix-degrading proteins like chymases and tryptases activating metalloproteinases, and expression of cytokines, proinflammatory substances, and growth factors.[35]

Atherosclerosis is an inflammatory disease;[36] in unstable angina, the inflammatory reaction is extreme. The exact reasons are unclear, and may be partly immunologic. Suggested candidate antigens for stimulation of inflammation have included non-infectious moieties such as modified LDL (low density lipoprotein) and, more recently, antigens derived from intracellular pathogens such as cytomegalovirus and *Chlamydia pneumoniae*, generating cytokines from distant or local infectious disease.[37] The inflammatory process, coupled to plaque characteristics increasing vulnerability to rupture, leads to thrombus formation, myocardial ischemia, and clinically overt disease.

Platelet thrombus formation plays a particularly important role in the process of unstable angina. Circulating platelets adhere within seconds to the damaged endothelium with no need for previous activation, through receptor–ligand interactions. Glycoprotein

(GP)Ib/IX recognizes von Willebrand factor present in large quantities in the subendothelium, and GPIa/IIa reccognizes collagen. Platelet adhesion triggers intracellular signaling, increased cytosolic Ca^{++} content, shape change, release of potent vasoactive and proaggregant substances, and activation of the GPIIb/IIIa receptor.[38] The activated GPIIb/IIIa receptor recognizes and binds the RGD sequence of various moieties, particularly of fibrinogen, resulting in platelet crossbridging and platelet aggregation.[39] The activated platelets become the template for blood clot formation. Tissue factor present in the atherosclerotic plaque forms a complex with factor VIIa, to generate the tenase complex on the platelet surface, generate thrombin, and convert fibrinogen to fibrin.[40] P-selectin expressed on the platelet membrane attracts leukocytes, promoting the inflammatory reaction.[41] This pathophysiologic background explains the efficacy of antithrombotic treatment, while setting the basis for investigation of new therapies, targeting various steps of the interaction between the endothelium, platelets, coagulation factors, leukocyctes, adhesive proteins, cytokines, and growth factors.

MANAGEMENT

Acute therapy

The initial goals are to relieve pain, anxiety, and ischemia, and to decrease the substantial risk of MI and sudden death. The therapeutic approaches include: general measures, anti-ischemic therapies, antithrombotic therapies, mechanical revascularization, and hemodynamic supports.

CLINICAL EVALUATION AND THE CONCEPT OF EARLY RISK STRATIFICATION

The pace of initial evaluation and the intensity of treatment will be influenced by the prognosis of the ischemic syndrome as determined by the likelihood of the presence of coronary artery disease, the severity of the ischemia, and the underlying medical status of the patient. The patient who presents with some clinical features of UA may not actually have coronary artery disease. The TIMI-3A trial[19] performed angiography on 391 patients with UA or non-Q wave MI based upon current strict clinical criteria. The distribution of coronary stenosis $\geq 60\%$ in a major vessel was as follows: 0 vessel, 15%; 1 vessel, 27%; 2 vessel, 31%; 3 vessel, 20%; left main coronary artery ($\geq 50\%$), 4%. Clearly it is those patients who actually have coronary artery disease who are at risk, and the determinants of the likelihood of coronary artery disease are therefore determinants of prognosis as well.[3]

Patients with a previous history of MI, resuscitated sudden death, angiographic stenosis, PTCA or CABG have coronary artery disease and are more likely to be experiencing ischemia. A prior history of characteristic ischemic pain precipitated by exertion and relieved by rest or nitroglycerin is strongly suggestive of coronary artery disease.[42,43] The presence of marked ST or T wave abnormalities, particularly transiently in association with chest pain, provides strong evidence for coronary artery disease,[17,44] as does the detection of transient S3 or S4 or mitral insufficiency.[45] The presence of coronary risk factors modestly increases the likelihood for coronary artery disease, while increasing age markedly does so.[3]

A second major element in determining prognosis is the pattern of pain and associated manifestations of myocardial ischemia.[46,47] Hence, prolonged rest pain (> than 20 minutes) confers a worse prognosis than a pattern of crescendo exertional pain, which in turn has a worse prognosis than the simple new onset of exertional angina without a rapidly progressive character. The presence of transient ST and T wave abnormalities with the pain worsens the prognosis,[15,25] as does the recurrence and persistence of episodes of ischemia once the patient is receiving intensive medical therapy in hospital.[3] A recent report describes the hospital outcomes of 1387 consecutive patients presenting to the emergency room of a large general hospital between 1989 and 1991.[9] Patients were managed aggressively with CCU care, extensive use of nitrates, beta-blockers, calcium antagonists, aspirin, and heparin. Patients with acceleration of previous exertional angina with no ECG changes had the best prognosis, whereas the chance of MI was doubled in the presence of transient ST or T wave abnormalities. Patients with new onset rest angina had a worse prognosis, and those with prolonged rest pain and ECG abnormalities had the worst prognosis, with an inhospital MI rate of 17.7% and a mortality rate of 6.4%.

Studies employing continuous ECG monitoring have demonstrated that ST segment shift is common and is highly predictive of subsequent ischemic events.[18,48–50] The incremental predictive value over that of abnormalities on the admitting ECG or in association with chest pain is unclear from these studies, and the appropriate clinical role of continuous ECG monitoring is uncertain. The prognosis is also worse when there is evidence of LV dysfunction during ischemic episodes, including a new or worsening mitral regurgitant murmur, an S3, or new or worsening rales.[3]

Thirdly, the prognosis is affected by a group of factors of importance to a patient at any stage in the evolution of coronary artery disease, including LV dysfunction, extensive coronary atherosclerosis, age, and comorbid conditions such as diabetes mellitus, chronic obstructive pulmonary disease, renal failure, cardiovascular disease, and malignancy.[3]

GENERAL MEASURES

The patient may present in a non-medical setting or by telephone, in the office, or in the hospital emergency room or ward. Those with the simple new onset of angina or mild exacerbation of previously stable angina, with no angina at rest, ECG changes, or hemodynamic abnormalities should be carefully assessed, initial treatment and educational materials provided, and medical follow-up planned, but they may generally be managed as outpatients with initial limitation of activities. High risk patients require admission to the CCU, generally to remain for about 24 hours following the last episode of rest pain. Patients at intermediate risk might go to the CCU, an intermediate care unit, or even to a regular ward depending on the availability of facilities and the specific level of risk.

Whatever the pathophysiology of the acute ischemia in a given patient, there is an imbalance of myocardial oxygen supply and demand, and restricted activities and rest in bed or a recliner chair will be helpful in reducing myocardial oxygen demand. Stool softeners are likely to be helpful. Emotional distress with its attendant increase in myocardial oxygen demand should be minimized by judicious control of environmental noise and light, supportive medical and nursing care, limitation and education of visitors, provision for restful sleep, and control of ischemic pain with intravenous narcotics and nitrates, and other specific anti-ischemic agents as appropriate. Nasal oxygen is routinely

R

Grade C

provided, particularly early in the emergency room or CCU course, although no evidence exists for a specific benefit in patients free of respiratory failure or severe hemodynamic dysfunction.

ANTI-ISCHEMIC THERAPIES

Nitroglycerin has been a mainstay in the therapy of UA since the prognostic importance was first recognized, and as longer acting nitrate preparations became available, these were incorporated into treatment regimens without rigorous comparisons to placebo. Studies of the use of IV nitroglycerin among patients with UA have been relatively small, of sequential or case-control design, and the dose regimens have varied considerably.[51] At least partial relief of anginal episodes is usually achieved, occasionally relief is complete, and absence of benefit is an infrequent observation. However, the trials have been of brief duration, generally a few days only, and problems of nitrate tolerance and recurrence of ischemic events emphasize that nitrates are not definitive therapy for UA beyond the acute phase. A trial comparing nitrate therapy and diltiazem[52] indicates that diltiazem is more effective in controlling angina and preventing ischemic events but these studies do not reflect clinical approaches that have employed long acting or intravenous nitroglycerin in combination with a beta-blocker or a rate-limiting calcium antagonist. The widespread use of oral, topical, and IV nitrates in UA is based upon reasonable extrapolation from pathophysiologic observations, case series, evidence of modest reduction of mortality in acute MI,[53–55] and extensive clinical experience using regimens developed in careful clinical studies.[53]

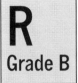

The beta-blockers were introduced in the 1960s and their effectiveness in the treatment of stable angina resulted in rapid acceptance for the management of unstable angina. There was remarkably little objective evidence for the efficacy of beta-blockers prior to their widespread use.[1] Subsequently, beta-blockers were evaluated in well designed studies. Muller et al.[56] evaluated a group of 126 patients hospitalized with UA (characterized by progressive or rest ischemic pain plus ECG changes with pain and documented coronary artery disease). Patients were randomly allocated to the addition to their regular therapy of either nifedipine or the combination of propranolol/isosorbide dinitrate, with appropriate placebos. The principal outcome was absence of recurrent chest pain for at least 48 hours, and the period of evaluation was 14 days. There was no overall difference between the two treatment regimens. However, in a post-hoc analysis of the data amongst the 59 patients not receiving beta-blocker on admission, the propranolol/isosorbide was more effective than the nifedipine in producing pain relief ($P<0.001$). Conversely, among the 67% of patients already receiving a beta-blocker on admission, nifedipine was more effective than augmentation of beta-blocker accompanied by isosorbide ($P=0.026$).

The HINT study[57] examined metoprolol and nifedipine in patients hospitalized with prolonged rest pain. The 338 patients who were not receiving beta-blocker on admission were randomly allocated to nifedipine, metoprolol, both, or neither in a double-blind placebo-controlled fashion. The outcome of AMI or recurrent angina with ST change within 48 hours occurred with the following frequencies: placebo (37%), nifedipine (47%), metoprolol (28%), nifedipine plus metoprolol (30%). Metoprolol was significantly more effective than nifedipine ($P<0.05$). The 177 patients already on a beta-blocker on admission were randomly allocated in double-blind fashion to nifedipine or placebo and treatment failure occurred in 51% of placebo and 30% of nifedipine ($P<0.05$).

Gottlieb et al.[58] studied 81 patients hospitalized with at least 10 minutes of ischemic chest pain at rest. All patients were receiving "optimal" doses of nitrates and nifedipine and were therefore treatment failures on this regimen. They were randomly allocated to the addition of either propranolol or placebo. In the first 4 days, propranolol resulted in a statistically significant reduction of recurrent rest angina episodes, duration of angina, nitroglycerin requirement, and ECG abnormalities. Although recurrences of rest angina remained less among the propranolol treated group over the next 4 weeks, the incidence of aortocoronary bypass, AMI, and sudden death was no different between the two groups.

Gerstenblith[59] evaluated patients hospitalized with prolonged pain accompanied by ECG abnormalities, and who had failed maximum treatment with propranolol and long acting nitrates. There were randomized to the addition of nifedipine or placebo, and the failure of medical treatment (sudden death, AMI, or bypass surgery) was less frequent with nifedipine than with placebo ($P=0.03$). The benefit was most marked among patients with ST segment elevation.

These trials suggest that among patients not receiving a beta-blocker on hospitalization, the institution of beta-blockade and the institution or maintenance of nitrates is more effective treatment than the institution of nifedipine. **Grade A** Amongst patients whose pain persists with optimal doses of nitrates and nifedipine, the addition of a beta-blocker is efficacious in the initial few days, although the incidence of ischemic outcomes (bypass surgery, AMI, sudden death) is not reduced. **Grade A** On the other hand, in patients hospitalized and already receiving a beta-blocker, then the addition of nifedipine is more effective than simply augmenting the beta-blocker dose. Recent data suggesting potentially harmful effects of short acting dihydropyridines[60] **Grade A** indicate that a more prudent choice for the addition to a beta-blocker would be a long acting dose preparation or an agent with an intrinsically long half-life such as amlodipine, although rigorous studies have not been conducted.

Diltiazem was compared to propranolol in a randomized single-blind study of patients hospitalized for crescendo rest or post-MI angina accompanied by ECG abnormalities.[61] Chest pain frequency was significantly reduced by both regimens, but there was no difference in efficacy. The 5-month follow-up was rather discouraging in both groups, with a high incidence of AMI, death, and bypass surgery, and few patients without bypass surgery were symptom free. Andre-Fouet et al.[62] randomized patients hospitalized with rest angina to diltiazem or propranolol in maximum tolerated doses. The agents were equally effective in reducing the frequency of daily anginal episodes, but in the subgroup with angina only at rest, diltiazem was efficacious whereas propranolol was not.

There is little rigorous evidence for the value of verapamil in unstable angina. Small placebo-controlled trials[63,64] demonstrated statistically significant reductions in the frequency of ischemia. Long term follow-up in these small trials[65] showed that in general ischemic pain continued to be well controlled but there was a high incidence of AMI and death.

In addition to reducing ischemic episodes, a reduction in MI would be desirable. Yusuf et al.[66] examined five trials involving about 4700 patients with threatened MI who were placed on intravenous beta-blocker followed by oral therapy for about a week. There was a modest 13% reduction in the risk of development of MI in this group. Meta-analysis of studies of calcium antagonists among patients with unstable angina shows no reduction of death or non-fatal MI.[66,67]

Diltiazem and verapamil appear to be effective as initial single agents in the management of UA, and diltiazem appears to be no different in efficacy from propranolol in one direct comparison. However, the meta-analytic data for benefit of beta-blocker but not calcium antagonists and the evidence for improved long term outcomes with beta-blocker therapy among survivors of myocardial infarction,[66] and those with chronic ischemia, support beta-blockers over rate-limiting calcium antagonists as the first choice therapy in patients with unstable angina. Nifedipine should not be the initial single agent for patients with UA.[56,57]

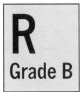

Among patients with variant angina, characterized by dramatic propensity for recurrent ischemia at rest accompanied by ST segment elevation, randomized placebo-controlled, double-blind trials of verapamil,[68–70] diltiazem,[71–74] and nifedipine[75–77] have demonstrated the efficacy of each of these agents in reduction of angina frequency. Several comparisons of calcium antagonist to beta-blockers have demonstrated greater efficacy with the calcium antagonists.[69,70,74] These agents are regarded as the therapy of choice for variant angina, although there is little direct comparative data with long acting nitrates.

ANTITHROMBOTIC THERAPIES

Clinical trials have conclusively demonstrated that antithrombotic therapy is highly effective to prevent the complications associated with progression of the intravascular thrombus leading to myocardial ischemia. The evidence is particularly conclusive with antiplatelet therapy.[78] It is also strong, although less so, with drugs acting on the coagulation system.[79] On the other hand, thrombolytic therapy has not been associated with clinical benefit, and trials have suggested that they may have a negative impact.[15]

These results are consistent with pathophysiology of the disease: platelets mediate first the acute response; thrombin is generated and entrapped in the clot, generating fibrin and mediating numerous cellular events.[80] It is more and more evident that UA is more than an acute condition, and often an exacerbation of an underlying disease with recurrent episodes of ischemia. The underlying activity may be the consequence of persisting procoagulant activity,[81] providing much potential for anticoagulant therapy. It may also be associated with incomplete repair of the thrombogenic substrate and control of the triggers to inflammation. Lysis of fibrin in these active plaques, not completely occlusive, may reactivate the underlying disease process, explaining the failure of thrombolytic therapy.

Antiplatelet therapy

Antiplatelet agents evaluated have been aspirin, prostacyclin, sulfinpyrazone, ticlopidine – and clopidogrel indirectly – and the GPIIb/IIIa antagonists. Aspirin has received unanimous approval and has become the gold standard for treatment, following numerous trials performed with the drug consistently showing benefit. Ticlopidine – and clopidogrel – is second line treatment in patients intolerant to aspirin; these thienopyridines are probably less effective during the acute phase and more useful in secondary prevention. No gain has been shown with prostacyclin; and there is no role for sulfinpyrazone. The GPIIIb/IIIa inhibitors used intravenously add significant benefit to aspirin and to heparin.

Aspirin has been tested in four conclusive trials. The Veterans Administration Study, performed between 1974 and 1981, included 1338 men hospitalized for UA within the previous week, manifested as crescendo or prolonged pain, or pain at rest.[82] The main analysis excluded 72 patients randomized with an evolving MI. Patients were randomly allocated to treatment with 324 mg of aspirin in an effervescent buffered powder (Alka-Seltzer) dissolved in water or to placebo. The principal outcome was death or MI over a 12-week treatment period. The rate of death or MI was reduced from 10.1% to 5.0% (51% risk reduction, $P = 0.0005$). By intention-to-treat analysis including the patients with a MI at entry, the reduction in death or MI was 41% ($P = 0.004$), and of mortality, 34% ($P = 0.17$). A follow-up of 86% of patients at one year revealed a reduction in mortality of 43% in the aspirin treated patients, from 9.6% to 5.5% ($P = 0.008$).

In the Canadian Multicenter Trial conducted between 1979 and 1984, 555 patients (73% men) with unstable angina were randomized before hospital discharge to aspirin (325 mg four times daily), sulfinpyrazone (200 mg four times daily), placebo, or both drugs.[83] In the efficacy analysis, the outcome of death or MI at 2 years was reduced from 17% to 8.6%, a risk reduction of 50.8% ($P = 0.008$). By intention-to-treat analysis, the risk reduction was 30% ($P = 0.072$); the outcome of death was reduced by 71% in the former analysis ($P = 0.004$), and by 43.4% in the latter ($P = 0.035$). Sulfinpyrazone had no significant effect or interaction with aspirin.

In the Montreal study, 479 patients were randomized during the acute phase of disease to aspirin (325 mg twice daily), heparin, both or neither in a 2×2 factorial design trial.[26] The study drugs were administered for a mean of 6 days. Aspirin reduced the risk of death or MI from 6.3% to 2.6%, a 63% risk reduction ($P = 0.04$). The RISC study randomized 945 patients to aspirin (80 mg daily), intravenous heparin (5000 U q 6 hours for 24 hours and 3750 U q 6 hours for 4 days), both or placebos.[25] Endpoints were assessed in 796 patients meeting the entry criteria. Aspirin, compared to no aspirin, reduced the rate of death or MI at 5 days from 5.8% to 2.55% ($P = 0.033$), at 7 days from 13.4% to 4.3% ($P = 0.0001$), and at 30 days from 17.1% to 6.5% ($P = 0.0001$).

The Antiplatelet Trialists' Collaboration meta-analysis of more than 100 000 patients randomized to antiplatelet therapy or placebo from 145 trials has shown a consistent reduction in cardiovascular events with antiplatelet therapy in patients at all levels of risk with cardiovascular diseases, including acute and old MI, stroke, stable angina, and unstable angina.[78] The odds of infarction, stroke or vascular death were reduced overall by more than 25%. In the 4000 patients with UA, vascular events after 6 months were reduced from 14% to 9% ($P < 0.00001$). Aspirin was by far the most frequently used antiplatelet drug in these trials.

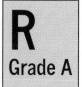

Aspirin possesses numerous physiologic effects, many of which are only partly characterized. The mechanism accounting for the benefit in UA is believed to be irreversible inhibition of the cyclo-oxygenase pathway in platelets, blocking formation of thromboxane A2 and platelet aggregation. This inhibition is total and irreversible with small doses of aspirin. The concomitant inhibition of prostacyclin generation by aspirin does not appear to limit significantly the protection afforded by aspirin. Consistently, infusion of prostacyclin has not resulted in benefit,[84] and drugs selectively inhibiting thromboxane synthase, or the thromboxane receptor or both, have not been shown to be superior to aspirin.

Ticlopidine, 250 mg twice a day, was compared in a randomized, open label trial of 652 unstable angina patients of either sex to conventional antianginal therapy without aspirin.[85] After a follow-up of 6 months, ticlopidine reduced by 46% the rate of fatal and non-fatal MI, from 13.6% to 7.3%. The benefit of ticlopidine in this study developed only after 2 weeks of treatment, consistent with the known delay of the drug to achieve full effect. Ticlopidine, unlike aspirin, does not block cyclo-oxygenase but interferes with the platelet activation mechanism mediated by adenosine diphosphate (ADP) and with transformation of the fibrinogen receptor GpIIb/IIIa, into its high affinity state. Clopidogrel is a thienopyridine closely related to ticlopidine. The drug was recently tested in the large CAPRIE trial with a total of 19 185 patients randomized to aspirin, 325 mg/day, or clopidogrel, 75 mg/day.[86] The population comprised subgroups of patients with atherosclerotic vascular disease manifested as either recent ischemic stroke, recent MI, or symptomatic peripheral disease. Follow-up extended between 1 and 3 years. The annual risk of ischemic stroke from MI, or vascular death was reduced by 8.7% in favor of clopidogrel from 5.83% to 5.32% ($P=0.043$). The relative risk was reduced by 23.8% ($P=0.00028$) in patients enrolled because of peripheral vascular disease, by 7.3% in patients enrolled because of stroke, but was increased by 5.03% ($P=0.66$) in patients enrolled following MI.

Abciximab, a monoclonal antibody blocking the GPIIb/IIIa receptor, is now approved for clinical use in high risk coronary angioplasty. A variety of synthetic inhibitors that compete reversibly with the RGD (or KGD) recognition site for fibrinogen, have also been developed. These drugs for intravenous use are eftifibatide, a cyclic heptapeptide, and tirofiban and lamifiban, two non-peptide inhibitors. Abciximab has been mainly investigated in coronary angioplasty. Its administration just before the procedure followed by a 12 hour infusion in the Evaluation of 7E3 in Preventing Ischemic Complications (EPIC) and Evaluation in PTCA to Improve Long Term Outcome with Abciximab GPIIb/IIIa Blockade (EPILOG) trials, has resulted in a significant reduction in the risk of procedure-related complications.[87,88] In the c7E3 Fab Antiplatelet Therapy in Unstable Refractory Angina (CAPTURE) trial involving 1265 patients, abciximab was administered for 20–24 hours before the angioplasty in patients with refractory unstable angina and for 1 hour after the procedure.[89] In this trial, abciximab, compared with placebo, reduced the rate of death and MI by 30 days from 15.9% to 11.3% ($P=0.012$). The drug was effective during the period of medical treatment before angioplasty; most events, however, and most benefit occurred during and immediately after the procedure.

Lamifiban was investigated in two dose-ranging studies. In the Canadian lamifiban study, 365 patients with UA were randomized double-blind to infusions of 1, 2, 4, or 5 µg/min of lamifiban or placebo. Lamifiban dose-dependently inhibited platelet aggregation.[90] Concomitant aspirin was administered to all patients and heparin to 28% of patients. Lamifiban compared with placebo reduced the risk of death, non-fatal MI, or the need for an urgent revascularization during the infusion period from 8.1% to 3.3% ($P=0.04$). At 1 month, death or non-fatal infarction occurred in 8.1% of patients with placebo and in 2.5% of patients with the two high doses ($P=0.03$). The larger PARAGON study with 2250 patients randomized between five study groups did not reproduce these results. The groups were low dose lamifiban with or without heparin, high dose lamifiban with or without heparin, and heparin alone. An excess event rate was observed at 30 days with the higher dose, especially when combined with heparin.[91] Follow-up, however, showed a significant reduction in the rate of death or MI after 6 months with the low dose with or without heparin.[91]

Tirofiban was investigated in two trials. The Platelet Receptor Inhibition for Ischemic Syndrome Management (PRISM) trial directly compared tirofiban to heparin in 3231 patients.[92] The primary composite endpoint of death, MI, and refractory ischemia measured at the end of a 48 hour infusion period was decreased by 36% with tirofiban ($P=0.007$). The benefit was not statistically significant after 1 week. After 30 days, however, death was significantly less frequent with tirofiban. The Platelet Receptor

Inhibition for Ischemic Syndrome Management in Patients Limited by Unstable Signs and Symptoms (PRISM-PLUS) trial documented a significant gain with tirofiban added to intravenous heparin compared with heparin alone in 1570 patients. The reduction in the primary endpoint of death, MI, and refractory ischemia at 7 days reached 32% (P=0.004) and in the risk of death and myocardial infarction 43% (P=0.006).[93] The gain appeared early and was sustained after 6 months. Tirofiban was administered for a mean duration of 73 hours in this trial, covering a period of 48 hours of medical treatment, subsequent coronary angiography, and angioplasty when performed.

The results of the Platelet IIb/IIIa in Unstable Angina: Receptor Suppression Using Integrilin™ (PURSUIT) trial were recently presented at the European Congress of Cardiology.[94] The trial has enrolled 9461 patients with UA and non-Q wave MI; by 30 days the rate of death or MI was reduced by 10% from 15.7% to 14.2%, a statistically significant reduction (P=0.042).

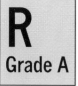

Altogether, these trials show efficacy of GPIIb/IIIa antagonism to prevent cardiac events in percutaneous coronary interventions and in UA. The benefits are additive to those of aspirin, and no trials have evaluated these drugs without aspirin. The data presently available suggest that heparin should also be used concomitantly. The arm testing tirofiban alone, with no heparin, in the PRISM-PLUS trial was dropped prematurely because of excess mortality; no excess was, however, observed in the other end points of the trial, such as myocardial infarction, and no excess mortality was observed with tirofiban alone in the PRISM trial.

The efficacy of aspirin has been well documented in UA. The drug is presently recommended in all patients unless a contraindication is present. Despite some limited efficacy as an antiplatelet agent, aspirin possesses a safety-efficacy profile and a cost-effectiveness ratio that will be extremely hard to equal. Grade A Ticlopidine can be used in patients intolerant to aspirin. Clopidogrel, when available, will be a better second choice considering its excellent safety profile compared with ticlopidine. Grade B The GPIIb/IIIa agents are also very effective and will have to be considered when they become available for clinical use. Grade A Other promising antiplatelet therapies are the oral GPIIb/IIIa inhibitors presently being investigated in large scale trials, the combination of aspirin and clopidogrel, and the inhibitors of platelet adhesion to von Willebrand factor.

Anticoagulants

Anticoagulants that have been evaluated during the acute phase of UA and non-Q wave MI are unfractionated heparin, the direct thrombin inhibitors, including recombinant hirudin and small synthetic peptides, and the low molecular weight heparins. Many promising new anticoagulants remain to be evaluated such as r-tissue factor pathway inhibitor, r-protein C, specific inhibitors of factor Xa, pentasaccharides, heparin cofactor 2, and others. Numerous recent trials of anticoagulants have documented their efficacy. Their effectiveness may be less striking when antiplatelet therapy is used concomitantly; yet clinical trials have documented additive gain. A limiting factor is rebound activity of the disease following their discontinuation, first described with heparin,[95] and subsequently with low molecular weight heparin[96] and recombinant hirudin.[97] Attempts are presently ongoing to prevent this reactivation using protocols of prolonged administration of low molecular weight heparin, oral anticoagulants, and oral inhibitors of the GPIIb/IIIa receptors. Results of small trials with antivitamin K are available and suggest that the therapy could be useful and worth investigating in large trials.

The first modern randomized, double-blind, controlled trial of heparin was published in 1981 by Telford and Wilson.[98] A total of 400 patients were randomized to heparin, atenolol, heparin plus atenolol, or placebo. An 80% reduction of the incidence of MI was reported by 7 days with heparin compared with no heparin. The impact of the trial was small because of a design problem, with 186 randomized patients (46% of the total population) withdrawn from the analysis because of incorrect recruitment. Subsequently, in 1986, Williams *et al.* published the results of a small trial of 102 patients randomized at hospital admission to treatment with heparin for 48 hours followed by warfarin for 6 months.[99] The randomization process was unusual since patients found to have MI at entry were dropped after randomization and the allocation code assigned to the next patient entering the study. At 6 months there were three MIs and one death in the treatment group, and three MIs and four deaths in the control group; recurrence of UA was observed in respectively three and 10 patients. Entering all events in the analysis, the risk reduction was 65% with treatment (*P*<0.05). The trial from Montreal has reintroduced heparin as standard treatment of UA.[26] The incidence of fatal and non-fatal MI was reduced from 7.5% to 1.2% (RR 85%, *P*=0.007), and of recurrent refractory ischemia from 19.7% to 9.6% (RR 51%, *P*=0.02). These risk reductions were greater than the risk reductions with aspirin alone, and the combination of aspirin with heparin added no additional benefit during the acute phase, although it prevented the clinical events associated with the discontinuation of the anticoagulant. An extension to this trial with randomization of additional patients to a total of 484 patients receiving heparin alone or aspirin alone confirmed a superiority of heparin with a risk reduction of 78% (*P*=0.035).[100] This study supports a benefit of heparin but cannot be considered as decisive, considering the limited power and a two sequential stage design.

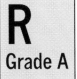

The RISC study of 945 men also compared aspirin, heparin, both, or placebo.[25] Heparin was initiated relatively late, after 24 hours, and used at relatively low dose with no titration. Heparin was not associated with a benefit in the study, but the combination of aspirin and of heparin resulted in a significant risk reduction in death and MI at 5 days. An open label trial involving 285 patients has compared aspirin alone, 150 mg, to the combination with heparin.[101] The primary endpoint of the trial, transient ST segment depression on continuous ECG monitoring, was not significantly modified by the combination therapy, although the total duration of ST segment shift was 2911 min compared with 4908 min with aspirin alone. The inhospital incidence of MI and of death was unusually high in this study at 29% and equally distributed in the two treatment groups; MI present at entry was included in the outcomes. The findings of this study contrast with another trial that had shown that only IV infusion of heparin, and not SC heparin, nor rt-PA nor aspirin, was effective to reduce the number and duration of ischemic episodes, as assessed by ST segment depression on ECG monitoring.[102] A small randomized double-blind study of 57 patients allocated to warfarin (INR 2–2.5) or placebo in addition to aspirin using repeated coronary angiography reported less progression after 10 weeks in the culprit lesion with coumadin (4% of patients vs 33%) and more regression (19% vs 9%).[103]

Another study of limited size, the ATACS trial, has randomized 214 patients with UA and non-Q wave MI not previously taking aspirin, to aspirin alone, 162.5 mg, or the combination of aspirin, 162.5 mg plus heparin titrated to aPTT, followed by coumadin (INR 2–2.5).[104] At 14 days, there was a significant reduction in the combined endpoint of death, MI, and recurrent ischemia in the combination group vs aspirin alone (10.5% vs 27%; *P*=0.004). The survival curves diverged mainly during the first few days of treatment. A meta-analysis by these authors of the three studies comparing combination

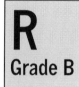

R

Grade B

therapy with aspirin alone showed a 56% reduction in the incidence of the hard endpoints of fatal and non-fatal MI with the combination therapy. A more recent meta-analysis of trials comparing combination heparin plus aspirin vs aspirin alone also supported a significant risk reduction of 33% with the combination.[105] The OASIS pilot study of hirudin vs heparin also compared a fixed dose regimen of 3 mg of coumadin in 309 patients, or a moderate dose titrated to an INR of 2–2.5 in 197 patients, for 6 months after the acute phase.[97] Aspirin was recommended for all patients. The low intensity fixed dose of coumadin had no benefit; moderate intensity coumadin reduced the risk of death, MI, or refractory angina by 58% ($P=0.08$), and the need for rehospitalization for UA by 58% ($P=0.03$).

GUSTO-2b was a large trial of 12 142 patients comparing r-hirudin to heparin for the treatment of acute coronary syndromes.[106] The drugs were administered for 72 hours. In the 8011 patients with no ST segment elevation, the primary composite endpoint of death or MI at 30 days occurred in 8.3% of the patients on hirudin and in 9.3% of patients on heparin (odds ratio 0.90, 95% confidence limits 0.78–1.06, $P=0.22$). In this trial, a bolus dose of hirudin of 0.2 mg/kg was administered followed by an infusion dose of 0.1 mg/kg/h. This dose was selected following the excess bleeding rate observed in 2564 patients enrolled in GUSTO-2a with the originally planned dose of 0.6 mg/kg bolus and 0.2 mg/kg/h infusion, and in the 757 patients enrolled in TIMI-9A.[107,108] Other trials of moderate sample size with synthetic direct thrombin inhibitors also had failed to show clearly a trend to benefit with the intervention; one of these trials has used efegatran.[109] The OASIS pilot study tested a small dose of r-hirudin of 0.2 mg/kg bolus and 0.1 mg/kg/h infusion, and a moderate dose of 0.4 mg/h bolus and 0.15 mg/kg/h infusion versus heparin in 909 patients with UA or suspected acute MI without ST segment elevation.[97] At 7 days, 6.5% of patients in the heparin group, 4.4% in the low dose group, and 3.0% in the medium dose group suffered cardiovascular death, new MI, or refractory angina ($P=0.047$ heparin vs medium dose hirudin). The proportions with cardiovascular death, new MI, or refractory or severe angina were 15.6%, 12.5%, and 9.4%, respectively ($P=0.02$ for heparin vs medium dose). The rates of new MI were 4.9%, 2.6%, and 1.9%, respectively ($P=0.046$ heparin vs medium dose). Fewer patients underwent coronary artery bypass graft surgery in the two hirudin groups. After cessation of study treatments, there was an increase in ischemic events in the low dose hirudin group at 24 hours and at 5 days in the medium dose group. Minor bleeding rates were more frequent with hirudin, but there was no excess major bleeding. A large phase 3 trial of 10 000 patients is now testing the moderate dose.

Low molecular weight heparins present distinct advantages over unfractionated heparin. They can be administered subcutaneously once or twice a day, with no need for monitoring. They bind plasma proteins and endothelial cells less avidly resulting in anticoagulation that is more predictable. They also stimulate platelets less and are less often associated with heparin-induced thrombocytopenia.[110] These advantages have been well demonstrated in venous disease, and are now emerging in UA. A pilot open label study from Argentina of 219 patients with UA first suggested that the combination of a low molecular weight heparin with aspirin could be better than treatment with aspirin alone or in combination with standard heparin.[111] The Fragmin during Instability in Coronary Artery Disease (FRISC) study randomized 1506 patients with UA or non-Q wave MI to subcutaneous dalteparin twice daily or placebo.[96] After 6 days, the dose was reduced to once a day administration for 35–45 days. Dalteparin was significantly better than placebo, with a 63% risk reduction in death or MI during the first 6 days, confirming the efficacy of anticoagulant therapy. Although an excess of events was observed with the dose reduction, significant benefit was still present after 40 days. The Fragmin in Coronary Artery Disease (FRIC) trial compared dalteparin to standard heparin in 1482 patients.[112] The rate of death, MI, and recurrent ischemia was not statistically significant with the two heparin formulations, 9.3% with dalteparin and 7.6% with heparin (RR 1.18, 95% CL, 0.84–1.66); a trend to more death with dalteparin was, however, of concern. Subcutaneous administration in this trial for 45 days did not improve prognosis. The Efficacy and Safety of Subcutaneous Enoxaparin in Non-Q Wave Coronary Events Study (ESSENCE) trial compared enoxaparin twice daily to heparin administered during the hospital stay for 48 hours to 8 days (median of 2.6 days).[113] The low molecular weight heparin significantly reduced the rate of death, MI, and recurrent ischemia at 30 days from 23.3% to 19.8% ($P=0.014$), and the rate of death and MI from 7.7% to 6.2% ($P=0.08$). The results of this well designed trial are convincing. A TIMI trial is presently evaluating the potential benefit of more prolonged enoxaparin therapy. The cost-effectiveness of low molecular weight heparin vs standard heparin remains to be established, before recommending routine use.

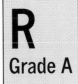

R
Grade A

ANGIOGRAPHY AND REVASCULARIZATION

Optimal medical therapy includes: CCU care with continuous ECG monitoring, bedrest, or minimal exertion, aspirin and heparin, and a combination of nitrates, beta-blockers, and calcium antagonists sufficient to prevent tachycardia and hypertension while avoiding major side effects. If there are recurrences of ischemic pain or silent ischemia in such patients at rest or with attempts at mobilization, optimal medical therapy may be considered to have failed, and such patients have a high incidence of MI and death.[9,25,114] The high risk and impressions of improved results from case series of PTCA and CABG have discouraged the conduct of controlled trials. The general approach has been to proceed to cardiac catheterization with a view to revascularization. Case series support the use of the intra-aortic balloon pump to stabilize patients before or during catheterization, as an aid to high risk PTCA, or as a way to sustain the patient until an operating room is available for a revascularization procedure.[115] The choice of PTCA vs CABG is generally governed by expert interpretation of case series.

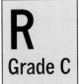

R
Grade C

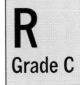

R
Grade C

With technical advances and increased safety of angiographic PTCA, and CABG procedures, a widespread practice developed, particularly in the US, of early routine angiography and revascularization among patients who had responded to medical therapy. TIMI-3B[15] was a randomized, controlled trial of an early invasive strategy (early coronary angiography followed by revascularization when the anatomy was suitable) with an early conservative strategy (coronary angiography only if initial medical therapy failed or functional testing revealed persisting residual ischemia, followed by revascularization when the anatomy was suitable). Tissue plasminogen activator was also evaluated in a factorial design. All patients were treated with bedrest, anti-ischemic medication, ASA, and heparin. The endpoint for the comparison of the two strategies was a composite of death, MI or an unsatisfactory symptom-limited exercise stress test at 6 weeks. Such an outcome occurred in 18.1% of patients assigned to the early conservative strategy and 16.2% of patients assigned to the early invasive strategy (NS). Although these major outcomes were not reduced by aggressive intervention, the average length of initial hospitalization, the incidence of rehospitalization within 6 weeks, and days of rehospitalization were all decreased in the early invasive group. Both strategies were judged to be safe and to constitute appropriate options for the treatment of patients with unstable angina.

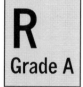

R

Grade A

The Veterans Affairs Non-Q Wave Infarction Strategies In-Hospital (VANQWISH) study,[116] reported at the March 1997 ACC meeting, randomized patients with non-Q wave MI to an early invasive strategy versus an early conservative strategy. There were 920 patients enrolled, among whom there were 21 inhospital deaths in the invasive arm and only 6 in the conservative arm. Following discharge there were respectively, 59 deaths and 53 deaths. The mean hospital length of stay was 9.5 days with the invasive strategy and 8.2 days with the conservative strategy. The investigation concluded that an initial conservative management strategy should be adopted to stratify non-Q wave MI patients, after which invasive procedures should be used electively and selectively.

Subacute therapy

RISK STRATIFICATION AND FUNCTIONAL ASSESSMENT

The TIMI-3B data indicate that patients whose ischemia is controlled by initial medical therapy do not routinely require angiography.[15] They may be evaluated by functional testing, with angiography and consideration for revascularization reserved for those with evidence of important residual ischemia. In the RISC trial,[16] of 740 men hospitalized with UA or non-Q wave MI, 51% experienced ≥ 1 mm of ST segment depression on a predischarge exercise test and had 18% 1-year incidence of MI or death, versus 9% in the 49% of patients without ST segment depression ($P<0.01$). When angina accompanied the ST segment depression the prognosis was still worse. It is generally considered to be prudent to wait for about 48 hours following control of ischemia before exercise stress testing. One study compared symptom-limited stress testing at 3–7 days following an episode of unstable angina or non-Q wave MI to a similar test done 1 month later.[117] Early testing was safe and predicted events that occurred over the first month and were relatively common, while the diagnostic and prognostic value of early versus later tests was similar. Accordingly, predischarge functional testing appears desirable. Exercise ECG is not helpful when there are ST segment abnormalities on the resting ECG and the use of radionuclide myocardial perfusion or LV function evaluation during exercise should be substituted. There are a number of studies among patients with UA, demonstrating substantially higher rates of MI and death among those with abnormal findings on stress ECG, stress perfusion, or stress LV function.[16,118] The radionuclide techniques have somewhat higher test accuracy than ECG stress testing and are often advocated for routine use, but comparative studies are generally compromised by small sample sizes.[119,120] Radionuclide techniques should probably be reserved for patients with resting ST segment abnormalities or when prognosis is not clear after an initial ECG stress test. Patients who are not able to exercise may be evaluated by pharmacologic stress testing employing vasodilators such as dipyridamole or inotropic agents such as dobutamine.[121] Echocardiographic measures of LV function during exercise or pharmacologic stress have not been rigorously assessed in patients with UA.

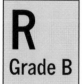

R

Grade B

MEDICAL THERAPY

Once patients have stabilized for about 48 hours in hospital, intravenous nitrate therapy is generally tapered with the substitution of oral or topical nitrates. The early efficacy of beta-blockers, and evidence for long-term benefits in patients following MI[122] and with stable ischemia suggests that the therapy should be continued indefinitely. Similar analogies appear reasonable if a rate-limiting calcium antagonist was chosen because of contraindications to a beta-blocker, although there is no good evidence for long term benefit in terms of major cardiovascular outcomes. If large doses of beta-blocker or calcium antagonists, or combined therapy were required for control of the ischemic episodes, judicious decrements of intensity are likely appropriate once the patient is fully mobilized and non-invasive testing has indicated that revascularization is not obligatory.

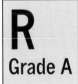

The evidence from the initial trials of aspirin for UA[82,83] demonstrated ongoing benefit for up to 2 years, consistent with evidence in survivors of MI and patients with stable angina.[78] Accordingly aspirin should be continued indefinitely. Ticlopidine should be reserved for patients intolerant of aspirin,[85] and consideration should be given to clopidogrel when it becomes available.[86] Heparin should be sustained for at least 48 hours following the resolution of acute ischemic episodes.[95] Ongoing therapy with low molecular weight heparin may improve ischemic outcomes, although the currently available data are not entirely clear.[96,109,111-113] Maintenance of GPII6/IIIa receptor inhibition with oral agents may eventually be indicated, although only preliminary data are available. Early attention to optimal management of coronary risk factors is prudent and vigorous long term management is likely to be advantageous (see Chapters 13, 14, 23 and 31).

Overall management – practical summary

Unstable angina encompasses a spectrum of symptomatic manifestations of ischemic heart disease, intermediate between stable angina and acute MI. The clinical picture is generally characterized by angina which is relatively severe, and of new onset, progressive severity, or occurring at rest. Variant angina, and angina in the early post-infarction period are included in the syndrome. The clinical diagnosis is based upon the presence of an unstable ischemic pain pattern, and accompanying evidence of coronary artery disease. The initial goals of therapy are to relieve pain, anxiety, and ischemia, and to decrease the substantial risk of MI and sudden death. The pace of initial evaluation and the intensity of treatment are influenced by the immediate prognosis, as determined by the likelihood of the presence of coronary artery disease, the severity of the ischemia, and the underlying medical status of the patient. The patient must be carefully assessed, but the management setting may vary from outpatient follow-up to hemodynamic monitoring in an intensive coronary care unit.

Correction of the imbalance of myocardial oxygen supply and demand is undertaken with reduced activities or bedrest, nitrates, and beta-blockers. Calcium antagonists are reserved for patients with contraindications to beta-blockers, or when beta-blocker therapy has failed to prevent recurrent or persistent ischemic episodes. Grade A If the patient is not already taking aspirin, a dose should immediately be chewed and swallowed. Grade A

Once it is clear that hospitalization is required, the patient should commence intravenous heparin, which should be sustained for at least 48 hours after the resolution of the unstable ischemic pattern. Low molecular weight heparin may prove to be more effective than heparin, and the addition of one of a variety of platelet glycoprotein IIB/IIIA inhibitors to heparin appears to reduce the incidence of important clinical outcomes. Grade B

411

Patients who fail to respond to medical therapy generally should undergo coronary angiography with a view to revascularization by angioplasty or surgical revascularization if possible. ⌊Grade A⌋ Those patients whose ischemic episodes are controlled medically may be managed using one of two general strategies. Coronary angiography may be undertaken to clearly define coronary anatomy and left ventricular function, followed by revascularization or ongoing medical therapy as appropriate. Alternatively, particularly when coronary angiographic and revascularization facilities are not readily available, medically controlled patients may be well managed by predischarge, or early postdischarge non-invasive evaluation for the presence of significant residual ischemia, reserving coronary angiography and potential revascularization for those who have evidence of important residual ischemia, or who have recurrences of unstable angina. Vigorous ongoing therapy with antianginal agents, aspirin, and optimal risk factor management is indicated.

REFERENCES

1 Cairns JA, Fantus IG, Klassen GA. Unstable angina pectoris. *Am Heart J* 1976;**92**:373–86.

2 Theroux P. Unstable angina: pathogenesis, diagnosis, and treatment. *Curr Probl Cardiol* 1993;March:163–231.

3 Braunwald E, Mark DB, Jones RH *et al. Unstable angina: diagnosis and management.* Clinical Practice Guideline, no. 10 (Agency for Health Care Policy and Research Publications No. 94–6–2). Rockville: US Department of Health and Human Services, 1994.

4 Sampson JJ, Eliaser M. The diagnosis of impending acute coronary occlusion. *Am Heart J* 1937;**13**:676–86.

5 Feil H. Preliminary pain in coronary thrombosis. *Am J Med Sci* 1937;**193**:42–48.

6 Fowler NO. "Preinfarctional" angina: a need for an objective definition and for a controlled clinical trial of its management. *Circulation* 1971;**44**:755–8.

7 Mark DB, Califf RM, Morris K *et al.* Clinical characteristics and long-term survival of patients with variant angina. *Circulation* 1984;**69**:880–8.

8 Bosch X, Theroux P, Waters DD *et al.* Early post infarction ischemia. Clinical, angiographic and prognostic significance. *Circulation* 1987;**75**:988–95.

9 Rizak DG, Healy S, Margulis A *et al.* A new clinical classification for hospital prognosis of unstable angina pectoris. *Am J Cardiol* 1995;**75**:993–7.

10 Braunwald E. Unstable angina. A classification. *Circulation* 1989;**80**:410–14.

11 Calvin JE, Klein LW, VanderBerg BJ *et al.* Risk stratification in unstable angina. Prospective validation of the Braunwald classification. *JAMA* 1995;**273**:136–41.

12 Van Miltenberg-vanZiji AJM, Simoons ML, Veerhoek RJ, Bossuyt PMM. Incidence and follow-up of Braunwald subgroups in unstable angina pectoris. *J Am Coll Cardiol* 1995;**25**:1286–92.

13 Hamm CW, Ravkilde J, Gerhardt W *et al.* The prognostic value of serum troponin T in unstable angina. *N Engl J Med* 1992;**327**:146–50.

14 Adams JE III, Bodor GS, Davila-Roman VG *et al.* Cardiac toponin I: a marker with high specificity for cardiac injury. *Circulation* 1993;**88**:101–16.

15 The TIMI-3B Investigators. Effects of tissue plasminogen activator and a comparison of early invasive and conservative strategies in unstable angina and non-Q wave myocardial infarction. Results of TIMI-3B trial. *Circulation* 1994;**89**:1545–56.

16 Larsson H, Jonasson T, Ringqvist I *et al.* Diagnostic and prognostic importance of ST recording after an episode of unstable angina or non-Q wave myocardial infarction. *Eur Heart J* 1992;**13**:207–12.

17 Pozen MW, D'Agostino RB, Selker HP *et al.* A predictive instrument to improve coronary-care-unit admission practices in acute ischemic heart disease. A prospective multicentre trial. *N Engl J Med* 1984;**310**:1273–8.

18 Langer A, Freeman MR, Armstrong PW. ST segment shift in unstable angina: pathophysiology and association with coronary anatomy and hospital outcome. *J Am Coll Cardiol* 1989;**13**:1495–502.

19 The TIMI-3A Investigators. Early effects of tissue-type plasminogen activator added to conventional therapy on the culprit coronary lesion in patients with ischemic cardiac pain at rest. Results of the Thrombolysis in Myocardial

Ischemia (TIMI-3A) Trial. *Circulation* 1993;**87**: 38–52.

20 Graves EJ. Detailed diagnosis and procedures. National Hospital Discharge Survey, 1992. National Center for Health Statistics. *Vital Health Statistics* 1994;ser. 13;no. 118.

21 National Center for Health Statistics, Collins JG. Prevalence of selected chronic conditions, United States, 1986–88. *Vital and Health Statistics* 1993; series 10,**182**:1–87.

22 National Center for Health Statistics, Kozak LJ, Moien M. Detailed diagnosis and surgical procedures for patients discharged from short-stay hospitals, United States, 1983. *Vital and Health Statistics* 1985;ser. 12;no. 82.

23 Cupples LA, D'Agostino RB. Survival following initial cardiovascular events: 30-year follow-up Framingham Heart Study, section 35. In: Kannel WB, Wolf PA, Garrison RJ, eds. *The Framingham Study: an epidemiological investigation of cardiovascular disease* (NIH pub. no. 88–2969). Bethesda: National Heart, Lung and Blood Institute, 1988.

24 Cairns J, Singer J, Gent M *et al*. One year mortality outcomes of all coronary and intensive care units with acute myocardial infarction, unstable angina or other chest pain in Hamilton, Canada, a city of 375 000 people. *Can J Cardiol* 1989;**5**: 239–46.

25 The RISC Group. Risk of myocardial infarction and death during treatment with low-dose aspirin and intravenous heparin in men with unstable coronary artery disease. *Lancet* 1990; **226**:827–30.

26 Theroux P, Waters D, Qiu S *et al*. Aspirin versus heparin to prevent myocardial infarction during the acute phase of unstable angina. *Circulation* 1993;**88**:2045–8.

27 Rafflenbeul W, Russel RO, Lichtlen PR. Angiographic anatomy of coronary arteries in unstable angina pectoris. In: Rafflenbeul W, Lichtlen PR, Balcon R, eds. *Unstable angina pectoris*. New York: Thieme-Stratton Inc, 1981, pp 51–7.

28 Maseri A, L'Abbate A, Baroldi G *et al*. Coronary vasospasm as a possible cause of myocardial infarction: conclusion derived from the study of "preinfarction" angina. *N Engl J Med* 1978;**299**: 1271–7.

29 Moise A, Theroux P, Taeymans Y *et al*. Unstable angina and progression of coronary atherosclerosis. *N Engl J Med* 1983;**309**:685–9.

30 Lesperance J, Theroux P, Liudon G, Waters D. A new look at coronary angiograms: plaque morphology as a help to diagnosis and to evaluate outcome. *Int J Cardiac Imaging* 1994; **10**:75–94.

31 Falk E. Unstable angina with fatal outcome: dynamic coronary thrombosis leading to infarction and/or sudden death: autopsy evidence of recurrent mural thrombosis with peripheral embolization culminating in total coronary occlusion. *Circulation* 1985;**71**: 699–708.

32 Davies MJ, Thomas A. Thrombosis and acute coronary artery lesions in sudden cardiac ischemic death. *N Engl J Med* 1984;**310**: 1137–40.

33 Fuster V, Badimon L, Badimon JJ *et al*. The pathogenesis of coronary artery disease and the acute coronary syndromes. *N Engl J Med* 1992; **326**:242–50.

34 Moreno PR, Falk E, Palacios IF *et al*. Macrophagics infiltration in acute coronary syndromes: implications for plaque rupture. *Circulation* 1994;**90**:775–8.

35 Kovanen PT, Kaartinen M, Paavonen T. Infiltrates of activated mast cells at the site of coronary atheromatous erosion or rupture in myocardial infarction. *Circulation* 1995;**92**: 1084–8.

36 Ross R. The pathgenesis of atherosclerosis: a perspective for the 1990s. *Nature* 1993;**362**: 801–9.

37 Gupta S, Leatham EW, Carrington D *et al*. Elevated *Chlamydia pneumoniae* antibodies, cardiovascular events, and azithromycine in male survivors of myocardial infarction. *Circulation* 1997;**96**:404–7.

38 Lefkovits J, Plow EF, Topol EJ. Platelet glycoprotein IIb/IIIa receptors in cardiovascular medicine. *N Engl J Med* 1995;**332**:1553–9.

39 Coller BS. Blockade of platelet GPIIb/IIIa receptors as an antithrombotic strategy. *Circulation* 1995;**92**:2372–80.

40 Ardissimo D, Merlin PA, Ariens R *et al*. Tissue-factor antigen and activity in human coronary atherosclerotic plaques. *Lancet* 1997;**349**: 769–71.

41 Ott I, Neumann FJ, Gawaz M, Schmitt M, Schomig A. Increased neutrophil-platelet adhesion in patients with unstable angina. *Circulation* 1996;**94**:1239–46.

42 Chaitman BR, Bourassa MG, David K *et al*. Angiographic prevalence of high-risk coronary artery disease in patient subgroups (CASS). *Circulation* 1981;**64**:360–7.

43 Pryor DB, Shaw L, McCants CB *et al*. Value of the history and physical in identifying patients at increase risk for coronary artery disease. *Ann Intern Med* 1993;**118**:81–90.

44 Ronan GW, Lee TH, Cook EF *et al*. Clinical characteristics and outcome of acute myocardial infarction in patients with initially normal or nonspecific electrocardiograms (a report from the Multicenter Chest Pain Study). *Am J Cardiol* 1989;**64**:1087–92.

413

45 Bosch X, Theroux P *et al.* Clinical and angiographic features and prognostic significance of early post infarction angina with and without electrocardiographic ECG signs of transient ischemia. *Am J Med* 1991;**91**: 493–501.

46 Califf RM, Mark DB, Harell EF *et al.* Importance of clinical measures of ischemia in the prognosis of patients with documented coronary artery disease. *J Am Coll Cardiol* 1988;**11**:20–6.

47 White LD, Lee TH, Cook EF *et al.* Comparison of the natural history of new onset and exacerbated chronic ischemic heart disease. The Chest Pain Study Group. *J Am Coll Cardiol* 1990;**16**:304–10.

48 Gottlieb SO, Weisfeldt MD, Oryang P *et al.* Silent ischemia as a marker of early unfavorable outcomes in patients with unstable angina. *N Engl J Med* 1986;**314**:1214–19.

49 Bugiardina R, Boughi A, Pozzati A *et al.* Relation of severity of symptoms to transient myocardial ischemia and prognosis in unstable angina. *J Am Coll Cardiol* 1995;**25**:597–604.

50 Nadamanee K, Intarachat V, Josephson MA *et al.* Prognostic significance of silent myocardial ischemia in patients with unstable angina. *J Am Coll Cardiol* 1987;**10**:1.

51 Orlander R. Use of nitrates in the treatment of unstable and variant angina. *Drugs* 1987;**33**: 131–9.

52 Gobel EJAM, Hautvast RWH, van Gilst WH *et al.* Randomized, double-blind trial of intravenous diltiazem versus glyceral tinitrate for unstable angina pectoris. *Lancet* 1995;**346**:1653–7.

53 Jugdutt Bl, Warnica JW. Intravenous nitroglycerin therapy to limit myocardial infarction size, expansions and complications. Effective timing, dosage and infarct location. *Circulation* 1988;**78**:906–20.

54 ISIS-4 A randomized factorial trial assessing early oral captopril, oral mononitrate, and intravenous magnesium sulphate in 58,050 patients with suspected myocardial infarction. *Lancet* 1995;**345**:669–85.

55 Gruppo Italiano per lo Studio della Sopravvivenze nell'Infarto Miocardico. GISSI-3: effects of lisinopril and transdermal glyceryl trinitrate single and together on 6-week mortality and ventricular function after acute myocardial infarction. *Lancet* 1994;**343**: 1115–22.

56 Muller JE, Turi ZG, Pearle DL *et al.* Nifedipine and conventional therapy for unstable angina pectoris: a randomized, double-blind comparison. *Circulation* 1984;**69**:728–39.

57 Holland Interuniversity Nifedipine/Metropolol Trial (HINT) Research Group. Early treatment of unstable angina in the coronary care unit: a randomized, double-blind, placebo controlled comparison of recurrent ischemia in patients treated with nifedipine or metropolol or both. *Br Heart J* 1986;**73**:331–7.

58 Gottlieb SO, Weisfeldt M, Ouyang P *et al.* Effect of the addition of propranolol to therapy with nifedipine for unstable angina pectoris. A randomized, double-blind, placebo-controlled trial. *Circulation* 1986;**73**:331–7.

59 Gerstenblith G, Ouyang P, Achuff SC *et al.* Nifedipine in unstable angina: a double-blind, randomized trial. *N Engl J Med* 1982;**306**:885–9.

60 Furberg CD, Psaty BM, Meye JV. Nifedipine. Dose-related increase in mortality in patients with coronary heart disease. *Circulation* 1995;**92**: 1326–31.

61 Théroux P, Taeymans Y, Morrissette D *et al.* A randomized study comparing propranolol and diltiazem in the treatment of unstable angina. *J Am Coll Cardiol* 1985;**5**:717–22.

62 Andre-Fouet X, Usdin JP, Gayet CH *et al.* Comparison of short-term efficacy of diltiazem and propranolol in unstable angina at rest. A randomized trial in 70 patients. *Eur Heart J* 1983;**4**:691–8.

63 Parodi O, Maseri A, Simonetti I. Management of unstable angina by verapamil. A double-blind crossover study in CCU. *Br Heart J* 1979;**41**: 167–74.

64 Mehta J, Pepine CJ, Day M, Guerrero JR, Conti CR. Short-term efficacy of oral verapamil in rest angina. A double-blind controlled trial in CCU patients. *Am J Med* 1981;**71**:977–82.

65 Scheidt S, Frishman WH, Packer M, Parodi O, Subramanian VB. Long-term effectiveness of verapamil in stable and unstable angina pectoris. One-year follow-up of patients treated in placebo-controlled double-blind randomized clinical trials. *Am J Cardiol* 1982;**50**:1185–90.

66 Yusuf S, Wittes J, Friedman L. Overview of results of randomized clinical trials in heart disease. II. Unstable angina, heart failure, primary prevention with aspirin, and risk factor modification. *JAMA* 1988;**260**:2259–63.

67 Held PH, Yusuf S, Furberg C. Calcium channel blockers in acute myocardial infarction and unstable angina: an overview. *Br Med J* 1989; **299**:1187–92.

68 Johnson SM, Mauritson DR, Willerson JT, Hillis LD. A controlled trial of verapamil for Prinzmetal's variant angina. *N Engl J Med* 1981; **304**:69–72.

69 Capucci A, Bracchetti D, Carini GC *et al.* Propranolol versus verapamil in patients with unstable angina. In: Zanchetti A, Krikler DM, eds. *Calcium antagonism in cardiovascular therapy. Experience with verapamil.* Amsterdam: Excerpta Medica, 1981, pp 69–72.

70 Parodi O, Simoneti I, Michelassi C *et al.* Comparison of verapamil and propranolol

therapy for angina pectoris at rest. A randomized, multiple-crossover, controlled trial in the coronary care unit. *Am J Cardiol* 1986; **57**:899–906.

71 Rosenthal SJ, Ginsburg R, Lamb IH, Baim DS, Schroeder JS. Efficacy of diltiazem for control of symptoms of coronary artery spasm. *Am J Cardiol* 1980;**46**:1027–32.

72 Pepine CJ, Feldman RL, Whittle J, Curry RC, Conti GR. Effect of diltiazem in patients with variant angina. A randomized double-blind trial. *Am Heart J* 1981;**101**:719–25.

73 Schroeder JS, Feldman RL, Giles TD *et al.* Multiclinic controlled trial of diltiazem for Prinzmetal's variant angina. *Am J Med* 1982; **72**:227–32.

74 Tilmant PY, LaBlanche JM, Thieuleux FA, Dupuis BA, Betrand ME. Detrimental effect of propranolol in patients with coronary arterial spasm countered by combination with diltiazem. *Am J Cardiol* 1983;**52**:230–3.

75 Previtali M, Salerno J, Tavazzi L *et al.* Treatment of angina at rest with nifedipine: a short-term controlled study. *Am J Cardiol* 1980;**45**:825–30.

76 Ginsburg R, Lab IH, Schroeder JS, Hu M, Harrison DC. Randomized double-blind comparison of nifedipine and isosorbide dinitrate therapy in variant angina pectoris due to coronary artery spasm. *Am Heart J* 1982;**103**: 44–8.

77 Hill JA, Feldman RI, Pepine CJ, Conti CR. Randomized double-blind comparison of nifedipine and isosorbide dinitrate in patients with coronary arterial spasm. *Am J Cardiol* 1982; **49**:431–8.

78 Antiplatelet Trialists' Collaboration. Collaborative overview of randomized trials of antiplatelet therapy – 1: Prevention of death, myocardial infarction, and stroke by prolonged antiplatelet therapy in various categories of patients. *Br Med J* 1994;**308**:81–106.

79 Oler A, Whooley MA, Oler J, Grady D. Adding heparin to aspirin reduces the incidence of myocardial and death in patients with unstable angina. *JAMA* 1996;**276**:811–15.

80 Coughlin SR, Vu TKH, Hung DT, Wheaton VI. Characterization of a functional thrombin receptor. *J Clin Invest* 1991;**89**:351–5.

81 Weitz JI, Huboch M, Massel D *et al.* Clot-bound thrombin is protected from inhibition by heparin-antithrombin III but is susceptible to inactivation by antithrombin III independent inhibitors. *J Clin Invest* 1990;**86**:385.

82 Lewis HD, Davis JW, Archibald DG *et al.* Protective effects of aspirin against myocardial infarction and death in men with unstable angina. *N Engl J Med* 1983;**313**:396–403.

83 Cairns JA, Gent M, Singer J *et al.* Aspirin, sulfinpyrazone, or both in unstable angina. *N Engl J Med* 1985;**313**:1369–75.

84 Theroux P, Latour JG, Diodati J *et al.* Hemodynamic, platelet, and clinical response to prostacycline in unstable angina pectoris. *Am J Cardiol* 1990;**65**:1084–9.

85 Balsano F, Rizzon P, Violi F *et al.* Antiplatlet treatment with ticlopidine in unstable angina. *Circulation* 1990;**82**:17–26.

86 CAPRIE Steering Committee. A randomized, blinded, trial of clopidogrel versus aspirin in patients at risk of ischaemic events. *Lancet* 1996; **348**:1329–39.

87 EPIC Investigators. Use of a monoclonal antibody directed against the platelet glycoprotein IIb/IIIa receptor in high-risk coronary angioplasty. *N Engl J Med* 1997;**336**:1689–96.

88 Platelet glycoprotein IIb/IIIa receptor blockade and low-dose heparin during percutaneous coronary revascularization. The EPILOG Investigators. *N Engl J Med* 1997;**336**:1689–96.

89 The CAPTURE Investigators. Randomized placebo-controlled trial of abciximab before and during coronary intervention in refractory unstable angina: the CAPTURE trial. *Lancet* 1997;**349**:1429–35.

90 Theroux P, Kouz S, Roy L *et al.* Platelet membrane receptor glycoprotein IIb/IIIa antagonism in unstable angina. The Canadian Lamifiban Study. *Circulation* 1996;**94**:899–905.

91 PARAGON. Results presented at the European Congress of Cardiology, Stockholm, Sweden, August 1997.

92 The Platelet Receptor Inhibition for Ischemic Syndrome Management in Patients Limited by Unstable Signs and Symptoms (PRISM) Trial. Results presented at the American College of Cardiology meeting, Anaheim, CA, March 1997.

93 The Platelet Receptor Inhibition for Ischemic Syndrome Management in Patients Limited by Unstable Signs and Symptoms (PRISM-PLUS) Trial. Results presented at the American College of Cardiology meeting, Anaheim, CA, March 1997.

94 The Platelet IIb/IIIa in Unstable Angina: Receptor Suppression Using Integrilin™ (PURSUIT) trial. Results presented at the European Congress of Cardiology, Stockholm, Sweden, August 1997.

95 Theroux P, Waters D, Lam J, Juneau M, McCans J. Reactivation of unstable angina after the discontinuation of heparin. *N Engl J Med* 1992; **327**:141–15.

96 The FRISC Study Group. Low-molecular-weight heparin during instability in coronary artery disease. *Lancet* 1996;**347**:561–8.

97 Organization to Assess Strategies for Ischemic Syndromes (OASIS) Investigators. Comparison

of the effects of two doses of recombinant hirudin compared with heparin in patients acute myocardial ischemia without ST segment elevation. *Circulation* 1997;**96**:769–77.

98 Telford AM, Wilson C. Trial of heparin versus atenolol in prevention of myocardial infarction in intermediate coronary syndrome. *Lancet* 1981;i:1225–8.

99 Williams DO, Kirby MG, McPherson K, Phear DM. Anticoagulant treatment in unstable angina. *Br J Clin Pract* 1986;**40**:114–6.

100 Theroux P, Waters D, Qiu S *et al*. Aspirin versus heparin to prevent myocardial infarction during the acute phase of unstable angina. *Circulation* 1993;**88**:2045–8.

101 Holdright D, Patel D, Cunningham D *et al*. Comparison of the effect of heparin and aspirin versus aspirin alone on transient myocardial ischemia and in-hospital prognosis in patients with unstable angina. *J Am Coll Cardiol* 1994; **24**:39–45.

102 Neri Serneri GG, Gensini GR, Poggesi L *et al*. Effect of heparin, aspirin or alteplase in reduction of myocardial ischemia in refractory unstable angina. *Lancet* 1990;**335**:615–18.

103 Williams MJA, Morson IM, Parker JH, Stewart RAH. Progression of the culprit lesion in unstable coronary artery disease with warfarin and aspirin versus aspirin alone: preliminary study. *J Am Coll Cardiol* 1997;**30**:364–9.

104 Cohen M, Adams PC, Parry G *et al*. and the Antithrombotic Theraphy in Acute Coronary Syndromes Research Group. Combination antithrombotic therapy in unstable rest angina and non-Q-wave infarction in nonprior aspirin users. *Circulation* 1994;**89**:81–8.

105 Oler A, Whooley MA, Oler J, Grady D. Adding heparin to aspirin reduces the incidence of myocardial infarction and death in patients with unstable angina. *JAMA* 1996;**276**:811–15.

106 The Global Use of Strategies to Open Occluded Coronary Arteries (GUSTO) IIb Investigators. A comparison of recombinant hirudin with heparin for the treatment of acute coronary syndromes. *N Engl J Med* 1996;**335**:775–82.

107 The Global Use of Strategies to Open Occluded Coronary Arteries (GUSTO) IIa Investigators. Randomized trial of intravenous heparin versus recombinant hirudin for acute coronary syndromes. *Circulation* 1994;**90**:1631–37.

108 Antman EM for the TIMI-9A Investigators. Hirudin in acute myocardial infarction. Safety report from the Thrombolysis and Thrombin Inhibition in Myocardial Infarction (TIMI) 9A trial. *Circulation* 1994;**90**:1624–30.

109 Results presented at the European Congress of Cardiology, Birmingham, UK, August 1996.

110 Hirsch J, Levine MN. Low molecular weight heparins. *Blood* 1992;**79**:1–17.

111 Gurfinkel EP, Manos E, Mejail RI *et al*. Low molecular weight heparin versus regular heparin or aspirin in the treatment of unstable angina and silent ischemia. *J Am Coll Cardiol* 1995;**26**:313–18.

112 Klein W, Buchwald A, Hillis SE *et al*. Comparison of low-molecular-weight heparin with unfractionated heparin acutely and with placebo for 6 weeks in the management of unstable coronary artery desease. *Circulation* 1997;**96**: 61–8.

113 Cohen M, Demers C, Gurfinkel EP *et al*. Low molecular weight heparin versus unfractionated heparin for unstable angina and non-Q-wave myocardial infarction. *N Engl J Med* 1997;**337**: 447–52.

114 Betriu A, Heras M, Cohen M, Fuster Y. Unstable angina outcome according to clinical presentation. *Am J Cardiol* 1992;**19**:1659–63.

115 Aroesty JM, Weintraub RM, Paulin S, O'Grady GP. Medically refractory unstable angina pectoris II. Hemodynamic and angiographic effects of intraaortic balloon counterpulsations. *Am J Cardiol* 1979;**43**:883–8.

116 Cody RJ. Results from late breaking clinical trials sessions at ACC 1997. *J Am Coll Cardiol* 1997; **30**:1–7.

117 Larsson H, Areskog M, Areskog NH *et al*. Should the exercise test (ET) be performed at discharge or one month later after an episode of unstable angina or non-Q-wave myocardial infarction? *Int J Card Imaging* 1991;**7**:7–14.

118 Moss AJ, Goldstein RE, Hall WJ *et al*. Detection and significance of myocardial ischemia in stable patients after recovery from an acute coronary event. Multicentre Myocardial Ischemic Research Group. *JAMA* 1993;**269**:2379–85.

119 Amanallah A, Bevegard S, Lindvall K *et al*. Early exercise thallium-201 single photon emission computed tomography in unstable angina: a prospective study. *Clin Physiol* 1992;**12**:607–17.

120 Marmur JD, Freeman MR, Langer A *et al*. Prognostic in medically stabilized unstable angina: Holter ST-segment monitoring compared with predischarge exercise thallium tomography. *Ann Intern Med* 1990;**113**:575–9.

121 Younis LT, Byers S, Shaw L *et al*. Prognostic value of intravenous dipyridamole thallium scintigraphy after an acute myocardial ischemic event. *Am J Cardiol* 1989;**64**:161–6.

122 Yusuf S, Peto R, Lewis J, Collins R, Sleight P. Beta blockade during and after myocardial infarction: an overview of the randomized trials. *Progr Cardiovasc Dis* 1985;**27**:335–71.

Part III
Specific cardiovascular disorders
iii: Acute myocardial infarction

JOHN A CAIRNS and BERNARD J GERSH

Grading of recommendations and levels of evidence used in *Evidence Based Cardiology*

GRADE A

Level 1a   Evidence from large randomized clinical trials (RCTs) or systematic reviews (including meta-analyses) of multiple randomized trials which collectively has at least as much data as one single well-defined trial.

Level 1b   Evidence from at least one "All or None" high quality cohort study; in which ALL patients died/failed with conventional therapy and some survived/succeeded with the new therapy (eg chemotherapy for tuberculosis, meningitis, or defibrillation for ventricular fibrillation); or in which many died/failed with conventional therapy and NONE died/failed with the new therapy (eg penicillin for pneumococcal infections).

Level 1c   Evidence from at least one moderate sized RCT or a meta-analysis of small trials which collectively only has a moderate number of patients.

Level 1d   Evidence from at least one RCT.

GRADE B

Level 2   Evidence from at least one high quality study of non-randomized cohorts who did and did not receive the new therapy.

Level 3   Evidence from at least one high quality case control study.

Level 4   Evidence from at least one high quality case series.

GRADE C

Level 5   Opinions from experts without reference or access to any of the foregoing (eg argument from physiology, bench research or first principles).

A comprehensive approach would incorporate many different types of evidence (eg RCTs, non-RCTs, epidemiologic studies, and experimental data), and examine the architecture of the information for consistency, coherence and clarity. Occasionally the evidence does not completely fit into neat compartments. For example, there may not be an RCT that demonstrates a reduction in mortality in individuals with stable angina with the use of beta-blockers, but there is overwhelming evidence that mortality is reduced following MI. In such cases, some may recommend use of beta-blockers in angina patients with the expectation that some extrapolation from post-MI trials is warranted. This could be expressed as Grade A/C. In other instances (e.g. smoking cessation or a pacemaker for complete heart block), the non-randomized data are so overwhelmingly clear and biologically plausible that it would be reasonable to consider these interventions as Grade A.

Recommendation grades appear either in a shaded margin box with an 'R' logo as shown, or within the text, for example Grade A .

Thrombolytic therapy

26

SANJEEV TREHAN
JEFFREY L. ANDERSON

IMPACT, PATHOPHYSIOLOGY, AND RATIONALE

Acute myocardial infarction (AMI) affects 900 000 individuals each year in the United States; 25% succumb. Over half of deaths occur outside of the medical care setting.[1] The impact of AMI is also large in Europe: the MONICA registry has reported 28-day mortality of 13–27%.[2] However, basic and clinical research efforts into AMI pathophysiology and therapy has been intense over the past 20 years, and impact on outcomes is growing.[3]

Herrick postulated 85 years ago that thrombosis-related coronary occlusion was a precipitating event in AMI.[4] However, not until 1980 did DeWood *et al.*[5] demonstrate this angiographically: complete occlusion was found in 87% of patients studied within 4 hours of symptom onset; its thrombotic nature was shown at emergent bypass surgery. A renewed focus on obstructing thrombosis and thrombolysis ensued.

The natural evolution of lipid laden atherosclerotic plaques may include plaque erosion or sudden rupture of an endothelial cap weakened by internal metalloproteinase activity.[6] Exposure to the blood stream of matrix elements, including collagen, and the intensely thrombogenic lipid core with its associated macrophage-derived tissue factor, stimulates platelet adhesion, activation, and aggregation; thrombin generation; and fibrin formation, causing vasospasm and formation of a platelet-rich clot. When these processes lead to reduction or interruption of coronary blood flow, myocardial cell death may occur.

In a canine model of coronary thrombotic occlusion and reperfusion, Reimer *et al.*[7,8] found that myocardial cell death began within 15 minutes of occlusion and proceeded rapidly in a wavefront from endocardium to epicardium. The extent of necrosis was modified by metabolic demands and collateral blood supply. Myocardial salvage could be achieved within a narrow time frame (≤ 3 hours) by releasing the occlusion. Salvage occurred in a reverse wavefront, from epicardium inwards. The time to restoration of coronary flow was the most important determinant of final infarct size; the presence of extensive collateral vessels also had a favorable impact. Myocardial salvage also has been demonstrated using positron emission tomography in experiments of streptokinase-induced reperfusion of thrombotic occlusion.[9]

EARLY OBSERVATIONAL AND CONTROLLED STUDIES

In 1933, Tillet and Garner reported their discovery of a streptococcal fibrinolysin.[10] Application of streptokinase to AMI was first reported in 1958:[11] intravenous streptokinase infusions could be given safely and treatment within 14 hours after symptom onset led to a more favorable hospital course than later treatment (at 20–72 hours), which was similar to no treatment. Between 1958 and 1979, at least 17 studies of IV streptokinase were published, but AMI pathophysiology was not well understood, study designs were poor, treatment was often delayed, and results were inconclusive and poorly accepted.[12-15] Foremost among these early studies was the 1979 European Corporative Study Group which reported in 1979:[12] 315 AMI patients were randomized to receive a 24-hour infusion of streptokinase (SK) or placebo. Six-month mortality was lower after SK (15.6% vs 30.6%, $P<0.01$). Bleeding was more frequent with SK but mostly minor.

With the establishment of the thrombotic nature of coronary occlusion,[5] Chazov,[16] Rentrop,[17,18] Ganz,[19] and several others[14,15] demonstrated the feasibility of clinical thrombolysis with intracoronary (IC) SK under angiographic monitoring in the period 1976–83. These mostly observational studies confirmed a high rate of coronary occlusion (>80%) during the early hours of AMI and the ability of IC SK to achieve early reperfusion ($\approx 75\%$ success).[15] It remained for randomized studies to clearly demonstrate efficacy and safety.

Anderson et al.[20] first reported a beneficial outcome after IC SK based on a randomized trial in 1983. Fifty patients were assigned to either IC SK or standard therapy after 2.7 hours of symptoms; SK was begun at an average of 4 hours, and reperfusion was achieved in 79% receiving SK an average of 30 minutes later. IC SK alleviated ischemic discomfort, prevented progression of heart failure, and led to improved functional (ejection fraction) recovery by hospital discharge; cardiac enzymes peaked earlier, ST segment elevations resolved more rapidly, and fewer Q waves developed than with standard (non-thrombolytic) coronary care. The results of echocardiographic wall motion and convalescent thallium perfusion studies also favored the SK group. A smaller concurrent randomized study treated patients later (at >6 hours) and showed relief of ischemic pain but found no improvement in global or regional myocardial function.[21]

Shortly thereafter, Kennedy et al.[22] reported on a survival benefit of IC SK in a larger randomized trial of 250 patients. Reperfusion was achieved in 69% of SK-treated patients vs 12% of controls. Thirty-day mortality was 3.7% in SK vs 11.2% in control patients ($P<0.02$). One-year mortality also was improved but only in the SK subgroup achieving complete reperfusion.[23] Additional evidence for survival benefit came from a Dutch study of 533 patients:[24] survival at one month (5.9% vs 11.7%) and at one year (8.6% vs 15.9%, $P<0.001$) were improved although interpretation was confounded by the initial use of intravenous (IV) SK in the last 117 patients. These favorable results were counterbalanced by variable results in other studies. Indeed, a meta-analysis of nine randomized trials of IC SK,[25] involving ≈ 1000 patients, found an 18% average mortality reduction but with wide confidence intervals (44% reduction to 19% increase, $P=NS$). The logistic difficulties and time delays inherent with IC SK administration and the less favorable results in broader clinical testing stimulated the re-evaluation of IV SK.

Schröder et al.[26] reawakened interest in IV SK with a report in 1983 of the feasibility of achieving early patency (in $\approx 60\%$) and favorable clinical outcomes with short-term (1 hour) infusions of SK in doses of 0.5 to 1.5 million units. Several small randomized

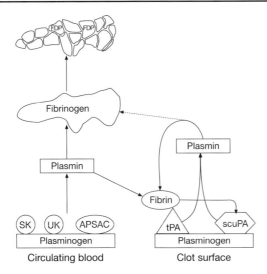

Figure 26.1 Schematic representation of the action of fibrinolytic enzymes. Streptokinase (SK), urokinase (UK), and anisoylated plasminogen streptokinase activator complex (APSAC) work predominantly on circulating plasminogen, whereas tissue type plasminogen activator (tPA) and single chain urokinase-type plasminogen activator (scuPA) are relatively clot-selective. (From Topol EJ: Clinical use of streptokinase and urokinase to treat acute myocardial infarction. *Heart Lung* 1987;**16**:760.)

trials of IC vs IV SK followed.[15,27–30] These demonstrated little difference in coronary patency at 24 hours and no significant difference in clinical outcome by route of SK administration. Bolstered by a favorable report on mortality and morbidity in a larger randomized study (ISAM),[31] intravenous administration became the preferred route for delivering thrombolysis in clinical trials by the mid-1980s. More definitive placebo-controlled and comparative mortality studies were to follow.

STANDARD THROMBOLYTIC AGENTS

General mechanisms of action and pharmacologic properties

Thrombolysis is mediated by plasmin, a non-specific serine protease that causes fibrinolysis by degrading clot-associated fibrin and fibrinogen. The thrombolytic (or "fibrinolytic") agents are all direct or indirect plasminogen activators that convert the proenzyme plasminogen to plasmin by cleaving the arginine 560–valine 561 bond (Figure 26.1). Plasmin degrades several proteins, including fibrin, fibrinogen, prothrombin, and factors V and VII. Fibrinolysis may disrupt a forming thrombus and lead to reperfusion. The thrombolytic agents may differ in several properties, including structure, fibrin-specificity, speed and duration of action, and antigenicity, as summarized in Table 26.1.

Streptokinase

Streptokinase (SK) was the first thrombolytic agent to be discovered and tested. It is a 415 amino acid bacterial protein that shares homology with serine proteases.[32,33] Upon

421

Table 26.1 Comparison of US FDA approved thrombolytic agents

	SK	APSAC	tPA (alteplase)	rPA (reteplase)
Dose	1.5 MU in 30–60 min	30 u in 5 min	100 mg in 90 min[a]	10 U + 10 U, 30 min apart
Circulating half-life (min)	~20	~100	~6	~18
Antigenic	Yes	Yes	No	No
Allergic reactions	Yes	Yes	No	No
Systemic fibrinogen depletion	Severe	Severe	Moderate	Moderate
Intracerebral hemorrhage	~0.4%	~0.6%	~0.7%	~0.8%
Patency (TIMI-2/3) rate, 90 min[b]	~51%	~70%	~84%	~83%
Lives saved per 100 treated	~3[c]	~3[c]	~4[d]	~4
Cost per dose (approx US dollers)	290	1700	2200	2200

[a] Accelerated tPA given as follows: 15 mg bolus, then 0.75 mg/kg over 30 min (maximum, 50 mg), then 0.50 mg/kg over 60 min (maximum 35 mg).
[b] Based on Granger *et al.*[45] and Bode *et al.*[95]
[c] Patients with ST elevation or BBB, treated <6 h.
[d] Based on the finding from the GUSTO trial[75] that tPA saves 1 more additional life per 100 treated than does SK.

injection, SK reacts immediately with plasminogen or plasmin on a 1:1 stoichiometric basis to form an SK–plasminogen or SK–plasmin complex; this activates a catalytic site for the cleavage of plasminogen to plasmin.[15,33] The SK–plasminogen complex can be autocatalytically cleaved to SK–plasmin, retaining its activity. The half-life of the SK complex is about 23 minutes *in vivo*. SK is antigenic and has little fibrin specificity, causing substantial systemic lytic effects in clinical doses.

Urokinase

Urokinase (UK) is a native protein, originally purified from urine, hence its name.[34] (It has subsequently been produced in renal cell cultures.) UK directly converts plasminogen to plasmin and has greater affinity for fibrin bound lys-plasminogen although it also has effects on circulating plasminogen and plasmin. It is non-antigenic and is cleared from the circulation, predominantly by the liver, with a half-life of 16 minutes.[35]

Anistreplase

Anisoylated plasminogen streptokinase activator complex or APSAC, the first "designer" agent, was synthesized by complexing streptokinase with lys-plasminogen and reversibly inactivating it by reacting it with the anisoyl group of a special reversible acylating agent.[36,37] It was tailored to allow rapid delivery, more rapid onset and prolonged duration of action (half-life, 90–105 min), and improved plasma stability and fibrin binding, compared with SK.[37]

Tissue-type plasminogen activator

Alteplase, or tPA, is believed to be the primary physiological (intrinsic) plasminogen activator.[38] The 527 amino acid glycoprotein tPA occurs as a single chain physiologically. It can be proteolytically cleaved to yield a two-subunit form, though both forms activate plasminogen with similar catalytic efficacy and biologic potency.[39] The relatively high fibrin-selectivity of tPA results in greater production of plasmin and fibrinolytic activity in the locale of the thrombus and less systemic plasminemia, fibrinogenolysis, and proteolysis than with SK. Non-antigenic and subject to inhibition by a circulating plasminogen activator inhibitor (PAI), tPA is rapidly cleared from the circulation with a half-life of about 5 minutes.[40]

Reteplase

Reteplase (rPA) is the first clinically available modified (mutant) tissue plasminogen activator.[41] Compared with tPA, rPA is non-glycosylated, smaller, less fibrin-specific (lower, more reversible binding affinity for fibrin), and has an extended half-life (13–16 min). The last feature allows for more convenient, double-bolus administration.

Single chain urokinase-type plasminogen activator (prourokinase)

In the early 1980s, a single chain form of urokinase (scuPA) was isolated from human urine and cell culture media and characterized biochemically as a proenzyme form of the active two chain enzyme (tcuPA). Prourokinase was of interest in part because it appeared to be more fibrin-specific than urokinase. This effect is now believed to be mediated by the preferential conversion of scuPA to active tcuPA at the fibrin surface.[42] The circulating half-life of natural and recombinant scuPA is 4 or 8 minutes respectively, with predominant hepatic clearance.[43]

EFFICACY OF INTRAVENOUS THROMBOLYTIC THERAPY

Effects on coronary artery patency

Because coronary reperfusion is the postulated mechanism of thrombolysis benefit in AMI, many angiographic studies have been undertaken to assess patency profiles of the infarct-related coronary artery after thrombolytic therapy.[44] Granger *et al.* recently summarized 14 124 angiographic observations from 58 studies (Figure 26.2).[45] Because the extent of myocardial salvage is time-dependent, early (60–90 min) patency has generally formed the primary endpoint in these studies. Without thrombolytic therapy, spontaneous perfusion early after ST elevation AMI occurs in only 15% and 21% at 60 and 90 minutes after study entry, respectively, and remains unchanged at 1 day, gradually increasing to about 60% by 3 weeks. All thrombolytic regimens improved early patency rates. At 60 and 90 minutes, streptokinase had the lowest rates (48%, 51%), APSAC and standard (3 hour) tPA infusions intermediate rates (about 60%, 70%), and accelerated (90 minute) tPA infusions the highest patency rates (74%, 84%). However, patency rates at ≥ 3 hours were similar for all regimens, and reocclusion rates were higher after tPA than non-fibrin-specific (systemically active) agents (13%

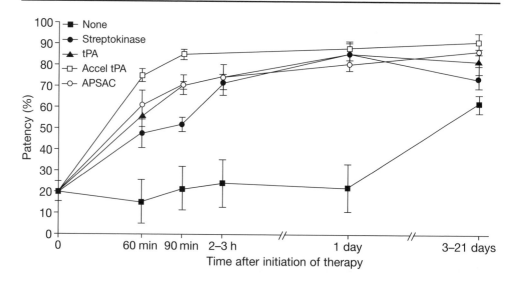

Figure 26.2 Pooled angiographic patency rates with 95% confidence intervals, over time after no thrombolytic agent, streptokinase, conventional dose tPA, accelerated dose tPA, and APSAC from 14 124 angiographic observations. (From Granger CB, White HD, Bates ER, Ohman EM, Califf RM. A pooled analysis of coronary arterial patency and left ventricular function after intravenous thrombolysis for acute myocardial infarction. *Am J Cardiol* 1994;**74**:1220–8.[45])

vs 8%) (*P*=0.002). It remained for the GUSTO angiographic study,[46] embedded within a larger comparative mortality study, to show that early but not late patency rates accurately predict mortality differences among AMI therapies (see below) and to provide direct support for the open artery hypothesis of thrombolytic benefit.

Effects on mortality

RANDOMIZED TRIALS WITH NON-THROMBOLYSIS CONTROLS

By the late 1980s, accumulating clinical trials data provided support for a survival benefit of IV thrombolysis.[47–49] The most important survival trials, comparing thrombolysis to placebo or standard non-thrombolysis care, are summarized in Figure 26.3.

The *Gruppo Italiano per lo Studio della Streptochinasi nell'Infarto Miocardico (GISSI)* study[50] was the first "definitive" mortality trial. Over 17 months, 11 806 AMI patients with ST elevation were randomized to receive 1.5 million units (MU) of IV SK over 1 hour or standard therapy. Aspirin was not routinely given, and coronary angiography, angioplasty, and bypass surgery were rarely used. Inhospital mortality was 10.7% in the SK group and 13.0% in the control group, a 17.6% risk reduction (*P*=0.0002, RR (relative risk)=0.81). A follow-up study showed that survival remained improved at 1–2 years.[51] Benefit was time-dependent and particularly large for treatment within 1 hour of symptom onset in an exploratory analysis (47% mortality reduction, RR 0.49, *P*=0.0001) but was not significant after 6 hours. Subgroup analyses specifically demonstrated benefit in patients with anterior infarction (RR 0.75), with no previous MI (RR 0.75), with Killip class I or II (RR 0.80), and with age <65 years (RR 0.72), although a trend favored improved survival in more elderly patients.

424

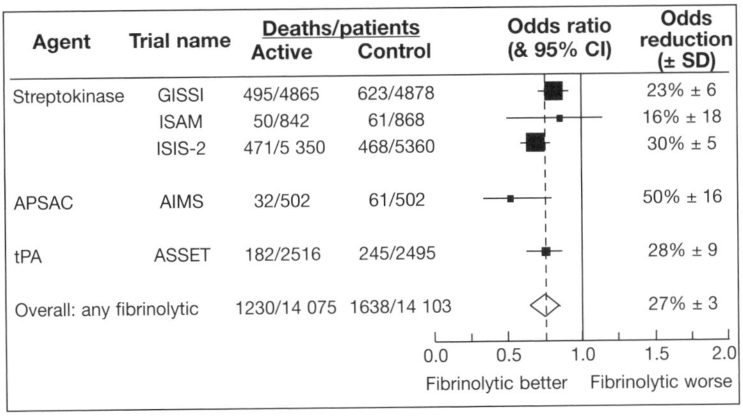

Agent	Trial name	Deaths/patients		Odds ratio (& 95% CI)	Odds reduction (± SD)
		Active	Control		
Streptokinase	GISSI	495/4865	623/4878		23% ± 6
	ISAM	50/842	61/868		16% ± 18
	ISIS-2	471/5 350	468/5360		30% ± 5
APSAC	AIMS	32/502	61/502		50% ± 16
tPA	ASSET	182/2516	245/2495		28% ± 9
Overall: any fibrinolytic		1230/14 075	1638/14 103		27% ± 3

0.0 0.5 1.0 1.5 2.0

Fibrinolytic better   Fibrinolytic worse

Figure 26.3 Reduction in the odds of early death among ST elevation AMI patients treated within 6 hours; overview from five largest randomized control trials of thrombolytic therapy versus placebo. (From Granger CB, Califf RM, Topol EJ. Thrombolytic therapy for acute myocardial infarction. *Drugs* 1992;**44**:293.)

The *Second International Study of Infarct Survival (ISIS-2)*[52] followed. ISIS-2 used a 2×2 factorial design to assess the effects of IV SK (1.5 MU), aspirin (162.5 mg), both, or neither (placebos) in patients with *suspected* AMI within 24 hours of symptom onset. Over 33 months, 17 187 patients were randomized. The 35-day vascular mortality rate was 13.2% for the double placebo group. The odds of dying were reduced by aspirin alone by 23% ($2P < 0.00001$), by SK alone by 25% ($2P < 0.00001$), and additively by the combination: 42% ($2P < 0.00001$). When SK and aspirin were given early (within 4 hours of symptom onset), a 53% reduction in mortality was achieved. Benefits were time-dependent, although less so than in GISSI. ISIS-2 demonstrated lower mortality rates with SK and aspirin in several patient subgroups beyond those shown in GISSI (SK alone), including those presenting with bundle branch block (14.1% vs 27.7%), inferior infarction (6.8% vs 10.2%), and age >60 years (11.5% vs 18.8%). After ISIS-2, aspirin became a routine part of clinical trials and practice regimens.

The *APSAC Intervention Mortality Study (AIMS)*[53,54] was a randomized, double-blind, placebo-controlled trial of APSAC (30 U) in AMI patients under age 70 with ST elevation and symptoms of <6 hours' duration. The trial was stopped early after enrolling 1258 patients because of a large treatment benefit. Aspirin was not used, but intravenous heparin was begun 6 hours after APSAC, and patients were later transferred to warfarin anticoagulation which was given for at least 3 months. APSAC reduced 30-day mortality from 12.2% to 6.4% (odds reduction (OR) 51%, $P = 0.0006$) and 1-year mortality from 17.8% to 11.1% (OR 43%, $P = 0.0007$). Virtually all patient subgroups benefited. The need for adjunctive IV heparin was not addressed by the AIMS design. However, the first Duke University Clinical Cardiology Study (DUCCS-1)[55] randomly assigned AMI patients treated with APSAC to receive IV heparin or no heparin. There were no differences in clinical endpoints other than a higher rate of bleeding in heparin-treated patients.

The *Anglo-Scandinavian Study of Early Thrombolysis (ASSET)*[56] evaluated the effects of tPA (alteplase) with heparin versus heparin alone (aspirin was not given) within a randomized, double-blind, placebo-controlled design. ASSET enrolled 5013 patients within 5 hours of suspected AMI (no ECG criteria were required). Therapies were tPA (100 mg IV over 3 hours) plus heparin (5000 U IV bolus, then 1000 U/h), or placebo

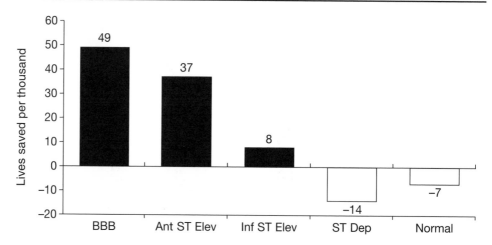

Figure 26.4 The effect of thrombolytic therapy on mortality (lives saved per 1000 treated) in various patient subsets classified according to admission ECG. Patients presenting with bundle branch block and anterior ST segment elevations derived most benefit from thrombolytic therapy. Patients with inferior ST segment elevation derived much less benefit, while those with ST depression or normal ECG did not benefit. (Based on data from FTT Collaborative Group.[57])

plus heparin. The 30-day mortality was lower in the tPA than the placebo group (7.2% vs 9.8%, $P = 0.0011$). Hemorrhagic risk was acceptable.

The *Fibrinolytic Therapy Trialists' (FTT) Collaborative Group*[57] pooled data from nine controlled thrombolytic trials that had randomized 1000 or more patients with suspected AMI and reported on their overall outcome. The database consisted of 58 600 patients of whom 6177 (10.7%) died, 564 (1.0%) had strokes, and 436 had major non-cerebral bleeds. The 45 000 patients who presented with ST elevation or bundle branch block (BBB) had an absolute mortality reduction of 30 per 1000 for treatment within the first 6 hours, 20 per 1000 for hours 7–12, and a statistically uncertain benefit of 13 per 1000 beyond 12 hours.

The large size of the FTT Group database provided the statistical strength to analyze the benefits of thrombolysis in subsets of patients although heterogeneity among trials may affect the validity of the conclusions. When analyzed by presenting ECG (Figure 26.4), proportional mortality reductions were observed for those with ST elevation (21%, $P < 0.000001$) and bundle branch block (BBB) obscuring ST segment analysis (25%, $P < 0.01$). The magnitude of benefit varied by location of ST elevation, being greater for those with anterior (37 lives saved per 1000 treated) compared with inferior (8 per 1000) or other (27 per 1000) sites. The absolute benefit was greater in those with greater absolute risk, e.g. BBB (49 lives saved per 1000 treated) and anterior ST elevation (37 per 1000). There was no significant mortality benefit in patients who presented with normal ECGs or ST depression, for which a slight adverse trend was noted (7 and 14 more deaths per 1000, respectively).

The magnitude of absolute and proportional mortality reductions also were dependent on time to therapy from symptom onset (Figure 26.5). For those with ST elevation or BBB, the absolute benefit (by time to therapy) was 39 (at 0–1 h), 30 (>1–3 h), 27 (>3–6 h), 21 (>6–12 h), and 7 (>12–24 h) lives saved per 1000 treated.

Other studies have indicated proportionally greater benefits for therapy within 1 hour.[58,59] Boersma *et al.*[59] reappraised very early therapy based on a large database

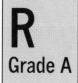

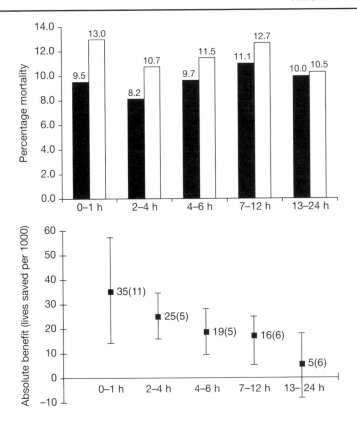

Figure 26.5. The effect of thrombolytic therapy on mortality in various patient subsets with suspected AMI classified according to time from symptom onset to treatment: (*above*) mortality rates in the fibrinolytic group (black bars) vs control groups (white bars); (*below*) absolute benefit (lives saved per 1000 treated, standard deviation in parentheses) by time to presentation. (Based on data from FTT Collaborative Group.[57])

(50 246 patients, derived from all randomized trials of 100 or more patients published between 1983 and 1993; many more patients were included who received prehospital or facilitated emergency department therapy). They found that absolute mortality reduction for treatment within 1 hour of symptom onset was 65 per 1000. The delay/benefit relation (Figure 26.6) was non-linear.

The FTT Collaborative Group analysis suggested that advanced age is not a contraindication to thrombolytic therapy.[57] For patients over age 75, proportionate mortality reduction was less (the trend to benefit was not significant), although absolute mortality reduction was still worthwhile, when compared with younger patients (Figure 26.7).

The FTT study[57] suggested that proportional mortality reduction was little influenced by systolic blood pressure (SBP) or heart rate. However, hypotension (SBP <100 mmHg) was associated with greater AMI risk and the absolute mortality reduction with therapy was larger (60 per 1000, P<0.001) (Figure 26.8). The benefits of thrombolytics were also confirmed for other high risk groups, including those with prior MI (absolute reduction, 15/1000) and diabetes (absolute reduction, 37/1000) (Figure 26.9).

While there is no doubt regarding the efficacy of thrombolytic therapy early after the onset of AMI, the benefit after 6 hours is less certain. The Late Assessment of Thrombolytic

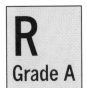

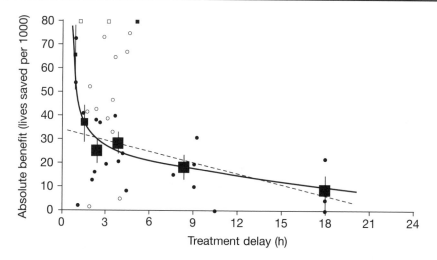

Figure 26.6 Absolute 35-day mortality reduction vs treatment delay: small closed dots, information from trials included in FTT analysis; open dots, information from additional trials; small squares, data beyond scale of X/Y cross. The linear $(34.7 - 1.6X)$ and non-linear $(19.4 - 0.6X + 29.3X^{-1})$ closed regression lines are fitted within these data, weighted by the inverse of the variance of the absolute benefit at each data point. The black squares denote the average effects in six time-to-treatment groups (areas of squares inversely proportional to the variance of absolute benefits described). (From Boersma E, Maas ACP, Deckers JW *et al.* Early thrombolytic treatment in acute myocardial infarction: Reappraisal of the golden hour. *Lancet* 1996;**348**:771–5.[59])

Efficacy (LATE) study[60] enrolled 5711 patients with symptoms and ECG evidence of AMI between 6 and 24 hours and randomized them to tPA (100 mg over 3 h) or placebo. The intention to treat survival analysis revealed a 25.6% relative reduction in mortality (8.9% vs 11.9%, $P = 0.02$, CI 6.3%–45%) for the pre-specified subgroup of patients treated with tPA within 12 hours. The 12–24 h subgroup showed a non-significant trend to benefit with tPA (8.7% vs 9.2%, mortality rate). The South American EMERAS collaborative group[61] treated 4534 patients with IV SK or placebo up to 24 hours after onset of suspected AMI and reported a non-significant trend towards a lower death rate with SK patients treated between hours 7 and 12 (11.7% SK vs 13.2% placebo, 14% relative risk reduction, CI 12%–33%). These trials, while not definitive by themselves, have established, together with other late treatment trials,[57] the rationale for treating patients up to 12 hours after the onset of AMI if they have persistent symptoms and ECG changes.

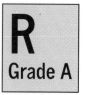

RISKS OF THROMBOLYTIC THERAPY

Bleeding

Thrombolytic agents are associated with an increased risk of bleeding. Fortunately, bleeding is usually minor and often (70%) at sites of vascular puncture. However, life-threatening hemorrhage may occur, including intracranial hemorrhage (ICH), which carries a fatality rate of 44–75%,[62–65] and survivors often have disability. The risk of ICH is about 0.5%, but varies with patient characteristics, the thrombolytic agent, and adjunctive antithrombotic therapy.[65–69] In ISIS-3,[67] non-cerebral bleeds were reported

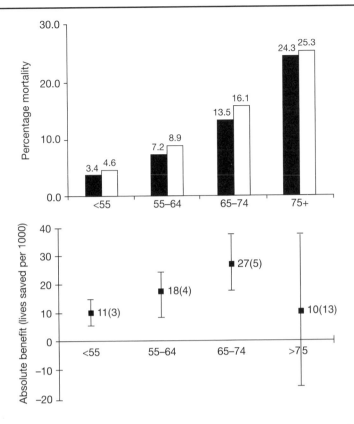

Figure 26.7 The effect of thrombolytic therapy on mortality in various patient subsets classified according to age: (*above*) mortality in each subgroup of fibrinolytic treated (black bars) vs placebo treated (white bars) patients; (*below*) absolute benefit (lives saved per 1000 treated, standard deviation in parentheses) with confidence intervals. (Based on data from FTT Collaborative Group.[57])

in 5.4% after APSAC, 5.2% after tPA, and 4.5% after SK; transfusion was required in 1.0%, 0.8%, and 0.9%, respectively. For individual drugs, ICH rates were about 0.4% with SK, 0.6% with APSAC, and 0.7% with tPA.[66-69] In the FTT group report,[57] thrombolytic therapy (mostly SK) was associated with four additional strokes per 1000 treated, with two additional deaths per 1000. An "early hazard" on day 1 (five additional deaths per 1000) was later compensated for by net benefit; contributing to early hazard were therapy-related ICH and ventricular rupture.

Simoons *et al.*[68] reviewed seven sources to develop a large database of patients who experienced ICH after thrombolytic therapy. Multivariate analysis identified four independent predictors of increased ICH risk: age >65 years (OR 2.2, CI 1.4–3.5), weight <70 kg (OR 2.1, CI 1.3–3.2), hypertension on admission (OR 2.0, CI 1.2–3.2), and use of tPA (alteplase) (OR 1.6, CI 1.0–2.5). ICH was 0.26% for SK treatment in the absence of risk factors, and 0.96%, 1.32%, and 2.17% with 1, 2 or 3 risk factors. The GUSTO-1 group[69] analyzed a database of 592 strokes in 41 021 patients and identified seven factors to be predictors of ICH: advanced age, lower weight, history of cerebrovascular disease, history of hypertension, higher systolic or diastolic pressure on presentation, and randomization to tPA (vs SK). Interestingly, the incidence of non-cerebral bleeding was higher with SK than tPA.[70]

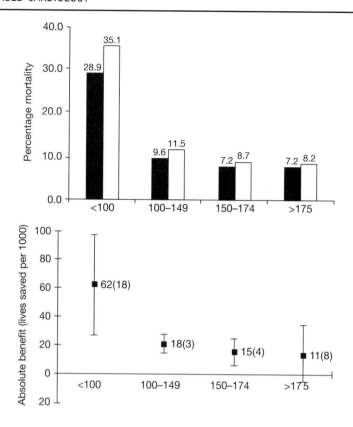

Figure 26.8 The effect of thrombolytic therapy on mortality in various patient subsets classified according to their systolic blood pressure: (*above*) mortality in fibrinolytic treated (black bars) and placebo treated (white bars) patients vs systolic blood pressure at presentation; (*below*) absolute benefit (lives saved per 1000 treated, standard deviation in parentheses) with confidence intervals vs systolic blood pressure at presentation. (Based on data from FTT Collaborative Group.[57])

ICH rates also increase with aggressive adjuvant antithrombotic regimens of heparin or hirudin. The GUSTO-2A, TIMI-9A, and the HIT-3 trials[71–73] were all stopped prematurely and reconfigured because of excessive hemorrhage. With lower doses of antithrombins, hemorrhage rates subsequently decreased.

Allergy, hypotension, and fever

Streptokinase and APSAC are antigenic and may be allergenic. Fortunately, serious anaphylaxis and bronchoconstriction after SK and APSAC are rare (<0.2–0.5%).[52,53,57,67,74–76] In ISIS-3,[67] any allergic-type reaction was reported after SK in 3.6%, APSAC in 5.1%, and tPA (duteplase) in 0.8%. Most were minor: only 0.3%, 0.5%, and 0.1%, respectively, required treatment. Angioneurotic and periorbital edema have been reported after SK or APSAC, and rarely hypersensitivity vasculitis, serum sickness or renal failure due to interstitial nephritis have been reported, especially after repeat administration.[76–78] Purpuric rashes also have been described after APSAC therapy.[54,76]

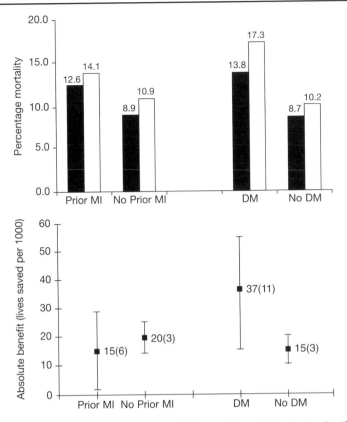

Figure 26.9 The effect of thrombolytic therapy on mortality on various patient subsets classified by presence of prior myocardial infarction or diabetes: (*above*) mortality in fibrinolytic treated (black bars) and placebo treated (white bars) patients; (*below*) the absolute benefit (lives saved per 1000, standard deviation in parentheses) with confidence intervals vs presence of prior MI and diabetes (DM). (Based on data from FTT Collaborative Group.[57])

Hypotension occurred in ISIS-3 in a similar percentage receiving SK (11.8%) and APSAC (12.5%), and less commonly after tPA (7.1%);[67] only half of these episodes required treatment. The acute hypotension may be related more to systemic release of bradykinin, a vasodilator, than an antigenic reaction.

Fever has been reported in 5–30% of SK treated and 5–10% of APSAC treated patients. Delayed-type hypersensitivity response may be one mechanism of fever and and usually responds to acetaminophen. Other reported complications have included splenic rupture,[79] aortic dissection,[80] and cholesterol embolization;[81] the role of thrombolytic therapy in these is uncertain.

COMPARATIVE THROMBOLYTIC TRIALS

After establishing the general utility of thrombolysis, the next phase of clinical trials focussed on comparing and optimizing thrombolysis-based drug regimens. The salient features of the major comparative trials GISSI-2/International, ISIS-3, and GUSTO-1 are presented in Table 26.2.

Table 26.2 Clinical endpoints in comparative thrombolytic trials

Endpoints	GISSI-2/international[82]		ISIS-3[67]			GUSTO-1[75]		
	SK (n=10 396)	tPA (10 372)	SK (13 607)	tPA (13 569)	APSAC (13 599)	SK (20 173)	tPA[a] (10 344)	SK+tPA (10 328)
Death (%)	8.5	8.9	10.6	10.3	10.5	7.3	6.3*	7.0
Reinfarction (%)	3.0	2.6	3.5	2.9*	3.6	3.7	4.0	4.0
Any stroke (%)	0.9	1.3*	1.0	1.4*	1.3	1.3	1.6	1.7
Hemorrhagic stroke (%)	0.3	0.4	0.2	0.7*	0.6	0.5	0.7*	0.9
Non-CNS bleeds (%)	0.9	0.6*	4.5	5.2*	5.4	6.0	5.4*	6.1

* $P<0.05$; statistical comparisons are only listed for SK vs tPA.
[a] Accelerated dose tPA.

The *GISSI-2/International Study Group* trial randomized 20 891 patients with AMI <6 h old and ST elevation to IV tPA (alteplase, 100 mg/3 h) or SK (1.5 MU/1 h).[82] A second randomization was to subcutaneous heparin (12 500 U twice daily) beginning 12 hours later or no heparin. Aspirin and atenolol were given as standard therapies unless contraindicated. Inhospital mortality was similar in the SK (8.5%) and tPA (8.9%) groups (P=NS). Intracranial hemorrhage rates were 0.5% and 0.8%, respectively; other major bleeds were most frequent with combined SK and heparin. At 35 days, the combined endpoint of death or severe left ventricular dysfunction also did not differ by thrombolytic (22.5% vs 23.1%, respectively).[83] Delayed, subcutaneous heparin added little benefit (RR 0.95, CI 0.86–1.04).

The *Third ISIS study (ISIS-3)*[67] randomized 41 299 patients with suspected AMI <24 h old to receive SK (1.5 MU/1 h), tPA (duteplase 0.6 MU/kg/4 h) or APSAC (30 U/3 min). Aspirin (162 mg/day) was given to all patients, with the first tablet given and chewed on admission. A second randomization was to subcutaneous heparin (12 500 U, 4 hours after beginning thrombolytics and b.i.d.) or no heparin. The median time to treatment was 4.0 hours; 88% of patients had "clear" treatment indications: presentation within 6 hours and ST elevation. The mortality at 35 days was similar among the three treatment regimens: SK=10.6%, APSAC=10.5%, and tPA=10.3%. In those with clear indications, rates were 10.0%, 9.9%, and 9.6%, respectively (NS). Six-month survival data also showed no differences among regimens. The addition of subcutaneous heparin tended to improve 1 week mortality modestly (7.4% vs 7.9%, P=0.06) at the expense of increased bleeding rates, but the mortality difference diminished by 35 days (10.3% vs 10.6%, P=NS).

In comparing thrombolytic regimens, GISSI-2 and ISIS-3 may be limited:[84] heparin was given subcutaneously and to only 1/2 of patients after a delay of 4–12 hours (probably suboptimal for short-acting, relatively fibrin-specific tPA), treatment was relatively late (mean times >4 hours), entry did not require ST elevation (ISIS-3), and tPA was not front-loaded. Indeed, several angiographic trials have shown higher patency rates with tPA when intravenous heparin was used in addition to aspirin[85–88] and with rates superior to those reported for SK.[41,44,88] Also, subcutaneous heparin (12 500 U b.i.d.) results in a mean activated partial thromboplastin time (aPTT) of only 35 seconds at 24–36 hours,[89] which may be suboptimal.[89,90]

These concerns led to *the Global Use of Streptokinase and tPA for Occluded Coronary Arteries (GUSTO) study*.[75] GUSTO enrolled 41 021 patients with AMI <6 h old and ST elevation and randomized them to: (1) IV SK 1.5 MU/1 h with SC heparin 12 500 U q 12 h starting 4 h after SK; (2) IV SK with IV heparin, 5000 U bolus then 1000 U/h, titrating aPTT to 60–85 seconds; (3) "accelerated dose" tPA (15 mg bolus, 0.75 mg/kg – maximum 50 mg – over 30 minutes, then 0.50 mg/kg – maximum 35 mg – over 60 minutes, for a maximum of 100 mg over 90 minutes) and IV heparin as per the SK regimen; or (4) a combination of tPA 1.0 mg/kg and SK 1.0 MU, administered concurrently over 60 minutes, with IV heparin.

The primary endpoint, 30-day mortality, was lowest with accelerated tPA with IV heparin (6.3%), representing a 14% risk reduction ($P = 0.001$) compared with the two SK strategies (7.3%), which did not differ. Combined tPA and SK gave an intermediate outcome. The risk of hemorrhagic stroke was higher with tPA (0.7%) than SK (0.5%), but the combined endpoint of death or disabling stroke favored tPA (6.9% vs 7.8%, $P = 0.006$).

The GUSTO authors suggest that these data provide a basis for preferring tPA over SK, especially for high risk patients. However, others disagree with the selective emphasis on adjunctive heparin and accelerated regimen for tPA, and contend that when ISIS-3, GISSI-2 and GUSTO-1 results are taken together, the differences in net clinical outcome between fibrinolytic agents are not significant.[91]

The *TPA-Eminase AMI study (TEAM-3)*[92] compared APSAC with standard dose tPA in about 300 AMI patients. Patency rates at 1 day were similar and high (>90%) with both therapies, but the convalescent left ventricular ejection fraction was greater in the tPA group.

The *TPA-APSAC Patency Study (TAPS)*[93] was an angiographic comparison of accelerated tPA and APSAC in 421 AMI patients. TPA gave superior 60 minute (73% vs 60%, $P = 0.05$), and 90 minute (84% vs 70%, $P = 0.0007$) patency rates; also, normal (TIMI grade 3) early flow rates were more frequently achieved with tPA (72% vs 54% at 90 min). On the other hand, reocclusion within 1–2 days occurred more frequently after tPA (10% vs 3%), and patency rates at ≥ 1 day did not differ. Bleeding was more frequent with APSAC, which was given with aggressive IV heparin.

The *Fourth Thrombolysis in Myocardial Infarction (TIMI-4) trial*[94] also compared APSAC and accelerated dose tPA, as well as the combination of tPA and APSAC, in 382 AMI patients. All groups received aspirin and IV heparin. The "unsatisfactory outcome" endpoint was defined as the composite of any of the following through hospital discharge: death (all causes), severe congestive heart failure, cardiogenic shock, low ejection fraction, reinfarction or reocclusion, TIMI grade flow <2, major hemorrhage, or severe anaphylaxis. Front loaded tPA tended to have fewer unsatisfactory outcomes (41%) than APSAC (49%) or combination therapy (54%), and the patency profile was superior (e.g., 90 min TIMI grade 3 flow rates were tPA = 60%, APSAC = 43%, $P < 0.01$).

INJECT (The International Joint Efficacy Comparison of Thrombolytics) trial[41] evaluated the new mutant thrombolytic reteplase (rPA), a non-glycosylated deletion mutant of the wild type tPA, for equivalence against SK in a 6010 patient double-blind, randomized trial. Mortality rates at 35 days were 9.0% for rPA and 9.5% for SK, a non-significant difference (0.5% absolute reduction; 95% CI -1.98% to $+0.96\%$). On this basis "equivalence" was established and rPA approved. Reteplase was next compared angiographically with tPA. In *RAPID 2 (Reteplase vs Alteplase Patency Investigation During acute myocardial infarction)*[95] 90 minute infarct-related artery

433

patency in 324 patients was 83% with rPA vs 73% with tPA, $P=0.03$, and TIMI grade 3 rates were 60% vs 45%, $P=0.01$. On this basis, a comparative mortality trial, GUSTO-3, was undertaken. Recently completed, GUSTO-3 randomized about 15 000 patients 2:1 to rPA, two 10 mg IV injections 30 minutes apart, or accelerated tPA (alteplase). In GUSTO-3, no survival advantage for rPA was found (30 day mortality 7.5% with rPA, 7.2% with tPA).[96] Earlier, a double bolus regimen of tPA (50 mg + 50 mg administered 30 minutes apart) also had been reported to establish improved patency compared with the accelerated tPA infusion regimen,[97] but a later study failed to show superiority and, in fact was discontinued due to increased bleeding.[98] Thus, no regimens have yet surpassed accelerated tPA with IV heparin in terms of mortality reductions.

INDICATIONS FOR THROMBOLYTIC THERAPY IN AMI

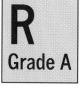

Based on the wealth of clinical trials information forthcoming over the past decade, "evidence based" guidelines for the use of thrombolysis in AMI have recently been established by the American College of Chest Physicians,[99] the European Society of Cardiology,[100] and the American College of Cardiology/American Heart Association's Joint Committee on Management of AMI.[1] The most recent, detailed recommendations are those of ACC/AHA (Table 26.3). Thrombolytic therapy is strongly recommended (class 1 indication; strong scientific basis) for those with suggestive clinical features (ischemic chest discomfort etc.) and ST elevation (>0.1 mV, ≥ 2 contiguous ECG leads) or BBB (obscuring ST segment analysis), time to therapy ≤ 12 hours, and age <75 years. Thrombolytic therapy is also generally recommended (class 2a indication; scientific basis suggestive but less firm) for these same ECG findings and age >75 years (in the absence of contraindications). Therapy is considered possibly effective (i.e., consider selected use) (class 2b indication; scientific basis weak, opinion divided) for these ECG findings but time 12–24 hours or blood pressure on presentation >180 mmHg systolic and/or >110 mmHg diastolic associated with a high risk AMI. Thrombolysis is not indicated (class 3 indication; no evidence of benefit or possibility of harm) for those with ST depression (at any time) or those with ST elevation (or BBB) but time to therapy >24 hours and ischemic pain resolved.

SELECTION OF A THROMBOLYTIC REGIMEN

The decision to use thrombolytic therapy should be based on the risk of the AMI and a benefit versus risk analysis of therapy, together with a consideration of available health care resources (cost). In the United States, tPA has become the dominant thrombolytic, whereas in Europe, SK is most frequently used. A number of algorithms for selecting the reperfusion regimen (i.e., a specific thrombolytic regimen or primary PTCA) have been proposed.[99,101–104] All await prospective testing and validation. Of these, the guidelines of the ACCP appear to the authors to be the most reasonable and evidence based.[99] Aspirin is recommended with all regimens, but heparin (or other antithrombotic) therapy is more controversial, given the relatively weak database, as reviewed above.[67,75,82,83,91,105]

Table 26.3 Guidelines for management of acute myocardial infarction

	Prerequisites for considering thrombolytic therapy	Choice/time of thrombolytic agent	Adjuvant therapy
ACC/AHA 1996	**Class I: (Available evidence for efficacy and benefit)** 1 ST elevation, time to therapy less than 12 h and age <75 years 2 BBB with history suggestive of MI **Class IIa: (Weight of evidence favors use/efficacy and benefit)** 1 ST elevation, age >75 years **Class IIb: (Usefulness/efficacy is less well established)** 1 ST elevation, time to therapy 12–24 h 2 SBP >180 mmHg, or DBP >110 mmHg with high risk MI **Class III (Evidence for harm)** 1 ST elevation, time to therapy >24 h, pain resolved 2 ST segment depression	**No specific recommendations** In patients with large area of infarction, early after symptom onset, and at low risk for ICH may consider the use of tPA. In smaller infants with smaller potential of survival benefit and if a greater risk of ICH exists, SK may be the choice **Door to needle time** less than 30 min	**Aspirin** 160–325 mg/d **Beta-blockers** unless contraindicated or CHF **ACE inhibitors** for anterior MI, CHF or EF <40% (alternatively; all patients, reassess need for continued therapy at 6 weeks). **IV heparin** treatment with tPA and non-ST elev. MI **SC heparin** If SK or APSAC unless at high risk for thromboembolism, when IV heparin is preferred
ACCP 1995	**(A) Certainty of diagnosis of acute MI** (a) At least 0.5 h of chest pain and (b) ST elevation or complete bundle branch block **(B) Timing post-MI onset** (a) Presenting within 6 h and, (b) Perhaps from 7 to 12 h (c) Not recommended beyond 12 h **(C) Patient subgroups** (a) Anterior or inferior infarction (b) First or subsequent MI (c) All age groups, including those >75 years	1 **tPA** should be considered if patient meets all the criteria: age less than 75, anterior or bad prognosis inferior infarction, less than 6 h from onset, or has history of prior exposure to SK or APSAC 2 All other patients without characteristics in (1) may be treated with **SK or APSAC or tPA** 3 Patients treated within 7–12 h may be given SK or APSAC or tPA. SK is the least expensive	**Aspirin** 160–325 mg/d **Beta-blockers** **IV heparin** with tPA, IV heparin with SK, APSAC only if high risk for systemic or venous thromboembolism. **SC heparin** 7500 U b.i.d. for low risk with SK or APSAC **ACE inhibitors** for large infarction, reduced EF, hypertension or CHF
ESC 1996	**All patients, unless there are contraindications** With clinical history and ST elevation or BBB within 12 h of symptom onset Thrombolytics should not be given in patients with normal ECG, T wave changes or ST depression, or infarction of >12 h unless there is evidence for ongoing ischemia	**No specific recommendations. Choice** based on individual assessment of risk, availability and cost-benefit **Call to needle time** <90 min **Door to needle time** <20 min	**Aspirin** 75 mg/d or higher **Beta-blockers** in patients without contraindications and those considered not low risk **ACE inhibitors** in all patients, with reevaluation at 4–6 weeks **IV heparin** with tPA No recommendation with SK, APSAC or urokinase

CHF, congestive heart failure; EF, ejection fraction; ICH, intracerebral hemorrhage.

THROMBOLYTIC AGENT

In the spirit of the ACCP (and ACC/AHA) guidelines,[1,99] accelerated dose tPA with IV heparin and aspirin may be recommended as the first choice regimen for high risk AMI patients who also have the potential for a large therapeutic benefit, i.e., anterior AMI, BBB-related AMI, or poor-prognosis inferior AMI (i.e., with right ventricular involvement or with anterior reciprocal ST depression, or with lateral and posterior extension), time <6 hours, and age <75 years (older patients have greater mortality risk, but also have greater bleeding risk and derive less proportionate and absolute benefit from therapy). Because of greater efficacy and similar safety, the accelerated (90 minute) tPA regimen is now always preferred over the previous "standard" (3 hour) regimen whenever tPA is selected. Some systems may wish to select tPA only when all criteria are met, and others with one or two. In all other patients, any of the approved thrombolytic regimens could be justified, with SK preferred when risk of intracranial hemorrhage is great or when cost is an important consideration, and tPA preferred with a history of prior SK or APSAC exposure (for at least ≥ 2 years and preferably indefinitely because of persistent neutralizing antibodies) or when modest incremental benefit is valued (as in younger, more active patients). The role of reteplase is not addressed in the guidelines; its mortality benefits appear to be intermediate between those of SK and tPA, with improved convenience in certain settings but with cost comparable to tPA. Primary PTCA may now be viewed as an alternative to thrombolysis in certain circumstances that are later addressed.

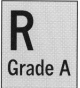

ANTIPLATELET THERAPY

Current guidelines strongly recommend (class 1 indication) aspirin on admission as antiplatelet therapy in a dose of 162–325 mg, preferrably chewed, then continued in the same dose once daily (enteric coated form is popular) indefinitely.[1]

ANTITHROMBOTIC THERAPY

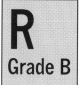

Intravenous heparin is recommended as standard therapy with tPA,[1,99] beginning concurrently with tPA and given for 48 hours, with a target aPTT at ≥ 12 hours after thrombolytics of 50–75 seconds ($1\frac{1}{2}$ to 2 times control).[90] This is achieved with a bolus of 70 U/kg (≈ 5000 U for a 70 kg person), then 15 U/kg per hour (≈ 1000 U/h). The aPTT is checked 6 hours after starting heparin and after dose changes. A nomogram for adjusting heparin to achieve aPTT goals has been published.[1]

However, IV heparin is not recommended with systemically active (non-fibrin-selective) agents, such as SK and APSAC, especially within 6 hours of thrombolysis.[1] Rather, IV heparin is viewed as probably effective (class 2a indication) in patients who are at high risk for coronary thrombosis or systemic thromboembolism (e.g., those with large or anterior MI, atrial fibrillation, previous embolus, or known left ventricular thrombus).[1,99] For other patients, subcutaneous heparin (7500–12 500 U twice daily until ambulatory) is viewed as possibly effective (class 2b indication).[1]

NEWER ANTIPLATELET AGENTS

Antibodies, peptides, and small molecules have been developed that block the platelet membrane IIb/IIIa glycoprotein (GP) fibrinogen receptor. These compounds have potent antiplatelet aggregatory effects and are being tested in the acute ischemic syndromes.[106-109] The role of abciximab, a monoclonal chimeric antibody against GP IIb/IIIa, is being tested as conjunctive therapy with lower doses of SK or tPA (to facilitate reperfusion and reduce reocclusion) in a current clinical trial (TIMI-14). Given the critical role of platelets in coronary arterial thrombosis, this combination regimen has substantial theoretical appeal as an approach to improving thrombolytic reperfusion.

NEWER ANTITHROMBOTICS

An important adjunctive role for the newer antithrombotic agents used with thrombolytics, including fractionated (low molecular weight) heparins and direct antithrombins such as hirudin and hirulog,[110-112] as replacements for unfractionated heparin, has not yet been established, especially with tPA. In a subanalysis of the GUSTO-2b study,[112] 30 day death/reinfarction was lower (9.6%) with hirudin as the adjunct to SK than with heparin (14.7%, $P = 0.01$). This finding needs to be prospectively validated.

CURRENT USE OF THROMBOLYTICS

The National Registry of Myocardial Infarction (NRMI) perhaps best tracks the use of reperfusion therapies in the United States (1470 hospitals). In its second phase, between June 1994 and July 1996, NRMI-2 registered 330 928 patients with AMI.[113] Overall, 37% received reperfusion therapy. Of these, 82% received thrombolytics and 18% were treated with primary PTCA or immediate bypass surgery. Specifically, thrombolytic therapy was given to 72% of the 31% of AMI patients deemed ideal candidates for thrombolysis (note that 41% presented at >6 hours, 25% had non-diagnostic ECGs, and 3% had contraindications).

Utilization experience in Europe suggests that 35% (range 13% to 52%) of AMI patients receive thrombolytics;[99] age is listed as the most frequent limitation to therapy.[114]

THROMBOLYSIS VS PRIMARY PTCA: CONTROLLED TRIALS AND OBSERVATIONAL EXPERIENCE

EARLY CONTROLLED TRIALS

Percutaneous transluminal coronary angioplasty (PTCA) has been successfully evaluated as a primary therapy (without adjunctive thrombolysis) for achieving reperfusion in AMI. In seven small, early randomized trials (1154 total patients), primary PTCA resulted in a favorable 6-week mortality rate when compared with thrombolysis (SK or standard dose regimen tPA) (OR 0.56; 95% CI 0.33–0.94).[115] The impact on the combined endpoint of death or non-fatal MI was also favorable (OR. 0.53; 95% CI 0.35–0.80). The early studies, though promising, raised concerns about study design and generalizability.

OBSERVATIONAL EXPERIENCE

In contrast, the broad (but non-randomized) experience of NRMI-2 reported a better outcome in 9000 AMI patients given thrombolysis than PTCA (hospital mortality, 4.9%

vs 7.4%); this result remained even when shock patients were excluded (4.1% vs 5.6%).[116] The better controlled Seattle-based MITI Registry found a virtually identical inhospital (≈ 6%) and 1 year mortality rate among 3600 patients treated with either reperfusion strategy.[117]

GUSTO-2b

In the GUSTO-2b angioplasty substudy, 1138 thrombolysis-eligible patients were randomized to receive either primary PTCA or accelerated dose tPA. In GUSTO-2b,[118] mortality (5.7% vs 7.0%, $P = 0.37$) and combined event rates (death, reinfarction or disabling stroke) (9.6% vs 13.6%, $P = 0.03$) were somewhat lower with angioplasty, although mortality differences were not significant. In an analysis by time to treatment, a relative benefit of PTCA was primarily observed in those treated >4 hours from symptom onset.[118,119] When earlier studies are included with GUSTO-2b, an advantage of PTCA is suggested,[120] but the conclusion is limited by the heterogeneity of thrombolytic regimens and study designs.

EXPLAINING THE "PTCA PARADOX"

Depending on the database, primary PTCA is better,[115] worse,[116] or similar to thrombolytic therapy.[117,118] The "paradox" of better PTCA results in clinical trials than in general practice may be explained by operator and system-dependent factors for PTCA and by design issues for thrombolysis.[121] Earlier trials were disadvantaged for thrombolysis by suboptimal regimens (SK or standard-dose tPA and higher than optimal heparin doses). Given the time dependence of salvage in AMI, delays in therapy may result in poor outcomes for PTCA in broad use; the average delay to thrombolysis in the United States is ≈ 40 minutes, whereas delays to PTCA in practice average >2 hours. Further, PTCA success is decreased and death and emergency bypass surgery increased in centers (<200–300 PTCA cases per year) and by operators (<75 per year) with low volumes.[122, 123] For optimal outcomes, thrombolysis is preferred in centers without PTCA capability or with low volumes or without surgical backup, and PTCA is a reasonable (or preferred) alternative in high volume centers with a dedicated primary PTCA program.

INDICATIONS FOR PRIMARY PTCA IN AMI

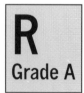

R
Grade A

The ACC/AHA guidelines for AMI management[1] recommend primary PTCA as an alternative to thrombolytic-eligible patients, but only if performed in a timely fashion (in <60–90 min) by individuals skilled in PTCA (>75 cases) supported by experienced personnel in high volume centers (>200 PTCAs per year). Also, primary PTCA is probably useful in eligible AMI patients with a thrombolysis contraindication and in shock patients, and is possibly useful in patients who do not qualify for thrombolysis for other reasons (controlled studies in these patient groups are lacking).[1]

NEW AND INVESTIGATIONAL THROMBOLYTIC AGENTS

Efforts to develop more efficient, effective, safe, and conveniently dosed thrombolytics continue.

Reteplase (rPA), a recently approved, mutant tPA, was discussed above.

TNK-plasminogen activator (TNK-PA) is a modified tPA with amino acid substitutions at three sites: at amino acid 103, threonine (T) is replaced by asparagine, adding a glycosylation site; at site 117, asparagine (N) is replaced by glutamine, removing a glycosylation site; at a third site, four amino acids (lysine [K], histidine, arginine and arginine) are replaced by four alanines. The result is a molecule with a prolonged half-life (allowing single bolus administration), increased fibrin specificity, and increased resistance to PAI-1. TNK-PA has been studied in small to moderate sized phase I and II trials,[124] with phase III trials being planned.

Lanoteplase (nPA) is a tPA mutant with deletions of the epidermal growth factor, the fibronectin finger domain, and the amino acid 117 glycosylation site; it is given by bolus injection. Phase I and II trials have been completed[125] and phase III trials are planned.

Staphylokinase is a 136 amino-acid single chain protein with fibrin-specific thrombolytic potential secreted by *Staphylococcus aureus* and produced for medical use by recombinant DNA technology.[126] In the small STAR (staphylokinase-recombinant) trial,[127] staphylokinase showed at least equivalent reperfusion potential and greater fibrin-specificity than accelerated dose tPA. Staphylokinase is antigenic, inducing neutralizing antibodies within 1 week.

Saruplase is a recombinant unglycosylated full length human form of single chain urokinase-type plasminogen activator (scuPA). Saruplase has undergone clinical testing, including comparative angiographic studies with SK and tPA. Saruplase achieves more rapid coronary patency than SK with less bleeding.[128] Saruplase showed a comparable safety profile to alteplase in a comparative angiographic study.[129] Glycosylated scuPA (*prourokinase*) is highly fibrin-specific and has shown promise in clinical angiographic trials.[130]

Whether the "ceiling" of the thrombolytic reperfusion profile, currently established by accelerated dose tPA (90 minute total and complete patency rates of 85% and 60%, respectively), can be broken with any of these or other newer fibrinolytics, or whether combinations of fibrinolytics with other therapies, such as the antiplatelet GP IIb/IIIa inhibitors, will be required to further optimize reperfusion therapy, remains to be determined.[131]

REFERENCES

1 Ryan TJ, Anderson JL, Antman EM *et al.* ACC/AHA guidelines for the management of patients with acute myocardial infarction. Report of the American College of Cardiology/American Heart Association Task Force on Practice Guidelines (Committee on Management of Acute Myocardial Infarction). *J Am Coll Cardiol* 1996; **28**:1328–428.

2 Tunstall-Pedoe H, Kuulasmaa K, Amouyel P *et al.* Myocardial infarction and coronary death in the World Health Organization MONICA Project. *Circulation* 1994;**90**:583–612.

3 Hunink MGM, Goldman L, Tosteson ANA *et al.* The recent decline in mortality from coronary heart disease, 1980–1990. The effect of secular trends in risk factors and treatment. *JAMA* 1997; **277**:535–42.

4 Herrick JB Clinical features of sudden obstruction of the coronary arteries. *JAMA* 1912;**59**:220–8.

5 DeWood MA, Spores J, Notske R *et al.* Prevalence of total coronary occlusion during the early hours of transmural myocardial infarction. *N Engl J Med* 1980;**303**:897–902.

6 Shah PK, Falk E, Badimon JJ *et al.* Human monocyte-derived macrophages induce collagen breakdown in fibrous caps of atherosclerotic plaques. Potential role of matrix-degrading metalloproteinases and implications for plaque rupture. *Circulation* 1995;**92**:1565–9.

7 Reimer KA, Jennings RB. The wavefront phenomenon of myocardial ischemic cell death. *Lab Invest* 1979;**40**:633–44.

8 Reimer KA, Lowe JE, Rasmussen MM *et al.* The wavefront phenomenon of ischemic cell death: myocardial infarct size versus duration of coronary occlusion in dogs. *Circulation* 1977; **56**:786–94.

9 Bergmann SR, Lerch RA, Fox KA *et al.* Temporal dependence of beneficial effects of coronary thrombolysis characterized by positron tomography. *Am J Med* 1982;**73**:573–81.

10 Tillet WS, Garner RL. The fibrinolytic activity of hemolytic streptococci. *J Exp Med* 1933;**58**: 485–502.

11 Fletcher AP, Alkjaersig N, Smyrniotis FE *et al.* Treatment of patients suffering from early acute myocardial infarction with massive and prolonged streptokinase therapy. *Trans Assoc Am Phys* 1958;**71**:287–97.

12 European Corporative Study Group for Streptokinase Treatment in Acute Myocardial Infarction. Streptokinase in Acute Myocardial Infarction. *N Engl J Med* 1979;**301**:797–802.

13 Sharma GVRK, Cella G, Parisi AF *et al.* Thrombolytic therapy. *N Engl J Med* 1982;**306**: 1268.

14 Anderson JL. Intravenous thrombolysis and other antithrombotic therapy. In: JL Anderson, ed. *Acute myocardial infarction: New management strategies*. Rockville, Md: Aspen Publishers, 1987, pp.185–217.

15 Anderson JL, Smith BR. Streptokinase in acute myocardial infarction. In: Anderson JL, ed. *Modern management of acute myocardial infarction in the community hospital*. New York: Marcel Dekker, 1991, pp 187–215.

16 Chazov EI, Matveeva LS, Mazaev AV *et al.* Intracoronary administration of fibrinolysin in acute myocardial infarct (In Russian). *Ter Arkh* 1976; **48**:8–19.

17 Rentrop KP, Blanke H, Karsch KR *et al.* Acute myocardial infarction: intracoronary application of nitroglycerine and streptokinase. *Clin Cardiol* 1979;**2**:354–63.

18 Rentrop KP, Blanke H, Karsch KR *et al.* Selective intracoronary thrombolysis in acute myocardial infarction and unstable angina pectoris. *Circulation* 1981;**63**:489–99.

19 Ganz W, Buchbinder N, Marcus H *et al.* Intracoronary thrombolysis in evolving myocardial infarction. *Am Heart J* 1981;**101**: 4–14.

20 Anderson JL, Marshall HW, Bray BE *et al.* A randomized clinical trial of intracoronary streptokinase in the treatment of acute myocardial infarction. *N Engl J Med* 1983;**308**: 1312–18.

21 Khaja F, Walton JA, Brymer JF *et al.* Intracoronary fibrinolytic therapy in acute myocardial infarction: report of a prospective randomized trial. *N Engl J Med* 1983:**309**:1477.

22 Kennedy JW, Ritchie JL, Davis KB *et al.* Western Washington randomized trial of intracoronary streptokinase in acute myocardial infarction. *N Engl J Med* 1983;**309**:1477–82.

23 Kennedy JW, Ritchie JL, Davis KB *et al.* The Western Washington randomized trial of intracoronary streptokinase in acute myocardial infarction: a 12-month follow-up report. *N Engl J Med* 1985;**312**:1073–8.

24 Simoons ML, Serruys PW, van den Brand M *et al.* Improved survival after early thrombolysis in acute myocardial infarction. *Lancet* 1985;**ii**: 578–82.

25 Yusuf S, Wittes J, Friedman L. Overview of results of randomized clinical trials in heart disease. I: treatments following myocardial infarction. *JAMA* 1988;**260**:2088–93.

26 Schröder R, Biamino G, Von-Leitner ER *et al.* Intravenous short term infusion of streptokinase in acute myocardial infarction. *Circulation* 1983: **67**:536–48.

27 Rogers WJ, Mantle JA, Hood WP *et al.* Prospective randomized trial of intravenous and intracoronary streptokinase in acute myocardial infarction. *Circulation* 1983:**68**:1051–61.

28 Anderson JL, Marshall HW, Askins JC *et al.* A randomized trial of intravenous and intracoronary streptokinase in patients with acute myocardial infarction. *Circulation* 1984; **70**:606.

29 Alderman EL, Jutzy KR, Berte LE *et al.* Randomized comparison of intravenous versus intracoronary streptokinase for myocardial infarction. *Am J Cardiol* 1984;**54**:14.

30 Valentine RP, Pitts DE, Brooks-Brunn JA *et al.* Intravenous vs intracoronary streptokinase in acute myocardial infarction. *Am J Cardiol* 1985; **55**:309–12.

31 ISAM Study Group. A prospective trial of intravenous streptokinase in acute myocardial infarction (ISAM): mortality, morbidity, and infarct size at 21 days. *N Engl J Med* 1986;**314**: 1465.

32 Jackson KW, Tang J. Complete amino acid sequence of streptokinase and its homology with serine proteases. *Biochemistry* 1982;**21**:6220.

33 Sherry S, Marder VJ. Streptokinase. In: Messerli FH, ed. *Cardiovascular drug therapy*, 2nd edn. Philadelphia: WB Saunders, 1996, pp 1521–52.

34 Bell WR Jr. Clinical applications of urokinase, the first tissue plasminogen activating thrombolytic agent. In: Anderson JL, ed. *Modern management of acute myocardial infarction in the community hospital*. New York: Marcel Dekker. 1991, pp 251–87.

35 Sherry S, Gustafson E. The current and future use of thrombolytic therapy. *Ann Rev Pharmacol Toxicol* 1985;**25**:413.

36 Ferres H. Preclinical pharmacologic evaluation of anisoylated plasminogen streptokinase activator complex. *Drugs* 1987;**33**(Suppl 3): 33–50.

37 Anderson JL, Califf RM. Anisoylated plasminogen-streptokinase activator complex (APSAC). In: Messerli FH, ed. *Cardiovascular drug therapy*, 2nd edn. Philadelphia: WB Saunders, 1996, pp 1553–67.

38 Tiefenbrunn AJ. Tissue-type plasminogen activator. In: Messerli FH, ed. *Cardiovascular drug therapy*, 2nd edn. Philadelphia: WB Saunders, 1996, pp 1567–77.

39 Rijken DC, Hoylaerts M, Collen D. Fibrinolytic properties of one-chain and two-chain human extrinsic (tissue-type) plasminogen activator. *J Biol Chem* 1982;**257**:2920.

40 Lucore CL, Sobel BE. Interactions of tissue-type plasminogen activator with plasma inhibitors and their pharmacologic implications. *Circulation* 1988;**77**:660.

41 International Joint Efficacy Comparison of Thrombolytics. A randomized double blind comparison of reteplase double bolus administration with streptokinase in patients with acute myocardial infarction (INJECT): a trial to investigate equivalence. *Lancet* 1995; **346**:329–36.

42 Lijnen HR, Van Hoef B, De Cock F *et al.* The mechanism of plasminogen activation and fibrin dissolution by single-chain urokinase-type plasminogen activator in a plasma mileu *in vitro*. *Blood* 1989;**73**:1864.

43 Van de Werf F, Vanhaecke J, De Geest H *et al.* Coronary thrombolysis with recombinant single-chain urokinase-type plasminogen activator (rscu-PA) in patients with acute myocardial infarction. *Circulation* 1986;**74**:1066.

44 Chesebro JH, Knatterud G, Roberts R *et al.* Thrombolysis in Myocardial Infarction (TIMI) Trial, phase I: comparison between intravenous tissue plasminogen activator and intravenous streptokinase. *Circulation* 1987;**76**:142–54.

45 Granger CB, White HD, Bates ER, Ohman EM, Califf RM. A pooled analysis of coronary arterial patency and left ventricular function after intravenous thrombolysis for acute myocardial infarction. *Am J Cardiol* 1994;**74**:1220–8.

46 GUSTO Angiographic Investigators. The effects of tissue plasminogen activator, streptokinase, or both on coronary patency, ventricular function and survival after acute myocardial infarction. *N Engl J Med* 1993;**329**:1615–22.

47 Yusuf S, Collins R, Peto R *et al.* Intravenous and intracoronary fibrinolytic therapy in acute myocardial infarction: overview of results on mortality, reinfarction and side effects from 33 randomized controlled trials. *Eur Heart J* 1985; **6**:556–85.

48 Yusuf S, Wittes J, Friedman L. Overview of results of randomized clinical trials in heart disease: I. Treatments following myocardial infarction. *JAMA* 1988;**260**:2088–93.

49 Yusuf S, Sleight P, Held P *et al.* Routine medical management of acute myocardial infarction. Lessons from overviews of recent randomized controlled clinical trials. *Circulation* 1990; **82**(Suppl II):II-117–II-134.

50 Gruppo Italiano per lo Studio della Streptochinasi nell'Infarto Miocardico (GISSI). Effectiveness of intravenous thrombolytic treatment in acute myocardial infarction. *Lancet* 1986;**i**:397–402.

51 Gruppo Italiano Per lo Studio della Streptochinasi nell'Infarto Miocardico (GISSI). Long term effects of intravenous thrombolysis in acute myocardial infarction. Final report of the GISSI study. *Lancet* 1987;**ii**:871–7.

52 The Second International Study of Infarct Survival Collaborative Group (ISIS-2). Randomized trial of intravenous streptokinase, oral aspirin, both or neither among 17,187 cases of suspected acute myocardial infarction. *Lancet* 1988;**ii**:349–60.

53 The APSAC Intervention Mortality Study (AIMS) Trial Study Group. Effect of intravenous APSAC on mortality after acute myocardial infarction: Preliminary report of a placebo-controlled clinical trial. *Lancet* 1988;**i**:546–9.

54 The APSAC Intervention Mortality Study (AIMS) Trial Study Group. Long-term effects of intravenous anistreplase in acute myocardial infarction: final report of the AIMS study. *Lancet* 1990;**335**:427–31.

55 O'Connor CM, Meese R, Carney R *et al.* A randomized trial of intravenous heparin in conjunction with an istreplase (anisoylated plasminogen streptokinase activator complex) in acute myocardial infarction. The Duke University Clinical Cardiology Study (DUCCS) 1. *J Am Coll Cardiol* 1994;**23**:11–18.

56 The Anglo-Scandinavian Study of Early Thrombolysis (ASSET). Trial of tissue plasminogen activator for mortality reduction in acute myocardial infarction. *Lancet* 1988;**i**: 349–60.

57 Fibrinolytic Therapy Trialists' (FTT) Collaborative Group. Indications for fibrinolytic therapy in suspected acute myocardial infarction: collaborative overview of early mortality and major morbidity results of all randomized trials of more than 1000 patients. *Lancet* 1994;**343**:311–22.

58 Gersh BJ, Anderson JL. Thrombolysis and myocardial salvage. Results of clinical trials and the animal paradigm – parodoxic or predictable? *Circulation* 1993;**88**:296–306.

59 Boersma E, Maas ACP, Deckers JW *et al.* Early thrombolytic treatment in acute myocardial infarction: reappraisal of the golden hour. *Lancet* 1996;**348**:771–5.

60 LATE Study Group. Late assessment of thrombolytic efficacy (LATE) study with alteplase 6–24 hours after onset of acute myocardial infarction. *Lancet* 1993;**342**:759–66.

61 EMERAS (Estudio Multicentrico Estreptoquinasa republicas de America del Sur) Collaborative Group. Randomized trial of late thrombolysis in patients with suspected acute myocardial infarction. *Lancet* 1993;**342**:767–72.

62 Kase CS, Pessin MS, Zivin JA *et al.* Intracranial hemorrhage following thrombolysis with tissue plasminogen activator. *Am J Med* 1992;**92**: 384–90.

63 De Jaegere PP, Arnold AP, Balk AH *et al.* Intracranial hemorrhage in association with thrombolytic therapy: incidence and clinical predictive factors. *J Am Coll Cardiol* 1992;**20**: 289–94.

64 Carlson S, Aldrich MS, Greenburg HS *et al.* Intracerebral hemorrhage complicating intravenous tissue plasminogen activator treatment. *Arch Neurol* 1988;**45**:1070–3.

65 Anderson JL, Karagounis LA, Allen A *et al.* Older age and elevated blood pressure are risk factors for intracerebral hemorrhage after thrombolysis. *Am J Cardiol* 1991;**68**:166–70.

66 Maggioni AP, Franzosi MG, Santoro E *et al.* The risk of stroke with acute myocardial infarction after thrombolytic and antithrombotic treatment. *N Engl J Med* 1992;**327**:1–6.

67 ISIS-3 Collaborative Group. A randomized comparison of streptokinase vs tissue plasminogen activator vs anistreplase and of aspirin plus heparin vs aspirin alone among 41 299 cases of suspected acute myocardial infarction. *Lancet* 1992;**339**:753.

68 Simoons MI, Maggioni AP, Knatterud G *et al.* Individual risk assessment for intracranial hemorrhage during thrombolytic therapy. *Lancet* 1993;**342**:523–8.

69 Gore JM, Granger CG, Simoons ML *et al.* Stroke after thrombolysis. Mortality and functional outcomes in the GUSTO-1 trial. *Circulation* 1995; **92**:2811–18.

70 Berkowitz SD, Granger CB, Pieper KS *et al.* Incidence and predictors of bleeding after contemporary thrombolytic therapy for myocardial infarction. *Circulation* 1997;**95**(11): 2508–16.

71 The Global Use of Strategies to Open Occluded Coronary Arteries (GUSTO) 2a Investigators. Randomized trial of intravenous heparin versus recombinant hirudin for acute coronary syndromes. *Circulation* 1994;**90**:1631–7.

72 Antman EM. Hirudin in acute myocardial infarction: safety report from the Thrombolysis and Thrombin Inhibition in Myocardial Infarction (TIMI)-9A trial. *Circulation* 1994;**90**: 1624–30.

73 Neuhaus KL, vonEssen R, Tebbe U *et al.* Safety observations from the pilot phase of the randomized r-Hirudin for Improvement of Thrombolysis (HIT-III) study. *Circulation* 1994; **90**:1638–42.

74 Thayer CF. Results of the post marketing surveillance program on streptokinase. *Curr Ther Res* 1981;**30**:129.

75 The GUSTO Investigators. An international randomized trial comparing four thrombolytic strategies for acute myocardial infarction. *N Engl J Med* 1993;**329**:673–82.

76 Johnson ES, Cregeen RJ. An interim report of the efficacy and safety of anisoylated plasminogen streptokinase activator complex (APSAC). *Drugs* 1987;**33**(Suppl 3):298–311.

77 Totty WG, Romano T, Benian GM *et al.* Serum sickness following streptokinase therapy. *AJR* 1982;**138**:143.

78 Manoharan A, Ramsay D, Davis S *et al.* Hypersensitivity vasculitis associated with streptokinase. *Aust NZ J Med* 1986;**16**:815.

79 Weiner MD, Ong LS. Streptokinase and splenic rupture. *Am J Med* 1989;**86**:249.

80 Blankenship JC, Almquist AK. Cardiovascular complications of thrombolytic therapy in patients with a mistaken diagnosis of acute myocardial infarction. *J Am Coll Cardiol* 1989; **14**:1579.

81 Queen M, Biem J, Moe GW *et al.* Development of cholesterol embolization syndrome after intravenous streptokinase for acute myocardial infarction. *Am J Cardiol* 1990;**65**:1042.

82 The International Study Group. In-hospital mortality and clinical course of 20 891 patients with suspected acute myocardial infarction randomised between alteplase and streptokinase with or without heparin. *Lancet* 1990;**336**:71–5.

83 Gruppo Italiano per lo Studio della Sopravvivenza nell'Infarto Miocardico (GISSI Study Group). GISSI-2: a factorial randomised trial of alteplase versus streptokinase and heparin versus no heparin among 12 490 patients with acute myocardial infarction. *Lancet* 1990;**336**:67–71.

84 Anderson JL, Karagounis LA. Does intravenous heparin or time-to-treatment/reperfusion explain differences between GUSTO and ISIS-3 results? *Am J Cardiol* 1994;**74**;1057–60.

85 de Bono DP, Simoons ML, Tijssen J *et al.* Effect of early intravenous heparin on coronary patency, infarct size, and bleeding complications after alteplase thrombolysis: results of a randomized

double blind European Cooperative Study Group trial. *Br Heart J* 1992;**67**:122–8.

86 Hsia J, Hamilton WP, Kleiman N *et al.* A comparison between heparin and low-dose aspirin as adjunctive therapy with tissue plasminogen activator for acute myocardial infarction: Heparin-Aspirin Reperfusion Trial (HART) Investigators. *N Engl J Med* 1990;**323**: 1433–7.

87 Bleich SD, Nichols TC, Schumacher RR *et al.* Effect of heparin on coronary arterial patency after thrombolysis with tissue plasminogen activator in acute myocardial infarction. *Am J Cardiol* 1990;**66**:1412–17.

88 Verstraete M, Bory M, Collen D for the ECSG group. Randomized trial of intravenous recombinant tissue type plasminogen activator versus intravenous streptokinase in acute myocardial infarction. Report from ECSG for tissue type plasminogen activator. *Lancet* 1985; **i**:842–7.

89 Turpie AGC, Robinson JG, Doyle GJ *et al.* Comparison of high dose subcutaneous heparin to prevent left ventricular mural thrombus with acute transmural anterior myocardial infarction. *N Engl J Med* 1989;**320**:352–8.

90 Granger CB, Hirsch J, Califf RM *et al.* Activated partial thromboplastin time and outcome after thrombolytic therapy for acute myocardial infarction: results from the GUSTO-I trial. *Circulation* 1996;**93**:870–8.

91 Collins R, Peto R, Baigent C *et al.* Aspirin, heparin and fibrinolytic therapy in suspected acute myocardial infarction. *N Engl J Med* 1997;**336**: 847–60.

92 Anderson JL, Becker LC, Sorensen SG *et al.* for the TEAM-3 Investigators. Anistreplase versus alteplase in acute myocardial infarction: comparative effects on left ventricular function, morbidity, and 1 day patency. *J Am Coll Cardiol* 1992;**20**:753–66.

93 Neuhaus KL, Von Essen R, Tebbe U *et al.* Improved thrombolysis in acute myocardial infarction with front-loaded administration of alteplase: results of the rt-PA-APSAC Patency Study (TAPS). *J Am Coll Cardiol* 1992;**19**: 885–91.

94 Cannon CP, McCabe CH, Diver DJ *et al.* Comparison of front loaded recombinant tissue plasminogen activator, anistreplase and combination thrombolytic therapy for acute myocardial infarction: results of the Thrombolysis in Myocardial Infarction (TIMI)-4 Trial. *J Am Coll Cardiol* 1994;**24**:1602–10.

95 Bode C, Smalling RW, Berg G *et al.* Randomized comparison of coronary thrombolysis achieved with double-bolus reteplase (recombinant plasminogen activator) and front-loaded,

accelerated alteplase (recombinant tissue plasminogen activator) in patients with acute myocardial infarction. *Circulation* 1996;**94**: 891–8.

96 The Global Use of Strategies to Open Occluded Coronary Arteries (GUSTO-3) Investigators. A comparison of reteplase with alteplase for acute myocardial infarction. *N Engl J Med* 1997;**337**: 1118–23.

97 Purvis JA, McNeill AJ, Siddiqui RA *et al.* Efficacy of double bolus alteplase in achieving complete reperfusion in the treatment of acute myocardial infarction. *J Am Coll Cardiol* 1994;**23**:6–10.

98 Van de Werf F, for the COBALT Investigators. Randomized study of continuous infusion vs double bolus administration of alteplase (rt-PA): the COBALT trial. *Circulation* 1996;**94**(Suppl) I-89.

99 Fourth American College of Chest Physicians consensus conference on antithrombotic therapy. *Chest* 1995;**108**(Suppl):225S–522S.

100 Report of a Task Force of the European Society of Cardiology. Acute myocardial infarction: pre-hospital and in-hospital management. *Eur Heart J* 1996;**17**:43–63.

101 Martin GV, Kennedy JW. Choice of thrombolytic agent. In Julian D, Braunwald E, eds. *Management of acute myocardial infarction.* London: WB Saunders, 1994, pp 71–105.

102 Fuster V. Coronary thrombolysis: a perspective for the practicing physician. *N Engl J Med* 1993; **329**:723–5.

103 Simoons ML, Arnold AE. Tailored thrombolytic therapy: a perspective. *Circulation* 1993;**88**: 2556–64.

104 White HD. Selecting a thrombolytic agent. *Cardiol Clin* 1995;**13**:347–54.

105 Collins R, MacMahon S, Flather M *et al.* Clinical effects of anticoagulant therapy in suspected acute myocardial infarction: a systematic overview of randomized trials. *Br Med J* 1996; **313**:652–9.

106 The EPIC Investigators. Use of monoclonal antibody directed against platelet glycoprotein IIb/IIIa receptor in high risk angioplasty. *N Engl J Med* 1994;**330**:956–61.

107 Simoons ML. Refractory unstable angina: reduction of events by c-7E3; the CAPTURE Study. Presented at the American College of Cardiology Annual Scientific Session, Orlando, Fl, March 1996.

108 Lincoff AM. Evaluation of PTCA to improve long-term outcomes by c7E3 glycoprotein IIb/IIIa receptor blockade (EPILOG). Presented at the American College of Cardiology Annual Scientific Session, Orlando, FL, March 1996.

109 White HD. Platelet Receptor Inhibition for Ischemic Syndrome Management (PRISM).

Presented at the American College of Cardiology Annual Scientific Session, Anaheim, CA, March 1997.·

110 Fragmin during Instability in Coronary Artery Disease (FRISC) Study Group. Low-molecular weight heparin during instability in coronary artery disease. *Lancet* 1996;**347**:561–8.

111 Cohen M. Efficacy and Safety of Subcutaneous Enoxaparin in Non-Q-Wave Coronary Events (ESSENCE Study). Presented at the 69th Scientific Session of the American Heart Association, New Orleans, LA, November 1996.

112 Metz BK, Granger CB, White HD *et al.* Streptokinase and hirudin reduces death and reinfarction in acute myocardial infarction compared with streptokinase and heparin: results from GUSTO 2b. *Circulation* 1996;**94**(8 Suppl I):I-430.

113 HV Barron. NRMI-2. (Written communication to the authors.)

114 Ketley D, Woods KL. Age limits the use of thrombolytic drugs for acute myocardial infarction in most European countries. *Eur Heart J* 1995;**16**(Abstr Suppl):10.

115 Michels KB, Yusuf S. Does PTCA in acute myocardial infarction affect mortality and reinfarction rates? A quantitative overview (meta-analysis) of randomized clinical trials. *Circulation* 1995;**91**:476–85.

116 Tiefenbrunn AJ, Chandra NC, French WJ *et al.* for the Second National Registry for Myocardial Infarction (NRMI-2) Investigators. Experience with primary PTCA compared to alteplase in patients with acute myocardial infarction (abstr). *Circulation* 1995;**92**(Suppl I):I-138.

117 Every NR, Parsons LS, Hlatky M, Martin JS, Weaver WD. A comparison of thrombolytic therapy with primary angioplasty for acute myocardial infarction. *N Engl J Med* 1996;**335**:1253–60.

118 The Global Use of Strategies to Open Occluded Coronary Arteries in Acute Coronary Syndromes (GUSTO IIb) Angioplasty Substudy Investigators. A clinical trial comparing primary coronary angioplasty with tissue plasminogen activator for acute myocardial infarction. *N Engl J Med* 1997;**336**:1621–8.

119 Granger CB, Phillips HR, Betriu A *et al.* Direct angioplasty may be less advantageous in patients presenting early after symptom onset: results from GUSTO 2b. *J Am Coll Cardiol* 1997;**29**(2A):366A.

120 Simes JR, Weaver DW, Ellis SG *et al.* Overview of randomized clinical trials of primary PTCA and thrombolysis in acute myocardial infarction. *Circulation* 1996;**94**(8 Suppl I):I-331.

121 Anderson JL, Karagounis LA, Muhlestein JB. Explaining discrepant mortality results between primary percutaneous transluminal coronary angioplasty and thrombolysis for acute myocardial infarction. *Am J Cardiol* 1996;**78**:934–9.

122 Jollis JG, Peterson ED, Nelson CL *et al.* Relationship between physician and hospital coronary angioplasty volume and outcome in elderly patients. *Circulation* 1997;**95**(11):2485–91.

123 Ellis SG, Weintraub W, Holmes D *et al.* Relation of operator volume and experience to procedural outcome of percutaneous coronary revascularization at hospitals with high interventional volumes. *Circulation* 1997;**95**(11):2479–84.

124 Cannon CP, Meccabech, Gibson CM *et al.* TNK tissue plasminogen activator in acute myocardial infarction. Results in the Thrombolysis in Myocardial Infarction (TIMI)-10A dose ranging trial. *Circulation* 1997;**95**:351–6.

125 den Heijer P. Intravenous nPA for treating infarcting myocardium early (InTIME). Presented at the American College of Cardiology 46th Annual Scientific Session, Anaheim, CA, March 1997.

126 Collen D, Lijnen HR. Staphylokinase, a fibrin specific plasminogen activator with therapeutic potential. *Blood* 1994;**84**:680–6.

127 Vanderschueren S, Barrios L, Kerdsinchai P *et al.* A randomized trial of recombinant staphylokinase versus alteplase for coronary artery patency in acute myocardial infarction. *Circulation* 1995;**92**:2044–9.

128 PRIMI study group: randomized double blind trial of recombinant pro-urokinase against streptokinase in acute myocardial infarction. *Lancet* 1989;**i**:863–8.

129 Bar FW, Mayer MJ, Vermeer F *et al.* Comparison of saruplase and altepase in acute myocardial infarction. *Am J Cardiol* 1997;**79**:727–32.

130 Weaver WD, Hartmann JR, Anderson JL *et al.* for the Prourokinase Study Group. New recombinant glycosylated prourokinase for treatment of patients with acute myocardial infarction. *J Am Coll Cardiol* 1994;**24**:1242–8.

131 Anderson JL. Why does thrombolysis fail? Breaking through the reperfusion ceiling. *Am J Cardiol* 1997 (in press).

Mechanical reperfusion strategies in patients presenting with acute myocardial infarction

27

NATHAN R. EVERY,
W. DOUGLAS WEAVER

INTRODUCTION

The use of mechanical reperfusion strategies to treat occluded coronary arteries in the setting of acute myocardial infarction (AMI) was first established in the early 1970s. At that time the pathophysiology of ST segment elevation AMI had been well established. In most instances, acute thrombus formation in the setting of pre-existing coronary artery disease resulted in myocardial cell death. Removal of the thrombus and establishment of coronary patency could decrease ischemia and limit cell death, thereby minimizing infarct size. Prior to the use of thrombolytic therapy and the widespread availability of coronary angioplasty, reperfusion was performed using coronary bypass surgery with surprisingly good results.[1,2] Due to the invasive nature of this strategy, efforts were made to provide pharmacological clot lysis in the form of thrombolytic therapy. Randomized controlled trials in large numbers of AMI patients showed substantial reduction in mortality by the use of thrombolytic therapy.[3,4]

Despite improvements in thrombolytic regimens and dosing, there remain distinct limitations to this therapy. First, many patients with ST segment elevation are ineligible for this treatment due to risks of bleeding.[5] Second, despite choosing optimal candidates for thrombolysis, there remained a small (<1%) but real risk of devastating intracranial bleed.[6] Third, thrombolysis did not always establish normal (TIMI-3) coronary blood flow.[7,8] Finally, after establishment of coronary patency, there remains the risk of reocclusion.[7,9] It has become clear that as the potency of the thrombolytic agents increases (improvements in TIMI-3 flow), the risk of bleeding also increases.

The limitations in treating AMI patients with thrombolytic therapy began to be addressed in the 1980s as the technology for percutaneous transluminal coronary angioplasty (PTCA) improved. Primary PTCA, or angioplasty performed in the setting of AMI as an alternative to thrombolysis, appeared to address some of the limitations of thrombolytic therapy. First, there are patients with contraindications to thrombolytic therapy (for example, high risk of bleeding) who may benefit from acute reperfusion therapy and are, in general, eligible for primary PTCA. Primary PTCA also has the advantage of allowing the definition of coronary and ventricular anatomy, thereby permitting earlier triage of patients to surgery in the case of mechanical complications of acute infarction or continued ischemia and earlier discharge of uncomplicated patients without further predischarge functional testing. Mechanical reperfusion has the advantage of greater establishment of TIMI-3 flow due to direct visualization of coronary arteries with mechanical treatments for complete occlusion, high thrombus burden, and residual stenosis. Finally, the risk of intracranial bleeding is substantially less in primary PTCA patients.[10,11]

Although improvements in TIMI-3 flow and lower risk of bleeding represent distinct theoretical advantages of primary PTCA, there remain several puzzling inconsistencies in the way acute reperfusion works. For example, the newly approved thrombolytic agent rPA (reteplase) appears to have better TIMI-3 flow at 90 minutes than tPA (alteplase) (63% vs 49%) without any obvious benefit in patient survival.[12,13] Further, randomized controlled trials of primary PTCA versus thrombolytic therapy have not demonstrated a convincing effect on postinfarct myocardial salvage.[14] In fact, the major benefit of a primary PTCA approach may be in a reduction of reinfarction by modification of myocardial stunning or reperfusion injury.[15]

Despite these advantages, limitations exist to the universal application of primary PTCA as a treatment strategy. The performance of primary angioplasty requires both access to a tertiary medical center and skilled operators and staff. Less than 20% of US hospitals have the capability to perform primary PTCA. It is unknown whether patients can be transferred to centers having this capability without loss of benefit from initial treatment with thrombolytic therapy. In addition, the time from hospital admission to treatment is often slower in patients treated with primary PTCA. There is strong (albeit indirect) evidence from the controlled thrombolysis trials that delays in the time to treatment can lead to a reduction in effectiveness and higher mortality rates.[3–5,16–18]

Recent reports have also questioned whether the results obtained in the early PTCA trials can by replicated in the community hospital setting.[19–21] There may be a learning curve and results from more general settings do not appear to replicate those reported in the randomized trials. Primary angioplasty always imposes some delay in the initiation of therapy and requires technical expertise far beyond that necessary to administer thrombolytic therapy.

Lessons from randomized trials in thrombolytic therapy have shown that there are two key factors in reducing AMI mortality in patients with ST segment elevation: faster treatment of patients[3,5] and establishment of TIMI-3 flow.[22] In comparing thrombolytic therapy to primary angioplasty, thrombolysis has the advantage of faster delivery of treatment in most hospital settings. While most would agree that delivery of the thrombolytic agent cannot be equated with opening the artery with mechanical intervention, there does seem to be a time advantage for thrombolytic therapy. On the other hand, primary angioplasty has the advantage of more reliable establishment of TIMI-3 flow. Core lab TIMI-3 flow rates for tPA in the GUSTO trial were 54%[7] in comparison with TIMI-3 flow rates of 73% in the GUSTO-2 trial of primary angioplasty.[10]

446

THE USE OF BYPASS SURGERY IN THE SETTING OF AMI

Prior to the wide availability and use of either thrombolytic therapy or primary angioplasty, some centers were using bypass surgery for mechanical revascularization in the acute setting of myocardial infarction with surprisingly good results. During the mid 1970s bypass surgery was the only available means for acute reperfusion. DeWood *et al.* reported on their experience with 187 patients treated with early coronary bypass surgery.[1] In this observational study, all patients under 65 years of age who presented with ST segment elevation underwent cardiac catheterization. After exclusion of 28 patients (comorbidity, diffuse or no coronary disease), 187 patients were treated with bypass surgery and 200 were treated medically. Although treatment was not randomly assigned, the groups were well balanced in terms of age, prior history, and presenting signs and symptoms. Hospital and long term mortality was lower in the bypass patients (5.8% vs 11.5%, $P=0.08$ in hospital; 11.7% vs 20.5%, $P<0.03$ at 56 months). In surgical patients placed on cardiopulmonary bypass within 6 hours of symptoms, hospital mortality was 2%. Similar results have been reported in 261 patients treated with acute bypass surgery at the Iowa Heart Center (hospital mortality 5.7%).[23] These findings, however, are limited by the fact that the comparisons between surgical and medical therapy were not randomized. Patients were excluded from the surgical cohort due to coronary anatomy, comorbidity as well as shock. Thus, these excellent results are probably not generalizable to the larger population of acute infarct patients.

In addition, obstacles to wider use of acute bypass are substantial. First, most hospitals are not able to perform acute bypass surgeries. Not only does this procedure require the availability of the operating room, but also highly trained and readily available personnel. Second, time to treatment was slow owing to delay for patient preparation and to get the patient on a bypass pump. Although the use of bypass surgery as a primary reperfusion strategy has decreased substantially, the growth in the use of acute PTCA has resulted in a small number of patients with indications for acute bypass surgery. In rare patients who undergo catheterization, the decision is made that bypass surgery is a more appropriate reperfusion choice. These are patients with anatomy not suitable for PTCA or with left main coronary disease most suitably treated with acute bypass surgery. In the PAMI Trial, 4.6% of patients randomized to primary angioplasty underwent emergency bypass due to high risk characteristics of the coronary lesion.[11] In the trial by Zijlstra *et al.*, 6% underwent bypass.[24] Outcome in this subgroup of patients was not reported; however, overall mortality rates including acute bypass patients were less than 3% in either study.

American College of Cardiology/American Heart Association practice guidelines for the treatment of AMI recommend acute bypass surgery only in the case where catheter based intervention has failed or is not feasible.[25] Class I recommendations for urgent/emergent bypass in the setting of AMI include those patients with failed PTCA with persistent pain or hemodynamic instability, persistent or recurrent ischemia refractory to medical therapy in candidates not eligible/suitable for catheter based intervention, or in the setting of a surgical repair for ventricular septal defect (VSD) or mitral valve insufficiency. Class II indications include cardiogenic shock or failed angioplasty in patients with a small amount of myocardium at risk.

447

Table 27.1 Description of the trials comparing primary PTCA and intravenous thrombolysis

Author	Lytic agent	Patient population description	Duration of symptoms (h)	Primary follow-up period	No. patients PTCA	No. patients TTX	Time to RX (min)	
							PTCA	TTx
DeWood[26]	Duteplase 4 h	ST↑ <76 yr	<12	30 days	46	44	294	258
Grines[11]	tPA 3 h	ST↑	<12	Dscharge	195	200	60	32
Zijlstra[24]	1.5 mU SK × 1 h	ST↑ <76 yr	<6	Discharge	152	149	62	30
Gibbons[14]	Duteplase 4 h	ST↑ <80 yr	<12	Discharge	47	56	45	20
Ribeiro[27]	1.2 mU SK × 1 h	ST↑ <75 yr	<6	Discharge	50	50	238	179
Zijlstra[24]	1.5 mU SK × 1 h	ST↑ Low risk	<6	30 days	45	50	68	30
Ribichini[29]	tPA 90 min	Inf. MI Ant. ST↓ <80 yr	<6	Discharge	41	42	40[a]	33[a]
Grinfeld[30]	1.5 mU SK × 1 h	ST↑	<12	30 days	54	58	63[a]	18[a]
GUSTO-2[7]	tPA 90 min	ST↑ LBBB	<12	30 days	565	573	72[a]	114[a]
Garcia[31]	tPA 90 min	Ant. MI	5	30 days	95	94	69	84
Total					1290	1316		

PTCA, percutaneous transluminal coronary angioplasty; TTx, thrombolysis; arrow indicates ST segment elevated or depressed; LBBB, left bundle branch block.
[a] From randomization.

RANDOMIZED CONTROLLED TRIALS: PRIMARY PTCA vs THROMBOLYTIC THERAPY

Multiple small to moderate sized randomized controlled trials comparing thrombolytic therapy with primary angioplasty have been performed (Table 27.1).[10,11,14,24,26-32] These trials can be divided by thrombolytic regimen used. In total, there were 2606 patients randomized in all of the trials. Of those allocated to receive thrombolytic therapy, 307 patients were assigned streptokinase, 300 received either a 3 or 4 h infusion of tPA, and 709 were allocated to the "accelerated" infusion regimen of tPA. Two of the "accelerated" tPA trials restricted enrollment to high risk patients, that is, only those with evidence of anterior infarction or inferior location accompanied by ST depression in the precordial ECG leads.[29,31] Entry criteria for time to treatment was 6 h or less for 768 of the patients enrolled (29%) and 1838 patients (71%) were enrolled in trials that included symptoms for up to 12 h (Table 27.1).

Table 27.2 Mortality at end of study period: primary PTCA vs thrombolysis

Study	PTCA	Thrombolysis	Odds ratio (95% CI)
SK trials			
Zijlstra[24]	3/152 (2.0%)	11/149 (7.4%)	0.25 (0.04–0.99)
Ribeiro[27]	3/50 (6.0%)	1/50 (2.0%)	3.13 (0.24–1.67)
Grinfeld[30]	5/54 (9.3%)	6/58 (10.3%)	0.88 (0.20–3.73)
Zijlstra[24]	1/45 (2.2%)	0/150 (0.0%)	
3–4 h tPA trials			
DeWood[26][a]	3/46 (6.5%)	2/44 (4.6%)	1.47 (0.16–18.3)
Grines[11]	5/195 (2.6%)	13/200 (6.5%)	0.38 (0.11–1.16)
Gibbons[14][a]	2/47 (4.3%)	2/56 (3.6%)	1.20 (0.08–17.1)
Accelerated tPA trials			
Ribichini[29]	0/41 (0%)	1/42 (2.4%)	0.00 (0.0–19.6)
Garcia[31]	3/95 (3.2%)	10/94 (10.6%)	0.27 (0.04–1.12)
GUSTO-2[7]	32/565 (5.7%)	40/573 (7.0%)	0.80 (0.48–1.32)
Total	57/1290 (4.4%)[b]	86/1316 (6.5%)[b]	0.66 (0.46–0.94)

[a] Duteplase.
[b] Percentages are pooled result and odds ratio calculated by exact method using all trials.

Table 27.3 Mortality and reinfarction at end of study period: meta-analysis of trials comparing primary PTCA with thrombolysis treatment

Study	PTCA	Thrombolysis	Odds ratio
SK trials			
Zijlstra[24]	5/152 (3.2%)	23/149 (15.4%)	0.19 (0.05–0.52)
Ribeiro[27]	5/50 (10%)	2/50 (4%)	2.67 (0.41–29.1)
Grinfeld[30]	6/54 (11.1%)	7/58 (12.1%)	0.91 (0.23–3.42)
Zijstra[24]	1/45 (2.2%)	8/50 (16.0%)	0.1 (0.00–0.97)
3–4 h tPA trials			
DeWood[26][a]	3/48 (6.5%)	2/44 (4.5%)	1.47 (0.16–18.3)
Grines[11]	10/195 (5.1%)	24/200 (12.0%)	0.40 (0.16–0.89)
Gibbons[14][a]	3/47 (6.3%)	5/56 (8.9%)	0.70 (0.10–3.82)
Accelerated tPA trials			
Ribichini[29]	0/41 (0%)	1/42 (2.4%)	0.00 (0.0 –19.5)
Garcia[31]	7/95 (7.4%)	14/94 (14.9%)[a]	0.50 (0.25–1.02)
GUSTO-2[7]	54/565 (9.6%)	70/573 (12.2%)	0.76 (0.51–1.12)
Total	94/1290 (7.2%)[b]	156/1316 (11.3%[b])	0.58 (0.44–0.76)

[a] Duteplase.
[b] Percentages are pooled result and odds ratio calculated by exact method using all trials.

Tables 27.2 and 27.3 show the mortality rates and the combined mortality and reinfarction rates for primary angioplasty versus thrombolysis. There were four small trials that compared streptokinase to primary PTCA. Mortality rates were not substantially different with either treatment regimen. However using the combined endpoint of mortality or recurrent AMI, three of the four trials appeared to favor primary angioplasty. One trial, carried out by Ribeiro *et al.*, trended in favor of streptokinase, but time to treatment in both the thrombolysis and primary PTCA groups was substantially longer than in the other trials.[27]

There were three trials that compared a 3–4 h infusion of tPA with primary PTCA. The largest trial in this group was performed by the PAMI investigators.[11] In that trial, there was a trend towards improved hospital mortality in patients treated with primary angioplasty and significant decrease in the combined endpoint of mortality plus reinfarction (OR 0.40, 95% CI 0.16–0.89). The two smaller single-center trials did not replicate these results.[14,26]

The largest randomized comparison of thrombolysis and primary PTCA was performed by the GUSTO investigators as part of the GUSTO-2 comparison of hirudin vs heparin in patients with AMI.[10] In that substudy, 1138 ST segment elevation patients were randomized to accelerated tPA vs primary PTCA and also randomized to hirudin vs heparin in a 2×2 design (the substudy is known as GUSTO–2b). This trial may be more representative of community practice than the previously reported trials where primary angioplasty was performed only in specialized centers. In addition, GUSTO-2 tested what most believe to be the best thrombolytic regimen (front loaded alteplase) delivered in an optimal fashion. In this trial, the incidence of the primary endpoint (death, non-fatal reinfarction, and non-fatal disabling stroke at 30 days) was 9.6% in the angioplasty group and 13.7% in the tPA group ($P = 0.03$).[10] By 6-month follow-up, however, there was no difference in the incidence of the composite endpoint (14.1% vs 16.1% $P = $ NS). From GUSTO-2b, we conclude that primary PTCA is a reasonable alternative to thrombolytic therapy and may result in improved patient outcomes in centers that can efficiently perform this procedure. However, improvements in hospital outcome observed in this trial were smaller than those reported in earlier trials, and those differences diminished by 6-month follow-up.

Subgroup analyses in GUSTO-2b illustrate that much of the benefit noted in patients treated with primary PTCA was observed in the elderly. This may be a result of two factors: the elderly tend to present later after symptoms of AMI, when thrombolytic therapy is less efficacious, and there is a higher risk of bleeding in the elderly, particularly intracranial bleeding that occurs with the use of thrombolytic therapy. Another subgroup who also seemed to benefit from primary PTCA were those patients who presented late after symptom onset (greater than 4 h). The advantage of primary PTCA in this setting may be due to the fact that "older" clots become more resistant to lytic agents and therefore more amenable to an angioplasty strategy.

The rate of stroke and intracranial bleeding is also an important endpoint when comparing thrombolytic therapy to primary PTCA. In nearly all of the cited randomized trials, stroke is lower in patients treated with primary PTCA. Rates of stroke in patients treated with primary PTCA range from 0 to 2.2% and in thrombolysis treated patients from 0 to 3.5%. In the GUSTO-2 trial, stroke in primary PTCA patients was 1.1% compared with a rate of 1.9% in thrombolysis patients. Stroke rates in patients treated with thrombolytic therapy in the randomized trials (thrombolytic therapy vs primary PTCA) are, in general, higher than those reported in the thrombolysis "mega-trials" such as GUSTO-1. This higher observed stroke rate may be due to differences in lytic dose and/or patient selection, but in the PAMI trial in particular, the high stroke rate in lytic treated patients may help to explain the poor overall outcome in thrombolysis treated patients. These data have led some investigators to suggest that primary PTCA is the preferable strategy in those patients at high risk for stroke (for example, older age or presentation with hypertension).

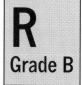

R
Grade B

Simes *et al.* pooled the results of all of the randomized trials.[33] Using total mortality as the endpoint, the pooled mortality at the end of the study period in those receiving thrombolytic therapy was 6.5% and was 4.4% for those treated by primary PTCA (OR 0.66, 95% CI 0.46–0.94; $P = 0.02$). Because of small numbers of patients studied to date, the precision of the estimate for the treatment effect of primary PTCA on mortality is still quite uncertain, with it accounting for as few as four to as many as 35 additional lives saved per thousand patients treated. Using death and reinfarction as the endpoint, the pooled data also favored primary PTCA. When all of the studies were combined, the pooled rate of death or non-fatal reinfarction was reduced in patients allocated to treatment by primary PTCA from 11.3% to 7.2% (OR 0.58, 95% CI 0.44–0.76).

Although there does appear to be a benefit from the use of primary angioplasty vs thrombolytic therapy when combining trials, there are several caveats. First, nearly all of the trials were performed in "expert centers" with high AMI and interventional volumes. Perhaps the most generalizable trial was GUSTO-2b, which was the largest trial and showed the smallest treatment benefit with primary angioplasty. In addition, the total number of patients (2606) and deaths (143) is probably too small to accurately estimate the comparative treatment effects with death as an endpoint. Previous experience in the setting of magnesium therapy in AMI showed that reliance on small trials with rare endpoints and even meta-analyses may lead to false conclusions.[34–36]

Finally, very little long term outcome data has been reported. One-year data from the Zijlstra trial appeared to show maintenance of benefit from primary angioplasty in terms of mortality and repeat hospitalizations.[37] On the other hand, 6-month follow-up data reported from the GUSTO-2b investigators have shown a diminished benefit from primary angioplasty in comparison with the 30-day principal endpoint.[10]

OBSERVATIONAL STUDIES

Although randomized controlled trials give critical information about treatment efficacy, they often lack effectiveness data. That is, in high volume and expert centers, primary PTCA appears to reduce mortality in comparison with thrombolytic therapy. The randomized trials do not tell us whether these results can be replicated in the average community setting. This question of effectiveness is particularly relevant with primary angioplasty where multiple observational studies have shown substantial variation in hospital morbidity and mortality ranging from studies that replicate results from the PAMI investigators[38] to centers where the institution of a primary angioplasty program has resulted in treatment delays with high emergent bypass surgery for failed PTCAs and higher than expected mortality.[19,20] Therefore, in this setting we must rely on observational studies to evaluate effectiveness.

There have been two large observational studies that have evaluated the effectiveness of primary angioplasty in comparison with thrombolytic therapy in the community setting. In Seattle's MITI Registry of 12 331 patients with AMI, short and long term outcomes in 1050 patients treated with primary PTCA were compared to 2095 patients treated with thrombolytic therapy.[39] In that study, primary angioplasty patients were treated at a combination of three high volume and seven lower volume centers. There was no difference in hospital or long term mortality (Figure 27.1) between patients treated with thrombolytic therapy vs primary angioplasty (hospital mortality 5.6% vs 5.5%, $P = 0.93$; long term adjusted hazard ratio = 0.95; 95% CI 0.8–1.2). There was

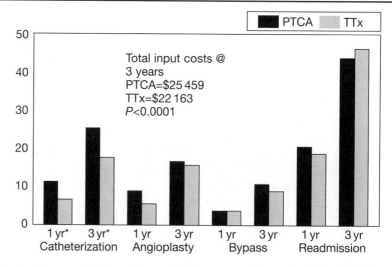

Figure 27.1 Postdischarge resource utilization in 1050 patients treated with primary angioplasty (PTCA) and 2095 patients treated with thrombolytic therapy (TTx). At 1- and 3-year follow-up, patients treated with primary angioplasty underwent more procedures and had higher costs than thrombolysis patients. $^*P<0.05$.

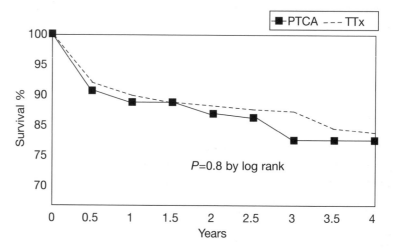

Figure 27.2 Cumulative survival in 1050 patients treated with primary angioplasty (PTCA) and 2095 patients treated with thrombolytic therapy (TTx). There was no difference in unadjusted long term survival between cohorts.

also no difference in mortality in a high risk subset of patients (age greater than 70 years, or anterior infarct location, or heart rate greater than 100 bpm) treated with either therapy. Procedure use and costs were lower in patients treated with thrombolytic therapy both at the time of hospital discharge and after 3-year follow-up (33% fewer coronary angiograms, 20% fewer coronary angioplasties and 14% lower costs at 3-year follow-up).

This observational study was the first to report long term follow-up on a large number of patients treated with primary angioplasty. Probably the most surprising finding was that primary PTCA patients underwent more procedures after discharge than thrombolysis patients (Figure 27.2). This finding may be a result of an overall more

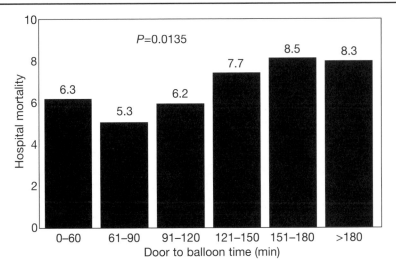

Figure 27.3   Hospital mortality as a function of time from hospital admission to balloon dilation in 6381 patients treated with primary PTCA in the Second National Registry of Myocardial Infarction (NRMI-2).

invasive strategy employed by physicians who prefer primary angioplasty. In addition, since all primary angioplasty patients underwent coronary angioplasty during the index admission (compared to 32% of thrombolytic therapy patients), the chance of clinical restenosis and repeat cardiac procedures is probably greater in the primary angioplasty cohort.

The other large report of community experience with primary angioplasty comes from the Second National Registry of Myocardial Infarction (NRMI-2), whose findings were very similar to those seen in the MITI Registry.[40] In that study, Tiefenbrunn *et al.* compared hospital outcome in 4939 primary PTCA patients with 24 705 patients treated with tPA. Thrombolysis patients were treated more quickly (42 minutes vs 111 minutes, $P<0.0001$, time from presentation to treatment). There was no difference in hospital mortality (5.4% vs 5.2% in PTCA and thrombolysis respectively) or reinfarction (2.9% vs 2.5%). There was no difference in mortality after multivariate adjustment for measured differences in baseline characteristics.

Although there is a strong association between time to treatment and mortality in patients treated with thrombolytic therapy, there is very little evidence addressing this question in primary PTCA patients. Cannon *et al.* addressed this question using data from NRMI-2.[41] In that study, hospital mortality in primary PTCA patients was calculated as a function of time from symptom onset to treatment. There was indeed a correlation between time from symptom onset to treatment and hospital mortality, with increased mortality observed after 90 minutes (Figure 27.3). This study provides indirect support for the American College of Cardiology/American Heart Association guideline that suggests door to balloon times of less than 60–90 minutes in primary PTCA patients. The NRMI-2 investigators have also provided observational data that addresses the question of patient transfer. Preliminary data from that Registry suggest that the transfer of patients for primary angioplasty requires an additional 1.5–2.0 h of transfer arrangement and transport time added on to the 1.0–1.5 h of arrival to dilation time. Whether or not transfer for primary PTCA is an acceptable alternative to thrombolytic therapy is unknown, but it is unlikely that a mortality advantage for primary PTCA could be maintained when an additional 1–2 h of transport is added to time to treatment.

These observational studies probably give a reasonable indication of the effectiveness of primary angioplasty in the community setting. Results in both groups of patients were excellent, however, results in angioplasty patients were somewhat worse and results in thrombolysis patients somewhat better than those reported in the randomized clinical trials. This is consistent with the hypothesis that it is more difficult to replicate trial results of a procedure than it is with a drug. Although the exact reasons for the higher observed mortality in primary PTCA patients in these observational studies is unknown, we might speculate that this may be associated with several factors. First, the average community hospital has, in all likelihood, lower interventional and AMI volume than those centers that participated in the randomized trials. In patients undergoing angioplasty in the elective setting of AMI there is a clear correlation between angioplasty volume and outcome.[42] Second, time to treatment in angioplasty patients in these cohort studies was also slower than those reported in the randomized trials. The time from emergency room arrival to balloon angioplasty was substantially longer in these observational studies (1.7–2.3 h) in comparison with the randomized trials (1.2–1.5 h). This slower treatment time in the community setting may help to explain the higher observed mortality in primary angioplasty patients.[21]

Finally, it should be noted that in all of these observational studies, there may be selection bias in treatment assignments. For example, if higher risk patients were chosen to receive primary PTCA in some centers, hospital mortality might be higher in primary PTCA patients as a result of that selection bias. Although major sources of selection bias such as shock on admission could be measured and adjusted for in these observational studies, more subtle bias cannot be adjusted without randomization. Thus, results from observational studies are limited by selection bias, whereas results from randomized trials may be limited in this setting due to issues of generalizability. It is critical for physicians and hospitals to measure their own performance in the treatment of infarct patients using baseline characteristics, time to treatment, and reinfarction and mortality rates as quality markers.

RESOURCE USE AND COST-EFFECTIVENESS OF PRIMARY PTCA

It has been suggested that the use of primary PTCA may be a more cost-effective means of reperfusion despite the potentially higher upfront cost.[14,37,43,44] This ratio depends on stable estimates of both costs and effectiveness, which may be difficult to calculate in this setting. In terms of costs, there still is relatively little carefully collected and generalizable data comparing long-term costs, rehospitalization and utilization rates in the current fast changing era of reperfusion and decreased length of hospital stay.[14,37,39,45,46] Of those available, costs seem comparable and there are reports showing both higher and lower rates of subsequent procedure utilization in the following year in patients initially treated by PTCA. In the MITI Registry, patients treated with primary PTCA were more likely to undergo catheterization and coronary angioplasty after hospital discharge.[39] This was a somewhat surprising finding since these patients all underwent a revascularization procedure as part of the index hospitalization. In that study, primary angioplasty patients incurred 13% higher costs than thrombolysis patients. In the other study with long-term follow-up, DeBoer *et al.* reported long term follow-up of patients enrolled in the Zwolle Trial and reported higher subsequent procedure use and costs in patients initially treated with thrombolytic therapy.[37] This may be a reflection of different practice styles by US vs European physicians. Most recently, the PAMI investigators have shown that primary PTCA patients who are classified as low risk after AMI treatment can be triaged to a "step-down unit" and a shorter length-of-stay with considerable short-term cost savings.

Most of these reports rely on hospital bills or costs calculated from Medicare cost to charge ratios. This methodology does not take into account critical differences in marginal costs depending on the services available and hospital volume at a particular medical center. In a study of the costs of primary PTCA, based on Kaiser insurance data, Lieu et al. used modeling to illustrate variation in marginal costs of primary angioplasty.[47] These investigators showed that the costs of primary angioplasty ranged from $1600 per case to >$9700 depending on whether an interventional program was already in place. Performing primary PTCA in centers with existing interventional programs, oncall staff and bypass facilities is relatively inexpensive. The costs of starting a new program with onsite surgical back-up in urban areas with excess capacity is probably prohibitive.[48]

As we have illustrated in the previous sections, an estimate of effectiveness is also difficult. Previous cost-effectiveness analyses have utilized data from the two largest efficacy trials available at the time and assumed a large (40–50%) reduction in mortality rate in patients treated by PTCA.[43] This appears to be an overestimate, and based on GUSTO-2b results, estimate of benefit may be much less. Thus, from the data that is presently available, we feel that there is lack of precision in both the cost and effectiveness measures of this ratio and therefore estimates of cost-effectiveness of primary angioplasty may be too imprecise to influence policy decisions.

CONCLUSIONS AND RECOMMENDATIONS

Recent American College of Cardiology/American Heart Association AMI guidelines have listed the use of primary PTCA as a class 1 indication *as an alternative to thrombolytic therapy only if performed in a timely fashion by individuals skilled in the procedure* and *supported by experienced personnel in high volume centers.*[25] There is presently no good evidence as to the minimum number of procedures or the maximum recommended time to dilatation to help define this recommendation. The guidelines have utilized procedure volume data from both elective and emergent PTCA studies in the setting of AMI to suggest an operator volume of greater than 75 PTCA procedures per year and hospital volume of greater than 200 PTCA procedures per year. There is less clear evidence as to what is the maximal door to balloon time in patients treated with primary PTCA. Observational studies have shown a relationship between treatment delay and higher mortality in primary PTCA patients, but whether or not the more stringent door to treatment time of less than 30–60 minutes is applicable in this setting is unknown.[41] In the absence of such evidence, we agree with the American College of Cardiology/ American Heart Association guidelines that suggest a door to dilation time of less than 60–90 minutes.

For patients who present with shock in the setting of AMI, there are observational studies that support the use of primary angioplasty.[49,50] It also seems reasonable to extrapolate from the thrombolysis studies that there would be benefit for reperfusion in patients with contraindications to thrombolytic therapy. Thus, although there is no randomized controlled trial evidence, we would also recommend a class 2 indication

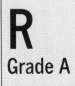

R

Grade A

for the use of primary angioplasty in patients with contraindications to thrombolytic therapy (e.g. risk of bleeding) and patients in shock.

Mechanical revascularization and thrombolytic therapy are different but effective choices for acute reperfusion in ST segment elevation AMI. The choice of therapy is based on multiple factors depending on patient, physician and hospital characteristics. If patients are eligible for both treatments, it seems reasonable to allow institutional experience and expertise to dictate treatments with rapid treatment being the primary goal.

Acute reperfusion: treatment recommendations

- Primary PTCA may be used as an alternative to thrombolysis if:

  Performed quickly (<90 min after hospital arrival) Grade A

  Performed by skilled operator and staff Grade A

  Performed in a high volume center Grade A

- Primary PTCA should be considered in:

  Patients with contraindications to thrombolytic therapy Grade B

  Patients at high risk for intracranial bleeding Grade B

  Patients presenting in shock Grade B

Thus, in a hospital without onsite catheterization facilities, a thrombolytic therapy program may be the most effective. On the other hand, a hospital with high interventional and AMI volumes may wish to pursue a primary angioplasty strategy. In our experience, written treatment protocols are extremely useful. These protocols must involve the emergency department, the coronary care unit, the catheterization lab and the cardiologists. Using protocols, delay is minimized and patient treatment and outcomes are optimized.

Finally it is important to recognize that there will be innovations in both primary PTCA and thrombolytic therapy technology that may influence treatment decisions in the future. There are several new thrombolytic agents both approved (reteplase)[13] and in trials (nPA[51] and TNK tPA[52]). These agents have the advantage of being either single or double bolus and therefore may be easier and quicker to deliver. Although TIMI-3 flow rates as high as 68% have been reported in phase 2 trials, whether or not the efficacy of these new agents is superior to tPA remains to be seen. Also in investigation is the combination of a lytic agent with platelet IIb/IIIa receptor antagonist. Phase 2 studies of the combination of tPA and integrelin have shown TIMI–3 flow rates of 68%.[53]

Technology for the use of primary PTCA is also changing and is under active investigation. Several observational studies have shown that it is safe to implant coronary stents in the setting of AMI.[54–56] The recently completed PAMI Stent Pilot Trial has shown excellent short term results with the heparin coated stent in this setting.[55] In addition, the use of platelet IIb/IIIa receptor antagonists in the setting of primary PTCA may reduce clot burden.[57] These new technologies have the potential to improve short term angioplasty outcome and improve long term results as well.

REFERENCES

1 DeWood MA, Spores J, Notske RN et al. Medical and surgical management of acute myocardial infarction. *Am J Cardiol* 1979;**44**:1356–64.

2 Phillips SJ, Zeff RH, Skinner JR et al. Reperfusion protocol and results in 738 patients with evolving myocardial infarction. *Ann Thorac Surg* 1986;**41**: 119–25.

3 Fibrinolytic Therapy Trialist's (FTT) Collaborative Group. Indications for fibrinolytic therapy in suspected acute myocardial infarction: collaborative overview of early mortality and major morbidity results from all randomized trials of more than 1,000 patients. *Lancet* 1994;**343**: 311–22.

4 The GUSTO Investigators. An international randomized trial comparing four thrombolytic strategies for acute myocardial infarction. *N Engl J Med* 1993;**329**:673–82.

5 Weaver WD, Cerqueira M, Hallstrom AP et al. for the Myocardial Infarction Triage and Intervention Project Group. Prehospital-initiated versus hospital-initiated thrombolytic therapy. The Myocardial Infarction Triage and Intervention trial. *JAMA* 1993;**270**:1211–16.

6 Gore JM, Granger CB, Simoons ML et al. Stroke after thrombolysis. Mortality and functional outcomes in the GUSTO-I trial. Global use of Strategies to Open Occluded Coronary Arteries. *Circulation* 1995;**92**(10):2811–18.

7 The GUSTO Angiographic Investigators. The effects of tissue plasminogen activator, streptokinase, or both on coronary-artery patency, ventricular function, and survival after acute myocardial infarction. *N Engl J Med* 1993; **329**:1615–22.

8 TIMI Study Group. The Thrombolysis in Myocardial Infarction (TIMI) Trial, Phase 1 findings. *N Engl J Med* 1985;**312**:932–7.

9 Gibson CM, Cannon CP, Piana RN et al. Angiographic predictors of reocclusion after thrombolysis: results from the Thrombolysis in Myocardial Infarction (TIMI) 4 trial. *J Am Coll Cardiol* 1995;**25**(3):582–9.

10 GUSTO IIb. A clinical trial comparing primary coronary angioplasty with tissue plasminogen activator for acute myocardial infarction. *N Engl J Med* 1997;**336**:1621–8.

11 Grines CL, Browne KF, Marco J et al. A comparison of immediate angioplasty with thrombolytic therapy for acute myocardial infarction. The Primary Angioplasty in Myocardial Infarction Study Group. *N Engl J Med* 1993;**328**:673–9.

12 Smalling RW, Bode C, Kalbfleisch J et al. More rapid, complete, and stable coronary thrombolysis with bolus administration of reteplase compared with alteplase infusion in acute myocardial

infarction. RAPID Investigators. *Circulation* 1995; **91**(11):2725–32.

13 Topol E. GUSTO III. *J Am Coll Cardiol* 1997;**30**:1.

14 Gibbons RJ, Holmes DR, Reeder GS et al. for the Mayo Coronary Care Unit and Catheterization Laboratory Groups: Immediate angioplasty compared with the administration of a thrombolytic agent followed by conservative treatment for myocardial infarction. *N Engl J Med* 1993;**328**:685–91.

15 Laster SB, Ohnishi Y, Saffitz JE, Goldstein JA. Effects of reperfusion on ischemic right ventricular dysfunction. Disparate mechanisms of benefit related to duration of ischemia. *Circulation* 1994; **90**(3):1398–409.

16 Late Assessment of Thrombolytic Efficacy (LATE) study with alteplase 6–24 hours after onset of acute myocardial infarction. *Lancet* 1993;**342**: 759–66.

17 EMERAS (Estudio Multicentrico Estreptoquinasa Republicas de America del Sur) Collaborative Group. Randomized trial of late thrombolysis in patients with suspected acute myocardial infarction. *Lancet* 1993;**342**:767–72.

18 Kleiman NS, White HD, Ohman EM et al. Mortality within 24 hours of thrombolysis for myocardial infarction: the importance of early reperfusion. The GUSTO Investigators, Global Utilization of Streptokinase and Tissue Plasminogen Activator for Occluded Coronary Arteries. *Circulation* 1994; **90**:2658–65.

19 Caputo RP, Loez JJ, Stoler RC et al. The effect of institutional experience on the outcome of primary angioplasty for acute myocardial infarction. *J Am Coll Cardiol* 1996;62A.

20 Patel S., Reese C., O'Connor RE, Doorey AJ. Adverse outcomes accompanying primary PTCA for acute myocardial infarction – dangers of delay. *J Am Coll Cardiol* 1996;62A.

21 Anderson JL, Karagounis LA, Muhlestein JB. Explaining discrepant mortality results between primary percutaneous transluminal coronary angioplasty and thrombolysis for acute myocardial infarction. *Am J Cardiol* 1996;**78**(8): 934–9.

22 Simes RJ, Topol EJ, Holmes DR et al. for the GUSTO-I Investigators. Link between the angiographic substudy and mortality outcomes in a large randomized trial of myocardial reperfusion. Importance of early and complete infarct artery reperfusion. *Circulation* 1995;**91**:1923–8.

23 Phillips SJ, Zeff RH, Skinner JR et al. Reperfusion protocol and results in 738 patients with evolving myocardial infarction. *Ann Thorac Surg* 1986;**41**: 119–25.

24 Zijlstra F, de Boer MJ, Hoornje JC et al. A comparison of immediate coronary angioplasty with intravenous streptokinase in acute

myocardial infarction. *N Engl J Med* 1993;**328**: 680–4.

25 Ryan TJ, Anderson JL, Antman EM *et al.* ACC/ AHA guidelines for the management of patients with acute myocardial infarction: report of the American College of Cardiology/American Heart Association Task Force on Practice Guidelines (Committee on Management of Acute Myocardial Infarction). *J Am Coll Cardiol* 1996;**28**:1328–428.

26 DeWood MA. Direct PTCA vs intravenous t-PA in acute myocardial infarction: results from a prospective randomized trial. Thrombolysis and interventional therapy in acute myocardial infarction. George Washington University: VI Symposium, 1990, pp 28–9.

27 Ribeiro EE, Silva LA, Carneiro R *et al.* Randomized trial of direct coronary angioplasty versus intravenous streptokinase in acute myocardial infarction. *J Am Coll Cardiol* 1993;**22**:376–80.

28 Boer JM, van Hout B, Liem A *et al.* Primary coronary angioplasty versus systemic thrombolysis in acute anterior myocardial infarction: in-hospital results from a prospective randomized trial. *Eur Heart J* 1993;**14**:118 (abstract).

29 Ribichini F, Steffenino G, Dellavalle A *et al.* Primary angioplasty versus thrombolysis in inferior acute myocardial infarction with anterior ST-segment depression: a single-center randomized study. *J Am Coll Cardiol* 1996;**27**: 221A (abstract).

30 Grinfeld L, Berrocal D, Belardi J *et al.* Fibrinolytics vs primary angioplasty in acute myocardial infarction (FAP): a randomized trial in a community hospital in Argentina. *J Am Coll Cardiol* 1996;**27**:222A (abstract).

31 Garcia E, Elizaga J, Soriano J *et al.* Hospital Gregorio Maranon, Madrid Spain. Primary angioplasty versus thrombolysis with t-PA in the anterior myocardial infarction: results from a single center trial. *J Am Coll Cardiol* 1997;**389A**: Suppl A (abstract).

32 Michels KB, Yusuf S. Does PTCA in myocardial infarction affect mortality and reinfarction rates? A quantitative overview of the randomized clinical trials. *Circulation* 1995;**91**:476–85.

33 Simes JR, Weaver WD, Ellis SG, Grines CL. Overview of the randomized trials of primary PTCA and thrombolysis in acute myocardial infarction. *Circulation* 1996;I-330.

34 Woods KL, Fletcher S, Roffe C, Haider Y. Intravenous magnesium sulphate in suspected acute myocardial infarction: results of the second Leicester Intravenous Magnesium Intervention Trial (LIMIT-2). *Lancet* 1992;**349**:1553–8.

35 Antman EM, Lau J, Kupelnick B, Mosteller F, Chalmers TC. A comparison of results of meta-analyses of randomized control trials and recommendations of clinical experts. Treatments for myocardial infarction. *JAMA* 1992;**268**: 240–8.

36 ISIS-4. A randomized factorial trial assessing early oral captopril, oral mononitrate, and intravenous magnesium sulphate in 58 050 patients with suspected acute myocardial infarction. *Lancet* 1995;**345**:669–85.

37 deBoer MJ, vanHout BA, Liem AL *et al.* A cost-effective analysis of primary coronary angioplasty versus thrombolysis for acute myocardial infarction. *Am J Cardiol* 1995;**76**:830–3.

38 Zahn R, Vogt A, Neuhaus K-L *et al.* for the ALKK Study Group Angioplasty in acute myocardial infarction in clinical practice: results in 4625 patients from the ALKK Angioplasty Registry. *J Am Coll Cardiol* 1997;**29**:15A.

39 Every NR, Parson LS, Hlatky M *et al.* for the MITI Investigators. A comparison of thrombolytic therapy with primary coronary angioplasty for acute myocardial infarction. *N Engl J Med* 1996; **335**:1253–60.

40 Tiefenbrunn AJ, Chandra NC, French WJ, Gore JM, Rogers WJ. Clinical experience with primary PTCA compared with alteplase (rtPA) in patients with acute myocardial infarction. A report from the Second National Registry of Myocardial Infarction (NRMI–2). (Submitted for publication in *Circulation*) 1996.

41 Cannon CP, Braunwald E. Time to reperfusion: the critical modulator in thrombolytic and primary angioplasty. *J Thromb Thrombol* 1996;**3**:109–17.

42 Ritchie J, Phillips D, Luft H. Coronary angioplasty. Statewide experience in California. *Circulation* 1993;**88**:2735–43.

43 Goldman L. Cost and quality of life: thrombolysis and primary angioplasty. *J Am Coll Cardiol* 1995; **25**(Supplement):38S–41S.

44 Stone G, Grines C, Rothbaum D *et al.* Analysis of the relative costs and effectiveness of primary angioplasty versus tissue-type plasminogen activator: the Primary Angioplasty in Myocardial Infarction: (PAMI) trial. The PAMI Trial Investigators. *J Am Coll Cardiol* 1997;**29**:901–7.

45 Mark D, O'Neill W, Brodie B *et al.* Baseline and 6-month costs of primary angioplasty therapy for acute myocardial infarction: results from the Primary Angioplasty Registry. *J Am Coll Cardiol* 1995;**26**:688–95.

46 Reeder G, Bailey K, Gersh B *et al.* Cost comparison of immediate angioplasty versus thrombolysis followed by conservative therapy for acute myocardial infarction: a randomized prospective trial. *Mayo Clin Proc* 1994;**69**:87–9.

47 Lieu TA, Lundstrom RJ, Ray GT *et al.* The cost of primary angioplasty for acute myocardial infarction. *J Am Coll Cardiol* 1996;**28**(4):882–9.

48 Ramsdale D, Grech E: Experience of primary angioplasty in the United Kingdom. *Br Heart J* 1995;**73**:414–16.

49 Lee L, Bates ER, Pitt B *et al*. Percutaneous transluminal coronary angioplasty improves survival in acute myocardial infarction complicated by cardiogenic shock. *Circulation* 1988;**78**:1345–51.

50 Hockman JS, Boland J, Sleeper LA *et al*. Current spectrum of cardiogenic shock and effect of early revascularization on mortality: results of an international registry. SHOCK Registry Investigators. *Circulation* 1995;**91**:873–81.

51 Den Heijer P. Intravenous nPA for treating infarcting myocardium early (In Time). *J Am Coll Cardiol* 1997;**30**:5.

52 Cannon CP, McCabe CH, Gibson CM *et al*. TNK-tissue plasminogen activator in acute myocardial infarction. Results of the TIMI 10A dose-ranging trial. *Circulation* 1997;**95**:351–6.

53 Ohman E, Kleiman N, Gacioch G *et al*. Combined accelerated tissue-plasminogen activator and platelet glycoprotein IIb/IIIa integrelin receptor blockage with integrelin in acute myocardial infarction. Results of a randomized, placebo-controlled, dose-ranging trial. IMPACT-AMI Investigators. *Circulation* 1997;**95**:846–54.

54 Grines C, Morice M, Mattos L *et al*. A prospective multicenter trial using the JJIS heparin-coated stent for primary reperfusion of acute myocardial infarction. *J Am Coll Cardiol* 1997;**29**:389A.

55 Stone G, Brodie B, Griffin J *et al*. Safety and feasibility of primary stenting in acute myocardial infarction-in-hospital and 30 day results of the PAMI stent pilot trial. *J Am Coll Cardiol* 1997;**29**:389A.

56 Ganim M, Wong P, Grover R *et al*. Superiority of coronary stenting compared to balloon angioplasty in acute myocardial infarction. *J Am Coll Cardiol* 1997;**29**:456A.

57 Lefkovits J, Ivanhoe R, Califf R *et al*. for the EPIC Investigators. Effects of platelet glycoprotein IIb/IIIa receptor blockage by a chimeric monoclonal antibody (abciximab) on acute and six-month outcomes after percutaneous transluminal coronary angioplasty for acute myocardial infarction. *Am J Cardiol* 1996;**77**:1045–51.

28 Adjunctive antithrombotic therapy for acute myocardial infarction

John K. French,
Harvey D. White

INTRODUCTION

The paradigm for the treatment of reperfusion-eligible patients[1] with acute myocardial infarction (AMI) is complete restoration of normal coronary blood flow to the infarct-related artery as soon as possible.[2,3] Left ventricular function and early survival are related to the frequency with which a particular therapeutic regimen achieves early (90 minute) TIMI-3 (thrombolysis in acute myocardial infarction[4]) grade flow.[5] In addition, sustained patency is associated with enhanced late survival.[6] Among reperfusion-eligible patients, complete and sustained infarct-related artery patency may be achieved by a combination of thrombolytic, antiplatelet, and antithrombin agents and/or in conjunction with reperfusion with angioplasty.

Patients without ST elevation or bundle branch block on the presenting electrocardiogram represent 30–35% of patients who have a discharge diagnosis of myocardial infarction.[7,8] A beneficial role of reperfusion therapies in these patients has not been confirmed by evidence from the randomized controlled trials, and in patients with ST depression thrombolytic therapy may be harmful.[9,10] The role of reperfusion therapies in patients presenting later than 12 hours with ST elevation requires further definition[9,11] though the magnitude of any treatment benefit is likely to be modest.[9]

This chapter will examine the evidence base for the use of adjunctive antithrombin therapies, in patients with AMI both with and without reperfusion therapy.

MECHANISM OF CORONARY THROMBOSIS

The common pathogenic basis for the clinical presentation of patients with acute ischemic syndromes is rupture of an atherosclerotic plaque, with release of tissue factor,

460

Direct   **Indirect**

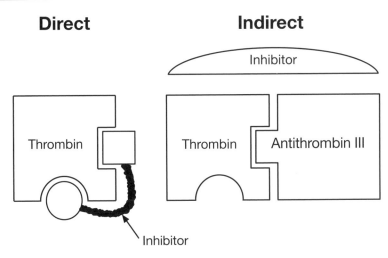

Figure 28.1 Thrombin inhibitors. Direct thrombin inhibitors such as hirulog and hirudin bind to both the catalytic and antithrombin III binding sites of thrombin, directly inhibiting each function. Indirect thrombin inhibitors such as heparin affect the functions of thrombin indirectly by binding at different sites.

exposure of collagen and release of lipid leading to activation of intrinsic and extrinsic coagulation pathways, which result in thrombus formation.[12,13] In patients with unstable angina or non-Q wave infarction ruptured plaques comprise mainly white, subocclusive, thrombi composed mostly of platelets. Patients who have ST elevation on the presenting electrocardiograph usually have an occlusive thrombus predominantly composed of red cells enmeshed in fibrin strands.

Epidemiological observations have shown prothrombotic factors, including increased blood levels of fibrinogen, are associated with an increased risk of suffering a myocardial infarction.[14,15] Thus, it has been postulated[14] that some patients may be predisposed to arterial thromboses because of either genetic or physiological abnormalities of coagulation–thrombotic and/or fibrinolytic pathways.

MECHANISM OF ACTION OF HEPARIN

Heparin, the clinical prototypic antithrombin agent, is a heterogeneous glycoprotein with the molecular mass varying between 5000 and 30 000 kD (mean 15 kD). Upon binding to antithrombin III, heparin forms a complex that inhibits the actions of thrombin (Figure 28.1) and factors IXa, Xa, and XIa. The varying molecular masses of commercial preparations of heparin result in incomplete (approximately one-third) stoichiometric binding to antithrombin III, and hence unpredictable pharmacokinetics and pharmacodynamics, i.e. anticoagulant effect.[16] Low molecular weight heparins have lower mean molecular mass and do not have 18 saccharide moieties, resulting in effective inhibition of factor Xa but not concurrent binding to thrombin and antithrombin. At least 18 saccharides are required in a heparin molecule for simultaneous binding of thrombin and antithrombin III. At heparin concentrations that prolong activated partial thromboplastin times (aPTT) to twice normal, there is only 20–40% inhibition of clot-bound thrombin activity.[17] The heparin–antithrombin III complex is relatively inaccessible to factor Xa in the prothrombinase complex, and it is also inhibited by

461

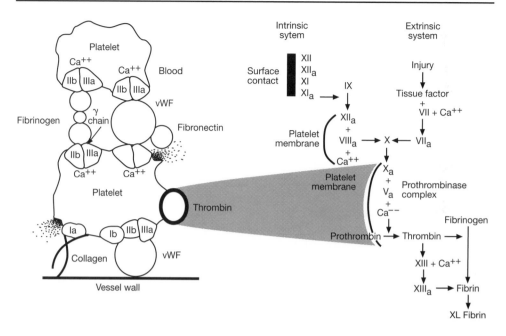

Figure 28.2 Interactions between platelets and thrombotic, coagulation, and fibrinolytic pathways. Biochemical interactions between platelet membrane receptors, vessel wall, and adhesive macromolecules during platelet adhesion and aggregation (*left*). Also depicted are the intrinsic and extrinsic systems of the coagulation cascade and their interaction with the platelet membrane (*right*), such as via the prothrombinase complex, the activator complex for thrombin. Coronary thrombosis is associated with both platelet and coagulation processes. Ca^{++} = calcium, vWF = von Willebrand factor, Ia = glycoprotein Ia, Ib = glycoprotein Ib, IIb/IIIa = glycoprotein IIb/IIIa, XL = cross-linked. (Modified from Stein *et al.* Antithrombotic therapy in cardiac disease: an emerging approach based on pathogenesis and risk. *Circulation* 1989;**80**:1502, with permission.)

fibrin monomer II. Heparin binds to several other plasma proteins including platelet factor 4, vitronectin, fibronectin, and von Willebrand factor, the latter resulting in inhibition of platelet function.

PROCOAGULANT STATE AFTER ADMINISTRATION OF THROMBOLYTIC THERAPY

Administration of either streptokinase or tissue plasminogen activator (tPA) produces a procoagulant state, with activation of platelets either by plasmin activating the thrombin receptor[18] or by plasmin triggering thrombin generation through activation of factor V (Figure 28.2).[19] The amount of thrombin activity induced by thrombolytic agents is directly related to the extent of free plasmin activity (Figure 28.3).[20] Administration of streptokinase results in the breakdown of circulating fibrinogen and an increase in fibrin degradation products, which have anticoagulant effects. However, because streptokinase induces extensive plasmin activity, it may be associated with more marked procoagulant effects than fibrin-specific agents such as tPA, which activate plasminogen less.[20] The exposure of clot-bound thrombin acts as a nidus for further thrombosis.

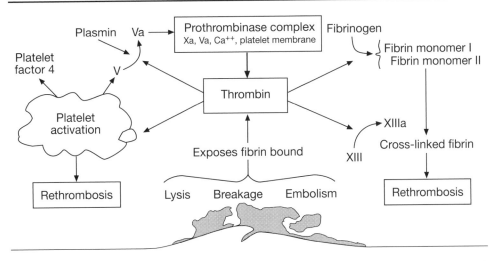

Figure 28.3 Clot lysis and thrombin generation. Disturbance of thrombus by lysis (endogenous or exogenous), mechanical breakage (including coronary angioplasty), or spontaneous embolism exposes thrombin bound to fibrin. Thrombin activates platelets, activates factor V to Va (which leads to generation of more thrombin via the prothrombinase complex), converts fibrinogen to fibrin I and fibrin II, and activates factor XIII to XIIIa (which cross-links fibrin). These processes combine to produce rethrombosis. Heparin may only partially prevent rethrombosis because factor Xa within the prothrombinase complex is protected from heparin–antithrombin III, platelet factor 4 neutralizes heparin, and fibrin monomer II inhibits heparin–antithrombin III. (Modified with permission from Webster *et al.* Antithrombotic therapy in acute myocardial infarction in *Current Topics in Cardiology – acute myocardial infarction* eds BJ Gersh and SH Rahimtoola 1990; Elsevier.)

Levels of fibrinopeptide A, a non-specific marker of thrombin activity, increase after administration of either streptokinase or tPA,[21,22] possibly due to release of coagulation factors bound to clot or to re-exposure of the core of the ruptured plaque. Lower levels of fibrinopeptide A have been associated with higher infarct-related artery patency after administration of thrombolytic therapy.[23,24]

EFFECT OF HEPARIN ON INFARCT ARTERY PATENCY

Angiographic studies, that compared the administration of heparin to aspirin showed heparin improved infarct-related artery patency by 18–81 hours following thrombolytic therapy with tPA.[25–27]

Two small cohort studies and one small trial have examined the effect on 90 minute TIMI-3 flow of a large single bolus of heparin. Fifty patients given heparin as a single intravenous bolus of 300U/kg with aspirin prior to planned primary angioplasty achieved 36% TIMI-3 flow at 90 minutes. This patency rate compares with 10% TIMI-3 flow in historic controls.[28] In another observational study, which used a 10–15 000 U bolus of heparin 25%, TIMI-3 flow was achieved at 70 minutes in 158 patients.[29] However, these findings were not confirmed in a preliminary report of the HEAP randomized trial, which found only 19% patency (11% TIMI-3) in 400 patients randomized to either high dose IV heparin (20 000–30 000 U) or low dose IV heparin (0–5000 U).[30]

In patients treated with streptokinase and aspirin, administration of a 5000 U bolus of heparin followed by an infusion of 1000 U/hour produced significantly lower

463

fibrinopeptide A levels and faster reperfusion, as judged by enzyme criteria, than delayed administration of SC heparin.[31] In the GUSTO-1 hemostasis substudy, IV heparin attenuated the increase in fibrinopeptide A seen after administration of streptokinase, aspirin and SC heparin. A 10 000 U bolus of heparin given following the administration of 200 mg of aspirin and streptokinase increased patency to 77% compared to 60% in controls at ≤ 90 minutes, as judged by ST-segment monitoring in the preliminary results of the Optimization Study of Infarct Reperfusion Investigated by ST Monitoring (OSIRIS).[32] Patients randomized to receive immediate IV heparin compared to saline, with heparin upon completion of the streptokinase infusion, had earlier and lower creatine kinase-MB peaks and earlier reperfusion as judged by ST segment monitoring; antiplatelet therapy commenced at the cessation of heparin infusion.[33]

ADJUNCTIVE SUBCUTANEOUS HEPARIN

In the Studio sulla Calciparina nell-Angina e nella Trombosi Ventricolare nell'Infarto (SCATI) trial 433 patients receiving streptokinase, without routine aspirin, were randomized to either control or a 2000 U heparin bolus followed 9 hours later by 12 500 U given SC twice daily.[34] Hospital mortality was reduced from 8.8% in the control group to 4.6% in the heparin group ($P = 0.05$).

Several large trials with clinical endpoints have evaluated SC heparin regimens in conjunction with aspirin and thrombolytic therapy.[35–37] The Gruppo Italiano per lo Studio della Sopravvivenza nell'Infarto Miocardico (GISSI-2) trial enrolled 20 891 patients randomized to receive either SC heparin 12 500 U twice daily throughout hospitalization or control, beginning 12 hours after aspirin (160–325 mg), and the initiation of thrombolytic therapy (either streptokinase or tPA). Hospital mortality rate was reduced to 5.4% with aspirin plus heparin compared to 6.0% with aspirin alone ($P < 0.05$).

In ISIS-3[35] 41 299 patients were given 162 mg of enteric coated aspirin, crushed or chewed, and randomized to receive one of three thrombolytic regimens (streptokinase, duteplase or anisoylated plasminogen streptokinase activator complex – APSAC) plus either 12 500 U of SC heparin every 12 hours begun 4 hours after initiation of thrombolytic therapy, or control.

During the scheduled heparin treatment period there was a trend towards mortality reduction from 7.9% to 7.4% with heparin ($P = 0.06$), which may represent a benefit of 5 lives saved per 1000 patients treated. As 12% of patients randomized to receive heparin received none and 25% of patients randomized to receive no heparin were actually given either IV heparin (14%) or high dose SC heparin, a benefit of about 7 lives saved per 1000 patients treated may accrue from "actual" use of SC heparin.[35] Following the period of randomization to receive heparin (7 days), there were slightly more deaths in the heparin group.

Overall, combining data from GISSI-2 and ISIS-3 at 35 days, the prespecified endpoint, allocation to SC heparin was associated with 2 fewer deaths and 2 fewer non-fatal reinfarctions per 1000 patients treated, at the expense of 3 transfusions and 0.3 non-fatal disabling strokes (Table 28.1).

After administration of SC heparin absorption is variable, with a delay of up to 24 hours before there is significant prolongation of the aPTT.[38] Hence, SC heparin cannot

Table 28.1 Overview of the addition of delayed subcutaneous heparin in the ISIS-3 and GISSI-2 trials for 1000 patients treated at 35 days

	ISIS-3	GISSI-2	Combined
Benefit			
Mortality reduction	2.8	1.0	2.2[a]
Reduced non-fatal reinfarction	1.8	1.9	1.8
Risk			
Transfusion	2.6	4.5	3.2
Total non-fatal stroke	0.5	0.6	0.6[b]

[a] Figures do not sum because of rounding.
[b] Half had fully recovered at discharge.

potentially affect the major mechanism of benefit of thrombolytic therapy, i.e. TIMI flow grade at 90 minutes.

META-ANALYSES OF HEPARIN TRIALS

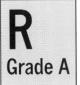

In a meta-analysis of trials involving 5459 patients randomized to receive either heparin or no antithrombotic therapy in the absence of routine aspirin (14% received thrombolysis), mortality (at a mean of 10 days) was reduced 25% (95% CI 10–37%) from 14.9% to 11.4% (*P* = 0.002).[39] Reinfarction was not reduced (8.3% vs 6.8%, *P* = 0.1), but stroke was reduced from 2.1% to 1.1% (*P* = 0.01) and pulmonary embolism from 3.8% to 2.0% (*P* ≤ (0.001).[39]

A total of 68 000 patients treated with aspirin and 93% with thrombolytic therapy have been entered in randomized trials examining various heparin regimens.[40] In patients randomized to receive heparin, mortality was reduced from 9.1% to 8.6% (95% CI 0–10%, *P*<0.05), reinfarction from 3.3% to 3.0% (*P*<0.05), and pulmonary embolism from 0.4% to 0.3% (*P*<0.05).

COMPARISON OF INTRAVENOUS HEPARIN TO CONTROL

Four trials[27,32,41,42] have randomized patients treated with aspirin to receive IV heparin or control therapy following thrombolysis (Table 28.2). There were no significant differences in rates of death or reinfarction. At least five times as many patients would have required randomization to detect clinically meaningful differences of 15%[43] in either endpoint.

The evaluation of the potential beneficial effect of IV heparin after thrombolysis has been confounded in trials because of the frequent addition of elective IV heparin in the control or placebo treatment arms. It is appropriate to conclude that there is a paucity of information comparing IV heparin with placebo following thrombolytic therapy with either streptokinase or tPA.

Table 28.2 Intravenous heparin in the presence of aspirin and thrombolysis

	Death (%)		Reinfarction (%)		Bleeding (%)	
	Control	Heparin	Control	Heparin	Control	Heparin
ISIS-2 pilot (n=626)[42]	6	8	5	1	1	0
ECSG (n=1296)[27]	3	2	10	10	NA	NA
OSIRIS (n=256)[32]	11	9	1	2	4	6
DUCCS (n=250)[41]	9	12	4	9	8	15
	4.8%	4.9%	3.3%	3.2%	4.5%	7.1%

NA, not available.

COMPARISON OF INTRAVENOUS HEPARIN TO SUBCUTANEOUS HEPARIN

In GUSTO, 20 173 patients were randomized to receive streptokinase and either SC or IV heparin with no difference in clinical endpoints, but 36% of the patients randomized to receive SC heparin also received IV heparin. This reduced the power of the study to detect a difference between these two treatment randomizations to 71%. The use of IV heparin for cardiac catheterization, which occurred in 54% of patients, was not counted in this crossover. Thus the comparison of the heparin regimens in the GUSTO trial was between patients randomized to receive IV heparin and patients randomized to receive the ISIS-3 regimen of SC heparin delayed 4 hours after thrombolytic therapy,[35] plus aggressive use of IV heparin. It is perhaps not surprising that no difference was seen in clinical endpoints. However, at 5–7 days, infarct-related artery patency (TIMI-2–3 flow) was 84% in patients randomized to receive IV heparin compared with 72% in patients randomized to receive SC heparin (P<0.05). This difference may well translate into long term clinical benefit, as patency of the infarct-related artery is an independent long term prognostic factor.[6]

Irrespective of the thrombolytic agent an aPTT of 50–70 seconds at 12 hours was associated with the lowest mortality in GUSTO-1,[44] and 50% of patients receiving SC heparin and streptokinase had aPTTs below this range. Thus, it could be argued that only with appropriate IV heparin could most patients achieve an aPTT of 50–70 seconds at 12 hours after intravenous streptokinase.

Adjunctive IV heparin may have a role to play in patients with cardiogenic shock. In GUSTO-1[45] the lowest mortality in patients with cardiogenic shock (54%) was in patients randomized to receive streptokinase and IV heparin. Mortality was 58% in patients randomized to receive streptokinase and SC heparin, and 63% in patients randomized to receive tPA and IV heparin. If such a benefit was statistically robust it could translate into 40 lives saved per 1000 patients treated if intravenous rather than SC heparin was used with streptokinase, and possibly 56 lives saved per 1000 if streptokinase and IV heparin are used in cardiogenic shock rather than an accelerated tPA regimen with IV heparin.[45]

EVIDENCE BASED RECOMMENDATIONS FOR ADJUNCTIVE HEPARIN THERAPY

Our personal approach is to use aspirin and IV heparin with both tPA and streptokinase for both anterior and inferior infarctions. Based on the data from the overview, the totality of data indicates a possible saving of 22 lives per 10 000 patients treated, together with 18 infarctions prevented at a cost of 32 transfusions (which are not a major complication) and 3 non-fatal disabling strokes. It is acknowledged that this is a value judgment. This recommendation is also based on mortality data from the GUSTO-1 cohort which showed that optimal aPTT was 50–70 seconds at 12 hours after thrombolytic therapy, regardless of the choice of agent.

For selective fibrinolytic agents such as tPA it can be recommended that patients receive IV heparin commencing with a 5000 U bolus, followed by an infusion for 48 hours to maintain the aPTT in the above range, based on data from small randomized angiographic studies, cohort data, and relative fibrin specificity. The evidence, albeit imperfect, favours the use of aspirin and adjunctive IV heparin with tPA.

Recommendations for IV heparin as an adjunct to less fibrin specific agents such as streptokinase are similar. While the GUSTO trials show no clinical benefit of randomization to receive IV heparin compared with SC heparin, there is the caveat that 36% of patients randomized to receive SC heparin also received IV therapy. Because of the delay in achieving an aPTT 1.5–2 times normal with SC heparin, we recommend that all patients should receive IV heparin. Based on the concept that the benefit rate is likely to be greater in patients with anterior infarction than in patients with inferior infarction, a recommendation could also be made that patients with anterior infarction should be treated but not patients with inferior infarcts. However, the increased patency rate at 5–7 days with intravenous, compared with SC, heparin in GUSTO[5] suggests a potential mechanistic benefit for IV heparin for all patients.

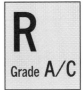

ADJUNCTIVE DIRECT THROMBIN INHIBITORS

A number of direct antithrombins have been shown in animal models to accelerate lysis of platelet rich thrombi, and animal studies have suggested these agents are effective at limiting infarct size.[46-49]

Hirudin

Hirudin is a leech-derived protein with 65 amino acids. It is renally excreted so blood levels may increase in patients with renal impairment. The three initial clinical trials comparing hirudin with heparin[50-52] in patients with AMI were stopped early because of increased intracerebral bleeding in both patients randomized to receive hirudin (2.1%) and patients randomized to receive heparin (1.3%). Both TIMI-9 and GUSTO-2 were recommended using lower doses of heparin (5000 U bolus and 1000 U/h infusion) or hirudin (0.2 mg bolus and 0.1 mg/h infusion) (Table 28.3). These trials included a total of 6054 patients who were thrombolytic-eligible (excluding 1138 patients who were randomized to receive primary angioplasty or tPA). At the doses of hirudin or heparin

Table 28.3 Antithrombin regimens in TIMI-9 and GUSTO-2

	GUSTO-2	TIMI-9	HIT-3
Heparin			
a* Bolus	5000 U	5000 u	70 U/kg
infusion	1000 U/h 96 h	1000 U/h 96 h	15 U/kg/h
	(≥ 80 kg 1300 U/h)	(≥ 80 kg 1300 U/h	
b* Bolus	5000 U	5000 U	
infusion	1000 U/h 3–5 days	1000 U/h 96 h	
	(aPTT 60–85 s)	(aPTT 55–85 s)	
Hirudin			
a* Bolus	0.6 mg/kg	0.6 mg/kg	0.4 mg/kg
infusion	0.2 mg/kg 96 h	0.2 mg/kg 96 h	0.15 mg/kg ≥ 48 h
b* Bolus	0.1 mg/kg	0.1 mg/kg	
infusion	0.1 mg/kg 3–5 days	0.1 mg/kg 96 h	
	(aPTT 60–85 s)	(aPTT 55–85 s)	

* a and b refer to treatment regimens in parts a and b of the GUSTO-2 and TIMI-9 studies; HIT-3 did not adjust its regimen.

Table 28.4 Clinical outcomes in patients with ST elevation in GUSTO-2b and TIMI-9B

	Hirudin	Heparin	Odds ratio	P
Death				
GUSTO-2b	99/1526 (6.5%)	92/1526 (6.0%)	0.93 (0.69–1.24)	0.60
TIMI-9B	76/1450 (5.1%)	90/1507 (6.0%)	1.18 (0.86–1.61)	0.31
SK[a]	59/1005 (5.9%)	57/972 (5.9%)	1.0 (0.69–1.46)	0.99
tPA[a]	116/2006 (5.8%)	125/2061 (6.1%)	1.05 (0.81–1.36)	0.72
Total	175/3011 (5.8%)	182/3033 (6.0%)	1.03 (0.83–1.28)	0.77
Death and MI				
GUSTO-2b	157/1526 (10.3%)	184/1526 (12.1%)	0.84 (0.67–1.05)	0.12
TIMI-9B	144/1507 (9.6%)	141/1485 (9.5%)	1.00 (0.79–1.28)	0.98
SK[a]	92/972 (9.5%)	110/1005 (10.9%)	0.85 (0.64–1.14)	0.28
tPA[a]	209/2061 (10.1%)	215/2006 (10.7%)	0.94 (0.77–1.15)	0.55
Total	301/3033 (9.9%)	325/3011 (10.8%)	0.91 (0.77–1.08)	0.27

[a] Investigator choice of thrombolytic agent.

in GUSTO-2b and TIMI-9B, there was less major bleeding, but there was no statistically significant treatment effect in the individual or combined studies in the ST elevation strata on the primary endpoint of death and myocardial infarction at 1 month (Table 28.4). However, the studies combined do not exclude a possible reduction of death or MI of up to 22% from hirudin.[53,54] Also, there was a 14% reduction in reinfarction ($P = 0.02$).

In GUSTO-2b 1977 patients received streptokinase according to their physician's preference. In this derived subgroup there was a beneficial effect of hirudin for the composite endpoint of death and reinfarction at 30 days (14.9% vs 9.1%, $P = 0.009$). The mortality amongst patients randomized to receive hirudin was 5.0% compared to 7.6% for heparin ($P = 0.09$). The relative reduction in reinfarction in the hirudin group was 50% (8.4% vs 4.2%, $P=0.004$). In TIMI-9B, which randomized 1072 patients treated with streptokinase, the same magnitude of effect (Table 28.4), was not reported. Whether these differences may relate to the timing of adjunctive therapy after administration of thrombolysis or other factors remains to be determined, as hirudin or heparin was commenced at a mean 34 and 50 minutes after administration of thrombolytic therapy in GUSTO-2b and TIMI-9B respectively. In a smaller study the OASIS investigators[55] enrolled 18% of 909 patients with MI, without ST elevation, and randomized patients to 72 hours of IV therapy with either heparin (5000 U bolus, 1200 U/h infusion (1000 U/h infusion if <60 kg) to maintain aPTT between 60–100 seconds; or two hirudin doses (0.2 U/kg bolus and 0.10 U/kg/h infusion (low) or 0.4 U/kg bolus and 0.15 U/kg/h infusion (medium). Fewer patients randomized to receive hirudin had cardiovascular death, new MI or refractory angina (4.4% low dose, 3% medium dose) compared with heparin (6.5%, $P=0.27$ vs low dose; $P=0.047$ vs medium dose). Hirudin does not block ongoing thrombin generation, and it is possible that different dosing regimens or a longer duration of treatment could have been more beneficial.

Hirulog

Hirulog is a 20 amino acid synthetic peptide that directly inhibits free and clot-bound thrombin, and when used in appropriate regimens as an adjuvant during thrombolytic therapy may prevent clot formation and extension and facilitate clot lysis. Hirulog is only 20% renally excreted, and has a half-life of 36 minutes compared with 2–3 hours for hirudin. Because of these differences, the two agents may have different risk–benefit ratios.

No large clinical trials have been performed in AMI with adjunctive hirulog therapy. The first Hirulog Early Reperfusion/Occlusion (HERO) trial treated patients presenting within 12 hours with AMI with aspirin and streptokinase and examined TIMI grade 3 flow at 90–120 minutes after randomization to receive either heparin, low dose hirulog, or high dose hirulog (Table 28.5).[56] In patients presenting within 3 hours in the high dose hirulog groups, TIMI-3 was 70% compared with 52% with heparin ($P=0.02$). Given the established relationship between improved 90 minute TIMI-3 flow and mortality,[3] and that the magnitude of hirulog effect seen in HERO is similar to that achieved with heparin plus tPA compared to streptokinase in GUSTO-1, it is reasonable to hypothesize that hirulog may improve mortality outcomes in AMI as adjunctive therapy to streptokinase. This hypothesis is currently being tested in HERO-2.

ANTITHROMBINS AND CORONARY ANGIOPLASTY

Following the exposure of thrombogenic material during coronary angioplasty, there is marked platelet activation and thrombin generation. A multicenter study of 4098 patients has been performed with the direct thrombin inhibitor hirulog in patients undergoing 'high risk' angioplasty,[57] including patients with postinfarction angina. Amongst this prespecified subgroup of patients with postinfarction angina, those

Table 28.5 Angiographic and clinical outcomes in HERO-1

Drug	TIMI-3 patency 90–120 min	Reocclusion (TIMI-2–3 to 0–1) 48 h	All stroke (hemorrhagic)	ReMI in hospital 35 days	Death in hospital 35 days	All cardiac[a] in hospital 35 days	Major bleeding/ transfusion[b]
Heparin (n=140)	35%	5/71 (7%)	2 (0)	12 (8.6%)	9 (6.4%)	25 (17.9%)	26 (19%)
Hirulog low (n=136)	46%	4/86 (4.6%)	0	8 (5.9%)	8 (5.9%)	19 (14%)	12 (9%) (P<0.02)
Hirulog high (n=136)	48% (P=0.024)	1/75 (1.3%)	2 (1)	6 (4.4%)	6 (4.4%)	17 (12.5%)	14 (10%) (P=NS)

[a] Death, myocardial infarction, cardiogenic shock.

[b] Fall in Hb >30 g/l, transfusion ≥2 units, retroperitoneal or intracranial: femoral artery catheterization site accounted for 42% of major bleeding in the heparin group, 40% in low dose hirulog group and 38% high dose hirulog in group 3.

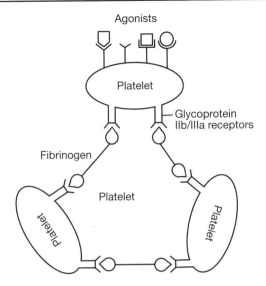

Figure 28.4 Glycoprotein IIb/IIIa receptors and platelet aggregation. Platelets are activated to aggregate by several mechanisms including high shear stress. The most common mechanism is the binding of an agonist (>90 described) to an external receptor which activates signal transduction pathways. This leads to the glycoprotein IIb/IIIa receptor binding fibrinogen which binds to other platelet(s).

randomized to receive hirulog had a reduction in periprocedural infarction compared with patients randomized to receive heparin (2.0% vs 5.1% $P=0.04$). The combined endpoint of death, MI, or bypass surgery (2.6% vs 6.2% $P=0.03$) was also reduced by hirulog in this prespecified subgroup. There was less bleeding in the hirulog group (3.0% vs 11.1%, $P<0.01$), though the heparin regimen aimed to maintain the ACT between 300 and 350 seconds.

ANTIPLATELET AGENTS

Aspirin

In considering the advances in antiplatelet therapy it is important to reflect on the impact of aspirin, which inhibits the cyclooxygenase-I pathway of platelet activation (Figure 28.4). In a meta-analysis aspirin has been shown to reduce the early mortality in patients with acute infarction by approximately one-third, preventing approximately 40 deaths per 1000 patients treated.[58]

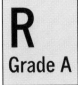

The major evidence for the benefit of aspirin, in association with thrombolytic therapy, is in the ISIS-2 study. This study randomized patients in a placebo controlled double blind manner to IV streptokinase (1.5×10^6 U over 1 hour) or aspirin 160 mg daily immediately, continued for 1 month or both or neither in 17 187 patients with suspected acute myocardial infarction presenting within 24 hours of symptom onset. Aspirin reduced the vascular mortality by 23% at 1 month, and when added to intravenous streptokinase the total reduction in this endpoint was 42%. In addition to the effects of aspirin on vascular mortality in ISIS-2, there was a significant reduction in non-fatal reinfarction (odds ratio 51%) and non-fatal stroke (49%). The benefit of aspirin combined with streptokinase was particularly apparent in patients aged over 70 years, with an absolute reduction of 8% in total mortality (from 23.8 to 15.8%, $P<0.001$). The earlier studies of adjunctive therapy in acute infarction were not powered to show significant effects of aspirin on mortality.[42,59,60]

A meta-analysis in 1992 suggested aspirin reduces reocclusion in the first 2 weeks after infarction.[61] It is perhaps surprising, in view of the effect of aspirin on reinfarction, that there is no convincing evidence that aspirin inhibits late reocclusion.[62,63] The dose of aspirin is important, as there is evidence that gastrointestinal bleeding is increased by increased doses. The bulk of the evidence in favor of a short term benefit of aspirin is from ISIS-2 in which 160 mg daily was used. The earlier studies used higher doses and current recommendations are for an initial dose of 150–325 mg. As cyclooxygenase is normally inhibited by chronic therapy in doses above 40 mg daily, on theoretical grounds any dose above this should be satisfactory. However, the CARS Study[64] which included patients post infarction had lower rates of events in patients taking 160 mg compared with 80 mg of aspirin (with 1 or 3 mg of warfarin; INR ≤ 1.4). Thus it is uncertain what the appropriate (minimum) daily dose for chronic therapy should be.

Aspirin reduces death and non-fatal myocardial infarction in patients presenting with the acute coronary syndrome non-Q wave infarction/unstable angina.[58] Ongoing aspirin therapy also prevents a similar number of deaths over 2 years in patients with a past history of myocardial infarction.[58]

Interestingly, it has been suggested that one of the mechanisms of aspirin's beneficial effect may be anti-inflammatory with a possible reduction of plaque rupture, as it has been recently shown that patients with an elevated C-reactive protein level benefit most.[65]

Glycoprotein IIb/IIIa receptor inhibitors

Inhibition of the glycoprotein IIb/IIIa receptor blocks the final common site of several signal transduction pathways leading to platelet aggregation (Figure 28.4). In current clinical use or in clinical trials are two main types of this drug class: (1) peptides and peptidomimetics and (2) abciximab, initially developed as a human–mouse chimeric monoclonal antibody to the Fc portion of the glycoprotein IIb/IIIa receptor.

Abciximab

Abciximab has been evaluated as an adjunctive agent to angioplasty in several studies including EPIC,[66] CAPTURE[67] and EPILOG.[68] The EPIC[66] study examined the efficacy of abciximab in patients undergoing "high risk", including postinfarction, angioplasty. The primary endpoint was the composite endpoints of death, MI, the need for coronary surgery, repeat angioplasty or stent deployment or intra-aortic balloon to treat ischemia at 30 days. The major benefits in EPIC were in patients who received a bolus and infusion therapy, though this group had the highest rate of major bleeding and the need for transfusion 17% vs 7% ($P<0.01$).

The study did not have sufficient statistical power to determine outcomes in patients with acute ischemic syndromes in general and, in particular, patients with MI. In a subgroup of 64 patients with AMI undergoing angioplasty (44 primary, 22 rescue) there was a trend towards a reduction in the primary composite endpoint (4.5% vs 26.1% $P=0.06$).

The EPILOG study tested lower doses of heparin with bolus and infusions of abciximab; bleeding was less frequent. The 30-day endpoint of death and non-fatal MI was 3.8% in patients randomized to receive low dose heparin and abciximab, compared with 9.1% for those randomized to receive standard heparin and abciximab ($P<0.01$).[68]

The CAPTURE[67] study had a slightly different design to the above studies as patients with unstable angina received 18–24 hours of abciximab prior to angioplasty. CAPTURE showed similar efficacy of abciximab as in EPIC with the 30-day composite endpoint of death/MI reduced from 9.0% to 4.3%, ($P=0.01$).

Administration of abciximab prior to planned primary angioplasty has been reported in a pilot study to achieve TIMI grade 2–3 flow in 46% of patients.[69]

Eptifibatide

In the IMPACT–AMI study patients were treated with tPA, aspirin, and IV heparin and various doses of the peptide eptifibatide (integrelin).[70] Increased TIMI-3 flow rates, compared with placebo, were achieved with the highest dose of integrelin (39% to 66%, $P=0.007$). However, this dose-escalation study contained small patient numbers (180 patients with five doses, including placebo).

Lamifiban

The non-peptide lamifiban has also been evaluated in two studies.[71,72] Using ST segment monitoring to assess patency non-invasively following aspirin and streptokinase or tPA, lamifiban had higher infarct-artery patency defined as ST elevation <200 μV compared to placebo (77% vs 56%, $P=0.019$).[71]

Tirofiban

The non-peptide IIb/IIIa receptor antagonist tirofiban has recently been shown in the Platelet Receptor Inhibition in Acute Ischemic Syndrome Management (PRISM) trial on a background of aspirin therapy to reduce cardiovascular events (death, MI, and ischemia requiring revascularization) in 821 patients presenting with non-Q wave MI compared with heparin therapy.[73] There was a 35% reduction of the composite primary endpoint in these patients at 48 hours (10.0% vs 6.0%, $P=0.007$).[73]

Low molecular weight heparins

Low molecular weight heparins block ongoing thrombin generation as they are potent inhibitors of factor Xa. Factor Xa inhibition is dose dependent and significant inhibition occurs at a comparatively lower dose of lower molecular weight heparin than with standard heparin and thus potentially has a lower risk of bleeding. Low molecular weight heparin also is not inactivated by platelet factor 4 and stimulates release of tissue factor pathway inhibitor from endothelium. In patients with non-Q wave MI/ unstable angina, the TIMI-11A investigators in an open label dose-ranging study[74] have recently found rates of major bleeding of 6.5% and 1.9% in patients receiving 1.2 and 1.0mg/kg enoxaparin SC twice daily, respectively. The lower dose is currently being evaluated in the phase III TIMI-11B study. The possible clinical benefit of lower molecular weight heparin in the management of patients with AMI presenting with ST elevation (or bundle branch block) is currently also being tested as adjunctive therapy to accelerated tPA.

Other newer antithrombins

Other direct antithrombins are undergoing phase II and III studies including, argatroban, inogatran, efegatran, and D-Phe-Pro-Arg-CH$_2$Cl.

Novel anticoagulants that inhibit early stages of the coagulation pathway have been shown experimentally to be effective adjuncts to thrombolytic therapy.[75–77] By complexing with factor VIIa, tissue factor catalyzes the extrinsic activation of factor X and the intrinsic activation of factor IX. Inhibition of tissue factor inhibits the amplification of thrombin formation by preventing the formation of the prothrombinase complex. Recombinant tissue factor pathway inhibition has been shown in dogs to decrease reocclusion after thrombolysis with tPA.

Evidence based recommendations for new antithrombins

The available data does not provide compelling evidence that specific thrombin inhibitors hirudin and hirulog are superior to heparin as adjuncts to thrombolytic therapy. In patients undergoing "high risk", including postinfarction, angioplasty, the data are strong. They have clearly been shown to be as effective as heparin and are easier to administer without the need to monitor aPTT.

There are no trial data regarding clinical outcomes in thrombolytic-eligible patients with ST elevation randomized to receive glycoprotein IIb/IIIa inhibitors or placebo. In a small number of patients undergoing "high risk" angioplasty, including postinfarction, glycoprotein IIb/IIIa antagonists were superior to conventional treatment. These agents have shown a trend to be better than heparin in patients with non-Q wave MI. Further data are required before firm recommendations can be made.

FUTURE DIRECTIONS

In spite of the progress in the understanding of the mechanistic aspects of adjunctive antithrombin therapies in acute ischemic syndromes, particularly reperfusion-eligible patients, many questions remain unanswered. These include whether the dose of existing thrombolytic agents should be modified in combination with either antithrombin agents or glycoprotein IIb/IIIa inhibitors including oral agents, to achieve optimal patency rates with acceptable bleeding risks, particularly intracranial hemorrhage.

Comparisons of percutaneous revascularization techniques including stenting and thrombolytic regimens in the presence of IIb/IIIa antagonists need to be evaluated, and optimal therapies in non reperfusion-eligible patients need to be further defined.

Key points

- There is ongoing thrombin generation in acute ischemic syndromes.
- Thrombolytic therapy results in a procoagulant state.
- Heparin has proven efficacy in the absence of aspirin.
- In the presence of aspirin heparin has a modest affect.
- There is a paucity of data in respect of IV heparin.
- Heparin has several limitations as an antithrombin, including variable pharmacokinetics and pharmacodynamics, relative lack of efficacy on clot bound thrombin and inhibition of only one pathway of platelet activation.
- The new adjunctive antithrombins hirudin and hirulog have a narrow window of benefit/risk.
- The efficacy of hirudin may not have been optimally tested because of its delayed administration after thrombolytic therapy.
- Glycoprotein IIb/IIIa receptor antagonists are effective agents in patients with postinfarction angina undergoing angioplasty. Their use as adjuncts to thrombolytic therapy may require dosage adjustment(s) due to bleeding risks.

REFERENCES

1 French JK, Williams BF, Hart HH et al. Prospective evaluation of eligibility for thrombolytic therapy in acute myocardial infarction. Br Med J 1996; 312:1637–41.

2 The TIMI Study Group. The Thrombolysis in Myocardial Infarction (TIMI) Trial: Phase I findings. N Engl J Med 1985;312:932–6.

3 Simes RJ, Topol EJ, Holmes DR et al. Link between the angiographic substudy and mortality outcomes in a large randomized trial of myocardial reperfusion: importance of early and complete infarct artery reperfusion. Circulation 1995;91:1923–8.

4 Chesebro JH, Knatterud G, Roberts R et al. Thrombolysis in Myocardial Infarction (TIMI) Trial, Phase I: a comparison between intravenous tissue plasminogen activator and intravenous streptokinase: clinical findings through hospital discharge. Circulation 1987;76:142–54.

5 The GUSTO Angiographic Investigators. The effects of tissue plasminogen activator, streptokinase, or both on coronary-artery patency, ventricular function, and survival after acute myocardial infarction. N Engl J Med 1993; 329:1615–22.

6 White HD, Cross DB, Elliott JM, Norris RM, Yee TW. Long term prognostic importance of patency of the infarct-related coronary artery after thrombolytic therapy for acute myocardial infarction. Circulation 1994;89:61–7.

7 ISIS-2 (Second International Study of Infarct Survival) Collaborative Group. Randomised trial of intravenous streptokinase, oral aspirin, both, or neither among 17 187 cases of suspected acute myocardial infarction: ISIS-2. Lancet 1988;ii: 349–60.

8 French JK, White HD. Data on eligibility for thrombolytic treatment can indeed be generalised (Letter). Br Med J 1997;314:301–2.

9 Fibrinolytic Therapy Trialists' (FTT) Collaborative Group. Indications for fibrinolytic therapy in suspected acute myocardial infarction: collaborative overview of early mortality and major morbidity results from all randomised trials of more than 1000 patients. Lancet 1994;343: 311–22.

10 The TIMI-IIIB Investigators. Effects of tissue plasminogen activator and a comparison of early invasive and conservative strategies in unstable angina and non-Q-wave myocardial infarction: results of the TIMI IIIB Trial. Circulation 1994; 89:1545–56.

11 LATE Study Group. Late Assessment of Thrombolytic Efficacy (LATE) study with alteplase 6–24 hours after onset of acute myocardial infarction. Lancet 1993;342:759–66.

12 Davies MJ, Thomas AC. Plaque fissuring: the cause of acute myocardial infarction, sudden ischemic death, and crescendo angina. Br Heart J 1985; 53:363–73.

13 Falk E. Unstable angina with fatal outcome: dynamic coronary thrombosis leading to infarction and/or sudden death: autopsy evidence

of recurrent mural thrombosis with peripheral embolization culminating in total vascular occlusion. *Circulation* 1985;**71**:699–708.

14 Meade TW, Brozovic M, Chakrabarti RR *et al.* Haemostatic function and ischaemic heart disease: principal results of the Northwick Park Heart Study. *Lancet* 1986;**ii**:533–7.

15 Kannel WB, Wolf PA, Castelli WP, D'Agostino RB. Fibrinogen and risk of cardiovascular disease: the Framingham study. *JAMA* 1987;**258**:1183–6.

16 Hirsh J, Raschke R, Warkentin TE *et al.* Heparin: mechanism of action, pharmacokinetics, dosing considerations, monitoring, efficacy, and safety. *Chest* 1995;**108**:258S–275S.

17 Weitz JI, Hudoba M, Massel D, Maraganore J, Hirsh J. Clot-bound thrombin is protected from inhibition by heparin–antithrombin III but is susceptible to inactivation by antithrombin III-independent inhibitors. *J Clin Invest* 1990;**86**:385–91.

18 Eisenberg PR, Miletich JP. Induction of marked thrombin activity by pharmacologic concentrations of plasminogen activators in nonanticoagulated whole blood. *Thromb Res* 1989;**55**:635–43.

19 Lee CD, Mann KG. Activation/inactivation of human coagulation factor V by plasmin. *Blood* 1989;**73**:185–90.

20 Eisenberg PR. Role of heparin in coronary thrombolysis. *Chest* 1992;**101**(Suppl 4): 131S–139S.

21 Eisenberg PR, Sherman LA, Jaffe AS. Paradoxic elevation of fibrin peptide A after streptokinase: evidence for intense thrombosis despite intense fibrinolysis. *J Am Coll Cardiol* 1987;**10**:527–9.

22 Eisenberg PR, Sherman LA, Rich M *et al.* Importance of continued activation of thrombin reflected by fibrinopeptide A to the efficacy of thrombolysis. *J Am Coll Cardiol* 1986;**7**:1255–62.

23 Gulba DC, Barthels M, Westhoff-Bleck M *et al.* Increased thrombin levels during thrombolytic therapy in acute myocardial infarction: relevance for the success of therapy. *Circulation* 1991;**83**: 937–44.

24 Rapold HJ, de Bono D, Arnold AER *et al.* Plasma fibrinopeptide A levels in patients with acute myocardial infarction treated with alteplase: correlation with concomitant heparin, coronary artery patency, and recurrent ischemia. *Circulation* 1992;**85**:928–34.

25 Hsia J, Hamilton WP, Kleiman N *et al.* A comparison between heparin and low-dose aspirin as adjunctive therapy with tissue plasminogen activator for acute myocardial infarction. *N Engl J Med* 1990;**323**:1433–7.

26 Bleich SD, Nichols TC, Schumacher RR *et al.* Effect of heparin on coronary arterial patency after thrombolysis with tissue plasminogen activator in acute myocardial infarction. *Am J Cardiol* 1990; **66**:1412–17.

27 de Bono DP, Simoons ML, Tijssen J *et al.* Effect of early intravenous heparin on coronary patency, infarct size, and bleeding complications after alteplase thrombolysis: results of a randomised double blind European Cooperative Study Group trial. *Br Heart J* 1992;**67**:122–8.

28 Verheugt FWA, Marsh RC, Veen G, Bronzwaer JGF, Zijlstra F. Megadose bolus heparin as reperfusion therapy for acute myocardial infarction: results of the HEAP pilot study (abstract). *Circulation* 1995;**92**:1–415.

29 Wharton TP, McNamara NS, Schmitz JM *et al.* Early coronary patency after high-dose heparin without thrombolytic therapy in 158 patients with acute myocardial infarction (abstract). *Circulation* 1996;**94**(Suppl I):I–553.

30 Hoorntje JCA. Megadose of heparin before primary PTCA. In: The George Washington University 13th International Workshop, Orlando, Florida, 8 November, 1997.

31 Galvani M, Abendschein DR, Ferrini D *et al.* Failure of fixed dose intravenous heparin to suppress increases in thrombin activity after coronary thrombolysis with streptokinase. *J Am Coll Cardiol* 1994;**24**:1445–52.

32 Col J, Decoster O, Hanique G *et al.* Infusion of heparin conjunct to streptokinase accelerates reperfusion of acute myocardial infarction: results of a double blind randomized study (OSIRIS) (abstract). *Circulation* 1992;**86**:I–259.

33 Melandri G, Branzi A, Semprini F *et al.* Enhanced thrombolytic efficacy and reduction of infarct size by simultaneous infusion of streptokinase and heparin. *Br Heart J* 1990;**64**:118–20.

34 The SCATI (Studio sulla Calciparina nell'Angina e nella Trombosi Ventricolare nell'Infarto) Group. Randomised controlled trial of subcutaneous calcium-heparin in acute myocardial infarction. *Lancet* 1989;**ii**:182–6.

35 ISIS-3 (Third International Study of Infarct Survival) Collaborative Group. ISIS-3: a randomised comparison of streptokinase vs tissue plasminogen activator vs anistreplase and of aspirin plus heparin vs aspirin alone among 41 299 cases of suspected acute myocardial infarction. *Lancet* 1992;**339**:753–70.

36 Gruppo Italiano per lo Studio della Sopravvivenza nell'Infarto Miocardico. GISSI-2: a factorial randomised trial of alteplase versus streptokinase and heparin versus no heparin among 12 490 patients with acute myocardial infarction. *Lancet* 1990;**336**:65–71.

37 The GUSTO Investigators. An international randomized trial comparing four thrombolytic strategies for acute myocardial infarction. *N Engl J Med* 1993;**329**:673–82.

38 Turpie AGG, Robinson JG, Doyle DJ *et al.* Comparison of high-dose subcutaneous heparin to prevent left ventricular mural thrombosis in patients with acute transmural anterior myocardial infarction. *N Engl J Med* 1989;**320**: 352–8.

39 Collins R, MacMahon S, Flather M *et al.* Clinical effects of anticoagulant therapy in suspected acute myocardial infarction: systematic overview of randomised trials. *Br Med J* 1996;**313**:652–9.

40 Collins R, Peto R, Baigent C, Sleight P. Aspirin, heparin, and fibrinolytic therapy in suspected acute myocardial infarction (review). *N Engl J Med* 1997;**336**:847–60.

41 O'Connor CM, Meese R, Carney R *et al.* for the DUCCS Group. A randomized trial of heparin in conjunction with anistreplase (anisoylated plasminogen streptokinase activator complex) in acute myocardial infarction: the Duke University Clinical Cardiology Study (DUCCS). *J Am Coll Cardiol* 1994;**23**:11–18.

42 Collins R, Conway M, Alexopoulos D *et al.* for the ISIS Pilot Study Investigators. Randomised factorial trial of high-dose intravenous streptokinase, of oral aspirin and of intravenous heparin in acute myocardial infarction. *Eur Heart J* 1987;**8**:634–42.

43 Topol EJ, Califf RM, Van de Werf F *et al.* Perspectives on large-scale cardiovascular clinical trials for the new millenium. *Circulation* 1997; **95**:1072–82.

44 Granger CB, Hirsh J, Califf RM *et al.* Activated partial thromboplastin time and outcome after thrombolytic therapy for acute myocardial infarction: results from the GUSTO-1 Trial. *Circulation* 1996;**93**:870–8.

45 Holmes DR, Califf RM, Van de Werf F *et al.* Difference in countries' use of resources and clinical outcome for patients with cardiogenic shock after myocardial infarction: results from the GUSTO Trial. *Lancet* 1997;**349**:75–8.

46 Maraganore JM, Bourdon P, Jablonski I, Ramachandran KL, Kenton JW. Design and characterization of hirulogs: a novel class of bivalent peptide inhibitors of thrombin. *Biochemistry* 1990;**29**:7095–101.

47 Collen D, Matsuo O, Stassen JM, Kettner C, Shaw E. *In vivo* studies of a synthetic inhibitor of thrombin. *J Lab Clin Med* 1982;**99**:76–83.

48 Yasuda T, Gold HK, Yaoita H *et al.* Comparative effects of aspirin, a synthetic thrombin inhibitor and a monoclonal antiplatelet glycoprotein IIb/IIIa antibody on coronary artery reperfusion, reocclusion and bleeding with recombinant tissue-type plasminogen activator in a canine preparation. *J Am Coll Cardiol* 1990;**16**:714–22.

49 Haskel EJ, Prager NA, Sobel BE, Abendschein DR. Relative efficacy of antithrombin compared with antiplatelet agents in accelerating coronary thrombolysis and preventing early reocclusion. *Circulation* 1991;**83**:1048–56.

50 The Global Use of Strategies to Open Occluded Coronary Arteries (GUSTO) IIa Investigators. Randomized trial of intravenous heparin versus recombinant hirudin for acute coronary syndromes. *Circulation* 1994;**90**:1631–7.

51 Antman EM for the TIMI-9A Investigators. Hirudin in acute myocardial infarction: safety report from the Thrombolysis and Thrombin Inhibition in Myocardial Infarction (TIMI) 9A trial. *Circulation* 1994;**90**:1624–30.

52 Neuhaus K, Van Essen R, Tebbe U *et al.* Safety observations from the pilot phase of the randomized r-Hirudin for Improvement of Thrombolysis (HIT-III) Study: a study of the Arbeitsgemeinschaft Leitender Kardiologischer Krankenhausärzte (ALKK). *Circulation* 1994;**90**: 1638–42.

53 Antman EM for the TIMI-9B Investigators. Hirudin in acute myocardial infarction: Thrombolysis and Thrombin Inhibition in Myocardial Infarction (TIMI) 9B Trial. *Circulation* 1996;**94**:911–21.

54 The Global Use of Strategies to Open Occluded Coronary Arteries (GUSTO) IIb Investigators. A comparison of recombinant hirudin with heparin for the treatment of acute coronary syndromes. *N Engl J Med* 1996;**335**:775–82.

55 Organization to Assess Strategies for Ischemic Syndromes (OASIS) Investigators. Comparison of the effects of two doses of recombinant hirudin compared with heparin in patients with acute myocardial ischemia without ST elevation: a pilot study. *Circulation* 1997;**96**:769–77.

56 White HD, Aylward PE, Frey M *et al.* A randomized, double-blind comparison of hirulog versus heparin in patients receiving streptokinase and aspirin for acute myocardial infarction (HERO). *Circulation* 1997;**96**:2155–61.

57 Bittl JA, Strony J, Brinker JA *et al.* Treatment with bivalirudin (hirulog) as compared with heparin during coronary angioplasty for unstable or postinfarction angina. *N Engl J Med* 1995;**333**: 764–9.

58 Antiplatelet Trialists' Collaboration. Collaborative overview of randomised trials of antiplatelet therapy – I: prevention of death, myocardial infarction, and stroke by prolonged antiplatelet therapy in various categories of patients. *Br Med J* 1994;**308**:81–106.

59 Elwood PC, Williams WO. A randomized controlled trial of aspirin in the prevention of early mortality in myocardial infarction. *J R Coll Gen Pract* 1979;**29**:413–16.

60 Verheugt FW, Kupper AJ, Galema TW, Roos JP. Low dose aspirin after early thrombolysis in

anterior wall acute myocardial infarction. *Am J Cardiol* 1988;**61**:904–6.

61 Roux S, Christeller S, Ludin E. Effects of aspirin on coronary reocclusion and recurrent ischemia after thrombolysis: a meta-analysis. *J Am Coll Cardiol* 1992;**19**:671–7.

62 Meijer A, Verheugt FWA, Werter CJPJ, Lie KI, van der Pol JMJ, van Eenige MJ. Aspirin versus coumadin in the prevention of reocclusion and recurrent ischemia after successful thrombolysis: a prospective placebo-controlled angiographic study: results of the APRICOT Study. *Circulation* 1993;**87**:1524–30.

63 White HD, French JK, Hamer AW, Brown MA, Williams BF, Ormiston JA *et al.* Frequent reocclusion of patient infarct-related arteries between 4 weeks and 1 year: effects of antiplatelet therapy. *J Am Coll Cardiol* 1995;**25**:218–23.

64 Coumadin Aspirin Reinfarction Study (CARS) Investigators. Randomised double-blind trial of fixed low-dose warfarin with aspirin after myocardial infarction. *Lancet* 1997;**350**:389–96.

65 Ridker PM, Cushman M, Stampfer MJ, Tracy RP, Hennekens CH. Inflammation, aspirin, and the risk of cardiovascular disease in apparently healthy men. *N Engl J Med* 1997;**336**:973–9.

66 The EPIC (Evaluation of IIb/IIa Platelet Receptor Antagonist (7E3) in Preventing Ischemic Complications) Investigators. Use of a monoclonal antibody directed against the platelet glycoprotein IIb/IIIa receptor in high-risk coronary angioplasty. *N Engl J Med* 1994;**330**:956–61.

67 The CAPTURE (Chimeric 7E3 Antiplatelet. Therapy in Unstable Angina Refractory to Standard Treatment) Investigators. Randomised placebo-controlled trial of abciximab before and during coronary intervention in refractory unstable angina: the CAPTURE study. *Lancet* 1997;**349**:1429–35.

68 The EPILOG (Evaluation of PTCA to Improve Long-term Outcome by c7E3 GPIIb/IIIa Receptor Blockade) Investigators. Platelet glycoprotein IIb/IIIa receptor blockade and low-dose heparin during percutaneous coronary revascularization. *N Engl J Med* 1997;**336**:1689–96.

69 Gold HK, Garabedian HD, Dinsmore RE *et al.* Restoration of coronary flow in myocardial infarction by intravenous chimeric 7E3 antibody without exogenous plasminogen activators: observations in animals and humans. *Circulation* 1997;**95**:1755–9.

70 Ohman EM, Kleiman NS, Gacioch G *et al.* Combined accelerated tissue-plasminogen activator and platelet glycoprotein IIb/IIIa integrin receptor blockade with integrilin in acute myocardial infarction: results of a randomized, placebo-controlled, dose-ranging trial. *Circulation* 1997;**95**:846–54.

71 Moliterno DJ, Harrington RA, Krucoff MW *et al.* More complete and stable reperfusion with platelet IIb/IIIa antagonism plus thrombolysis for acute myocardial infarction: the PARADIGM trial (abstract). *Circulation* 1996;**94**(Suppl I):I–553.

72 PARAGON Investigators. A randomized trial of potent platelet IIb/IIIa antagonism, heparin, or both in patients with unstable angina: the PARAGON Study (abstract). *Circulation* 1996; **94**(Suppl I):I–553.

73 White HD, on behalf of the Platelet Receptor Inhibition in Ischemic Syndrome Management (PRISM) Study Investigators. The Platelet Receptor Inhibition in Ischemic Syndrome Management (PRISM) Study. Proceedings of the American College of Cardiology 46th Annual Scientific Sessions, Anaheim, Ca.

74 The TIMI IIA Trial Investigators. Dose ranging trial of enoxaparin for unstable angina: results of TIMI IIA. *J Am Coll Cardiol* 1997;**29**:1474–82.

75 Abendschein DR, Meng YY, Torr-Brown S, Sobel BE. Maintenance of coronary patency after fibrinolysis with tissue factor pathway inhibitor. *Circulation* 1995;**92**:944–9.

76 Sitko GR, Ramjit DR, Stabilito II *et al.* Conjunctive enhancement of enzymatic thrombolysis and prevention of thrombotic reocclusion with the selective factor Xa inhibitor, tick anticoagulant peptide. *Circulation* 1992;**85**:805–15.

77 Gruber A, Harker LA, Hanson SR, Kelly AB, Griffin JH. Antithrombotic effects of combining activated protein C and urokinase in non-human primates. *Circulation* 1991;**84**:2454.

Pain relief, general management, and other adjunctive treatments

29

ALDO P MAGGIONI,
ROBERTO LATINI,
GIANNI TOGNONI,
PETER SLEIGHT

The prognosis of patients admitted to hospital with acute myocardial infarction (AMI) has improved greatly since the introduction of reperfusion therapies into clinical practice. Several trials testing different thrombolytic agents, aspirin, and more recently, primary PTCA have shown that mortality can be reduced by 20–30% when these therapies are begun in the first few hours after the onset of symptoms of AMI. The favourable effects were proportional to the patency rates obtained. Although there is no objective evidence for mortality reduction, pain relief, oxygen, bedrest, and adjunctive therapies should be considered to reduce clinical symptoms and further improve prognosis.

PAIN RELIEF

The relief of pain is a priority in patients with AMI, not only for humane reasons, but also because pain activates the sympathetic nervous system increasing cardiac work and myocardial oxygen consumption. Two approaches are used: (a) reduction of ischemia and (b) direct analgesia. Nitroglycerin by the sublingual route or by IV infusion is the most commonly used drug to reduce pain due to ischemia (see Nitrates below). Few controlled data are available, so the recommendations are based mainly on empiricism and personal expertise.

Among direct analgesics, morphine is the drug of choice, while meperidine and pentazocine can be substituted in patients with documented hypersensitivity to morphine. Morphine, besides its analgesic effect, has useful hemodynamic actions, including peripheral vasodilation without a decrease of left ventricular filling pressure. This action, together with central reduction of tachypnea, can be particularly useful in patients with pulmonary edema.[1–4]

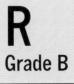

Effective analgesia should not be delayed because of the fear of masking the effects of anti-ischemic therapy with recommended agents (i.e. thrombolytics, beta-blockers, aspirin, nitrates). Morphine is given at doses of 4–8 mg IV and repeated every 5–15 minutes in doses of 2–8 mg until pain is relieved. Morphine also reduces anxiety, thereby decreasing metabolic demands of the heart during the early critical phase. The decrease in heart rate resulting from the reduction of sympathetic tone and the vagomimetic action of morphine contributes to the reduction of anxiety. Usually opioids are sufficient and tranquillizers are not needed.

Adverse reactions to morphine such as severe vomiting, hypotension, and respiratory depression may limit its administration. Hypotension (i.e. systolic blood pressure <100 mmHg) can be minimized by keeping the patient supine with elevated lower extremities. In the case of excessive bradycardia, atropine may be administered intravenously (0.5–1.5 mg). Depression of respiration seldom occurs and can be treated with intravenous naloxone (0.1–0.2 mg, repeated after 15 minutes if necessary). Nausea and vomiting, if disturbing, may be treated with a phenothiazine.

A double-blind randomized trial on 69 patients[5] showed that inhaled nitrous oxide can decrease pain in the absence of hemodynamic changes or other major adverse events.

The widespread use of reperfusion therapy early after AMI has decreased the intensity and duration of pain, which is largely due to ongoing cardiac ischemia. The additional use of IV beta-blockers[6,7] further decreases the extent of pain by reducing cardiac work.

New approaches to analgesia after AMI include synthetic and semisynthetic analgesics like fentanyl and sufentanyl and thoracic epidural anesthesia, but clinical experience is too limited to recommend regimens and modalities.

GENERAL MANAGEMENT

Oxygen

R

Grade B

Experimental studies have shown that breathing oxygen could decrease myocardial injury;[8] moreover, in patients with AMI the administration of oxygen reduced ST segment elevation.[9] It is assumed that oxygen breathing might improve the ventilation/perfusion mismatch which may be seen in AMI patients. Arterial Po_2 is reduced for about 48 h in many uncomplicated cases of AMI.[10]

There are no objective randomized trials on the benefit of oxygen breathing after AMI. However, in the presence of severe hypoxemia oxygen is recommended, while in uncomplicated cases its use should probably be limited to the first day or less.

Oxygen therapy is indicated if monitored oxygen saturation is lower than 90%. In complicated AMI, with severe heart failure, pulmonary edema or mechanical complications, supplemental oxygen is not sufficient and continuous positive pressure breathing or tracheal intubation with mechanical ventilation are sometimes required.[11]

Excessive oxygen can cause systemic vasoconstriction with a consequent increase in cardiac workload, an important consideration in uncomplicated patients.

Bedrest

Bedrest has been traditionally advised for patients with AMI on the assumption that it would decrease cardiac workload. However, it is now recognized that the intensive use of recommended treatments (i.e. thrombolysis, intravenous beta-blockade, aspirin) allows a much shorter stay in bed for AMI patients. This may decrease the risk of thromboembolism and help to prevent the adverse effects of deconditioning.[12]

Prophylactic use of lidocaine (lignocaine)

The observation that life threatening arrhythmias occur within the first 24–48 hours of onset of AMI in a substantial proportion of patients led to the hypothesis that the prophylactic administration of lidocaine could prevent or reduce the incidence of ventricular fibrillation and resulting early mortality.[13]

However, an overview of 14 controlled trials testing the effects of prophylactic lidocaine (administered by the intramuscular or IV route) on a total of 9155 patients confirmed a significant reduction of 35% in the rate of ventricular fibrillation, but a strong trend to an increase of 38% in early mortality (OR 1.38, 95% CI 0.98–1.95).[14] The increase in mortality appeared to be caused by bradyarrhythmias, advanced atrioventricular block and asystole. In view of these findings, prophylactic lidocaine is no longer considered as a standard treatment in patients with AMI, but is reserved for those patients who have already experienced ventricular fibrillation (VF).

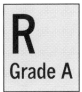

OTHER ADJUNCTIVE TREATMENTS (Table 29.1)

We will now discuss adjunctive drug therapy with beta-blockers, ACE inhibitors, nitrates, magnesium, and calcium-antagonists. The results of published randomized trials which were of adequate size to show reliable data in terms of mortality, together with overviews of the data, will be summarized. We will also indicate areas of doubt.

Beta-blockers

RATIONALE

Beta-blockers reduce oxygen demand by lowering heart rate and blood pressure and decreasing myocardial wall stress, thereby limiting infarct size, reducing cardiac rupture, and improving ventricular function and mortality.[15] By their beta-adrenergic antagonist properties, they can also prevent the life-threatening ventricular arrhythmias which are related to the increased adrenergic activity occurring in the first hours after the onset of AMI.[16]

EVIDENCE FROM TRIALS AND OVERVIEWS OF EARLY IV BETA-BLOCKADE

Studies testing the effects of early IV beta-blockade on the mortality of patients with AMI show consistent results.[17] Available data on more than 27 000 patients from 27 trials show that the mortality rate of the patients allocated to the active treatment was significantly reduced by about 14% in comparison with placebo-allocated patients (from 4.3% to 3.7%; in absolute terms, 6 lives saved per 1000 patients treated with beta-blockers).[18] The largest study testing this treatment, the ISIS-1 trial, showed that the

Table 29.1 Other adjunctive therapies: summary of evidence

	Study	n	Follow-up duration	Mortality (%)		P value	NNT
				Treated	Control		
Beta-blockers							
ISIS-1[19]	LSRCT	16 027	7 d	3.9	4.6	0.04	143
Sleight et al.[18]	OV	27 536	7 d	3.7	4.3	0.03	167
ACE inhibitors							
Early unselected strategy							
GISSI-3[32]	LSRCT	19 394	42 d	6.4	7.2	0.03	125
ISIS-4[33]	LSRCT	58 050	35 d	7.2	7.7	0.02	200
ACE-i MICG[35]	OV	98 469	30 d	7.1	7.6	0.004	200
Late selected strategy							
SAVE[36]	LSRCT	2 231	42 mth (mean)	20.4	24.6	0.019	24
AIRE[37]	LSRCT	2 006	15 mth (mean)	17.0	23.0	0.002	17
TRACE[38]	LSRCT	1 749		34.7	62.3	0.001	13
Nitrates							
Yusuf et al.[49]	OV	3 041	Inhospital	13.3	18.9	0.002	18
GISSI-3[32]	LSRCT	19 394	42 d	6.5	6.9	NS	—
ISIS-4[33]	LSRCT	58 050	35 d	7.3	7.5	NS	—
Overview[33]	OV	81 908	35 d	7.4	7.7	0.03	333
Calcium antagonists							
Teo et al.[56]	OV	20 342	—	9.6	9.3	NS	—
Magnesium							
Teo et al.[61]	OV	1 301	Inhospital	3.8	8.2	0.001	23
LIMIT-2[62]	LSRCT	2 316	28 d	7.8	10.4	0.04	42
ISIS-4[33]	LSRCT	58 050	35 d	7.6	7.2	NS	—
Overview[33]	OV	61 860	35 d	7.6	7.5	NS	—

LSRCT, large scale randomized clinical trials; OV, overview; NNT, number of patients needed to treat to save 1 life.

mortality reduction by atenolol treatment in patients with AMI was concentrated in the first day or two from the onset of AMI symptoms.[19] Further, this study suggested that reduction in cardiac rupture and cardiac arrest were the most notable changes in early death associated with beta-blocker therapy.[20] These observations may be considered as the rationale for the combined use of beta-blockers and thrombolytics, which are both known to reduce mortality. In particular, in the first few days from the onset of AMI, beta-blockers may reduce cardiac rupture, the incidence of which may be increased by thombolytic induced hemorrhage of infarcted myocardium.[21,22]

RECOMMENDATIONS

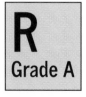

R
Grade A

All patients with AMI, in the absence of specific contraindications, should be treated with beta-blockers within 24 hours from the onset of symptoms and treatment should be continued for at least 2 years. Clear contraindications are pulmonary edema, asthma, hypotension, bradycardia or advanced atrioventricular block. Even in the absence of trials of adequate size testing specifically the effects of the combination of beta-blockers and thrombolytics, pathophysiological premises, observational data, and the few controlled studies suggest that this treatment should be considered in association with reperfusion treatment with thrombolysis. In the GISSI-2 trial IV atenolol was used in conjunction with thrombolytics in 48% of the patients.

LACK OF RANDOMIZED TRIALS OF EARLY BETA-BLOCKADE IN THE ERA OF REPERFUSION

The trials testing the effects on mortality of beta-blockers in patients with AMI were conducted in the early 1980s, before the widespread use of reperfusion therapy. Trials formally testing the effects of the combination of beta-blockers and thrombolytics are few and underpowered to provide reliable data in terms of mortality reduction. The only data available are from the TIMI-2B trial, in which 1434 patients, all treated with tPA and aspirin, were randomized to receive immediate or delayed (6–8 days) oral metoprolol.[23] Total mortality rate at 6 and 42 days was not significantly decreased by the immediate treatment, but the number of deaths was smaller, and the rate of non-fatal reinfarction was reduced in the group receiving immediate metoprolol.

LONG TERM USE

The effects of beta-blocker therapy started after the acute phase of myocardial infarction (5–28 days from the onset of symptoms) have been tested among more than 35 000 patients not receiving a reperfusion therapy in several placebo-controlled trials.[24] Overall, long term mortality and reinfarction was reduced by 20–25%.

Timolol, metoprolol, and propranolol were the most extensively studied drugs.[25–27] In the Norwegian Multicenter Study,[25] patients allocated to timolol showed a 39% mortality reduction and a 28% reinfarction reduction. The initial benefit persisted for at least 72 months in the patients who continued timolol treatment after trial termination. Similar results have been obtained by the Beta-Blocker Heart Attack Trial (BHAT),[26] in which 3837 patients were allocated to propranolol or placebo. After 25 months of treatment overall mortality was reduced by 28%. Subgroup analysis showed that the beneficial effects of beta-blockers were apparent among the various subgroups, but the magnitude of the benefit was greater in high risk patients, i.e. those with large or anterior AMI or with signs or symptoms of moderate left ventricular dysfunction.

Definite contraindications to beta-blocker therapy are pulmonary edema, asthma, severe hypotension, bradycardia or advanced atrioventricular block. Evidence from trials and overviews suggests that all patients with AMI who do not have clear contraindications should be treated with intravenous beta-blockers within 24 hours from the onset of symptoms. If tolerated, the treatment should be continued for at least 2–3 years, and perhaps longer.

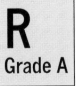

Despite the clear evidence of benefit, observational studies showed that in clinical practice beta-blockers are generally underused, only 36–42% of patients receiving a beta-blocker at discharge.[28]

A debate is still open about whether beta-blockers should be prescribed to all patients without contraindications or whether they should be given only to the patients at moderate to high risk who have the most to gain from a long term treatment.

ACE inhibitors

RATIONALE

The rationale behind this strategy is based mainly on the fact that activation of the renin–angiotensin system occurs during the very early phase of MI, carrying deleterious consequences, including an increase of peripheral resistance and heart rate, decrease of coronary perfusion, and alteration in endogenous fibrinolytic activity.[29,30]

EVIDENCE FROM TRIALS AND OVERVIEWS

After the disappointing results of the CONSENSUS-2 trial,[31] which did not show a benefit from enalapril treatment, the results of GISSI-3 and ISIS-4 studies were published.[32,33] In the GISSI-3 trial, 6-week total mortality was significantly lower in the patients treated with lisinopril: 6-week lisinopril treatment significantly reduced mortality from 7.2% to 6.4% (in absolute terms 8 lives saved per 1000 treated patients).[32]

The favorable results on mortality shown by the GISSI-3 study have been confirmed by the larger ISIS-4 trial. During the first 5 weeks there were 2088 (7.19%) deaths recorded among 29 028 captopril-allocated patients compared with 2231 (7.69%) among 29 022 patients allocated placebo.[33] This 7% relative reduction in total mortality was statistically significant ($2P = 0.02$) and corresponded in absolute terms to 5 fewer deaths per 1000 patients treated with captopril for 1 month. The reduction in total mortality shown by CCS-1[34] was similar to that demonstrated by the larger GISSI-3 and ISIS-4 trials, but statistical significance was not achieved, presumably because of inadequate sample size.

An overview of the trials testing an early unselected approach with ACE inhibitors in patients with AMI has been recently presented.[35] Information was available for 98 496 patients. This overview showed that immediate treatment is safe, well tolerated and that it produces a small, but significant reduction of 30-day mortality. This benefit is quantifiable as about 5 extra lives saved for every 1000 patients treated with ACE inhibitors early after the onset of AMI.

With respect to the safety profile, persistent hypotension and renal dysfunction were (as expected) reported significantly more often in the patients treated with ACE inhibitors than in corresponding controls.

The overview also confirmed the important benefit achievable with early ACE inhibitor treatment. Of the total 239 lives saved by early ACE inhibitor treatment, 200 were saved in the first week after AMI.

The "selective" strategy of starting ACE inhibitors some days after AMI only in patients with clinical heart failure and/or objective evidence of left ventricular dysfunction was tested in three trials (SAVE, AIRE, TRACE), involving about 6000 patients overall.[36–38] These trials consistently showed that long term ACE inhibitor treatment in this selected population of patients was associated with a significant reduction of mortality.

CONTROVERSY: ASPIRIN AND ACE INHIBITORS

It has been proven that part of the hypotensive/unloading effect of ACE inhibitors is attributable to increased synthesis of vasodilatory prostaglandins such as PGE_2.[39]

Some experimental findings have shown that the concomitant administration of salicylate reduced the effectiveness of ACE inhibitors in patients with congestive heart failure.[40,41] However, the appropriateness of extrapolating these data to clinical practice is questionable since: (a) the SOLVD investigators have recently concluded that aspirin use was beneficial in both symptomatic and asymptomatic patients with left ventricular dysfunction, (b) more recent studies have reached opposite conclusions on the interaction between ACE–aspirin in post-AMI patients with heart failure[42] and (c) in relatively unselected AMI patients enrolled in the GISSI-3 trial there was a beneficial effect from ACE inhibitors although almost all patients received aspirin.[43] In conclusion, it seems that the pharmacologic interaction between salicylates and ACE inhibitors is devoid of major clinical relevance in the setting of AMI, both in terms of reduction of the unloading effect of ACE inhibitors and in terms of adverse effects on renal function. Therefore in the absence of adequate data from randomized controlled trials (RCTs), both ACE inhibitors and aspirin may be safely administered in the early phase of AMI. Since patients with left ventricular (LV) dysfunction have a mortality rate of about 50% if they experience a new infarction, prevention with aspirin should not be abandoned on the basis of inadequate data.

RECOMMENDATIONS

ACE inhibitor treatment should be started during the first day following AMI in most patients after timely and careful observation of the patient's hemodynamic and clinical status, and after administration of routinely recommended treatments (thrombolysis, aspirin and beta-blockers). If echocardiography shortly before discharge shows LV dysfunction, the treatment should be continued for a long period of time. In the patients showing neither clinical symptoms nor objective evidence of LV dysfunction, the treatment can be stopped and ventricular function re-evaluated after an adequate period of time.

R
Grade A

The main contraindications to early ACE inhibitor treatment are hypotension, bilateral renal artery stenosis, severe renal failure or a history of cough or angioedema attributed to previous treatment with ACE inhibitors. Caution is needed in patients on prior high dose diuretic (>50 mg furosemide/day).

NEED FOR ACE INHIBITOR TREATMENT IS LESS CLEAR IN LOW RISK PATIENTS

The most debated issue raised after the publication of the GISSI-3, ISIS-4, and CCS-1 trials was how to integrate the results of early ACE inhibitor use with the impressive results of the selective approach, where ACE inhibitors are started some days after AMI, only in the patients at high risk such as those with signs or symptoms of LV dysfunction. The consensus of a meeting of investigators in the field[44] was that if the hemodynamics were satisfactory AMI patients could benefit from earlier treatment than that used in SAVE, AIRE, and TRACE. There was still some disagreement whether *all* patients should be treated or just clinically high risk patients.

The role of long term treatment with ACE inhibitors for secondary prevention among patients with preserved LV function is currently being tested in large scale randomized clinical trials.

Nitrates

RATIONALE

Experimental and clinical studies showed that nitrates can reduce oxygen demand and myocardial wall stress during AMI by reducing pre- and afterload.[45] Further, nitrates can increase coronary blood supply to the ischemic muscle by reducing coronary vasospasm.[46] These favorable effects have been demonstrated in both animals and humans, to reduce infarct size and improve left ventricular function.[47,48]

EVIDENCE FROM TRIALS AND OVERVIEWS

Controlled clinical trials and overviews provide conflicting results. At the beginning of the 1980s, Yusuf *et al.* carried out a meta-analysis of seven small trials testing IV nitroglycerin and three trials testing IV nitroprusside. Overall, the results on 2041 patients showed that nitrate treatment was able to reduce mortality by about 35%.[49]

More recently, the effects of different nitrate treatments in patients with AMI has been tested in two large scale mortality trials enrolling more than 77 000 patients, receiving currently recommended concomitant therapies (90% received aspirin and about 70% thrombolysis).[32,33] Both trials showed that routine nitrate use does not produce an improvement in survival, either in the total population of patients with AMI or in the subgroups at different risk of death. A large number of patients allocated to the control groups in these trials received out-of-protocol nitrate treatment because of a specific indication (angina, heart failure, hypertension), possibly obscuring a true benefit in terms of mortality reduction. Accordingly the ISIS-4 investigators analyzed the effects of nitrates in the subgroup of patients not receiving out-of-protocol nitrate treatment. The results of this subanalysis confirmed the main results of the study.[33]

A further trial, ESPRIM, of the nitric oxide donor molsidomine also failed to show any mortality benefit in AMI patients.[50] A further overview of all existing data (the first ten small trials plus the two recent large scale studies) confirms the negative results in terms of mortality reduction.[33]

RECOMMENDATIONS

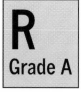

R

Grade A

Nitrates are not a recommended treatment for all patients with AMI. However, nitrates are confirmed to be well tolerated even in the context of the other treatments (beta-blockers, aspirin, thrombolysis, ACE inhibitors), suggesting that their utilization, limited to the patients with specific indications such as angina or pump failure, is safe and likely beneficial in the treatment of ischemic chest pain and pump failure. Definite data on the short term mortality benefit of IV nitroglycerin started in the first 24 hours after the beginning of AMI symptoms are not available.

UNCLEAR INTERACTION WITH ACE INHIBITORS

The results of the GISSI-3 trial suggest that nitrates can produce some additive beneficial effect when used in combination with ACE inhibitors but this was not seen on ISIS-4. Additional trials should be conducted to confirm or reject this hypothesis.

Calcium-channel blockers

RATIONALE

Calcium-channel blockers can reduce oxygen demand by lowering blood pressure and reducing contractility;[51] verapamil and diltiazem also reduce heart rate.[52] These mechanisms could be beneficial in patients during AMI.

EVIDENCE FROM TRIALS AND OVERVIEWS

Trials testing nifedipine at different dosages either in the acute phase of MI or after discharge showed a non-significant increase of mortality.[53] Controlled clinical trials testing calcium-channel blockers other than dihydropyridines, such as diltiazem or verapamil, have also found no significant reduction of mortality. However, the DAVIT-2 trial did show a 20% reduction of the combined endpoint of cardiovascular mortality and reinfarction.[54] Similarly, the largest trial testing diltiazem showed a 23% reduction of deaths from cardiac causes and reinfarction in the subgroup of patients without signs of pulmonary congestion, while in the subgroup of patients with pulmonary congestion a 41% increase of these events was observed.[55] An overview of the 24 trials testing any kind of calcium-channel blocker in patients with AMI showed a non-significant increase of mortality of about 4%.[56]

RECOMMENDATIONS

Since individual trials and overviews revealed no statistically significant evidence of harm or benefit in terms of mortality reduction, these drugs are not recommended as standard therapy in patients in the acute phase of MI. Verapamil or diltiazem may be useful after MI in patients intolerant of beta-blockade. Despite the consistent negative results of trials and overviews, the rate of use of calcium-channel blockers remains high.[28,57]

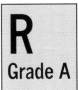

NEWER DRUGS

Few data are available concerning the effects either of long-acting nifedipine or of newer, more selective dihydropyridines, such as felodipine or amlodipine or of new agents from this class of drugs, such as mibefradil. New trials of these drugs are planned or under way.

Magnesium

RATIONALE

In experimental models of AMI, high plasma levels of magnesium can prevent extensive myocardial damage, possibly through inhibition of the inward current of calcium in ischemic cardiac cells, and the reduction of coronary tone.[58,59] Infusion of magnesium in experimental models of AMI can increase the threshold for malignant arrhythmias, reducing the occurrence of ventricular fibrillation.[60] In humans, high plasma levels of magnesium reduce peripheral vascular resistance and increase cardiac output without affecting myocardial oxygen consumption. Thus, infusions of magnesium started early during AMI could reduce infarct size, prevent life threatening arrhythmias and improve survival.

EVIDENCE FROM TRIALS AND OVERVIEWS

Conflicting results have been provided by the trials in which intravenous infusion of magnesium has been tested. A first overview by Teo *et al.* of seven trials among about 1300 patients showed that mortality was reduced by 58% (from 8.2% to 3.8%) by an early intravenous infusion of magnesium.[61] The greatest part of the benefit was due to the reduction of life threatening ventricular arrhythmias. These favourable data encouraged the conduct of a large single centre study, LIMIT-2, in which 2316 patients were randomized to receive IV magnesium or placebo.[62] This study showed that the 28-day mortality rate was significantly reduced by 24% ($2P = 0.04$) (but with a lower confidence interval near zero). No difference was observed in terms of ventricular arrhythmias, but surprisingly a reduction in clinical heart failure was observed. More recently the results of the ISIS-4 trial on more than 58 000 patients did not confirm that intravenous magnesium can reduce mortality.[33] As expected, the current overview of all the existing data is dominated by the results of ISIS-4.[33]

RECOMMENDATIONS

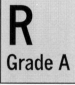

Intravenous magnesium cannot be recommended for routine use for patients with AMI. Its use should be limited to the patients with specific indications (i.e. patients with ventricular arrhythmias and prolonged QT interval, or those with high blood pressure not controlled by usual therapy).

A NEW TRIAL

Experimental studies suggested in animal models that magnesium is effective only if administered before thrombolysis, thereby preventing reperfusion injury.[63,64] This hypothesis is supported by animal models of AMI and by the LIMIT-2 trial which showed a reduction of the cases of heart failure after magnesium infusion.

Even though the ISIS-4 trial showed that magnesium treatment was not effective in any of the studied subgroups of patients, including those treated with thrombolysis within 6 hours from the onset of symptoms, the possibility that magnesium treatment can limit reperfusion injury after recanalization therapy has not been formally tested.

Because of this disparity between ISIS-4 and LIMIT-2, a further trial (MAGIC) is planned in selected patients.

CONCLUSIONS

The therapeutic approaches discussed in the chapter can provide benefits only to patients who survive long enough to reach a monitored bed. The potential reduction of mortality obtainable with the use of evidence based therapies is applicable to only about half of the population of patients suffering an AMI.[65]

Besides research efforts aimed at designing new strategies to further improve survival, the challenges are several:

1. To broaden the correct use of evidence based treatments for the patients reaching the hospital.
2. To apply these or new treatments to the subgroup of patients generally excluded from randomized clinical trials (elderly, patients with comorbidities, etc.).
3. To reduce the number of patients who die before reaching the hospital.

APPENDIX: LONG TERM USE OF ASPIRIN AFTER THE ACUTE PHASE OF MYOCARDIAL INFARCTION

Besides the favorable effects in terms of mortality reduction when used in the first 24 h from the onset of symptoms of AMI,[66] long term use of aspirin in the postinfarction period also results in a significant reduction of morbidity and mortality.

The Antiplatelet Trialists' Collaborative Group reviewed all the long term trials of antiplatelet agents in secondary prevention.[67] Six randomized, placebo-controlled trials tested the effects of aspirin started between 1 week and 7 years after the initial infarct. Vascular mortality, non-fatal reinfarction and non-fatal stroke rates were significantly reduced respectively by 13%, 31%, and 42% among the patients allocated to aspirin in comparison with the placebo-allocated patients. The beneficial effects on major vascular events were apparent in all subgroups examined.

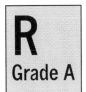

The overview also shows that, although other antiplatelet agents, such as dipyridamole or sulphinpyrazone, have been used in postinfarct patients, there is no evidence that they can be more efficacious than aspirin alone.

The benefits of aspirin were seen to be similar in the trials which evaluated doses from 160 mg to 1500 mg daily. These observations suggest that it is reasonable to recommend aspirin at 160–325 mg/day, starting early after the onset of symptoms of AMI and continuing for a long period of time (probably lifelong). A trial in patients with stable angina recently showed that lower doses of aspirin (75 mg daily) were associated with a significant reduction of 34% of non-fatal MI and sudden death.[68] These data suggest that lower doses of aspirin can be effective with fewer side effects.

REFERENCES

1 Roth A, Keren G, Gluck A, Braun S, Laniado S. Comparison of nalbuphine hydrochloride versus morphine sulfate for acute myocardial infarction with elevated pulmonary artery wedge pressure. *Am J Cardiol* 1988;**62**:551–5.

2 Semenkovich CF, Jaffe AS. Adverse effects due to morphine sulfate. Challenge to previous clinical doctrine. *Am J Med* 1985;**79**:325–30.

3 Timmis AD, Rothman MT, Henderson MA, Geal PW, Chamberlain DA. Haemodynamic effects of intravenous morphine in patients with acute myocardial infarction complicated by severe left ventricular failure. *Br Med J* 1980;**280**:980–2.

4 Nielsen JR, Pedersen KE, Dahlstrom CG *et al.* Analgesic treatment in acute myocardial infarction. A controlled clinical comparison of morphine, nicomorphine and pethidine. *Acta Med Scand* 1984;**215**:349–54.

5 Thompson PL, Lown B. Nitrous oxide as an analgesic in acute myocardial infarction. *JAMA* 1976;**235**:924–7.

6 Waagstein F, Hjalmarson A. Double blind study of the effect of cardioselective beta-blockade on chest pain in acute myocardial infarction. *Acta Med Scand* 1975;**587**:201–8.

7 Ramsdale DR, Faragher EB, Bennett DH *et al.* Ischemic pain relief in patients with acute myocardial infarction by intravenous atenolol. *Am Heart J* 1982;**103**(4pt1):459–67.

8 Maroko PR, Radvany P, Braunwald E, Hale SL. Reduction of infarct size by oxygen inhalation following acute coronary occlusion. *Circulation* 1975;**52**:360–8.

9 Madias JE, Hood WB Jr. Reduction of precordial ST-segment elevation in patients with anterior myocardial infarction by oxygen breathing. *Circulation* 1976;**53**(Suppl I):I-198–I-200.

10 Fillmore SJ, Shapiro M, Killip T. Arterial oxygen tension in acute myocardial infarction: serial analysis of clinical state and blood gas changes. *Am Heart J* 1970;**79**:620–9.

11 Aubier M, Trippenbach T, Roussos C. Respiratory muscle fatigue during cardiogenic shock. *J Appl Physiol* 1981;**51**:499–508.

12 Coats AJS, Adamopoulos S, Meyer TE, Conway J, Sleight P. Effects of physical training of chronic heart failure. *Lancet* 1990;**335**:63–6.

13 Lie KI, Wellens HJJ, Downar E, Durrer D. Observations on patients with primary ventricular fibrillation complicating acute myocardial infarction. *Circulation* 1975;**52**:755–9.

14 MacMahon S, Collins R, Peto R, Koster RW, Yusuf S. Effects of prophylactic lidocaine in suspected acute myocardial infarction: an overview of results from the randomized, controlled trials. *JAMA* 1988;**260**:1910–16.

15 Yusuf S, Sleight P, Rossi PRF *et al*. Reduction in infarct size, arrhythmias, chest pain and morbidity by early intravenous beta-blockade in suspected acute myocardial infarction. *Circulation* 1983;**67**(pt2):32–41.

16 Rossi PRF, Yusuf S, Ramsdale D *et al*. Reduction of ventricular arrhythmias by early intravenous atenolol in suspected acute myocardial infarction. *Br Med J* 1983;**286**:506–10.

17 Yusuf S, Peto R, Lewis J, Collins R, Sleight P. Beta-blockade during and after myocardial infarction: an overview of the randomized trials. *Prog Cardiovasc Dis* 1985;**27**:335–43.

18 Sleight P (for ISIS Study Group). Beta blockade early in acute myocardial infarction. *Am J Cardiol* 1987;**60**:6A–12A.

19 ISIS-1 (First International Study of Infarct Survival) Collaborative Group. Randomised trial of intravenous atenolol among 16 027 cases of suspected acute myocardial infarction. ISIS-1. *Lancet* 1986;**ii**:57–66.

20 ISIS-1 (First International Study of Infarct Survival) Collaborative Group. Mechanisms for the early mortality reduction produced by beta-blockade started early in acute myocardial infarction: ISIS-1. *Lancet* 1988;**i**:921–7.

21 Mauri F, DeBiase AM, Franzosi MD *et al*. GISSI: analisi delle cause di morte intraospedaliera. *G Ital Cardiol* 1987;**17**:37–44.

22 Honan MB, Harrell FE, Reimer KA *et al*. Cardiac rupture, mortality and the timing of thrombolytic therapy: a meta-analysis. *J Am Coll Cardiol* 1990;**16**:359–67.

23 Roberts R, Rogers WJ, Mueller HS *et al*. Immediate versus deferred beta-blockade following thrombolytic therapy in patients with acute myocardial infarction: results of the Thrombolysis in Myocardial Infarction (TIMI) II-B Study. *Circulation* 1991;**83**:422–37.

24 Yusuf S, Lessem J, Jha P, Lonn E. Primary and secondary prevention of myocardial infarction and strokes: an update of randomly allocated controlled trials. *J Hypertens* 1993;**11**(Suppl 4): S61–S73.

25 The Norwegian Multicenter Study Group. Timolol-induced reduction in mortality and reinfarction in patients surviving acute myocardial infarction. *N Engl J Med* 1981;**304**: 801–7.

26 Beta-Blocker Heart Attack Trial Research Group. A randomized trial of propranolol in patients with acute myocardial infarction. I. Mortality results. *JAMA* 1982;**247**:1707–14.

27 Hjalmarson A, Elmfeldt D, Herlitz J *et al*. Effect on mortality of metoprolol in acute myocardial infarction: a double-blind randomised trial. *Lancet* 1981;**ii**:823–7.

28 Rogers WJ, Bowlby LJ, Chandra NC *et al*. Treatment of myocardial infarction in the United States (1990 to 1993): observations from the National Registry of Myocardial Infarction. *Circulation* 1994;**90**:2103–14.

29 Liang CS, Gavras H, Black J, Sherman LG, Hood WB Jr. Renin–angiotensin system inhibition in acute myocardial infarction in dogs. Effects on systemic hemodynamics, myocardial blood flow, segmental myocardial function and infarct size. *Circulation* 1982;**66**:1249–55.

30 Ertl G, Kloner RA, Alexander RW, Braunwald E. Limitation of experimental infarct size by an angiotensin-converting enzyme inhibitor. *Circulation* 1982;**65**:40–8.

31 Swedberg K, Held P, Kjekshus J *et al*., CONSENSUS II Study Group. Effects of the early administration of enalapril on mortality in patients with acute myocardial infarction. *N Engl J Med* 1992;**327**: 678–84.

32 Gruppo Italiano per lo Studio della Supravvivenza nell'Infarto Miocardico. GISSI-3: effects of lisinopril and transdermal glyceryl trinitrate singly and together on 6-week mortality and ventricular function after acute myocardial infarction. *Lancet* 1994;**343**:1115–22.

33 ISIS-4 Collaborative Group. ISIS-4: A randomised factorial trial assessing early oral captopril, oral mononitrate, and intravenous magnesium sulphate in 58 050 patients with suspected acute myocardial infarction. *Lancet* 1995;**345**:669–85.

34 Chinese Cardiac Study Collaborative Group. Oral captopril versus placebo among 13 634 patients

with suspected acute myocardial infarction: interim report from the Chinese Cardiac Study (CCS-1). *Lancet* 1995;**345**:686–7.

35 ACE-Inhibitor MI Collaborative Group. Evidence for early beneficial effect of ACE-inhibitors started within the first day in patients with AMI: results of a systematic overview among about 100 000 patients. *Circulation* 1996;**94**:I-90.

36 Pfeffer MA, Braunwald E, Moyé LA *et al.* Effect of captopril on mortality and morbidity in patients with left ventricular dysfunction after myocardial infarction. Results of the survival and ventricular enlargement trial (SAVE). *N Engl J Med* 1992; **327**:669–77.

37 The Acute Infarction Ramipril Efficacy (AIRE) Study Investigators. Effect of ramipril on mortality and morbidity of survivors of acute myocardial infarction with clinical evidence of heart failure. *Lancet* 1993;**342**:821–8.

38 The Trandolapril Cardiac Evaluation (TRACE) Study Group. A clinical trial of the angiotensin-converting-enzyme inhibitor trandolapril in patients with left ventricular dysfunction after myocardial infarction. *N Engl J Med* 1995;**333**: 1670–6.

39 Swartz SL, Williams GH, Hollenberg NK *et al.* Captopril-induced changes in prostaglandin production. Relationship to vascular responses in normal man. *J Clin Invest* 1980;**65**:1257–64.

40 Hall D, ZeitlerH, Rudolph W. Counteraction of the vasodilator effect of enalapril by aspirin in severe heart failure. *J Am Coll Cardiol* 1992;**20**:1549–55.

41 Pitt B, Yusuf S, for the SOLVD Investigators, University of Michigan Medical Center. Studies of left ventricular dysfunction (SOLVD): subgroup results (abstract). *J Am Coll Cardiol* 1992;**19**: 215A.

42 Baur LHB, Schipperheyn JJ, van der Laarse A *et al.* Combining salicylate and enalapril in patients with coronary artery disease and heart failure. *Br Heart J* 1995;**73**:227–36.

43 GISSI-3 Investigators, ANMCO and M. Negri Institute. Aspirin does not affect circulatory or renal effects of lisinopril early after myocardial infarction. *Circulation* 1993;**88**:I-556.

44 Latini R, Maggioni AP, Flather M *et al.* ACE-inhibitor use in patients with myocardial infarction. Summary of evidence from clinical trials. *Circulation* 1995;**92**:3132–7.

45 Jugdutt BI, Becker LC, Hutchins GM *et al.* Effect of intravenous nitroglycerin on collateral blood flow and infarct size in the conscious dog. *Circulation* 1981;**63**:17–28.

46 Hackett D, Davies G, Chierchia S, Maseri A. Intermittent coronary occlusion in acute myocardial infarction: value of combined thrombolytic and vasodilator therapy. *N Engl J Med* 1987;**317**:1055–9.

47 Jugdutt BI, Warnica JW. Intravenous nitroglycerin therapy to limit myocardial infarction size, expansion, and complications: effect of timing, dosage and infarct location. *Circulation* 1988;**78**: 906–19.

48 Jugdutt BI, Sussex BA, Tymchak WJ, Warnice JW. Intravenous nitroglycerin in the early management of acute myocardial infarction. *Cardiovasc Rev Rep* 1989;**10**:29–35.

49 Yusuf S, Collins R, MacMahon S, Peto R. Effect of intravenous nitrates on mortality in acute myocardial infarction: an overview of the randomised trials. *Lancet* 1988;**i**:1088–92.

50 The European Study of Prevention of Infarction with molsidomine (ESPRIM) Group. The ESPRIM trial: short-term treatment of acute myocardial infarction with molsidomine. *Lancet* 1994;**344**: 91–7.

51 Kloner RA, Braunwald E. Effects of calcium antagonists on infarcting myocardium. *Am J Cardiol* 1987;**59**:84–94B.

52 Opie LE, Buhler FR, Fleckenstein A *et al.* Working group on classification of calcium antagonists for cardiovascular disease. *Am J Cardiol* 1987;**60**: 630–2.

53 Yusuf S, Furberg CD. Effects of calcium channel blockers on survival after myocardial infarction. *Cardiovasc Drugs Ther* 1987;**1**:343–4.

54 The Danish Study Group on Verapamil in Myocardial Infarction. Effect of verapamil on mortality and major events after acute myocardial infarction (the Danish Verapamil Infarction Trial II – DAVIT II). *Am J Cardiol* 1990;**66**:779–85.

55 The Multicenter Diltiazem Postinfarction Trial Research Group. The effect of diltiazem on mortality and reinfarction after myocardial infarction. *N Engl J Med* 1988;**319**:385–92.

56 Teo KK, Yusuf S, Furberg CD. Effects of prophylactic antiarrhythmic drug therapy in acute myocardial infarction: an overview of results from randomized controlled trials. *JAMA* 1993;**270**:1589–95.

57 Zuanetti G, Latini R, Avanzini F *et al.* on behalf of the GISSI Investigators. Trends and determinants of calcium antagonist usage after acute myocardial infarction (the GISSI experience). *Am J Cardiol* 1996;**78**:153–7.

58 Vormann J, Fischer G, Classen HG, Thoni H. Influence of decreased and increased magnesium supply on the cardiotoxic effects of epinephrine in rats. *Arzneimittelforschung* 1983;**33**:205–10.

59 Turlapaty PDMV, Altura BM. Magnesium deficiency produces spasms of coronary arteries: relationship to etiology of sudden death ischemic heart disease. *Science* 1980;**208**:198–200.

60 Watanabe Y, Dreifus LS. Electrophysiological effects of magnesium and its interactions with potassium. *Cardiovasc Res* 1972;**6**:79–88.

61 Teo KK, Yusuf S, Collins R, Held PH, Peto R. Effect of intravenous magnesium in suspected acute myocardial infarction: overview of randomized trials. *Br Med J* 1991;**303**:1499–503.

62 Woods KL, Fletcher S, Roffe C, Haider Y. Intravenous magnesium sulphate in suspected acute myocardial infarction: results of the second Leicester Intravenous Magnesium Intervention Trial (LIMIT-2). *Lancet* 1992;**339**:1553–8.

63 Herzog WR, Schlossberg ML, MacMurdy KS *et al.* Timing of magnesium therapy affects experimental infarct size. *Circulation* 1995;**92**: 2622–6.

64 Christensen CA, Rieder MA, Silvestein EL, Gencheff NE. Magnesium sulfate reduces myocardial infarct size when administered before but not after coronary reperfusion in a canine model. *Circulation* 1995;**92**:2617–21.

65 Tunstall-Pedoe H, Morrison C, Woodward M, Fitzpatrick B, Watt G. Sex difference in myocardial infarction and coronary deaths in the Scottish MONICA population of Glasgow 1985 to 1991. Presentation, diagnosis, treatment and 28-day case fatality of 3991 events in men and 1551 events in women. *Circulation* 1996;**93**:1981–92.

66 ISIS-2 (Second International Study of Infarct Survival) Collaborative Group. Randomized trial of intravenous streptokinase, oral aspirin, both, or neither among 17 187 cases of suspected acute myocardial infarction: ISIS-2. *Lancet* 1988;**2**: 349–60.

67 Antiplatelet Trialists' Collaboration. Secondary prevention of vascular disease by prolonged antiplatelet treatment. *Br Med J* 1988;**296**: 320–31.

68 Becker RC. Antiplatelet therapy in coronary heart disease: emerging strategies for the treatment and prevention of acute myocardial infarction. *Arch Pathol Lab Med* 1993;**117**:89–96.

Complications after myocardial infarction

30

DAVID WATERS,
GOHAR JAMIL

Most of the complications of myocardial infarction (MI) are related to the extent and the location of myocardial damage. Mechanical complications include acute and chronic heart failure, cardiogenic shock, ventricular aneurysm, right ventricular infarction and failure, mitral regurgitation due to papillary muscle dysfunction or rupture, rupture of the interventricular septum and rupture of the free wall of the left ventricle. The important electrical complications are ventricular fibrillation, ventricular tachycardia, atrial fibrillation, sinus bradycardia, sinus arrest, and heart block at the level of the atrioventricular node or below. A common and important category of complication that is frequently neglected is the psychosocial and socioeconomic complications of MI; indeed, depression after MI is a powerful independent predictor of mortality within the first few months.[1]

Other chapters in this book cover the topics of left ventricular dysfunction and heart failure (Part III (vii)), ventricular arrhythmias (Part III (v)), bradyarrhythmias (Part III (vi)) and atrial fibrillation (Part III (iv)). Although these conditions may occur as complications of MI, they commonly have other etiologies; in some patients the cause is uncertain and in others it is multifactorial. When complications of MI are chronic and relatively common, such as left ventricular (LV) dysfunction, heart failure or ventricular arrhythmias, they lend themselves to study with controlled clinical trials. However, clinical trials are more difficult to accomplish for many of the acute complications of MI, and thus much of the evidence upon which treatment decisions for these complications are based is either derived from uncontrolled observations or extrapolated from other clinical situations. Within these constraints, this chapter will cover the clinical features and management of the major complications of acute MI.

LEFT VENTRICULAR DYSFUNCTION AND FAILURE

Pathophysiology

Acute transmural MI results in akinesis or dyskinesis of the affected segment of the left ventricle within seconds after coronary occlusion, well before the myocytes are irreversibly damaged. Stroke volume decreases in proportion to the size of the involved segment. Cardiac output may be sustained by a catecholamine-mediated increase in heart rate and augmented contractility in the non-infarcted myocardium. LV end-diastolic pressure increases, sometimes to levels that cause pulmonary congestion or pulmonary edema. The left ventricle remodels over the ensuing hours, days and months, particularly when the infarct is large and the location anterior. Remodeling is associated with an increase in end-diastolic and end-systolic volumes, an increase in the sphericity of the ventricle, and systolic bulging and thinning of the infarct zone.[2] These adaptations allow the left ventricle to maintain a normal or nearly normal stroke volume in spite of a depressed ejection fraction (EF), but increase wall stress and often lead to progressive heart failure.

Autopsy studies indicate that MIs that involve greater than 40% of the left ventricle are usually fatal, but that acute and chronic adaptive mechanisms usually permit survival when less than 30% of the ventricle is infarcted.[3] A threshold such as this can be reached as a consequence of one large infarction or multiple smaller ones. Echocardiographic evidence from infarct survivors hospitalized in an intensive care unit shows that up to 60–80% of the left ventricle may be akinetic or severely hypokinetic in those with a history of multiple infarctions.[4]

Assessment

Markers of LV dysfunction are strong predictors of short and long term outcome after MI. In one commonly cited study,[5] mortality during a postdischarge follow-up of 22 months was 3% in patients with an EF above 0.40, 12% when the EF was between 0.20 and 0.40, and 47% when it was below 0.20. Indirect markers of severe LV dysfunction in the acute phase of infarction include basilar rales, a third heart sound, and sinus tachycardia; each of these is a powerful predictor of increased mortality. Killip and Kimball[6] devised a simple classification which stratifies MI patients from low to very high risk based upon signs of heart failure detected on physical examination.

The Forrester classification comprises four categories defined according to the presence or absence of pulmonary congestion and peripheral hypoperfusion.[7] An advantage of this classification is that it can be based upon either physical findings or measurements of cardiac output and LV filling pressure derived from invasive monitoring. In addition, the category defines the optimal therapy: patients with pulmonary congestion without hypoperfusion need diuretics and other measures that lower filling pressure, while patients with hypoperfusion without pulmonary congestion are often volume-depleted and benefit from fluid replacement.[8] When both pulmonary congestion and peripheral hypoperfusion coexist, vasodilators have the potential to correct both perturbations; however, their utility in these circumstances is often limited by hypotension. Inotropic drugs and mechanical support with intra-aortic balloon pumping are then indicated, but neither treatment provides a long term solution to the underlying problem of a left ventricle too damaged to support the circulation.

In some patients the clinical classification is misleading; for example, pulmonary rales may not be present when the LV filling pressure is elevated, or signs of peripheral hypoperfusion may be absent when the cardiac index is slightly below the normal range. In spite of these discrepancies between physical findings and hemodynamic measurements, none of the available evidence suggests that hemodynamic monitoring leads to better outcomes in any subset of patients with MI. In fact, in both postinfarction patients[9] and in a wider range of critically ill patients in intensive care units,[10] right heart catheterization for hemodynamic monitoring correlates strongly with a higher mortality even after adjusting for other prognostic variables. This association may be spurious, due to a failure to identify and adjust for all relevant variables. The mechanism whereby right heart catheterization might increase mortality is speculative.[11] A randomized trial of hemodynamic monitoring has been recommended[11] but has not been done.

Treatment

Most of the studies supporting specific treatments for acute heart failure use short-term hemodynamic measurements as endpoints. For example, furosemide has been shown to reduce elevated LV filling pressures without adversely affecting cardiac output.[12] Drugs that are predominantly arterial vasodilators, such as nitroprusside, increase cardiac output and reduce filling pressure with very little decrease in arterial pressure.[13] The main effect of nitroglycerin is venodilation, so that it reduces filling pressure more than arterial pressure, and usually causes a fall in cardiac output and a reflex increase in heart rate.[14]

A concern with any treatment for heart failure in the acute phase of MI is how it might influence infarct size. Thus, inotropic drugs are avoided unless they are essential to support arterial pressure and renal perfusion. Although the hemodynamic response to nitroprusside is usually preferable to the response to nitroglycerin, nitroglycerin may increase collateral blood flow to the infarct zone and thus limit infarct size, particularly if heart rate is controlled.[15] Some drugs appear to increase mortality in the acute phase of MI by unpredictably causing severe hypotension and compromising coronary perfusion in the presence of critical coronary disease. This mechanism may explain why nifedipine increased mortality in SPRINT-2,[16] and why intravenous enalaprilat may have increased mortality in CONSENSUS-II (Cooperative New Scandinavian Enalapril Survival Study).[17]

Vasodilators, specifically nitroglycerin and ACE inhibitors, have been shown to influence postinfarction remodeling in a favorable way, by limiting the increases in LV end-systolic and end-diastolic volumes and the bulging and thinning in the infarct zone. A major component of the survival benefit from ACE inhibitors post infarction may be the effect of these drugs on remodeling. The fact that remodeling begins soon after the onset of infarction is a justification for beginning intravenous nitroglycerin or an ACE inhibitor early, even when these drugs are not required to correct a hemodynamic abnormality.

Eight large randomized, placebo-controlled trials[17–24] have assessed the effect of an ACE inhibitor on mortality after MI. ACE inhibitors unequivocally reduce mortality overall, and the benefit appears to be the greatest among patients with depressed LV

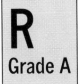

495

function, overt heart failure, or anterior infarction. Whether low risk postinfarction patients with normal EFs derive benefit from ACE inhibitors is still controversial. In the only trial that did not show a mortality benefit, CONSENSUS-II, treatment was begun early with an intravenous ACE inhibitor. Therefore, it seems reasonable in practice to withhold therapy until the patient exhibits stable hemodynamics.

Digitalis may provide limited benefit to the acute postinfarction patient with heart failure when the left ventricle is already dilated and damaged due to previous infarctions or other conditions, but use of this drug carries more risk than benefit when heart failure complicates a large infarction in a previously healthy ventricle.[25] Digoxin reduced the rate of hospitalization for heart failure, but did not decrease or increase total mortality, in a large randomized trial of patients with chronic heart failure, 70% of whom had ischemic heart disease as the primary cause.[26]

The best treatment for heart failure after MI is prevention. Therapies that reduce MI size either by re-establishing coronary perfusion, such as thrombolytic therapy or primary angioplasty, or to a lesser extent, by reducing myocardial oxygen consumption, such as beta-blockers, reduce mortality in part because they reduce infarct size. Furthermore, therapies that prevent reinfarction also reduce mortality and patients with reinfarction have a higher incidence of heart failure and other complications.

Patients with heart failure after MI may have myocardium that is stunned[27] or even hibernating.[28] Stunned myocardium has been successfully reperfused but has not regained its normal contractile function; improvement can be expected over the ensuing days or weeks, leading to improvement in overall ventricular function. Hibernating myocardium is underperfused and non-contractile, but is not infarcted; with revascularization its function will gradually improve. Hibernating myocardium is more commonly found in association with unstable angina than with MI; however, its identification post infarction can lead to an improvement in ventricular function, and presumably survival, with successful revascularization.[29]

CARDIOGENIC SHOCK

The severest form of heart failure is cardiogenic shock, a syndrome characterized by hypotension and peripheral hypoperfusion, usually accompanied by high LV filling pressures. The hypoperfusion is expressed clinically as mental obtundation or confusion, cold, clammy skin, and oliguria or anuria. When cardiogenic shock is not secondary to a correctable cause, such as arrhythmia, bradycardia, hypovolemia or a mechanical defect, short term mortality is 80% or higher, depending upon the strictness of the definition. Cardiogenic shock is the commonest cause of inhospital mortality after MI.[30] Old age, diabetes, previous infarction and extensive current infarction as assessed either by enzymatic or electrocardiographic criteria are factors commonly associated with cardiogenic shock.[30]

Inotropic drugs and intra-aortic balloon pumping are used to stabilize patients with cardiogenic shock. Although satisfactory clinical trials to document their value are lacking, both of these interventions improve cardiac output, at least temporarily.[31,32] A careful search should be made for treatable causes and circulatory parameters that may not be optimal, such as heart rate, oxygenation, hematocrit or wasted cardiac output due to heat loss or the cost of breathing.

Early administration of thrombolytic therapy reduces the occurrence of cardiogenic shock.[33] However, the large clinical trials of thrombolytic therapy did not include many patients with severe heart failure or shock and did not show benefit in this group.[34] Observational studies suggest that coronary arteriography followed by emergency revascularization reduces the mortality of patients with cardiogenic shock after MI. For example, the 30-day mortality was 38% in 406 patients who underwent early angiography and were usually revascularized, most often with angioplasty, compared to 62% in the 1794 patients without early angiography in the GUSTO-1 Trial.[35] This benefit persisted after adjustment for baseline differences (odds ratio 0.43, 95% CI 0.34–0.54, $P = 0.0001$). A controlled clinical trial of coronary angioplasty in cardiogenic shock is currently under way.[36] This therapy is most likely to be lifesaving when it is applied early. Theoretically, benefit accrues not only from restoring blood flow to the infarct zone but also from revascularizing ischemic or hibernating myocardium, and thereby improving its function.

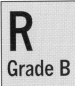

R
Grade B

VENTRICULAR ANEURYSM

A ventricular aneurysm is a thin walled, non-contractile region of the left ventricle composed of fibrous tissue and necrotic muscle, sometimes containing viable myocardium.[37] Ventricular aneurysms develop most commonly after large transmural anterior MIs, although in 5–15% of cases the site is inferior or posterior.[38] A ventricular aneurysm may cause no problems, but they are often associated with heart failure because they put the left ventricle at a mechanical disadvantage by stealing stroke volume with each systolic bulge. Although ventricular aneurysms are mainly composed of electrically dead tissue, the myocardium around the aneurysm is often arrhythmogenic, and ventricular tachycardia late after infarction is commonly associated with an aneurysm.

A ventricular aneurysm also provides a nidus for the development of an intracavitary thrombus. Although early autopsy studies indicated that thrombus was present in approximately half of all ventricular aneurysms,[39] the risk of a clinical embolic event, based on four observational studies, is approximately 5%.[39,40] The risk of thromboembolism after infarction is greatest within the first few weeks, as discussed below, and is less in patients with chronic ventricular aneurysms.

On physical examination a ventricular aneurysm can often be palpated as a dyskinetic region either adjacent to the apical impulse or as a part of it. A third heart sound and signs of heart failure may also be detected. A non-specific marker of an aneurysm is ST segment elevation that persists weeks after the acute phase of infarction. Echocardiography can delineate LV aneurysms as well as left ventriculography and has a higher sensitivity in the detection of thrombus.[41]

Surgical removal is indicated for patients with heart failure that is difficult to control medically, for patients with recurrent ventricular tachycardia not controlled by other means, and for patients with embolic episodes in spite of adequate anticoagulation.[39] The size of the aneurysm and the function of the remaining myocardium must be carefully assessed preoperatively to ensure that the left ventricle will function adequately after surgery. Aneurysmectomy is often performed at the time of coronary bypass surgery, and coronary bypass of severe lesions almost always accompanies aneurysmectomy.

A pseudoaneurysm is a rare complication of MI that develops when a myocardial rupture is sealed off by surrounding adherent pericardium. The aneurysmal sac may progressively enlarge but maintains a narrow neck, in contrast to an ordinary ventricular aneurysm.[42] Diagnosis can be made by echocardiography or left ventriculography and treatment consists of surgical repair.

CARDIAC THROMBOEMBOLISM

Left ventricular thrombi develop in up to 40% of patients with large anterior transmural MIs[43–45] but much less frequently in infarcts that are smaller or at another site. If left untreated, up to 15% of thrombi will dislodge and result in a symptomatic embolic event.[45–47] Overall, 1.5–3.6% of patients with MIs suffer a complicating stroke, most often from a dislodged mural thrombus.[48,49] Emboli are more common within the first few months after infarction than later, and with large, irregular shaped thrombi, particularly those with frond-like appendages.[46,47] Echocardiography should be performed within the first few days after MI, particularly large anterior transmural infarctions, to look for thrombus as well as to assess ventricular function. When thrombus is visualized by echocardiography, the risk ratio for embolization is 5.45 (95% CI 3.0–9.8) according to a meta-analysis.[50]

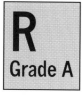

Anticoagulation with heparin followed by warfarin for 6 months has been shown to reduce the incidence of thromboembolism in patients with documented intracavitary thrombus (OR 0.14, 95% CI 0.04–0.52).[50] The benefits in terms of reduction of embolic potential outweigh the risks of hemorrhage with anticoagulation. Anticoagulation also prevents thrombus formation (OR 0.32, 95% CI 0.20–0.52), but antiplatelet drugs do not.[50]

RIGHT VENTRICULAR INFARCTION AND FAILURE

Right ventricular (RV) infarction typically occurs in association with inferior or posterior MI, as a consequence of total occlusion of the right coronary artery proximal to its marginal branches.[51] In patients with a left dominant coronary system, a proximal circumflex occlusion can produce the same picture. RV infarction was diagnosed in 54% of patients with inferior MI in one typical series.[52] RV involvement is much less common in anterior infarction, with 13% being the highest incidence reported.[53] Isolated RV infarction accounts for less than 3% of all cases of infarction and usually results from a non-dominant right coronary or marginal branch occlusion, or in association with severe RV hypertrophy in the absence of coronary disease.[51]

The pathophysiology of RV failure due to infarction involves several mechanisms that are different than those accounting for LV failure due to infarction.[51] The right ventricle is thin-walled, is perfused in both systole and diastole, and receives a generous collateral blood supply.[51,54] Extensive RV infarction induces RV dilation and an increase in intrapericardial pressure; as a consequence LV filling and cardiac output are reduced.[55] The loss of septal contraction due to infarction, the loss of the atrial contribution to RV filling due to atrial dysfunction or atrioventricular block, and the lack of an adequate venous return due to volume depletion or vasodilators may act singly or in combination to reduce RV output.[51,56,57] These factors are relevant to the treatment of RV infarction.

The diagnosis of RV infarction is virtually certain when a patient with inferior MI exhibits hypotension, clear lung fields and an elevated jugular venous pressure; however, the sensitivity of this combination of findings is less than 25%.[51,58] A RV gallop, atrioventricular dissociation and signs of tricuspid regurgitation are commonly found in the presence of RV infarction.[51] Jugular venous distension on inspiration (Kussmaul's sign) has been reported to be a sensitive and specific sign of RV infarction.[59] The hemodynamic features of RV infarction may disappear with volume depletion or may emerge only after volume loading.[59]

ST segment elevation in V_{4R} (a RV lead) has been reported to have a sensitivity of 70% and a specificity of nearly 100% for the diagnosis of RV infarction when the electrocardiogram is recorded within the first hours after the onset of symptoms.[51] Echocardiography commonly reveals wall motion abnormalities of the right ventricle and interventricular septum, and RV dilation.[51] Bowing of the interatrial septum toward the left atrium indicates that the right atrial pressure exceeds the left atrial pressure, and is a marker of a poor prognosis.[60] Detection by radionuclide right ventriculography of a low RVEF and a segmental wall motion abnormality had a sensitivity of 92% and a specificity of 82% for identifying hemodynamically significant RV infarction in one study.[59]

Volume loading is the first step in the treatment of hypotension due to RV infarction.[51] This treatment often normalizes blood pressure and increases cardiac output;[56] however, when it fails to do so, an inotropic drug such as dobutamine should be initiated.[51] High degree atrioventricular bock and atrial fibrillation have been reported to complicate one-half and one-third of RV infarctions respectively.[51] The maintenance of atrioventricular synchrony is often critical to the maintenance of a satisfactory cardiac output; when atrioventricular block or atrial fibrillation causes a low cardiac output syndrome, atrioventricular pacing or cardioversion should be used promptly to treat these complications.[51] Successful thrombolysis appears to reduce the incidence of RV infarction.[51] Patients with inferior MI in TIMI-II were less likely to have RV involvement when the culprit artery was patent as compared to patients with persistent occlusion.[61]

The inhospital mortality when RV infarction complicated inferior MI was 31%, compared to 6% when RV involvement was absent, in one series of 200 consecutive cases.[62] RV dysfunction almost always resolves in survivors during the first few weeks.[51] Some studies have shown that RV infarction is an independent predictor of long term prognosis, while others have not demonstrated a difference in long term mortality between patients with and without this complication.[51]

ACUTE MITRAL REGURGITATION

MI, particularly when associated with any significant degree of LV dilation, deforms the geometry of the left ventricle and often interferes with normal function of the mitral valve apparatus. Additionally, the papillary muscles, because of their subendocardial location, are particularly vulnerable to myocardial ischemia or infarction. The posteromedial papillary muscle is involved more often than the anterolateral muscle because the latter receives its blood supply from both branches of the left coronary artery, whereas the former is supplied mainly by the circumflex.[63] The spectrum of mitral regurgitation complicating MI ranges from mild to severe; the mild forms are common and can result from ventricular dilation, changes in cavity geometry or papillary muscle dysfunction.[64] In an animal model, hypokinesis of the ventricular segment overlying the papillary muscle is sufficient to cause mitral regurgitation, without annular dilation, mitral valve prolapse, segmental dyskinesis or LV dilation.[65] The most severe form results from complete rupture of the head of a papillary muscle and usually leads quickly to severe heart failure or cardiogenic shock. Severe mitral regurgitation is a rare complication of MI, but 19% of postinfarction patients who undergo left ventriculography[66] and 39% of those who undergo Doppler echocardiography[67] show evidence of some degree of mitral regurgitation.

Severe mitral regurgitation may produce a loud pansystolic murmur maximal at the apex, with radiation to the axilla; however, if LV function is severely impaired or if left atrial pressure is very high, the murmur may be unremarkable or entirely absent. A third heart sound and signs of LV failure are usually present. Echocardiography will usually show severe mitral regurgitation by Doppler and a flail mitral leaflet is often seen with papillary muscle rupture. However, in some cases echocardiography is non-diagnostic. Nevertheless, the presence of cardiogenic shock or severe failure with preserved LV function usually indicates that an important mechanical complication is present, and further investigation should be urgently pursued. If the mitral regurgitation is acute in its onset, the left atrium should not be greatly enlarged, and the pulmonary capillary wedge pressure tracing should exhibit large v waves. Large v waves are neither highly sensitive nor highly specific for severe chronic mitral regurgitation,[68] but the correlation between giant v waves and severe acute mitral regurgitation is stronger.[69]

Diagnosing acute severe mitral regurgitation as a complication of infarction is important because mitral valve replacement can be lifesaving. Urgent echocardiography followed by coronary arteriography and left ventriculography is essential when this condition is suspected. Arterial dilators such as nitroprusside can be very useful to improve hemodynamic status temporarily, because by reducing afterload they may reduce the regurgitant fraction and increase effective stroke volume.[70]

Observational data suggest that surgery should be performed acutely, even in patients who appear to stabilize with medical therapy, because subsequent deterioration is usual, abrupt, and unpredictable.[71] The perioperative mortality associated with mitral valve surgery for postinfarction papillary muscle rupture was 27% in one series, but two-thirds of the survivors were still alive at 7 years.[71] Patients with a low preoperative EF had the highest short term and long term mortality.

The more common form of mitral regurgitation, without papillary muscle rupture, is an independent predictor of cardiovascular mortality in postinfarction patients: in the cohort from the SAVE trial undergoing early angiography after MI, the relative risk was 2.00 (95% CI 1.28–3.04).[66] Thrombolytic therapy may decrease the incidence of significant mitral regurgitation after MI.[72] In selected patients with mitral regurgitation in the acute phase of MI, reperfusion with thrombolytic therapy or angioplasty often produces dramatic improvement in the severity of mitral regurgitation,[73] presumably due to improvement in the underlying wall motion abnormality. The indications for valve surgery for chronic mitral regurgitation are similar for patients without coronary disease and for patients who have had a MI, but the risk is much higher in coronary patients.[74] Preoperative ventricular function is the strongest predictor of both perioperative and long term survival.[74]

VENTRICULAR SEPTAL RUPTURE

Rupture of the interventricular septum is an infrequent complication, occurring in 2% of 1264 consecutive acute MI patients in one series.[75] When septal rupture complicates anterior infarction, the defect is usually apical and involves one direct perforation; inferior infarctions more often involve the posterior or basal septum and are more often complex, serpiginous defects.[76] The median time of onset of rupture was at 2.5 days in one study[76] and 7 days in another.[75] Most patients with septal rupture develop signs of acute right and left sided heart failure and a loud pansystolic murmur at the left sternal border. However, if cardiogenic shock is present, the murmur may be unimpressive or even absent. Echocardiography with Doppler color flow mapping is very sensitive and specific in the diagnosis of this condition; this technique also localizes the defect accurately and provides important prognostic information.[77] The diagnosis can also be made by right heart catheterization, which demonstrates an oxygen step-up at the level of the right ventricle.

Successful treatment of septal rupture requires surgical closure, and early closure is now recognized to yield better results than attempting to wait for days or weeks until the conditions for surgery improve, because unpredictable deterioration occurs even in patients who appear to be stabilized with medical treatment.[78,79] Medical treatment includes vasodilators if tolerated, and intra-aortic balloon pumping. Even when most patients undergo surgical repair, inhospital or 30-day mortality remains high: 43%,[79] 55%,[78] 56%,[75] and 59%[80] in four large series.

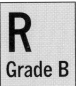

FREE WALL RUPTURE

Rupture of the free wall of the left ventricle is an almost uniformly fatal complication of MI that now probably accounts for 10–20% of inhospital deaths.[81] Older patients with anterior infarctions, hypertension on admission and marked or persistent ST elevation are at highest risk for rupture.[82] The usual presentation is sudden collapse, associated electrical–mechanical dissociation, and failure to respond to cardiopulmonary resuscitation. However, in some patients ventricular rupture is subacute, allowing time for ante-mortem diagnosis.[83] Premonitory symptoms of chest discomfort, a sense of impending doom and intermittent bradycardia signal impending myocardial rupture in many cases,[84] and if recognized, can lead to lifesaving surgery.[85] Persistently positive or newly positive T waves due to localized pericardial involvement are characteristic of impending rupture.[84] Echocardiography reveals some fluid within the pericardium and early signs of tamponade in many patients before complete rupture occurs, and large effusions and severe tamponade when rupture is complete.[83]

In one recent report[86] of 81 consecutive patients presenting with acute hypotension due to cardiac tamponade, with electrical mechanical dissociation in 72, 19 survived with medical management alone. Medical management consisted of prolonged bedrest, blood pressure control with beta-blockers and pericardiocentesis as needed for tamponade. In spite of this report, surgery remains the recommended treatment for this condition.

PERICARDITIS

Pericarditis occurs within the first week and involves approximately 25% of patients with Q wave infarctions.[87] Pericardial pain differs from myocardial ischemic pain in that it is sharper, is not relieved by nitroglycerin and may be influenced by position. A cardiac rub may be present but is not found in half of patients with typical symptoms and should not be required for diagnosis or treatment.[87] The pain associated with pericarditis may cause tachycardia, hypertension and ventricular arrhythmias; atrial and ventricular arrhythmias may be directly due to pericarditis. On the other hand, the only evidence of pericarditis in many patients is a transient pericardial rub, with no symptoms.

High dose aspirin and non-steroidal anti-inflammatory drugs are recommended to treat the symptoms of pericarditis,[88] although no studies have been done to document their efficacy. A single intravenous bolus of a steroid (e.g. Solu-cortef 500 mg) is more likely to relieve the pain within 1 or 2 hours, and if only a single dose is given, will not cause the adverse effects associated with steroid use.[88] Thrombolytic therapy reduces the incidence of pericarditis by approximately half.[87]

A pericardial effusion can be detected by echocardiography in one-quarter of patients with acute Q wave MI.[89,90] This finding correlates with the presence of heart failure and a poor prognosis.[89,90] A pericardial rub is present in less than half of patients with a pericardial effusion.[90] Cardiac tamponade is a rare complication of thrombolytic therapy for acute MI, being reported in 4 of 392 consecutively treated patients in one series.[91]

In 1956 Dressler described a distinct form of postinfarction pericarditis occurring 2–11 weeks after the acute event.[92] The full syndrome includes prolonged or recurrent positional pleuritic chest pain, fever, pulmonary infiltrates or a small pulmonary effusion, an increased sedimentation rate, and a pericardial friction rub. These findings are now most commonly seen among patients recovering from cardiac surgery, and are rare after MI.[87]

VENTRICULAR ARRHYTHMIAS

The acute phase: ventricular fibrillation

The risk of dying from acute MI is highest in the first few hours, and most of these deaths are due to ventricular fibrillation. This knowledge and the development of external defibrillation and cardiopulmonary resuscitation led to the creation of Coronary Care Units (CCUs) in the 1960s. The prophylactic administration of intravenous lidocaine (lignocaine) was shown to decrease the risk of ventricular fibrillation by 35% and was widely used, despite the fact that it did not reduce mortality.[93] The incidence of ventricular fibrillation in CCUs has progressively declined over the past 30 years, so that 400 patients would have to be treated with lidocaine to prevent one episode of ventricular fibrillation.[94] Routine use of this drug has therefore been generally abandoned because the risks outweigh the benefit.

Intravenous magnesium reduces infarct size and the risk of ventricular fibrillation in experimental animals when it is administered very early after the onset of MI.[95] A clinical trial involving 2316 patients randomized to early magnesium or placebo showed a significant 24% reduction in mortality; however, a trial in 58 050 patients showed a slight but non-significant increase in mortality in magnesium-treated patients.[95] Proponents of magnesium therapy claim that the timing of the start of the infusion – 3 hours in the small trial and 8 hours in the large trial – accounts for the different

R
Grade A

results.[95] Although this controversy remains unresolved, magnesium is not routinely used in the acute phase of MI.

After hospital discharge: ventricular extrasystoles

Frequent ventricular extrasystoles during the recovery phase of MI have long been recognized as an independent risk factor for subsequent mortality, a relationship that persists in the current era of thrombolysis.[96] However, suppression of ventricular arrhythmias has consistently failed to improve survival. A meta-analysis of 138 randomized trials of prophylactic antiarrhythmic drug therapy involving 98 000 postinfarction patients was reported by Teo et al.[97] in 1993. The mortality of patients randomized to receive Class I agents was increased (OR 1.14, 95% CI 1.01–1.28, P = 0.03). In the Cardiac Arrhythmia Suppression Trial (CAST),[98] mortality was significantly higher in postinfarction patients with ventricular arrhythmias randomized to Class IC drugs, even though these drugs effectively suppressed ventricular extrasystoles. Subsequently, the SWORD study was stopped after enrollment of only 3400 of the planned 6400 high risk survivors of MI because of an excess mortality (4.6% vs 2.7%, P = 0.005) in patients randomized to D-sotalol.[99]

Two randomized clinical trials, each with more than 1000 postinfarction patients with either frequent or repetitive ventricular extrasystoles (CAMIAT)[100] or an EF of 0.40 or less (EMIAT),[101] have compared amiodarone to placebo. EMIAT reported no difference in mortality between treatment groups but CAMIAT reported a decrease in the primary endpoint, a composite of resuscitated ventricular fibrillation or arrhythmic death (3.3% vs 6.0%, RR 48%, 95% CI 4–72%). A trend toward decreased all-cause mortality was seen. A limitation of amiodarone therapy is the high incidence of serious adverse effects seen with long term therapy. The clinical trial evidence that is now available does not appear to be strong enough to recommend amiodarone therapy to MI survivors with asymptomatic ventricular extrasystoles or a depressed EF. However, patients with symptomatic ventricular tachycardia as a long term complication of MI often benefit from amiodarone therapy.

The implanted defibrillator reduced total mortality over 27 months in MADIT, a small randomized clinical trial in a specific high risk subgroup of postinfarction patients.[102] Eligible patients had an EF of 0.35 or less, a documented episode of unsustained ventricular tachycardia, and inducible, non-suppressible ventricular tachyarrhythmia during electrophysiologic study. The risk ratio for total mortality was 0.46 (95% CI 0.26–0.82).

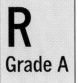

The AVID (Amiodarone Versus Implantable Defibrillators) study compared the implanted cardiac defibrillator to therapy with amiodarone or sotalol guided by Holter or electrophysiologic study in patients with ventricular fibrillation or ventricular tachycardia with a low EF, or patients with ventricular tachycardia and hemodynamic compromise.[99] Not all AVID patients had had a recent infarction. The study goal was to enroll 1200 patients; however, the trial was halted early, in April 1997, because of a statistically significant benefit of defibrillator therapy compared to drugs.[99]

Overall, the evidence indicates that Class I antiarrhythmic drugs should not be used to treat ventricular extrasystoles or unsustained ventricular tachycardia post infarction. The implanted defibrillator appears to be the treatment of choice in specific subgroups at high risk for sudden cardiac death. Beta-blockers reduce total mortality and the incidence of reinfarction by one-quarter in postinfarction patients.[99]

ATRIAL FIBRILLATION

Atrial fibrillation can present as a complication of MI or can be a pre-existing condition. In a database of more than 40 000 patients with MI treated with thrombolytic therapy, atrial fibrillation was present on admission in 2.5% and developed during hospitalization in an additional 7.9% of cases.[103] Patients with atrial fibrillation more often had underlying three vessel disease and an incompletely patent infarct-related artery. Inhospital stroke developed more often in patients with atrial fibrillation: 3.1% compared to 1.3% ($P=0.0001$).[103] Atrial fibrillation was more likely to complicate the inhospital course of older patients with larger infarctions, worse Killip class and higher heart rates. The unadjusted mortality was higher at 30 days (14.3% vs 6.2%, $P=0.0001$) and at 1 year (21.5% vs 8.6%, $P=0.0001$) in patients with atrial fibrillation. The adjusted 30-day mortality ratio was 1.3 (95% CI 1.2–1.4).[103]

The onset of atrial fibrillation is usually after the first hospital day, and the usual underlying causes are heart failure, pericarditis and atrial ischemia, with heart failure being by far the most common.[104] Atrial fibrillation may also precipitate heart failure because either the rapid ventricular rate or the loss of the atrial kick reduces ventricular filling. When atrial fibrillation develops within the first 3 hours after the onset of chest pain, occlusion of the circumflex coronary artery proximal to its left atrial branch should be considered.[105]

Treatment consists of rate control with a beta-blocker, often in combination with digitalis. The underlying cause should also be treated and heparin should be started or continued. Sinus rhythm usually returns spontaneously when the underlying cause is controlled, usually within 24 hours. If atrial fibrillation persists, cardioversion is usually indicated. In patients with chronic atrial fibrillation who develop MI, coronary embolus should be considered as a potential cause and anticoagulation should be continued.

HEART BLOCK AND CONDUCTION DISTURBANCES

Complete atrioventricular block occurred in 7.7% of patients with inferior MI in one large series.[106] Prolongation of the PR interval and Mobitz type I second degree atrioventricular block occur more often and represent incomplete block. Atrioventricular block in the setting of inferior MI can usually be treated successfully with intravenous atropine or temporary transvenous pacing. However, it is both an indicator of a larger infarct size and an independent predictor of inhospital mortality. Patients with inferior infarction complicated by complete heart block had higher inhospital mortality rates than did those without this complication: 42% vs 14% ($P<0.01$) in one study, with an adjusted odds ratio of 2.7 (95% CI 1.6–4.6).[106] In another series the inhospital mortality rate was also higher (24.2% vs 6.3%, $P<0.001$), but at hospital discharge the survivors had similar clinical characteristics to patients without atrial fibrillation, and a similar mortality rate during the next year.[107]

Complete heart block complicating acute anterior infarction usually signifies extensive myocardial damage and is associated with a very high mortality for that reason. In one series patients with anterior infarction experienced a 63% inhospital mortality rate with, and a 19% mortality rate without complete heart block.[106] Transvenous pacing is required urgently because the escape rhythm is below the level of the atrioventricular node and is therefore unstable and usually very slow (20–40 bpm). Prophylactic pacing should be considered when right bundle branch block and left anterior hemiblock develop within the first few hours of a large anterior infarction. If the patient survives, this type of complete heart block usually regresses; however, permanent pacing appears to be indicated because of the risk of complete heart block causing death after hospital discharge.[108]

The development of left or right bundle branch block as a complication of MI is a marker of a larger infarct size and a higher mortality after hospital discharge,[109] but is not an indication for pacing. On the other hand, left anterior hemiblock denotes neither a larger infarct size nor a worse prognosis.[110]

Sinus bradycardia is often seen during the first few hours of inferior MI, and is caused by an increase in vagal tone. Sinus arrest with prolonged pauses occurs much less frequently; patients with this finding often have latent or coexisting sick sinus syndrome. Atropine is used to treat sinus bradycardia. Some patients with prolonged sinus arrest may need temporary or permanent pacing.

POSTINFARCTION ANGINA AND MYOCARDIAL ISCHEMIA

Angina occurs during hospitalization after MI in approximately 20% of cases and is predictive of a worse prognosis.[111,112] Ischemia at a distance is more dangerous than ischemia within the infarct zone,[112] but both indicate that a severe stenosis is present with viable but jeopardized myocardium distal to it. Non-Q wave infarction, previous angina and multiple coronary risk factors are predictors of inhospital, postinfarction angina.[111] Patients with this complication have more extensive coronary disease at arteriography and are more likely to develop infarct extension during hospitalization: the incidence was 28% compared to 2.4% in one study.[111]

Exercise testing or pharmacologic provocation are commonly used in postinfarction patients to uncover evidence of myocardial ischemia, and increased risk.[113] This strategy appears to be more cost-effective than the strategy of performing coronary arteriography on all patients after MI.[114] Postinfarction ischemia can also be detected with ambulatory electrocardiographic monitoring done before hospitalized discharge, and in one study was associated with a one-year mortality rate that was three-fold higher than the rate among patients without ischemia on monitoring.[115]

Coronary bypass surgery[116] and coronary angioplasty[117] relieve symptoms in almost all patients with postinfarction angina, with low complication rates, but whether these therapies prevent coronary events and reduce mortality is less well documented. The Danish Trial in Acute MI (DANAMI) randomized 503 patients with inducible ischemia after thrombolytic therapy for MI to an invasive strategy, with coronary bypass surgery or angioplasty done in 82% of cases, or to a conservative strategy.[118] After 2.4 years of follow-up, mortality was 3.6% in the invasive group and 4.4% in the conservative group ($P=$NS). MI had recurred in 5.6% of the invasive group and in 10.5% of the conservative group ($P=0.038$), and far fewer hospitalizations for unstable angina were observed in the invasive group (17.9% vs 29.5%, $P<0.00001$). It appears reasonable to extrapolate these results to postinfarction patients who have not received thrombolytic therapy.

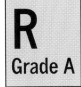

R

Grade A

PSYCHOSOCIAL COMPLICATIONS

An estimated 20–50% of postinfarction patients have high levels of psychosocial stress, including anxiety, depression, denial, hostility, and social isolation.[120] These problems are often compounded by uncertainty surrounding issues such as return to work and lifestyle recommendations. Depression is an independent predictor of mortality after MI.[1] A clear explanation of the expected course of events by the physician and other health care workers can alleviate much of the anxiety surrounding an acute coronary event. In 10–20% of cases, some form of intervention is required because symptoms persist or worsen. Depressed patients may benefit from consultation with a psychiatrist or psychologist, and socially isolated patients often improve with support therapy such as a visiting nurse.

The effect of a specific nursing intervention designed to improve the psychological and social status of postinfarction patients was assessed in the Montreal Heart Attack Readjustment Trial (M-HART).[121] The 1376 patients were randomized to usual care or to a treatment plan consisting of nurse visits and telephone calls to patients exhibiting high levels of psychological stress. The intervention had no effect on mortality in men, and was associated with an increased mortality in women that was of borderline statistical significance ($P = 0.069$). Further studies are needed to ascertain what role stress reduction therapy should play in survivors of MI.

Cardiac rehabilitation programs provide psychological and social support to patients after MI, in addition to education about risk factors and their modification. Randomized clinical trials of formal exercise programs postinfarction have not yielded definitive results individually, but an overview that included 36 trials involving 4554 patients was suggestive of benefit.[122] After an average follow-up of 3 years, the odds ratio was 0.80 for total mortality (95% CI 0.66–0.96) but the rate of non-fatal reinfarction was not reduced.

REFERENCES

1 Frasure-Smith N, Lesperance F, Talajic M. Depression and 18-month prognosis after myocardial infarction. *Circulation* 1995;**91**: 999–1005.

2 Pfeffer MA, Braunwald E. Ventricular remodeling after myocardial infarction. Experimental observations and clinical implications. *Circulation* 1990;**81**:1161–72.

3 Page DL, Caulfield JB, Kastor JA, DeSanctis RW, Saunders CA. Myocardial changes associated with cardiogenic shock. *N Engl J Med* 1971;**285**: 133–7.

4 Fisher JP, Picard MH, Mikan JS *et al*. Quantitation of myocardial dysfunction in ischemic heart disease by echocardiographic endocardial surface mapping: correlation with hemodynamic status. *Am Heart J* 1995;**129**:1114–21.

5 The Multicenter Postinfarction Research Group. Risk stratification and survival after myocardial infarction. *N Engl J Med* 1983;**309**:331–6.

6 Killip T, Kimball JT. Treatment of myocardial infarction in a coronary care unit: a two year experience with 250 patients. *Am J Cardiol* 1967; **20**:457–64.

7 Forrester JS, Diamond G, Chatterjee K, Swan HJC. Medical therapy of acute myocardial infarction by application of hemodynamic subsets. *N Engl J Med* 1976;**295**:1356–62,1404–14.

8 Forrester JS, Waters DD. Hospital treatment of congestive heart failure: management according to hemodynamic profile. *Am J Med* 1979;**65**: 173–80.

9 Zion MM, Balkin J, Rosenmann D *et al*. Use of pulmonary artery catheters in patients with acute myocardial infarction: analysis of experience in 5841 patients in the SPRINT Registry. *Chest* 1990;**98**:1331–5.

10 Connors AF, Speroff T, Dawson N *et al*. The effectiveness of right heart catheterization in the initial care of critically ill patients. *JAMA* 1996; **276**:889–97.

11 Dalen JE, Bone RC. Is it time to pull the pulmonary artery catheter? *JAMA* 1996;**276**: 916–18.

12 Dikshit K, Vyden JK, Forrester JS *et al.* Renal and extrarenal hemodynamic effects of furosemide in congestive heart failure after myocardial infarction. *N Engl J Med* 1973;**288**:1087–90.

13 Chatterjee K, Parmley WW, Ganz W *et al.* Hemodynamic and metabolic responses to vasodilator therapy in acute myocardial infarction. *Circulation* 1973;**48**:1183–93.

14 Williams DO, Amsterdam EA, Mason DT. Hemodynamic effects of nitroglycerin in acute myocardial infarction. Decrease in ventricular preload at the expense of cardiac output. *Circulation* 1975;**51**:421–7.

15 Armstrong PW, Walker DC, Burton JR, Parker JO. Vasodilator therapy in acute myocardial infarction. A comparison of sodium nitroprusside and nitroglycerin. *Circulation* 1975;**52**: 1118–22.

16 Goldbourt U, Behar S, Reicher-Reiss H *et al.* Early administration of nifedipine in suspected acute myocardial infarction: the Secondary Prevention Reinfarction Israeli Nifedipine Trial 2 Study. *Arch Intern Med* 1993;**153**:345–53.

17 Swedberg K, Held P, Kjekshus J *et al.* Effects of the early administration of enalapril on mortality in patients with acute myocardial infarction. *N Engl J Med* 1992;**327**:678–84.

18 Chinese Cardiac Study Collaborative Group. Oral captopril vs placebo among 13634 patients with suspected acute myocardial infarction: interim report from the Chinese Cardiac Study (CCS-1). *Lancet* 1995;**345**:686–7.

19 Pfeffer MA, Braunwald E, Moye LA *et al.* Effect of captopril on mortality and morbidity in patients with left ventricular dysfunction after myocardial infarction. Results of the Survival and Ventricular Enlargement Trial. *N Engl J Med* 1992;**327**:669–77.

20 Gruppo Italiano per lo Studio della Sopravvivenza nell'Infarto Miocardico. GISSI-3: effects of lisinopril and transdermal glyceryl trinitrate singly and together on 6-week mortality and ventricular function after acute myocardial infarction. *Lancet* 1994;**343**: 1115–22.

21 The Acute Infarction Ramipril Efficacy (AIRE) Study Investigators. Effect of ramipril on mortality and morbidity of survivors of acute myocardial infarction with clinical evidence of heart failure. *Lancet* 1993;**342**:821–8.

22 Ambrosioni E, Borghi C, Magnani B. The effect of angiotensin-converting-enzyme inhibitor zofenopril on mortality and morbidity after anterior myocardial infarction. *N Engl J Med* 1995;**332**:80–5.

23 ISIS-IV Collaborative Group. A randomized factorial trial assessing early oral captopril, oral mononitrate and intravenous magnesium sulphate in 58 050 patients with suspected acute myocardial infarction. *Lancet* 1995;**345**: 669–85.

24 Kober L, Torp-Pedersen C, Carlsen JE *et al.* A clinical trial of the angiotensin-converting-enzyme inhibitor trandolapril in patients with left ventricular dysfunction after myocardial infarction. *N Engl J Med* 1995;**333**:1670–6.

25 Van Veldhuisen DJ, de Graeff PA, Remme WJ. Value of digoxin in heart failure and sinus rhythm: new features of an old drug? *J Am Coll Cardiol* 1996;**28**:813–19.

26 The Digitalis Investigation Group. The effect of digoxin on mortality and morbidity in patients with heart failure. *N Engl J Med* 1997;**336**: 525–33.

27 Bolli R. Myocardial 'stunning' in man. *Circulation* 1992;**86**:1671–91.

28 Braunwald E, Rutherford JD. Reversible ischemic left ventricular dysfunction: evidence for the "hibernating myocardium". *J Am Coll Cardiol* 1986;**8**:1467–70.

29 Shivalkar B, Maes A, Borgers M *et al.* Only hibernating myocardium invariably shows early recovery after coronary revascularization. *Circulation* 1996;**94**:308–15.

30 Goldberg RJ, Gore JM, Alpert JS *et al.* Cardiogenic shock after acute myocardial infarction. Incidence and mortality from a community wide perspective, 1975–1988. *N Engl J Med* 1991; **325**:1117–22.

31 Richard C, Ricome JL, Rimailho A, Bottineau G, Auzepy P. Combined hemodynamic effects of dopamine and dobutamine in cardiogenic shock. *Circulation* 1983;**67**:620–6.

32 Scheidt S, Wilner G, Mueller H *et al.* Intra-aortic balloon counterpulsion in cardiogenic shock. Report of a co-operative clinical trial. *N Engl J Med* 1973;**288**:979–84.

33 AIMS Trial Study Group. Effect of intravenous APSAC on mortality after acute myocardial infarction: preliminary report of a placebo-controlled clinical trial. *Lancet* 1988;**i**:545–9.

34 Bates ER, Topol EJ. Limitations of thrombolytic therapy for acute myocardial infarction complicated by congestive heart failure and cardiogenic shock. *J Am Coll Cardiol* 1991;**18**: 1077–84.

35 Berger PB, Holmes DR, Stebbins AL *et al.* for the GUSTO-1 Investigators. Impact of an aggressive invasive catheterization and revascularization strategy on mortality in patients with cardiogenic shock in the Global Utilization of Streptokinase and Tissue Plasminogen Activator for Occluded Coronary Arteries (GUSTO-1) Trial. *Circulation* 1997;**96**:122–7.

36 Hochman JS, Boland J, Sleeper LA *et al.* Current spectrum of cardiogenic shock and effect of early

revascularization on mortality. Results of an international registry. *Circulation* 1995;**91**: 873–81.

37 Schlichter J, Hellerstein HK, Katz LN. Aneurysm of the heart: a correlative study of 102 proved cases. *Medicine* 1954;**33**:43–86.

38 Ba'albaki HA, Clements SD. Left ventricular aneurysm: a review. *Clin Cardiol* 1989;**12**:5–13.

39 Cohen M, Packer M, Gorlin R. Indications for left ventricular aneurysmectomy. *Circulation* 1983; **67**:717–22.

40 Lapeyre AC, Steele PM, Kazmier FJ *et al.* Systemic embolism in chronic left ventricular aneurysm: incidence and the role of anticoagulation. *J Am Coll Cardiol* 1985;**6**:534–8.

41 Sechtem U, Theissen P, Heindel W *et al.* Diagnosis of left ventricular thrombi by magnetic resonance imaging and comparison with angiocardiography, computed tomography and echocardiography. *Am J Cardiol* 1989;**64**: 1195–9.

42 Roberts WC, Morrow AG. Pseudoaneurysm of the left ventricle: an unusual sequel of myocardial infarction and rupture of the heart. *Am J Med* 1967;**43**:639–54.

43 Vecchio C, Chiarella F, Lupi G, Bellotti P, Domenicucci S. Left ventricular thrombus in anterior acute myocardial infarction after thrombolysis. A GISSI-2 connected study. *Circulation* 1991;**84**:512–19.

44 Nihoyannopoulos P, Smith GC, Maseri A, Foale RA. The natural history of left ventricular thrombus in myocardial infarction: a rationale in support of masterly inactivity. *J Am Coll Cardiol* 1989;**14**:903–11.

45 Funke Küpper AJ, Verheugt FWA, Peels CH, Galema TW, Roos JP. Left ventricular thrombus incidence and behavior studied by serial two-dimensional echocardiography in acute anterior myocardial infarction: left ventricular wall motion, systemic embolism and oral anticoagulation. *J Am Coll Cardiol* 1989;**13**: 1514–20.

46 Stratton JR, Resnick AD. Increased embolic risk in patients with left ventricular thrombi. *Circulation* 1987;**75**:1004–11.

47 Keren A, Goldberg S, Gottlieb S *et al.* Natural history of left ventricular thrombi: their appearance and resolution in the post-hospital period of acute myocardial infarction. *J Am Coll Cardiol* 1990;**15**:790–800.

48 Konrad MS, Coffey CE, Coffey KS *et al.* Myocardial infarction and stroke. *Neurology* 1984;**34**: 1403–9.

49 Vaitkus PT, Berlin JA, Schwartz JS, Barnathan ES. Stroke complicating acute myocardial infarction: a meta-analysis of risk modification by anticoagulation and thrombolytic therapy. *Arch Intern Med* 1992;**152**:2020–4.

50 Vaitkus PT, Barnathan ES. Embolic potential, prevention and management of mural thrombus complicating anterior myocardial infarction: a meta-analysis. *J Am Coll Cardiol* 1993;**22**: 1004–9.

51 Kinch JW, Ryan TJ. Right ventricular infarction. *N Engl J Med* 1993;**330**:1211–17.

52 Zehender M, Kasper W, Kauder E *et al.* Eligibility for and benefit of thrombolytic therapy in inferior myocardial infarction: focus on the prognostic importance of right ventricular infarction. *J Am Coll Cardiol* 1994;**24**:362–9.

53 Cabin HS, Clubb KS, Wackers FJT, Zaret BL. Right ventricular myocardial infarction with anterior wall left ventricular infarction: an autopsy study. *Am Heart J* 1987;**113**:16–23.

54 Farrer-Brown G. Vascular pattern of myocardium of right ventricle of human heart. *Br Heart J* 1968;**30**:679–86.

55 Goldstein JA, Vlahakes GJ, Verrier ED *et al.* The role of right ventricular systolic dysfunction and elevated intrapericardial pressure in the genesis of low output in experimental right ventricular infarction. *Circulation* 1982;**65**:513–22.

56 Goldstein JA, Vlahakes GJ, Verrier ED *et al.* Volume loading improves low cardiac output in experimental myocardial infarction. *J Am Coll Cardiol* 193;**2**:270–8.

57 Goldstein JA, Barzilai B, Rosamond TL, Eisenberg PR, Jaffe AS. Determinants of hemodynamic compromise with severe right ventricular infarction. *Circulation* 1990;**82**:359–68.

58 Dell'Italia LJ, Starling MR, O'Rourke RA. Physical examination for exclusion of hemodynamically important right ventricular infarction. *Ann Intern Med* 1983;**99**:608–11.

59 Dell'Italia LJ, Starling MR, Crawford MH *et al.* Right ventricular infarction: identification by hemodynamic measurements before and after volume loading and correlation with noninvasive techniques. *J Am Coll Cardiol* 1984; **4**:931–9.

60 López-Sendón J, López de Sá E, Roldán I *et al.* Inversion of the normal interatrial septum convexity in acute myocardial infarction: incidence, clinical relevance and prognostic significance. *J Am Coll Cardiol* 1990;**15**:801–5.

61 Berger PB, Ruocco NA, Ryan TJ *et al.* Frequency and significance of right ventricular dysfunction during inferior wall left ventricular myocardial infarction treated with thrombolytic therapy (results from the Thrombolysis in Myocardial Infarction [TIMI] II trial). *Am J Cardiol* 1993;**71**: 1148–52.

62 Zehender M, Kasper W, Kauder E *et al.* Right ventricular infarction as an independent predictor of prognosis after acute inferior myocardial infarction. *N Engl J Med* 1993;**328**: 981–8.

63 Shelburne JC, Rubinstein D, Gorlin R. A reappraisal of papillary muscle dysfunction: correlative clinical and angiographic study. *Am J Med* 1969;**46**:862–71.

64 Izumi S, Miyatake K, Beppu S *et al.* Mechanism of mitral regurgitation in patients with myocardial infarction: a study using real-time two-dimensional Doppler flow imaging and echocardiography. *Circulation* 1987;**76**:777–85.

65 Kono T, Sabbah HN, Rosman H *et al.* Mechanism of functional mitral regurgitation during acute myocardial ischemia. *J Am Coll Cardiol* 1992; **19**:1101–5.

66 Lamas GA, Mitchell GF, Flaker GC *et al.* Clinical significance of mitral regurgitation after acute myocardial infarction. *Circulation* 1997;**96**: 827–33.

67 Barzilai B, Gessler C, Pérez JE, Schaab C, Jaffe AS. Significance of Doppler-detected mitral regurgitation in acute myocardial infarction. *Am J Cardiol* 1988;**61**:220–3.

68 Fuchs RM, Heuser RR, Yin FCP, Brinker JA. Limitations of pulmonary wedge *v* waves in diagnosing mitral regurgitation. *Am J Cardiol* 1982;**49**:849–54.

69 Baxley W, Kennedy JW, Field B, Dodge HT. Hemodynamics in ruptured chordae tendinae and chronic rheumatic mitral regurgitation. *Circulation* 1973;**48**:1288–94.

70 Chatterjee K, Parmley WW, Swan HJC *et al.* Beneficial effects of vasodilator agents in severe mitral regurgitation due to dysfunction of subvalvular apparatus. *Circulation* 1973;**47**: 684–90.

71 Kishon Y, Oh JK, Schaff HV *et al.* Mitral valve operation in postinfarction rupture of a papillary muscle: immediate results and long-term follow-up of 22 patients. *Mayo Clin Proc* 1992;**67**: 1023–30.

72 Leor J, Feinberg MS, Vered Z *et al.* Effect of thrombolytic therapy on the evolution of significant mitral regurgitation in patients with a first inferior myocardial infarction. *J Am Coll Cardiol* 1993;**21**:1661–6.

73 Hickey MS, Smith R, Muhlbaier LH *et al.* Current prognosis of ischemic mitral regurgitation. Implications for future management. *Circulation* 1988;**78**(Suppl I):I-51–I-59.

74 Replogle RL, Campbell CD. Surgery for mitral regurgitation associated with ischemic heart disease. Results and strategies. *Circulation* 1989; **79**(Suppl I):I-122–I-125.

75 Moore CA, Nygaard TW, Kaiser DL, Cooper AA, Gibson RS. Postinfarction ventricular septal rupture: the importance of location of infarction and right ventricular function in determining survival. *Circulation* 1986;**74**:45–55.

76 Edwards BS, Edwards WD, Edwards JE. Ventricular septal rupture complicating acute myocardial infarction: identification of simple and complex types in 53 autopsied hearts. *Am J Cardiol* 1984;**54**:1201–5.

77 Helmcke F, Mahan EF, Nanda NC *et al.* Two-dimensional echocardiography and Doppler color flow mapping in the diagnosis and prognosis of ventricular septal rupture. *Circulation* 1990;**81**:1775–83.

78 Lemery R, Smith HC, Giuliani ER, Gersh BJ. Prognosis in rupture of the ventricular septum after acute myocardial infarction and role of early surgical intervention. *Am J Cardiol* 1992; **70**:147–51.

79 Hill JD, Stiles QR. Acute ischemic ventricular septal defect. *Circulation* 1989;**79**(Suppl I):I-112–I-115.

80 Montoya A, McKeever L, Scanlon P *et al.* Early repair of ventricular septal rupture after infarction. *Am J Cardiol* 1980;**45**:345–8.

81 Reddy SG, Roberts WC. Frequency of rupture of the left ventricular free wall or ventricular septum among necroscopy cases of fatal acute myocardial infarction since introduction of coronary care units. *Am J Cardiol* 1989;**63**: 906–11.

82 Figueras J, Curos A, Cortadellas J, Sans M, Soler-Soler J. Relevance of electrocardiographic findings, heart failure, and infarct site in assessing risk and timing of left ventricular free wall rupture during acute myocardial infarction. *Am J Cardiol* 1995;**76**:543–7.

83 López-Sendón J, Gonzalez A, López de Sá E *et al.* Diagnosis of subacute left ventricular wall rupture after acute myocardial infarction: sensitivity and specificity of clinical, hemodynamic and echocardiographic criteria. *J Am Coll Cardiol* 1992;**19**:1145–53.

84 Oliva PB, Hammill SC, Edwards WD. Cardiac rupture: a clinically predictable complication of acute myocardial infarction: a report of 70 cases with clinical-pathological correlations. *J Am Coll Cardiol* 1993;**22**:720–6.

85 Bashour T, Kabbani SS, Ellertson DG, Crew J, Hanna ES. Surgical salvage of heart rupture: report of two cases and review of the literature. *Ann Thorac Surg* 1983;**36**:209–13.

86 Figueras J, Cortadellas J, Evangelista A, Soler-Soler J. Medical management of selected patients with left ventricular free wall rupture during acute myocardial infarction. *J Am Coll Cardiol* 1997;**29**:512–18.

87 Oliva PB, Hammill SC, Talano JV. Effect of definition on incidence of postinfarction pericarditis. Is it time to redefine postinfarction pericarditis? *Circulation* 1994;**90**:1537–41.

88 Roberts R, Morris D, Pratt CM, Alexander RW. Pathophysiology, recognition, and treatment of acute myocardial infarction and its

complications. In: Schlant RC, Alexander RW, eds. *Hurst's the heart*, 8th edn. New York: McGraw Hill, p 1152.

89 Pierard LA, Albert A, Henrard L *et al.* Incidence and significance of pericardial effusion in acute myocardial infarction as determined by two-dimensional echocardiography. *J Am Coll Cardiol* 1986;**8**:517–20.

90 Sugiura T, Iwasaka T, Takayama Y *et al.* Factors associated with pericardial effusion in acute Q wave myocardial infarction. *Circulation* 1990; **81**:477–81.

91 Renkin J, De Bruyne B, Benit E *et al.* Cardiac tamponade early after thrombolysis for acute myocardial infarction: a rare but not reported hemorrhagic complication. *J Am Coll Cardiol* 1991;**17**:280–5.

92 Dressler W. A post-myocardial-infarction syndrome: preliminary report of a complication resembling idiopathic, recurrent, benign pericarditis. *JAMA* 1956;**160**:1379–83.

93 MacMahon S, Collins R, Peto R, Koster RW, Yusuf S. Effects of prophylactic lidocaine in suspected acute myocardial infarction: an overview of the results from the randomized, controlled trials. *JAMA* 1988:**260**:1910–16.

94 Antman EM, Berlin JA. Declining incidence of ventricular fibrillation in myocardial infarction. Implications for the prophylactic use of lidocaine. *Circulation* 1992;**86**:764–73.

95 Baxter GF, Sumeray MS, Walker JM. Infarct size and magnesium: insights into LIMIT-2 and ISIS-4 from experimental studies. *Lancet* 1996;**348**: 1424–6.

96 Maggioni AP, Zuanetti G, Franzosi MG *et al.* Prevalence and prognostic significance of ventricular arrhythmias after myocardial infarction in the fibrinolytic era. GISSI-2 Results. *Circulation* 1993;**87**:312–22.

97 Teo K, Yusuf S, Furberg CD. Effects of prophylactic antiarrhythmic drug therapy in acute myocardial infarction: an overview of results from randomized controlled trials. *JAMA* 1993;**270**:1589–95.

98 Echt DS, Liebson PR, Mitchell B *et al.* Mortality and morbidity in patients receiving encainide, flecainide, or placebo. The Cardiac Arrhythmia Suppression Trial. *N Engl J Med* 1991;**324**: 781–8.

99 Domanski MJ, Zipes DP, Schron E. Treatment of sudden cardiac death. Current understandings from randomized trials and future research directions. *Circulation* 1997;**95**:2694–99.

100 Cairns JA, Connolly SJ, Roberts R, Gent M. Randomised trial of outcome after myocardial infarction in patients with frequent or repetitive ventricular premature depolarisations: Canadian Amiodarone Myocardial Infarction

Arrhythmia Trial (CAMIAT). *Lancet* 1997;**349**: 675–82.

101 Julian DG, Camm AJ, Frangin G *et al.* Randomised trial of the effect of amiodarone on mortality in patients with left-ventricular dysfunction after recent myocardial infarction: European Myocardial Infarction Amiodarone Trial (EMIAT). *Lancet* 1997;**349**:667–74.

102 Moss AJ, Hall J, Cannom DS *et al.* Improved survival with an implanted defibrillator in patients with coronary disease at high risk for ventricular arrhythmia. Multicenter Automatic Defibrillation Implantation Trial (MADIT) *N Engl J Med* 1996;**335**:1933–40.

103 Crenshaw BS, Ward SR, Granger CB *et al.* for the GUSTO-1 Trial Investigators. Atrial fibrillation in the setting of acute myocardial infarction: the GUSTO-1 experience. *J Am Coll Cardiol* 1997;**30**: 406–13.

104 Sugiura T, Iwasaka T, Takahashi N *et al.* Factors associated with atrial fibrillation in Q wave anterior myocardial infarction. *Am Heart J* 1991; **121**:1409–12.

105 Hod H, Lew AS, Keltai M *et al.* Early atrial fibrillation during evolving myocardial infarction: a consequence of impaired left atrial perfusion. *Circulation* 1987;**75**:146–50.

106 Goldberg RJ, Zevallos JC, Yarzebski J *et al.* Prognosis of acute myocardial infarction complicated by complete heart block (the Worcester Heart Attack Study). *Am J Cardiol* 1992;**69**:1135–41.

107 Nicod P, Gilpin E, Dittrich H *et al.* Long-term outcome in patients with inferior myocardial infarction and complete atrioventricular block. *J Am Coll Cardiol* 1988;**12**:589–94.

108 Atkins JM, Leshin SJ, Blomqvist G, Mullins CB. Ventricular conduction blocks and sudden death in acute myocardial infarction. Potential indications for pacing. *N Engl J Med* 1973;**288**: 281–4.

109 Ricou F, Nicod P, Gilpin E, Henning H, Ross J. Influence of right bundle branch block on short- and longterm survival after acute anterior myocardial infarction. *J Am Coll Cardiol* 1991; **17**:858–63.

110 Bosch X, Theroux P, Roy D, Moise A, Waters DD. Coronary angiographic significance of left anterior fascicular block. *J Am Coll Cardiol* 1985; **5**:9–15.

111 Bosch X, Theroux P, Waters DD, Pelletier GB, Roy D. Early postinfarction ischemia: clinical, angiographic, and prognostic significance. *Circulation* 1987;**75**:988–95.

112 Schuster EH, Bulkley BH. Early post-infarction angina. Ischemia at a distance and ischemia in the infarct zone. *N Engl J Med* 1981;**305**: 1101–5.

113 Waters DD, Bosch X, Bouchard A *et al.* Comparison of clinical variables and variables derived from a limited predischarge exercise test as predictors of early and late mortality after myocardial infarction. *J Am Coll Cardiol* 1985; **5**:1–8.

114 Dittus RS, Roberts SD, Adolph RJ. Cost-effectiveness of patient management alternatives after uncomplicated myocardial infarction: a model. *J Am Coll Cardiol* 1987;**10**:869–78.

115 Gill JB, Cairns JA, Roberts RS *et al.* Prognostic importance of myocardial ischemia detected by ambulatory monitoring early after myocardial infarction. *N Engl J Med* 1996;**334**:65–70.

116 Levine FH, Gold HK, Leinbach RC *et al.* Safe early revascularization for continuing ischemia after acute myocardial infarction. *Circulation* 1979;**60**:I-5–I-9.

117 De Feyter PJ, Serruys PW, Soward A *et al.* Coronary angioplasty for early postinfarction unstable angina. *Circulation* 1986;**74**:1365–70.

118 Madsen JK, Grande P, Saunamäki K *et al.* Danish multicenter randomized study of invasive vs conservative treatment in patients with inducible ischemia after thrombolysis in acute myocardial infarction (DANAMI). *Circulation* 1997;**96**:748–55.

119 Gibson RS, Beller GA, Gheorghiade M *et al.* The prevalence and clinical significance of residual myocardial ischemia 2 weeks after uncomplicated non-Q wave infarction: a prospective natural history study. *Circulation* 1986;**73**:1186–98.

120 Balady G, Fletcher BJ, Froelicher ES *et al.* Cardiac rehabilitation programs. A statement for healthcare professionals from the American Heart Association. *Circulation* 1994;**90**: 1602–10.

121 Cody RJ. Results from late breaking clinical trials sessions at ACC '97. *J Am Coll Cardiol* 1997;**30**: 1–7.

122 O'Connor GT, Buring JE, Yusuf S *et al.* An overview of randomized trials of rehabilitation with exercise after myocardial infarction. *Circulation* 1989;**80**:234–44.

31 An integrated approach to the management of patients after the acute phase of myocardial infarction

DESMOND G. JULIAN

THE CHANGING DEFINITIONS AND PROGNOSIS OF MYOCARDIAL INFARCTION AND UNSTABLE ANGINA

It is now difficult to establish the "natural history" of acute coronary events, as both diagnostic methods and management have changed greatly over the past 30 years. Until the development of coronary care in the early 1960s, there was no effective treatment for myocardial infarction and the reported inhospital mortality of the condition was in the region of 25–30%.[1] Over the next decade, the fatality fell to about 15–20%, largely as a consequence of cardiopulmonary resuscitation and the abandonment of undesirable practices, such as prolonged bedrest and the excessive use of inotropic drugs.[2] There was little further improvement in outcome until the introduction of thrombolysis and aspirin usage in the late 1980s, and there has been a further improvement with the use of ACE inhibitors, so that the current inhospital mortality varies between 3 and 20%, largely depending upon the age of the patient.[3] Some of the apparent improvement may be due to changing diagnostic criteria, as modern tests identify many smaller infarctions that were not detected previously. Diagnostic criteria for unstable angina have also changed, as cases that would be previously have classified under this category have been recategorized as non-Q wave infarction. Longer term prognosis is largely determined by the severity of myocardial damage as measured by left ventricular ejection fraction or wall motion index. Other important risk factors include age, complex arrhythmias, lipid levels, diabetes, and the response to stresses such as exercise.

512

MANAGEMENT OF THE POSTINFARCTION PATIENT

Treatment of the postinfarction patient can be divided into two categories – secondary prevention and the management of specific complications. Secondary prevention has been studied in many large and well conducted trials and it is possible to arrive at some firm conclusions as to the optimal programme. By contrast, the management of complications has seldom been submitted to randomized controlled trials, mainly for the reason that it may not be ethical to use placebo when treating seriously ill patients. Even in this context, however, two or more active treatments can be compared, but this has not often been done.

SECONDARY PREVENTION TRIALS

DIET AND DIETARY SUPPLEMENTS

Although it is usual practice to advise patients after myocardial infarction to adhere to a lipid lowering diet, no trials to date have shown this to be effective. Nonetheless, as drug trials have demonstrated the beneficial effect of lipid lowering on morbidity and mortality, it seems prudent to advise a diet that would have a similar effect. It has been found if 60% of saturated fats are replaced by other fats and if 60% of the dietary cholesterol is avoided, this would reduce blood total cholesterol level by about 0.8 mmol/l (10–15%),[4] sufficient to achieve a level below 5mmol/l in many of those with "average" cholesterol levels.

Encouraging data have been provided from three studies in which an increase in the use of omega-3 fatty acids was tested. One study[5] suggested that advising the consumption of fatty fish at least twice a week reduced the risk of reinfarction and death. In a study from India,[6] it was claimed that patients taking a diet high in fiber, omega-3 fatty acids, antioxidants and vitamins had a 42% reduction in cardiac death and a 45% reduction in total mortality at one year compared with a control group on a standard "low fat" diet. In the recent but prematurely terminated Lyon Heart Study,[7] there was reported to be a 70% reduction in myocardial infarction, coronary mortality, and total mortality after 2 years. Each of these trials is open to quite severe criticism but, in the absence of any evidence of harm, it is not unreasonable to recommend increased consumption of fatty fish, nuts, vegetables, and fruit.

SMOKING

It has not been possible to conduct randomized studies of smoking cessation after myocardial infarction but observational studies show that those who quit smoking have a mortality in the succeeding years less than half that of those who continue to do so.[8] This is, therefore, potentially the most effective of all secondary prevention measures. Unfortunately, resumption of smoking is common after return home and it is important to establish methods which will prevent this. A randomized study has demonstrated the effectiveness of a program in which specially trained nurses maintained contact with patients over several months.[9]

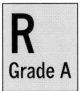

513

CARDIAC REHABILITATION

Two systematic reviews of exercise based rehabilitation trials concluded that these reduced mortality after infarction by 20–25%.[10,11] These claims must be viewed with caution as no single trial has shown a significant benefit, and there has been no evidence of a reduction in reinfarction. Furthermore, it is difficult to be sure that any benefits achieved were due to exercise rather than the other components of a rehabilitation program, which include improved medical attention. Nonetheless, there is no doubt that such programs improve exercise performance and a sense of wellbeing and can be justified on that basis.

ANTIPLATELET AND ANTICOAGULANT TREATMENT

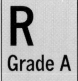

The Antiplatelet Trialists Collaboration[12] meta-analysis demonstrated about a 25% reduction in reinfarction and death in postinfarction patients. In the trials analysed, aspirin dosages ranged from 75 to 1500 mg daily. There is some evidence that the lower dosages are effective and produce fewer adverse effects. Because few patients have contraindications to aspirin therapy, it is appropriate for most postinfarction survivors. A recent trial of clopidogrel in 11 630 survivors of myocardial infarction[13] failed to show any difference between this drug and aspirin in terms of death or reinfarction, although it appears superior to aspirin in patients with peripheral vascular disease. It had few side effects and can be considered an alternative for those who cannot be prescribed aspirin.

Trials undertaken before the widespread use of aspirin showed that oral anticoagulants were effective in preventing reinfarction and death in the months and years after myocardial infarction.[14,15] The patients in these trials were randomized at least 2 weeks after the index infarction. The role of routine early oral anticoagulation following acute myocardial infarction is less clear and has only recently been evaluated after thrombolytic therapy.[16,17] In such patients there is no clear benefit over antiplatelet therapy. The addition of low dose warfarin to low dose aspirin conferred no benefit in the Coumadin Aspirin Reinfarction Study (CARS).[18]

Patients with left ventricular aneurysm, atrial fibrillation or echocardiographically proven left ventricular thrombus, however, may benefit from early oral anticoagulation, but large randomized trials in this field are lacking. The ambulant use of subcutaneous heparin may be helpful,[19] but the results should be confirmed in more studies.

BETA-BLOCKERS

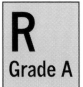

Several trials and meta-analyses have demonstrated that beta-adrenoceptor blocking drugs reduce mortality and reinfarction by 20–25% in those who have recovered from acute myocardial infarction.[20,21] Of the individual beta-blockers, only propranolol, metoprolol, timolol, and acebutolol have been shown to improve prognosis, but studies with other beta-blockers, although not significant, are compatible with a comparable effect. About one-quarter of postinfarction patients have contraindications to beta-blockade because of uncontrolled heart failure, respiratory disease or other conditions. Of the remainder, perhaps half can be defined as of low risk,[21,22] in whom beta-blockade exerts only a marginal benefit, bearing in mind the minor though sometimes troublesome side effects. Beta-blockers are most clearly indicated in the higher risk patient without contraindications.

CALCIUM ANTAGONISTS

Trials with dihydropyridine calcium antagonists[23] have failed to show a benefit in terms of improved prognosis after myocardial infarction.

One trial with verapamil[24] suggested that it prevented reinfarction and death. Trials with diltiazem[25] have failed to show a reduction in mortality; indeed, it was increased in those with impaired left ventricular function. However, there is some rather tenuous evidence that this drug may prevent reinfarction.[26]

NITRATES

Oral or transdermal nitrates did not improve prognosis in the first few weeks after myocardial infarction in the ISIS-4[27] and GISSI-3[28] trials. A recent study from Japan[29] has reported an increase in cardiac events in those receiving nitrates (6.6%) compared with those in the control group (3.1%). These results must be treated with caution because the trial was not blinded, there are doubts about the randomization technique and several different regimens of nitrate therapy were used.

ANGIOTENSIN CONVERTING ENZYME (ACE) INHIBITORS

Several trials have established that ACE inhibitors reduce mortality after acute myocardial infarction.[30-33] In the SAVE (Survival and Ventricular Enlargement) trial,[30] patients who survived the acute phase of infarction were recruited to receive captopril or placebo if they had an ejection fraction less than 40% on nuclear imaging, and if they were free of manifest ischemia on an exercise test. No mortality benefit was seen in the first year, but there was a 19% mortality reduction in 3–5 years of follow-up (from 24.6 to 20.4%). Fewer reinfarctions and less heart failure were, however, seen even within the first year.

R

Grade A

In the AIRE trial,[31] postinfarction patients were randomized to ramipril or placebo after a myocardial infarction that had been complicated by the clinical or radiological features of heart failure. At an average of 15 months later, the mortality was reduced from 22.6% to 16.9% (a 27% reduction). In the TRACE study,[32] patients were randomized to trandolapril or placebo if they had left ventricular (LV) dysfunction as demonstrated by a wall motion index of 1.2 or less. At an average follow-up of 108 weeks, the mortality was 34.7% in the treated group and 42.3% in the placebo group. In the SMILE (Survival of Myocardial Infarction Long-Term Evaluation) study,[33] 1556 patients with anterior myocardial infarction were randomized to zofenopril or placebo within 24 hours of onset, the treatment being continued for 6 weeks. At one year, the mortality rate was significantly lower in the zofenopril group (10.0%) than in the placebo group (14.1%). These studies provide powerful evidence of the effectiveness of ACE inhibitors in patients who have experienced heart failure in the acute event, even if no features of this persist, who have an ejection fraction of less than 40%, or a wall motion index of 1.2 or less, provided there are not contraindications. Analysis of the results of these studies indicates that ACE inhibitors are beneficial in patients with poor LV function even if they have not experienced heart failure, but also in those who have suffered from heart failure even if their LV function is relatively good. The SMILE study suggests that ACE inhibitor therapy may be appropriate for anterior infarction even in the absence of poor ventricular function. As discussed in Chapter 29, there is a case for administering ACE inhibitors to all patients with acute infarction from admission, provided there are no contraindications. Against such a policy is the increased incidence of hypotension and renal failure in those receiving ACE inhibitors in the acute stage, and the small benefit in those at relatively low risk, such as patients with small inferior infarctions. With the very early use of ACE inhibitors, consideration should be given to discontinuing these agents at 4–6 weeks if the clinical course has been uncomplicated and the ejection fraction greater than 40%.

ANTIARRHYTHMIC DRUGS

Trials of antiarrhythmic drugs after myocardial infarction have proved disappointing. A meta-analysis of 18 trials of Class I drugs showed a significant 21% increase in mortality.[34] The Survival with Oral d-Sotalol trial[35] of the Class III drug d-sotalol was stopped because of an increased mortality.

Amiodarone has been studied in four trials. Two small trials were favorable, but the two larger trials – EMIAT[36] and CAMIAT[37] – failed to demonstrate a reduction in total mortality. However, there was a reduction in arrhythmic death in these studies, and a pooling of results from amiodarone trials will show a non-significant trend towards lower total mortality. Unlike the other Class I and III antiarrhythmic drugs, amiodarone does not appear to have an important proarrhythmic effect, but its use is limited by its significant side effects.

LIPID LOWERING AGENTS

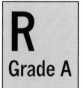

The Scandinavian Simvastatin Survival Study (4S)[38] clearly demonstrated the benefits of lipid lowering in a population of 4444 anginal and/or postinfarction patients with serum cholesterol levels of 5.5–8.0 mmol/l (212–308 mg/dl) after dietary measures had been tried. Overall mortality at a median of 5.4 years was reduced by 30% (from 12 to 8%). This represented 33 lives saved per 1000 patients treated over this period. There were substantial reductions in coronary mortality, and in the need for coronary bypass surgery. Older patients appeared to benefit as much as younger patients. Relatively few women were recruited, perhaps accounting for the failure to show a significant reduction in mortality but coronary events were reduced as they were in men.

In the Cholesterol and Recurrent Events (CARE) trial,[39] 4159 postmyocardial infarction patients with "average" cholesterol levels were randomized to pravastatin or placebo at least 3 months after the acute event. During the trial, which lasted 5 years, 13.2% of the placebo group and 10.2% of the treatment group ($P = 0.003$) experienced a primary endpoint (fatal coronary event or non-fatal myocardial infarction). There was also a reduction in stroke and in the need for coronary artery bypass surgery and angioplasty. The effects appeared to be greater in women than in men, and in those with higher low density lipoprotein (LDL) levels. Indeed, no benefit was shown in patients with LDL levels below 125 mg/dl (3.25 mmol/l). These trials firmly establish the use of statins in postmyocardial infarction patients with "average" or high lipid levels. It seems prudent to try dietary methods of lipid modification first. Furthermore, patients with lipid abnormalities other than those studied in these trials (e.g. hypertriglyceridemia) might benefit from other lipid lowering regimens.

PERCUTANEOUS TRANSLUMINAL CORONARY ANGIOPLASTY

The role of PTCA in preventing recurrent infarction and death when performed in the days after myocardial infarction remains uncertain. The SWIFT (Should We Intervene

Following Thrombolysis)[40] and TIMI-2[41] trials failed to show any benefit in terms of recurrent infarction and death in thrombolysed patients. Recently, however, the Danish Acute Myocardial Infarction (DANAMI) Trial[42] has been reported. In this trial, 1008 survivors of a first acute infarction in whom ischemia could be induced were randomized to catheterization and revascularization or standard medical therapy. There were significantly fewer non-fatal infarctions in the $2\frac{1}{2}$-year follow-up period in those who underwent revascularization, as well as a reduction in hospitalization and a reduction in medical costs.

TREATMENT OF THE COMPLICATIONS OF MYOCARDIAL INFARCTION

CARDIAC FAILURE

On the basis of the trials with ACE inhibitors described above and the results of the CONSENSUS,[43] and Studies of Left Ventricular Dysfunction[44] trials, ACE inhibitors should be given to patients in heart failure without contraindications in addition to diuretics and, perhaps, digitalis. The use of diuretics and digitalis is largely based on observational studies.

ANGINA PECTORIS

There have been few randomized studies of the therapy of angina after infarction. The DANAMI[42] study referred to above suggests that PTCA and coronary artery bypass surgery have an important role in controlling symptoms and improving prognosis.

LIFE-THREATENING ARRHYTHMIAS

As mentioned above, the use of antiarrhythmic drugs is potentially hazardous in the postinfarction patient. However, the findings of the EMIAT[36] and CAMIAT[37] studies have shown that amiodarone is relatively free of arrhythmogenesis, and is effective in preventing sudden death in high risk patients without life threatening arrhythmias. It seems an appropriate therapy for those with such arrhythmias.

The place of implantable defibrillators in the postinfarction patient with arrhythmias remains uncertain, although recent trials have been encouraging. In the Multicenter Automatic Defibrillator Implantation Trial (MADIT),[45] 202 patients with prior myocardial infarction, together with an ejection fraction of 0.35 or less, unsustained ventricular tachycardia, and non-suppressible ventricular tachycardia on electrophysiologic study, were randomly assigned to an implantable defibrillator or conventional medical therapy. At an average follow-up of 27 months, there were 15 deaths in the defibrillator group and 39 deaths in the conventionally treated group ($P=0.009$).

In the Antiarrhythmics Versus Implantable Defibrillators (AVID) trial,[46] in which there were some postinfarction patients, half of those included had experienced ventricular fibrillation and the other half serious ventricular tachycardia. After one year, patients in the defibrillator group experienced a nearly 38% reduction in deaths compared with the placebo group. It is evident that an implantable defibrillator is highly effective in the types of patient included in these studies, but its eventual place in the prevention of sudden death following myocardial infarction remains to be determined.

MANAGEMENT OF THE UNSTABLE ANGINA PATIENT AFTER THE ACUTE PHASE

ANTIPLATELET AND ANTICOAGULANT THERAPY

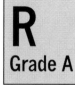

R Grade A

As reported in Chapter 25, the effectiveness of aspirin and anticoagulants in the acute phase of unstable angina has been demonstrated in randomized clinical trials. Théroux et al.,[47] have shown that it is unwise to discontinue heparin, in the absence of an antiplatelet agent. In the US Veterans Administration Study trial of aspirin reported by Lewis et al.,[48] the intention-to-treat analysis demonstrated a risk reduction in the primary endpoint of death and myocardial infarction of 41% at 12 weeks. At longer term follow-up, mortality was 5.5% in the aspirin group compared with 9.6% in the control group. In the Canadian Multicenter Trial,[49] cardiac death was reduced by aspirin from 9.7% to 4.3%. No benefit was observed with sulphapyrazone. In a non-blinded trial of ticlopidine,[50] death and infarction occurred in 13.6% of the control group compared with 7.6% in the treated group at 6 months. These trials make it evident that long-term treatment after unstable angina should include an antiplatelet agent.

The added effect of an anticoagulant is less clear. In the Antithrombotic Therapy in Acute Coronary Syndromes (ATACS) study,[51] aspirin alone was compared with aspirin with intravenous heparin for 3–4 days, followed by warfarin. The primary outcome of death, myocardial infarction and recurrent angina was observed in 27% of the aspirin group compared with 10% in the anticoagulant group ($P = 0.004$). However, the difference was no longer significant at 12 weeks. In the Fragmin during Instability in Coronary Artery Disease (FRISC) study,[52] aspirin alone was compared with aspirin combined with low molecular weight heparin. While at 6 days the rate of death and myocardial infarction was 4.8% and 1.8% respectively ($P = 0.001$), the difference at 10.7% and 8.0% respectively was no longer significant at 40 days ($P = 0.07$).

In the Effectiveness and Safety of Subcutaneous Enoxaparin in non-Q wave coronary events (ESSENCE) trial,[53] low molecular weight heparin was compared with unfractionated heparin in patients with unstable angina or non-Q wave myocardial infarction. Treatment lasted between 2 and 8 days, but a significant 16% reduction in the composite endpoint of death, myocardial infarction or recurrent angina was observed up to 30 days. Early experiences with glycoprotein IIb/IIIa antagonists are promising, but the published evidence is still inadequate to make recommendations as to their use. It is evident, however, that considerable improvements in the management of the acute coronary syndromes are on the horizon.

ANTI-ISCHEMIC DRUGS

R Grade A

There have been few randomized controlled studies of anti-ischemic drugs in the context of unstable angina. Observational studies have shown the effectiveness of both oral and intravenous nitrates, but no prognostic information is available on the use of these agents. The Holland Interuniversity Nifedipine/ Metoprolol Trial[54] provided evidence that metoprolol was superior to nifedipine in preventing recurrent ischemia and myocardial infarction in patients who had not previously been on a beta-blocker, whereas the combination was superior in patients who had had this prior therapy. This study and that of Gerstenblith et al.[55] suggest that nifedipine alone should not be administered in unstable angina, and that a beta-blocker (with nitrates) should be the first line of treatment in this condition, with the addition of a calcium antagonist if myocardial ischemia persists or recurs.

PTCA AND CABG

These interventional methods are widely used after unstable angina and observational studies suggest that they are highly effective in relieving symptoms in those with refractory or recurrent angina but their effect on prognosis is not established. In the TIMI-3B study,[56] 1473 patients with unstable angina or non-Q wave myocardial infarction were randomized, according to a factorial design, to (1) tissue plasminogen activator (tPA) versus placebo and (2) to an early invasive strategy (early coronary angiography followed by revascularization) versus an early conservative strategy (coronary angiography followed by revascularization if medical treatment failed). There was no difference in the primary outcome of death, myocardial infarction or an unsatisfactory symptom-limited exercise stress test at 6 weeks. In fact, only 61% of the "invasive" group were revascularized at 6 weeks, compared with 48% of the "conservative" group (about 25% of both groups underwent coronary bypass surgery).

PTCA was compared with CABG in unstable angina patients in a subset of the CABRI trial.[57] There was no significant difference in the death and myocardial infarction rates at the end of one year, although more patients in the surgical group were symptom-free.

In the Veterans Affairs Non-Q Wave Infarction Strategies in Hospital (VANQWISH) trial,[58] patients with non-Q wave myocardial infarction were randomized to an invasive or a conservative strategy. In the former, cardiac catheterization was carried within 3–7 days, and, subsequently, PTCA or coronary artery bypass surgery was carried out according to the coronary anatomy. A total of 920 patients were randomized. Death and myocardial infarction occurred in 7.8% of the invasive arm and 5.7% of the conservative arm at hospital discharge ($P = 0.012$). An initial conservative approach seems appropriate in this context.

Limitations of the evidence available

While randomized clinical trials provide the most reliable evidence of efficacy, their findings may not readily be applied to a wide spectrum of patients with the given condition, particularly if the entry criteria are very rigidly defined. Furthermore, even though the internal validity may be beyond question, few trials are sufficiently powered to permit reliable estimates of effect in subgroups, such as women, the elderly, and in relation to concomitant therapy. The latter problem is compounded by the fact that there may be interactions between effective agents, as is suspected between aspirin and ACE inhibitors.

Subgroup analysis is rightly suspect, although it is important to differentiate between "proper subgroups" (based on baseline characteristics) and "improper subgroups" which are based on findings after entry into the trial.[59] Analysis of proper subgroups may be of great importance, particularly when there are marked differences in risk in various baseline characteristics so that even if the effect of therapy is relatively the same whatever the risk, the absolute effect will be very different. In postinfarction and post-unstable angina patients it is possible to define high, medium, and low risk patients on quite simple clinical and investigational criteria, and the probable effect of the secondary preventive treatment can then be estimated. Thus, one can anticipate little benefit from beta-blockers or ACE inhibitors in a patient with a small inferior first infarction who has had no complications in the acute phase, whereas the patient who has had heart failure which has been brought under control remains at high risk and would benefit from both these therapies.

A further problem with applying trial results to practice is that of adherence to therapy. There is abundant evidence that compliance falls off if therapies have to be taken more than twice a day and when more than three types of drug are prescribed. It is now commonplace for patients to be given five or more drug therapies, and several widely recommended drugs (for example, captopril) have to be taken three or more times a day.

Increasingly, the cost of therapies is being critically scrutinized. An outstanding example is that of the statins, which are now being recommended for most patients with manifest coronary disease. As pointed out by Yusuf and Anand,[60] based on the 4S study, the cost-effectiveness of this therapy in high risk individuals is very favorable. Pedersen et al.[61] have concluded that the drug costs of treatment are largely offset by savings that result from fewer hospitalizations and less need for revascularization.

These estimates were made on assumptions from the United States. They will be very different in countries with substantially lower hospitalization costs but are also very sensitive to the cost of the drug.

Both compliance issues and health economic considerations argue for economy in the prescription of drugs, which will influence the integrated approach to management.

AN INTEGRATED APPROACH TO POSTMYOCARDIAL INFARCTION AND UNSTABLE ANGINA PATIENTS

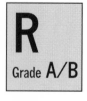

As far as secondary prevention is concerned, it is possible to base therapy on the results of well conducted randomized clinical trials. However, one must bear in mind that it may not be feasible to undertake randomized trials with regard to certain lifestyle factors, such as smoking and diet, nor can patients with major remediable symptoms be subjected to placebo-controlled trials. One can, however, advise the cessation of smoking based on strong observational data, and recommend a "Mediterranean" diet, knowing that it is probably beneficial and unlikely to have any harmful effects. The same is true of exercise-based rehabilitation programs.

Aspirin should be administered to all patients with these diagnoses, unless contraindicated. Clopidogrel is an acceptable alternative. Beta-blockers should be considered in all patients, but the risks and benefits should be carefully weighed up in those at low risk. Calcium antagonists and nitrates should be prescribed for symptomatic reasons only, the former should probably be avoided in those with heart failure or poor left ventricular function.

ACE inhibitors should be prescribed for all patients (except those with contraindications) who have been or are in heart failure, as well as those who have poor left ventricular function. Patients with average or raised lipid levels should first be treated by dietary means, but appropriate lipid modifying therapy should be given if an adequate fall in LDL is not achieved.

PTCA and CABG should be considered in patients with recurrent angina or easily provoked ischemia. Such patients should have coronary angiography and the choice of treatment determined by the anatomical and functional findings.

Evidence based therapys for postinfarction patients

- Smoking cessation **Grade A**.
- Lipid lowering diet **Grade C**.
- Lipid lowering drugs if diet fails **Grade A**.
- Aspirin for all patients without contraindications **Grade A**. Other antiplatelet agents (e.g. clopidogrel) if aspirin contraindicated **Grade A**.
- Beta-blockers, particularly for high risk patients, in the absence of contraindications **Grade A**.
- ACE inhibitors for all patients with severely impaired left ventricular function or heart failure **Grade A**.

Evidence based therapy for patients with unstable angina or non-Q wave myocardial infarction

- Aspirin or other antiplatelet agent for all patients **Grade A**.
- Heparin (fractionated or unfractionated) **Grade A**.
- Beta-blockers for all patients for whom they are not contraindicated **Grade A**.
- Calcium antagonists added if beta-blockers alone are not effective **Grade A**.

REFERENCES

1 Norris RM, Caughey OE, Mercer CJ, Scott PJ. Prognosis after myocardial infarction. Six year follow-up. *Br Heart J* 1974;**36**:786–90.

2 De Vreede JJM, Gorgels APM, Verstaaten GMP, Vermeer F, Dassen WRM, Wellens HJJ. Did prognosis after acute myocardial infarction change during the past 50 years? A meta-analysis. *J Am Coll Cardiol* 1991;**18**:698–706.

3 Maynard C, Weaver WD, Litwin PF *et al*. Hospital mortality in acute myocardial infarction in the era of reperfusion therapy. *Am J Cardiol* 1993;**72**: 877–92.

4 Clarke R, Frost C, Collins R, Appleby P, Peto R. Dietary lipids and blood cholesterol: quantitative meta-analysis of metabolic ward studies. *Br Med J* 1997;**314**:112–17.

5 Burr ML, Fehily AM, Gilbert JF *et al*. The effects of changes in fat, fish and fibre intakes on death and myocardial infarction: diet and reinfarction trial. *Lancet* 1989;**ii**:757–81.

6 Singh RB, Rastogi SS, Verma T *et al*. Randomised controlled trial; of cardioprotective diet in patients with acute myocardial infarction: results of one year follow-up. *Br Med J* 1992;**304**:1015–19.

7 de Lorgeril M, Renaud S, Mamelle N *et al*. Mediterranean alpha-linolenic acid-rich diet in secondary prevention of coronary heart disease. *Lancet* 1994;**343**:1454–9.

8 Åberg A, Bergstrand R, Johansson S *et al*. Cessation of smoking after myocardial infarction. Effects on mortality after 10 years. *Br Heart J* 1983;**49**:416–22.

9 Taylor CB, Houston-Miller N, Killen JD, De Busk RF. Smoking cessation after acute myocardial infarction: effect of a nurse-managed intervention. *Ann Intern Med* 1990;**113**:118–32.

10 O'Connor GT, Buring JE, Yusuf S *et al*. An overview of randomized trials of rehabilitation with exercise after myocardial infarction. *Circulation* 1989;**80**: 234–44.

11 Oldridge NB, Guyatt GH, Fischer MD, Rimm AA. Cardiac rehabilitation after myocardial infarction: combined experience of randomized trials. *JAMA* 1988;**260**:945–50.

12 Antiplatelet Trialists' Collaboration. Collaborative overview of randomised trials of antiplatelet therapy. I. Prevention of death, myocardial infarction, and stroke by therapy in various categories of patients. *Br Med J* 1994;**308**: 81–106.

13 CAPRIE Steering Committee. A randomised, blinded, trial of clopidogrel versus aspirin in

patients at risk of ischaemic events (CAPRIE). *Lancet* 1996;**348**:1329–39.

14 Smith P, Arnesen H, Holme I. The effect of warfarin on mortality and reinfarction after myocardial infarction *N Engl J Med* 1990;**323**:147–52.

15 Anticoagulants in the Secondary Prevention of Events in Coronary Thrombosis (ASPECT) Research Group. Effect of long-term oral anticoagulant treatment on mortality and cardiovascular morbidity after myocardial infarction. *Lancet* 1994;**343**:499–503.

16 Meijer A, Verheugt FWA, Werter CJPJ *et al.* Aspirin versus coumadin in the prevention of reocclusion and recurrent ischemia after successful thrombolysis: a prospective placebo-controlled angiographic study: results of the APRICOT Study. *Circulation* 1993;**87**:1524–30.

17 Julian DG, Chamberlain DA, Pocock SJ for the AFTER Study Group. A comparison of aspirin and anticoagulation following thrombolysis for myocardial infarction. *Br Med J* 1996;**313**: 1429–31.

18 Coumadin Aspirin Reinfarction Study (CARS) Investigators. Randomised double-blind trial of fixed-dose warfarin with aspirin after myocardial infarction. *Lancet* 1997;**350**:389–96.

19 Neri Serneri GG, Gensini GF, Carnovali M *et al.* Effectiveness of low-dose heparin in prevention of myocardial reinfarction. *Lancet* 1987;**i**:937–42.

20 Yusuf S, Lessem J, Jha P, Lonn E. Primary and secondary prevention of myocardial infarction and strokes: an update of randomly allocated controlled trials. *J Hypertens* 1993:**11**(Suppl 4): S61–S73.

21 The Beta-Blocker Pooling Project Research Group. The Beta-Blocker Pooling Project (BBPP): subgroup findings from randomized trials in post infarction patients. *Eur Heart J* 1988;**9**:8–16.

22 Furberg CD, Hawkins CM, Lichstein F. Effect of propranolol in postinfarction patients with mechanical and electrical complications. *Circulation* 1983;**69**:761–5.

23 Yusuf S, Held P, Furberg C. Update of effects of calcium antagonists in myocardial infarction or angina in light of the second Danish Verapamil Infarction Trials (DAVIT-II) and other recent studies. *Am J Cardiol* 1991;**67**:1295–7.

24 The Danish Study Group on Verapamil in Myocardial Infarction. Effect of verapamil on mortality and major events after myocardial infarction (the Danish Verapamil Infarction Trial II-DAVIT II). *Am J Cardiol* 1990;**66**:779–85.

25 The Multicenter Diltiazem Postinfarction Trial Research Group. The effect of diltiazem on mortality and reinfarction after myocardial infarction. *N Engl J Med* 1988;**319**:385–92.

26 Gibson RS, Boden WE, Theroux P *et al.* Diltiazem and reinfarction in patients with non-Q wave infarction. *N Engl J Med* 1986;**315**:423–9.

27 ISIS-4 (Fourth International Study on Infarct Survival) Collaborative group. ISIS-4: a randomised factorial trial assessing early oral captopril, oral mononitrate and intravenous magnesium in 58 000 patients with suspected acute myocardial infarction. *Lancet* 1995;**345**: 669–85.

28 Gruppo Italiano per lo Studio della Sopravvivenza nell'infarto Miocardico. GISSI-3. Effects of lisinopril and transdermal nitrate singly and together on 6-week mortality and ventricular function after acute myocardial infarction. *Lancet* 1994;**343**:1115–22.

29 Ishikawa K, Kanamasa K, Ogawa I *et al.* Long-term nitrate treatment increases cardiac events in patients with healed myocardial infarction. *Jap Circulation J* 1996;**60**:779–88.

30 Pfeffer MA, Braunwald E, Moyé LA *et al.* Effect of captopril on mortality and morbidity in patients with left ventricular dysfunction after myocardial infarction. *N Engl J Med* 1992;**327**:669–77.

31 AIRE (Acute Infarction Ramipril Efficacy) Investigators. Effect of ramipril on mortality and morbidity of survivors of acute myocardial infarction with clinical evidence of heart failure. *Lancet* 1993;**342**:821–8.

32 Kober L, Torp-Pedersen C, Carlsen JE *et al.* A clinical trial of the angiotensin converting enzyme inhibitor trandolapril in patients with left ventricular dysfunction after myocardial infarction. *N Engl J Med* 1995;**333**:1670–6.

33 Ambrosioni E, Borghi C, Magnani B. The effect of angiotensin-converting enzyme inhibitor zofenopril on mortality and morbidity after anterior myocardial infarction. The Survival of Myocardial Infarction Long-Term Evaluation (SMILE) Study Investigators. *N Engl J Med* 1995; **332**:80–5.

34 Teo KK, Yusuf S, Furberg CD. Effects of prophylactic antiarrhythmic drug therapy in acute myocardial infarction: an overview of results from randomized controlled trials. *JAMA* 1993;**270**:1589–95.

35 Waldo AL, Camm AJ, deRuyter H *et al.* Effect of d-sotalol on mortality in patients with left ventricular dysfunction after recent and remote myocardial infarction. *Lancet* 1996;**348**:7–12.

36 Julian DG, Camm AJ, Frangin G *et al.* Randomised trial of effect of amiodarone on mortality in patients with left ventricular dysfunction after recent myocardial infarction: EMIAT European Myocardial Infarct Amiodarone Trial Investigators. *Lancet* 1997;**349**:667–74.

37 Cairns JA, Connolly SJ, Roberts R, Gent M. Randomised trial of outcome after myocardial infarction in patients with frequent or repetitive ventricular premature depolarisations: CAMIAT. Canadian Amiodarone Myocardial Infarction

Arrhythmia Trial Investigators. *Lancet* 1997;**349**: 675–82.

38 Scandinavian Simvastatin Survival Study Group. Randomised trial of cholesterol lowering in 4444 patients with coronary heart disease: the Scandinavian Simvastatin Survival Study (4S). *Lancet* 1994;**344**:1383–9.

39 Sacks FM, Pfeffer MA, Moye LA *et al.* The effect of pravastatin on coronary events after myocardial infarction in patients with average cholesterol levels. *N Engl J Med* 1996;**335**:1001–9.

40 SWIFT (Should we intervene following thrombolysis?) Study Group. SWIFT trials of delayed elective intervention v conservative treatment after thrombolysis with anistreplase in acute myocardial infarction. *Br Med J* 1991;**302**: 555–60.

41 The TIMI Study Group. Comparison of invasive and conservative strategies after treatment with intravenous tissue plasminogen activator in acute myocardial infarction: results of the Thrombolysis in Myocardial Infarction (TIMI) Phase II trial. *N Engl J Med* 1989;**320**:618–27.

42 Saunamäki K *et al.* on behalf of the Danami Study Group. Danish multicenter randomized study of invasive versus conservative treatment in patients with inducible ischaemia after thrombolysis in acute myocardial infarction (DANAMI). *Circulation* 1997;**96**:748–55.

43 The CONSENSUS Trial Study Group. Effects of enalapril on mortality in severe congestive failure. *N Engl J Med* 1987;**316**:1429–35.

44 The SOLVD Investigators. Effect of enalapril on survival in patients with reduced left ventricular ejection fractions and congestive heart failure. *N Engl J Med* 1991;**325**:293.

45 Moss AJ, Hall WJ, Cannom DS *et al.* Improved survival with an implanted defibrillator in patients with coronary disease at high risk for ventricular arrhythmia. *N Engl J Med* 1996;**335**:1933–40.

46 The Anti-arrhythmics Vs Implantable Defibrillator (AVID) Study. Awaiting publication.

47 Théroux P, Ouimet H, McCans J *et al.* Aspirin, heparin or both to treat unstable angina. *N Engl J Med* 1988;**319**:1105–11.

48 Lewis HD, Davis J, Archibald D, Steinke W *et al.* Protective effects of aspirin against acute myocardial infarction and death in men with unstable angina. *N Engl J Med* 1983;**309**: 396–403.

49 Cairns J, Gent M, Singer J, Finnie K *et al.* Aspirin, sulphinpyrazone or both in unstable angina: results of a Canadian Multicenter trial. *N Engl J Med* 1985;**313**:1369–75.

50 Balsano F, Rizzon P, Violoi F *et al.* Antiplatelet treatment with ticlopidine in unstable angina. *Circulation* 1990;**82**:17–26.

51 Cohen M, Adams P, Parry G *et al.* on behalf of the Antithrombotic Therapy in Acute Coronary Syndromes Research Group. Combination antithrombotic therapy in unstable angina and non-Q wave infarction in non-prior aspirin users: primary end-points from the ATACS trial. *Circulation* 1994;**89**:81–8.

52 Fragmin during Instability in Coronary Artery Disease (FRISC) Study Group. Low molecular weight heparin during instability in coronary artery disease. *Lancet* 1996;**347**:561–8.

53 Cohen M, Demers C, Gurfinkel EP *et al.* A comparison of low-molecular weight heparin with unfractionated heparin for unstable coronary artery disease. *N Engl J Med* 1997;**337**:447–52.

54 The Holland Interuniversity Nifedipine/ Metoprolol Trial (HINT) research group. Early treatment of unstable angina in the coronary unit: a randomised double blind placebo-controlled comparison of recurrent ischaemia in patients treated with nifedipine or metoprolol or both. *Br Heart J* 1986;**56**:400–13.

55 Gerstenblith G, Oyang P, Achuff SC *et al.* Nifedipine in unstable angina. A double-blind, randomized trial. *N Engl J Med* 1982;**306**:885–9.

56 TIMI-3-B Investigators. Effects of tissue plasminogen activator and a comparison of early invasive and conservative strategies in unstable angina and non-Q wave infarction. *Circulation* 1994;**89**:1545–56.

57 Bertrand ME, Simon RL, Rlckards AF, Serruys PW on behalf of the CABRI investigators. Angioplasty versus surgery in patients with unstable angina and multivessel disease: a CABRI subgroup analysis. *Circulation* 1996;**94** (Suppl 1):435.

58 Veterans Affairs Non-Q Wave Infarction Strategies in Hospital trial (VANQWISH) In Press.

59 Yusuf S, Wittes J, Probstfield J, Tyroler HA. Analysis and interpretation of treatment effects in subgroups of patients in randomized clinical trials. *JAMA* 1991;**266**:93–8.

60 Yusuf S, Anand S. Cost of prevention. The case of lipid-lowering. *Circulation* 1996;**93**:1774–6.

61 Pedersen TR, Kjekshus J, Berg K *et al.* Cholesterol lowering and the use of healthcare resources. *Circulation* 1996;**93**:1796–1802.

Part III
Specific cardiovascular disorders
iv: Atrial fibrillation and supraventricular tachycardia

A JOHN CAMM and JOHN A CAIRNS, Editors

Grading of recommendations and levels of evidence used in *Evidence Based Cardiology*

GRADE A

Level 1a   Evidence from large randomized clinical trials (RCTs) or systematic reviews (including meta-analyses) of multiple randomized trials which collectively has at least as much data as one single well-defined trial.

Level 1b   Evidence from at least one "All or None" high quality cohort study; in which ALL patients died/failed with conventional therapy and some survived/succeeded with the new therapy (eg chemotherapy for tuberculosis, meningitis, or defibrillation for ventricular fibrillation); or in which many died/failed with conventional therapy and NONE died/failed with the new therapy (eg penicillin for pneumococcal infections).

Level 1c   Evidence from at least one moderate sized RCT or a meta-analysis of small trials which collectively only has a moderate number of patients.

Level 1d   Evidence from at least one RCT.

GRADE B

Level 2   Evidence from at least one high quality study of non-randomized cohorts who did and did not receive the new therapy.

Level 3   Evidence from at least one high quality case control study.

Level 4   Evidence from at least one high quality case series.

GRADE C

Level 5   Opinions from experts without reference or access to any of the foregoing (eg argument from physiology, bench research or first principles).

A comprehensive approach would incorporate many different types of evidence (eg RCTs, non-RCTs, epidemiologic studies, and experimental data), and examine the architecture of the information for consistency, coherence and clarity. Occasionally the evidence does not completely fit into neat compartments. For example, there may not be an RCT that demonstrates a reduction in mortality in individuals with stable angina with the use of beta-blockers, but there is overwhelming evidence that mortality is  reduced following MI. In such cases, some may recommend use of beta-blockers in angina patients with the expectation that some extrapolation from post-MI trials is warranted. This could be expressed as Grade A/C. In other instances (e.g. smoking cessation or a pacemaker for complete heart block), the non-randomized data are so overwhelmingly clear and biologically plausible that it would be reasonable to consider these interventions as Grade A.

Recommendation grades appear either in a shaded margin box with an 'R' logo as shown, or within the text, for example Grade A.

Atrial fibrillation: antiarrhythmic therapy

32

HARRY J. G. M. CRIJNS,
ISABELLE C. VAN GELDER,
ROBERT G. TIELEMAN,
WIEK H. VAN GILST

DEFINITION OF THE ARRHYTHMIA

There is no consensus concerning classifications and terminologies used to characterize atrial fibrillation, especially its temporal pattern. For the purpose of this chapter we will use a classification of atrial fibrillation based on the 3P division recently proposed by Sopher and Camm.[1] Atrial fibrillation is paroxysmal if the duration is short (usually less than 2–7 days) and the arrhythmia terminates spontaneously or after an antiarrhythmic drug. In contrast, persistent atrial fibrillation lasts longer than 2–7 days and usually it can only be terminated by an electrical cardioversion rather than drugs. Eventually, atrial fibrillation may become permanent, i.e. restoration of sinus rhythm has failed or is considered not feasible (Table 32.1).

Table 32.1 Classification of atrial fibrillation

Type	Duration and character	Therapeutic strategy
Paroxysmal	<2–7 days, frequently <24 hours Spontaneous conversion occurs frequently	Conversion and prevention with Class IC or III AADs and/or Rate control therapy during paroxysm
Persistent	>2–7 days Usually electrical cardioversion needed to restore sinus rhythm	Electrical cardioversion ± AADs + warfarin pericardioversion
Permanent	Restoration of sinus rhythm not feasible	Control of the ventricular rate + warfarin or aspirin

AADs, antiarrhythmic drugs.

NATURAL HISTORY AND PATHOPHYSIOLOGY

Natural history

Atrial fibrillation is the most common cardiac arrhythmia and the incidence increases with age. The Framingham Heart Study showed that the biennial prevalence ranged from 6.2 and 3.8 cases per 1000 in men and women aged 55–64 years, respectively, up to 75.9 and 62.8 per 1000 in men and women aged 85–94 years. Men were 1.5 times more likely to develop atrial fibrillation than women.[2]

Patients with atrial fibrillation are characterized in both sexes by a higher age, the presence of diabetes, hypertension, congestive heart failure, and valve disease. Coronary artery disease is a risk factor for atrial fibrillation only in men.[2] Other predictors are cardiomyopathy and obesity. Echocardiographic predictors include large atria, diminished left ventricular function, and increased left ventricular wall thickness. In the past, rheumatic heart disease was the most common cause of atrial fibrillation, but at present more patients have atrial fibrillation on the basis of coronary artery disease and systemic hypertension.

Mechanisms of atrial fibrillation

Moe and coworkers[3] postulated that atrial fibrillation is maintained by multiple re-entering wavelets circulating randomly in the myocardium and that the stability of the fibrillatory process depends on the average number of wavelets. This hypothesis was confirmed experimentally by Allessie and colleagues,[4] who estimated that the critical number of wavelets to sustain atrial fibrillation was approximately four to six. Atrial fibrillation may also present itself as a focal arrhythmia amenable to ablation. It then occurs in the absence of heart disease in relatively young patients.

Atrial fibrillation has the tendency to become more persistent over time. This is illustrated by the fact that about 30% of patients with paroxysmal atrial fibrillation eventually will develop persistent atrial fibrillation.[5] Also, pharmacological and electrical cardioversion, and maintenance of sinus rhythm thereafter become more difficult the longer the arrhythmia exists.[6,7] This relates to progression of the underlying disease and possibly also to electrical remodeling of the atria.[8]

Modulating factors

The onset and persistence of atrial fibrillation may be modulated by the autonomic nervous system. Coumel and coworkers distinguished vagal and adrenergic atrial fibrillation.[9] However, the distinction between both mechanisms is not always clear. This implies that it is more appropriate to speak of autonomic imbalance rather than either an increased vagal or an increased sympathetic tone.

VAGALLY MEDIATED ATRIAL FIBRILLATION

Vagally mediated atrial fibrillation occurs more frequently in men than in women, usually at a younger age (30–50 years). It only rarely progresses to permanent atrial fibrillation and it predominantly occurs in the absence of structural heart disease.[9] Attacks occur at night, end in the morning, and neither emotional stress nor exertion trigger the arrhythmia. On the contrary, when patients feel that atrial fibrillation may start (repeated atrial extrasystoles), some observe that they can prevent an arrhythmia by doing exercise. The arrhythmia frequently starts after exercise or stress. Rest, the postprandial state, and alcohol are other precipitating factors. The pathophysiological mechanism may relate to vagally induced shortening of the atrial refractory period.

ADRENERGIC TONE IN ATRIAL FIBRILLATION

Adrenergic atrial fibrillation is more frequently associated with structural heart disease (ischemic heart disease) than its vagal counterpart.[9] Typically, it occurs during day time and is favored by stress, exercise, tea, coffee or alcohol. Attacks terminate often within a few minutes. It is less frequently observed than vagal atrial fibrillation. The underlying mechanism is unknown.

CLINICAL IMPACT

Atrial fibrillation causes palpitations, chest pain, dyspnea, and fatigue. Some patients experience presyncope or even drop attacks, especially at arrhythmia onset or termination. All patients with longer lasting atrial fibrillation develop left ventricular dysfunction, even those without underlying heart disease. This is often indicated as tachycardiomyopathy. Conversely, many patients with atrial fibrillation have pre-existent heart failure. Furthermore, atrial fibrillation is associated with excess thromboembolic complications, especially in the elderly.

Hemodynamic consequences and mortality

Atrial fibrillation reduces cardiac output and may lead to heart failure.[10,11] Apart from loss of atrial kick, excessive rate response and rhythm irregularity, two other pathogenetic factors should be mentioned, i.e. progression of underlying cardiovascular disease and development of tachycardia-related cardiomyopathy.[12] In fact, associated heart disease creates the background hemodynamic derangement which is modulated by the other factors. Tachycardiomyopathy may occur in the absence of heart disease and it may be concealed, i.e. heart failure due to tachycardiomyopathy cannot be distinguished from that due to the underlying cardiovascular disease, but may be demonstrable only after restoration of sinus rhythm or adequate rate control.[12,13]

Several cohort and retrospective studies have shown that the relative risk of death in subjects with atrial fibrillation is roughly twice that found in subjects in sinus rhythm.[10,11,14] The reduced survival relates to progression of the underlying cardiovascular disease and stroke. The prognostic impact of atrial fibrillation in patients with heart failure is still uncertain.[15,16]

Progressive increase of atrial size

Atrial enlargement is a cause but also a consequence of atrial fibrillation.[17,18] Atrial enlargement is associated with an increased risk for thromboembolic complications and a high arrhythmia recurrence rate following cardioversion. In addition, drugs used to convert the arrhythmia may be less effective. Restoration of sinus rhythm may reverse the process of atrial enlargement, even in patients with mitral valve disease.[19]

Increased number of thromboembolic complications

Atrial fibrillation is the most common cardiac cause of systemic emboli, usually cerebrovascular.[20] In the presence of atrial fibrillation, the risk of stroke shows an approximately five-fold increase unrelated to age.[20] The proportion of atrial fibrillation-related stroke increases significantly with age from 6.7 for ages 50–59 years to 36.2 for ages 80–89 years. The risk for stroke in lone atrial fibrillation is still uncertain. The cardiac embolus often results in occlusion of a major cerebral artery. The ensuing infarct is often large and may be fatal.[21] Apart from symptomatic strokes, atrial fibrillation has been associated with an increased risk of silent strokes.[21] Risk factors for stroke in atrial fibrillation include rheumatic heart disease, age >65 years, hypertension, previous stroke or transient ischemic attack, and diabetes, recent heart failure, and echocardiographic atrial or ventricular enlargement.[20,22,23]

ANTIARRHYTHMIC THERAPY OF ATRIAL FIBRILLATION

Essentially, there are three antiarrhythmic strategies: acute pharmacological termination; drug prevention in paroxysmal atrial fibrillation and persistent atrial fibrillation post cardioversion; and control of the ventricular rate during a paroxysm of atrial fibrillation or during the presence of persistent or permanent atrial fibrillation. Drug treatment to convert or prevent atrial fibrillation aims at prolonging the wavelength or reducing the triggers for atrial fibrillation. The former can be achieved by Class IA or III antiarrhythmic drugs or even the Class IC drugs flecainide and propafenone which prolong refractoriness at fast cycle lengths. The latter, for example, through beta-blockers in the case of adrenergic atrial fibrillation.

Paroxysmal atrial fibrillation

Defining the temporal pattern of atrial fibrillation requires a careful history, an electrocardiogram, and frequently a 24-hour Holter monitor. This implies that the definite pattern cannot always be established on the first consultation. Which strategy will be chosen in the individual patient should depend on the frequency of the paroxysms, the triggers for the arrhythmia, the accompanying symptoms, and the underlying heart disease. The three possible strategies for the pharmacological treatment of paroxysmal atrial fibrillation will be discussed below (Table 32.2).

ACUTE CONVERSION OF PAROXYSMAL ATRIAL FIBRILLATION

If the arrhythmia is not self-limiting, antiarrhythmic drugs can be administered to restore sinus rhythm. Figure 32.1 shows conversion rates on placebo and the different

Table 32.2 Drug treatment of atrial fibrillation: summary

Type	Strategy	Drugs	Recommendation level
Paroxysmal	1 Terminate paroxysm	1 Class IC AAD IV or oral	Grade A
		or procainamide IV	Grade B
		Class IA, IC in WPW	Grade B
		Class III drugs in atrial flutter	Grade B
		Amiodarone in hemodynamically compromised patients (cardioversion)	Grade B
	2 Prevent paroxysm	2 Class IC or III AAD[a]	Grade B
		amiodarone (first choice in hemodynamically compromised patients)	Grade B
		Disopyramide/flecainide in vagally induced AF	Grade B
		Beta-blockers in adrenergically induced AF	Grade B
	3 Rate control during paroxysm	3 Digitalis	Grade B
		±	
		Beta-blockers	
		±	
		Calcium-channel blockers	
Persistent	Serial cardioversion	DC electrical cardioversion[b]	Grade A
	±	±	Grade B
	Serial antiarrhythmic drug therapy	Sotalol (initiate in hospital)	
	+	Class IC drug (not in patients with significant structural heart disease)	Grade B
	Patient counselling (report to hospital at recurrence)		
		Amiodarone (first choice in hemodynamically compromised patients)	Grade B
Permanent	Accept AF, rate control therapy:	Digitalis	Grade A
		±	
	if duration AF >36 months	Beta-blockers	
	or	±	
	age >70 years and NYHA III + IV	Calcium-channel blockers	
	or		
	after failure of serial cardioversion therapy		
Post surgery	1 Prevent AF	1 Beta-blockers	Grade A
		±	
		Digitalis	
	2 Terminate AF	2 Class IC AAD IV	Grade A

[a] Quinidine associated with proarrhythmia. [b] Drugs usually ineffective.
WPW, Wolff–Parkinson–White syndrome.

531

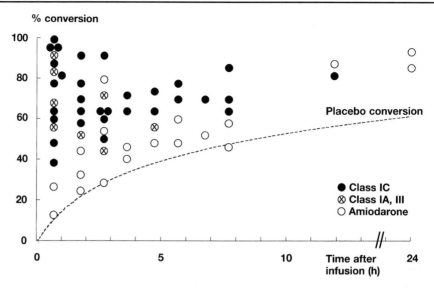

Figure 32.1 Conversion of paroxysmal atrial fibrillation (<3 days). Conversion rates in relation to time after start of the infusion found in studies investigating the efficacy of Class IC (flecainide and propafenone), Class IA and III drugs (procainamide, quinidine, sotalol, ibutilide, dofetilide) and amiodarone are presented. The curve indicating placebo conversion was constructed from placebo conversion rates found in the above studies. Class IC drugs appear most efficacious. Note the late onset of conversion on amiodarone. (Modified after Fresco et al.[6])

antiarrhythmic drugs in recent onset atrial fibrillation. It demonstrates that with time the cumulative conversion rate increases both on placebo and drugs. Although the different data points do not concern direct comparisons, it is clear that drugs facilitate conversion and that Class IC drugs are most effective compared to agents from Class III.[6] Thus, Class IC drugs are first choice therapy for conversion of an acute paroxysm of atrial fibrillation. Conversion rates up to 90% are found 1 hour after intravenous flecainide or propafenone. Both flecainide and propafenone can also be administered orally with success rates over 70% at 8 hours. Class III antiarrhythmic drugs perform less well, especially in terms of acute (i.e. <1 hour) conversion. However, as far as late conversion has been studied, quinidine and amiodarone may produce sinus rhythm in over 80% within 24 hours. An advantage of amiodarone (but not quinidine) is its ability to lower ventricular rates before conversion, whereas Class IC drugs and quinidine may increase the ventricular rate. However, in patients suffering from His Purkinje system disease both Class IA and Class IC drugs may cause atrioventricular conduction disturbances. Although Class IC drugs may be considered first choice therapy for atrial fibrillation because of their earlier conversion, amiodarone is especially recommended in hemodynamically compromised patients since it is less negatively inotropic.[24] For acute conversion, sotalol must be considered ineffective. This has only become apparent after the drug has been used as an "active" comparator in trials studying new Class III agents. On the other hand, sotalol is effective for the *prevention* of atrial fibrillation. This discrepancy relates to its property to prolong the refractory period predominantly at *lower* atrial rates, but not during rapid atrial fibrillation, due to its so-called reverse use dependency. The newer Class III drug ibutilide is also less effective than Class IC drugs with maximal early conversion rates of 47%.[25] In contrast, Class III antiarrhythmic drugs, including ibutilide, are more effective than Class IC drugs for the conversion of atrial flutter.[25,26] The availability of studies on the efficacy of procainamide and disopyramide are limited, precluding definite conclusions. Procainamide has been found to convert at least 65% of the patients with atrial fibrillation within approximately 1 hour. Its lack of efficacy (compared to Class IC drugs) may relate to the rather low dose used in the procainamide studies: up to a maximum of 1 gram in 30 minutes, sometimes followed by a low maintenance infusion.

Digitalis, beta-blockers, and calcium-channel blockers are ineffective for the acute conversion of atrial fibrillation.[6,27,28]

Oral amiodarone and quinidine are also successful in restoring sinus rhythm in approximately 50% of patients with *persistent* atrial fibrillation (>3 weeks). However, especially quinidine and also disopyramide and Class IC drugs may be associated with uncontrolled ventricular rate due to enhanced atrioventricular conduction while the patient is still in atrial fibrillation. In addition, chronic drug therapy while in atrial fibrillation may not be safe out-of-hospital because of the risk of torsade de pointes at conversion (Class IA and III drugs, except for amiodarone which exhibits a rather low proarrhythmia rate).

Self-administered oral drug conversion may be applied if the patient is clinically stable and if the agent has been shown safe and effective in that patient.[6]

PREVENTION OF PAROXYSMAL ATRIAL FIBRILLATION

Paroxysmal atrial fibrillation is a chronic disease: the first attack will not be the last in over 90% of patients, despite antiarrhythmic prophylaxis. As a consequence the endpoint of treatment used in controlled drug studies has been "attack-free rate" or "time to first recurrence". Therefore, when considering drug efficacy, it might be more appropriate to focus on quality of life but firm data concerning this issue are available only for His bundle ablation. In this respect, it is important to note that up to 50% of patients discontinue drug therapy for loss of quality of life due to side effects and drug inefficacy. Moreover, too many studies looked at drug effects in mixed populations, including both paroxysmal and persistent atrial fibrillation. Finally, older drugs like procainamide have not been tested extensively in appropriate placebo-controlled studies. Useful data concerning these agents have or will become available only after they have been used as active comparators in studies on Class IC and the new Class III drugs. Therefore, this paragraph contains clinically useful conclusions which, however, are not all evidence based.

If attacks occur frequently, chronic prophylaxis can be effective after removal of precipitating factors, such as caffeine, alcohol, stress, and adequate treatment of underlying diseases like myocardial ischemia, thyrotoxicosis, and heart failure. Class IC antiarrhythmic drugs are highly effective but should not be given to individuals with clinical features resembling the CAST high risk group (i.e. patients with a previous myocardial infarction).[29,30] In a placebo-controlled, crossover study Anderson and colleagues included 53 patients with two or more attacks of atrial fibrillation within a 4-week baseline period.[29] The median dose of flecainide was 300 mg, which is well above the clinical dose currently instituted (150–200 mg daily). During therapy with flecainide, the median time to the first recurrence was significantly prolonged (15 vs 3 days, $P<0.001$). Similarly, the time interval between subsequent attacks lengthened, from 6 to 27 days during flecainide compared to placebo ($P<0.001$). The efficacy of flecainide was maintained during a mean follow-up of 17 months.[30] Also propafenone

Table 32.3 Review of controlled studies on maintenance of sinus rhythm after cardioversion of persistent atrial fibrillation using different antiarrhythmic drugs

Study (1st author)	Year	Patients (n)	Duration AF (mth; mean)	Age (yr; mean)	Underlying heart disease (%) CAD	VHD	SH	Lone AF
Quinidine vs no treatment								
1 Södermark	1975	176	<36	58	35	27	9	8
2 Byrne-Q	1970	92	<120	54	16[b]	56	—[b]	20
3 Hillestad	1971	100	?	54	10	70	?	8
4 Lloyd	1984	53	<36	46	11	70	5	6
5 Boissel	1981	212	?	?	1	70	4	20
6 Hartel	1970	175	?	?	18	30	2	11
Disopyramide 450–500 mg vs no treatment								
7 Karlson	1988	90	4[a]	60	16	13	13	40
Procainamide 3000 mg vs propranolol 60 mg								
8 Szekely	1970	166–23	NA	NA	8	78	NA	5
Flecainide 150–300 mg vs no treatment								
9 Van Gelder	1989	73	6–11[a]	58	27	37	10	18
Propafenone 900 mg vs disopyramide 750 mg								
10 Crijns	1996	56	5[a]	60	12	28	16	40
Sotalol 160–320 mg vs quinidine sulfate 1200 mg								
11 Juul-Möller	1990	183	5	59	16	6	26	≤ 52
Sotalol 320–950 mg (mean 335 ± 18) vs propafenone 450–900 mg (mean 737 ± 177)								
12 Reimold	1993	53[c]	55	61	16	30	19	19
Amiodarone 2000 mg/week vs quinidine 1200 mg								
13 Vitolo	1981	54	79%<6	53	56	44	0	0

continued

is effective, especially the lower dose (600 mg daily). A higher dose of propafenone causes significantly more adverse events.[31] Quinidine is as effective as flecainide but quinidine is less well tolerated. Naccarelli included 239 patients randomized to flecainide (maximum dose 300 mg) or quinidine (maximum dose 1500 mg/day) and followed them for 12 months. Inadequate response caused 10% and 12% terminations of the drug, respectively. However, 30% of the quinidine patients stopped the drug due to adverse effects, versus only 18% of the flecainide group.[32] Placebo-controlled data on sotalol and amiodarone are lacking and data on the new Class III drugs like dofetilide are not yet available. In one open label comparison of sotalol and propafenone in a mixed population with paroxysmal and persistent atrial fibrillation, 37% and 30% of the patients were attack-free during 1 year.[33] Concerning amiodarone, the evidence available suggests that it is effective but has a relatively high incidence of side effects.[34]

Table 32.3 *continued*

Study	Follow-up (mth)	Patients in SR at 1 mth (%)		Patients in SR at 6 mth (%)		Stat. sig.	Death on (n/n)		Drug-related death
		AA	Ctrl	AA	Ctrl		AA	Ctrl	
1	12	90	50	51	28	Yes	5/91	2/75	0
2	12	NA	NA	54	16	Yes	1/45	0/43	1
3	12	60	46	40	21	Yes	1/48	0/52	0
4	6	70	82	48	39	No	2/26	0/25	1
5	3	NA	NA	75[d]	56[d]	Yes	2/103	1/104	1
6	3	NA	NA	69[d]	41[d]	Yes	1/88	0/87	1
7	12	70	39	54	30	Yes	2/44	0/46	0
8	12	66	61[e]	25	13	No	NA	NA	NA
9	12	70	54	49	36	No	0/36	0/37	0
10	6	76	71[f]	55	67	No	0	0	0
11	6	80	70[g]	49	42[g]	No	1/97	1/86[g]	0[i]
12	12	61	59[h]	37	30[h]	No	2/28	0/25	2[j]
13	6	NA	NA	83	43[g]	Yes	0/28	0/26[g]	0

AF, atrial fibrillation; CAD, coronary artery disease; VHD, valvular heart disease; SH, systemic hypertension; SR, sinus rhythm; Lone AF, atrial fibrillation without underlying heart disease; AA, antiarrhythmic drug; CTR, control group; Stat. sig., statistically significant.

[a] Median value.

[b] Ischemic and/or hypertensive heart disease.

[c] For persistent atrial fibrillation only.

[d] Follow-up 3 months.

[e] Control drug: propranolol.

[f] Control drug: disopyramide.

[g] Long acting quinidine.

[h] Control drug: propafenone.

[i] Two severe proarrhythmias on each drug early after start of the drug.

[j] Sudden deaths (one documented torsade de pointes) after recent dosage increase.

Modified from Crijns *et al.*,[37] where details of the studies are given.

In patients suffering from vagally induced atrial fibrillation beta-blockers and digitalis should be avoided as these drugs may provoke attacks. Quinidine, disopyramide, and flecainide may be effective due to their vagolytic effect. Propafenone is also considered ineffective due to its beta-blocking properties.

In patients with adrenergic-dependent atrial fibrillation, underlying cardiac disorders should be treated. After that, patients usually benefit from a beta-blocker. Class IA and IC drugs are generally ineffective although some patients may respond to propafenone. At this point it should be stressed that firm data concerning this issue are missing since unequivocal identification of vagal or adrenergic atrial fibrillation may be impossible. This has precluded large, controlled studies on drug efficacy in predominantly vagally or adrenergically induced atrial fibrillation.

CONTROL OF THE VENTRICULAR RATE DURING PAROXYSMAL ATRIAL FIBRILLATION

Digitalis, beta-blockers or calcium-channel blockers may be necessary to control the ventricular rate when a relapse occurs. This holds especially in hemodynamically

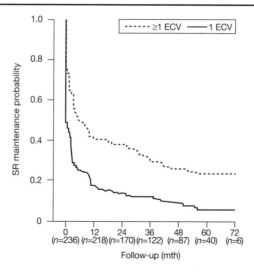

Figure 32.2 Kaplan–Meier plots depicting the probability of maintenance of sinus rhythm (SR) after serial electrical cardioversions (≥1 ECV) compared to a single cardioversion without drug prescription (1 ECV). *n*, number of patients at risk during serial cardioversion therapy. (From Van Gelder *et al.*[7] with permission.)

compromised patients who may decompensate during the attack. These agents may also prevent rate-dependent proarrhythmias (rapid atrioventricular conduction, excessive QRS widening and ventricular tachycardia) of Class IA and IC drugs during a recurrence of atrial fibrillation, but conclusive data on this issue are lacking.[35] If amiodarone or sotalol are used to prevent atrial fibrillation, addition of conventional rate control drugs is not necessary. Controlling the ventricular rate in patients with paroxysmal atrial fibrillation in the setting of a sick sinus syndrome may be impossible without implanting an artificial pacemaker. This relates to possible sinus node or atrioventricular conduction disturbances caused by negative chronotropic drugs. In Wolff–Parkinson–White syndrome complicated by atrial fibrillation acute rate control (as well as conversion to sinus rhythm) may be achieved by procainamide or flecainide.[36]

Prevention of recurrences of persistent atrial fibrillation

Persistent atrial fibrillation does not disappear spontaneously and is difficult to terminate with drugs. First choice therapy for restoration of sinus rhythm is DC electrical cardioversion. However, the Achilles' heel of cardioversion is that atrial fibrillation frequently relapses if left untreated. Recurrences happen predominantly during the first month after cardioversion (Table 32.3, Figure 32.2).[37] Preliminary data from our institution indicate that there is a vulnerable period which is confined even to the first week after the shock.

The notion that about 50% of patients will maintain sinus rhythm for over 1 year after cardioversion should be taken with caution since most studies show a progressive pattern of relapses but do not give information beyond 1 year. After a single shock (without prophylactic drugs) the 4-year arrhythmia-free survival rate presumably does not exceed 10%.[7] This means that most patients need prophylactic therapy after cardioversion. However, even when using a serial antiarrhythmic approach only around 30% of patients maintain sinus rhythm for 4 years (Figure 32.2).[7]

Most prophylactic drugs are equally effective, except for amiodarone which appears to be more efficacious. Quinidine has been studied most frequently. A meta-analysis of six controlled trials showed that quinidine was superior to no treatment (50% vs 25% of the patients remained in sinus rhythm during one year, respectively). However, the total mortality was significantly higher in the quinidine group: 12 of 413 patients (2.9%) vs 3 of 387 patients (0.8%), respectively, $P<0.05$.[38] Also a recent registry demonstrated a relatively high incidence of sudden death with quinidine.[39] Of 570 patients aged younger than 65 years, 6 patients died suddenly, all shortly after restoration of sinus rhythm. These findings make it questionable whether there is still a role for quinidine in the prophylaxis of atrial fibrillation.

Only a few controlled trials evaluated the Class IC drugs flecainide and propafenone and the Class III drug sotalol, showing that they are comparable to Class IA drugs (Table 32.3). However, differences may be observed in the adverse event profile which may guide the choice for one particular drug (see below). In general, Class IC drugs and sotalol are better tolerated than Class IA drugs and amiodarone. On the other hand, all except amiodarone cause significant proarrhythmia. Minimal prospective comparative data of amiodarone are available but a favorable outcome has been reported when amiodarone is instituted as a last resort agent. The drug is particularly useful in atrial fibrillation complicated by heart failure. Unfortunately, its use is limited by potentially severe non-cardiac side effects. However, low dose amiodarone (200 mg daily) is effective and gives only few adverse events.[40] Gosselink et al. included 89 patients with chronic atrial fibrillation who had failed previous treatment aimed at maintenance of sinus rhythm. These patients were treated with a mean dose of amiodarone of 204 ± 66 mg. Actuarially, 53% of these patients were still in sinus rhythm after a follow-up of 3 years. Adverse events occurred in 3 patients and were a reason for discontinuation in only 1 patient.[40]

Beta-blockers are only effective in preventing early but not late recurrences,[41] presumably by suppressing adrenergic-dependent premature beats in the early phase after cardioversion. It is uncertain when to start beta-blockade and which patients benefit. Obviously, these issues warrant further evaluation.

CLINICAL FACTORS DETERMINING ARRHYTHMIA OUTCOME

Patients prone to recurrences have a long previous arrhythmia duration (>1–3 years), high age (>60–75 years), large left atrial size (>55 mm, long axis on echocardiogram) or rheumatic mitral valve disease. In addition, a low functional capacity ($\geq$ NYHA III) portends a poor arrhythmia prognosis.[7,37] Obviously, some of the parameters are interrelated, e.g. duration of the arrhythmia and atrial size.

Rate control in permanent atrial fibrillation

The aim of rate control in permanent atrial fibrillation is to improve quality of life and to prevent heart failure. This is achieved by digitalis, calcium channel blockers and beta-blockers. The evidence in favor of sotalol (distinct from common beta-blockade) or amiodarone as rate slowing agents is lacking. Quality of life data before and after treatment are sparse. However, His bundle ablation studies indicate that quality of life may increase significantly.[42]

There is no accepted definition for adequate rate control at rest or exercise. In addition, the optimal heart rate may vary from one patient to the other. In general, a heart rate below 90 beats per minute at rest and below 110 beats per minute during light and moderate exercise is usually accepted. Peak exercise heart rate should remain below the normal value for the patient corrected for age and sex.

In permanent atrial fibrillation, digoxin usually provides rate control at rest. Due to sympathetic overdrive it may, however, not prevent excessive heart rate increase during daily life exercise. Therefore, it is especially useful in elderly patients with a low level of activity and should be titrated primarily on resting heart rate. On the other hand, beta-blockers but also verapamil and diltiazem may reduce peak heart rate too much, thereby limiting the exercise tolerance and quality of life. These agents may be titrated to provide control of both resting and daily life exercise heart rate. In active patients it is necessary to monitor peak exercise heart rate which should not be blunted too much by drugs. Especially in these patients combined drug therapy may be indicated.

Digoxin is accepted as primary rate control treatment in atrial fibrillation complicated by heart failure, but this advice lacks a solid scientific basis. In the light of the positive studies on beta-blockers in heart failure it seems worthwhile to evaluate their rate controlling effects in this setting.

Atrial fibrillation after cardiac surgery

Atrial fibrillation after cardiac surgery occurs in up to 30% of the patients, predominantly during the first 4 days, and significantly increases the inhospital stay. Independent predictors include a higher age, male sex, a previous history of atrial fibrillation or congestive heart failure and a longer cross-clamp time.[43]

For the prevention of post-cardiac surgery atrial arrhythmias beta-blockers are most effective. However, data of a large number of studies reveal that despite beta-blockade up to 10% of the patients may suffer from these arrhythmias.[44,45] Beta-blockade should always be started or continued as soon as possible after cardiac surgery. Evidence exists that adding digoxin to beta-blocker therapy may further reduce the occurrence of atrial arrhythmias.[44] Sotalol seems to have no clear advantages above beta-blockade alone. In a randomized study, both low dose propranolol (40 mg daily) and low dose sotalol (120 mg daily) were comparably effective in reducing the incidence of atrial fibrillation to 14 and 19%, respectively.[46] Neither digoxin alone nor verapamil reduced atrial arrhythmias after surgery.[45] The efficacy of Class IA and IC antiarrhythmic drugs has only seldom been studied. So far, these drugs cannot be recommended for this indication. In contrast, magnesium (administered intravenously during the first 4 days) reduced the number of episodes of atrial fibrillation significantly (12 vs 42 episodes, $P<0.02$).[47] Understanding the favorable effects of magnesium is difficult. It may, however, relate to the obtained correction of reduced magnesium levels which have been frequently observed after surgery. Alternatively, the stimulating effects of magnesium on the sodium/potassium pump may act beneficially by inducing a calcium-channel blocking effect. Although amiodarone has been reported to be effective in lowering the incidence of atrial fibrillation after surgery, adverse events, especially bradycardia, have been reported to limit its feasibility.[48] Amiodarone started immediately after surgery intravenously (15 mg/kg during 24 hours), followed by a daily oral dose of 600 mg for another 5 days reduced the incidence of atrial arrhythmias (8% vs 20%, $P=0.07$).

Significantly fewer patients on amiodarone required treatment of arrhythmias (6 vs 14, $P = 0.05$). However, the observed increased incidence of bradycardia (all during the first 24 hours) necessitating chronotropic support or pacing (13 patients in the amiodarone group versus 5 placebo-treated patients, respectively) is a potential disadvantage of prophylactic amiodarone treatment.[48] A lower loading dose and starting later after surgery may possibly reduce these adverse events.

Alternatively, antiarrhythmic therapy may be started at onset of the arrhythmia. There are only a few controlled studies. Flecainide and propafenone seem to be most effective. One placebo-controlled study and several non-randomized studies showed the efficacy of propafenone.[49,50] Gentili *et al.* administered propafenone intravenously (2 mg/kg in 10 minutes) in 50 patients suffering from atrial fibrillation. Sinus rhythm was restored in 35 patients (70%).[50] Sotalol and disopyramide show lower conversion rates, whereas verapamil and digitalis are ineffective.[49] The role of amiodarone has not been studied extensively in this respect.

Persistent and permanent atrial fibrillation in the setting of heart failure

In patients suffering from atrial fibrillation in the setting of heart failure treatment should be aimed initially at adequate treatment of heart failure. Thereafter, electrical cardioversion may be considered in younger patients with a short arrhythmia duration who have been successfully recompensated. In case of an early relapse (<6 months after the last shock) recardioversion should be performed after pretreatment with amiodarone.[40] Class IA and IC drugs should be avoided.[16] Repeated cardioversions with intervals longer than 6 months between each shock are an appropriate manner to prevent progression of heart failure. If cardioversion is unsuccessful or early recurrences occur despite loading with amiodarone patients should receive adequate control of the heart rate (see above). If heart rate remains uncontrolled despite drugs, His bundle ablation with implantation of a VVIR pacemaker may be useful. In patients with atrial fibrillation undergoing cardiac surgery for heart failure related to valvular disease, additional arrhythmia surgery may be contemplated.[51]

Tolerability and safety of antiarrhythmic drugs

The most important adverse effects of drugs used in atrial fibrillation are ventricular proarrhythmia, heart failure, enhanced atrioventricular nodal conduction and exacerbation of sick sinus syndrome (or atrioventricular conduction disturbances). The latter may be the basis for atrial fibrillation and can be unmasked by all antiarrhythmic drugs, including digitalis.

Ventricular proarrhythmia includes new onset ventricular fibrillation, ventricular tachycardia or torsade de pointes. Class IA and III drugs predominantly cause polymorphic ventricular tachycardia or torsade de pointes,[52,53] and Class IC drugs, incessant monomorphic ventricular tachycardias and ventricular fibrillation.[54,55] In contrast to the quinidine-like drugs, ventricular proarrhythmia or sudden death due to Class IC drugs is virtually absent in patients *without* overt heart disease. Patients treated with quinidine or sotalol may experience sudden death especially *early* after onset of therapy or after dosage increases.[39,53] Amiodarone shows a low incidence of torsade de pointes and may even be instituted after proarrhythmic events on Class IA drugs. Electrocardiographic signs, potentially useful in the prediction of proarrhythmia with Class IA and III drugs, include acute and excessive QT prolongation, pause-related TU wave changes, and increased QT dispersion. Torsade de pointes may occur, especially if there is a pre-existing QT prolongation, and is enhanced by bradycardia (e.g. occurring after sudden conversion of "rapid" atrial fibrillation to "slow" sinus rhythm). Late proarrhythmia may occur after addition of drugs, like diuretics or during intercurrent bradycardia. Recently, it was demonstrated that women are more susceptible than men.[56] Ventricular proarrhythmia with Class IC drugs should be expected in patients with previous sustained ventricular tachycardia and in those with structural heart disease receiving a high dose. It occurs predominantly late after institution of the drug, and especially during higher heart rates. In this respect, it is considered useful to perform an exercise test after institution of the drug. During higher heart rates conduction slowing may become more prominent. Excessive broadening of the QRS complex during high heart rates may be a marker of future ventricular proarrhythmia necessitating dose reduction or termination of the drug.

Patients using Class IA and IC drugs may experience high ventricular rates during breakthrough atrial fibrillation or flutter. These agents do not suppress and may even augment atrioventricular conduction by anticholinergic stimulation. AV conduction is further reinforced by exercise and anxiety. Therefore patients using these drugs prophylactically must be cautioned to avoid exercise during a recurrence of atrial fibrillation. Digoxin, a beta-blocker or a calcium-channel blocker may be added but there are no clinical data to support this approach.

Depending on dose and duration of therapy, especially Class IA and IC drugs may cause heart failure mainly through cardiodepression. Disopyramide allegedly has the largest negative inotropic effects and may cause heart failure early but also late (months) after initiation, especially in patients with a history of cardiac insufficiency. The other Class IA drugs, as well as beta-blockers (including sotalol) and calcium-channel blockers, rarely cause heart failure in patients with atrial fibrillation. Heart failure induced by amiodarone has not been described.

CONCLUSION

Rational antiarrhythmic treatment of atrial fibrillation starts with establishing whether one is dealing with the paroxysmal, persistent or permanent subtype. Only then the goal of treatment can be identified: to restore sinus rhythm with the option of prophylactic drug treatment or to adopt atrial fibrillation as the dominant rhythm. Antiarrhythmic treatment is further guided by the duration of the arrhythmia, the tendency for recurrence after conversion, and the potential side effects of drugs. At some stage during treatment, rate control is useful in all three subtypes of atrial fibrillation but especially in the *permanent* form. The termination of *paroxysmal* atrial fibrillation is enhanced by intravenous drugs. For fibrillation Class IC drugs are first choice whereas Class III drugs may effectively terminate atrial flutter. Restoration of sinus rhythm in *persistent* atrial fibrillation is most effectively achieved by electrical cardioversion but to reduce postshock recurrence usually antiarrhythmics are indispensable. Despite drugs, the latter approach will at best postpone progression from persistent to permanent atrial fibrillation.

Most patients cannot be cured from atrial fibrillation: almost all will experience recurrence of the arrhythmia earlier or later after the first attack despite drug treatment. Therefore the primary goal of treatment is to reduce morbidity (and possibly also mortality) rather than simply mending the rhythm at any price. Currently, rhythm and rate control strategies are being evaluated concerning their effect on morbidity and mortality. These studies may help to better define the role of the different antiarrhythmic treatments.

Acknowledgment

Isabelle C. Van Gelder is supported by the Dutch Heart Foundation, grant 94.014.

REFERENCES

1 Sopher SM, Camm AJ. Atrial fibrillation – maintenance of sinus rhythm versus rate control. Am J Cardiol 1996;77:24A–38A.

2 Benjamin EJ, Levy D, Vaziri SM et al. Independent risk factors for atrial fibrillation in a population-based cohort. The Framingham study. JAMA 1994;271:840–4.

3 Moe GK. On the multiple wavelet hypothesis of atrial fibrillation. Arch Int Pharmacodyn Ther 1962;140:183–8.

4 Allessie MA, Lamers WJEP, Bonke FIM, Hollen SJ. Experimental evaluation of Moe's multiple wavelet hypothesis of atrial fibrillation. In: Zipes DP, Jalife J, eds. Cardiac electrophysiology and arrhythmias. New York: Grune and Stratton, 1985, pp 265–75.

5 Godtfredsen J. Atrial fibrillation. Etiology, course and prognosis. A follow-up study of 1212 cases. Thesis, University of Copenhagen, 1975.

6 Fresco C, Proclemer A, on behalf of the PAFIT-2 Investigators. Management of recent onset atrial fibrillation. Eur Heart J 1996;17(Suppl C): C41–C47.

7 Van Gelder IC, Crijns HJGM, Tieleman RG et al. Value and limitation of electrical cardioversion in patients with chronic atrial fibrillation – importance of arrhythmia risk factors and oral anticoagulation. Arch Intern Med 1996;156: 2585–92.

8 Wijffels MCEF, Kirchhof CJHJ, Dorland R, Allessie MA. Atrial fibrillation begets atrial fibrillation. A study in awake chronically instrumented goats. Circulation 1995;92:1954–68.

9 Coumel P. Neural aspects of paroxysmal atrial fibrillation. In Falk RH, Podrid PJ, eds. Atrial fibrillation: mechanisms and management. New York: Raven Press, 1992, pp 109–25.

10 Krahn AD, Manfreda J, Tate RB, Mathewson FAL, Cuddy TE. The natural history of atrial fibrillation:

incidence, risk factors, and prognosis in the Manitoba follow-up study. Am J Med 1995;98: 476–84.

11 Önundarson PT, Thorgeirsson G, Jonmundsson E, Sigfusson N, Hardarson Th. Chronic atrial fibrillation – epidemiologic features and 14 years follow-up: a case control study. Eur Heart J 1987; 8:521–7.

12 Crijns HJGM, Van den Berg MP, Van Gelder IC, Van Veldhuisen DJ. Management of atrial fibrillation in the setting of heart failure. Eur Heart J 1997; 18(Suppl C):C45–C49.

13 Van Gelder IC, Crijns HJGM, Blanksma PK et al. Time course of hemodynamic changes and improvement of exercise tolerance after cardioversion of chronic atrial fibrillation unassociated with cardiac valve disease. Am J Cardiol 1993;72:560–6.

14 Kannel WB, Abbott RD, Savage DD, McNamara PM. Epidemiologic features of chronic atrial fibrillation. N Engl J Med 1982;306:1018–22.

15 Carson PE, Johnson GR, Dunkman WB et al. The influence of atrial fibrillation on prognosis in mild to moderate heart failure: the V-HeFT studies. Circulation 1993;87(Suppl VI):VI-102–VI-110.

16 Stevenson WG, Stevenson LW, Middlekauff HR et al. Improving survival for patients with atrial fibrillation and advanced heart failure. J Am Coll Cardiol 1996;28:1458–463.

17 Keren G, Etzion T, Sherez J et al. Atrial fibrillation and atrial enlargement in patients with mitral stenosis. Am Heart J 1987;114:1146–55.

18 Sanfilippo AJ, Abascal VM, Sheehan M et al. Atrial enlargement as a consequence of atrial fibrillation. Circulation 1990;82:792–7.

19 Gosselink ATM, Crijns HJGM, Hamer JPM, Hillege H, Lie KI. Changes in atrial dimensions after cardioversion: role of mitral valve disease. J Am Coll Cardiol 1993;22:1666–72.

20 Wolf PA, Abbott RD, Kannel WB. Atrial fibrillation: a major contributor to stroke in the elderly. Arch Intern Med 1987;147:1561–4.

21 Petersen P. Thromboembolic complications of atrial fibrillation and their prevention: a review. *Am J Cardiol* 1990;**65**:24C–28C.

22 The Stroke Prevention in Atrial Fibrillation investigators. Predictors of thromboembolism in atrial fibrillation: I. Clinical features of patients at risk. *Ann Intern Med* 1992;**116**:1–5.

23 The Stroke Prevention in Atrial Fibrillation investigators. Predictors of thromboembolism in atrial fibrillation: II. Echocardiographic features of patients at risk. *Ann Intern Med* 1992;**116**: 6–12.

24 Hou Z-Y, Chang M-S, Chen C-Y *et al.* Acute treatment of recent-onset atrial fibrillation and flutter with a tailored dosing regimen of intravenous amiodarone. A randomized, digoxin-controlled study. *Eur Heart J* 1995;**16**:521–8.

25 Stambler BS, Wood MA, Ellenbogen KA *et al.* and the Ibutilide repeat dose study investigators. Efficacy and safety of repeated intravenous doses of ibutilide for rapid conversion of atrial flutter or fibrillation. *Circulation* 1996;**94**:1613–21.

26 Crijns HJGM, Van Gelder IC, Kingma JH *et al.* Atrial flutter can be terminated by a class III antiarrhythmic drug but not by class IC drug. *Eur Heart J* 1994;**15**:1403–8.

27 Falk RH, Knowlton AA, Bernard SA, Gotlieb NE, Battinelli NJ. Digoxin for converting recent-onset atrial fibrillation to sinus rhythm. *Ann Intern Med* 1987;**106**:503–6.

28 Noc M, Stajer D, Horvat M. Intravenous amiodarone versus verapamil for acute conversion of paroxysmal atrial fibrillation to sinus rhythm. *Am J Cardiol* 1990;**65**:679–80.

29 Anderson JL, Gilbert EM, Alpert BL *et al.* Prevention of symptomatic recurrences of paroxysmal atrial fibrillation in patients initially tolerating antiarrhythmic therapy. *Circulation* 1989;**80**:1557–70.

30 Anderson JL, Platt ML, Guarnieri T *et al.* and the flecainide supraventricular tachycardia study group. Flecainide acetate for paroxysmal supraventricular arrhythmias. *Am J Cardiol* 1994; **74**:578–84.

31 UK Propafenone PSVT Study Group. A randomized, placebo-controlled trial of propafenone in the prophylaxis of paroxysmal supraventricular tachycardia and paroxysmal atrial fibrillation. *Circulation* 1995;**92**:2250–7.

32 Naccarelli GV, Dorian P, Hohnloser SH, Coumel P, for the flecainide multicenter atrial fibrillation group. Prospective comparison of flecainide versus quinidine for the treatment of paroxysmal atrial fibrillation/flutter. *Am J Cardiol* 1996;**77**: 53A–59A.

33 Reimold SC, Cantillon CO, Friedman PL, Antman EM. Propafenone versus sotalol for suppression of recurrent symptomatic atrial fibrillation. *Am J Cardiol* 1993;**71**:558–63.

34 Horowitz LN, Spielman SR, Greenspan AM *et al.* Use of amiodarone in the treatment of persistent and paroxysmal atrial fibrillation resistant to quinidine therapy. *J Am Coll Cardiol* 1985;**6**: 1402–7.

35 Marcus FI. The hazard of using type IC antiarrhythmic drugs for the treatment of paroxysmal atrial fibrillation. *Am J Cardiol* 1990; **66**:366–7.

36 Crozier I. Flecainide in the Wolff–Parkinson–White syndrome. *Am J Cardiol* 1992;**70**: 26A–32A.

37 Crijns HJGM, Gosselink ATM, Van Gelder IC *et al.* Drugs after cardioversion to prevent relapses of chronic atrial fibrillation. In: Kingma JH, van Hemel NM, Lie KI, eds. *Atrial fibrillation, a treatable disease?* Dordrecht: Kluwer Academic Publishers, 1992, pp 105–48.

38 Coplen SE, Antman EM, Berlin JA, Hewitt P, Chalmers TC. Efficacy and safety of quinidine therapy for maintenance of sinus rhythm after cardioversion. A meta-analysis of randomized control trials. *Circulation* 1990;**82**:1106–16.

39 Carlsson J, Tebbe U, Rox J *et al.* for the ALKK study group. Cardioversion of atrial fibrillation in the elderly. *Am J Cardiol* 1996;**78**:1380–4.

40 Gosselink ATM, Crijns HJ, Van Gelder IC *et al.* Low-dose amiodarone for maintenance of sinus rhythm after cardioversion of atrial fibrillation or flutter. *JAMA* 1992;**267**:3289–93.

41 Szekely P, Sideris DA, Batson GA. Maintenance of sinus rhythm after atrial defibrillation. *Br Heart J* 1970;**32**:741–6.

42 Brignole M, Gianfranchi L, Menozzi C *et al.* Influence of atrioventricular junction radiofrequency ablation in patients with chronic atrial fibrillation and flutter on quality of life and cardiac performance. *Am J Cardiol* 1994;**72**: 242–6.

43 Mathew JP, Parks R, Savino JS *et al.* for the Multicenter Study of Perioperative Ischaemia Research Group. Atrial fibrillation following coronary artery bypass graft surgery. *JAMA* 1996; **276**:300–6.

44 Kowey PR, Taylor JE, Rials SJ, Marinchak RA. Meta-analysis of the effectiveness of prophylactic drug therapy in preventing supraventricular arrhythmia early after coronary artery bypass grafting. *Am J Cardiol* 1992;**69**:963–5.

45 Andrews TC, Reimold SC, Berlin JA, Antman EM. Prevention of supraventricular arrhythmias after coronary artery bypass surgery. A meta-analysis of randomized trials. *Circulation* 1991;**84**(Suppl III):III-236–III-244.

46 Suttorp MJ, Kingma JH, Tjon Joe Gin RM *et al.* Efficacy and safety of low and high dose sotalol versus propranolol in the prevention of supraventricular tachyarrhythmias early after

coronary artery bypass surgery. *J Thorac Cardiovasc Surg* 1990;**100**:921–6.

47 Fanning WJ, Thomas CS Jr, Roach A *et al*. Prophylaxis of atrial fibrillation with magnesium sulfate after coronary artery bypass grafting. *Ann Thorac Surg* 1991;**52**:529–33.

48 Butler J, Harriss DR, Sinclair M, Westaby S. Amiodarone prophylaxis for tachycardias after coronary artery surgery: a randomised, double blind, placebo controlled trial. *Br Heart J* 1993; **70**:56–60.

49 Groves PH, Hall RJC. Review article. Atrial tachyarrhythmias after cardiac surgery. *Eur Heart J* 1991;**12**:458–63.

50 Gentili C, Giordano F, Alois A, Massa E, Bianconi L. Efficacy of intravenous propafenone in acute atrial fibrillation complicating open-heart surgery. *Am Heart J* 1992;**123**:1225–8.

51 Crijns HJGM, Van Gelder IC, Van der Woude HJ *et al*. Efficacy of serial electrical cardioversion therapy in patients with chronic atrial fibrillation after valve replacement and implications for

surgery to cure atrial fibrillation. *Am J Cardiol* 1996;**78**:1140–4.

52 Hohnloser SH, Van Loo A, Baedeker F. Efficacy and proarrhythmic hazards of pharmacologic cardioversion of atrial fibrillation: prospective comparison of sotalol versus quinidine. *J Am Coll Cardiol* 1995;**26**:852–8.

53 Jackman WM, Friday KJ, Andersen JL *et al*. The long QT syndromes: a critical review, new clinical observations and a unifying hypothesis. *Prog Cardiovasc Dis* 1988;**31**:115–72.

54 Falk RH. Flecainide-induced ventricular tachycardia and fibrillation in patients treated for atrial fibrillation. *Ann Intern Med* 1989;**111**:107–11.

55 Flaker GC, Blackshear JL, McBride R *et al*. on behalf of the Stroke Prevention in Atrial Fibrillation Investigators. Antiarrhythmic drug therapy and cardiac mortality in atrial fibrillation. *J Am Coll Cardiol* 1992;**20**:527–32.

56 Lehmann MH, Hardy S, Archibald D, Quart B, MacNeilx DJ. Sex differences in risk of torsade de pointes with *d,l*-sotalol. *Circulation* 1996;**94**: 2534–41.

33 Atrial fibrillation: antithrombotic therapy

JOHN A. CAIRNS

DEFINITIONS, INCIDENCE, AND NATURAL HISTORY

Although oral anticoagulant prophylaxis against embolic stroke in rheumatic atrial fibrillation had been in wide use, it remained for the Framingham study[1-5] to demonstrate that the annual incidence of stroke was similar among patients with rheumatic and non-rheumatic atrial fibrillation. These observations, together with evidence of the greater safety of lower dose warfarin,[6,7] prompted the initiation of several well designed randomized controlled trials of anticoagulant and antiplatelet therapy of non-rheumatic atrial fibrillation (see Table 33.1). Non-rheumatic atrial fibrillation was generally defined by the exclusion of echocardiographic mitral stenosis. The terms non-valvular atrial fibrillation and non-rheumatic atrial fibrillation are not entirely synonymous although they are often used interchangeably. The term non-rheumatic atrial fibrillation is generally preferred.

In the Framingham study,[4] patients were stratified according to the presence or absence of rheumatic heart disease, and the risk of stroke was adjusted for age and blood pressure. In comparison with patients without atrial fibrillation, the risk ratio for stroke was 17.6 for those with rheumatic atrial fibrillation and 5.6 for those with non-rheumatic atrial fibrillation. However, the absolute annual rate of stroke was virtually the same in the two groups (4.5% per year for the rheumatic atrial fibrillation group and 4.2% per year for the non-rheumatic atrial fibrillation group). The most reliable

Table 33.1 Non-rheumatic atrial fibrillation trial designs

Trial	Sample size	Warfarin	INR	Aspirin
BAATAF	420	Open	1.5–2.7	
CAFA	383	Blind	2.0–3.0	
SPINAF	536	Blind	1.5–2.5	
AFASAK	1007	Open	2.8–4.2	75 mg/day
SPAF	1330	Open	2.0–4.5	325 mg/day

INR, international normalized ratio.
BAATAF, Boston Area Anticoagulation Trial for Atrial Fibrillation; CAFA, Canadian Atrial Fibrillation Anticoagulation; SPINAF, Stroke Prevention in Nonrheumatic Atrial Fibrillation; AFASAK, Copenhagen Atrial Fibrillation Aspirin Anticoagulation; SPAF, Stroke Prevention in Atrial Fibrillation.

Table 33.2   Non-rheumatic atrial fibrillation trial outcomes: warfarin

	Ischemic stroke				Major bleed
	Control per 1000 pt/yr	Warfarin per 1000 pt/yr	Risk reduction (RR) (%)	Reduction per 1000 pt/yr	Increase per 1000 pt/yr
BAATAF	30	4	87	26	2
CAFA	38	26	32	12	15
SPINAF	43	9	79	34	6
AFASAK	50	32	36	18	8
SPAF	70	23	67	47	−1
Overview	45	14	68	31	3

and current information comes from an analysis of the placebo groups in the recent clinical trials[8–13] where the annual incidence of stroke ranged from 3% to 7%, and the annual incidence of stroke plus other systemic emboli ranged from 3% to 7.4% (see Table 33.2). Patients were selected for entry into these trials based upon a variety of criteria, including the absence of contraindications to warfarin and in some instances to aspirin, and the willingness to participate in a clinical trial. Hence, generalizations to a wider population must be made cautiously, but it is likely that these rates of stroke and other systemic embolism are reasonably close to those in the general population. In early case series, 50–70% of embolic stroke resulted in either death or severe neurologic deficit[14] and in the recent randomized trials as many as half the strokes resulted in death or permanent disability.

Several cohort studies[14] have demonstrated a reasonably consistent reduction of annual stroke risk among patients with paroxysmal or transient atrial fibrillation compared to those with chronic atrial fibrillation. The recent clinical trials have not been helpful in further delineating the relative risk of systemic embolization among patients with paroxysmal versus chronic atrial fibrillation.

The term "lone atrial fibrillation" is generally used to describe patients who have atrial fibrillation in the absence of other demonstrable heart disease.[14] The definition is frequently extended to require the exclusion of diabetes mellitus and hypertension, and, in some series, an age younger than 60 years is required to fulfill the criteria. In general, stroke rates are much lower among patients with lone atrial fibrillation, and discrepancies amongst them are most likely explained by differences in age, the presence of cardiovascular risk factors, and the chronicity of atrial fibrillation.[15,16] Studies suggest that as the study population ages, a decreasing proportion of patients with atrial fibrillation is free of other heart disease.

ANTITHROMBOTIC MANAGEMENT

Anticoagulant therapy

Five randomized controlled trials of warfarin versus control or placebo have been reported (Tables 33.1, 33.2). The trials generally enrolled patients with chronic atrial fibrillation detected on a routine or screening electrocardiogram (mean age 69 years). AFASAK[11] and SPINAF[10] excluded patients with intermittent atrial fibrillation, whereas the proportion of intermittent atrial fibrillation was 7% in CAFA,[9] 16% in BAATAF,[8] and 34% in SPAF.[13] Previous stroke or transient ischemic attack was infrequent. Treatment allocation was randomized in all trials. There was a double-blind comparison of warfarin to placebo in CAFA and SPINAF, and an open label comparison in BAATAF. AFASAK compared warfarin, aspirin, and aspirin placebo. SPAF allocated patients as warfarin-eligible (group 1) and warfarin-ineligible (group 2). Group 1 patients were randomized to open label warfarin or usual therapy; Group 2 patients were randomized to open label warfarin, aspirin, or aspirin placebo. The INR range in these trials varied from 1.2–2.5 to 2.8–4.2.

Four of the trials were stopped early by their Data and Safety Monitoring Boards because interim analyses were strongly positive, whereas the fifth[9] was stopped early because of the strongly positive results from two other trials. The primary outcomes varied somewhat among the trials. However, it is possible to determine the rates of ischemic stroke and major bleeding (intracranial, transfusion of ≥ 2 units, hospitalization) from each trial, to make comparisons and to pool the results. The Atrial Fibrillation Investigators overview[17] was a collaborative prospective meta-analysis which provides reliable summary data, based on individual patient information. The overall risk of ischemic stroke was 4.5% per year, identical to that documented in the Framingham study. This was reduced to 1.4% per year with warfarin, a reduction of 31 strokes for every 1000 patients treated ($P<0.001$). A major concern with warfarin is hemorrhage, which was carefully documented in each trial. The rate of major hemorrhage with warfarin was 1.3% per year versus 1% per year in control, an increase of 3 major hemorrhages per 1000 patients treated, including an excess of intracranial hemorrhage of 2 per year for every 1000 patients treated. Hence, the overall picture is one of major benefit from warfarin, with only a modest increase in the risk of major hemorrhage and cerebral hemorrhage.

The European Atrial Fibrillation Trial compared warfarin, aspirin, and placebo among patients with non-rheumatic atrial fibrillation who had experienced a transient ischemic attack (TIA) or stroke within the preceding 3 months.[18] The risk of recurrence of stroke was 12% among the placebo patients, dramatically higher than the 4.5% annual risk in the overall population of patients with non-rheumatic atrial fibrillation. The relative risk reduction on warfarin was 66% ($P<0.001$), virtually identical to that calculated in the overview of the five major randomized controlled trials, but the absolute reduction of strokes was much greater (80 per year per 1000 versus 31 per year per 1000) because of the high baseline risk of stroke in this population. Major bleeding was more frequent (excess of 21 per year per 1000), but the risk benefit ratio was strongly in favor of warfarin over placebo.

Additional analyses from the five trials have provided useful data on the prognostic stratification of patients in regard to risk of stroke.[17] The Atrial Fibrillation Investigators overview has demonstrated that the statistically significant multivariate predictors of stroke are previous stroke or TIA, increasing age, history of hypertension, congestive heart failure, or myocardial infarction, and diabetes. The Stroke Prevention in Atrial Fibrillation investigators have also demonstrated that echocardiographic increased left atrial size and LV dysfunction are important determinants of the risk of stroke.[19] The annual risk of stroke is about 4.5% among the group of patients with non-rheumatic atrial fibrillation. However, patients under 60 years of age with no risk factors have an annual risk of <1% (there were no strokes among 112 such patients in the Atrial

R

Grade A

R

Grade A

R

Grade A

Table 33.3 Non-rheumatic atrial fibrillation trial outcomes: aspirin

| | Ischemic stroke | | | | Major bleed |
	Control per 1000 pt/yr	Aspirin per 1000 pt/yr	RR (%)	Reduction per 1000 pt/yr	Increase per 1000 pt/yr
AFASAK	50	42	16	8	4
SPAF	58	32	44	26	2
EAFT	120	100	17	20	2
Overview			21		

Fibrillation Investigators' overview). Patients of any age with no echocardiographic or clinical risk factors have a risk of only 1%, whereas this risk rises to 5% with the presence of enlarged left atrium or LV dysfunction and to 7.2% with the presence of congestive heart failure, previous stroke, or hypertension. When two or three clinical risk factors are present, the annual risk of stroke rises to 17.6%.[19,20]

The short term risk of stroke appears to be higher among patients with recent onset atrial fibrillation than among those in whom atrial fibrillation has been present for more than 1–2 years.[21,22] Among patients with atrial fibrillation who have experienced an embolic event, the risk of recurrence in subsequent months appears to be considerably higher than the overall incidence. The high rate of recurrence, although not observed in every study, suggested there is some urgency in initiating anticoagulation following the occurrence of embolic stroke in patients with atrial fibrillation. However, such therapy can increase the risk for hemorrhagic transformation of an embolic brain infarction. Based on a review of the literature and the results of the only available randomized clinical trial, the cerebral embolism study group recommended anticoagulation therapy for patients with small and moderate sized embolic infarcts if a CT scan performed 24 hours from stroke onset did not show hemorrhage. In patients with large infarction, it was recommended that anticoagulant therapy be delayed until the CT scan was performed at 7 days to exclude delayed hemorrhage.[14,23]

Grade B

Aspirin therapy

Comparisons of aspirin to placebo resulted in somewhat less impressive risk reduction for stroke of about 16% (NS) in AFASAK,[11,12] 44% ($P=0.02$) in SPAF,[13] and 17% (NS) in the European Atrial Fibrillation Trial (EAFT)[18] (Table 33.3). A meta-analysis of these trials found an overall reduction of 21% ($P=0.05$) in the rate of ischemic stroke by aspirin compared to placebo.[24] Hence, aspirin can be expected to reduce the risk of ischemic stroke with a relative risk reduction of perhaps one-third that of warfarin with a low risk of major bleeding.

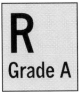

Grade A

Aspirin vs warfarin

The SPAF II trial studied 715 patients aged 75 years or less and 385 patients aged over 75 years, with each group randomly allocated warfarin or aspirin.[25] The incidence of

Table 33.4 Non-rheumatic atrial fibrillation trial outcomes: warfarin vs aspirin

Trial	Ischemic stroke			
	Warfarin per 1000 pt/yr	ASA per 1000 pt/yr	RR (%)	Reduction per 1000 pt/yr
SPAF-2	18	26	31	8
AFASAK	15	38	50	19
EAFT	40	104	62	64
Overview			48	

ischemic stroke was less with warfarin than aspirin in each group (*P*=NS), but intracranial hemorrhage was more frequent on warfarin and the overall rate of stroke was little different on warfarin compared to aspirin. The rate of all strokes with residual deficit was lower with warfarin than aspirin in the ≤75-year-old group (*P*=NS), but was slightly higher in the >75-year-old group (*P*=NS) (mean age 80 years). When patients with clinical risk factors (congestive heart failure, increased blood pressure, previous stroke) were examined, there was a strong trend toward more reduction of stroke with warfarin than aspirin in both the under-75 and over-75 years age groups. In an attempt to better delineate the relative benefits of warfarin vs aspirin, particularly in patients at high risk of stroke, the SPAF III trial was undertaken.[26] Patients at high risk of embolic stroke because of impaired LV function, systolic hypertension, prior thromboembolism, or who were female and aged over 75 were randomly allocated warfarin, INR 2–3 or warfarin 1–3 mg per day plus aspirin 325 mg per day. This trial was discontinued early after a mean follow up of 1.2 years because the rate of the composite primary outcome of ischemic stroke or systemic embolus was significantly higher in those given combination therapy versus those given adjusted dose warfarin (7.9% versus 1.9% per year, risk increase 216%, *P*<0.0001). Rates of disabling stroke and of the composite of ischemic stroke, systemic embolus or vascular death were also significantly and markedly increased. The rates of major bleeding were similar in the two treatment groups. It is clear that in high risk patients, targeting INR in the range of 1.2–1.5 does not provide adequate protection against thromboembolism.

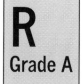

R

Grade A

Direct comparisons of warfarin and aspirin were undertaken in AFASAK,[11,12] SPAF II[25] and EAFT[18] (Table 33.4). The risk reductions for stroke with warfarin were AFASAK 51% (NS), SPAF II 32% (NS) and EAFT 62% (*P*=0.001). When the three trials comparing warfarin to aspirin are looked at in aggregate there is a statistically significant benefit of warfarin compared to aspirin (relative RR 49%, *P*<0.001).[27] Major bleeding had occurred at a rate of 2.8% per year on warfarin, 0.9% per year on aspirin, and 0.7% per year on placebo.

Risk of hemorrhage

The efficacy of warfarin for the prevention of ischemic stroke must be balanced against the risk of major hemorrhage, particularly cerebral hemorrhage which is usually fatal. The risk of major hemorrhage is related to the intensity of anticoagulation, patient age, and fluctuation of INR.[28,29] It is likely that the risk of major hemorrhage is higher in clinical practice than in the rigorous setting of a clinical trial.[28,29] The 3.1% absolute reduction of ischemic stroke observed in the initial five randomized controlled trials was accompanied by an absolute excess risk of major hemorrhage of only 0.3%. The INR ranged from a low of 1.5 to a high of 4.5. The most widely recommended INR range for patients with NRAF is 2.0–3.0, with a target of 2.5.[30] However, the greatest reductions in the rate of ischemic stroke were observed in the two trials with the lowest INR ranges.[8,10] In SPAF II,[25] the greater efficacy of warfarin over aspirin for the prevention of ischemic stroke was outweighed by excess cerebral hemorrhage in the patients over age 75 years (mean 80 years), suggesting that a somewhat lower INR might be preferable. On the other hand, analysis of the INR levels in relation to ischemic stroke and cerebral hemorrhage in EAFT (mean patient age 71 years)[31] found no treatment effect below an INR of 2.0, most major bleeding complications occurred at an INR of 5.0 or above, and the rate of thromboembolic events was lowest at an INR from 2.0 to 3.9. The authors recommended a target INR of 3.0, with values below 2.0 and above 5.0 to be avoided.

For most patients who are candidates for warfarin, an INR range of 2.0–3.0 with a target of 2.5 appears optimal.[30] However, those with a previous TIA or minor stroke may benefit from a somewhat higher range of 2.0–3.9 with a target of 3.0,[31] while those at higher risk of cerebral hemorrhage, particularly patients over the age of 75, may benefit from a somewhat lower INR range of 1.6–2.5 with a target of 2.0.

Cardioversion

The principal determinant of systemic embolism in non-rheumatic atrial fibrillation is the atrial fibrillation itself rather than any other underlying heart disease. Accordingly, cardioversion of patients with atrial fibrillation and maintenance of sinus rhythm have a strong rationale for the prevention of stroke and systemic embolism. Although there is no reliable information in the literature that cardioversion via electrical or pharmacologic means reduces the risk for systemic embolism, these goals remain an expectation along with a resolution of symptoms related to the atrial fibrillation itself. The strongest predictor of initial and persistent success with cardioversion is short duration of the atrial fibrillation before cardioversion. In general, it may be expected that atrial fibrillation that occurs in conjunction with a viral illness, with alcohol or other pharmacologic excess, or in association with thyrotoxicosis or pulmonary embolus has a high likelihood of reversion with persistence of sinus rhythm. The rate of initial success in restoring sinus rhythm ranges from 76% to 100%, but persistence of sinus rhythm during the next 12 months is noted in 25–81% of patients only.[32–35] Although with chronic antiarrhythmic drug therapy maintenance of sinus rhythm is more likely, a meta-analysis of six randomized, placebo-controlled trials of quinidine therapy[33] revealed a statistically significant tripling of mortality during treatment. Other reviews of the use of Class I antiarrhythmic therapy in ischemic heart disease indicate a statistically significant excess in mortality.[36] Grade A Antiarrhythmic therapy does not appear to be justified in an attempt to prevent embolic events.

Although no study has clearly documented the incidence of systemic embolism following electrical cardioversion, an increased incidence is likely. The best available study,[37] using a prospective cohort design, demonstrated a reduction of postcardioversion systemic embolism from 5.3% to 0.8% among anticoagulated patients. Grade B Other

Table 33.5 Choice of antithrombotic therapies for patients with non-rheumatic atrial fibrillation

Clinical risk factors	Age		
	<65 yr	65–75 yr	>75 yr
No	Aspirin definite	Aspirin >warfarin INR target 2.5	Consider warfarin >aspirin INR target 2.0
Yes	Warfarin definite INR target 2.5	Warfarin definite INR target 2.5	Warfarin Consider INR target 2.0

studies of less rigorous design have also indicated benefit from anticoagulation. It is generally stated that a newly formed thrombus will become organized and adherent to the left atrial wall within 2 weeks of formation. Accordingly, anticoagulation is usually recommended for about 3 weeks before cardioversion.[30] Evidence exists that even after successful electroversion, atrial contraction may not normalize for some weeks, and therefore, maintenance of anticoagulation for about 4 weeks following cardioversion seems prudent.[30,38,39] New onset atrial fibrillation is generally not thought to warrant anticoagulation if cardioversion is undertaken within 48 hours of its onset. The commencement of intravenous heparin immediately upon diagnosis may be prudent, while decisions as to the appropriateness of electrical cardioversion and the preparation for the procedure are undertaken. Emergency cardioversion may be required because of ischemia or hemodynamic compromise in some situations, and if atrial fibrillation has been present for more than 48 hours, heparinization may offer some benefit before cardioversion.

The potential role of transesophageal echocardiography (TEE) for the detection of atrial thrombi and simplification and shortening of anticoagulation regimens in association with cardioversion has recently been studied in a consecutive series of 230 patients.[40] Atrial thrombi were detected in 15%. Of 196 patients without thrombi, 95% were successfully cardioverted without prolonged anticoagulation and none had a clinical thromboembolic event. The Assesment of Cardioversion Using Echocardiography (ACUTE) Pilot Study[41] was a multicenter, randomized controlled trial designed to compare TEE-guided cardioversion with conventional management of cardioversion. There were 62 patients assigned to TEE-guided cardioversion preceded by brief heparinization and followed by at least 4 weeks of warfarin. There were 64 patients assigned to 3 weeks of warfarin, followed by cardioversion and at least 4 further weeks of warfarin. There were no embolic events in the TEE group, and one in the conventional therapy group, while time to cardioversion was shorter in the TEE group. Since the ongoing requirement for anticoagulation following successful cardioversion remains uncertain and the sensitivity and practical availability of TEE in community settings are likely to be less than in university centers, it is not clear which approach is preferable. A large randomized trial is addressing the comparative advantages of TEE-guided cardioversion and the conventional approach.

SUMMARY RECOMMENDATIONS

Patients with persisting atrial fibrillation should generally receive chronic antithrombotic therapy with warfarin or aspirin (Table 33.5). Young patients with atrial fibrillation in the absence of other cardiac abnormality and who are free of a history of hypertension, cerebral vascular disease, congestive heart failure or diabetes mellitus are at very low risk of thrombi embolic events. Aspirin is generally preferable to warfarin, and even no antithrombotic therapy may be acceptable. Warfarin is more effective than aspirin for the prevention of embolic strokes, but the risk of major hemorrhage, including cerebral hemorrhage, is greater. Accordingly, its use should generally be confined to patients who have a substantial risk of embolic stroke. The optimal INR for most patients is 2.0–3.0, with a target of 2.5. Very elderly patients have a higher risk of cerebral hemorrhage while taking warfarin, and it is possible that the optimal risk–benefit ratio may be achieved with an INR range of 1.6–2.5, with a target of 2.0, although some authorities would recommend a target of 2.5 for all patients.

The most powerful predicator of cerebral embolism is previous TIA or stroke, but substantial increased risk is also associated with a history of congestive heart failure, hypertension or diabetes mellitus and echocardiographic evidence of left atrial enlargement or left ventricular dysfunction. The risk–benefit ratio of warfarin is improved among such patients.

Patients undergoing cardioversion should generally receive oral anticoagulation for about 3 weeks prior to the procedure and for 4 weeks after. If the atrial fibrillation has been present for less than 48 hours, initial heparin therapy before cardioversion, followed by 4 weeks of warfarin therapy after cardioversion are likely sufficient. New algorithms involving the use of transesophageal detection of left atrial thrombi in conjunction with cardioversion are being evaluated.

Current trials are attempting to determine relative benefits of warfarin, lower dose of warfarin, warfarin plus aspirin, and aspirin alone in various categories of patients. These trials include AFASAK-II, SPAF III, and PATAF (Primary Prevention of Arterial Thromboembolism in Patients with Atrial non-Rheumatic Fibrillation in general practice).

REFERENCES

1 Kannel WB, Abbott RD, Savage DD *et al.* Coronary heart disease and atrial fibrillation: the Framingham Study. *Am Heart J* 1983;**106**: 389–96.

2 Kannel WB, Abbot RD, Savage DD *et al.* Epidemiologic features of chronic atrial fibrillation: the Framingham Study. *N Engl J Med* 1982:**306**:1018–22.

3 Wolf PA, Abbott RD, Kannel WB. Atrial fibrillation: a major contributor to stroke in the elderly. *Arch Intern Med* 1987;**147**:1561–4.

4 Wolf PA, Dawber TR, Thomas E Jr *et al.* Epidemiologic assessment of chronic atrial fibrillation and risk of stroke: the Framingham Study. *Neurology* 1978;**28**:973–7.

5 Wolf PA, Kannel WB, McGee DL *et al.* Duration of atrial fibrillation and eminence of stroke: the Framingham Study. *Stroke* 1983;**14**:664–7.

6 Hull R, Hirsh J, Jay R *et al.* Different intensities of oral anticoagulant therapy in the treatment of proximal-vein thrombosis. *N Engl J Med* 1982; **307**:1676–81.

7 Turpie AGG, Gunstensen J, Hirsh J *et al.* Randomised comparison of two intensities of oral anticoagulant therapy after tissue heart valve replacement. *Lancet* 1988;**i**:1242–5.

8 The Boston Area Anticoagulation Trial of Atrial Fibrillation Investigators. The effect of low-dose warfarin on the risk of stroke in patients with nonrheumatic atrial fibrillation. *N Engl J Med* 1990;**323**:1505–11.

9 Connolly SJ, Laupacis A, Gent M *et al.* for the CAFA Study Coinvestigators. Canadian Atrial Fibrillation Anticoagulation (CAFA) Study. *J Am Coll Cardiol* 1991;**18**:349–55.

10 Ezekowitz MD, Bridgers SL, James KE *et al.* Warfarin in the prevention of stroke associated with nonrheumatic atrial fibrillation. *N Engl J Med* 1992;**327**:406–12.

11 Petersen P, Boysen G, Godtfredsen J *et al.* Placebo-controlled, randomised trial of warfarin and aspirin for prevention of thromboembolic complications in chronic atrial fibrillation: the Copenhagen AFASAK study. *Lancet* 1989;**i**: 175–9.

12 Petersen P, Boysen G. Letter to Editor. *N Engl J Med* 1990;**323**:482.

13 Stroke Prevention in Atrial Fibrillation Investigators. Stroke prevention in atrial fibrillation study: final results. *Circulation* 1991; **84**:527–39.

14 Cairns JA, Connolly SJ. Nonrheumatic atrial fibrillation: risk of stroke and role of antithrombotic therapy. *Circulation* 1991;**84**: 469–81.

15 Brand FN, Abbott RD, Kannel WB *et al.* Characteristics and prognosis of lone atrial fibrillation: 30-year follow-up in the Framingham Study. *JAMA* 1985;**254**:3449–53.

16 Kopecky SL, Gersh BJ, McGoon MD *et al.* The natural history of lone atrial fibrillation: a population-based study over three decades. *N Engl J Med* 1987;**317**:669–74.

17 Atrial Fibrillation Investigators. Risk factors for stroke and efficiency of antithrombotic therapy in atrial fibrillation analysis of pooled later from five randomized controlled trials. *Arch Intern Med* 1994;**154**:1449–57.

18 EAFT (European Atrial Fibrillation Trial) Study Group. Secondary prevention in non-rheumatic atrial fibrillation after transient ischemic attack or minor stroke. *Lancet* 1993;**342**:1255–62.

19 The Stroke Prevention in Atrial Fibrillation Investigation. Prevention of thromboembolism in atrial fibrillation: II Echocardiographic features of patients at risk. *Ann Intern Med* 1992;**116**:6–12.

20 The Stroke Prevention in Atrial Fibrillation Investigation. Prevention of thromboembolism in atrial fibrillation: I Clinical features of patients at risk. *Ann Intern Med* 1992;**116**:1–5.

21 Petersen P, Godtfredsen J. Embolic complications in paroxysmal atrial fibrillation. *Stroke* 1986;**17**: 622–6.

22 Wolf PA, Kannel WB, McGee DL *et al.* Duration of atrial fibrillation and eminence of stroke: the Framingham Study. *Stroke* 1983;**14**:664–7.

23 Cerebral Embolism Study Group. Cardioembolic stroke, early anticoagulation, and brain hemorrhage. *Arch Intern Med* 1987;**147**:636–40.

24 Atrial Fibrillation Investigators. The efficiency of aspirin in patients with atrial fibrillation: analysis of pooled data from three randomized trials. *Arch Intern Med* 1997 (in press).

25 Stroke Prevention in Atrial Fibrillation Investigators. Warfarin versus aspirin for prevention of thromboembolism in atrial fibrillation. Stroke Prevention in Atrial Fibrillation II Study. *Lancet* 1994;**343**:687–91.

26 Stroke Prevention in Atrial Fibrillation Investigators. Adjusted-dose warfarin versus low-intensity, fixed-dose warfarin plus aspirin for high-risk patients with atrial fibrillation: the Stroke Prevention in Atrial Fibrillation III randomized clinical trial. *Lancet* 1996;**348**:633–8.

27 Albers GW. Atrial fibrillation and stroke. Three new studies, three remaining questions. *Arch Intern Med* 1994;**154**:1443–8.

28 Hylek EM, Singer DE. Risk factors for intracranial hemorrhage in patients taking warfarin. *Ann Intern Med* 1994;**120**:897–902.

29 Fihu SD, Callahan CM, Martin DC *et al.* The risk for and severity of bleeding complications in elderly patients treated with warfarin. *Ann Intern Med* 1996;**124**:970–9.

30 Laupacis A, Albers G, Dalend *et al.* Antithrombotic therapy in atrial fibrillation. *Chest* 1995;**108**: 3528–95.

31 The European Atrial Fibrillation Trial Study Group. Optimal oral anticoagulant therapy in patients with nonrheumatic atrial fibrillation and recent cerebral ischemia. *N Engl J Med* 1995;**333**: 5–10.

32 Brodsky MA, Allen BJ, Capparelli EV *et al.* Factors determining maintenance of sinus rhythm after chronic atrial fibrillation with left atrial dilatation. *Am J Cardiol* 1989;**63**:1065–8.

33 Coplen SE, Antman EM, Berlin JA *et al.* Prevention of recurrent atrial fibrillation by quinidine: a meta-analysis of randomized trials (abstract). *Circulation* 1989;**80**(Suppl II):II-633.

34 Dittrich HC, Erickson JS, Schneiderman T *et al.* Echocardiographic and clinical predictors for outcome of elective cardioversion of atrial fibrillation. *Am J Cardiol* 1989;**63**:193–7.

35 Lundstrom T, Ryden L. Chronic atrial fibrillation: long-term results of direct current conversion. *Acta Med Scand* 1988;**223**:53–9.

36 Teo KK, Yusuf S, Furberg CD. Effects of prophylactic antiarrhythmic drug therapy in acute myocardial infarction: an overview of results from the randomized controlled trials. *JAMA* 1993;**270**:1589–95.

37 Bjerkelund CJ, Orning OM. The efficacy of anticoagulant therapy in preventing embolism related to DC electrical conversion of atrial fibrillation. *Am J Cardiol* 1969;**23**:208.

38 Manning WJ, Leeman DE, Gotch PJ *et al.* Pulsed Doppler evaluation of atrial mechanical function after electrical cardioversion of atrial fibrillation. *J Am Coll Cardiol* 1989;**13**:617–23.

39 Padraig GO, Puleo PR, Bolli R *et al.* Return of atrial mechanical function following electrical cardioversion of atrial dysrhythmias. *Am Heart J* 1990;**120**:353–9.

40 Manning WJ, Silverman DI, Keightly CS *et al.* Transesophageal echocardiographically facilitated early cardioversion from atrial fibrillation using short-term anticoagulation – five results of a prospective 4.5 year study. *J Am Coll Cardiol* 1995;**25**:1354–61.

41 Klein AL, Grimm RA, Black IW *et al.* Cardioversion guided by transesophageal echocardiography: the ACUTE Pilot Study. *Ann Intern Med* 1997;**126**: 200–9.

Atrial fibrillation: non-pharmacologic therapies

34

Andrew E. Epstein,
G. Neal Kay

The burden of atrial fibrillation is carried not only by patients, but also by society. From the pioneering epidemiologic studies begun in Framingham, Massachusetts, atrial fibrillation has become recognized not only as the most common arrhythmia recorded in the elderly, but also one associated with important morbidity, mortality, and cost.[1-3] By the age of 75 years, over 10% of the population are affected.[1] In patients over 75 years of age with atrial fibrillation, there are yearly increases in mortality (estimated as high as 70%), stroke (70%), and medical costs ($2500 in men and $1700 in women).[4]

The importance of antithrombotic therapy is now undisputed,[5] and various options are available for antiarrhythmic drug therapy either to maintain sinus rhythm or to control the ventricular response in patients in whom sinus rhythm cannot be restored or maintained. Although the role of antiarrhythmic drug therapy has been the subject of intense debate, and it is unknown whether strategies designed to maintain sinus rhythm or simply to control the ventricular response in atrial fibrillation result in greater survival and less morbidity,[6] this chapter is directed at the non-pharmacologic therapy of atrial fibrillation, usually when drug therapy has failed. The various surgical procedures directed at atrial fibrillation, the implantable atrial defibrillator, AV node ablation, and the catheter-based Maze procedure will be discussed.

SURGICAL THERAPY

There are no randomized, controlled trials comparing surgical therapy with others. Indeed, most patients chosen for surgical intervention have failed standard therapies directed at rate and rhythm control. Thus, most reports represent clinical series, and data base analyses.

The ideal surgical procedure designed to treat atrial fibrillation should restore normal sinus rhythm, AV synchrony, normal hemodynamics, atrial transport function, and a graded exercise response. The patient should be symptomatically improved with resolution of palpitations and the feeling of rhythm irregularity. Finally, the vulnerability to thromboembolism should be corrected.

The first surgical intervention directed at atrial fibrillation was cryosurgical ablation of the His bundle followed by implantation of a pacemaker.[7] As will be discussed, catheter ablation of the His bundle with pacemaker implantation has replaced this procedure for patients in whom interruption of AV conduction is deemed appropriate. Although electrical disconnection of the atria and ventricles corrects the feeling of an irregular heart beat, atrial transport is not restored, and anticoagulation must be continued because the atria remain in fibrillation with the attendant risk of thromboembolism.

In 1980, surgical isolation of the left atrium was undertaken to treat atrial fibrillation.[8] Although sinus rhythm is restored and abnormal hemodynamics are largely corrected, the risk of thromboembolism continues because the isolated left atrium is either electrically silent, asynchronous with left and right ventricular contraction, or it continues to fibrillate. Similarly, in the "corridor" procedure for the surgical treatment of atrial fibrillation, both the right and left atria are isolated and an electrical corridor is constructed between the sinus node, AV node, and ventricles.[9] Thus, the sinus node drives the ventricles and provides a regular heart rate. However, since the right and left atria are isolated from the ventricles, the atrial contribution to ventricular filling (the "atrial kick") is absent, AV asynchrony and the hemodynamic abnormalities persist, and the risk for thromboembolism is not corrected.

To overcome the problems associated with His bundle ablation, left atrial isolation, and the corridor procedure, Cox et al. developed the "Maze" procedure.[10-13] The principle underlying the operation is that strategically placed incisions render the atria incapable of generating electrical impulses from any point that can return to the same point without crossing a suture line. In addition, the operation provides a route by which sinus-generated impulses can reach the AV node and thereby drive ventricular contraction.

The details of the Maze procedure are not the subject of this chapter. However, in brief, the operation consists of amputating both atrial appendages and isolating the pulmonary veins. Atrial incisions are made that interrupt conduction circuits within the atria, and direct the sinus impulse from the sinus node to the AV node. Following the operation, sinus rhythm is restored, hemodynamics return to normal, and the vulnerability to thromboembolism is corrected by the re-establishment of sinus rhythm. Although a high incidence of sinus node dysfunction complicated early operations, the procedure has been revised (the Maze III operation) such that injury to the sinus node and its blood supply is decreased, and the need for pacemaker implantation markedly diminished.[14,15]

Most recent results with the Maze III operation are encouraging. The operation has been expanded to allow the possibility of its performance at the time of mitral valve repair and/or coronary revascularization. In Cox's first report of the revised Maze procedure,[14] there were 76 patients, with a mean age of 54 years, of whom 72% were male. Atrial fibrillation was paroxysmal in 58% and chronic in 42%. The duration of atrial fibrillation preoperatively was 9 years, 7% had a previous cardiac surgery, and 34% underwent concomitant cardiac surgery. The major modification of the Maze III operation was to move the left atrial dome incision more posteriorly which caused the atrial septotomy to be more posterior as well. These changes provide a more optimal surgical exposure, less injury to the sinus node, and the need for only one incision to the superior vena cava, thereby decreasing the need for pericardial patching and subsequent left atrial dysfunction. Of the first 76 patients reported, there were two early postoperative deaths: both were in 72-year-old males, one with black lung disease who died with respiratory insufficiency, and one who suffered a cardiac arrest that resulted from tamponade. Although atrial arrhythmias occur commonly in the first 3 months following the operation, these usually resolve. After the Maze III operation, only 1 of 65 patients evaluated had inappropriate resting bradycardia, 8 of 65 had inappropriate resting tachycardia, and 6 of 47 had a blunted chronotropic response. Since many of these patients have various degrees of the bradytachy syndrome, it should be expected that some will require postoperative pacing. Nevertheless, the need for postoperative pacing has decreased from 56% to 29% to 25% after the Maze I, II, and III procedures, respectively. At 3–6 months follow-up, 75% have sinus rhythm, 25% have an atrially paced rhythm, and 94% have restoration of left atrial function.

The Maze III operation demands a great deal of technical skill, and although it is being performed at an increasing number of institutions, the operation is challenging and its undertaking remains relatively confined to specialized cardiac centers. Nevertheless, the results of the St Louis Group have been replicated by other investigators. In 1993, McCarthy et al. claimed a "100%" cure in 13 of 14 patients who survived the operation (7% operative mortality).[16] In 1995, Morris et al. reported a 100% success rate in 37 patients of whom none needed a pacemaker postoperatively.[17] Kosakai et al. combined a Maze operation with simultaneous other open heart procedures in 101 patients with a 2% operative mortality, and the achievement of sinus rhythm in 82%. Of the remainder, all of whom had concomitant mitral valve disease, 4% had a junctional rhythm, and 14% had atrial fibrillation.[18]

DUAL CHAMBER PACING TO PREVENT ATRIAL FIBRILLATION

From empiric, non-randomized, and uncontrolled observations that dual chamber pacing is associated with a lower incidence of atrial fibrillation, atrial-based pacing techniques are in the process of being investigated for this purpose.[19–21] The mechanism of benefit is unknown, but may relate to prevention of slow heart rates in patients with bradycardia-dependent atrial fibrillation, or decreasing the dispersion of refractoriness in patients with marked inter- and intra-atrial conduction delays. Daubert et al. observed a low recurrence rate of atrial flutter and fibrillation in patients with severe interatrial conduction disturbances who underwent *biatrial* (right and left via the coronary sinus) pacing.[19] Saksena et al. have shown that *dual-site* right atrial pacing (from the high right atrium and from the posterior rim of the coronary sinus ostium) prolongs arrhythmia-free intervals in patients with drug-refractory paroxysmal atrial fibrillation.[20] Belham et al. showed that pacing from the proximal coronary sinus provides better pacing thresholds and avoids ventricular capture compared to pacing the distal coronary sinus.[21] Further work is required to demonstrate long-term lead stability, efficacy, and appropriate pacing and sensing.

R
Grade B

THE ATRIAL IMPLANTABLE DEFIBRILLATOR

With the successful use of implantable defibrillators to treat ventricular arrhythmias, the development of an atrial defibrillator was to be expected. As with surgery, however, there have been no controlled trials that compare efficacy, survival, quality of life, or cost in patients treated with implantable atrial defibrillators versus other therapies, either drug or surgical. The feasibility of internal cardioversion of atrial fibrillation has

R
Grade C

been recognized for over a decade, first being tested in animals and later in humans. Atrial fibrillation can often be converted with energies of 2 joules or less. However, although the defibrillation threshold for short duration, acute episodes of atrial fibrillation may be low, whether patients with chronic atrial fibrillation will also respond to low energies is less certain.[22] The major controversies surrounding the use of the implantable atrial defibrillator center on the risk of asynchronous shocks causing ventricular fibrillation and patient discomfort. When shocks of over 1 joule are given, patient discomfort can be important. Whereas patients with ventricular arrhythmias are likely to tolerate higher levels of pain since they recognize the life-saving nature of their device, such tolerance may not be enjoyed by patients with atrial arrhythmias which, if treated with anticoagulation by themselves, are associated with a low risk of death.

The problem of ventricular proarrhythmia resulting from atrial defibrillation shocks has been carefully studied in both animals and man.[22–26] The induction of ventricular fibrillation is rare, but must be placed in the context of proarrhythmia associated with the drug therapy of atrial fibrillation.[27,28] It is likely that the relative risk of proarrhythmia is probably smaller with device than drug treatment strategies.

Only a few implantable atrial defibrillators have been implanted worldwide,[29] and comparisons to other therapies are not available. The technology is in its infancy and its place in the management of atrial fibrillation has yet to be determined.

CATHETER ABLATION OF THE AV CONDUCTING SYSTEM

The feasibility of inducing complete AV block as a method for controlling rapid ventricular rates during atrial fibrillation was first demonstrated by Scheinman[30] and Gallagher.[31] Initially performed in the operating room with cryoablation[7] and later with direct current (DC) discharges from a catheter,[30–34] AV junctional ablation is now routinely performed using radiofrequency (RF) current.[35–40] Although conduction through the AV node can be modified by the application of RF current to the posterior inputs to the AV node in the region normally targeted for slow AV nodal pathway ablation, the standard technique of AV junctional ablation requires the implantation of a permanent pacemaker since complete interruption of AV conduction is produced.

The Percutaneous Cardiac Mapping and Ablation Registry[35] reported in 1987 the procedural outcome data from 55 centers performing DC catheter ablation of the AV conduction system in 495 patients. A voluntary registry without rigorous controls on data collection, this registry reported that third degree AV block was achieved in 64% of patients, successful modification of AV conduction without the need for antiarrhythmic drugs in 9%, resumption of AV conduction requiring antiarrhythmic drugs in 12%, and procedural failure in 15%. Complications of catheter ablation were frequent, including inhospital mortality in 23 patients (5%) with sudden death in 8 patients. New ventricular arrhythmias were observed in 29% and pacemaker-related complications were reported in 20 patients (4%). The French Cardiac Arrhythmia Working Group reported the results of AV junction ablation with DC shocks in 71 patients.[33] Sudden death occurred in 2 patients on days 1–3 after the procedure with 3 additional deaths from pacemaker infection (1 patient) or congestive heart failure (2 patients).

While several other small studies of DC discharges for ablation of the AV conduction system have been reported, the Catheter Ablation Registry was the first international, multicenter, prospective study of the safety and efficacy of this technique.[34] The Catheter

Ablation Registry included 136 patients in whom the technique of DC ablation was attempted to control supraventricular tachycardias, especially atrial fibrillation. Although complete AV block was induced in 113 of 136 patients (83%), complications were frequent and 8 patients died during hospitalization (including 5 deaths directly attributed to the procedure). Left ventricular dysfunction was a powerful predictor of inhospital mortality, with 5 of 8 deaths occurring in patients with a left ventricular ejection fraction (LVEF) <0.20, as compared with only 3 of 128 patients with LVEF ≥0.20 (P<0.01). Polymorphous ventricular tachycardia with QT interval prolongation was observed after ablation in 4 patients. Overall, torsades de pointes ventricular tachycardia or ventricular fibrillation were observed in 9 patients prior to discharge. The corrected QT intervals before (P<0.01) and after (P<0.01) ablation were strong predictors of the development of ventricular arrhythmias.

Following these initial reports using DC discharges, RF current has emerged as the preferred energy source for catheter ablation of the AV conduction system.[35–40] Huang et al. were the first to report the use of RF current to ablate the AV conduction system in canines.[35] Langberg et al. reported the importance of electrode size (3 mm length) to the success of RF catheter ablation, with complete heart block induced in 92% of patients as compared with only 50% with a standard diagnostic catheter.[37] Jackman et al. reported the pathologic findings related to RF ablation of the AV conduction system in 2 patients, with atrial necrosis extending to a depth of 5 mm in the proximal AV node and the full thickness of the proximal His bundle. Complete replacement of the conduction system with dense fibrotic tissue (1.5 × 1.3 cm in area) was observed in one patient who subsequently underwent heart transplantation.[38] Several authors have reported that RF catheter ablation successfully induces complete AV block in over 95% of patients with a risk of recurrent AV conduction in approximately 5–10% of patients.[36–40] The RF ablation procedure appears to be much safer than DC ablation, with lack of barotrauma and without the need for general anesthesia. Morady et al. performed a prospective, randomized comparison of DC and RF catheter ablation of the AV conduction system in 40 patients with drug-refractory atrial fibrillation or flutter.[39] Complete AV block was achieved in 65% of patients with DC ablation and 95% of patients assigned to RF ablation (P<0.05). An escape rhythm was observed in 78% of patients after DC and 85% after RF ablation, though the escape interval was significantly longer after DC than after RF ablation (2074 versus 1460 msec, P<0.05). There was one late sudden death after DC ablation but none after RF ablation.

The multicenter Ablate and Pace Trial (APT) was designed as a prospective registry of RF catheter ablation and permanent pacemaker implantation for the treatment of atrial fibrillation that was refractory to medical therapy.[40] The APT population included 156 patients with a mean age of 66 years with either paroxysmal (n=55), chronic (n=70), or recurrent (n=31) atrial fibrillation. Successful ablation of AV conduction was achieved in 155 of 156 patients (99.4%). Survival at 1 year of follow-up was 85.3%, with 5 of 23 deaths being sudden. Survival over the first year following ablation was significantly lower for patients with a baseline LVEF <0.45 (73%) than for patients with an LVEF >0.45 (88%, P=0.03).

Several authors have reported that catheter ablation of the AV conduction system and permanent pacemaker implantation are associated with improvement in quality of life and exercise capacity.[40–43] Kay et al. noted that the physical functioning and emotional wellbeing of 13 patients undergoing DC catheter ablation significantly improved as compared with baseline measurements. The treadmill exercise capacity and VO$_2$ max were also significantly improved after ablation in this small study.[41] In a large prospective study of patients undergoing catheter ablation of a wide variety of arrhythmias, Bubien et al. reported that quality of life was improved at 6 months after ablation as compared with baseline.[42] However, the baseline quality of life scores of patients with atrial fibrillation who were referred for AV junctional ablation were significantly lower than for patients with other forms of supraventricular arrhythmias undergoing RF ablation. In addition, although AV junctional ablation and permanent pacemaker implantation were followed by improvement in quality of life as compared with baseline measurements, quality of life scores remained far lower than for other groups of patients at the 6 month follow-up assessment. The APT trial found that the New York Heart Association (NYHA) functional class was significantly improved after ablation from a baseline mean value of 2.1 to 1.8 at 3 months and 1.9 at 12 months following the procedure ($P=0.0001$).[37] Quality of life as measured with the Health Status Questionnaire, the Quality of Life Index, and the Symptom Checklist-Frequency and Severity Scale was dramatically improved for this group of patients 12 months after ablation as compared with baseline measurements. There was no difference in maximal treadmill exercise duration (10.0 vs 11.6 min) or VO_2 max (1467 vs 1629 ml O_2) before as compared to 1 year after ablation. Similar improvements in quality of life have been reported by other authors.[43]

The effect of AV nodal ablation and permanent pacemaker implantation on ventricular function in patients with chronic atrial fibrillation and rapid ventricular rates has been studied by several authors.[44–47] Grogan et al. reported 10 patients with chronic atrial fibrillation and with severe left ventricular dysfunction (mean LVEF 0.25) who were initially considered to have an idiopathic dilated cardiomyopathy.[47] Following control of the ventricular rate, the mean LVEF increased to 0.52, suggesting that tachycardia-induced left ventricular dysfunction may be more prevalent than suspected. Heinz et al. studied 10 patients with drug refractory atrial fibrillation with an average ventricular rate >120 bpm. After catheter ablation of the AV conduction system, the left ventricular fractional shortening increased from 0.28 to 0.35 ($P=0.006$), with a concomitant reduction in the left ventricular end-systolic dimension.[44] The APT trial demonstrated that patients with chronic atrial fibrillation and a baseline LVEF <0.45 demonstrated significant improvement in left ventricular function after ablation from a mean of 0.31 at baseline to 0.41 12 months after ablation ($P=0.04$).[40] In contrast, patients with a baseline LVEF ≥0.45 demonstrated no change in left ventricular function after ablation. Similarly, patients with paroxysmal atrial fibrillation did not experience an improvement in LVEF after catheter ablation of AV conduction.

RF catheter modification of AV nodal conduction has been proposed as an alternative to AV node ablation and pacemaker implantation.[48–52] Target sites for RF energy delivery are typically in the basal portion of Koch's Triangle, from its midportion towards the tricuspid annulus to the coronary sinus ostium. Morady et al.[52] have provided favorable long term follow-up using this technique, reporting short term ventricular rate control in 50 (81%) of 62 patients without the induction of pathologic AV block. Ten (16%) had inadvertent high degree AV block. During 19 ± 8 months follow-up, 5 (10%) of 50 patients had a symptomatic recurrence of an uncontrolled rate during atrial fibrillation, and overall long term adequate rate control at rest and during exertion was achieved in 45 (73%) of 62 patients.[52] Others, however, have reported less favorable results, with as few as 5 (31%) of 16 patients reporting long term improvement.[53,54] Thus, the role of AV nodal modification as opposed to ablation remains uncertain.

In summary, catheter ablation of AV conduction and pacemaker implantation are associated with improved quality of life when performed for patients with medically refractory atrial fibrillation. These procedures are associated with the potential for

Table 34.1 Benefits of non-pharmacologic therapy options to treat atrial fibrillation

Procedure	Reference no.	Restores sinus rhythm	Restores hemodynamics	Decreases risk of stroke	Need for implantable device (pacemaker/ defibrillator)
Surgical AV node ablation	7	No	No	No	Yes
Left atrial isolation	8	No	No	No	No
Corridor procedure	9	Yes	No	No	No
Surgical Maze procedure	10–18	Yes	Yes	Yes	No (usually)
Dual or multiple site atrial pacing	19–21	Unknown	Unknown	Unknown	Yes
Implantable atrial defibrillator	22–29	Yes	Yes	Unknown	Yes
Catheter-based ablation of AV conduction	30–47	No	No	No	Yes
Catheter-based modification of AV conduction	48–54	No	No	No	No
Catheter-based Maze procedure	55, 56	Yes	Yes	Yes	No

ventricular arrhythmias and late sudden cardiac death. Whether these risks are increased in this population as compared with medically treated controls is unknown.

CATHETER ABLATION OF ATRIAL FIBRILLATION

Swartz reported the results of a catheter-based ablation procedure designed to reproduce many of the features of the surgical Maze III operation for the treatment of chronic atrial fibrillation.[55] The results suggest that atrial fibrillation can be interrupted by the application of RF current within the left atrium in at least 80% of patients by this technique. Although the technique has been reproduced by other centers with similar results, it remains a long procedure (mean 12.15 hours), with considerable fluoroscopic exposure (mean 2 hours) and the potential for complications. Swartz reported two occurrences of stroke among the first 38 patients, in addition to pulmonary and pericardial complications, urinary tract infections, and the risk of gastrointestinal bleeding. Other authors have reported that paroxysmal atrial fibrillation can sometimes be ablated successfully by a right atrial ablation procedure, though the chances of long term prevention of atrial fibrillation are quite low (<20%).[56] Thus, it appears that catheter ablation of atrial fibrillation is feasible but significant improvements in technique will be required before this treatment can be widely applied.

R

Grade C

CONCLUSIONS

In the absence of controlled clinical trials, much of the management of atrial fibrillation, both medical and interventional, is based on physician judgments made in concert with

Table 34.2 Indications for non-operative therapy options to treat atrial fibrillation (AF)

Procedure	Likelihood of procedural success	Patients likely to benefit from procedure	Desirability of procedure
Surgical AV node ablation	High	Not currently used. If patient needs AV node ablation and is having another cardiac surgical procedure, ablation and pacemaker implantation usually done as a separate procedure	Low
Left atrial isolation	Moderate–high	Not currently used	Low
Corridor procedure	Moderate	Not currently used	Low
Surgical Maze procedure	High	Patients with chronic or paroxysmal AF whose arrhythmia is refractory to medical therapy and who wish to avoid drug and/or pacemaker therapy. Ideal for those having other cardiac surgery with which Maze can be done concomitantly	Moderate–high
Dual or multiple site atrial pacing	Investigations in progress	Patients with paroxysmal AF whose arrhythmia is refractory to medical therapy and who wish to maintain sinus rhythm. Most have bradycardia as additional indication for pacemaker	Investigations in progress
Implantable atrial defibrillator	Investigations in progress	Patients with infrequent episodes of AF. Place in treatment of AF currently under investigation	Investigations in progress
Catheter-based ablation of AV conduction	High	Patients with chronic or paroxysmal AF whose arrhythmia is refractory to medical therapy and who wish to avoid surgical Maze procedure	High
Catheter-based modification of AV conduction	Moderate	Patients with chronic or paroxysmal AF whose arrhythmia is refractory to medical therapy and who wish to avoid surgical Maze procedure and/or pacemaker	Moderate–high
Catheter-based Maze procedure	Investigations in progress	Patients with chronic or paroxysmal AF whose arrhythmia is refractory to medical therapy and who wish to avoid drug therapy, surgical Maze procedure, or pacemaker	Investigations in progress

individual patients. Randomized controlled trials have clearly shown the benefit of systemic anticoagulation in the management of this disease, but whether strategies directed at rate control, rhythm control, and what method should be adopted based on estimates of improved survival, quality of life, and at a reasonable cost is unknown and untested. In the future, some of these questions will be answered by ongoing clinical trials. In contrast, some management strategies may never be compared with others. For the present, Tables 34.1 and 34.2 summarize the anticipated efficacy and appropriate populations that may benefit from the non-pharmacologic therapies for atrial fibrillation that have been described.

Levels of evidence for efficacy and safety of procedures to manage atrial fibrillation

Procedure	Level of evidence
• Surgical AV node ablation	Grade B
• Left atrial isolation	Grade B
• Corridor procedure	Grade B
• Surgical Maze procedure	Grade B
• Dual or multiple site atrial pacing	Grade B
• Implantable atrial defibrillator	Grade C
• Catheter-based ablation of AV conduction	Grade B
• Catheter-based modification of AV conduction	Grade B
• Catheter-based Maze procedure	Grade C

REFERENCES

1 Kannel WB, Abbott RD, Savage DD, McNamara PM. Coronary heart disease and atrial fibrillation: the Framingham Study. *Am Heart J* 1983;**106**: 389–96.

2 Cairns JA, Connolly SJ. Nonrheumatic atrial fibrillation. Risk of stroke and role of antithrombotic therapy. *Circulation* 1991;**84**: 469–81.

3 Camm AJ, Obel OA. Epidemiology and mechanism of atrial fibrillation and atrial flutter. *Am J Cardiol* 1996;**78**:3–11.

4 Wolf PA, Kannel WB, Baker CS, D'Agostino RB, Mitchell JB. Increased mortality, stroke and medical costs imposed by atrial fibrillation (Abstract). *J Am Coll Cardiol* 1996;**27**:312A.

5 The Atrial Fibrillation Investigators. Risk factors for stroke and efficacy of antithrombotic therapy in atrial fibrillation. Analysis of pooled data from five randomized controlled trials. *Arch Intern Med* 1994;**154**:1449–57.

6 The NHLBI AFFIRM Investigators. Atrial Fibrillation Follow-up Investigation of Rhythm Management – the AFFIRM Study design. *Am J Cardiol* 1997;**79**:1198–202.

7 Klein GJ, Sealy WC, Pritchett EL *et al.* Cryosurgical ablation of the atrioventricular node–His bundle: long-term follow-up and properties of the junctional pacemaker. *Circulation* 1980;**61**:8–15.

8 Williams JM, Ungerleider RM, Lofland GK, Cox JL. Left atrial isolation: a new technique for the treatment of supraventricular arrhythmias. *J Thorac Cardiovasc Surg* 1980;**80**:373–80.

9 Leitch JW, Klein G, Yee R, Guiraudon G. Sinus node–atrioventricular node isolation: long-term results with the "corridor" operation for atrial fibrillation. *J Am Coll Cardiol* 1991;**17**:970–5.

10 Cox, JL, Schuessler RB, Boineau JP. The surgical treatment of atrial fibrillation. I. Summary of the current concepts of the mechanisms of atrial flutter and atrial fibrillation. *J Thorac Cardiovasc Surg* 1991;**101**:402–5.

11 Cox JL, Canavan TE, Schuessler RB *et al.* The surgical treatment of atrial fibrillation. II. Intraoperative electrophysiologic mapping and description of the electrophysiologic basis of atrial flutter and atrial fibrillation. *J Thorac Cardiovasc Surg* 1991;**101**:406–26.

12 Cox JL, Schuessler RB, D'Agostino HJ *et al.* The surgical treatment of atrial fibrillation. III. Development of a definitive surgical procedure. *J Thorac Cardiovasc Surg* 1991;**101**:569–83.

13 Cox JL. The surgical treatment of atrial fibrillation. IV. Surgical technique. *J Thorac Cardiovasc Surg* 1991;**101**:584–92.

14 Cox JL, Boineau JP, Schuessler RB, Jaquiss RDB, Lappas DG. Modification of the maze procedure for atrial flutter and atrial fibrillation. I. Rationale and surgical results. *J Thorac Cardiovasc Surg* 1995;**110**:473–84.

15 Cox JL, Jaquiss RDB, Schuessler RB, Boineau JP. Modification of the Maze procedure for atrial flutter and atrial fibrillation. II. Surgical technique of the maze III procedure. *J Thorac Cardiovasc Surg* 1995;**110**:485–95.

16 McCarthy PM, Castle LW, Maloney JD *et al.* Initial experience with the maze procedure for atrial fibrillation. *J Thorac Cardiovasc Surg* 1993;**105**: 1077–87.

17 Morris JJ, Stanton MS, Hammill SC. The maze procedure: a reproducibly safe and effective cure for refractory nonvalvular atrial fibrillation (Abstract). *Circulation* 1995;**92**:1–264.

18 Kosakai Y, Kawaguchi AT, Isobe F *et al.* Modified maze procedure for patients with atrial fibrillation undergoing simultaneous open heart surgery. *Circulation* 1995;**92**:II-359–II-364.

19 Daubert C, Mabo P, Berder V, Gras D, Leclereq C. Atrial tachyarrhythmias associated with high

degree interatrial conduction block: prevention by permanent atrial resynchronization. *Eur J Cardiac Pacing Electrophysiol* 1994;**4**:35–44.

20 Saksena S, Prakash A, Hill M *et al.* Prevention of recurrent atrial fibrillation with chronic dual-site right atrial pacing. *J Am Coll Cardiol* 1996;**28**: 687–94.

21 Belham M, Bostock J, Bucknall C, Holt P, Gill J. Bi-atrial pacing for atrial fibrillation: where is the optimal site for left atrial pacing (Abstract). *PACE* 1987;**20**:1074.

22 Hillsley RE, Wharton JM. Implantable atrial defibrillators. *J Cardiovasc Electrophysiol* 1995;**6**: 634–48.

23 Ayers GM, Alferness CA, Ilina M *et al.* Ventricular proarrhythmic effects of ventricular cycle length and shock strength in a sheep model of transvenous atrial defibrillation. *Circulation* 1994; **89**:413–22.

24 Alt E, Schmitt C, Ammer R *et al.* Initial experience with intracardiac atrial defibrillation in patients with chronic atrial fibrillation. *PACE* 1994;**17**: 1067–78.

25 Griffin JC, Ayers GM, Adams J *et al.* Is the automatic atrial defibrillator a promising approach? *J Cardiovasc Electrophysiol* 1996;**7**: 1217–24.

26 Cooper RAS, Johnson EE, Wharton JM. Internal atrial defibrillation in humans. Improved efficacy of biphasic waveforms and importance of phase duration. *Circulation* 1997;**95**:1487–96.

27 Coplen SE, Antman EM, Berlin JA, Hewitt P, Chalmers TC. Efficacy and safety of quinidine therapy for maintenance of sinus rhythm after cardioversion. A meta-analysis of randomized control trials. *Circulation* 1990;**82**:1106–16.

28 Flaker GC, Blackshear JL, McBride R *et al.*, on behalf of the Stroke Prevention in Atrial Fibrillation Investigators. Antiarrhythmic drug therapy and cardiac mortality in atrial fibrillation. *J Am Coll Cardiol* 1992;**20**:527–32.

29 Lau CP, Tse HF, Lok NS *et al.* Initial clinical experience with an implantable human atrial defibrillator. *PACE* 1997;**20**:220–5.

30 Scheinman MM, Morady F, Hess DS, Gonzales R. Catheter induced ablation of the atrioventricular junction to control refractory supraventricular arrhythmias. *JAMA* 1982;**248**:851–5.

31 Gallagher JJ, Svenson RH, Kasell JH *et al.* Catheter technique for closed-chest ablation of the atrioventricular conduction system. A therapeutic alternative for the treatment of refractory supraventricular tachycardias. *N Engl J Med* 1982;**306**:194–200.

32 Evans GT, Scheinman MM, Zipes DP *et al.* The percutaneous cardiac mapping and ablation registry: summary of results. *PACE* 1987;**10**: 1395–9.

33 Lévy S, Bru P, Aliot E *et al.* JP, Long-term follow-up of atrioventricular junctional transcatheter electrical ablation. *PACE* 1988;**11**:1149–53.

34 Evans GT, Scheinman MM, Bardy G *et al.* Predictors of *in*-hospital mortality after DC catheter ablation of atrioventricular junction. Results of a prospective, international, multicenter study. *Circulation* 1991;**84**:1924–37.

35 Huang SK, Bharati S, Graham AR *et al.* Closed chest catheter desiccation of the atrioventricular junction using radiofrequency energy – a new method of catheter ablation. *J Am Coll Cardiol* 1987;**9**:349–58.

36 Yeung-Lai-Wah JA, Alison JF, Lonergan L *et al.* High success rate of atrioventricular node ablation with radiofrequency energy. *J Am Coll Cardiol* 1991;**18**:1753–8.

37 Langberg JJ, Chin M, Schamp DJ *et al.* Ablation of the atrioventricular junction with radiofrequency energy using a new electrode catheter. *Am J Cardiol* 1991;**67**:142–7.

38 Jackman WM, Wang X, Friday KJ *et al.* Catheter ablation of atrioventricular junction using radiofrequency current in 17 patients. Comparison of standard and large-tip catheter electrodes.*Circulation* 1991;**83**:1562–76.

39 Morady F, Calkins H, Langberg JJ *et al.* A prospective randomized comparison of direct current and radiofrequency ablation of the atrioventricular junction. *J Am Coll Cardiol* 1993; **21**:102–9.

40 Kay GN, Ellenbogen KA, Giudici M *et al.* and the APT Investigators. The Ablate and Pace Trial: a prospective study of catheter ablation of the AV conduction system and permanent pacemaker implantation for treatment of atrial fibrillation. *J Am Coll Cardiol* 1998; (in press).

41 Kay GN, Bubien, RS, Epstein AE, Plumb VJ. Effect of catheter ablation of the atrioventricular junction on quality of life and exercise tolerance in paroxysmal atrial fibrillation. *Am J Cardiol* 1988;**62**:741–4.

42 Bubien RS, Knotts-Dolson SM, Plumb VJ, Kay GN. Effect of radiofrequency catheter ablation on health-related quality of life and activities of daily living in patients with recurrent arrhythmias. *Circulation* 1996;**94**:1585–91.

43 Brignole M, Gianfranchi L, Menozzi C *et al.* Influence of atrioventricular junction radiofrequency ablation in patients with chronic atrial fibrillation and flutter on quality of life and cardiac performance. *Am J Cardiol* 1994;**74**: 242–6.

44 Heinz G, Siostrzonek P, Kreiner G, Göossinger H. Improvement in left ventricular systolic function after successful radiofrequency His bundle ablation for drug refractory, chronic atrial fibrillation and recurrent atrial flutter. *Am J Cardiol* 1992;**69**:489–92.

45 Twidale N, Sutton K, Bartlett L *et al*. Effects on cardiac performance of atrioventricular node catheter ablation using radiofrequency current for drug-refractory atrial arrhythmias. *PACE* 1993;**16**:1275–84.

46 Shinbane JS, Wood MA, Jensen DN *et al*. Tachycardia-induced cardiomyopathy: a review of animal models and clinical studies. *J Am Coll Cardiol* 1997;**29**:709–15.

47 Grogan M, Smith HC, Gersh BJ, Wood DL. Left ventricular dysfunction due to atrial fibrillation in patients initially believed to have idiopathic dilated cardiomyopathy. *Am J Cardiol* 1992;**69**:1570–3.

48 Feld GK, Fleck RP, Fujimura O *et al*. Control of rapid ventricular response by radiofrequency catheter modification of the atrioventricular node in patients with medically refractory atrial fibrillation. *Circulation* 1994;**90**:2299–307.

49 Williamson BD, Man KC, Dauod E *et al*. Radiofrequency catheter modification of atrioventricular conduction to control the ventricular rate during atrial fibrillation. *N Engl J Med* 1994;**331**:910–17.

50 Della Bella P, Carbucicchio C, Tondo C, Riva S. Modulation of atrioventricular conduction by ablation of the "slow" atrioventricular node pathway in patients with drug-refractory atrial fibrillation or flutter. *J Am Coll Cardiol* 1995;**25**:39–46.

51 Tebbenjohanns J, Pfeiffer D, Schumacher B *et al*. Slowing of the ventricular rate during atrial fibrillation by ablation of the slow pathway of AV nodal reentrant tachycardia. *J Cardiovasc Electrophysiol* 1995;**6**:711–15.

52 Morady F, Hasse C, Strickberger SA *et al*. Long-term follow-up after radiofrequency catheter modification of the atrioventricular node in patients with atrial fibrillation. *J Am Coll Cardiol* 1997;**27**:113–21.

53 Kreiner G, Heinz G, Siostrzonek P, Gössinger HD. Effect of slow pathway ablation on ventricular rate during atrial fibrillation. Dependence on electrophysiological properties of the fast pathway. *Circulation* 1996;**93**:277–83.

54 Canby RC, Román CA, Kessler DJ, Horton RP, Page RL. Selective radiofrequency ablation of the "slow" atrioventricular nodal pathway for control of the ventricular response to atrial fibrillation. *Am J Cardiol* 1996;**77**:1358–61.

55 Swartz JF. Presentation to the 17th Annual Scientific Sessions of the North American Society of Pacing and Electrophysiology (NASPE). Seattle, Washington, 17 May 1996.

56 Haïssaguerre M, Jaïs P, Shah DC *et al*. Right and left atrial radiofrequency catheter therapy of paroxysmal atrial fibrillation. *J Cardiovasc Electrophysiol* 1996;**7**:1132–44.

35 Supraventricular tachycardia: drugs vs ablation

R. W. F. CAMPBELL

Radiofrequency ablation is dramatically changing the management of many cardiac arrhythmias. More than anything else, it is forcing redefinition of cardiac arrhythmias. The term supraventricular tachycardia (SVT) is imprecise and, in many cases, an inaccurate descriptor. Accessory pathway tachycardias, which account for up to 40% of all SVTs, are as dependent upon the ventricle as they are upon supraventricular structures. The deficiencies of the descriptor SVT have prompted the use of narrow QRS tachycardia as a substitute label. Used as an ECG descriptor, it has merit but it is not synonymous with the arrhythmias classified as SVT. For instance, some forms of ventricular tachycardia may produce a narrow QRS complex (His bundle and some forms of fascicular tachycardia), whilst a variety of supraventricular tachycardias may produce broad QRS complexes as, for instance, when there is a bundle branch aberration and with Mahaim tachycardias and antidromic reciprocating tachycardias involving accessory pathways.

Improved understanding of arrhythmia mechanisms and anatomy are encouraging greater precision in describing arrhythmias. Whilst the catch-all phrases "SVT" and "narrow QRS tachycardia" will continue to be used as a convenient, crude grouping, arrhythmias should now be categorized by terms that indicate an electrophysiological mechanism and which define aspects of their anatomy. The following SVTs should be recognized: automatic atrial tachycardia, re-entrant atrial tachycardia, para atrioventricular (AV) nodal re-entry tachycardia – also known as AV nodal re-entrant tachycardia (AVNRT) and AV junctional tachycardia (AVJT) – orthodromic reciprocating tachycardia involving an accessory pathway, antidromic reciprocating tachycardia involving an accessory pathway, atriofascicular (Mahaim) tachycardia, atrial flutter, and atrial fibrillation. Further specifications are possible as, for instance, declaring the site of accessory pathways or the subtype of atrial flutter.

The issue of arrhythmia labeling is not pedantry. The therapeutic options for each of these defined arrhythmia types varies whether a drug or a non-pharmacological approach is considered. Combining descriptors of the electrical mechanism and anatomy is important in this regard. For the most part, drugs alter electrophysiological mechanisms whilst radiofrequency ablation alters the anatomy of the arrhythmogenic process. For radiofrequency ablation to succeed, the anatomy of the arrhythmia must be well understood and must contain some crucial small volume arrhythmia generator or arrhythmia conduit that is within the ablative capacity of currently delivered radiofrequency energy.

WHAT DO DRUGS OFFER?

Drug management of SVT alters the electrophysiological processes which either initiate the tachycardia or which contribute to its perpetuation. Drug therapy is palliative except in those rare situations where, through natural history, resolution of the arrhythmogenic process can be expected. Until 1969, when surgery was introduced for the management of patients with refractory arrhythmias based on accessory pathways,[1] drugs were the only therapeutic avenue for those arrhythmias that required treatment. As such, many of the studies investigating drug management of SVT were conducted over 20 years ago. Their design was appropriate for the time, but with increasing sophistication and improved understanding of biostatistics, many of these studies are flawed by present day standards.

There is much less information on the efficacy rates for drug management of tachycardias than is desirable. Table 35.1[2–10] shows the efficacy of antiarrhythmic drugs in studies selected either because they were comparative (usually with placebo) or they involved a large patient population. Very few of these studies were long term. In many, complete abolition of the arrhythmia was not achieved but success was declared by markedly fewer events which were better tolerated. Other measures of success have included, for instance, the more ready termination of tachycardia by vagal maneuvers when drug therapy is present. It is thus difficult to establish a general figure for antiarrhythmic drug success. Until recently, there have been relatively few randomized studies of drug therapy.[2,3,8,10] Even relatively modern studies have often involved small numbers of patients, have inadequately defined the treated arrhythmias and have combined different arrhythmia types. For instance, patients with atrial flutter are commonly considered in atrial fibrillation (AF) trials,[3] yet the basic electrophysiology of these two arrhythmias is very different. In Table 35.1, "SVT" (excluding AF and atrial flutter) results are reported as a composite; effects on specific arrhythmic subtypes are rarely provided.

The success of drug management may be mitigated by changes in the basic process of arrhythmogenesis, as, for instance, with progressive atrial fibrosis or with age-related changes in AV nodal function. Drug success is also dependent upon patient compliance. Antiarrhythmic drugs, which offer rhythm control, may be associated with unwanted effects that discourage continued dosing. Long term antiarrhythmic therapy, as is often required in SVT management, may be associated with an increasing risk of adverse effects contributing to cessation of therapy. This is a particular problem with amiodarone therapy.

WHAT DOES RADIOFREQUENCY ABLATION OFFER?

For most supraventricular tachycardias, radiofrequency (RF) ablation can offer a cure. By direct destruction of the arrhythmia generating site or by interruption of a re-entrant circuit, the arrhythmia can be completely and permanently abolished. RF ablation is

Table 35.1 Efficacy of antiarrhythmia drug management of SVTs – selected studies

Study	Arrhythmia	n	Therapy	Analysis period	Success rate (%)	U/E rate (%)	Comment
Pritchett et al., 1991[2]	"SVT"	14	Flecainide	1 mth	86	23–53	4 doses of flecainide. Attrition with 4 dose flecainide
		28	Placebo		29		
	PAF/A Flutter		Flecainide	1 mth	61	23–55	Statistically significant to placebo for both indications
			Placebo		7	31	
UK Propafenone PSVT Group, 1995[3]	"SVT"	52	Propafenone	3 mth	67–91	2–26	High and low dose crossover study
			Placebo		29–41	0–4	
	PAF	48	Propafenone	3 mth	60–96	3–40	Propafenone statistically significantly superior to placebo. Clinical U/E rate 34% placebo, 52–64% propafenone
			Placebo		30–32	3–4	
Chimienti et al., 1995[4]	"SVT"	72	Flecainide	12 mth	93	10	
		63	Propafenone		86	8	
	PAF	97	Flecainide	12 mth	77	16	
		103	Propafenone		75	14	
Hellestrand, 1996[5]	SVT	102	Flecainide	4 yr	87	9	Included: AF/A Flutter/slow-fast pAVNRT/ortho RT/AT Infants/neonates
Weindling et al., 1996[6]	SVT	106	Digoxin and/or propanolol	Up to 1 yr	70	0	Included: RT/para AVNRT/iar/ectopic AT
Podrid and Anderson, 1996[7]	SVT	480	Propafenone	14 mth	?	15	Randomized comparison. Included: RT, pAVNRT, AT
Dorian et al., 1996[8]	SVT	63	Flecainide	8 mth	86	19	
		58	Verapamil	8 mth	73	24	Included: AT/RT/AF/A Flutter
Hopson et al., 1996[9]	SVT		Flecainide	Up to 1 yr			Study terminated because of CAST
	PSVT	67			87	67	
	PAF	67			73	64	
	CAF	17			56	56	
Aliot et al., 1996[10]	AF/A Flutter	48	Flecainide	1 yr	62	9	Randomized comparison
		49	Propafenone		53	17	

For abbreviations used, see note to Table 35.2.

therefore a most attractive option but there are several detrimental factors to consider. Finding the appropriate place for a curative RF lesion may be difficult or even impossible. Success rates vary depending upon the arrhythmia mechanism and depending upon the skill and persistence of the electrophysiological team (Table 35.2).[11-21]

RF ablation is an invasive procedure and any such technique must carry some risk. Fatalities have been reported with RF ablation of supraventricular tachycardias. The currently reported rate of less than 2 per 1000 "SVT" procedures is low[22] but is still important in the context of treatment for conditions that do not threaten life. The most serious "common" complication is cardiac tamponade produced by cardiac perforation. This may occur in up to 7 per 1000 procedures.[22] Certain high risk situations for its occurrence can be identified, such as when delivering RF energy in the coronary sinus or in a coronary vein. Complications may also be related to operator experience.

Traditionally, RF ablation techniques have been employed for patients whose arrhythmias are not controlled by drug therapy. In only a few high risk situations, such as AF complicating Wolf–Parkinson–White syndrome, has RF ablation became a first line option. The remarkable success rates of RF ablation are changing clinical practice and it is likely that those with access to the technique will use it more aggressively for patients with symptomatic arrhythmias.

The high success rates for RF ablation have discouraged comparative studies against drug management. There is, in fact, no randomized comparative study of RF therapy versus medical treatment. The fact that high success rates of RF ablation are achieved, principally in patients who have already failed drug therapy, might argue its superiority in terms of rhythm control.

SPECIFIC ARRHYTHMIAS

The electrophysiology and anatomy of the various supraventricular tachycardias varies considerably. The relative merits of drugs and radiofrequency should be considered for each individual subtype. Regrettably, it is rare in arrhythmia drug trials for specific arrhythmias to be identified and for the effect of therapy on individual arrhythmia mechanisms to be reported.

Accessory pathway tachycardias

Accessory pathway arrhythmias have received considerable attention. Understanding the mechanism of accessory pathway tachycardias was a major advance which came quickly following the advent of clinical electrophysiological studies in the late 1960s. The pivotal role of an abnormal electrical connection between atria and ventricles and/or ventricles and atria was established.

DRUG MANAGEMENT

Very many antiarrhythmic drugs were tested using accessory pathway arrhythmias as an elegant clinical model.[23] The drugs investigated included quinidine, procainamide, disopyramide, flecainide, propafenone, digoxin, sotalol, verapamil, and diltiazem. These interventions revealed that accessory pathway arrhythmias could be controlled by

Table 35.2 Efficacy of RF ablative management of SVTs – selected studies

Study	Arrhythmia	n	Therapy	Analysis period	Success rate (%)	U/E rate (%)	Comment
Jackman et al., 1991[11]	APT	166	RF ablation	3.1 mth mean	99	1.8	
Van Hare et al., 1991[12]	AVNRT	4	RF ablation	1 wk	75	0	Pediatric population 10 months–17 years
Jackman et al., 1992[13]	APT	12			92	0	
	AVNRT	80	RF ablation	15.5 mth mean	100	6.3	
Sethi et al., 1992[14]	AVNRT	23	DC	11 mth	73	2/23	
Kay et al., 1993[15]	SVT		RF	6 mth			
	AVNRT	245			99	21	7% recurrence
	RT	363			95	1	6% recurrence
	TAT	20			100	0	15% recurrence
	A Flutter	13			77		6% recurrence
Sathe et al., 1993[16]	SVT						
	AVNRT	58	RF	9 mth	95	1/58	2/58 recurrence – flutter procedure RF cured
	RT	58	RF		85		
Haissaguerre et al., 1994[17]	RT	25	DC	10 mth	100	4	
		54	RF		100	4	
Kugler et al., 1994[18]	APT ⎫ AVNRT ⎬ AET ⎪ A Flutter ⎭	640	RF ablation	13.5 mth mean	83 83 92 67	3.7	Pediatric population 20 days to 21 years
Chen et al., 1996[18]	A Flutter	30	RF focal	3–6 mth	93	10	Comparison of two types of RF delivery
	A Flutter	30	RF linear		97	10	
Poty et al., 1996[20]	AT	36	RF	18 mth	86	—	Included: automatic/iar/sar/
Movsowitz et al., 1996[21]	A Flutter	32	RF	9 mth	97		

"SVT", supraventricular tachycardia; U/E, unwanted effects; PAF, paroxysmal atrial fibrillation; A Flutter, atrial flutter; AVNRT, AV nodal re-entry tachycardia; ortho RT, orthodromic reciprocating tachycardia; AT, atrial tachycardia; RT, reciprocating tachycardia; AF, atrial fibrillation; iar, intra-atrial re-entry; PSVT, paroxysmal supraventricular tachycardia; CAF, chronic atrial fibrillation; CAST, Cardiac Arrhythmia Suppression Trial; TAT, "true" atrial tachycardia; AET, atrial ectopic tachycardia; DC, direct current; RF, radiofrequency; sar, sinoatrial re-entry.

interventions that altered AV nodal physiology, accessory pathway physiology or perhaps even atrial or ventricular myocardial electrophysiology. Numerous electrophysiological concepts such as the "window of initiation" were explored. It was quickly recognized that autonomic tone could dramatically alter cardiac electrophysiology in a way that might either be antiarrhythmic or arrhythmogenic.[24] There are no studies of long term drug control but a short term "success" rate of 81% reported for the Class IC drug flecainide represents a reasonable estimate of what is possible.[25]

RF ABLATION

For almost 10 years, cardiac surgery had shown that destruction of the abnormal AV connection could permanently stop accessory pathway arrhythmias including the much feared pre-excited atrial fibrillation. The localized and localizable abnormality involved in accessory pathway arrhythmias created interest in the possibility of non-surgical pathway destruction by catheter-delivered energy. Initial approaches involved the delivery of DC energy but this was quickly supplanted by RF ablation. In even the earliest studies, success rates for accessory pathway ablation were as high as 99%.[11] With destruction of the pathway, reciprocating tachycardias could not occur and thus the procedure was curative. In patients with accessory pathways prone to attacks of atrial fibrillation, some continued to have bouts of atrial fibrillation but without the risk of excessive ventricular response rates. Large databases have revealed that RF ablation of accessory pathways is not without risk. Fortunately, fatal events are very uncommon (up to 2 per 1000).[22] Morbidity of the procedure is also important given that affected individuals are young and otherwise are usually free of disease. Serious morbid problems are uncommon but cardiac perforation may occur in up to 1% of procedures. Strokes can also occur, being reported in 11 of 2222 procedures.[22] Even given these problems, the success rate for ablation in terms of arrhythmia control are better than those achieved by drug therapy.

Not surprisingly, RF ablation is now considered first line management for patients with life threatening forms of accessory pathway arrhythmias and has long been indicated for those with drug refractory arrhythmias. The growth in availability of RF therapy is encouraging its use as first line management for patients with modest symptomatology and often before any drug trial.

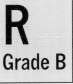

Para AV nodal re-entry tachycardia (AVNRT)

For many years this arrhythmia was considered to be completely contained within the AV node. Mapping during open heart surgery revealed that atrionodal connections constituting atrial inputs to the AV node were an integral part of the circuit supporting the arrhythmia. Like accessory pathways, these atrial inputs, particularly in the form of the slow pathway, are amenable to attack by RF ablation. In large series, success rates are between 80 and 100%,[13,18] with a current average being around 90%. RF therapy is usually used in the event of drug failure, but as experience improves, it is set to become first line therapy for those with severe and frequent symptoms. In most drug studies (Table 35.1) results for para AV nodal re-entry tachycardia are not separated from accessory pathway tachycardia, preventing accurate definition of arrhythmia drug success.

DRUG MANAGEMENT

The concept that para AV nodal re-entry tachycardia was a micro re-entrant circuit contained within the AV node prompted the use of digoxin and/or calcium entry blocker therapy. Clinical practice showed that other drugs including the Class IC agents also had a role. The arrhythmia is probably more difficult to manage than that based on accessory pathways and medical success rates of approximately 60% have been reported.[25] As with accessory pathways, medical success is not necessarily the same as complete abolition of the arrhythmia. Abbreviation of attack duration and reduced frequency of attacks have been used as surrogates for success.

RF ABLATION

The RF ablation success rate for managing para AV nodal re-entry tachycardia is probably marginally lower than that for accessory pathways ablation principally because there is a risk of AV nodal damage and a consequent need for permanent pacing. AV block has been reported in 6% of RF procedures directed at the fast pathway and in 2% directed at the now favored target, the slow pathway.[22] Given the location of the slow pathway, cardiac perforation by RF ablation is relatively rare.

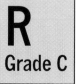

R

Grade C

As with accessory pathways, RF ablation of tissue responsible for para AV nodal re-entry is associated with a high success rate and a low morbidity and mortality. RF ablation offers a curative management with good long term results. Were it not for the risk of permanent damage to the AV node, then this option would be preferred over drug therapy, which is less effective. Current management is usually to try antiarrhythmic drug therapy (a Class IC drug is a reasonable choice) and to have a low threshold for changing the therapeutic strategy to RF ablation in the event of drug failure or intolerance.

True atrial tachycardia

The rarest forms of regular narrow QRS tachycardia are those due to either intra-atrial re-entry or automatic atrial tachycardias. They often exist in the setting of atrial disease.

DRUG MANAGEMENT

True atrial tachycardias are particularly resistant to drugs and often medical management is to control the resultant ventricular response rate rather than to abolish the arrhythmia itself. In a bid to suppress individual arrhythmias, a wide variety of antiarrhythmic agents have been used. There have been very few systematic reports of medical therapy directed against these arrhythmias and no experience has been large enough to offer comparative efficacy evaluations (medical success rates are probably no more than 50%), although there are isolated reports of impressive drug efficacy (e.g. an 83% success rate for flecainide[25]).

RF ABLATION

The micro re-entrant circuit or the automatic focus responsible for the two main types of true atrial tachycardia are, in theory, amenable to RF attack. The success rate is not as high as for the other forms of regular narrow QRS tachycardia. This reflects the varied anatomical basis of the arrhythmia. Nonetheless, overall success rates of 80–90% are possible.[15,18,20]

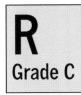

R

Grade C

Atrial flutter

Atrial flutter is a relatively uncommon arrhythmia. Information on its drug susceptibility is sparse, not just because of its rarity but because patients with this arrhythmia often are enrolled in AF studies and efficacy results against flutter are not separated from fibrillation. The electrophysiological mechanism of atrial flutter is now known to be quite different from that of atrial fibrillation and it is long overdue that this arrhythmia be given separate attention.[26] "Common" atrial flutter is based on a macro re-entrant circuit contained largely within the right atrium and depending crucially upon an area of slowed conduction near the tricuspid valve annulus and coronary sinus orifice. Not surprisingly, such a macro re-entrant circuit is difficult to influence with drug therapy.

DRUG MANAGEMENT

A wide range of antiarrhythmic drugs have been tried for the long term control of atrial flutter. The overall success rate for medical therapy is unknown as rarely are these patients separated from those with AF.[2,10] It is probably no more than 50%.[27] Pacing increases the medical success rate but only in so far as acute termination of the arrhythmia is concerned.[28]

RF ABLATION

RF ablation has a growing role to play in the management of atrial flutter. A series of interconnected lesions (a typical approach is from the inferior vena cava to the tricuspid annulus) can interrupt the macro re-entrant circuit of atrial flutter, with long term success rates of between 67% and 97% being reported.[15,18–20] This is probably much better than the results of drug therapy.

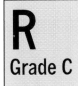

R

Grade C

Atrial fibrillation

AF is the commonest of the atrial arrhythmias and is due to multiple interlacing wavelets of re-entry. The arrhythmia is a major challenge for clinical management, which may seek to restore sinus rhythm, seek to maintain sinus rhythm or may be directed to rate control with continuation of AF. Many factors determine the success rate for medical therapy in restoring sinus rhythm, but overall rates of 80–90% have been reported.[25] A new approach is a single oral dose of drug; propafenone offers successful reversion in 57% of treated patients.[29]

Drug success rates for maintaining sinus rhythm in patients recently cardioverted or who have paroxysms are lower. Short term success rates of 80% are reported.[3] By one year, probably less than 50% of patients are either free of paroxysms or have maintained sinus rhythm, yet in selected patients, sinus rhythm may be maintained in over 70%.[4,9]

DRUG MANAGEMENT

Drug therapy to control ventricular response rates in permanent AF, a feature traditionally provided by digoxin monotherapy, has seemed relatively satisfactory. Clinicians, however, recognize that exercise and sympathetically modulated heart rate increases are not well controlled by digoxin alone. Surprisingly, there has been very little recent research in this area. Coadministration of a beta-blocker or a calcium antagonist has been suggested as bringing benefit. Rate control (an ill defined state) usually improves, but perhaps surprisingly, in only a few studies has effort performance improved.[30]

RF ABLATION

Ablative techniques currently have only a small part to play in AF but their role will likely dramatically expand. Total ablation of the AV node or its modification[27] are important strategies directed at rate control. Crude as it is, total AV node ablation with physiological pacing is associated with marked improvements in quality of life for selected patients.[31] The role of AV nodal modification, i.e. rate control without the need for pacing, is less secure. Only relatively small studies have been reported, again, in selected patients.[32] Success rates of about 75% are suggested, with total AV nodal block being produced in the remainder. Although this latter outcome is labeled a "failure", a pacemaker can be implanted and rate control secured. Studies are currently under way comparing drug vs RF strategies for AF rate control. Their results are not expected until 2001.

With the modest success of the surgical maze procedure,[33] attention has turned to the possibility of "curing" AF with catheter delivery of RF energy. Isolated case reports have suggested that this is possible.[17] Procedural times have been very long. In a very small subgroup of AF patients who appear to have a focal mechanism of their arrhythmia, RF ablation may have a greater role to play. As yet, only isolated, small series have been reported[34] and it would appear that this is a very uncommon mechanism for AF. For the present, medical management of AF would seem the superior option.

REFERENCES

1 Sealy WC, Hattler Jr BG, Blumenschein SD *et al*. Surgical treatment of Wolff–Parkinson–White syndrome. *Ann Thorac Surg* 1969;**8**:1–11.

2 Pritchett ELC, Datorre SD, Platt ML *et al*. Flecainide acetate treatment of paroxysmal supraventricular tachycardia and paroxysmal atrial fibrillation – dose response studies. *J Am Coll Cardiol* 1991;**17**:297–303.

3 UK Propafenone PSVT Study Group. A randomized, placebo-controlled trial of propafenone in the prophylaxis of paroxysmal supraventricular tachycardia and paroxysmal atrial fibrillation. *Circulation* 1995;**92**:2550–7.

4 Chimienti M, Cullen Jr MT, Casadei G for the Flecainide and Propafenone Italian Study Investigators. Safety of flecainide versus propafenone for the long-term management of symptomatic paroxysmal supraventricular tachyarrhythmias. Report from the Flecainide and Propafenone Italian Study (FAPIS) group. *Eur Heart J* 1995;**16**:1943–51.

5 Hellestrand KJ. Efficacy and safety of long-term oral flecainide acetate in patients with responsive supraventricular tachycardia. *Am J Cardiol* 1996; **77**(3):83A–88A.

6 Weindling SN, Saul JP, Walsh EP. Efficacy and risks of medical therapy for supraventricular tachycardia in neonates and infants. *Am Heart J* 1996;**131**(1):66–72.

7 Podrid PJ, Anderson JL. Safety and tolerability of long-term propafenone therapy for supraventricular tachyarrhythmias. The Propafenone Multicenter Study Group. *Am J Cardiol* 1996;**78**(4):430–4.

8 Dorian P, Naccarelli GV, Coumel P *et al.* A randomized comparison of flecainide versus verapamil in paroxysmal supraventricular tachycardia. The Flecainide Multicenter Investigators Group. *Am J Cardiol* 1996;**77**(3): 89A–95A.

9 Hopson JR, Buxton AE, Rinkenberger RL *et al.* Safety and utility of flecainide acetate in the routine care of patients with supraventricular tachyarrhythmias: results of a multicenter trial. The Flecainide Supraventricular Tachycardia Study Group. *Am J Cardiol* 1996;**77**(3):72A–82A.

10 Aliot E, Denjoy I, Attuel *et al.* Comparison of the safety and efficacy of flecainide versus propafenone in-hospital out-patients with symptomatic paroxysmal atrial-fibrillation/flutter. The Flecainide AF French Study Group. *Am J Cardiol* 1996;**77**(3):66A–71A.

11 Jackman WM, Wang XZ, Friday KJ *et al.* Catheter ablation of accessory atrioventricular pathways (Wolff–Parkinson–White syndrome) by radiofrequency current. *N Engl J Med* 1991;**324**(23): 1605–11.

12 Van Hare GF, Lesh MD, Scheinman M *et al.* Percutaneous radiofrequency catheter ablation for supraventricular arrhythmias in children. *J Am Coll Cardiol* 1991;**17**(7):1613–20.

13 Jackman WM, Beckman KJ, McClelland JH *et al.* Treatment of supraventricular tachycardia due to atrioventricular nodal reentry by radiofrequency ablation of slow-pathway conduction. *N Engl J Med* 1992;**327**:313–18.

14 Sethi KK, Singh B, Nair M *et al.* Catheter ablation of retrograde fast pathway in patients with atrioventricular nodal reentrant supraventricular tachycardia. *Indian Heart J* 1992;**44**(6):359–64.

15 Kay GN, Epstein AE, Dailey SM *et al.* Role of radiofrequency ablation in the management of supraventricular arrhythmias: experience in 760 consecutive patients. *J Cardiovasc Electrophysiol* 1993;**4**(4):371–89.

16 Sathe S, Vohra J, Chan W *et al.* Radiofrequency catheter ablation for paroxysmal supraventricular tachycardia: a report of 135 procedures. *Aust NZ J Med* 1993;**23**(3):317–24.

17 Haissaguerre M, Gencel L, Fischer B *et al.* Successful catheter ablation of atrial fibrillation. *J Cardiovasc Electrophysiol* 1994;**5**(12):1045–52.

18 Kugler JD, Danford DA, Deal BJ *et al.* Radiofrequency catheter ablation for tachyarrhythmias in children and adolescents. The Pediatric Electrophysiology Society. *N Engl J Med* 1994;**330**(21):1481–7.

19 Chen SA, Chiang CE, Wu TJ *et al.* Radiofrequency catheter ablation of common atrial flutter: comparison of electrophysiologically guided focal ablation technique and linear ablation technique. *J Am Coll Cardiol* 1996;**27**(4):860–8.

20 Poty H, Saoudi N, Haissaguerre M *et al.* Radiofrequency catheter ablation of atrial tachycardias. *Am Heart J* 1996;**131**(3):481–9.

21 Movsowitz C, Callans DJ, Schwartzman D *et al.* The results of atrial flutter ablation in patients with and without a history of atrial fibrillation. *Am J Cardiol* 1996;**78**(1):93–6.

22 Hindricks G. Complications of radiofrequency catheter ablation of arrhythmias. The Multicentre European Radiofrequency Survey (MERFS) investigators of the Working Group on Arrhythmias of the European Society of Cardiology. *Eur Heart J* 1993;**14**(12):1644–53.

23 Sellers TD, Campbell RWF, Bashore TM *et al.* Effects of procainamide and quinidine sulphate in the Wolff–Parkinson–White syndrome. *Circulation* 1977;**55**:15–22.

24 Crick JCP, Davies DW, Holt P *et al.* Effect of exercise on ventricular response to atrial fibrillation in Wolff–Parkinson–White syndrome. *Br Heart J* 1985;**54**:80–5.

25 Anderson JL, Jolivette DM, Fredell PA. Summary of efficacy and safety of flecainide for supraventricular arrhythmias (Review). *Am J Cardiol* 1988;**62**(6):62D–66D.

26 Waldo AL. Atrial flutter. New directions in management and mechanism. *Circulation* 1990; **81**(3):1142–3.

27 Geraets DR, Kienzle MG. Atrial fibrillation and atrial flutter (Review). *Clin Pharmacy* 1993; **12**(10):721–35.

28 Heldal M, Orning OM. Effects of flecainide on termination of atrial flutter by rapid atrial pacing. *Eur Heart J* 1993;**14**(3):421–4.

29 Botto GL, Bonini W, Broffoni T *et al.* Conversion of recent onset atrial fibrillation with single loading oral dose of propafenone: is in-hospital admission absolutely necessary? *PACE* 1996; **19**(11 Pt 2):1939–43.

30 Lang R, Klein HO, Weiss E *et al.* Superiority of oral verapamil therapy to digoxin in treatment of chronic atrial fibrillation. *Chest* 1983;**83**:491–9.

31 Fitzpatrick AP, Kourouyan HD, Siu A *et al.* Quality-of-life and outcomes after radiofrequency His-bundle catheter ablation and permanent pacemaker implantation – impact of treatment in paroxysmal and established atrialfibrillation. *Am Heart J* 1996;**131**:499–507.

32 Williamson BD, Man KC, Daoud E *et al.* Radiofrequency catheter modification of

atrioventricular conduction to control the ventricular rate during atrial fibrillation. *N Engl J Med* 1994;**331**(14):910–17.

33 Cox JL, Boineau JP, Schuessler RB *et al.* Modification of the Maze procedure for atrial flutter and atrial fibrillation. I. Rationale and surgical results. *J Thorac Cardiovasc Surg* 1995; **110**(2):473–84.

34 Jais P, Haissaguerre M, Shah DC *et al.* A focal source of atrial fibrillation treated by discrete radiofrequency ablation. *Circulation* 1997;**95**: 572–6.

Part III
Specific cardiovascular disorders
v: Ventricular arrhythmias

A John Camm, Editor

Grading of recommendations and levels of evidence used in *Evidence Based Cardiology*

GRADE A

Level 1a   Evidence from large randomized clinical trials (RCTs) or systematic reviews (including meta-analyses) of multiple randomized trials which collectively has at least as much data as one single well-defined trial.

Level 1b   Evidence from at least one "All or None" high quality cohort study; in which ALL patients died/failed with conventional therapy and some survived/succeeded with the new therapy (eg chemotherapy for tuberculosis, meningitis, or defibrillation for ventricular fibrillation); or in which many died/failed with conventional therapy and NONE died/failed with the new therapy (eg penicillin for pneumococcal infections).

Level 1c   Evidence from at least one moderate sized RCT or a meta-analysis of small trials which collectively only has a moderate number of patients.

Level 1d   Evidence from at least one RCT.

GRADE B

Level 2   Evidence from at least one high quality study of non-randomized cohorts who did and did not receive the new therapy.

Level 3   Evidence from at least one high quality case control study.

Level 4   Evidence from at least one high quality case series.

GRADE C

Level 5   Opinions from experts without reference or access to any of the foregoing (eg argument from physiology, bench research or first principles).

A comprehensive approach would incorporate many different types of evidence (eg RCTs, non-RCTs, epidemiologic studies, and experimental data), and examine the architecture of the information for consistency, coherence and clarity. Occasionally the evidence does not completely fit into neat compartments. For example, there may not be an RCT that demonstrates a reduction in mortality in individuals with stable angina with the use of beta-blockers, but there is overwhelming evidence that mortality is reduced following MI. In such cases, some may recommend use of beta-blockers in angina patients with the expectation that some extrapolation from post-MI trials is warranted. This could be expressed as Grade A/C. In other instances (e.g. smoking cessation or a pacemaker for complete heart block), the non-randomized data are so overwhelmingly clear and biologically plausible that it would be reasonable to consider these interventions as Grade A.

Recommendation grades appear either in a shaded margin box with an 'R' logo as shown, or within the text, for example Grade A.

Antiarrhythmic therapy in ventricular arrhythmias

36

Johannes Brachmann,
Thomas Hilbel

The pharmacologic therapy of ventricular arrhythmias is currently under discussion due to unfavorable results of recent clinical studies. After the negative results from the CAST I study with the Class IC antiarrhythmic drugs encainide and flecainide,[1] attention turned from sodium channel blockers to antiarrhythmic drugs that had a different, and presumably safer, mechanism of action by prolongation of repolarization. But the excess mortality of d-sotalol, a pure potassium-channel blocker, in the SWORD study[2] made the prophylactic use of antiarrhythmic agents more and more questionable. Thus the most significant side effect of antiarrhythmic drugs is their proarrhythmic potential.

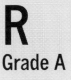

R
Grade A

In contrast, recent studies with amiodarone and dofetilide, which also prolong the action potential duration, showed more positive results, suggesting that a classification of antiarrhythmic drugs would be of some clinical value. The most commonly used classifications, of Vaughan-Williams[3] and the Sicilian Gambit,[4] are based on the effect of antiarrhythmic drugs on intracellular action potentials and receptors of normal heart muscle which has been expanded by drug action on ion channels of the cell membrane.

R
Grade A

Class I	Drugs with direct membrane action. Antiarrhythmic activity is manifest by an inhibition of the rapid inward sodium current ($I_{Na}+$). The kinetics of association and dissociation from channel proteins responsible for different drug action on QRS and QT duration are the basis for their subclassification.
Class IA	Depression of action potential upstroke, slow conduction, prolongation of repolarization (quinidine, procainamide, disopyramide).
Class IB	Little effect on upstroke in normal tissue, depression of upstroke in abnormal fibers, shortening of repolarization (lidocaine, mexiletine, diphenylhydantoin).
Class IC	Marked depression of upstroke depolarization, marked slowing of conduction, slight effect on repolarization (flecainide, propafenone, encainide, ajmalin, prajmalin, moricizine).
Class II	Beta-receptor blocking agents.

577

Class III Drugs that prolong repolarization (amiodarone, sotalol, dofetilide, azimilide, ibutilide), mostly potassium-channel blockers; ibutilide also inhibits the inactivation of the slow sodium inward current.

Class IV Calcium channel-blocking drugs (verapamil, diltiazem).

The antiarrhythmic activities of digoxin and adenosine are not covered within the Vaughan-Williams classification and are of little significance for ventricular arrhythmias.

Several drugs demonstrate multiple pharmacologic activity. Amiodarone, in addition to Class III activity also exerts Class I, II and IV action. Racemic sotalol also possesses Class II effects in addition to its Class III activity.

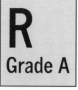

In order to provide improved antiarrhythmic drug therapy in the future, important questions remain to be solved. Is there any antiarrhythmic drug that is safe and prevents the occurrence of a life threatening arrhythmia resulting in reduction not only of sudden cardiac death but more importantly in lowering total mortality? This leads to the next question. Is there any invasive or non-invasive approach that is capable of predicting the outcome of antiarrhythmic drug therapy as well as prognosis of these cardiac conditions?

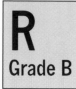

So far no study has evaluated the efficacy of any antiarrhythmic therapy to reduce total mortality by preventing life threatening recurrent ventricular tachycardia or ventricular fibrillation in a randomized, placebo-controlled design. Although CAMIAT (Canadian Amiodarone Myocardial Infarction Arrhythmia Trial) and EMIAT[5,6] (European Myocardial Infarct Amiodarone Trial) demonstrated that life threatening arrhythmias can be prevented in moderate risk patients by antiarrhythmic drug therapy, e.g. amiodarone, this effect was not accompanied by extending those patients lives' significantly. In clinical practice four different pharmacologic strategies for treatment of ventricular arrhythmias are considered appropriate based on existing clinical evidence:

1. Individualized antiarrhythmic drug therapy selected by non-invasive methods (mostly suppression of spontaneous ectopy during Holter recordings).
2. Individualized antiarrhythmic drug therapy selected by invasive methods (mostly suppression of ventricular tachyarrhythmias induced by programmed electrical stimulation).
3. Empiric beta-blocker therapy.
4. Empiric amiodarone therapy.

This variety of methods was also employed in the evaluation of specific antiarrhythmic drug strategies.

OUTCOME OF CLINICAL TRIALS USING CLASS I ANTIARRHYTHMIC AGENTS

Table 36.1 displays the results of recent studies. In the Cardiac Arrhythmia Suppression Trial (CAST) the effect of Class IC drugs versus placebo was investigated in asymptomatic patients with ventricular ectopy following myocardial infarction (MI).[1] The CAST trial was prematurely terminated, due to excess mortality in the treatment group with flecainide and encainide. Although the drugs suppressed spontaneous ventricular

Table 36.1   Results of recent antiarrhythmic drug trials

Study	Objective	Inclusion method	Outcome		
			Worse		Better
CAST[1]	Class IC post MI	VPC suppression by Holter MI (6 d–2 y) EF $\leq 55\%$ if MI ≤ 90 d EF $\leq 40\%$ if MI >90 d	Class IC	<	Placebo
CASH[7]	ICD vs drugs in SCD	Inducible VT/VF	Propafenone	<	ICD
ESVEM[8–10]	Holter vs PES in VT/VF	History of VT/VF, SCD or syncopy Holter ≥ 10 VPC/h on Holter and PES inducible VT	Class I	<	Sotalol
Steinbeck[11]	Beta-blocker vs EP guided drug therapy	Patients with inducible VT/VF	No significant difference		
SSSD[12]	Beta-blocker vs amiodarone vs control (no AAD)	Post MI (10–60 d) $20\% \leq EF \leq 45\%$ ≥ 3 VPCs/h Couplet or runs <15 beats	Metoprolol	<	Amiodarone Control
EMIAT[6]	Amiodarone post MI	Post MI EF $\leq 40\%$	Total mortality Placebo Arrhythmic mortality Placebo	n.s. <	Amiodarone Amiodarone
CAMIAT[5]	Amiodarone post MI	Post MI (6–45 d) ≥ 10 VPCs/h or ≥ 1 run of VT	Total mortality Placebo Arrhythmic mortality Placebo	n.s. <	Amiodarone Amiodarone
SWORD[2]	d-sotalol post MI	EF $\leq 40\%$ MI (6–42 d) or MI >42 d and NYHA class II, III	d-sotalol	<	Placebo
CASCADE[14,15]	Empiric amiodarone vs EP or Holter guided Class I therapy	Cardiac arrest survivors 46% received additional ICD therapy	Conventional therapy	<	Amiodarone
Böcker[13]	EP guided sotalol vs ICD in VT/VF	CAD and inducible VT/ VF or ICD after SCD (case-control study)	Sotalol	<	ICD
MADIT[22]	ICD vs drugs in non-sustained VT	Prior MI (>3 wk), non-sustained VT, EF $\leq 35\%$	Conventional therapy (71% amiodarone)	<	ICD
AVID[21]	ICD vs empiric amiodarone or EP guided sotalol in VT/VF	SCD, VT with syncope, Symptomatic VT with EF $\leq 40\%$	Amiodarone (85%) Sotalol (15%)	<	ICD

ICD, implantable cardioverter defibrillator; MI, myocardial infarction; CAD, coronary artery disease; EP, electrophysiological; PES, programmed electrical stimulation; SCD, sudden cardiac death; VF, ventricular fibrillaiton; VT, ventricular tachycardia; EF, ejection fraction; VPC, ventricular premature complex; n.s., not significant.

arrhythmias, they also increased all-cause mortality, most probably due to drug-induced proarrhythmias. Successful suppression of ventricular ectopy in the CAST study was assessed by the non-invasive approach using Holter monitoring. In this study, subgroup analysis demonstrated that patients with left ventricular ejection fraction[3] 30% or remote MIs (>90 days) had a very low risk of arrhythmic death. In the CAST-II study moricizine increased early mortality and had no protective long term effect in patients with LVEF <40%. In the Cardiac Arrest Study Hamburg (CASH) cardiac arrest survivors with inducible ventricular tachyarrhythmias were randomly assigned to receive either oral propafenone, amiodarone, metoprolol, or an implantable defibrillator.[7] The propafenone arm was prematurely stopped due to increased mortality. A significantly higher incidence of total mortality, sudden cardiac death (12%), and both cardiac arrest recurrence or sudden death (23%) was found in the propafenone group compared with the implantable defibrillator-treated patients (0%, P<0.05). Thus propafenone treatment was significantly less effective than implantable defibrillator treatment for prevention of malignant arrhythmias. However, the remaining study limbs have not yet been reported.

In the ESVEM trial (Electrophysiologic Study Versus Electrocardiographic Monitoring), serial antiarrhythmic drug testing guided either by non-invasive Holter monitoring or invasive electrophysiologic study with programmed electrical stimulation had similar clinical outcomes. Although analysis of different drug effects was not the primary objective of the ESVEM study, patients treated with the Class III (Class II) drug d,l-sotalol had improved outcome and a lower cost of therapy compared to all other six drugs with Class I effects.[8–10]

R

Grade A

OUTCOME OF CLINICAL TRIALS USING CLASS II ANTIARRHYTHMIC AGENTS

Beta-blockers have been consistently effective in reducing total mortality and sudden cardiac death following MI. However, less data are available concerning their efficacy in populations at high risk for malignant ventricular arrhythmias. In a randomized trial by Steinbeck et al.,[11] investigating patients with sustained ventricular tachycardia, beta-blockers were compared to individualized antiarrhythmic therapy based on programmed stimulation. No overall difference in mortality was detected between the two groups. However, the recurrence rate was high and the choice of drugs based on programmed electrical stimulation did not require suppression of inducibility. If this criterion was applied, successful drugs had a recurrence rate of only 20% compared to 45% using beta-blockers. In the CASH study (see above), metoprolol is still under investigation, indicating a potentially better outcome compared to propafenone. However, the efficacy of beta-blocking agents using programmed electrical stimulation is low. In contrast to most studies, the SSSD study (Spanish Study on Sudden Death),[12] conducted in patients with recent MI, depressed left ventricular function, and ventricular arrhythmias, demonstrated a significant excess total mortality of 15.4% in the metoprolol group compared to 7.7% in the control group (P≤0.006), while amiodarone exhibited a positive tendency (3.5%, n.s.). Although beta-blockers were not randomly assigned, it is noteworthy that there was an apparent positive interaction between beta-blockers and amiodarone, which deserves further investigation.

R

Grade A

OUTCOME OF CLINICAL TRIALS USING CLASS III ANTIARRHYTHMIC AGENTS

D,l-sotalol had greater efficacy compared to all other drugs with Class I effect (imipramine, mexiletine, pirmenol, procainamide, propafenone, quinidine), in the ESVEM trial, but appeared to be less effective than implantable cardiac defibrillator (ICD) therapy in patients with ventricular tachycardia/ventricular fibrillation (VT/VF) and coronary artery disease in a case-control study[13] of long term efficacy. In the d,l-sotalol group, VT/VF which was inducible in drug free programmed stimulation was suppressed by d, l-sotalol. d,l-sotalol treatment led to a marked reduction in arrhythmic events. Whereas 83% of the patients in the d,l-sotalol group were free of sudden death and non-fatal VT at 3 years, only 33% of the ICD patients did not receive appropriate ICD therapies ($P<0.005$). Actuarial rates for absence of sudden death and overall survival at 3 years were 85% and 75% in the d,l-sotalol group and 100% and 85% in the ICD group respectively ($P<0.005$, $P=0.02$). Thus, successful suppression of VT/VF by d,l-sotalol using programmed electrical stimulation is less effective than ICD device therapy. However, these results need to be confirmed in a prospective randomized trial.

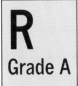

Although VT/VF can be successfully suppressed by the selective potassium-channel blocker d-sotalol, the SWORD study (Survival With ORal D-Sotalol) was terminated due to excess mortality in the d-sotalol group.[2] Patients with a left ventricular ejection fraction (LVEF) of 40% or less and either a recent (6–42 days) MI or symptomatic heart failure with a remote (>42 days) MI were randomly assigned to d-sotalol or placebo. The trial was stopped due to 78 deaths (5.0%) in the d-sotalol group compared with 48 deaths (3.1%) within the placebo group ($P=0.006$). The vast majority of excess deaths occurred in the group with relatively preserved LV function (EF = 31–40%) and remote MI, who had an extremely low risk of dying on placebo. This observation underlines the need for appropriate risk stratification to identify high risk patients in order to achieve positive results using drugs with a significant side effect profile.

The new pure Class III antiarrhythmic agents dofetilide and azimilide are currently undergoing clinical investigation. Preliminary results of the DIAMOND II study (Danish Investigation of Arrhythmia and MOrtality on Dofetilide) presented at the European Congress of Cardiology (Stockholm 1997) indicate that dofetilide did not affect the total mortality in high risk heart failure patients but reduced the incidence of atrial fibrillation and hospitalization due to heart failure.

Azimilide which inhibits the slow (I_{Ks}) and rapid (I_{Kr}) components of the potassium current will be tested in the ALIVE (Azimilide Post Infarct Survival Evaluation) trial, which will risk stratify patients using heart rate variability as an innovative approach.

Multiple clinical trials using amiodarone have been conducted. In most studies amiodarone was empirically administered as no unequivocal method for therapy control of long term amiodarone administration has been established.

The CASCADE (Cardiac Arrest in Seattle: Conventional versus Amiodarone Drug Evaluation) study[14,15] evaluated antiarrhythmic drug therapy in patients who had survived an episode of out-of-hospital ventricular fibrillation (VF) and who were thought to be at high risk for recurrence of VF. Therapy with empiric amiodarone was compared to therapy with other antiarrhythmic agents, guided by electrophysiologic testing and/or Holter recording. The study comprised 228 patients, 105 patients also received an ICD. In 113 patients, amiodarone was given empirically while 115 patients received conventional Class I antiarrhythmic drug therapy guided by Holter or programmed

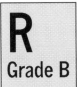

R

Grade B

stimulation. Most patients had coronary artery disease with prior MI, half of the population had a history of congestive heart failure with a mean overall LVEF of 35%. Survival was improved in patients treated with amiodarone compared to all other antiarrhythmic agents. After 2, 4 and 6 years, survival free of cardiac death, resuscitated VF, or syncopal defibrillation, was 82%, 66% and 53% with amiodarone therapy and 69%, 52% and 40% with conventional drug therapy respectively ($P = 0.007$). Survival free of cardiac death and sustained ventricular arrhythmias was 78%, 52%, and 41% with amiodarone therapy and 52%, 36%, and 20% with conventional drug therapy respectively ($P < 0.001$). Although patients with amiodarone had a significantly better outcome, the overall mortality was high, and discontinuation of amiodarone therapy even at low doses due to serious side effects such as thyroid disease and pulmonary toxicity, were common.

The GESICA trial investigated the use of amiodarone in a prospective randomized study in patients with heart failure and systolic dysfunction. The majority of 516 enrolled patients presented with non-ischemic cardiac disease, many of whom had Chagas disease. The study was prematurely terminated due to a significant reduction in total mortality by amiodarone. Presence of non-sustained ventricular tachycardia was related to an overall increased risk of death. However, amiodarone caused a significant risk reduction independent of the presence of spontaneous arrhythmias.[16] In contrast, amiodarone had no significant effect on all-cause mortality or sudden cardiac death in the CHF-STAT study.[17] Although the majority of these patients suffered from coronary heart disease, a subgroup with dilated cardiomyopathy in the amiodarone limb had a positive trend for improved prognosis. Thus, dilated cardiomyopathy rather than heart failure after myocardial infarction may be more suitable for prophylactic antiarrhythmic therapy with amiodarone, although prospective studies are needed for confirmation.

R

Grade A

In the CAMIAT[5] and the EMIAT[6] studies, the risk of arrhythmic events and arrhythmic mortality was reduced, but there was no significant difference in total and cardiac mortality. Possibly, both studies failed to enroll sufficient numbers of patients at high risk for sudden cardiac death due to broad inclusion criteria. In the BASIS (Basel Antiarrhythmic Study of Infarct Survival)[18] and the PAT (Polish Amiodarone Trial)[19] studies, amiodarone reduced mortality only in a subgroup of patients with LVEF exceeding $\geq 40\%$. In the recently published ATMA trial (Amiodarone Trials Meta-Analysis)[20] the individual data from 13 prophylactic amiodarone trials in patients with myocardial infarction or congestive heart failure were pooled for a meta-analysis. In the meta-analysis 6553 patients were randomly assigned treatment. Total mortality was reduced by 13% ($p = 0.030$) and arrhythmic/sudden death was reduced by 29% ($p = 0.0003$). There was no effect on non-arrhythmic deaths. The excess (amiodarone minus control) risk of pulmonary toxicity was 1% per year, excess risk of discontinuation was 14% by end of 2 years. So prophylactic amiodarone reduces the rate of arrhythmic/sudden death in high-risk patients with recent MI or CHF and this effect results in an overall reduction of 13% in total mortality.

By comparison, amiodarone appears to be currently the most effective antiarrhythmic agent despite its considerable side effects. However, in the MADIT (Multicenter Automatic Defibrillator Implantation Trial) and AVID (Antiarrhythmics versus Implantable Defibrillators) studies comparing the implantable defibrillator to antiarrhythmic drug treatment, device therapy with the ICD was significantly superior to pharmacologic treatment mostly consisting of amiodarone. In the AVID trial, patients with a history of VF or life threatening VT were randomly assigned to receive treatment with either a

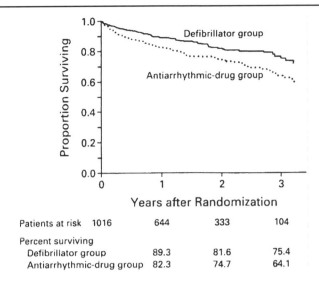

Figure 36.1 AVID survival curves.

defibrillator or with a drug – amiodarone (85%) or sotalol (15%). The objective of the study was to determine which strategy offered the greatest reduction in mortality.[21] All patients in each group were allowed to receive other drugs as needed, including beta-blockers, aspirin, and ACE inhibitors. In AVID, 1016 patients averaging 65 years were enrolled before the study was prematurely terminated, the AVID investigators had planned to recruit 1200 patients into the trial. Approximately half of the patients in the study had VT and the others, VF. After one year, patients in the defibrillator group experienced a 39% reduction in deaths compared to the group of patients on antiarrhythmic drugs. The defibrillator group showed a 27 and 31% reduction in deaths in years two and three, respectively (Figure 36.1). However, preliminary subgroup analysis showed no benefit for ICD therapy when LVEF was normal.

In the MADIT trial (Multicenter Automatic Defibrillator Implantation Trial)[22] prophylactic therapy with an implanted cardioverter–defibrillator was compared with conventional medical therapy: 196 patients with prior MI; a LVEF ≤ 0.35; a documented episode of asymptomatic non-sustained VT; and inducible, ventricular tachyarrhythmia on electrophysiologic study not suppressed by procainamide, were randomly assigned to receive an implanted defibrillator ($n=95$) or conventional medical therapy ($n=101$). During an average follow-up of 27 months, there were 15 deaths in the defibrillator group (11 from cardiac causes) and 39 deaths in the conventional therapy group (27 from cardiac causes). There was no evidence that amiodarone, beta-blockers or any other antiarrhythmic therapy had a significant influence on the observed hazard ratio.

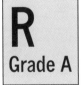

OUTCOME OF CLINICAL TRIALS USING CLASS IV ANTIARRHYTHMIC AGENTS

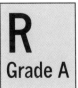

There have been no prospective trials evaluating calcium-channel blockers in patients with ventricular tachyarrhythmias. Data from postmyocardial infarction studies indicate a moderate preventive efficacy of verapamil (DAVIT II Danish Study Group on Verapamil

In Myocardial Infarction) and diltiazem (MDPIT Multicenter Diltiazem PostInfarction Trial Research Group) on mortality in subgroups with preserved left ventricular function and/or non-Q wave infarction.[23,24] In DAVIT II, however, verapamil tended to enhance spontaneous ventricular ectopy with significant increase of VPC count in the presence of heart failure or non-Q wave infarction.[25] Although verapamil does not appear to affect malignant ventricular arrhythmias in general, positive case reports were presented in idiopathic VT and in verapamil sensitive VT. In general, calcium-channel blockers are of little importance in the treatment of ventricular arrhythmias.

ANTIARRHYTHMIC AGENTS FOR TREATMENT OF UNEXPLAINED CARDIAC ARREST

Survivors of unexplained cardiac arrest have not been shown to be effectively treated by antiarrhythmic drugs and may therefore be candidates for primary ICD therapy.

CONCLUSION

In patients with prior MI at high risk for ventricular tachyarrhythmias, prophylactic therapy with an implanted defibrillator may be associated with improved survival compared to conventional medical therapy. Currently there is no preventive indication for antiarrhythmic drugs in asymptomatic patients following MI or with heart failure. In high risk patients, the use of the ICD appears to be superior to drugs for reducing total mortality. Risk stratification for selection of high risk patient subgroups is still under investigation.

The results of MADIT suggest that evaluation of non-suppressible ventricular tachyarrhythmias by programmed electrical stimulation may represent one potentially appropriate selection of high risk patients for ICD therapy.

REFERENCES

1 The Cardiac Arrhythmia Suppression Trial (CAST) Investigators. Preliminary report: effect of encainide and flecainide on mortality in a randomized trial of arrhythmia suppression after myocardial infarction. N Engl J Med 1989;321: 406–12.

2 Waldo AL, Camm AJ, deRuyter H et al. Effect of d-sotalol on mortality in patients with left ventricular dysfunction after recent and remote myocardial infarction. The SWORD Investigators (Survival With Oral d-Sotalol). Lancet 1996;348: 7–12.

3 Vaughan-Williams EM. A classification of antiarrhythmic actions reassessed after a decade of new drugs. J Clin Pharmacol 1984;23:129–47.

4 Rosen MR, Schwartz PJ. The Sicilian Gambit a new approach to the classification of antiarrhythmic drugs based on their actions on arrhythmogenic mechanisms. Circulation 1991;84:1831–51.

5 Cairns JA, Connolly SJ, Roberts R, Gent M. Randomised trial of outcome after myocardial infarction in patients with frequent or repetitive ventricular premature depolarisations: CAMIAT (Canadian Amiodarone Myocardial Infarction Arrhythmia Trial Investigators). Lancet 1997; 349:675–82.

6 Julian DG, Camm AJ, Frangin G et al. Randomised trial of effect of amiodarone on mortality in patients with left-ventricular dysfunction after recent myocardial infarction (EMIAT). Lancet 1997;349:667–74.

7 Siebels J, Cappato R, Ruppel R, Schneider MA, Kuck KH. Preliminary results of the Cardiac Arrest Study Hamburg (CASH). Am J Cardiol 1993; 72(16):109F–113F.

8 Mason JW, The ESVEM Investigators. A comparision of electrophysiologic testing with

Holter monitoring to predict antiarrhythmic drug efficacy for ventricular tachyarrhythmias. *N Engl J Med* 1993;**329**:445–51.

9 Mason JW, The ESVEM Investigators. A comparision of seven antiarrhythmic drugs in patients with ventricular tachyarrhythmias. *N Engl J Med* 1993;**329**:452–8.

10 Mason JW, Marcus FI, Bigger JT *et al*. A summary and assessment of the findings and conclusions of the ESVEM trial. *Prog Cardiovasc Dis* 1996; **38**(5):347–58.

11 Steinbeck G, Andresen D, Bach P *et al*. A comparison of electrophysiologically guided antiarrhythmic drug therapy with β-blocker therapy in patients with symptomatic, sustained ventricular tachycardia. *N Engl J Med* 1992;**327**: 987–92.

12 Navarro-Lopez F, Cosin J, Marrugat J, Guindo J, Bayes-de-Luna A. Comparison of the effects of amiodarone versus metoprolol on the frequency of ventricular arrhythmias and on mortality after acute myocardial infarction (SSSD Investigators: Spanish Study on Sudden Death). *Am J Cardiol* 1993;**72**:1243–48.

13 Böcker D, Haverkamp W, Block M *et al*. Comparison of d,l-sotalol and implantable defibrillators for treatment of sustained ventricular tachycardia or fibrillation in patients with coronary artery disease. *Circulation* 1996; **94**:151–7.

14 Greene HL, CASCADE Investigators. The CASCADE Study: randomized antiarrhythmic drug therapy in survivors of cardiac arrest in Seattle. *Am J Cardiol* 1993;**72**:70F–74F.

15 Dolack GL. Clinical predictors of implantable cardioverter-defibrillator shocks (results of the CASCADE trial) (Cardiac Arrest in Seattle, Conventional versus Amiodarone Drug Evaluation). *Am J Cardiol* 1994;**73**:237–41.

16 Doval HC, Nul DR, Grancelli HO *et al*. Randomized trial of low-dose amiodarone in severe heart failure. *Lancet* 1994;**344**:493–8.

17 Singh SN, Fletcher RD, Fisher SG *et al*. Amiodarone in patients with congestive heart failure and ventricular arrhythmia. *N Engl J Med* 1995;**333**:77–82.

18 Burkart F, Pfisterer M, Kiowski W, Follath F, Burckhardt D. Effect of antiarrhythmic therapy on mortality in survivors of myocardial infarction with asymptomatic complex ventricular arrhythmias (Basel Antiarrhythmic Study of Infarct Survival: BASIS). *J Am Coll Cardiol* 1990; **19**:1711–18.

19 Ceremuzynski L, Kleczar E, Krzeminska-Pakula M *et al*. Effect of amiodarone on mortality after myocardial infarction: a double-blind, placebo-controlled, pilot study (PAT). *J Am Coll Cardiol* 1992;**20**:1056–62.

20 Amiodarone Trials Meta-Analysis Investigators. Effect of prophylactic amiodarone on mortality after acute myocardial infarction and in congestive heart failure: meta-analysis of individual data from 6500 patients in randomised trials. *Lancet* 1997;**350**:1417–1424.

21 National Institute of Health. NHLBI stops arrhythmia study – implantable cardiac defibrillators reduce deaths. National Institute of Health, News Release, Monday 14 April, 1997.

22 Moss AJ, Hall WJ, Cannom DS *et al*. Improved survival with an implanted defibrillator in patients with coronary disease at high risk for ventricular arrhythmia. *N Engl J Med* 1996;**335**:1933–40.

23 The Multicenter Diltiazem Postinfarction Trial Research Group. The effect of diltiazem on mortality and reinfarction after myocardial infarction. *N Engl J Med* 1988;**319**:385–92.

24 The Danish Study Group on Verapamil in Myocardial Infarction. Secondary prevention with verapamil after myocardial infarction. *Am J Cardiol* 1990;**66**:331–401.

25 Jespersen CM, Vaage Nilesn M. Ventricular arrhythmias in patients recovering from myocardial infarction: do residual myocardial ischemia and anti-ischemic medical intervention influence the one-month prevalence? (The Danish Study Group on Verapamil in Myocardial Infarction). *Clin Cardiol* 1993;**16**:109–14.

585

37 Non-pharmacologic therapy for sustained ventricular tachycardia and ventricular fibrillation

STUART J. CONNOLLY

Recurrent sustained ventricular tachycardia (VT) and ventricular fibrillation (VF) are life-threatening conditions which are difficult to prevent. Pharmacologic therapy, the only therapy available until the early 1980s, is only partially effective. Since that time non-pharmacologic approaches have become increasingly important in the management of these disorders. Two main non-pharmacologic therapies for VT and VF are currently in use to prevent recurrences of sustained VT and VF. These are the implantable cardioverter defibrillator (ICD), and surgical or catheter ablation of the anatomic site of VT in the myocardium.

ICD THERAPY

The ICD is, by far, the non-pharmacologic therapy which is most widely used and the only non-pharmacologic therapy which has been subjected to rigorous validation. The ICD was developed in the 1970s and was first implanted in a patient in 1980. Since then there have been many refinements to the initial technology and refinements continue to occur at a brisk pace. At present the typical ICD includes a multi programmable generator capable of delivering multiple defibrillating/cardioverting direct current shocks. It is usually implanted subclavicularly and its housing serves as one of the defibrillation electrodes. Most often a single lead for defibrillation, tachycardia detection and pacing is inserted via the subclavian or cephalic vein into the right ventricular apex. The fundamental therapy is the direct current shock capable of cardioversion/defibrillation. Overdrive pacing therapy for the termination of VT and bradycardia pacing are available. Therapy can be tiered so that if overdrive pacing fails to convert VT or transforms it to a more malignant arrhythmia, defibrillation/cardioversion can be deployed subsequently.

586

Detection of VT or VF is achieved by automatic counting of the heart rate. Automatic gain control allows the device to detect VF as well as VT. Most devices now also allow additional refinements for arrhythmia detection using programmable criteria for abruptness of onset of tachycardia and for stability of tachycardia rate to exclude either sinus tachycardia or atrial fibrillation. Major recent refinements are reduction in size and addition of atrial electrodes which allow dual chamber pacing as well as use of the atrial electrogram to improve the specificity of VT and VF detection.

Implantation is generally done under anesthesia in the operating room or the electrophysiology lab, with intraoperative testing for pacing and defibrillation thresholds. The operative mortality with modern endocardial systems is <1%.[1,2] The ICD is associated with a number of adverse experiences. The rate of infection with non-thoracotomy systems is 0.6–4.1%.[3] A troublesome complication is the painfulness of virtually all cardioversion/defibrillator shocks. The availability of overdrive pacing therapy, which is painless, reduces the frequency of these shocks but many patients still require shocks periodically.[4]

ICD therapy has achieved considerable sophistication in detection and treatment of VT and VF. There is no doubt that it is an effective therapy for termination of episodes of VT and VF. This has been clear for many years from the fact that VT or VF, artificially induced in hospital, can be reliably terminated by the ICD. Modern ICDs now provide ECG collection and telemetry ability that allows inspection of the cardiac electrograms immediately before and after discharges of the ICD. It is now possible to directly confirm the success of the ICD against episodes of spontaneously occurring VT and VF. Thus it is safe to conclude that the ICD is a very effective therapy for many episodes of VT and VF.

Assessment of ICD efficacy

Assessment of the overall effectiveness of the ICD is made complex by the fact that VT and VF, in the vast majority of patients, are not isolated conditions but late complications of ischemic heart disease or cardiomyopathy. In fact VT and VF only rarely occur in the absence of serious structural heart disease. The vast majority of patients with VT or VF have multivessel coronary artery disease and have had previous myocardial infarction, with the result that these patients have extensive myocardial fibrosis. During the 1990s there has been considerable debate on the issue of whether ICD therapy is effective for prolonging life in patients with VT and VF. The typical patient receiving an ICD is at risk of dying not only from recurrence of VT or VF but also from recurrent myocardial infarction and congestive heart failure. Prevention of recurrent VF or VT may have little impact on survival in these patients as they are just as likely to die from another complication of their ischemic heart disease. Thus while the ICD is clearly effective against VT and VF episodes, it is not obvious that it prolongs life in the average patient treated. Furthermore, amiodarone provides a pharmacologic strategy that is at least moderately successful at reducing the risk of arrhythmic death in high risk patients.[5] Thus one of the key questions about ICD therapy has become whether or not it improves survival in patients with VT/VF when compared to best medical therapy.

Beginning in the late 1980s and early 1990s, a number of randomized clinical trials evaluating the ICD were initiated. Some have been reported and others are nearing completion. Prior to these trials, the best available data regarding the overall efficacy of the ICD were non-randomized comparisons of patients receiving or not receiving an ICD for management of recurrent VT or VF.[6,7] Although these tended to point towards a benefit from the ICD, the potential for bias in these studies was such that they were not reliable evidence.

The trials evaluating ICD therapy are diverse but can be broadly divided into two groups according to the target population treated: (1) patients with previous sustained VT or VF or (2) patients without VT or VF but at high risk for arrhythmic death. Trials targeted at the first group can be thought of as secondary prevention or treatment studies, whereas those targeted at the second group are primary prevention or prophylactic studies.

The patient who has survived an episode of out-of-hospital cardiac arrest is at high risk of dying if the episode was not associated with recent myocardial infarction or a correctible cause such as electrolyte abnormality.[8] Natural history studies from the 1970s placed this risk at over 20% in the first year.[8] Recent improvements in care for ischemic heart disease and left ventricular dysfunction have undoubtably reduced this risk, but it is still substantial. These patients, in whom a single recurrence of arrhythmia is likely to be fatal, are prime candidates for ICD study. The patient with sustained VT may, on the other hand, experience degrees of symptoms varying from none at all to cardiac arrest, depending upon the rate of VT and the integrity of cardiac pump function.

ICD treatment trials

There are three randomized trials which evaluate the ICD as a treatment for patients with previous documented sustained VT or VF. The Cardiac Arrest Study Hamburg (CASH)[9] has enrolled only the patient with prior VF, whereas the Canadian Implantable Defibrillator Study (CIDS)[10] and the Antiarrhythmic vs Implantable Defibrillator (AVID)[11] study have enrolled both patients with prior VF as well as patients with hemodynamically unstable VT. CASH was planned as a 400 patient study with four treatment arms – ICD, amiodarone, metoprolol, propafenone. The propafenone arm was terminated prematurely due to excessive mortality compared to the other treatments. Enrollment of 100 patients into each of the other three arms was completed early in 1997. The final results are expected in 1998. CIDS randomized 658 patients to receive or not to receive an ICD; patients not receiving the ICD all were treated with amiodarone. CIDS completed enrollment in January 1997 and will report final results in the Spring of 1998.

AVID is the first of these three trials to report its results. There were 1016 patients randomized to receive either an ICD or drug therapy, which was specified as either amiodarone or sotalol. Drug therapy was randomly allocated in patients eligible for either drug. Forty-five per cent of patients had VF and the rest had VT. Only 13 of 509 patients randomized to drug therapy actually were discharged from hospital on sotalol. The mean dose of amiodarone at one year was 331 mg/day and 87% of patients remained on amiodarone at one year. There was a marked imbalance in beta-blocker use between ICD and amiodarone patients, with 45% of ICD patients receiving this therapy compared to 13% of drug therapy patients.

In the AVID study there was a reduction in mortality with the ICD. Over a mean follow-up of 18 months, crude death rates were $15.8 \pm 3.2\%$ for the ICD vs $24.0 + 3.7\%$ for drugs ($P < 0.02$). The relative risk reductions at 1, 2 and 3 years were $39 \pm 20\%$,

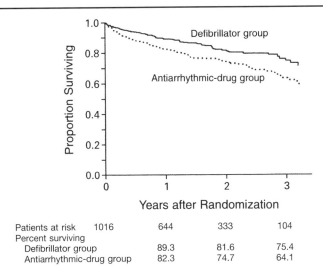

Patients at risk	1016	644	333	104
Percent surviving				
Defibrillator group		89.3	81.6	75.4
Antiarrhythmic-drug group		82.3	74.7	64.1

Figure 37.1 Overall survival, unadjusted for base-line characteristics. Survival was better among patients treated with the implantable cardioverter-defibrillator (*P*<0.02, adjusted for repeated analyses (n = 6)). Reproduced with permission from the Antiarrhythmics Versus Implantable Defibrillators (AVID) investigators. A comparison of antiarrhythmic drug therapy with implantable defibrillators in patients resuscitated from near-fatal ventricular arrhythmias. *N Engl Journal Med* 1997;**337**:1576–83.

27 ± 21% and 31 ± 21% (± 95% confidence intervals). An analysis of the efficacy of the ICD adjusting for small imbalances in baseline features and concomitant therapy had little effect on the main result. There was no identified subgroup in whom there was a significantly greater or lesser effect of the ICD. The average unadjusted lifetime extension conferred by the ICD at 3 years was 3.2 months. (See Figure 37.1.)

This study provides strong evidence that the ICD prolongs life compared to carefully administered drug therapy. The fact that the vast majority of drug treatment patients actually received amiodarone and stayed on the drug during follow-up is a major strength of the study because amiodarone is the only drug, other than beta-blockers, for which there is evidence from randomized controlled trials of a beneficial effect on arrhythmia death and overall mortality.[11] The treatment effect is quite large in terms of relative risk reduction (approximately one-third) but the prolongation of life is modest, only just over 3 months. The 95% confidence interval is quite broad and the results are consistent with a relative reduction as small as only about 10%, which would translate into a prolongation in life of a few weeks. Considering the substantial costs of therapy initiation with the ICD and the higher rate of re-hospitalization with the ICD compared to amiodarone (60% vs 56%, *P* = 0.04), it is likely that the cost per year of life saved will be very high. Preliminary analysis of cost data from AVID place the incremental cost of ICD therapy (over drug therapy) at US$114 917 per year of life saved.[12]

The results of CIDS and CASH will be complimentary to AVID, providing much longer average duration of follow-up and more than doubling the number of events. A meta-analysis of the three trials will provide the most accurate assessment of the true benefit of the ICD. CIDS and CASH will be important because if they support the findings of AVID, the confidence interval will tighten, giving greater security in the conclusions of AVID. These trials will very likely be consistent with AVID but may give different point estimates of the treatment effect. There is some concern, however, that AVID has

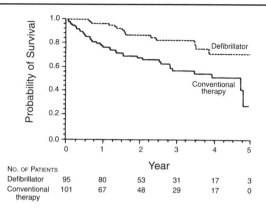

Figure 37.2   MADIT survival curves.

overestimated the benefit of the ICD. Trials that terminate prematurely due to observation of a benefit have a tendency, in general, to overestimate the benefit. There was also an imbalance in AVID in the use of beta-blocker therapy, which favored the ICD treatment limb. Meta-analysis will also be valuable because, by means of pooling data, it may also be able to identify subgroups of patients with substantially greater or lesser benefit from the ICD. This would be important because it would allow resources to be directed most appropriately.

At present when managing a patient with life-threatening sustained VT or VF, the balance of evidence now favours ICD therapy over amiodarone. The ICD is thus in general the preferred therapy. In light of the modest prolongation of life conferred by the ICD and its high cost, where resources are limited, amiodarone is still a reasonable therapy.

R
Grade A

Prophylactic ICD trials

Two randomized trials have evaluated the ability of the ICD to reduce the risk of death in patients, without prior sustained ventricular tachyarrhythmia, but at high risk of sudden death from VT or VF: the Multicenter Automatic Defibrillator Implantation Trial (MADIT)[13] and the Coronary Artery Bypass Graft (CABG)-Patch Trial.[14] The rationale for these trials is based on the finding that patients with severe left ventricular dysfunction are at high risk for sudden death and may benefit from ICD therapy. Both trials used further risk stratification to enrich the study populations with patients thought to be at very high risk of VT and VF.

In MADIT, patients with left ventricular ejection fraction $\leq 35\%$ were further screened by programmed ventricular stimulation. Patients found to have inducible VT or VF became eligible for the study if inducibility of the tachycardia could not be suppressed by procainamide. There were 196 patients randomized to either receive an ICD or "conventional" therapy. Conventional therapy was not specified. Amiodarone and beta-blockers, the only proven effective drugs against VT and VF, were used predominantly but sporadically (in 45% and 5%, respectively, of "conventional" patients at last contact). The trial was prematurely terminated when about 75% of patients had been enrolled due to an apparent clear benefit of ICD treatment. The hazard ratio was 0.46 (95% CI 0.26, 0.82; $P=0.009$) indicating a greater than 50% reduction in death with ICD

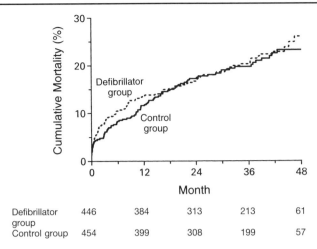

| Defibrillator group | 446 | 384 | 313 | 213 | 61 |
| Control group | 454 | 399 | 308 | 199 | 57 |

Figure 37.3 Kaplan-Meier analysis of the probability of death according to study group in the CABG-Patch Trial. By April 30 1997, 95 deaths had occurred in the control group and 101 in the defibrillator group. By four years of follow-up, the actuarial mortality was 24% in the control group and 27% in the group assigned to implanted-defibrillator therapy (P=0.64). The numbers below the figure show the numbers of patients at risk. Reproduced with permission from Bigger, for the CABG Patch-Trial Investigators.[14]

therapy. When cause of death was examined, the ICD reduced not only arrhythmic death (13 vs 3), but there appeared to be reduction in non-arrhythmic cardiac death (13 vs 7) and deaths of unknown cause (6 vs 0), which is not explained and not biologically plausible. There was a marked imbalance in the use of beta-blocker therapy in favour of the ICD group, but this did not explain the benefit observed with the ICD. (See Figure 37.2.)

The rationale for the CABG-Patch Trial was developed at a time when a thoracotomy was required for implantation of an ICD. Patients requiring CABG, who were identified to be at high risk of sudden death, were thought to be good candidates for prophylactic ICD implantation because the detrimental effect of a major surgical procedure to implant the ICD was already accounted for. Thus in the CABG-Patch Trial, patients scheduled for CABG with LVEF ≤35% were further stratified for risk of arrhythmic death by signal-averaged ECG. High risk patients were randomized to receive or not receive an ICD at the time of CABG surgery.

The trial identified 1422 eligible patients, enrolled 1055 and randomized 900 – 446 to ICD and 454 to control. Use of antiarrhythmic drugs was similar between the two groups. There were 52 patients randomized to ICD who either never received a device or who had it removed. There were 196 deaths (101 in the ICD group and 95 in the control group) for a crude mortality rate of 21.8% during an average follow-up of 32 ± 16 months. The hazard ratio was 1.07 (95% CI 0.81, 1.42), indicating no benefit from the ICD in this patient population. (See Figure 37.3.)

Can the discrepancy between the results of the CABG-Patch Trial and MADIT be resolved? The degree of difference in the hazard ratios is substantial (1.07 vs 0.46) and there is little overlap in the 95% confidence intervals, which were 0.26–0.82 for MADIT and 0.81–1.46 for the CABG-Patch Trial. Thus the difference in results is unlikely to be due to the play of chance. The 24 month actuarial mortality in the CABG-Patch Trial was 18%, whereas in MADIT it was almost twice as high at 32%. It was intermediate at 24% in AVID. It is possible that the CABG-Patch Trial did not select patients at high enough risk of arrhythmic death or that CABG surgery reduced the risk of arrhythmic death to a substantial degree so that there were few deaths potentially responsive to ICD therapy. It will be useful to assess the ratio of arrhythmic to non-arrhythmic deaths in the two studies. Electrophysiologic testing was used to further stratify patients in MADIT and it is possible that this is an important aspect of the observed difference in hazard ratios. Electrophysiologic testing may select a group at especially high risk for arrhythmic death. In MADIT, however, only 13 of 29 deaths in the conventional treatment group were clearly arrhythmic in nature, suggesting that this population was not particularly enriched for risk of arrhythmic death.

The role of ischemia in the pathogenesis of arrhythmic death is poorly understood. It is clearly possible that the CABG surgery performed in the CABG-Patch Trial patients played a role in preventing arrhythmic death and thus removed the substrate upon which the ICD has its effect.

In summary, the results of the two trials now published evaluating the efficacy of the ICD for prolonging life in high risk patients provide a mixed picture; a striking benefit was observed in MADIT (the smallest of the two), and no benefit in the CABG-Patch Trial. The evidence supporting prophylactic ICD implantation in high risk patients is not at present sufficiently compelling for it to be recommended.

R

Grade A

SURGICAL AND CATHETER ABLATION OF VT

In the 1970s and 1980s it became apparent that monomorphic VT can be localized to specific areas of the ventricular myocardium. This provided the opportunity to surgically remove or isolate the anatomic site of tachycardia. During the 1980s a variety of surgical approaches to mapping and ablating the anatomical site of VT in diseased myocardial tissue were developed and validated.[15,16] The advent of the ICD, however, has relegated the surgical approach to the sidelines of VT management. There is little doubt that the surgical approach to VT can, in highly selected patients, remove the focus of VT and provide excellent quality of life; the major drawback is operative mortality. While early series of patients reported unacceptable mortality, more recent series, by means of improved patient selection and operative technique, have reported operative mortality between 0 and 7%.[17–19] Suppression of inducible VT is acceptable at 72–92%. Nonetheless, the role of VT surgery has become very minor due to the ease and effectiveness of the ICD, which has an operative mortality of <1%[1,2] and which can be applied with much less surgical skill to a virtually unselected patient population. No randomized comparisons of surgical to pharmacologic or device therapy have been done and none is likely in the near future. The technique should only be offered where mortality of <1% and an excellent cure rate of VT can be assured.

Radiofrequency catheter ablation of sites of origin of VT is a less invasive means of achieving anatomic control of VT. This technique is based upon the same insight that inspired surgical ablation of VT, that in many patients the mechanism of VT is intramyocardial re-entry.[20] Radiofrequency energy delivered by means of a catheter is directed to target sites identified by endocardial mapping. There has been success with catheter ablation in the treatment of idiopathic VT. Idiopathic VT occurs in otherwise normal hearts and can often be localized by endocardial mapping to the right ventricular outflow tract or to the posteroinferior aspect of the left ventricular septum.[21–23] In the small series reported, success rates for ablation of idiopathic VT are good (85–100%).[21–23]

However, both types of VT are often sensitive to drug therapy (beta-blocker and calcium-channel blocker),[22] and no controlled comparisons have been reported. Complications are rare but can include perforation and death. For these rare conditions catheter ablation can be considered effective and it is reasonable treatment, especially where there is an inadequate response to medical therapy.

For the vast majority of VT patients who have myocardial disease secondary to coronary artery stenosis, the use of catheter ablation techniques is investigational. In such patients where VT is often related to large re-entry circuits in scarred myocardium, the small lesions created by RF ablation may be inadequate. Furthermore, many patients have multiple morphologies of VT and it is often not possible to abolish them all. Current limitations of mapping technologies confine this approach to patients with well-tolerated slow VT. Small series report success rates varying from 40 to 75%.[24,25] No randomized comparisons of this therapy against pharmacologic or device therapy are reported. Recurrent symptomatic VT in a patient already treated with an ICD and pharmacologic therapy, is a situation where catheter ablation offers the possibility of improved quality of life.

CORONARY ARTERY BYPASS GRAFT SURGERY

Acute myocardial ischemia can cause VF. Thus it has been hypothesized that coronary artery bypass graft (CABG) surgery can prevent sudden death. Autopsy studies of patients with sudden death indicate a high prevalence of apparently fresh thrombus in coronary arteries, suggesting recent acute myocardial infarction.[26] Analysis of the Coronary Artery Surgery Study (CASS) revealed a lower risk of sudden cardiac death in patients randomized to CABG surgery than in medically treated patients (1.6% vs 4.9%).[27] Similarly, in the CASS registry where treatment was not randomly allocated, the sudden death rate was 4.9% in 5258 medically treated patients and 1.6% in surgically treated patients.[28] Several non-randomized series suggest that CABG surgery reduces inducible ventricular arrhythmia and long term spontaneous recurrence of VT or VF.[29-31] There have, however, been no controlled studies of CABG surgery in patients with VT or VF. There is little evidence to support CABG surgery as the primary therapy for prevention of recurrent cardiac arrest. Where there is normal left ventricular function and high grade coronary stenosis and an absence of inducible ventricular arrhythmia, such an approach can be considered.

Recommendations

Grade A

1 ICD is indicated for patients with a cardiac arrest, ventricular fibrillation, or hemodynamically unstable sustained ventricular tachycardia (VT) (where there is no correctible precipitating cause). This is very expensive therapy and where cost constraints exist, amiodarone is an alternative.

2 Due to conflicting results from two clinical trials, in general ICD is not recommended as prophylactic therapy, there is evidence from one small RCT supporting ICD use in post-myocardial infarction patients with left ventricular ejection fraction $\leq 35\%$, unsustained VT and inducible, non-suppressable VT.

Grade C

3 In general map-guided ablation of the site of origin of VT is not recommended, with the exception being idiopathic VT where radiofrequency catheter ablation is a reasonable alternative to medical therapy.

4 CABG surgery is not recommended as primary therapy for VT or VF.

REFERENCES

1 Strickberger SA, Hummel JD, Daoud E *et al.* Implantation by electrophysiologists of 100 consecutive cardioverter defibrillators with nonthoracotomy lead systems. *Circulation* 1994; **90**:868–72.

2 The PCD Investigator Group. Clinical outcome of patients with malignant ventricular tachyarrhythmias and a multiprogrammable implantable cardioverter-defibrillator implanted with or without thoracotomy: an international multicenter study. *J Am Coll Cardiol* 1994; **23**: 1521–30.

3 Shepard RB, Epsten AE. ICD infection avoidance: science, art, discipline. In: Kroll MW, Lehmann MH, eds. *Implantable cardioverter defibrillator therapy: the engineering–clinical interface.* Norwell MA: Kluwer Academic Press, 1996, pp 365–88.

4 Rosenqvist M. Pacing techniques to terminate ventricular tachycardia. *PACE* 1995; **18**:592–8.

5 Amiodarone trials meta-analysis investigators. The effect of prophylactic amiodarone on mortality after acute myocardial infarction and in congestive heart failure: meta-analysis of individual patient data on 6500 patients from randomized trials. *Lancet* (in press).

6 Manolis AS, Tan-Deguzman W, Lee MA *et al.* Clinical experience in seventy-seven patients with implantable cardioverter defibrillator. *Am Heart J* 1989; **118**:445–50.

7 Pinski SL, Sgarbossa EB, Maloney JD, Trohman RG. Survival in patients declining implantable cardioverter defibrillators. *Am J Cardiol* 1991; **68**: 800–1.

8 Baum RS, Alvarez H, Cobb LA. Survival after resuscitation from out-of-hospital ventricular fibrillation. *Circulation* 1974; **50**:1231–5.

9 Siebels J, Cappato R, Ruppel R *et al.* and the CASH Investigators. Preliminary results of the cardiac arrest study Hamburg (CASH). *Am J Cardiol* 1993; **72** (Suppl):109F–13F.

10 Connolly SJ, Gent M, Roberts RS on behalf of the CIDS Co-Investigators. *Am J Cardiol* 1993; **72** (Suppl):103F–8F.

11 The AVID Investigators. A comparison of antiarrhythmic drug therapy with implantable defibrillators in patients resuscitated from near-fatal sustained ventricular arrhythmias. *N Engl J Med* (in press).

12 Larson GC, McAnulty JH, Hallstrom A *et al.* Hospitalization charges in the Antiarrhythmics Versus Implantable Defibrillators (AVID) Trial: the AVID economic analysis study (abstract). *Circulation* 1997 (in press).

13 Moss AJ, Hall WJ, Cannom DS *et al.* for the Multicenter Automatic Defibrillator Implantation Trial Investigators. Improved survival with an implantable defibrillator in patients with coronary artery disease at high risk for ventricular arrhythmias. *N Engl J Med* 1996; **335**:1933–40.

14 Bigger JT, for the CABG Patch-Trial Investigators. Prophylactic use of implanted cardiac defibrillators in patients at high risk for ventricular arrhythmias after coronary artery bypass graft surgery *N Engl J Med* 1997; **337**: 1569–75.

15 Mason JW, Buda AJ, Stinson EB, Harrison DC. Surgical therapy of ventricular tachyarrhythmias in ischemic heart disease using conventional techniques. In: Birks W, Loogen F, Schulte HD, Seipel L eds. *Medical and surgical management of tachyarrhythmia* Berlin: Springer Verlag, 1980; p 175.

16 Ostermeyer J, Breithard TG, Gorgrefe M *et al.* Surgical treatment of ventricular tachycardias: complete versus partial encircling endocardial ventriculotomy. *J Thorac Cardiovasc Surg* 1984; **87**:517–25.

17 Mickleborough LL, Mizuno S, Downar E, Gray GC. Late results of operation for ventricular tachycardia. *Ann Thorac Surg* 1992; **54**:832–9.

18 Rastegar H, Link MS, Foote CB, Wang PJ, Manolis AS, Estes M. Perioperative and long-term results with mapping-guided subendocardial resection and left ventricular endoaneurysmorrhaphy. *Circulation* 1996; **94**:1041–8.

19 Page PL, Cardinal R, Shenasa M *et al.* Surgical treatment of ventricular tachycardia. Regional cryoablation guided by computerized epicardial and endocardial mapping. *Circulation* 1989; **80** (Suppl 1):124–34.

20 Ganz LI, Stevenson WG. Catheter mapping and ablation of ventricular tachycardia. *Coronary Artery Disease* 1996; **7**:29–35.

21 Coggins DL, Lee RJ, Sweeney J *et al.* Radiofrequency catheter ablation as a cure for idiopathic ventricular tachycardia of both left and right ventricular origin. *J Am Coll Cardiol* 1994; **23**:1333–41.

22 Belhassen B, Shapira I, Pelley A, Copperman I, Kauli N, Laniado S. Idiopathic recurrent sustained ventricular tachycardia responsive to verapamil: an ECG-electrophysiologic entity. *Am Heart J* 1984; **108**:1034–6.

23 Klein LS, Shih HT, Hackett FK, Zipes DP, Miles WM. Radiofrequency catheter ablation of ventricular tachycardia in patients without structural heart disease. *Circulation* 1992; **85**: 1666–74.

24 Ginska BD, Cao K, Schaumann A, Dorszewski A, Muhlen F, Kreuzer H. Catheter ablation of ventricular tachycardia in 136 patients with coronary artery disease: results and long term follow-up. *J Am Coll Cardiol* 1994; **24**:1506–14.

25 Stevenson WG, Kahn H, Sager P *et al.* Identification of re-entry circuit sites during

catheter mapping and radiofrequency catheter ablation of ventricular tachycardia late after myocardial infarction. *Circulation* 1993;**88:** 1647–70.

26 Davies MJ, Thomas A. Thrombosis and acute coronary artery lesions in sudden cardiac ischemic death. *N Engl J Med* 1984;**310:**1137–40.

27 Alderman EL, Bourassa MG, Cohen LS *et al.* for the CASS Investigators. Ten-year follow-up of survival and myocardial infarction in the randomized Coronary Artery Surgery Study. *Circulation* 1990;**82:**1629–46.

28 Holmes DR, Davis KB, Mock MB *et al.* and participants in the Coronary Artery Surgery Study. The effect of medical and surgical treatment on subsequent sudden cardiac death

in patients with coronary artery disease: a report from the coronary artery surgery study. *Circulation* 1986;**73:**1263–86.

29 Kelly P, Ruskin JN, Vlahakes GJ *et al.* Surgical coronary revascularization in survivors of prehospital cardiac arrest: its effect on inducible ventricular arrhythmias and long-term survival. *J Am Coll Cardiol* 1990;**15:**267–73.

30 Autschbach R, Falk V, Gonska BD, Dalichau H. The effect of coronary bypass graft surgery for prevention of sudden cardiac death: recurrent episodes after ICD implantation and review of literature. *PACE* 1994;**17:**552–8.

31 Kron IL, Lerman BB, Haines DE, Flanagan TL, DiMarco JP. Coronary artery bypass grafting in patients with ventricular fibrillation. *Ann Thorac Surg* 1989;**48:**85–9.

Part III
Specific cardiovascular disorders
vi: Management of bradyarrhythmias

A JOHN CAMM, Editor

Grading of recommendations and levels of evidence used in *Evidence Based Cardiology*

GRADE A

Level 1a   Evidence from large randomized clinical trials (RCTs) or systematic reviews (including meta-analyses) of multiple randomized trials which collectively has at least as much data as one single well-defined trial.

Level 1b   Evidence from at least one "All or None" high quality cohort study; in which ALL patients died/failed with conventional therapy and some survived/succeeded with the new therapy (eg chemotherapy for tuberculosis, meningitis, or defibrillation for ventricular fibrillation); or in which many died/failed with conventional therapy and NONE died/failed with the new therapy (eg penicillin for pneumococcal infections).

Level 1c   Evidence from at least one moderate sized RCT or a meta-analysis of small trials which collectively only has a moderate number of patients.

Level 1d   Evidence from at least one RCT.

GRADE B

Level 2   Evidence from at least one high quality study of non-randomized cohorts who did and did not receive the new therapy.

Level 3   Evidence from at least one high quality case control study.

Level 4   Evidence from at least one high quality case series.

GRADE C

Level 5   Opinions from experts without reference or access to any of the foregoing (eg argument from physiology, bench research or first principles).

A comprehensive approach would incorporate many different types of evidence (eg RCTs, non-RCTs, epidemiologic studies, and experimental data), and examine the architecture of the information for consistency, coherence and clarity. Occasionally the evidence does not completely fit into neat compartments. For example, there may not be an RCT that demonstrates a reduction in mortality in individuals with stable angina with the use of beta-blockers, but there is overwhelming evidence that mortality is  reduced following MI. In such cases, some may recommend use of beta-blockers in angina patients with the expectation that some extrapolation from post-MI trials is warranted. This could be expressed as Grade A/C. In other instances (e.g. smoking cessation or a pacemaker for complete heart block), the non-randomized data are so overwhelmingly clear and biologically plausible that it would be reasonable to consider these interventions as Grade A.

Recommendation grades appear either in a shaded margin box with an 'R' logo as shown, or within the text, for example Grade A.

Impact of pacemakers: when and what kind?

38

WILLIAM D. TOFF,
A. JOHN CAMM

The development and implementation of the first fully implantable cardiac pacemaker in 1958 transformed the outlook for patients with symptomatic bradycardia and Stokes–Adams attacks.[1] The first pacemaker recipient is still alive and during the four decades since he received his initial implant many millions of patients have benefited from this dramatically effective form of treatment. Technological advances and innovation have enabled the development of increasingly sophisticated pacing systems, better able to simulate the normal cardiac activation sequence, and a wide variety of different pacing modes is now available.

Initially, pacemakers were only implanted for atrioventricular (AV) block, but their use was soon extended to the management of symptomatic bradycardia associated with sinus node disease. In recent years, improved understanding of pathophysiological mechanisms has prompted the assessment of pacemaker therapy in a number of other conditions such as neurocardiogenic syncope, hypertrophic cardiomyopathy, and paroxysmal atrial fibrillation. With the emergence of new indications for pacing and the availability of a vast array of different pacing modes and techniques, an evidence based approach to the practice of cardiac pacing has become increasingly important.

GOALS OF CARDIAC PACING

The fundamental aims of cardiac pacing are to relieve symptoms, to improve the quality of life and, in some instances, to prolong survival. The achievement of these aims is mediated by improvements in hemodynamic function and functional capacity, reduction in cardiovascular morbidity, and prevention of sudden death. Any consideration of the indications for pacing and selection of the appropriate pacing mode must have regard to all of these factors and their interrelations, which are summarized in Figure 38.1. Hemodynamic differences between alternative pacing modes do not always translate into significant differences in clinical utility and a comprehensive assessment of outcome in clinical trials is therefore essential. It is important to note that inappropriate pacing

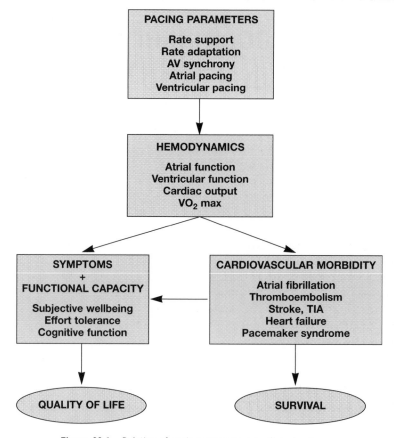

Figure 38.1 Relation of pacing parameters to clinical outcome.

or complications from pacing may result in new or worse symptoms and increased cardiovascular morbidity. This is perhaps best exemplified by the pacemaker syndrome which is most often seen during ventricular pacing in the presence of retrograde ventriculoatrial conduction. The syndrome has aptly been described as an iatrogenic condition.[2]

CURRENT PACING PRACTICE

It is estimated that about 400 000 pacemakers per annum are implanted worldwide,[3] but there is considerable national and regional variation in the implant rate. In the United Kingdom, there are currently 270 new implants per million population[4] as compared with 370 per million in Europe and 434 per million in the United States.[5] These variations may partly reflect differences in the age distribution and morbidity of the relevant populations but availability of resources and variations in standards of medical care and attitudes towards pacing may also be relevant. There has also been some suggestion, in the past, of inappropriate and excessive pacemaker implantation.[6]

In an effort to define appropriate pacing practice, a joint task force sub-committee of the American College of Cardiology (ACC) and the American Heart Association (AHA) published guidelines for permanent pacemaker implantation in 1984.[7] These were updated and revised in 1991[8] and again in 1998[9] (Table 38.1). The guidelines follow an evidence based approach and include grading of the evidence supporting each recommendation. With regard to the indications for pacing, the following classification is used: Class I – conditions for which there is evidence and/or general agreement that pacing is beneficial, useful and effective; Class II – conditions for which there is conflicting evidence and/or a divergence of opinion about the usefulness/efficacy of pacing; Class III – conditions for which there is evidence and/or general agreement that pacing is not useful/effective and in some cases may be harmful. Class II is subdivided into Class IIa – weight of evidence/opinion is in favour of usefulness/efficacy and Class IIb – usefulness/efficacy is less well established by evidence/opinion. It is recognized that, although applicable to the "average" patient, recommendations for specific conditions may require modification to take account of patient co-morbidity, limited life expectancy, and other factors which only the implanting physician can evaluate appropriately.

A working party of the British Pacing and Electrophysiology Group (BPEG) also published recommendations for pacemaker prescription in 1991.[10] These advocated general principles to guide pacemaker mode selection and made specific recommendations for optimal and alternative pacing modes in various clinical settings (Table 38.2). The recommendations regarding mode selection have, however, been criticized and attention has been drawn to their reliance on observational data from retrospective studies rather than prospective randomized clinical trials.[11] Attention has also been drawn to the financial implications of the recommendations, implementation of which might increase pacing budgets by up to 75%.[12] For whatever reason, it is clear that the BPEG recommendations have not been universally adopted in the United Kingdom[13] and there is evidence of ageism, with the preferential use of optimal pacing modes only in younger patients.[14]

General principles of pacemaker mode selection

1   The ventricle should be paced if there is actual or threatened atrioventricular block.
2   The atrium should be paced/sensed unless contraindicated.
3   Rate response is not essential if the patient is inactive or has a normal chronotropic response.
4   Rate hysteresis may be valuable if the bradycardia is intermittent.

Based on recommendations of a working party of the British Pacing and Electrophysiology Group[10]

Against this background, it is pertinent to review the evidence concerning the indications for pacing and pacemaker mode selection in order fully to comprehend the basis for rational, evidence based pacing practice. It is important to note that there have been no randomized trials to assess the efficacy of pacing in the treatment of symptomatic AV block. The absence of any satisfactory alternative therapy and the overwhelming evidence of symptom relief from observational studies over four decades render such a trial unethical and unneccessary. In the assessment of new indications for pacing and alternative pacing modes, however, observational data require critical evaluation and, where inconclusive, should be supplemented by data from carefully designed clinical trials.

Table 38.1 ACC/AHA Guidelines: indications for permanent cardiac pacing[9]

Condition	Class I	Class IIa	Class IIb	Class III
Acquired AV block (adults):				
First degree		First degree AV block with symptoms suggestive of "pacemaker syndrome" and alleviation of symptoms with temporary AV pacing (B)	Marked first degree AV block (PR>0.3 s) in patients with LV dysfunction and symptoms of CHF in whom a more physiologic AV interval results in hemodynamic improvement (C)	Asymptomatic first degree AV block (B)
Second degree	Second degree AV block (any type or level) with associated symptomatic bradycardia (B)	Asymptomatic type I second degree block at intra- or infra-His levels found incidentally at EPS (B) Asymptomatic type II second degree AV block (B)		Asymptomatic type I second degree block at the supra-His (AV node) level (B,C)
Third degree (CHB)	CHB associated with any of: (a) Symptomatic bradycardia (C) (b) Need for drugs causing symptomatic bradycardia (C) (c) Documented asystole ≥3 s or escape rate <40/min in awake, symptom-free patients (B,C) (d) Post ablation of AV junction (B,C) (e) Post operative AV block not expected to resolve (C) (f) Neuromuscular disease (e.g. myotonic dystrophy) (B)	Asymptomatic CHB at any anatomic site, with average, awake, ventricular rates ≥40/min (B,C)		AV block that is expected to resolve and is unlikely to recur (e.g. drug toxicity, Lyme disease) (B)
Chronic bifascicular or trifascicular block	Associated with intermittent CHB (B) Associated with type II second degree AV block (B)	Syncope not proven due to AV block when other likely causes, such as VT, have been excluded (B) Incidental finding at EPS of markedly prolonged HV interval (>100 ms) in asymptomatic patient (B) Incidental finding at EPS of pacing-induced infra-His block that is not physiologic (B)	None	Fascicular block without AV block or symptoms (B) Fascicular block with first degree AV block without symptoms (B)

AV block after the acute phase of myocardial infarction (MI)	Persistent second degree AV block in the His–Purkinje system with bilateral bundle branch block or third degree AV block within or below the His-Purkinje system after acute MI (B) Transient advanced (second or third degree) infranodal AV block and associated bundle branch block. If the site of block is uncertain, an EPS may be necessary (B) Persistent and symptomatic second or third degree AV block (C)	None	Persistent second or third degree AV block at the AV node level (B)	Transient AV block in the absence of intraventricular conduction defects (B) Transient AV block in the presence of isolated left anterior fascicular block (B) Acquired left anterior fascicular block in the absence of AV block (B) Persistent first degree AV block in the presence of bundle branch block that is old or age indeterminate (B)
Sinus node dysfunction (SND)	SND with documented symptomatic bradycardia including frequent symptomatic sinus pauses (including iatrogenic bradycardia due to essential long term drug therapy with no acceptable alternative) (C) Symptomatic chronotropic incompetence (C)	SND, occurring spontaneously or as a result of necessary drug therapy, with heart rates <40/min when a clear association between significant symptoms consistent with bradycardia and the actual presence of bradycardia has not been documented (C)	Chronic heart rates <30/min whilst awake, in minimally symptomatic patients (C)	SND in asymptomatic patients, including those in whom substantial sinus bradycardia (<40/min) is due to long term drug treatment SND in patients in whom symptoms suggestive of bradycardia are clearly documented not to be associated with a slow heart rate SND with symptomatic bradycardia due to non-essential drug therapy

continued

Table 38.1 *continued*

Condition	Class I	Class IIa	Class IIb	Class III
Hypersensitive carotid sinus syndrome and neurally mediated syncope	Recurrent syncope caused by carotid sinus stimulation; minimal carotid sinus pressure induces ventricular asystole of >3 s duration in the absence of any medication that depresses the sinus node or AV conduction (C)	Recurrent syncope without clear, provocative events and with a hypersensitive cardioinhibitory response (C) Syncope of unexplained origin when major abnormalities of sinus node function or AV conduction are discovered or provoked at EPS	Neurally mediated syncope with significant bradycardia reproduced by head-up tilt with or without isoproterenol or other provocative maneuvers (B)	Hyperactive cardioinhibitory response to carotid sinus stimulation in the absence of symptoms Vague symptoms, such as dizziness or light-headedness, or both, with a hyperactive cardioinhibitory response to carotid sinus stimulation Recurrent syncope, lightheadedness or dizziness in the absence of cardioinhibitory response Situational vasovagal syncope in which avoidance behavior is effective
Tachycardia prevention	Sustained pause-dependent VT, with or without prolonged QT, in which the efficacy of pacing is thoroughly documented (C)	High risk patients with congenital long QT syndrome (C)	AV re-entrant or AV node re-entrant supraventricular tachycardia not responsive to medical or ablation therapy (C) Prevention of symptomatic, drug refractory atrial fibrillation (C)	Frequent or complex ventricular ectopic activity without sustained VT in the absence of the long QT syndrome Long QT syndrome due to reversible causes
Hypertrophic cardiomyopathy	Class I indications for sinus node dysfunction or AV block as above (C)	None	Medically refractory, symptomatic hypertrophic cardiomyopathy patients with significant resting or provoked LV outflow obstruction (C)	Asymptomatic or medically controlled patients Symptomatic patients without evidence of LV outflow obstruction
Dilated cardiomyopathy	Class I indications for sinus node dysfunction or AV block as above (C)	None	Symptomatic, drug refractory dilated cardiomyopathy with prolonged PR interval when acute hemodynamic studies have demonstrated hemodynamic benefit (C)	Asymptomatic dilated cardiomyopathy Symptomatic dilated cardiomyopathy when patients are rendered asymptomatic by drug therapy Symptomatic ischemic cardiomyopathy

604

After cardiac transplantation	Symptomatic bradyarrhythmia or chronotropic incompetence that is not expected to resolve and meets other Class I indications for permanent pacing (C)	None	Symptomatic bradyarrhythmia or chronotropic incompetence that, although transient, may persist for months and require intervention	Asymptomatic bradyarrhythmia post cardiac transplantation
Children and adolescents	Sinus node dysfunction with correlation of symptoms during age-inappropriate bradycardia (B)	Asymptomatic sinus bradycardia in a child with complex congenital heart disease where the resting heart rate is <35/min or ventricular pauses >3 s occur (C)	Asymptomatic sinus bradycardia in an adolescent with congenital heart disease where the resting heart rate is <35/min or ventricular pauses >3 s occur (C)	Asymptomatic sinus bradycardia in an adolescent where the longest R–R interval is <3 s and the minimum rate >40/min (C)
	Advanced second or third degree AV block associated with symptomatic bradycardia, CHF or low cardiac output (C)	Bradycardia-tachycardia syndrome needing chronic antiarrhythmic therapy other than digitalis (C)		Asymptomatic type I second degree AV block (C)
	Congenital CHB with a wide QRS escape rhythm or ventricular dysfunction (B)	Congenital CHB, beyond the first year of life, with an average heart rate <50/min, or with abrupt ventricular pauses two or three times the basic cycle length (B)	Congenital CHB in an asymptomatic neonate, child or adolescent with an acceptable rate, narrow QRS complex and normal ventricular function (B)	
	Congenital CHB in the infant with a ventricular rate <50–55/min or with congenital heart disease and a ventricular rate <70/min (B,C)			
	Post-operative advanced second or third degree AV block that is not expected to resolve, or persists at least 7 days after cardiac surgery (B,C)	Long QT syndrome with 2:1 or third degree AV block (B)	Transient postoperative CHB that reverts to sinus rhythm with residual bifascicular block (C)	Transient postoperative AV block with return of normal AV conduction within 7 days (B)
	Sustained pause-dependent VT, with or without prolonged QT, in which the efficacy of pacing is thoroughly documented (B)			Asymptomatic postoperative bifascicular block, with or without first degree AV block (C)

CHB, complete heart block; CHF, congestive heart failure; EPS, electrophysiology study; VT, ventricular tachycardia.
The grade of evidence supporting each recommendation is indicated in parentheses: (A) data derived from multiple randomized clinical trials involving a large number of individuals; (B) data derived from limited number of trials involving comparatively small number of patients or from well designed data analyses of non-randomized studies or observational data registries; (C) recommendation based on consensus opinion of experts. For explanation of classification scheme, see text.

Based on Gregoratos *et al*.[9]

Table 38.2 Recommended pacemaker modes

Diagnosis	Optimal	Alternative	Inappropriate
SND	AAIR	AAI	VVI/VDD
AVB	DDD	VDD	AAI/DDI
SND + AVB	DDDR/DDIR	DDD/DDI	AAI/VVI
Chronic AF + AVB	VVIR	VVI	AAI/DDD/VDD
CSS	DDI	DDD/VVI + hysteresis	AAI/VDD
MVVS	DDI	DDD	AAI/VVI/VDD

SND, sinus node disease; AVB, atrioventricular block; AF, atrial fibrillation; CSS, carotid sinus syndrome; MVVS, malignant vasovagal syndrome.

Interpretation of mode acronyms:

First letter:	Chamber(s) paced	A, atrium; V, ventricle; D, atrium and ventricle
Second letter:	Chamber(s) sensed	A, atrium; V, ventricle; D, atrium and ventricle
Third letter:	Response to sensing	I, inhibition; T, triggering; D, inhibition and triggering
Fourth letter:	Additional functions	R, adaptive rate

Based on recommendations of the British Pacing and Electrophysiology Group.[10]

CONVENTIONAL INDICATIONS FOR PACING

The principal indication for cardiac pacing is to relieve or prevent symptoms associated with bradycardia. In high grade AV block, however, there is evidence that survival may also be improved by pacing, even in the absence of symptoms, and pacing should be considered on prognostic grounds alone.

The symptoms associated with bradycardia include manifestations of limited cardiac output (tiredness, exercise intolerance, breathlessness, oedema or chest discomfort), relative cerebral ischemia (transient dizziness, light-headedness, pre-syncope or syncope), and uncoordinated cardiac contraction (palpitation, neck or abdominal pulsation). Where significant symptoms are clearly associated with documented bradycardia, the requirement for pacing will rarely be in doubt. In other contexts, the cause of symptoms may be unclear and it is important to note that the most common symptoms are non-specific and prevalent in the elderly population, even in the absence of bradycardia.

Remediable causes of bradycardia such as acute myocardial ischemia, electrolyte imbalance, hypothyroidism or drug toxicity should always be considered before proceeding to cardiac pacing. In some instances, drugs that depress sinus node function or AV conduction may be essential and pacing may be required to enable their continued use.

The most common causes of bradycardia requiring pacing are impaired impulse formation, as in sinus node disease, or a disturbance of cardiac conduction, as in AV block. In the United Kingdom, sinus node disease accounts for about 43% of primary implants and AV block or other conduction disturbance for about 50%.[13] The remainder includes patients paced for a variety of conditions, including carotid sinus syndrome, cardio-inhibitory forms of neurocardiogenic syncope and others. The pattern is different in the United States, where sinus node disease accounts for over 50% of primary implants and AV block for about 34%.[5] The reasons for this disparity are unclear but it may reflect different perceptions regarding the indications for pacing.

Atrioventricular block

FIRST DEGREE AV BLOCK

Isolated prolongation of the PR interval may be seen as a normal variant in healthy young subjects. In this context, it is most likely due to autonomic influences and has no prognostic significance.[15] In older subjects, PR prolongation is more often associated with underlying pathology, such as conducting system fibrosis or coronary artery disease but it does not usually give rise to symptoms and pacing is not generally indicated.

Occasionally, however, symptoms may arise if the PR interval is markedly prolonged. Atrial systole may then closely follow delayed ventricular systole from the previous cycle, resulting in a comparable hemodynamic disturbance to that seen in the pacemaker syndrome caused by retrograde VA conduction during ventricular pacing. The phenomenon may be accentuated during exercise as the atrial rate increases and the PR interval fails to shorten appropriately. This has been referred to as the "pacemaker syndrome without a pacemaker"[16] or the "pseudo-pacemaker syndrome"[17] and a favorable response to dual chamber pacing has been reported.[16–18] In symptomatic patients with first degree AV block, the response to temporary dual chamber pacing should be assessed. If clinical and hemodynamic improvement can be demonstrated by restoration of a physiologic AV interval, permanent dual chamber pacing should be considered.[19,20] Symptomatic first degree AV block with a demonstrable improvement during temporary dual chamber pacing may reasonably be considered at least a Class II[19] and perhaps even a Class I[20] indication for pacing.

SECOND DEGREE AV BLOCK

When second degree AV block of any type is associated with clearly attributable symptoms, pacing is indicated. In the absence of symptoms, the situation is more complex. Prognosis is thought to relate to the site of block, proximal block at the level of the AV node being more benign than distal block in the His–Purkinje system.[21] The ECG classification into Mobitz type I (Wenckebach), Mobitz type II or advanced (2:1, 3:1 or 4:1) second degree AV block is purely descriptive and the site of block cannot always be inferred although electrophysiologic studies have shown that type I block is most commonly proximal whereas type II block is almost always distal.[22] In the past, type I second degree AV block has often been regarded as benign but evidence from the Devon Heart Block and Bradycardia Survey in the United Kingdom[23] suggests that, even in asymptomatic patients, survival is significantly improved by pacing. Although this was a non-randomized, observational study, it constitutes the best available evidence and published opinion suggests that pacing should be considered in asymptomatic type I second degree AV block, particularly in older patients with structural heart disease.[24,25] In young subjects, however, asymptomatic type I second degree AV block occurring during sleep or associated with athletic training is more likely to reflect high resting vagal tone and pacing is unnecessary.[26,27]

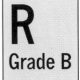

COMPLETE AV BLOCK

In symptomatic complete AV block, pacing usually, although not invariably, improves the symptoms and should always be considered. Irrespective of symptoms, however, untreated acquired complete heart block is associated with significantly impaired survival. Overall mortality may exceed 50% at one year, the outlook being worst in older patients (>80 years) and those with associated non-rheumatic structural heart disease.[28] Male sex and a history of syncope have also been associated with a worse outlook in some studies[29] but there is conflicting evidence regarding syncope.[30] Transient AV block carries a more favorable prognosis, with a one-year mortality of 36%, compared with 70% in patients with permanent AV block,[28] but a significant proportion of patients (38–39% over median follow-up of 36–54 months) progress to permanent AV block and become pacemaker-dependent when paced.[31]

Observational studies of outcome in paced patients during the early days of cardiac pacing suggested that pacing in complete AV block could improve survival to approach that of a similar age- and sex-matched group.[29,32] Mortality was higher in those with a history of myocardial infarction but not influenced by pre-pacing QRS duration or morphology, ventricular rate (dichotomized about 40/min) or whether AV block was intermittent or constant.[32] In a more recent study of patients aged ≥ 65 years, paced for symptomatic, high grade AV block, overall survival was less than expected for an age- and sex-matched cohort.[33] However, in patients aged <80 years without structural heart disease, survival was normal. Congestive heart failure, chronic obstructive pulmonary disease, age, syncope, insulin-dependent diabetes and male gender emerged as independent predictors of increased mortality. There have been no prospective randomized trials to assess the impact of pacing on survival but the high mortality of untreated complete AV block, the prevalence of symptoms, and the strength of the data from observational studies suggest that such a trial is neither ethical nor necessary. The vast majority of patients with complete AV block should be paced, whether or not they have symptoms.

R
Grade A

CONGENITAL COMPLETE AV BLOCK

The natural history and management of congenital complete AV block in infancy and childhood is beyond the scope of this review. In patients surviving to adulthood, the prognosis has previously been regarded as benign, based largely on retrospective studies of small series of patients.[34] More recent data concerning long term follow-up (7–30 years) of 102 patients with isolated congenital complete AV block, who survived without symptoms to the age of 15 years, suggests a less favorable outlook.[35] Stokes–Adams attacks occurred in 27 patients, of whom 8 died (6 during the first attack) and 6 others required cardiac resuscitation. All survivors received pacemakers. A further 8 patients had repeated fainting spells requiring pacing and 27 others were paced for other reasons (fatigue, effort dyspnea, dizziness, ectopics during exercise, mitral regurgitation or slow ventricular rates). Of 40 patients followed for 30 years, only 4 remained asymptomatic without pacing. The only significant predictor of risk was QT_c prolongation, which was seen in 7 patients, all of whom had Stokes–Adams attacks and 3 of whom died. In contrast to previous studies, low ventricular rates, widened QRS complexes, poor chronotropic response to exercise and ectopics were not predictive of future Stokes–Adams attacks or death. These data appear to support the authors' recommendation of prophylactic pacing in adolescents and adults with congenital complete AV block, even without symptoms, notwithstanding the fact that a number of questions remain unanswered.[36]

R
Grade B

FASCICULAR BLOCK

In asymptomatic subjects with unifascicular block (right bundle branch block, left anterior hemiblock or left posterior hemiblock), the risk of progression to high grade AV block is remote[37] and pacing is not indicated. In asymptomatic bifascicular block (left bundle branch block or right bundle branch block with left anterior or posterior hemiblock), the risk of progression to high grade AV block is in the region of 2% per annum. Prognosis is principally determined by the presence or absence of underlying structural heart disease and prophylactic pacing is not routinely indicated.[38] Progression to high grade AV block is more commonly seen in patients with a history of syncope but should not be presumed to be the cause without further assessment. If high grade AV block is documented, pacing is mandatory. When the cause of syncope remains unclear, an electrophysiology study may help to identify patients likely to benefit from pacemaker implantation. A prolonged HV interval >100 ms and His–Purkinje block during atrial pacing have high specificity for prediction of subsequent progression to high grade AV block.[39,40] Unfortunately, these are rare findings and thus of low sensitivity. Less marked HV prolongation (>70 ms) is more common but its significance is uncertain.[41] Sensitivity for disclosure of latent high grade AV block may be markedly enhanced by the use of intravenous disopyramide during the study but this is not advised in patients with impaired left ventricular function.[42] The electrophysiology study may also be of value to identify inducible ventricular tachycardia which is a relatively common finding in patients with bundle branch block and a history of syncope.[43] This argues strongly against the empiric use of permanent pacing in this context. However, in patients with bifascicular block and a history of syncope for which no other cause is apparent despite thorough evaluation, including an electrophysiology study, empiric pacing may be the most expeditious course. This strategy is principally justified for relief of symptoms as pacing does not appear to influence mortality or the incidence of sudden death in this context.[38,39]

ATRIOVENTRICULAR AND BUNDLE BRANCH BLOCK AFTER MYOCARDIAL INFARCTION

Transient conduction disturbance is a relatively common complication of acute myocardial infarction. The acute management and indications for temporary cardiac pacing are beyond the scope of this review and will not be considered further. The long term prognosis is principally determined by the extent of myocardial injury. When AV block complicates inferior myocardial infarction, it typically resolves within a few days and rarely persists beyond 2 or 3 weeks. In anterior infarction, however, AV block may reflect extensive septal necrosis and the prognosis is poor despite pacing.[44] Patients with high grade AV block persisting for more than 3 weeks after myocardial infarction should be considered for permanent pacing.

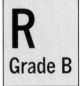

The occurrence of an intraventricular conduction disturbance (apart from isolated left anterior hemiblock) in patients with acute myocardial infarction identifies a group with poor short term and long term prognosis and an increased risk of sudden death.[45] The poor prognosis in this group, however, is mainly attributable to a high incidence of malignant ventricular arrhythmia, pump failure, and electromechanical dissociation, rather than progressive conduction disturbance. A prospective study of 50 patients randomized to pacing or control groups and followed for 5 years showed no significant difference in survival.[46] However, evidence from a retrospective multicenter study of patients with bundle branch block complicating myocardial infarction, indicates that

Grade C

transient high degree AV block during the acute phase is associated with a high incidence of recurrent AV block and sudden death that may be reduced by pacemaker implantation.[47,48] The risk appears to be particularly high in patients with right bundle branch block and left anterior hemiblock.[48,49]

MODE SELECTION IN AV BLOCK

The essential requirement in AV block is that the ventricle be paced. When sinus rhythm and chronotropic competence are preserved, dual chamber pacing with atrial tracking will ensure the maintenance of AV synchrony and physiologic rate adaptation. When sinus rhythm is absent or when chronotropic incompetence is present, an extrinsic sensor may be used to provide rate-adaptation with either ventricular or dual chamber pacing, as appropriate.

Grade A

Both dual chamber pacing[50–52] and adaptive rate single chamber pacing[53–55] have been shown to offer benefits in terms of improved hemodynamics, increased treadmill exercise tolerance and reduced symptoms when compared with single rate ventricular pacing in small randomized crossover trials. The mean patient age in most of these trials was younger than the typical paced population but similar benefits have recently been reported in patients aged 75 years or over.[56] Nonetheless, the long term clinical benefit of physiologic pacing in the elderly has been questioned.[11] Quality of life studies have yielded conflicting results although physiologic pacing does appear to offer advantages in terms of symptoms and there is considerable evidence of patient preference for physiologic modes.[57] Single chamber ventricular pacing is associated with an increased risk of pacemaker syndrome. The true incidence of this complication is unknown but estimated to be between 7 and 20%.[2] It has, however, been suggested that a subclinical form may be present in many apparently asymptomatic patients.[58] Data from a retrospective review of outcome in patients paced single or dual chamber has suggested that dual chamber pacing may confer a survival advantage in a subset of patients with congestive heart failure.[59] A more recent case-control study has confirmed this finding but showed no difference in overall survival.[60]

Grade B

The clinical impact and cost utility of single and dual chamber pacing are currently being compared in two large scale prospective randomized trials.[61] The Canadian Trial of Physiologic Pacing (CTOPP)[62] is comparing outcomes in 2566 patients of all ages (>18 years) paced for either AV block or sinoatrial disease. The United Kingdom Pacing and Cardiovascular Events (UKPACE) trial[63] is of similar design and size (2000 patients) but concerns only elderly patients (≥70 years) with AV block. It is anticipated that these studies will greatly strengthen the evidence base for mode selection in AV block. In the meantime, adherence to published guidelines[10] (see p. 601) is recommended.

Sinoatrial disease

Sinoatrial disease encompasses a wide spectrum of arrhythmia including sinus bradycardia, sinus arrest, sinoatrial block, sick sinus syndrome and the tachycardia–bradycardia syndrome in which paroxysmal atrial tachyarrhythmia alternates with bradycardia. The prognosis in sinoatrial disease is generally good unless myocardial ischemia, heart failure or systemic embolism are present.[64] Permanent pacing is indicated for the relief of symptoms that are due to bradycardia. Every effort should be made to establish a causal relationship by recording an ECG during symptoms although this may not always be possible. Occasionally, drugs needed to control tachyarrhythmia may cause or exacerbate bradycardia and pacing may be required to facilitate their continued use.

The first and only randomized trial to assess the efficacy of pacing in sick sinus syndrome has recently been reported.[65] One hundred and seven patients with symptomatic sick sinus syndrome were randomized to receive either no treatment, oral theophylline or permanent DDDR pacing. Patients were excluded in very severe cases, defined as symptomatic resting sinus rate<30/min, sinus pauses >3 s or heart failure refractory to treatment with ACE inhibitors and diuretics. During a mean follow-up period of 19 months, both pacing and theophylline were associated with a lower incidence of heart failure compared with the untreated patients (3%, 3% and 17% respectively) but only pacing was associated with a significantly lower incidence of syncope (6%, 17% and 23% respectively). It is noteworthy that 14 of the 16 patients who were syncopal during follow-up had a history of syncope at randomization. During follow-up, 51% of patients in the control group and 42% in the theophylline group were withdrawn from the study due to syncope, overt heart failure, poorly tolerated paroxysmal tachyarrhythmia, patient wishes or drug side effects. There were no significant differences in NYHA class or symptom scores (fatigue, dizziness, and palpitation) between the groups either at baseline or after 3 months. The untreated controls showed subjective improvement, with a significant reduction of dizziness and a trend towards decreased fatigue. These findings were associated with significant increases in resting, mean and maximum heart rates, emphasizing the unpredictable natural history of the condition and the possibility of spontaneous improvement. Pacing remains the treatment of choice for patients with symptomatic sick sinus syndrome. In the absence of long term follow-up data to confirm efficacy and safety, theophylline or other pharmacologic means of chronotropic support cannot be recommended.

R

Grade A

Pacing does not appear to improve survival in sinoatrial disease[66] and it is not generally indicated in asymptomatic patients. Such patients, however, should be followed closely to assess progression. Athletically trained subjects may have sinus rates as low as 30/min during sleep with pauses of almost 3 s.[67] These findings usually reflect high vagal tone and do not require pacing in the absence of symptoms. If lower rates or longer pauses are observed during sleep or if similar findings occur during the day, particularly if there is evidence of progression with time, prophylactic pacing may be justified on empiric grounds although there are no supportive data.

R

Grade B/C

MODE SELECTION IN SINOATRIAL DISEASE

In isolated sinoatrial disease, rate support can be achieved by atrial, ventricular or dual chamber pacing. Current guidelines[10] recommend the avoidance of single chamber ventricular pacing. Small crossover studies comparing ventricular with dual chamber pacing have reported less favorable hemodynamics, worse symptomatology, and an increased risk of pacemaker syndrome.[57,68–70] Numerous retrospective studies also suggest that ventricular pacing is associated with an increased risk of atrial fibrillation, heart failure, and thromboembolism.[64,71] There is also evidence of increased mortality in ventricular paced patients.[72] Attention has been drawn to the confounding effect of selection bias on data derived almost exclusively from retrospective studies and the need for prospective randomized trials has been stressed.[61,71]

The first prospective trial was reported from Denmark in 1994.[73] In this study, 225 patients with sick sinus syndrome were randomized to either AAI or VVI pacing and followed for a mean of 3.3 years. Neither the incidence of atrial fibrillation or stroke nor survival differed significantly between the two groups, although the incidence of a combined endpoint of stroke plus peripheral embolism was significantly lower in the atrial paced group. Only 2 of 115 patients in the VVI group required upgrade for severe pacemaker syndrome. Extended follow-up of the same group of patients after a mean period of 5.5 years has subsequently been reported.[74] The previously identified benefits of atrial pacing were enhanced, with a significantly lower incidence of atrial fibrillation, thromboembolism and heart failure in the atrial paced group. All-cause mortality and mortality due to cardiovascular causes were also significantly lower in the atrial paced group. After adjustment for other pre-implant variables, there was a significant association between ventricular pacing and cardiovascular death but only a non-significant trend towards increased overall mortality. A further study from the same group is now in progress to compare AAIR and DDDR pacing in patients with sinus node disease.[75]

R

Grade A

Preliminary results from a second randomized study, the Pacemaker Selection in the Elderly (PASE) trial, have recently been reported.[76,77] This included 163 patients with sinus node disease, all aged ≥ 65 years, randomized to either DDDR or VVIR pacing. At one year, there were interesting trends in clinical endpoints suggesting benefit for DDDR pacing but none achieved statistical significance. A large scale trial, the Mode Selection Trial in Sinus Node Dysfunction (MOST), is currently in progress.[61] This will randomize 2000 patients, aged ≥ 21 years, implanted with DDDR pacemakers, to programming in either DDDR or VVIR mode with follow-up for a minimum of 1.5 years. The Canadian Trial of Physiologic Pacing (CTOPP)[62] also includes patients with sinus node disease randomized to either physiologic (AAI/AAIR or DDD/DDDR) or ventricular (VVI/VVIR) pacing and followed for a minimum of 2 years. A number of other trials are also in progress to assess the ability of physiologic pacing to prevent atrial fibrillation.[61] These include the Systematic Trial of Pacing to Prevent Atrial Fibrillation (STOP-AF)[78] which will randomize approximately 350 patients aged ≥ 18 with sick sinus syndrome, implanted with dual chamber pacemakers, to programming in either atrial based (AAI or DDD) or ventricular pacing modes. The study, which uses sequential trial methodology to allow greater power with a limited sample size, includes an adaptive rate arm for patients with chronotropic incompetence. The primary endpoint is permanent atrial fibrillation resistant to DC cardioversion. Secondary outcomes include congestive heart failure, pacemaker syndrome, change of mode for lead problems, and death.

R

Grade A

Pending the outcome of these prospective trials, adherence to current guidelines is recommended. In sinoatrial disease, atrial based pacing is preferable. When AV conduction is intact, single chamber adaptive rate atrial (AAIR) pacing is regarded as the optimal mode[10] as it preserves both atrioventricular synchrony and a normal ventricular activation pattern. Retrospective analysis of pooled data from 28 studies has shown a low risk of subsequent AV block (0.6% per annum)[79] and this is supported by data from the recent prospective study.[73,74] Dual chamber pacing may thus be unnecessary for most patients although some physicians prefer to implant a DDDR pacing system with programming to AAIR mode, a mode conversion option or AV search hysteresis. When a single chamber atrial pacing system is proposed, assessment of AV conduction at the time of implant to ensure preservation of 1:1 conduction during atrial pacing at 140/min is customary and prudent although its predictive value is unproven.[79] When AV block coexists with sinoatrial disease, dual chamber pacing in DDDR mode is recommended. In patients with a history of paroxysmal atrial tachyarrhythmia, DDI pacing is preferable to avoid rapid ventricular tracking. The recent introduction of mode-switching pacemakers capable of switching from DDD/DDDR to DDI/DDIR mode on detection of atrial tachyarrhythmia has offered an attractive alternative.

NEW INDICATIONS FOR PACING

Neurocardiogenic syncope

Neurocardiogenic syncope describes the clinical syndromes of syncope resulting from inappropriate autonomic responses, manifested as abnormalities in the control of peripheral vascular resistance and heart rate.[80] It is thought to account for the largest proportion of faints in clinical practice. The most common forms are carotid sinus syndrome and vasovagal syncope but other related syndromes include cough, deglutition, and micturition syncope. The pathophysiologic mechanisms are not fully understood but carotid sinus massage[81,82] and tilt-table testing[83] have emerged as useful diagnostic tools in carotid sinus syndrome and vasovagal syncope respectively, enabling abnormal reflex responses to be categorized as cardioinhibitory (asystole >3 s, bradycardia or AV block), vasodepressor (fall in systolic blood pressure >50 mmHg) or mixed. This has invited assessment of the utility of cardiac pacing which might be expected to benefit patients with predominantly cardioinhibitory or mixed responses.

Early reports of pacing in carotid sinus syndrome confirmed its efficacy in some patients but persistent symptoms were seen in those in whom there was a significant vasodepressor response or hypotension during ventricular pacing.[84] The latter was improved by AV sequential pacing and it was suggested that this was the appropriate mode in patients with mixed responses. Attention has been drawn to the variable natural history of the condition, which may remit spontaneously, and the importance of a control group when evaluating therapy has been emphasized.[85] A prospective randomized trial of pacing in patients with severe carotid sinus syndrome has subsequently been reported.[86] Sixty patients were randomized to pacing (VVI in 18 and DDD in 14 patients) or no therapy (28 patients). During a mean follow-up of 36 months, syncope recurred in 16 (57%) of the non-paced group and only 3 (9%) of the paced group. Nineteen patients (68%) in the unpaced group were eventually paced because of the severity of symptoms. Pacing is now the treatment of choice in all but the most mild forms of carotid sinus syndrome. Recent evidence suggests that carotid sinus syndrome is underdiagnosed and that comprehensive assessment of patients presenting with syncope, dizziness or falls may identify a significant number of otherwise unrecognized patients who may benefit from pacing.[87]

R
Grade A

Pacing has also been evaluated in the so-called "malignant" form of vasovagal syndrome, characterized by recurrent syncope with only brief or absent prodromal symptoms. Evidence from several studies using temporary pacing during tilt-table testing indicates that pacing rarely prevents vasovagal syncope. The limited efficacy of pacing reflects the fact that hypotension precedes the onset of bradycardia in most patients. However, dual chamber pacing does attenuate the evolution of the final and most extreme degrees of hypotension and may thereby prolong the symptomatic presyncopal period in selected patients with a documented cardioinhibitory component.[88] A retrospective review of 37 patients receiving predominantly dual chamber implanted pacemakers, followed for a mean of 50.2 months, reported symptomatic improvement in 89% with 62% remaining free of syncope and 27% completely asymptomatic. The collective syncopal burden was reduced from 136 to 11 episodes per year.[89] This was an uncontrolled study but two multicenter prospective randomized trials have subsequently been initiated.

The North American Vasovagal Pacemaker Study[90] randomized patients with a history of frequent syncope and a positive (cardioinhibitory) tilt test to receive either DDI pacing with a pacemaker incorporating a specialized rate drop sensing algorithm, or no pacing. The rate drop sensing algorithm is designed to detect the characteristic pattern of onset of bradycardia that is seen in vasovagal syndrome. The fall in heart rate is typically more marked than occurs with natural diurnal fluctuation yet less precipitous than that seen at the onset of complete AV block or asystole. On detection of a characteristic rate drop, pacing commences with a high initial intervention rate that gradually decreases.[91] The North American study was stopped towards the end of a 2-year pilot phase (May 1997) due to substantial benefit in the paced group. Syncope recurred in only 4 of 24 paced patients (16.7%) but in 13 of 22 unpaced patients (59.1%).[92] A second trial, coordinated by the Vasovagal International Study (VASIS) Group, is ongoing.[93] In this trial, 200 patients are to be randomized to receive either DDI pacing with hysteresis or no pacing, with follow-up for a minimum of 1 year, the main endpoint being time to recurrence of syncope.

The available data indicate that pacing may be beneficial in selected patients with malignant vasovagal syndrome but further data are required to clarify the relative efficacy of pharmacologic therapy, such as beta-blockers, disopyramide, scopolamine, alpha-agonists, selective serotonin reuptake inhibitors and others, which although largely disappointing, have been of benefit to some patients.[94] In the meantime, it would seem prudent to reserve pacing (outside the context of clinical trials) for patients with severe symptoms refractory to conservative measures and drug therapy.

R

Grade A

Hypertrophic cardiomyopathy

The ability of pacing at the right ventricular apex to reduce the left ventricular outflow tract (LVOT) gradient in patients with hypertrophic obstructive cardiomyopathy has been recognized for over 30 years.[95] The benefits are thought to be due to eccentric or abnormal activation of the septum which may increase the LVOT diameter and decrease systolic anterior movement of the mitral valve during systole. A recent resurgence of interest has been prompted by the availability of sophisticated dual chamber pacemakers able to optimize ventricular filling by preservation of AV synchrony and maximize ventricular capture by the programming of a short AV delay. In some cases, drug therapy or ablation of the AV node may be required to prolong intrinsic AV conduction for maintenance of optimal LA-LV timing, whilst permitting maximal right ventricular pre-excitation by pacing.

Initial clinical studies showed encouraging results over the short and medium term with decreased symptoms and improved exercise capacity associated with reductions of LVOT gradient in the region of 60%.[96-99] Three prospective randomized trials have subsequently been completed. All used a similar design with blinded crossover between active (DDD) and inactive (AAI backup at 30/min) pacing modes after 3 months. A study performed at the Mayo Clinic[100] enrolled 21 patients with severe symptoms, refractory to drug therapy. The LVOT gradient decreased to a mean of 55 mmHg during DDD pacing, compared with 76 mmHg at baseline and 83 mmHg during the AAI phase. Quality of life scores and exercise duration during DDD pacing were significantly improved from baseline but not significantly different from those during the AAI phase. Overall, 63% of patients had symptomatic improvement during DDD pacing but 42% also improved during the AAI phase. In 5%, symptoms were worse during DDD pacing. The symptomatic improvement during the AAI phase suggests that there is an important placebo effect associated with pacemaker implantation, underscoring the importance of randomized trials in assessing this form of treatment. The European Pacing In Cardiomyopathy (PIC) study reported similar findings in a larger group of 83 similarly selected patients.[101] LVOT gradient decreased to a mean of 30 mmHg during DDD pacing compared with 59 mmHg at baseline. Exercise duration was not significantly increased, except for a sub-group of patients with more severely limited exercise tolerance (<10 minutes of the Bruce protocol) during the inactive (AAI backup) phase. Dyspnea, angina and functional class improved during active pacing compared with the inactive phase and 95% of patients preferred pacing. A placebo effect was once again seen, with significant improvement in symptoms compared to baseline even during the inactive AAI backup phase. Subsequent activation of pacing, however, resulted in significant improvement in symptoms and quality of life scores and, conversely, inactivation resulted in significant deterioration. A third study, the Multicentre Pacing Therapy for Hypertrophic Cardiomyopathy (M-PATHY) trial, has yet to report.

The role of dual chamber pacing in the management of patients with hypertrophic obstructive cardiomyopathy is presently unclear. It may benefit some patients with significant symptoms refractory to drug therapy and obviate or delay the need for surgery but there is no evidence that it reduces the risk of sudden death or alters the long term clinical course. The response to temporary dual chamber pacing in the acute setting does not predict long term outcome and is therefore of no value in patient selection.[99,102] An intriguing finding is the observation, in some series, of geometrical and functional changes, suggesting that left ventricular remodelling may occur after prolonged pacing. Decreased thickness of the anterior septum and the anterolateral wall of the left ventricle have been reported, with persistence of at least partial gradient reduction on pacemaker inhibition, for a period related to the duration of pacing.[102–104] These controversial findings require further elucidation and a measured approach is recommended pending the results of further prospective randomized trials and long term follow-up.[105]

Dilated cardiomyopathy

It has been suggested that dual chamber pacing with a short AV delay might improve cardiac function in dilated cardiomyopathy by improving the relation between atrial and ventricular systole, thereby decreasing presystolic mitral and tricuspid regurgitation and increasing ventricular filling time.[106] Initial hemodynamic and clinical studies yielded encouraging results[106–108] but others have failed to show any significant benefit.[109,110] It might be anticipated that patients with first-degree heart block would be most likely to benefit and this has been confirmed in hemodynamic[111] and short term clinical studies.[109] Other criteria that may predict benefit from short AV delay pacing in

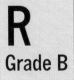

this context include prolonged QRS duration, functional mitral regurgitation ≥ 450 ms, ventricular filling time <200 ms and early cessation of transmitral flow with concomitant diastolic mitral regurgitation on Doppler echocardiography.[113,114] During temporary pacing, responders will have an increase in systolic blood pressure and an increase in mitral regurgitation velocity (indicating a higher left ventricular systolic pressure and lower left atrial pressure), but despite these findings, the clinical outcome with pacing cannot be predicted with certainty.[114]

Recent interest has focussed on the use of multi-site, three or four chamber pacing with synchronized biventricular activation in an atrial tracking (VDD) mode with optimized AV delay. Hemodynamic and clinical improvements have been reported in a small number of patients with end-stage heart failure.[115] In this mode of pacing, the left ventricular electrode is placed either transvenously in the lateral coronary vein or by a thoracoscopic technique on the posterolateral wall of the left ventricle. Biatrial synchronization is also used in the presence of interatrial conduction delay. A number of randomized clinical trials are in progress in Europe and the USA to assess the efficacy of biventricular DDD pacing in dilated cardiomyopathy. In the Pacing Therapy in Congestive Heart Failure (PATH-CHF) trial,[116] right or left univentricular pacing is compared with biventricular pacing using a randomized crossover study design. An epicardial left ventricular pacing lead is implanted by mini-thoracotomy and the optimal univentricular pacing mode and AV delay are determined by intra-operative testing. The Multi-site Stimulation in Cardiomyopathy (MUSTIC) trial[117] uses a blinded crossover between active and inactive pacing to assess biventricular pacing with one lead at the right ventricular apex and the other – the left ventricular lead, in the posterior coronary vein. Septal movement is optimized by varying the pacing sites during placement. Alternative pacing sites have also been assessed, such as the right ventricular outflow tract (paced either alone or in synchrony with the right ventricular apex). Benefit has been reported in acute hemodynamic studies and results from clinical studies are awaited.[118] At the present time, in the absence of other indications, pacing in dilated cardiomyopathy should be regarded as an experimental technique pending further data from controlled studies.

Atrial fibrillation

The possible influence of mode selection on the incidence of atrial fibrillation when pacing in sick sinus syndrome has been discussed above as has the occasional need for pacing to permit antiarrhythmic drug therapy. The limited success of drug therapy in suppressing paroxysmal atrial fibrillation has prompted the assessment of various pacing strategies, even in patients with no other indication for pacemaker implantation. In selected patients with the vagally mediated, pause-dependent, form of atrial fibrillation, permanent atrial rate support has been shown to be of benefit although concomitant drug therapy may still be required.[119] In a broader context, the use of atrial based pacing to prevent paroxysmal atrial fibrillation in patients selected for ablation of the AV node is under evaluation in a prospective randomized trial (Antiarrhythmic Effects of Atrial-based Pacing Pre- and Post-AV Node Ablation – PA³).[120] Patients receive a DDDR pacemaker 3 months prior to ablation and are randomized to receive either atrial pacing or no pacing. Following ablation, a second phase of the trial compares the efficacy of continued atrial pacing in DDDR/DDIR mode with VDD pacing in the suppression of atrial fibrillation.

It has been postulated that reduced dispersion of refractoriness might decrease the propensity to paroxysmal AF in susceptible patients. Dual site atrial pacing in DDDR mode, with leads in the high right atrium and at the coronary sinus os, has been reported to increase the arrhythmia-free interval and to offer greater benefit than single site pacing.[121] The technique is currently under evaluation in a prospective randomized trial (Dual Site Atrial Pacing to Prevent AF – DAPPAF).[122] Others have reported encouraging results of biatrial synchronization in patients with advanced interatrial conduction delay and drug refractory atrial flutter and fibrillation.[123,124] Pacing leads were positioned in the right atrium and within the mid or distal coronary sinus to pace right and left atria simultaneously in triggered (AAT) mode. This strategy is also under evaluation in a prospective randomized trial (Synchronized Biatrial Pacing – SYNBIAPACE).[117]

In permanent atrial fibrillation, pacing may be required when there is coexisting AV block or sinoatrial disease with bradycardia and occasionally to facilitate the use of antiarrhythmic medication. Pacing, usually in adaptive rate ventricular (VVIR) mode, is also required after radiofrequency ablation of the AV node when this is used to effect control of the ventricular rate. It is thought that the benefits of this form of treatment accrue not only from rate control but also from the regularity of paced ventricular activation. In patients with dilated cardiomyopathy and permanent atrial fibrillation, pharmacologic therapy and ablation with pacing are currently being compared in a multicenter prospective randomized trial, the Dilated Cardiomyopathy and Atrial Fibrillation (DCAF) trial.[125]

Long QT syndrome

Patients with the long QT syndrome are at high risk of syncope and sudden death, usually due to polymorphic ventricular tachycardia. There are compelling data from observational studies[126,127] and from the International Long QT Syndrome Registry[128,129] indicating that cardiac pacing, with concomitant beta-blockade, may reduce the rate of recurrent syncope and sudden death. The Registry data, from 124 patients who were paced for the long QT syndrome, indicate approximately a 50% reduction in the incidence of cardiac events. Interpretation of the data is confounded by the initiation or increase of beta-blockers at the time of pacing in some patients. However, 30 patients were identified in whom a pacemaker was implanted after failure of beta-blockers but without an increase in drug dosage. In this subset, there was a significant reduction in the incidence of syncope, confirming the independent benefit of pacing. It is important to note that pacing should not be implemented without concomitant beta-blocker therapy and that beta-blockers should not be stopped. Of the 10 Registry patients in whom beta-blockers were withdrawn after pacemaker implantation, 3 died suddenly during 2 years follow-up. The benefit of pacing is thought to be due to the prevention of bradycardia and pauses together with rate-related shortening of the QT interval. Unfortunately, for pacing to be effective, relatively high rates (>80/min) may be required with the attendant disadvantage of reduced battery life and the potential risk of tachycardia-induced cardiomyopathy.[130] Pacing should be considered as an adjuvant to beta-blockade in all patients with long QT syndrome and high grade AV block and whenever there is evidence of pause-dependent malignant arrhythmias.

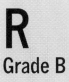

R

Grade B

Post-cardiac transplantation

Bradycardia, usually due to transient sinus node dysfunction or AV block, may occur in almost two-thirds of patients in the first few weeks following orthotopic cardiac transplantation.[131] Recovery from transient AV block usually occurs within 16 days but transient sinus node dysfunction may persist for several weeks and the optimal time for consideration of permanent pacemaker implantation is uncertain.[132] In some cases, temporary treatment with oral theophylline may avert the need for permanent pacing.[133] The proportion of transplant recipients receiving permanent pacing for persistent bradycardia ranges from 4% to 29% in different centres.[131,132,134–136] The variation may reflect differences in the incidence of bradycardia and the criteria for permanent pacing although differences in surgical technique may also be relevant.[136] In paced transplant recipients, bradycardia often resolves and pacemaker usage decreases during the first few months.[132,137] Deferring consideration of permanent pacing until 3 weeks after transplantation may mean that some patients with transient sinus node dysfunction are spared unnecessary pacemaker implantation. Deferral is also associated with a commensurate increase in pacemaker usage in those paced. However, even with this strategy, less than half of those using their pacemakers at 3 months continue to do so at 6 months and there are no clear predictive factors to guide patient selection.[132]

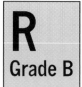

R

Grade B

Following heterotopic cardiac transplantation, the donor's and recipient's hearts beat independently of one another, the denervated donor heart typically beating at a faster rate. Competitive contraction of the two hearts may be deleterious and left ventricular function in the recipient heart is improved when the two hearts beat out of phase. Acute studies have shown that paced linkage of the two hearts to produce consistent counterpulsation may result in significant functional improvement.[138] This technique has recently been evaluated in a chronic study using permanent dual chamber pacemakers with the atrial channel connected to the donor atrium and the 'ventricular' channel connected to the recipient atrium.[139] Paced linkage was associated with significant improvements in symptoms, general health, energy, levels of activity and maximum cardiac output in the donor heart.

Arrhythmia diagnosis

In recent years, the increasing sophistication and memory capacity of cardiac pacemakers has introduced the possibility of an important diagnostic role. In patients with syncope, the cause of which remains unknown after appropriate investigation, implantation of a pacemaker with diagnostic capabilities may enable the occurrence and cause of bradycardia to be identified whilst providing a therapeutic safety net.[140] Single chamber diagnostic devices capable of detecting the occurrence of bradycardia have been available for several years and dual chamber devices with diagnostic algorithms are now also available and enable the mechanism of bradycardia to be identified in many cases.[141]

In patients with known or suspected tachyarrhythmia, the Holter and telemetry functions of dual chamber pacemakers may be used to facilitate arrhythmia diagnosis. They also enable the frequency and natural history to be determined and the efficacy of antiarrhythmic therapy to be assessed.[142] In devices with the capability of switching from atrial tracking modes to non-tracking modes on detection of atrial tachyarrhythmia, mode switch counters may serve a similar function, whilst the change in mode avoids the risk of rapid paced ventricular rates.

CONCLUSIONS

The role of cardiac pacing in symptomatic bradycardia is well established yet many questions remain regarding appropriate mode selection in the conditions for which it is most often used, namely AV block and sinoatrial disease. Technological advances and innovation have greatly expanded the possibilities for sophisticated pacing with better emulation of normal physiology, yet for many of these developments, evidence of clinical utility comes predominantly from observational studies and retrospective reviews with their attendant methodologic limitations. In recent years, improved diagnostic techniques have increased understanding of the pathophysiology of other conditions, identifying many possible new roles for pacing as a therapeutic modality. The advent of large scale clinical trials to the field of cardiac pacing offers an opportunity both to test well constructed hypotheses regarding established indications and to evaluate new ones in order to provide a solid evidence base to guide future practice.

REFERENCES

1 Elmqvist R, Senning A. An implantable pacemaker for the heart. In: Smith CN, ed. *Medical electronics* (Proceedings of the Second International Conference on Medical Electronics, Paris, 1959). London: Illiffe, 1960, pp 253–54.

2 Travill CM, Sutton R. Pacemaker syndrome: an iatrogenic condition. *Br Heart J* 1992;**68**: 163–6.

3 Barold SS, Zipes DP. Cardiac pacemakers and antiarrhythmic devices. In: Braunwald E, ed. *Heart disease. A textbook of cardiovascular medicine*, 5th edn. Philadelphia: WB Saunders, 1997, pp 705–41.

4 Cunningham AD, Morley-Davies AJ, Rowland E, Rickards AF. Cardiac pacemaker, ICD and ablation procedures in the UK and Ireland. *Eur J Cardiac Pacing Electrophysiol* 1995;**5**:259–64.

5 Bernstein AD, Parsonnet V. Survey of cardiac pacing and defibrillation in the United States in 1993. *Am J Cardiol* 1996;**78**:187–96.

6 Greenspan AM, Kay HR, Berger BC *et al.* Incidence of unwarranted implantation of permanent cardiac pacemakers in a large medical population. *N Engl J Med* 1988;**318**: 158–63.

7 Frye RL, Collins JJ, DeSanctis RW *et al.* Guidelines for permanent cardiac pacemaker implantation, May 1984: A report of the Joint American College of Cardiology/American Heart Association Task Force on Assessment of Cardiovascular Procedures (Sub-committee on

Pacemaker Implantation). *Circulation* 1984;**70**: 331A–339A.

8 Dreifus LS, Fisch C, Griffin JC *et al.* Guidelines for Implantation of Cardiac Pacemakers and Antiarrhythmia Devices. A report of the American College of Cardiology/American Heart Association Task Force on Assessment of Diagnostic and Therapeutic Cardiovascular Procedures (Committee on Pacemaker Implantation). *Circulation* 1991;**84**:455–67.

9 Gregoratos G, Cheitlin MD, Conill A *et al.* ACC/ AHA Guidelines for Implantation of Cardiac Pacemakers and Antiarrhythmia Devices. A Report of the American College of Cardiology/ American Heart Association Task Force on Practice Guidelines (Committee on Pacemaker Implantation). *J Am Coll Cardiol* 1998 (in press).

10 Clarke M, Sutton R, Ward D *et al.* Recommendations for pacemaker prescription for symptomatic bradycardia: report of a working party of the British Pacing and Electrophysiology Group. *Br Heart J* 1991;**66**: 185–91.

11 Petch M. Who needs dual chamber pacing? *Br Med J* 1993;**307**:215–6.

12 de Belder MA, Linker NJ, Jones S, Camm AJ, Ward DE. Cost implications of the British Pacing and Electrophysiology Group's recommendations for pacing. *Br Med J* 1992; **305**:861–5.

13 National Pacemaker Database (United Kingdom and Ireland). Annual Report 1995. London: British Pacing and Electrophysiology Group.

14 Aggarwal RK, Ray SG, Connelly DT, Coulshed DS, Charles RG. Trends in pacemaker mode

prescription 1984–1994: a single centre study of 3710 patients. *Heart* 1996;**75**:518–21.

15 Bexton RS, Camm AJ. First degree atrioventricular block. *Eur Heart J* 1984;**5**(Suppl A):107–9.

16 Chirife R, Ortega DE, Salazar AL. "Pacemaker syndrome" without a pacemaker. Deleterious effects of first-degree AV block. *RBM* 1990;**12**(3): 22.

17 Zornosa JP, Crossley GH, Haisty WK Jr *et al.* Pseudo-pacemaker syndrome: a complication of radiofrequency ablation of the AV junction. *PACE* 1992;**15**:590.

18 Mabo P, Varin C, Vauthier M. Deleterious hemodynamic consequences of isolated long PR intervals: correction by DDD pacing. *Eur Heart J* 1992;**13**:225.

19 Barold SS. Indications for permanent cardiac pacing in first-degree AV block: class I, II, or III? *PACE* 1996;**19**:747–51.

20 Wharton JM, Ellenbogen KA. Atrioventricular conduction system disease. In: Ellenbogen KA, Kay GN, Wilkoff BL, eds. *Clinical cardiac pacing.* Philadelphia: WB Saunders, 1995, pp 304–20.

21 Dhingra RC, Denes P, Wu D *et al.* The significance of second degree atrioventricular block and bundle branch block. *Circulation* 1974;**49**: 638–46.

22 Puech P, Grolleau R, Guimond C. Incidence of different types of AV-block and their localisation by His bundle recordings. In: Wellens HJJ, Lie KI, Janse MJ, eds. *The conduction system of the heart: structure, function and clinical implications.* Philadelphia: Lea & Febiger, 1976, pp 467–84.

23 Shaw DB, Kekwick CA, Veale D, Gowers J, Whistance T. Survival in second degree atrioventricular block. *Br Heart J* 1985;**53**: 587–93.

24 Campbell RWF. Chronic Mobitz type I second degree atrioventricular block: has its importance been underestimated? *Br Heart J* 1985;**53**: 585–6.

25 Connelly DT, Steinhaus DM. Mobitz type I atrioventricular block: an indication for permanent pacing? *PACE* 1996;**19**:261–4.

26 Grossman M. Second degree heart block with Wenckebach phenomenon: its occurrence over a period of several years in a young healthy adult. *Am Heart J* 1958;**56**:607–10.

27 Meytes I, Kaplinsky E, Yahini JH, Hanne-Papara N, Neufeld HN. Wenckebach A-V block: a frequent feature following heavy physical training. *Am Heart J* 1975;**90**:426–30.

28 Johansson BW. Complete heart block. A clinical hemodynamic and pharmacological study in patients with and without an artificial pacemaker. *Acta Med Scand* 1966;**180**(Suppl 451):1–127.

29 Edhag O, Swahn Å. Prognosis of patients with complete heart block or arrhythmic syncope who were not treated with artificial pacemakers. *Acta Med Scand* 1976;**200**:457–63.

30 Rosenqvist M, Nordlander R. Survival in patients with permanent pacemakers. *Cardiol Clin* 1992; **10**:691–703.

31 Rosenqvist M, Edhag KO. Pacemaker dependence in transient high grade atrioventricular block. *PACE* 1984;**7**:63–70.

32 Ginks W, Leatham A, Siddons H. Prognosis of patients paced for chronic atrioventricular block. *Br Heart J* 1979;**41**:633–6.

33 Shen WK, Hammill SC, Hayes DL *et al.* Long-term survival after pacemaker implantation for heart block in patients ≥ 65 years. *Am J Cardiol* 1984;**74**:560–4.

34 Campbell M, Emanuel R. Six cases of congenital heart block followed for 34–40 years. *Br Heart J* 1966;**59**:587–90.

35 Michaëlsson M, Jonzon A, Riesenfeld T. Isolated congenital complete atrioventricular block in adult life. *Circulation* 1995;**92**:442–9.

36 Friedman RA. Congenital AV block. Pace me now or pace me later? *Circulation* 1995;**92**: 283–5.

37 Rowlands DJ. Left and right bundle branch block, left anterior and left posterior hemiblock. *Eur Heart J* 1984;**5**(Suppl A):99–105.

38 McAnulty JH, Rahimtoola SH, Murphy E *et al.* Natural history of "high-risk" bundle branch block. Final report of a prospective study. *N Engl J Med* 1982;**307**:137–43.

39 Scheinman MM, Peters RW, Sauvé J MJ *et al.* Value of the H–Q interval in patients with bundle branch block and the role of prophylactic permanent pacing. *Am J Cardiol* 1982;**50**: 1316–22.

40 Dhingra RC, Wyndham C, Bauernfeind RA *et al.* Significance of block distal to His bundle induced by atrial pacing in patients with chronic bifascicular block. *Circulation* 1979;**60**: 1455–64.

41 Ward DE, Camm AJ. Atrioventricular conduction delays and block. In: Ward DE, Camm AJ, eds. *Clinical electrophysiology of the heart.* London: Edward Arnold, 1987, pp 79–93.

42 Englund A, Bergfeldt L, Rosenqvist M. Disopyramide stress test: a sensitive and specific tool for predicting impending high degree atrioventricular block in patients with bifascicular block. *Br Heart J* 1995;**74**:650–5.

43 Click RL, Gersch BJ, Sugrue DD *et al.* Role of electrophysiologic testing in patients with symptomatic bundle branch block. *Am J Cardiol* 1987;**59**:817–23.

44 Ginks WR, Sutton R, Oh W, Leatham A. Long-term prognosis after acute anterior infarction

with atrioventricular block. *Br Heart J* 1977;**39**: 186–9.

45 Col JJ, Weinberg SL. The incidence and mortality of intraventricular conduction defects in acute myocardial infarction. *Am J Cardiol* 1972;**29**: 344–50.

46 Watson RDS, Glover DR, Page AJF *et al.* The Birmingham trial of permanent pacing in patients with intraventricular conduction disorders after acute myocardial infarction. *Am Heart J* 1984;**108**:496–501.

47 Hindman MC, Wagner GS, JaRo M *et al.* The clinical significance of bundle branch block complicating acute myocardial infarction. 1. Clinical characteristics, hospital mortality and one-year follow-up. *Circulation* 1978;**58**: 679–88.

48 Hindman MC, Wagner GS, JaRo M *et al.* The clinical significance of bundle branch block complicating acute myocardial infarction. 2. Indications for temporary and permanent pacemaker insertion. *Circulation* 1978;**58**: 689–99.

49 Ritter WS, Atkins J, Blomqvist CG, Mullins CB. Permanent pacing in patients with transient trifascicular block during acute myocardial infarction. *Am J Cardiol* 1976;**38**:205–8.

50 Kruse I, Arnman K, Conradson T-B, Rydén L. A comparison of the acute and long-term hemodynamic effects of ventricular inhibited and atrial synchronous ventricular inhibited pacing. *Circulation* 1982;**65**:846–55.

51 Perrins EJ, Morley CA, Chan SL, Sutton R. Randomised controlled trial of physiological and ventricular pacing. *Br Heart J* 1983;**50**:112–17.

52 Boon NA, Frew AJ, Johnston JA, Cobbe SM. A comparison of symptoms and intra-arterial ambulatory blood pressure during long term dual chamber atrioventricular synchronous (DDD) and ventricular demand (VVI) pacing. *Br Heart J* 1987;**58**:34–9.

53 Benditt DG, Mianulli M, Fetter J *et al.* Single-chamber cardiac pacing with activity-initiated chronotropic response: evaluation by cardiopulmonary exercise testing. *Circulation* 1987;**75**:184–91.

54 Lipkin DP, Buller N, Frenneaux M *et al.* Randomised crossover trial of rate responsive Activitrax and conventional fixed rate ventricular pacing. *Br Heart J* 1987;**58**:613–16.

55 Smedgård P, Kristensson B-E, Kruse I, Rydén L. Rate-responsive pacing by means of activity sensing versus single rate ventricular pacing: a double-blind cross-over study. *PACE* 1987;**10**: 902–15.

56 Hargreaves MR, Channon KM, Cripps TR, Gardner M, Ormerod OJM. Comparison of dual chamber and ventricular rate responsive pacing

in patients over 75 with complete heart block. *Br Heart J* 1995;**74**:397–402.

57 Linde C. How to evaluate quality-of-life in pacemaker patients: problems and pitfalls. *PACE* 1996;**19**:391–7.

58 Sulke N, Dritsas A, Bostock J *et al.* "Subclinical" pacemaker syndrome: a randomised study of symptom free patients with ventricular demand (VVI) pacemakers upgraded to dual chamber devices. *Br Heart J* 1992;**67**:57–64.

59 Alpert MA, Curtis JJ, Sanfelippo JF *et al.* Comparative survival after permanent ventricular and dual chamber pacing for patients with chronic high degree atrioventricular block with and without preexistent congestive heart failure. *J Am Coll Cardiol* 1986;**7**:925–32.

60 Linde-Edelstam C, Gullberg B, Norlander R *et al.* Longevity in patients with high degree atrioventricular block paced in the atrial synchronous or the fixed rate ventricular inhibited mode. *PACE* 1992;**15**:304–13.

61 Lamas GA. Pacemaker mode selection and survival: a plea to apply the principles of evidence based medicine to cardiac pacing practice. *Heart* 1997;**78**:218–20.

62 Connolly SJ. Personal communication.

63 Toff WD, Skehan JD, de Bono DP, Camm AJ. The United Kingdom Pacing and Cardiovascular Events (UKPACE) trial. *Heart* 1997;**78**:221–3.

64 Sutton R, Kenny RA. The natural history of sick sinus syndrome. *PACE* 1986;**9**:1110–14.

65 Alboni P, Menozzi C, Brignole M *et al.* Effects of permanent pacemaker and oral theophylline in sick sinus syndrome. The THEOPACE study: a randomized controlled trial. *Circulation* 1997; **96**:260–6.

66 Shaw DB, Holman RR, Gowers JI. Survival in sinoatrial disorder (sick-sinus syndrome). *Br Med J* 1980;**280**:139–41.

67 Talan DA, Bauernfeind RA, Ashley WW, Kanakis C Jr, Rosen KM. Twenty-four hour continuous ECG recordings in long-distance runners. *Chest* 1982;**82**:19–24.

68 Rediker DE, Eagle KA, Homma S, Gillam LD, Harthorne JW. Clinical and hemodynamic comparison of VVI versus DDD pacing in patients with DDD pacemakers. *Am J Cardiol* 1988;**61**: 323–9.

69 Mitsuoka T, Kenny RA, Au Yeung T *et al.* Benefits of dual chamber pacing in sick sinus syndrome. *Br Heart J* 1988;**60**:338–47.

70 Hummel J, Barr E, Hanich R *et al.* DDDR pacing is better tolerated than VVIR in patients with sinus node disease. *PACE* 1990;**13**:504.

71 Camm AJ, Katritsis D. Pacing for sick sinus syndrome – a risky business? *PACE* 1990;**13**: 695–9.

72 Rosenqvist M, Brandt J, Schuller H. Long-term pacing in sinus node disease: effects of

stimulation mode on cardiovascular morbidity and mortality. *Am Heart J* 1988;**116**:16–22.

73 Andersen HR, Thuesen L, Bagger JP, Vesterlund T, Thomsen PE. Prospective randomised trial of atrial versus ventricular pacing in sick-sinus syndrome. *Lancet* 1994;**344**:1523–8.

74 Andersen HR, Nielsen JC, Thomsen PEB *et al.* Long-term follow-up of patients from a randomised trial of atrial versus ventricular pacing for sick sinus syndrome. *Lancet* 1997; **350**:1210–16.

75 Andersen HR. Personal communication.

76 Lamas G, Stambler B, Mittelman R *et al.* Clinical events following DDDR versus VVIR pacing: results of a prospective trial. *PACE* 1996;**19**: 619.

77 Stambler B, Ellenbogen K, Pinsky S *et al.* Development of post-implant atrial fibrillation (AFIB) during DDDR versus VVIR pacing in the PASE trial. *PACE* 1996;**19**:619.

78 Charles RG, McComb JM. Systematic trial of pacing to prevent atrial fibrillation (STOP-AF). *Heart* 1997;**78**:224–5.

79 Rosenqvist M, Obel IWP. Atrial pacing and the risk for AV block: is there a time for change in attitude? *PACE* 1989;**12**:97–101.

80 Quan KJ, Carlson MD, Thames MD. Mechanisms of heart rate and arterial blood pressure control: implications for the pathophysiology of neurocardiogenic syncope. *PACE* 1997;**20**: 764–74.

81 Morley CA, Sutton R. Carotid sinus syncope. *Int J Cardiol* 1984;**6**:287–93.

82 Brignole M, Menozzi C. Methods other than tilt testing for diagnosing neurocardiogenic (neurally mediated) syncope. *PACE* 1997;**20**: 795–800.

83 Kenny RA, Ingram A, Bayliss J, Sutton R. Head-up tilt: a useful test for investigating unexplained syncope. *Lancet* 1986;**i**:1352–5.

84 Morley CA, Perrins EJ, Grant P *et al.* Carotid sinus syncope treated by pacing. Analysis of persistent symptoms and role of atrioventricular sequential pacing. *Br Heart J* 1982;**47**:411–18.

85 Sugrue DD, Gersh BJ, Holmes DR, Wood DL, Osborn MJ, Hammill SC. Symptomatic "isolated" carotid sinus hypersensitivity: natural history and results of treatment with anticholinergic drugs or pacemaker. *J Am Coll Cardiol* 1986;**7**: 158–62.

86 Brignole M, Menozzi C, Lolli G, Bottoni N, Gaggioli G. Long-term outcome of paced and nonpaced patients with severe carotid sinus syndrome. *Am J Cardiol* 1992;**69**:1039–43 .

87 Dey AB, Bexton RS, Tynan MM, Charles RG, Kenny RA. The impact of a dedicated "syncope and falls" clinic on pacing practice in Northeastern England. *PACE* 1997;**20**:815–17.

88 Petersen MEV, Sutton R. Cardiac pacing for vasovagal syncope: a reasonable therapeutic option? *PACE* 1997;**20**:824–6.

89 Petersen MEV, Chamberlain-Webber R, Fitzpatrick AP *et al.* Permanent pacing for cardioinhibitory malignant vasovagal syndrome. *Br Heart J* 1994;**71**:274–81.

90 Sheldon RS, Gent M, Roberts RS, Connolly SJ. North American Vasovagal Pacemaker Study: study design and organisation. *PACE* 1997;**20**: 844–8.

91 Sutton R, Petersen MEV. First steps towards a pacing algorithm for vasovagal syncope. *PACE* 1997;**20**:827–8.

92 Sheldon RS. Personal communication.

93 Sutton R. Personal communication.

94 Raviele A, Themistoclakis S, Gasparini G. Drug treatment of vasovagal syncope. In: Blanc JJ, Benditt D, Sutton R, eds. *Neurally mediated syncope: pathophysiology, investigations, and treatment.* Armonk, NY: Futura, 1996, pp 113–17.

95 Bourdarias JP, Lockhart A, Ourbak P *et al.* Hemodynamique des cardiomyopathies obstructives. *Arch Mal Coeur* 1964;**57**:737–8.

96 McDonald K, McWilliams E, O'Keefe B *et al.* Functional assessment of patients treated with permanent dual-chamber pacing as a primary treatment for hypertrophic cardiomyopathy. *Eur Heart J* 1988;**9**:893–8.

97 Fananapazir L, Cannon RO, Tripodi D, Panza JA. Impact of dual-chamber permanent pacing in patients with obstructive hypertrophic cardiomyopathy with symptoms refractory to verapamil and beta-adrenergic blocker therapy. *Circulation* 1992;**85**:2149–61.

98 Jeanrenaud X, Goy JJ, Kappenberger L. Effects of dual-chamber pacing in hypertrophic obstructive cardiomyopathy. *Lancet* 1992;**339**: 1318–23.

99 Slade AKB, Sadoul N, Shapiro L *et al.* DDD pacing in hypertrophic cardiomyopathy: a multicentre clinical experience. *Heart* 1996;**75**:44–9.

100 Nishimura RA, Trusty JM, Hayes DL *et al.* Dual-chamber pacing for hypertrophic cardiomyopathy: a randomized, double-blind, crossover trial. *J Am Coll Cardiol* 1997;**29**: 435–41.

101 Kappenberger L, Linde C, Daubert C *et al.* Pacing in hypertrophic obstructive cardiomyopathy. A randomized crossover study. *Eur Heart J* 1997; **18**:1249–56.

102 Daubert JC. Pacing and hypertrophic cardiomyopathy. *PACE* 1996;**19**:1141–2.

103 Fananapazir L, Epstein ND, Curiel RV, Panza JA, Tripodi D, McAreavey D. Long-term results of dual-chamber (DDD) pacing in obstructive hypertrophic cardiomyopathy: evidence for

progressive symptomatic and haemodynamic improvement and reduction of left ventricular hypertrophy. *Circulation* 1994;**90**:2731–42.

104 Pavin D, Gras D, De Place C, Leclercq C, Mabo P, Daubert C. Long-term effect of DDD pacing in patients with hypertrophic obstructive cardiomyopathy: is there a left ventricular remodelling? *PACE* 1996;**19**:680.

105 Spirito P, Seidman CE, McKenna WJ, Maron BJ. The management of hypertrophic cardiomyopathy. *N Engl J Med* 1997;**336**: 775–85.

106 Brecker SJD, Xiao HB, Sparrow J, Gibson D. Effects of dual-chamber pacing with short atrioventricular delay in dilated cardiomyopathy. *Lancet* 1992;**340**:1308–12.

107 Hochleitner M, Hörtnagl H, Fridrich L, Gschnitzer F. Long-term efficacy of physiologic dual-chamber pacing in the treatment of end-stage idiopathic dilated cardiomyopathy. *Am J Cardiol* 1992;**70**:1320–5.

108 Auricchio A, Sommariva L, Salo RW, Scafuri A, Chiariello L. Improvement of cardiac function in patients with severe congestive heart failure and coronary artery disease by dual chamber pacing with shortened AV delay. *PACE* 1993; **16**:2034–43.

109 Linde C, Gadler F, Edner M *et al.* Results of atrioventricular synchronous pacing with optimized delay in patients with severe congestive heart failure. *Am J Cardiol* 1995;**75**: 919–23.

110 Gold MR, Feliciano Z, Gottlieb SS, Fisher ML. Dual-chamber pacing with a short atrioventricular delay in congestive heart failure: a randomized study. *J Am Coll Cardiol* 1995;**26**: 967–73.

111 Nishimura RA, Hayes DL, Holmes DR Jr, Tajik AJ. Mechanism of hemodynamic improvement by dual-chamber pacing for severe left ventricular dysfunction: an acute Doppler and catheterisation hemodynamic study. *J Am Coll Cardiol* 1995;**25**:281–8.

112 Paul V, Cowell R, Morris-Thurgood J *et al.* First-degree heart block in heart failure: is this a class I indication for dual-chamber pacing? *PACE* 1995;**18**:906.

113 Brecker SJD, Gibson DG. What is the role of pacing in dilated cardiomyopathy? *Eur Heart J* 1996;**17**:819–24.

114 Glikson M, Hayes DL, Nishimura RA. Newer clinical applications of pacing. *J Cardiovasc Electrophysiol* 1997;**8**:1190–203.

115 Cazeau S, Ritter P, Lazarus A *et al.* Multi-site pacing for end-stage heart failure. *PACE* 1996; **19**:1748–57.

116 Auricchio A. Personal communication.

117 Daubert JC. Personal communication.

118 Buckingham TA, Candinas R, Schläpfer J *et al.* Acute hemodynamic effects of atrioventricular pacing at different sites in the right ventricle individually and simultaneously. *PACE* 1997; **20**:909–15.

119 Coumel P, Friocourt P, Mugica J, Attuel P, Leclerq JF. Long term prevention of vagal atrial arrhythmias by atrial pacing at 90/min: experience with 6 cases. *PACE* 1983;**6**:552–60.

120 Gillis AM. Personal communication.

121 Saksena S, Prakash, Hill M *et al.* Prevention of recurrent atrial fibrillation with chronic dual-site right atrial pacing. *J Am Coll Cardiol* 1996; **28**:687–94.

122 Saksena S. Personal communication.

123 Daubert C, Mabo P, Berder V. Arrhythmia prevention by permanent atrial resynchronization in advanced interatrial block. *Eur Heart J* 1990;**11**:237.

124 Daubert C, Mabo P, Berder V *et al.* Permanent dual atrium pacing in major interatrial conduction block: a four years experience. *PACE* 1993;**16**:885.

125 Saxon LA. Atrial fibrillation and dilated cardiomyopathy. *PACE* 1997;**20**:720–5.

126 Moss AJ, Liu JE, Gottlieb S *et al.* Efficacy of permanent pacing in the long QT syndrome. *Circulation* 1991;**84**:1524–9.

127 Eldar M, Griffin JC, Van Hare GF *et al.* Combined use of beta-adrenergic blocking agents and long-term cardiac pacing for patients with the long QT syndrome. *J Am Coll Cardiol* 1992;**20**:830–7.

128 Schwartz PJ. *The Long QT Syndrome*. New York: Futura, 1997, pp 78–83.

129 Zareba W, Priori SG, Moss AJ *et al.* Permanent pacing in the long QT syndrome patients. *PACE* 1997;**20**:1097.

130 Viskin S, Alla SR, Baron HV *et al.* Mode of onset of torsade de pointes in congenital long QT syndrome. *J Am Coll Cardiol* 1996;**28**:1262–8.

131 Jacquet L, Ziady G, Stein K *et al.* Cardiac rhythm disturbances early after orthotopic heart transplantation: prevalence and importance of the observed abnormalities. *J Am Coll Cardiol* 1990;**16**:832–7.

132 Holt ND, Tynan MM, Scott CD, Parry G, Dark JH, McComb JM. Permanent pacemaker use after cardiac transplantation: completing the audit cycle. *Heart* 1996;**76**:435–8.

133 Bertolet BD, Eagle DA, Conti JB, Mills RM, Belardinelli L. Bradycardia after heart transplantation: reversal with theophylline. *J Am Coll Cardiol* 1996;**28**:396–9.

134 Miyamoto Y, Curtiss EI, Kormos RL, Armitage JM, Hardesty RL, Griffith BP. Bradyarrhythmias after heart transplantation. *Circulation* 1990; **82**(Suppl IV):313–7.

135 DiBiase A, Tse TM, Schnittger I, Wexler L, Stinson EB, Valantine HA. Frequency and mechanism of

bradycardia in cardiac transplant recipients and need for pacemakers. *Am J Coll Cardiol* 1991; **67**:1385–9.

136 Heinz G, Kratochwill C, Schmid S *et al.* Sinus node dysfunction after orthotopic heart transplantation: the Vienna experience 1987–1993. *PACE* 1994;**17**:2057–63.

137 Scott CD, Omar I, McComb JM, Dark JH, Bexton RS. Long-term pacing in heart transplant recipients is usually unnecessary. *PACE* 1991; **14**:1792–6.

138 Morris-Thurgood J, Cowell R, Paul V *et al.* Hemodynamic and metabolic effects of paced linkage following heterotopic cardiac transplantation. *Circulation* 1994;**90**:2342–7.

139 Morris-Thurgood J, Paul VE, Dyke C *et al.* Chronic linkage after heterotopic heart transplantation. *Transplantation Proceedings* 1997;**29**:580.

140 Murdock CJ, Klein GJ, Yee R, Leitch JW, Teo WS, Norris C. Feasibility of long-term electro-cardiographic monitoring with an implanted device for syncope diagnosis. *PACE* 1991;**13**: 1374–8.

141 Lascault G, Barnay C, Cazeau S, Frank R, Medvedowsky JL. Preliminary evaluation of a dual chamber pacemaker with bradycardia diagnostic functions. *PACE* 1995;**18**:1636–43.

142 Cazeau S, Ritter P, Nitzsché R, Limousin M, Mugica J. Diagnosis of atrial arrhythmias using the Holter function of a new DDD pacemaker. *PACE* 1994;**17**:2106–13.

624

Syncope

39

DAVID G. BENDITT,
WILLIAM H. FABIAN,
KEITH G. LURIE

Syncope is defined as the sudden loss of both consciousness and postural tone with subsequent spontaneous recovery. Typically, syncopal episodes are brief; loss of consciousness rarely lasts longer than 20 or 30 seconds. However, in some forms of syncope there may be an extended premonitory period in which various symptoms offer warning of an impending syncopal event. Additionally, the postsyncope recovery phase may comprise an extended period of fatigue and listlessness. As a result, the total period of "syncope" may be reported to last many minutes in duration. As a rule, recovery from syncope is generally unassociated with retrograde amnesia and is accompanied by relatively prompt restoration of appropriate behavior and orientation. Syncope must be differentiated from other conditions which are accompanied by real or apparent loss of consciousness, such as seizures, sleep disturbances, accidents, and some psychiatric conditions.

To date, the evaluation and treatment of syncope has not been the subject of large scale clinical trials. Diagnostic strategies are based largely on experience derived from multiple relatively small independent studies, with certain issues being subject to "expert task force" review and recommendation by professional and/or scientific societies (e.g., the American College of Cardiology task force report on tilt-table testing published in 1996).[1] Similarly, recommendations regarding the treatment of specific disorders associated with syncope (e.g., sinus node dysfunction, AV block, vasovagal syncope) have been based on the compilation of numerous uncontrolled and often retrospective experiences. In several important clinical scenarios, such as acquired complete heart block and syncope associated with life-threatening ventricular tachyarrhythmias, evidence of treatment efficacy obtained in this manner appears to be well substantiated. On the other hand, in conditions such as neurally mediated vasovagal syncope, the efficacy of current treatments is far less certain and large scale studies are very much needed.

This chapter focusses on the principal clinical conditions associated with syncope. The primary objectives are:

1. to identify and prioritize the most common causes of syncope;
2. to outline a practicable strategy for evaluation of the syncope patient;
3. to define appropriate directions for treatment.

Throughout, an attempt has been made to characterize the status of current clinical evidence related to each of these topics.

EPIDEMIOLOGIC CONSIDERATIONS

With few exceptions, studies examining the frequency of syncope in the population encompass relatively small numbers of subjects. Further, these studies have tended to focus on select populations such as the military, or tertiary care medical centers, or solitary medical practices. Consequently, the true incidence of syncope in the population as a whole remains uncertain.

Reports suggest that syncope accounts for approximately 3% of emergency room visits and from 1 to 6% of general hospital admissions in the United States.[2-4] The Framingham Study, in which biennial examinations were carried out over a 26-year period in 5209 free-living individuals, reported the occurrence of at least one syncopal event in approximately 3% of men and 3.5% of women.[5] Further, while syncope occurred at virtually all ages, prevalence of syncope increased in older age groups. Additionally, among those who experienced syncope, recurrence of symptoms was reported to be very common. Several reports provide consistent estimates suggesting that syncope recurrences are to be expected in about 30% of individuals.[5-7]

CLASSIFICATION OF THE CAUSES OF SYNCOPE

A classification of the causes of syncope is given in the box on page 627. The causes are listed in approximate order of the frequency with which they occur in clinical practice (beginning with the most common cause – neurally mediated syncopal syndromes). However, the diagnostic problem is complicated by the fact that more than one cause often contributes to the clinical picture. For example, syncope in valvular aortic stenosis is not solely due to a narrowed orifice restricting cardiac output, but also inappropriate reflex vasodilation and/or primary cardiac arrhythmias. Similarly, syncope in association with certain brady- and tachyarrhythmias in part depends on neural reflex factors, for example the ability to initiate vasoconstriction in response to an arrhythmic stress.[8]

Neurally mediated syncopal syndromes

In the neurally mediated syncopal syndromes systemic hypotension occurs primarily as a result of inappropriate neural reflex activity. In certain cases syncope is the result of parasympathetically induced bradycardia or asystole (so-called cardioinhibition). In others, symptomatic hypotension is due primarily to inappropriate vasodilation (i.e., vasodepressor component). In the vast majority of these cases, however, both phenomena contribute.[1,8-11]

The vasovagal faint and carotid sinus syndrome are the most common forms of neurally mediated syncope. The vasovagal faint (also known as the "common faint") may be triggered by any of a variety of factors, including unpleasant sights, pain, extreme emotion, and prolonged standing. As a result, vasovagal syncope may often be suspected based on a typical medical history. However, often the history does not provide a definitive diagnosis. In such cases, tilt-table testing is the most important available supportive test.[1,8-11] Carotid sinus syndrome is the second most common form of the neurally mediated syncopal syndromes,[12,13] but it is often overlooked in clinical practice. The occurrence of syncope without warning in older persons should lead to consideration of carotid sinus syndrome. The condition is likely present when, during firm linear carotid sinus massage (usually best undertaken with the patient in the upright position), the development of asystole or paroxysmal AV block, and/or a marked drop in systemic arterial pressure result in reproduction of symptoms.[13] In the absence of symptom reproduction, a pause in the ventricular rhythm of 5 seconds or longer is probably sufficient to support the diagnosis.

Syncope: diagnostic classification

- **Neurally mediated syncopal syndromes**
  Vasovagal faint
  Carotid sinus syncope
  Cough syncope and related disorders
  Gastrointestinal, pelvic, or urologic origin
- **Orthostatic, dysautonomic, and drug-induced**
  Idiopathic orthostatic hypotension
  Shy–Drager's syndrome
  Diabetic neuropathy
  Drug-induced orthostasis
- **Primary cardiac arrhythmias**
  Sinus node dysfunction (including bradycardia/tachycardia syndrome)
  AV conduction system disease
  Paroxysmal supraventricular and ventricular tachycardias
  Implanted device (pacemaker, ICD) malfunction
- **Structural cardiovascular or cardiopulmonary disease**
  Cardiac valvular disease (e.g. aortic stenosis)
  Acute myocardial infarction/ischemia
  Obstructive cardiomyopathy
  Subclavian steal syndrome
  Pericardial disease/tamponade
  Pulmonary embolus
  Pulmonary hypertension
  Tetralogy of Fallot (syncope mimicks)
- **Cerebrovascular, neurologic, and psychiatric disturbances**
  Vascular steal syndromes
  Seizure disorders
  Panic attacks
  Hysteria
- **Miscellaneous syncope-like conditions**
  Hyperventilation (hypocapnia)
  Hypoglycemia
  Volume depletion (e.g. Addison's disease, pheochromocytoma)
  Hypoxemia

Neurally mediated syncopal syndromes

Emotional syncope (common or "vasovagal" faint, "malignant" vasovagal faint)
Carotid sinus syncope
Cough, sneeze syncope
Exercise, post-exercise variant
Gastrointestinal stimulation –
   swallow syncope, defecation syncope
Glossopharyngeal neuralgia
Postmicturition syncope
Raised intrathoracic pressure, airway stimulation –
   brass wind instrument-playing, weight-lifting
Miscellaneous conditions in which neurally mediated syncope may contribute: aortic stenosis, PSVT, atrial
   fibrillation

Orthostatic, dysautonomic, and drug-induced disturbances of blood pressure control

Abrupt assumption of upright posture often results in presyncopal symptoms. However, frank syncope may occur, especially in elderly or less physically fit individuals, or patients who are volume-depleted. Iatrogenic factors such as excessive diuresis or aggressive prescription of antihypertensives (e.g. vasodilators, beta-blockers) are probably the most important contributors to the development of posturally related syncope. Neuropathies associated with chronic diseases (e.g., diabetes) or toxic agents (e.g., alcohol) are also very common, whereas other forms of autonomic nervous system dysfunction are thought to be infrequent. In terms of the latter conditions, however, some of the more important include acute sympathetic neural dysfunction following infections (Guillain–Barré syndrome), multiple system atrophy (Shy–Drager syndrome), and familial dysautonomia (Riley–Day syndrome).[14–17] Perhaps, as these disturbances and their potentially subtle manifestations become more widely appreciated, they will be identified more often. Recently, Low et al.[15] reviewed their experience in 155 patients referred for assessment of suspected orthostatic hypotension. Findings in this referral population revealed that among the most severely affected symptomatic patients ($n =$ 90, mean age 64 years), pure autonomic failure accounted for 33%, multisystem atrophy 26%, and autonomic/diabetic neuropathy 31%.

Tilt-table testing facilities may be helpful in identifying patients susceptible to syncope associated with orthostatic hypotension. However, the diagnosis of the various forms of autonomic failure using tilt-table and other autonomic testing procedures,[16,17] require a level of experience which is currently available in relatively few centers.

Primary cardiac arrhythmias

Primary cardiac arrhythmias, that is those rhythm disturbances arising as a result of cardiac conduction system disturbances, anomalous electrical connections, or myocardial disease, are important causes of syncope. In general terms, the arrhythmias most often associated with syncope or near-syncope are the bradyarrhythmias accompanying

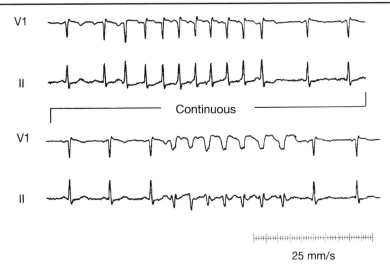

25 mm/s

Figure 39.1 Electrocardiographic recording during episodes of atrial tachycardia in a patient with recurrent dizziness and syncope. Electrophysiologic recordings during spontaneous arrhythmia demonstrated the atrial origin of both the narrow and wide QRS tachycardias. Systemic pressure fell precipitously at onset of each tachycardia episode.

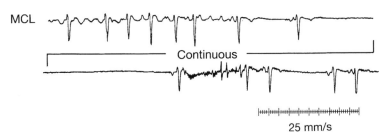

25 mm/s

Figure 39.2 Electrocardiographic recording during a spontaneous "dizzy" spell. A prolonged pause following spontaneous termination of atrial fibrillation is a typical feature of sinus node dysfunction.

sinus node dysfunction (also termed "sick sinus syndrome"[18]) or AV block, and the tachyarrhythmias of ventricular origin.

Sinus node dysfunction comprises various sinus node and/or atrial arrhythmias which result in persistent or intermittent periods of inappropriately slow (sinus bradycardia, sinus pauses, sinoatrial exit block) or fast heart beating (paroxysmal or persistent atrial fibrillation or atrial flutter)[18–20] (Figures 39.1, 39.2). In terms of syncope, it is the bradyarrhythmias which appear to be the more important culprits. For example, among 56 patients with either severe bradyarrhythmias or bradycardia–tachycardia syndrome described by Rubenstein et al.,[20] 25 (45%) presented with syncope and an additional 15 (27%) reported various presyncopal symptoms. In the vast majority of these cases (80%), bradyarrhythmias were considered to be the principal responsible rhythm disturbance.

For the most part sinus node dysfunction is closely associated with underlying structural disturbances in the atria (e.g., fibrosis, chamber enlargement). However extrinsic factors (e.g., autonomic nervous system influences, cardioactive drugs, metabolic disturbances) may also contribute. Of these, drug-induced disturbances (particularly beta-adrenergic receptor blockers, calcium-channel blockers, membrane-

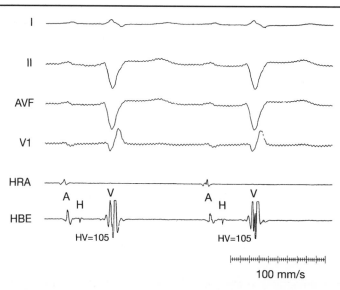

Figure 39.3 Electrocardiographic and intracardiac recordings illustrating a prolonged HV interval during sinus rhythm in a patient presenting with recurrent syncope. Electrophysiologic study findings suggested infra-His block as the most likely cause of syncope.

active antiarrhythmics, especially amiodarone, sotalol, flecainide, and propafenone, and the antiepileptic drug carbamazepine) are well characterized in the literature.[18,21,22]

Disturbances of AV conduction range from slowing of AV conduction (first degree AV block), to intermittent failure of impulse transmission (second degree AV block), to complete conduction failure (third degree AV block). For practical purposes, isolated first degree AV block is not a cause of syncope. However, first degree AV block in the presence of a wide QRS complex suggests more severe conduction system disease, and raises the possibility that higher grades of AV block may be occurring from time to time. Similarly, Mobitz type I second degree AV block is an unlikely cause of syncope. However, when second degree type I block occurs in the setting of a wide QRS, there is risk that periods of higher grade AV block may be causing symptoms. As a rule, however, it is the more severe forms of acquired AV block (that is, Mobitz type II block, "high grade" and complete AV block) which are most closely associated with syncopal symptoms. In these cases, the cardiac rhythm may become dependent on the subsidiary pacemaker sites. Syncope occurs (reported in 38–61%)[23,24] due to the often long delay before these pacemakers begin to "fire". In addition, they tend to have relatively slow rates (often 25–40 beats/min) and be unreliable. In contrast to acquired forms of AV block, congenital complete AV block has generally been considered to be more benign and less often the cause of syncope. Recently, however, this latter concept has been questioned. The detailed study by Michaelsson et al.[25] suggests that syncope is more common in this condition than had previously been suspected.

Syncope in patients with various forms of bundle branch block and fascicular blocks depends both on the risk of developing high grade or complete AV block, as well as on the risk of occurrence of ventricular tachyarrhythmias. As a rule, in chronic infranodal conduction system disease, such as most forms of bifascicular block, progression to more severe AV block is slow. However, risk increases the longer the duration of the HV interval (normal range 35–55 msec), and is particularly great for HV intervals >100 msec[26,27] (Figure 39.3). Nevertheless, despite clearcut evidence for severe

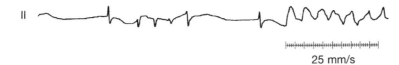

25 mm/s

Figure 39.4 Electrocardiographic recording illustrating polymorphous VT in a patient with recurrent syncope and presyncope. The arrhythmia morphology is suggestive of torsade de pointes. The underlying rhythm is junctional bradycardia with a long QT interval.

conduction system disease, syncope in these patients may still be the result of ventricular tachycardia.[27] Although the evidence is not unequivocal, invasive electrophysiologic testing is probably the most helpful way to address this concern in individual patients.

Ventricular tachyarrhythmias have been reported to be responsible for syncope in up to 20% of patients referred for electrophysiologic assessment. Risk factors favoring ventricular tachyarrhythmias as a cause of syncope include underlying structural heart disease, evident conduction system disease, and congenital or drug-induced long QT syndrome (Figure 39.4). Tachycardia rate, status of left ventricular function, and the efficiency of peripheral vascular reactivity determine whether the arrhythmia is of sufficient severity to account for syncopal symptoms.

Non-sustained ventricular tachycardia is a common finding during ambulatory electrocardiographic monitoring, especially in patients with structural heart disease. As a result, such a finding during the assessment of a syncope patient is not usually very helpful in the absence of documented concomitant symptoms. Nevertheless, in the absence of other causes of syncope, the potential role of non-sustained ventricular tachycardia may warrant additional testing (i.e., electrophysiologic study). Similarly perplexing is the appropriate approach to be taken when syncope occurs in patients with severe underlying left ventricular dysfunction (e.g., dilated cardiomyopathy). Recent evidence suggests that there is high risk for symptom recurrence and probably sudden death,[28,29] and prescription of prophylactic placement of an implantable cardioverter defibrillator (ICD) is becoming more frequently recommended.

The supraventricular tachycardias have been reported to be the cause of syncope in about 15% of patients referred for electrophysiologic evaluation.[30] The rate of the tachycardia, the volume status and the posture of the patient at time of onset of the arrhythmia, the presence of associated structural cardiopulmonary disease, and the integrity of reflex peripheral vascular compensation are key factors determining whether hypotension of sufficient severity to cause syncope occurs.[31] As a rule, if symptoms of syncope or presyncope do develop, they will be at the onset of a paroxysmal tachycardia prior to the possibility of adequate vascular compensation.

Structural cardiovascular or cardiopulmonary disease

The most common cause of syncope attributable to left ventricular disease is that which occurs in conjunction with acute myocardial ischemia or infarction. Other relatively common acute medical conditions associated with syncope include pulmonary embolism, and pericardial tamponade. As alluded to earlier, the basis of syncope in all of these conditions is multifactorial, including both the hemodynamic impact of the specific lesion as well as neurally mediated reflex effects (the latter being especially important in the setting of acute ischemic events).[8]

Syncope may also occur (and perhaps even be a presenting feature) in conditions in which there is fixed or dynamic obstruction to left ventricular outflow (e.g., aortic stenosis, hypertrophic obstructive cardiomyopathy).[8] In such cases, symptoms are often provoked by physical exertion, but may also develop if an otherwise benign arrhythmia should occur (e.g., atrial fibrillation). The basis for the faint may be in part inadequate blood flow due to the mechanical obstruction. However, especially in the case of valvular aortic stenosis, ventricular mechanoreceptor-mediated bradycardia and vasodilation is thought to be an important contributor.[8,32] In the case of obstructive cardiomyopathy, neural reflex mechanisms may also play a role, but the occurrence of atrial tachyarrhythmias (particularly atrial fibrillation) or ventricular tachycardia (even at relatively modest rates) is important.

On rare occasion subclavian "steal" syndrome or severe carotid artery disease may be the cause of syncope. Other even less common causes include left ventricular inflow obstruction in patients with mitral stenosis or atrial myxoma, right ventricular outflow obstruction, and right-to-left shunting secondary to pulmonic stenosis or pulmonary hypertension.

Cerebrovascular, neurologic, and psychiatric disturbances

Cerebrovascular disease and neurologic disturbances (e.g., seizure disorders) are rarely the cause of true syncope.[33,34] More often, these conditions result in a clinical picture which may be mistaken for syncope but can be distinguished by careful history taking and neurologic examination. However, on rare occasions certain seizure types (particularly temporal lobe seizures) may so closely mimic (or possibly even induce) neurally mediated reflex bradycardia and hypotension that differentiation from "true" syncope is difficult. In such cases a diagnostic EEG is necessary (recognizing that not all forms of epilepsy will be detected by EEG). More often, a number of important features help differentiate seizures from true syncope:

1. seizures tend to be positionally independent while syncope is most commonly associated with upright posture;
2. seizures are often preceded by an aura whereas syncope is not;
3. seizures are often immediately accompanied by convulsive activity and incontinence whereas in true syncope any abnormal motor activity is less severe and incontinence is unusual;[35]
4. seizures are typically followed by a confusional state while true syncope is typically followed by prompt restoration of mental state (although fatigue may persist).

Syncope may also be mimicked by anxiety attacks, hysteria or other psychiatric disturbances.[36] Anxiety attacks are frequently associated with hyperventilation and hypocapnia. Hysteria, however, tends to be characterized by its occurring in the presence of onlookers and being unassociated with marked alterations of heart rate, systemic pressure, or skin color. Currently, however, despite the apparent frequency of these conditions in patients referred for evaluation of "syncope",[36] they must be considered only after other conditions have been carefully excluded.

Occasionally, transient disturbances of cerebrovascular blood flow may initiate a true syncopal spell. For example, migraine with presumed cerebrovascular spasm may present with what appears to be a syncopal episode. In the latter case, other historical features of migraine and migraine susceptibility are usually sufficient to distinguish the diagnosis. On the other hand, it has recently been proposed that cerebrovascular spasm may be a cause of apparently "normotensive" syncope.[37,38] Currently, the evidence for this phenomenon is very limited. Nevertheless, if this proves to be the case, then it will be necessary to reassess the nature of the diagnosis in many patients, particularly those currently considered to be "psychogenic".

Miscellaneous causes

Severe hyperventilation resulting in hypocapnia and transient alkalosis may be the most frequent "syncope-like" condition in this category. In these patients, marked anxiety may be an important feature. Consequently, the association of emotional upset with the occurrence of syncope may make these individuals difficult to differentiate from some vasovagal fainters.

Metabolic and endocrine problems are rarely the cause of true syncope. More often these conditions may be responsible for confusional states or behavioral disturbances. Retrospectively, however, making a clearcut distinction between such symptoms and syncope may not be possible by history alone. As a rule though, unlike true syncope, conditions such as diabetic coma, or severe hypoxia or hypercapnia do not resolve in the absence of active therapeutic intervention.

STRATEGY FOR THE DIAGNOSTIC EVALUATION

The goal of diagnostic testing is to establish a sufficiently strong correlation between syncopal symptoms and detected abnormalities to permit assessment of prognosis and initiation of an appropriate treatment plan (Figure 39.5). To this end, the first step is to obtain a detailed medical history, including interviewing knowledgeable bystanders and relatives. Next, a physical examination along with certain basic tests (electrocardiogram and echocardiogram) should be undertaken to ascertain whether there is evidence of underlying structural heart disease. Exercise testing may be included if syncope occurred with exertion or if ischemic heart disease is suspected. Thereafter, the need for further specialized diagnostic testing will vary depending on a variety of factors, including: the certainty of the initial clinical impression, findings during physical examination, the number and frequency of syncopal events reported, the occurrence of injury or accident, family history of syncope or sudden death, and the potential risks associated with the individual's occupation (e.g., commercial vehicle driver, machine operator, professional athlete, sign painter, surgeon) or avocation (e.g., skier, swimmer).

As a rule, if structural heart disease is deemed to be absent by initial evaluation, then tilt-table testing is usually the most useful next diagnostic test since neurally mediated vasovagal syncope is by far the most frequent cause of syncope in this setting. On the other hand, if abnormal cardiac findings are identified, their functional significance should be characterized by hemodynamic and/or angiographic assessment. Furthermore, since cardiac arrhythmias are a common cause of syncope in patients with structural

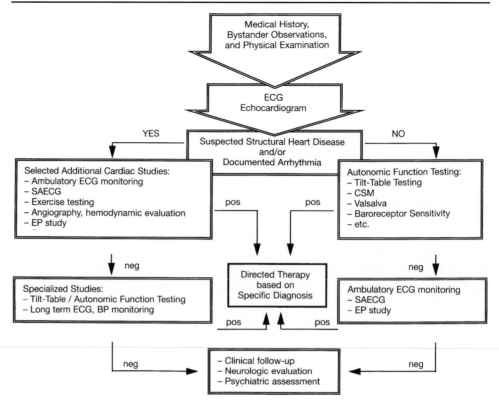

Figure 39.5 Schematic diagram illustrating a practicable strategy for the clinical evaluation of syncope. BP, blood pressure; CSM, carotid sinus massage; EP, electrophysiologic.

cardiac disease, assessing the patient's susceptibility to tachy- and bradyarrhythmias by various non-invasive (e.g., ambulatory electrocardiography, signal averaged electrocardiography – SAECG) and invasive electrophysiological testing is warranted. Reasonably strong evidence suggests that tilt-table testing would follow if the diagnosis remains in doubt.[1] Similarly, strong evidence supports the view that only infrequently should specialized neurologic studies be ordered early in the evaluation (e.g., if the history was more suggestive of a seizure disorder).[1,34,35]

Electrocardiographic recordings

Since cardiac arrhythmias are so frequently the cause of syncope, ECG documentation during a spontaneous syncopal event is highly desirable. In this regard, the 12-lead ECG is usually too brief to capture a specific cause. However, findings such as ventricular pre-excitation or QT interval prolongation may suggest a diagnosis. If feasible at all, obtaining ECG documentation during spontaneous symptoms necessitates prolonged ambulatory monitoring by "Holter" or "event" recorders. Exercise testing is usually of limited utility unless the syncopal events are clearly exertionally related by history. However, in rare instances exercise testing may permit detection of rate-dependent AV block, exertionally related tachyarrhythmias, or the exercise-associated variant of neurally mediated syncope.[8,39,40] Finally, although the SAECG cannot provide direct evidence for the cause of syncope, such testing may be helpful if "normal", by tending to exclude susceptibility to ventricular tachyarrhythmias in patients with ischemic heart disease.[41]

Imaging techniques

Although echocardiography rarely provides a definitive basis for syncope, it is a valuable imaging technique in the syncope patient given the importance of identifying structural heart disease in patients with syncope. Further, in some cases the echocardiogram may provide clues to the cause if, for example, hypertrophic obstructive cardiomyopathy, severe valvular aortic stenosis, an intracardiac tumor, or anomalous origin of one or more coronary arteries are detected. Ultrasound techniques also are appropriately employed to assess vascular disturbances detected on physical examination. Thus, assessment of the carotid and/or subclavian system may be a useful step in selected individuals. Other imaging modalities, such as radionuclide imaging, should be reserved for specific clinical indications.

Clinical electrophysiologic testing

Electrophysiologic testing for assessment of syncope has been the subject of many reports. Although there are no large randomized studies, there is strong evidence to indicate that electrophysiologic testing is most likely to be "diagnostic" in individuals with underlying structural heart disease.[30,42–46] For example, in a review by Camm and Lau,[30] testing was clearly more successful in patients with structural cardiac disease (71%) than in patients without (36%). However, care must be taken in interpreting findings of these studies. Fujimura et al.[47] summarized outcomes of electrophysiologic testing in syncope patients in whom bradyarrhythmias were known to be the cause of syncope. Among 21 syncopal patients with known symptomatic AV block or sinus pauses, electrophysiologic testing only correctly identified 3 of 8 patients with documented sinus pauses (sensitivity 37.5%), and 2 of 13 patients with documented AV block (sensitivity 15.4%). On the other hand, although firm evidence is lacking, the induction of reentry supraventricular or ventricular tachycardia in a syncope patient should be taken seriously. These arrhythmias are rarely innocent bystanders.

Head-up tilt-table testing

To date, the head-up tilt-table test is the only diagnostic tool subjected to sufficient clinical scrutiny to assess its effectiveness as a diagnostic tool in the evaluation of vasovagal syncope, and the evidence supporting its utility is convincing.[1] Such testing, especially when undertaken in the absence of drugs, appears to discriminate well between symptomatic patients and asymptomatic control subjects.[48–52] For example, de Mey and Enterling[48] reported only eight instances of hypotension bradycardia among 40 apparently normal subjects (20%). Similarly, during a 45 minute drug-free tilt at 60 degrees, Raviele et al.[50] noted that among 35 control subjects, none developed syncope. In regard to the potential impact of provocative pharmacologic agents on specificity of tilt testing, Natale et al.[53] found that tilt-table testing at 60, 70, and 80 degrees exhibited specificities of 92%, 92%, and 80% respectively when low doses of isoproterenol were used. In summary, there is very strong evidence to suggest that tilt-table testing at angles of 60–70 degrees, in the absence of pharmacologic provocation, exhibits a specificity of approximately 90%. In the presence of pharmacologic provocation, test specificity may be reduced, but nonetheless remains in a range which permits the test to be clinically useful.

The combination of tilt-table testing and invasive electrophysiologic testing has substantially enhanced diagnostic capabilities in syncope patients. Sra et al.[46] reported results of electrophysiologic testing in conjunction with head-up tilt testing in 86 consecutive patients referred for evaluation of unexplained syncope. Electrophysiologic testing was abnormal in 29 (34%) of patients, with the majority of these (21 patients) being inducible sustained monomorphic ventricular tachycardia. Among the remaining patients, head-up tilt testing proved positive in 34 (40%) cases, while 23 patients (26%) remained undiagnosed. In general, patients exhibiting positive electrophysiologic findings were older, more frequently male, and exhibited lower ventricular ejection fractions and higher frequency of evident heart disease than was the case in patients with positive head-up tilt tests or patients in whom no diagnosis was determined.

In a further evaluation of the combined use of electrophysiologic testing and head-up tilt testing in assessment of syncope, Fitzpatrick et al.[54] analyzed findings in 322 syncope patients. Conventional electrophysiologic testing provided a basis for syncope in 229 of 322 cases (71%), with 93 patients having a normal electrophysiologic study. Among the patients with abnormal electrophysiologic findings, AV conduction disease was diagnosed in 34%, sinus node dysfunction in 21%, carotid sinus syndrome in 10%, and an inducible sustained tachyarrhythmia in 6%. In the 93 patients with normal electrophysiologic studies, tilt-table testing was undertaken in 71 cases, and reproduced syncope, consistent with a vasovagal faint, in 53/71 (75%).

Neurologic studies

Conventional neurologic laboratory studies (EEG, head CT, and MRI) have had a relatively low yield in the syncope patient. Among the 433 syncope evaluations reviewed by Kapoor,[34] the EEG proved helpful in only two cases and cerebral angiography in two others. Consequently, specialized neurologic studies should be restricted to those situations in which other clinical observations suggest organic nervous system disease. On the other hand, given the importance of orthostatic and dysautonomic causes of syncope, an increasingly strong evidence base indicates that tilt-table testing and other tests of autonomic function have an important role to play.

TREATMENT

An accurate etiologic diagnosis is the key to successful prevention of syncopal symptoms. Thereafter, a wide range of pharmacologic and device therapy is available. The effectiveness of these varies, however, depending upon the specific diagnosis. Thus, the evidence supporting the utility of cardiac pacing in carotid sinus syncope and acquired AV block is substantial **Grade A/B**, whereas that favoring pharmacologic management in vasovagal syncope is much more arguable (Grade C with the possible exception of beta-adrenergic blockade – Grade B), inasmuch as large scale randomized controlled treatment trials have yet to be undertaken and virtually all reports (although numerous) are uncontrolled.

In the case of neurally mediated syncopal syndromes, and excluding for the most part carotid sinus syndrome, treatment strategies should if possible address trigger factors (e.g., suppressing the cause of cough in cough syncope). However, in many conditions such an approach is not feasible. Thus, for patients with vasovagal syncope (when recurrent or severe symptoms demand more than reassurance) a variety of pharmacologic approaches have been proposed but none is unequivocally substantiated in terms of long-term benefit. Beta-adrenergic blocking drugs, disopyramide, and to a lesser extent vasoconstrictor agents (e.g., midrodine) have been the agents of principal interest. "Volume expanders" (e.g., fluorocortisone, salt tablets), anticholinergics, and serotonin-reuptake inhibitors also find application in this setting. However, for any of these drugs only a small experience currently exists.[55–59] The few small controlled studies which have been reported (atenolol, cafedrine, disopyramide, scopolamine, and etilefrine) all have methodologic problems. Nonetheless, only one of these (the beta-adrenergic blocker, atenolol) has shown a drug benefit over 1 month follow-up.[59]

Cardiac pacing has proved highly successful in carotid sinus syndrome Grade B and is acknowledged to be the treatment of choice when bradycardia has been documented.[60] In contrast, experience with pacing in vasovagal syncope and other forms of neurally mediated syncope is more limited.[61,62] Nevertheless, in vasovagal syncope pacing may play a useful role in severe cases with recurring periods of symptomatic cardioinhibition (Grade B see below).

The treatment of patients with syncope due to orthostasis and/or dysautonomias is similar to that of the neurally mediated syncopal syndromes, apart from perhaps greater emphasis on physical maneuvers (e.g., anti-gravitational hose, elevation of the head of the bed at night).[63] The mainstay of pharmacologic treatment has been attempted chronic expansion of central circulating volume. To this end, increased salt in the diet, and/or use of salt retaining steroids (i.e., principally fludrocortisone) is usually the first step Grade B/C . Additional benefit has been reported with the use of agents such as erythropoietin, which increases blood volume. A second element in the strategy is reduction of the tendency for central volume to be displaced to the lower extremities with upright posture. To this end, vasoconstrictors have been employed, although with limited success due to the tendency for tachyphylaxis to develop Grade C . Of greatest current interest is midodrine, an agent which has prominent venoconstrictor properties.[64] Physical rehabilitation (gentle progressive increments of exercise), with enforced periods of increasing exposure to upright posture is also advisable. Cardiac pacing at relatively rapid rates may prove valuable in certain very difficult cases. The strongest evidence in this regard is derived from an interim analysis of findings from the North American Vasovagal Pacemaker Study reported in spring 1997 at the scientific sessions of the North American Society of Pacing and Electrophysiology (NASPE). The study was terminated earlier than originally anticipated due to having acheived a statistically significant endpoint result. In this study, the principal clinical endpoint was syncope recurrence.[65] Syncope patients qualified for inclusion if they had both a positive head-up tilt test and either or both of (1) at least six syncopal episodes preceding the tilt test; or (2) at least one syncope recurrence within 6 months of a positive tilt test. Additionally, during the tilt test, patients had to exhibit degrees of bradycardia exceeding certain pre-established thresholds.[65] At the time of the preliminary report, data were provided in

24 patients randomized to pacing (22 of 24 received devices), and 22 randomized to no pacemaker. Syncope recurrence occurred in 4/24 of the pacemaker group and 13/22 control patients, resulting in an actuarial 1-year rate of recurrent syncope of 18.5% for pacemaker patients and 59.7% for controls. A detailed assessment of these results cannot be provided until a complete report is published by the investigators. Nevertheless, the findings seem to provide solid (although in need of confirmation) support to the view that cardiac pacing can offer benefit to a select group of very symptomatic vasovagal fainters Grade A.

In the treatment of primary cardiac arrhythmias, especially the bradycardias and hypotensive tachyarrhythmias, strong clinical evidence supports the importance of treatment interventions for symptom prevention. The evidence unquestionably supports the importance of cardiac pacemaker therapy in patients with syncope due to bradyarrhythmias, whether due to sinus node dysfunction or AV conduction disturbances Grade B.[66–69] In the case of paroxysmal supraventricular tachyarrhythmias (PSVT), there is little in the way of long term follow-up studies examining the efficacy of conventional antiarrhythmic drug treatment when the presenting feature was syncope. However, at present such patients are no longer usually treated in that fashion due to the frequency of drug-related side effects, issues of compliance, expense, and the availability of effective alternatives. Specifically, transcatheter ablation has become a very cost-effective treatment option,[70] and in PSVT associated with syncope is probably the treatment of choice Grade B.

In the case of syncope due to ventricular tachycardia (VT), the almost ubiquitous presence of underlying left ventricular dysfunction increases the proarrhythmic risk associated with antiarrhythmic drug therapy (reported 5–15% incidence with Class I agents). Consequently, pharmacologic therapeutic strategies often involve early consideration of Class III agents (particularly amiodarone given a proarrhythmia risk of 2% or less). However, given the difficulty of assuring effective prophylaxis in this often high risk patient population, the use of both transcatheter ablation and implantable pacemaker cardioverter defibrillators (ICDs) are becoming increasingly important. Currently, ablation techniques are appropriate first choices in only a few forms of ventricular tachycardia, specifically symptomatic patients with right ventricular outflow tract tachycardia and bundle branch re-entry tachycardia Grade B. In the future ablation techniques may be used more extensively as mapping becomes easier and energy delivery systems evolve. In regard to implantable devices, prospective evaluation of ICD efficacy in syncope patients with poor left ventricular function is needed before concrete recommendations can be made. However, reports examining this issue retrospectively tend to provide support for early ICD implantation Grade B. Middlekauff et al.[71,72] noted that among patients with severe left ventricular dysfunction, the presence of a history of syncope was accompanied by a significantly higher 1-year mortality (65% vs 25% in comparable patients without syncope) and a greater tendency toward sudden death (45% of deaths vs 12% in comparable patients). Recently two prospective randomized ICD studies (MADIT and AVID) have been completed.[73,74] Both show reduction in total mortality compared to conventional therapy. In the context of the syncope patient, AVID is particularly pertinent as it included patients with symptomatic hypertensive ventricular tachyarrhythmias. Among more than 1000 patients included in AVID, there were reductions of total mortality by 38%, 26%, and 30% at 1, 2, and 3 years respectively. Thus ICDs are indicated in patients with poor left ventricles (EF $\leq 40\%$), ventricular tachyarrhythmias and syncope Grade A.

In the subset of patients in whom structural cardiovascular or cardiopulmonary disease are the cause of syncope, treatment is best directed at amelioration of the specific structural lesion or its consequences. Thus, in syncope associated with myocardial ischemia, pharmacologic therapy and/or revascularization is clearly the appropriate strategy in most cases. Similarly, when syncope is closely associated with surgically addressable lesions (e.g., valvular aortic stenosis, pericardial disease, atrial myxoma, congenital cardiac anomaly), a direct corrective approach is often feasible. On the other hand, when syncope is caused by certain difficult to treat conditions such as primary pulmonary hypertension or restrictive cardiomyopathy, it is often impossible to ameliorate the underlying problem adequately. Even modifying outflow gradients in hypertrophic cardiomyopathy (HOCM) is not readily achieved surgically. In the latter condition, the effectiveness of standard pharmacologic therapies remains uncertain, and despite ongoing controversy, recent success with cardiac pacing techniques offers considerable promise to symptomatic individuals.[75,76]

COST-EFFECTIVENESS ISSUES

Syncope occurs in all age groups. Consequently, lost productivity is an important consideration, and should be considered along with medical cost burden when evaluating the manner in which syncope is to be evaluated and treated. Unfortunately, most managed care providers in the United States have little reason to look beyond the immediate "up front" cost in dealing with these patients since at the present time most payers are not necessarily responsible for the long-term care of that individual. Whether national health care schemes (which are inherently responsible for long-term outcomes) are more sensitive to the larger economic impact is currently uncertain.

In 1982, Kapoor et al.[77] identified a need for a more cost-effective approach to the syncope evaluation. At that time, the average cost for evaluating syncope patients was estimated to be US$2600. However, since the actual etiology was determined in only relatively few cases, the real cost was far greater (approximately US$24 000 per specific diagnosis). Given inflation, and the more widespread proliferation of diagnostic imaging procedures, conventional electrophysiologic testing, and tilt-table testing, it is reasonable to assume that the per patient expenditure has increased at least two-fold in the past decade, an estimate approximately confirmed by Calkins et al.[78] On the other hand, given the marked improvement in the frequency with which a specific diagnosis is now obtained, the cost per specific diagnosis is probably considerably lower now than was the case in 1982.

CONCLUSIONS

Syncope is a common medical problem with multiple potential causes. A number of well documented clinical studies indicate that in the absence of appropriate treatment, syncope is associated with a relatively high recurrence rate. Further, many of these same reports provide strong evidence for the view that prognosis is of particular concern among the subset of syncope patients with underlying organic cardiac or vascular disease. Consequently, assessment of each patient must be thorough, with particular attention being paid to recognition and evaluation of structural cardiovascular problems.

When structural disease is thought likely, hemodynamic and angiographic studies are needed. In the absence of structural disease, syncope is more often neurally mediated in origin, and autonomic function testing (particularly tilt-table testing) should be an early step in the diagnostic strategy (see Figure 39.5). Specialized neurologic testing has proven useful in only a small minority of cases.

The treatment of syncope has not been the subject of thorough large scale clinical trials. Nevertheless, when structural cardiovascular disturbances or primary cardiac arrhythmias are the cause of syncope, appropriately directed therapy (e.g., valve replacement, pacemaker implantation) seems to be highly effective. On the other hand, documentation of treatment efficacy in vasovagal faints, orthostatic hypotension and dysautonomic states, and the various neurologic and psychiatric conditions which can mimic syncope, is much less well established.

Key points: the evaluation of the syncope patient

- The goals
    Establish a correlation between symptoms and abnormalities
    Assess prognosis
    Initiate appropriate treatment plan
- Key steps
    Obtain detailed medical history (including bystanders/relatives)
    Identify underlying structural heart disease
- Factors determining need for further tests
    Evidence for structural disease
    Certainty of the initial clinical impression
    Number and frequency of syncopal events
    Occurrence of injury or accident
    Family history of syncope or sudden death
    Occupation, avocation

Acknowledgment

The authors would like to thank Wendy Markuson and Barry L.S. Detloff for assistance in the preparation of the manuscript.

REFERENCES

1 Benditt DG, Ferguson DW, Grubb BP *et al*. Tilt-table testing for assessing syncope. An American College of Cardiology expert consensus document. *J Am Coll Cardiol* 1996;**28**(1):263–75.

2 Gendelman HE, Linzer M, Gabelman M *et al*. Syncope in a general hospital population. *NY State J Med* 1983;**83**:116–65.

3 Martin GJ, Adams SL, Martin HG *et al*. Prospective evaluation of syncope. *Ann Emerg Med* 1984;**13**: 499–504.

4 Wayne HH. Syncope: physiological considerations and an analysis of the clinical characteristics in 510 patient. *Am J Med* 1961;**30**:418–38.

5 Savage DD, Corwin L, McGee DL *et al*. Epidemiologic features of isolated syncope: the Framingham Study. *Stroke* 1985;**16**:626–9.

6 Kapoor WN, Karpf M, Wieand S *et al*. A prospective evaluation and follow-up of patients with syncope. *N Engl J Med* 1983;**309**:197–204.

7 Bass EB, Elson JJ, Fogoros RN *et al*. Long-term prognosis of patients undergoing electrophysiologic studies for syncope of unknown origin. *Am J Cardiol* 1988;**62**:1186–91.

8 Benditt DG, Goldstein MA, Adler S, Sakaguchi S, Lurie KG. Neurally mediated syncopal syndromes: pathophysiology and clinical evaluation. In: Mandel WJ, ed. *Cardiac arrhythmias* 3rd edn. Philadelphia: JB Lippincott, 1995, pp 879–906.

9 Kenny RA, Bayliss J, Ingram A, Sutton R. Head up tilt: a useful test for investigating unexplained syncope. *Lancet* 1986;**i**:1352–4.

10 Almquist A, Goldenberg IF, Milstein S *et al.* Provocation of bradycardia and hypotension by isoproterenol and upright posture in patients with unexplained syncope. *N Engl J Med* 1989;**320**: 346–51.

11 Sutton, R, Petersen M, Brignole M *et al.* Proposed classification for tilt induced vasovagal syncope. *Eur J Cardiac Pacing Electrophysiol* 1992;**2**:180–3.

12 Weiss S, Baker JP. The carotid sinus reflex in health and disease. Its role in the causation of fainting and convulsions. *Medicine* 1993;**12**: 297–354.

13 Almquist A, Gornick C, Benson DW Jr, Dunnigan A, Benditt DG. Carotid sinus hypersensitivity: evaluation of the vasodepressor component. *Circulation* 1985;**71**:927–36.

14 Bannister R. Chronic autonomic failure with postural hypotension. *Lancet* 1979;**ii**:404–6.

15 Low PA, Opfer-Gherking TL, McPhee BR *et al.* Prospective evaluation of clinical characteristics of orthostatic hypotension. *Mayo Clin Proc* 1995: **70**:617–22.

16 Low PA. Autonomic nervous system function. *J Clin Neurophys* 1993;**10**:14–27.

17 Weiling W, van Lieshout JJ. Investigation and treatment of autonomic circulatory failure. *Curr Opin Neurol Neurosurg* 1993;**6**:537–43.

18 Benditt DG, Sakaguchi S, Goldstein MA *et al.* Sinus node dysfunction: pathophysiology, clinical features, evaluation and treatment. In: Zipes DP, Jalife J, eds. *Cardiac electrophysiology. From cell to bedside*, 2nd edn. Philadelphia: WB Saunders, 1995, pp 1215–46.

19 Kaplan BM, Langendorf R, Lev M, Pick A. Tachycardia–bradycardia syndrome (so-called "sick sinus syndrome"). *Am J Cardiol* 1973;**26**: 497–508.

20 Rubenstein JJ, Schulman CL, Yurchak PM *et al.* Clinical spectrum of the sick sinus syndrome. *Circulation* 1972;**46**:5–13.

21 Benditt DG, Benson DW Jr, Dunnigan A *et al.* Drug therapy in sinus node dysfunction. In: Rapaport E, ed. *Cardiology update – 1984*. New York; Elsevier, 1984, pp 1215–46.

22 Linker NJ, Camm AJ. Drug effects on the sinus node. A clinical perspective. *Cardiovasc Drugs Ther* 1988;**2**:165–70.

23 Rowe JC, White PD. Complete heart block: a follow-up study. *Ann Intern Med* 1958;**49**: 260–70.

24 Penton GB, Miller H, Levine SA. Some clinical features of complete heart block. *Circulation* 1956; **13**:801–24.

25 Michaelsson M, Jonzon A, Riesenfeld T. Isolated congenital complete atrioventricular block in adult life. *Circulation* 1995;**92**:442–9.

26 Scheinman MM, Peters RW, Sauve MJ *et al.* Value of H–Q interval in patients with bundle branch block and the role of prophylactic permanent pacing. *Am J Cardiol* 1982;**50**:1316–22.

27 Dhingra RC, Denes P, Wu D *et al.* Syncope in patients with chronic bifascicular block. *Ann Intern Med* 1974;**81**:302–6.

28 Swerdlow CD, Winkle RA, Mason JW. Determinents of survival in patients with ventricular tachyarrhythmias. *N Engl J Med* 1983;**308**:1436–42.

29 Middelkauff HR, Stevenson WG, Stevenson LW, Saxon LA. Syncope in advanced heart failure: high risk of sudden death regardless of origin of syncope. *J Am Coll Cardiol* 1993;**21**:110–16.

30 Camm AJ, Lau CP. Syncope of undetermined origin: diagnosis and management. *Prog Cardiol* 1988;**1**:139–56.

31 Leitch JW, Klein GJ, Yee R *et al.* Syncope associated with supraventricular tachycardia: an expression of tachycardia or vasomotor response. *Circulation* 1992;**85**:1064–71.

32 Johnson AM. Aortic stenosis, sudden death, and the left ventricular baroreceptors. *Br Heart J* 1971; **33**:1–5.

33 Ross RT. *Syncope*. London: WB Saunders, 1988.

34 Kapoor W. Evaluation and outcome of patients with syncope. *Medicine* 1990;**69**:160–75.

35 Grubb BP, Gerard G, Rousch K *et al.* Differentiation of convulsive syncope and epilepsy with head up tilt table testing. *Ann Intern Med* 1991;**115**: 871–6.

36 Linzer M, Varia I, Pontinen M *et al.* Medically unexplained syncope: relationship to psychiatric illness. *Am J Med* 1992;**92**:18–25.

37 Grubb BP, Gerard G, Roush K *et al.* Cerebral vasoconstriction during head-upright tilt induced vasovagal syncope: a paradoxic and unexpected response. *Circulation* 1991;**84**:1157–64.

38 Njemanze PC. Cerebral circulation dysfunction and hemodynamic abnormalities in syncope during upright tilt test. *Can J Cardiol* 1993;**9**: 238–42.

39 Sakaguchi S, Shultz J, Remole C *et al.* Syncope associated with exercise, a manifestation of neurally mediated syncope. *Am J Cardiol* 1995; **75**:476–81.

40 Calkins H, Seifert M, Morady F. Clinical presentation and long term followup of athletes with exercise-induced vasodepressor syncope. *Am Heart J* 1995;**129**:1159–64.

41 Kuchar DL, Thorburn CW, Sammel NL. Signal-averaged electrocardiogram for evaluation of

recurrent syncope. *Am J Cardiol* 1986;**58**:949–53.

42 DiMarco JB, Garan H, Hawthorne WJ *et al.* Intracardiac electrophysiologic techniques in recurrent syncope of unknown cause. *Ann Intern Med* 1981;**95**:542–8.

43 Akhtar M, Shenasa M, Denker S, Gilbert CJ, Rizwi N. Role of cardiac electrophysiologic studies in patients with unexplained recurrent syncope. *PACE* 1983;**6**:192–201.

44 Morady F, Shen E, Schwartz A *et al.* Long-term follow-up of patients with recurrent unexplained syncope evaluated by electrophysiologic testing. *J Am Coll Cardiol* 1983;**2**:1053–9.

45 Denes P, Ezri MD. The role of electrophysiologic studies in the management of patients with unexplained syncope. *PACE* 1985;**8**:424–35.

46 Sra JS, Anderson AJ, Sheikh SH *et al.* Unexplained syncope evaluated by electrophysiologic studies and head-up tilt testing. *Ann Intern Med* 1991; **114**:1013–19.

47 Fujimura O, Yee R, Klein GJ *et al.* The diagnostic sensitivity of electrophysiologic testing in patients with syncope caused by bradycardia. *N Engl J Med* 1989;**321**:1703–7.

48 deMey C, Enterling D. Assessment of the hemodynamic responses to single passive head-up tilt by non-invasive methods in normotensive subjects. *Meth Find Exp Clin Pharmacol* 1986;**8**: 449–57.

49 Fitzpatrick A, Theodorakis G, Vardas P *et al.* The incidence of malignant vasovagal syndrome in patients with recurrent syncope. *Eur Heart J* 1991; **12**:389–94.

50 Raviele A, Gasparini G, DiPede F *et al.* Usefulness of head-up tilt test in evaluating patients with syncope of unknown origin and negative electrophysiologic study. *Am J Cardiol* 1990;**65**: 1322–7.

51 Grubb BP, Temesy-Armos P, Hahn H, Elliott L. Utility of upright tilt table testing in the evaluation and management of syncope of unknown origin. *Am J Med* 1991;**90**:6–10.

52 Grubb BP, Wolfe D, Samoil D *et al.* Recurrent unexplained syncope in the elderly: the use of head-upright tilt table testing in evaluation and management. *J Am Geriat Soc* 1992;**40**:1123–8.

53 Natale A, Akhtar M, Jazayeri M *et al.* Provocation of hypotension during head-up tilt testing in subjects with no history of syncope or presyncope. *Circulation* 1995;**92**:54–8.

54 Fitzpatrick A, Theodorakis G, Vardas P, Sutton R. Methodology of head-up tilt testing in patients with unexplained syncope. *J Am Coll Cardiol* 1991; **17**:125–30.

55 Fitzpatrick AP, Ahmed R, Williams S *et al.* A randomized trial of medical therapy in malignant vasovagal syndrome or neurally-mediated bradycardia/hypotension syndrome. *Eur J Cardiac Pacing Electrophysiol* 1991;**1**:199–202.

56 Brignole M, Menozzi C, Gianfranchi L *et al.* A controlled trial of acute and long-term medical therapy in tilt-induced neurally mediated syncope. *Am J Cardiol* 1992;**70**:339–42.

57 Morillo CA, Leitch JU, Yee R *et al.* A placebo-controlled trial of intravenous and oral disopyramide for prevention of neurally mediated syncope induced by head-up tilt. *J Am Coll Cardiol* 1993;**22**:1843–8.

58 Moya A, Permanyer-Miralda G, Sagrista-Sauleda J *et al.* Limitations of head-up tilt test for evaluating the efficacy of therapeutic interventions in patients with vasovagal syncope: results of a controlled study of etilefrine versus placebo. *J Am Coll Cardiol* 1995;**25**:65–9.

59 Mahananda N, Bhuripanyo K, Kangkagate C *et al.* Randomized double-blind placebo-controlled trial of oral atenolol in patients with unexplained syncope and positive upright tilt table results. *Am Heart J* 1995;**130**:1250–3.

60 Benditt DG, Remole S, Asso A *et al.* Cardiac pacing for carotid sinus syndrome and vasovagal syncope. In: Barold SS, Mugica J, eds. *New perspectives in cardiac pacing, 3.* Mount Kisco, NY: Futura, 1993, pp 15–28.

61 Benditt DG, Peterson M, Lurie K *et al.* Cardiac pacing for prevention of recurrent vasovagal syncope. *Ann Intern Med* 1995;**122**:204–9.

62 Petersen MEV, Chamberlain-Webber R, Fitzpatrick AP *et al.* Permanent pacing for cardioinhibitory malignant vasovagal syndrome. *Br Heart J* 1994; **71**:274–81.

63 Bannister R, Mathias C. Management of postural hypotension. In: Bannister R, ed. *Autonomic failure. A textbook of clinical disorders of the autonomic nervous system.* Oxford: Oxford University Press, 1988, pp 569–95.

64 Jankovic J, Gilden JL, Hiner BC, Brown DC, Rubin M. Neurogenic orthostatic hypotension: a double-blind placebo-controlled study with midodrine. *Am J Med* 1993;**95**:38–48.

65 Sheldon RS, Gent M, Roberts RS, Connolly SJ, on behalf of the NAVPAC Investigators. North American Vasovagal Pacemaker Study: study design and organization. *PACE* 1997;**20**: 844–8.

66 Perrins EJ, Astridge PS. Clinical trials and experience. In: Ellenbogen KA, Kay GN, Wilkoff BL, eds. *Clinical cardiac pacing.* Philadelphia: WB Saunders, 1995, pp 399–418.

67 Stangl K, Wirtzfeld A, Seitz K *et al.* Atrial stimulation (AAI): long-term follow-up of 110 patients. In: Belhassen B, Feldman S, Copperman Y, eds. *Cardiac pacing and electrophysiology* (Proceedings of the VIIIth World Symposium on Cardiac Pacing and Electrophysiology). Jerusalem: R&L Creative Communications, 1987, pp 283–5.

68 Rosenqvist M, Brandt J, Schuller H. Long-term pacing in sick sinus node disease: effects of stimulation mode on cardiovascular morbidity and mortality. *Am Heart J* 1988;**116**:16–22.

69 Andersen HR, Thuesen L, Bagger JP *et al.* Prospective randomised trial of atrial versus ventricular pacing in sick-sinus syndrome. *Lancet* 1994;**344**:1523–28.

70 Naccarelli GV, Dougherty AH, Jalal S, Shih H-T, Wolbrette D. Paroxysmal supraventricular tachycardia: comparative role of therapeutic methods – drugs, devices, and ablation. In: Saksena S, Luderitz B, eds. *Interventional electrophysiology: a textbook*, 2nd edn. Armonk, NY: Futura Publishing, 1996, pp 461–70.

71 Middelkauff HR, Stevenson WG, Stevenson LW, Saxon LA. Syncope in advanced heart failure: high risk of sudden death regardless of origin of syncope. *J Am Coll Cardiol* 1993;**21**:110–16.

72 Middelkauff HR, Stevenson WG, Saxon LA. Prognosis after syncope: impact of left ventricular function. *Am Heart J* 1993;**125**:121–7.

73 Moss AJ, Hall WJ, Cannon DS *et al.* Improved survival with an implanted defibrillator in patients with coronary disease at high risk for ventricular arrhythmia. *N Engl J Med* 1996;**335**:1933–40.

74 The AVID Investigators. Antiarrhythmics versus implantable defibrillators (AVID) – rationale, design, and methods. *Am J Cardiol* 1995;**75**: 470–5.

75 McKenna WJ, Deanfield J, Faruqui A *et al.* Prognosis in hypertrophic cardiomyopathy: role of age and clinical electrocardiographic and hemodynamic features. *Am J Cardiol* 1981;**47**: 532–8.

76 McAreavey D, Epstein ND, Fananapazir L. Dual chamber pacing is effective therapy for hypertrophic cardiomyopathy patients with provocable LV outflow tract obstruction and symptoms refractory to medical therapy (abstract). *J Am Coll Cardiol* 1994;**23**:11.

77 Kapoor W, Karpf M, Maher Y *et al.* Syncope of unknown origin: the need for a more cost-effective approach to its evaluation. *JAMA* 1982;**247**: 2687–91.

78 Calkins H, Byrne M, El-Atassi R *et al.* The economic burden of unrecognized vasodepressor syncope. *Am J Med* 1993;**95**:473–9.

Part III
Specific cardiovascular disorders
vii: Left ventricular dysfunction

SALIM YUSUF, Editor

Grading of recommendations and levels of evidence used in *Evidence Based Cardiology*

GRADE A

Level 1a   Evidence from large randomized clinical trials (RCTs) or systematic reviews (including meta-analyses) of multiple randomized trials which collectively has at least as much data as one single well-defined trial.

Level 1b   Evidence from at least one "All or None" high quality cohort study; in which ALL patients died/failed with conventional therapy and some survived/succeeded with the new therapy (eg chemotherapy for tuberculosis, meningitis, or defibrillation for ventricular fibrillation); or in which many died/failed with conventional therapy and NONE died/failed with the new therapy (eg penicillin for pneumococcal infections).

Level 1c   Evidence from at least one moderate sized RCT or a meta-analysis of small trials which collectively only has a moderate number of patients.

Level 1d   Evidence from at least one RCT.

GRADE B

Level 2   Evidence from at least one high quality study of non-randomized cohorts who did and did not receive the new therapy.

Level 3   Evidence from at least one high quality case control study.

Level 4   Evidence from at least one high quality case series.

GRADE C

Level 5   Opinions from experts without reference or access to any of the foregoing (eg argument from physiology, bench research or first principles).

A comprehensive approach would incorporate many different types of evidence (eg RCTs, non-RCTs, epidemiologic studies, and experimental data), and examine the architecture of the information for consistency, coherence and clarity. Occasionally the evidence does not completely fit into neat compartments. For example, there may not be an RCT that demonstrates a reduction in mortality in individuals with stable angina with the use of beta-blockers, but there is overwhelming evidence that mortality is  reduced following MI. In such cases, some may recommend use of beta-blockers in angina patients with the expectation that some extrapolation from post-MI trials is warranted. This could be expressed as Grade A/C. In other instances (e.g. smoking cessation or a pacemaker for complete heart block), the non-randomized data are so overwhelmingly clear and biologically plausible that it would be reasonable to consider these interventions as Grade A.

Recommendation grades appear either in a shaded margin box with an 'R' logo as shown, or within the text, for example Grade A .

Management of overt heart failure

40

BERT ANDERSSON,
KARL SWEDBERG

The cardiac muscle may be exposed to various hemodynamic, metabolic, or toxic conditions that eventually lead to the clinical syndrome of congestive heart failure. Given a certain severity, any cardiac disorder will ultimately lead to heart failure. Further, many non-cardiac disorders will result in heart failure, alone or in combination with cardiovascular conditions. Last, but not least, progressive deterioration of cardiac function with age further increases the susceptibility to develop heart failure. Taken together, the aforementioned circumstances, in a continuously aging population, explain why congestive heart failure is one of the most common, and most costly, diseases in Western society.

Congestive heart failure is a potentially lethal condition, and it has been evident during the past decade that whilst we are in possession of some drugs that may improve cardiac function and symptoms, some of those agents are simultaneously capable of impeding long term survival. Furthermore, as with other treatment traditions, we lack modern documentation about the oldest drugs, such as diuretics. In this chapter we intend to cover the present knowledge regarding evidence based medical therapies in congestive heart failure.

CARDIAC GLYCOSIDES

Digitalis is the oldest of the drugs used in the treatment of congestive heart failure today. It has been used for at least 200 years. Although all internists, general practitioners, and cardiologist have a profound experience with this drug, the mode of action is still partly unknown. The main action of the drug is thought to be exerted by action on the plasma membrane Na^+/K^+-ATPase, increasing intracellular concentrations of Na^+ and Ca^+. A variety of autonomic effects have been shown in acute experimental studies.

Acute effects in congestive heart failure

Older uncontrolled studies have suggested that digitalis produced beneficial hemodynamic effects in patients with decompensated heart failure, expressed as a decrease in pulmonary capillary wedge pressure, an increase in cardiac output, and a fall in heart rate.[1,2] It appears that the effect of digitalis on hemodynamics is dependent on the hemodynamic state of the patient. Whereas positive effects have been observed in decompensated heart failure, the effects in normal subjects are largely negligible.[3,4] Although the slowing of heart rate would be of benefit in diastolic heart failure without systolic dysfunction, there are no data to support the use of digoxin in diastolic heart failure. On the contrary, on a theoretical basis, the increase in intracellular Ca^+ and increase in contractility may be harmful to the hypertrophic heart. Although digoxin has been found to act synergistically in combination with different vasodilators, no such effects were seen in combination with dobutamin. Ferguson showed that acute administration of digitalis restored baroreceptor function and caused a decrease in sympathetic activity.[5,6] Goldsmith *et al.* were not able to reproduce these results with regard to norepinephrine kinetics or baroreceptor function.[7] Both increase and decrease in neurohormonal activity has been reported following acute digoxin administration.

Chronic digitalis therapy

The first double-blind placebo-controlled trial with chronic digoxin treatment was published in 1977.[8] In a crossover design, 46 patients were randomized, about one-third of which were in atrial fibrillation. Sixteen patients deteriorated while on placebo, eight of whom improved after being switched over to digoxin. In a 3-month trial Fleg *et al.* could not show any superior effect of digitalis treatment over placebo, although a majority of patients on digitalis deteriorated after discontinuation of the drug.[9] Improvement of myocardial function in patients with mild heart failure was demonstrated by Taggart *et al.*[10] Other studies have shown positive effects of digoxin on clinical heart failure symptoms, echocardiographic findings, and exercise capacity, in particular in patients with more advanced left ventricular dysfunction.[11–13]

The abovementioned trials were small, and the first larger study was the Captopril–Digoxin Multicenter Research Group trial.[14] In this study 300 patients with mild heart failure were compared using captopril, digoxin or placebo. Digoxin and captopril were equally effective in preventing hospitalization or an increase in diuretic dosages. Although digoxin-treated patients showed a significant increase in ejection fraction, in contrast to the captopril group, digoxin did not improve exercise capacity as much as captopril. In another study with 433 patients with mild heart failure, the German and Austrian Xamoterol Study Group investigated the effect of digoxin together with xamoterol and placebo. Digoxin improved clinical indices of heart failure but not exercise capacity.[15]

Several trials have used a withdrawal design for the placebo-treated patients. Di Bianco *et al.* compared digoxin to milrinone in a 3-month multicenter trial in 230 patients with moderate to severe heart failure.[16] The digoxin-treated patients showed a significant improvement in left ventricular function and exercise capacity compared to the placebo group. Furthermore, digoxin was significantly less prone to induce arrhythmias compared to milrinone.

In the PROVED trial a randomized double-blind withdrawal of digoxin was investigated in 88 patients with NYHA class II to III.[17] The placebo patients showed several signs of worsening heart failure as expressed by an increase in the need for diuretics and hospitalizations, and a impairment in exercise capacity and LV function. In a similar study – the RADIANCE trial – 178 patients with congestive heart failure were investigated during digoxin withdrawal compared to maintained digoxin therapy.[18] The results were also similar to the PROVED trial, with placebo patients showing a statistically significant deterioration in cardiac function, hospitalization, quality of life and exercise capacity.

It should be noted that the withdrawal study design is inferior compared to prospective treatment studies. Because of the selection of responders and exclusion of non-responders who have suffered from deterioration or even lethal arrhythmias during digoxin treatment, the study design will result in different answers.

The Digitalis Investigators Group (DIG) study is the largest study in congestive heart failure. It is the only survival study with digoxin. The effect of digoxin was studied in a multicenter, prospective, randomized, placebo-controlled, double-blind trial in 7788 patients with mild to moderate heart failure and sinus rhythm.[19] Among the investigated patients 6800 had signs of systolic dysfunction expressed as ejection fraction <45%. The remaining 998 patients might be considered to have diastolic dysfunction. There was no effect on the primary endpoint all-cause mortality (odds ratio 1.0). Digoxin reduced the number of hospitalizations from worsening heart failure. The result in these situations will often be neutral, as in the DIG study.

Documented value of digoxin

Proven indication: always acceptable
- Symptomatic left ventricular systolic heart failure and sinus rhythm. Symptomatic improvement, improved exercise capacity and decreased hospitalization for heart failure.
- Congestive heart failure with atrial fibrillation. Heart rate control.

Acceptable indication but of uncertain efficacy and may be controversial
- Symptomatic heart failure due to diastolic dysfunction.

Not proven: potentially harmful (contraindicated)
- Bradycardia and atrioventricular block.
- Significant ventricular arrhythmias.
- Renal dysfunction.
- Electrolyte disturbances, hypokalemia in particular.

Taken together, present data on digoxin suggest that this drug induces small but beneficial effects on cardiac function, morbidity, and symptoms. There is a neutral effect on all-cause mortality, with a possibly lower incidence of deaths due to worsening heart failure, balanced by an increase in arrhythmic and myocardial infarction deaths. However, the therapeutic window is narrow, and the potential risk for serious arrhythmias cannot be ignored.

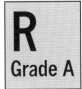

R
Grade A

DIURETICS

Fluid retention is a consistent finding in almost every patient with congestive heart failure. The need for reduction of blood volume in patients with edema was recognized several hundred years ago. Drugs with mild diuretic effects, such as mercury salts, carbonic anhydrase inhibitors, and thiazides, have been used. A more substantial way of inducing diuresis was achieved when the loop-diuretics were introduced, and this class of drugs has since been the cornerstone of heart failure treatment.[20] The compensatory fluid retention, as a response to lower cardiac output and reduced kidney perfusion,[21] might be of some benefit in restoring optimal preload in the earlier states of congestive heart failure. A further increase in intracavitary pressure increases wall stress in the myocardium with a parallel increase in oxygen consumption and energy expenditure. The elevation of venous pressure shifts the hydrostatic balance across the capillary wall toward a net filtration of fluid to the extracellular space, and finally to the formation of edema. The edema impairs the transportation of oxygen, nutritive substances and waste products, which ultimately leads to organ failure. In the case of pulmonary edema, the decrease in oxygen uptake affects all organs in the body. The decrease in renal blood flow stimulates the renin system, which leads to secretion of angiotensin and aldosterone. Other neurohormones that promote retention of sodium and water include vasopressin, norepinephrine, and prostaglandins.[22] Sodium excretion is promoted by atrial natriuretic factor, dopamine, and prostacyclin.

Acute neuroendocrine and hemodynamic effects

In patients with pulmonary edema, intravenous furosemide is normally followed by a prompt response and relief of symptoms. There have not been consistent findings regarding the mode of action of loop-diuretics in the acute phase of decompensated heart failure. The reduction in filling pressures occurs even before diuresis is initiated,[23-25] and has been attributed to vasodilation. However, also arterial vasoconstriction has been found, alone or in combination with venodilation.[26-28] Regarding cardiac output, an increase, no change, or a decrease has been reported. Although furosemide is the most thoroughly tested loop-diuretic, there are others available, including bumetanide,[29] ethacrynic acid,[30] piretanide,[31] and toresemide.[32] There is little information about the acute neuroendocrine effects of diuretics. The effects on vascular tone suggest signs of neuroendocrine modulation. Venodilation may be due to the release of renal vasodilator prostaglandins.[33]

Chronic neuroendocrine and hemodynamic effects

Most long term studies have involved a small number of patients and utilized a variety of drugs and doses. The first study to give information with oral diuretics was performed in a small number of patients with valvular heart disease.[24] Hydrochlorthiazide was administered and resulted in a reduction in weight, pulmonary artery pressure, arterial pressure, heart rate, and cardiac output at rest as well as during exercise. Results from other studies have yielded similar results, using different diuretics, including furosemide,[34] piretanide,[35] torasemide,[36] and amiloride.[37] Chronic neuroendocrine effects are less well studied. Oral furosemide treatment has been associated with a reduction in norepinephrine concentration and a profound increase in plasma renin activity, angiotensin, and plasma aldosterone concentration.[38,39]

Effects on survival

No study has been performed examining the effect of diuretics on long term survival. There has been some concern raised regarding the potential neurohormonal activation by diuretics. However, any longterm neuroendocrine activation has not been demonstrated. Further, it should be kept in mind that studies showing positive survival effects in heart failure – using ACE inhibitors, beta-blockers or vasodilators – have all used diuretics as background treatment.

Documented value of diuretics

Proven indication: always acceptable
- Symptomatic improvement in case of congestion. Improvement of exercise capacity.

Acceptable indication but of uncertain efficacy and may be controversial
- Long-term treatment in conjunction with other drugs for heart failure, such as ACE inhibitors, vasodilators and beta-blockers.

Not proven: potentially harmful (contraindicated)
- Heart failure without congestion or edema.
- Severe decompensated hypokalemia or hyperuricemia.

Clinical management

It is clear that diuretics reduce symptoms in congestive heart failure. The effect on symptoms has been formally tested in trials with furosemide and torasemide.[40,41] Further, it has been observed that the effects of ACE inhibitors may require the coadministration of diuretics.[42,43] Diuretics are also more effective in relieving edema and congestive symptoms than ACE inhibitors when given as single therapy.[44] Through an increase in urinary excretion of electrolytes, diuretics are prone to induce hypokalemia, hyponatremia, hypocalcemia, hypomagnesemia, and metabolic alkalosis.[45] The need for potassium supplement might be diminished by using potassium sparing diuretics, such as amiloride or aldosterone. The possible benefit to aldosterone is now formally tested in the RALES trial. A first dose-range study has been presented,[46] and a survival trial is under way. ACE inhibitors act synergistically with potassium sparing diuretics, which may produce hyperkalemia. The addition of a potassium sparing diuretic to a loop-diuretic will further increase diuresis. Additionally, the diuretic effect of a loop-diuretic is boosted by other diuretics acting at different sites in the nephron. Therefore, the combination of a loop-diuretic with a thiazide enhances the diuretic effect.

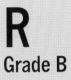

R
Grade B

It is difficult to foresee a future situation when diuretics are no longer needed in the treatment arsenal of congestive heart failure. Further, the obvious need for relief of edema and fluid retention will prevent the launching of any long term survival study. With reference to the multiple side effects produced by electrolyte disturbances it is advisable to keep the diuretic dosages as low as possible, and aim for combination therapies in which dosages are minimized.

VASODILATORS

Vasodilation reduces left ventricular afterload and preload, and these beneficial effects were observed in 1956,[47,48] but it was not until the 1970s that the concept was widely accepted.[49,50] The first drugs used were pure vasodilators, such as nitroprusside, nitroglycerin and phentolamine. Later, agents with combined effects were developed. Examples of combination therapies are the inotropic drugs with simultaneous vasodilation, such as dobutamine, and ACE inhibitors, which are reviewed in another section of this chapter.

Reduction of afterload and preload in congestive heart failure improves the left ventricular performance according to the Frank-Starling relation with less myocardial oxygen demand and increased cardiac output.[51,52] Further, vasodilation might reduce valvular regurgitation by means of afterload reduction. Vasodilation may improve organ dysfunction by acting directly on selected vascular beds, such as the coronary and the renal vasculature.

Acute vasodilator therapy

Nitroglycerin and nitroprusside are the drugs most commonly used for acute short term vasodilation therapy in heart failure.

NITROGLYCERIN

Nitroglycerin causes smooth muscle cell relaxation and vasodilation of arterial and venous vessels through action on guanylate cyclase and the generation of cyclic guanosine monophosphate.[53] Nitrates can be used as sublingual tablet, lingual-buccal spray, or as intravenous infusion. Administration causes reduction in left ventricular filling pressures within 3–5 minutes, mainly by venodilation and lowering of preload.[54–59] Further, nitroglycerin reduces systemic vascular resistance and afterload, with ensuing improvement in cardiac output. Although the effect of nitroglycerin on coronary blood flow has not been studied in congestive heart failure, it is conceivable that nitrate therapy favourably affects myocardial perfusion and oxygen supply/demand ratio.[60,61] Acute nitrate administration appears to be especially useful in cases of elevated filling pressures and ischemic conditions, such as in ischemic cardiomyopathy and myocardial infarction.

NITROPRUSSIDE

Nitroprusside generates nitric oxide and nitrosothiols, which stimulate guanylate cyclase to increase intracellular cGMP. The smooth muscle cell relaxation is rapidly induced after administration. Sodium nitroprusside is converted to cyanide, and is metabolized to thiocyanate. Thiocyanate may accumulate and lead to thiocyanate toxicity during prolonged nitroprusside therapy. As compared to nitroglycerin, nitroprusside is far more potent and causes a more pronounced arterial vasodilation.[57] The most prominent effect of nitroprusside is the arterial vasodilation with afterload reduction. There are minor effects on renal and hepatosplanchnic vasculature.[57] In contrast to nitroglycerin, nitroprusside may induce a coronary steal phenomenon.[62] Nitroprusside is best employed in cases of acute heart failure after cardiac surgery or myocardial infarction, or in waiting for a more definitive intervention, e.g., valvular surgery. Further, nitroprusside has been used to stabilize patients with chronic heart failure and to determine their optimal level of vasodilation.[63] Owing to its potent vasodilation property, nitroprusside may cause adverse hypotension, especially in cases of inadequate filling pressure. Thiocyanate and cyanide toxicity is rare during short term administration (≤ 3 µg/kg/min for less than 72 hours).

Hemodynamic effects of long term vasodilator therapy

NITRATES AND HYDRALAZINE

Oral nitroglycerin and hydralazine have been studied, either alone or in combination therapy. The effects on left ventricular function and hemodynamics are similar to the acute effects of vasodilators described above.[64–67]

Hydralazine was available as an antihypertensive agent when vasodilator therapy was adopted as a therapeutic strategy in congestive heart failure. Hydralazine acts as a dominant arterial vasodilator, but has probably also mild inotropic properties, which might be due to a reflex activation of sympathetic activity.[68,69] This inotropic action might be responsible for a less favorable effect on myocardial oxygen consumption counteracting the unloading effects of vasodilation.[70,71]

The addition of a nitrate to hydralazine causes a greater effect on the reduction in filling pressures than can be achieved by hydralazine alone.[72] In view of the beneficial action of nitrates on coronary dynamics, a nitrate should be added to hydralazine therapy in patients with significant coronary artery disease.[73] Although hydralazine-nitrate therapy was marginally superior to ACE inhibitor in improving exercise capacity, this combination displayed worse tolerability.[74]

CALCIUM-CHANNEL BLOCKERS

Besides its vasodilatory effect, the first generation calcium-blocker nifedipine possesses negative inotropic effects. Deleterious effects with regard to hemodynamics, neurohormonal activation and disease progression have been demonstrated in several trials.[75] Diltiazem has been associated with deterioration, no change, or improvement in hemodynamic function. In a postinfarction study patients with heart failure did not benefit from verapamil treatment, in contrast to patients without heart failure.[76] Furthermore, the effects of diltiazem were unfavorable in patients with congestive heart failure in conjunction with myocardial infarction in a large placebo-controlled trial in 1237 patients.[77] Second generation calcium-blockers have not been extensively studied in patients with heart failure, but there are indications of a risk for clinical deterioration with drugs such as nisoldipine and nicardipine.[78,79] The second generation calcium-blocker felodipine caused vasodilation and an increase in cardiac output during 8 weeks of treatment in a placebo-controlled trial.[80]

OTHER VASODILATORS

Other potent vasodilators, such as prazosin, minoxidil, and epoprosternol are discussed in the next section regarding survival. These drugs are currently not used in the long term management of chronic heart failure.

Effects on survival

HYDRALAZINE AND ISOSORBIDE DINITRATE

The V-HeFT I was the first placebo-controlled clinical trial to study the effect of a vasodilator on survival in patients with chronic heart failure. The study recruited 642 patients with mild to moderate heart failure, and randomized to receive placebo, prazosin hydrochloride, or the combination of hydralazine hydrochloride and isosorbide dinitrate. Two years after randomization, the survival in the hydralazine-isosorbide treated group was significantly better than the placebo group (P<0.028). For the entire follow-up, the difference was not significant (P=0.093). The mortality rate in the prazosin group was not different from the placebo group.[81]

The second V-HeFT study examined the efficacy of hydralazine and isosorbide with that of enalapril. There were 804 patients, randomized to the two treatment strategies. Two years after randomization, the all-cause mortality was 18% in the enalapril group as compared with 25% in the hydralazine-isosorbide group (P=0.016). For the total follow-up, the difference was not significant (P=0.08).

CALCIUM-CHANNEL BLOCKERS

Felodipine was studied in the V-HeFT III study, in which the effect on survival was neutral.[82] Amlodipine, a third generation calcium-channel blocker, was investigated in the PRAISE trial.[83] A total of 1153 patients with NYHA class III–IV were randomized, including 421 patients with non-ischemic dilated cardiomyopathy. The overall effect on mortality as well as on the combined endpoint mortality and hospitalization was neutral. Whereas the mortality was unchanged in the subgroup with ischemic heart failure, there were significantly fewer endpoints in the non-ischemic group treated with amlodipine as compared to patients on placebo (22% vs 35%, P<0.001). However, this was not expected prior to the conduct of the study and this hypothesis is being evaluated in a new study – PRAISE-2.

OTHER VASODILATORS

Flosequinan is a vasodilator with a combined venous and arterial effect, with a possible positive inotropic and chronotropic effect. A large multicenter trial (PROFILE) was launched to study the effects on survival in heart failure patients. However, this study had to be stopped prematurely, due to an increase in mortality in the flosequinan-treated patients.[84] Additionally, the prostacyclin epoprostenol might improve hemodynamics, but has been shown to have a less favourable effect on mortality in severe heart failure.[85]

Documented value of vasodilators

Proven indication: always acceptable
- Short-term reduction of afterload in cases with acute heart failure.
- The combination hydralazine–isosorbide dinitrate can be used for long term treatment in patients who do not tolerate ACE inhibitors.

Acceptable indication but of uncertain efficacy and may be controversial
- Third generation calcium-blockers may be used for symptomatic treatment in patients with non-ischemic etiology.

Not proven: potentially harmful (contraindicated)
- Other vasodilators than hydralazine–isosorbide dinitrate and amlodipine in non-ischemic cardiomyopathy may increase mortality during long term treatment.
- Occurrence of significant valvular stenosis.

Most vasodilators can improve hemodynamics on a short term basis. Besides the combination of hydralazine and isosorbide dinatrate, the long term effects of different vasodilators are either neutral or detrimental. The majority of studies have shown harmful effects with calcium-blockers in congestive heart failure, with the exception for amlodipine in a subgroup of patients with non-ischemic dilated cardiomyopathy. It is therefore suggested that vasodilators other than ACE inhibitors may be used to relieve symptoms and to acutely improve the hemodynamic condition. The effects on survival are less favorable as compared with ACE inhibitors, but hydralazine–isosorbide dinitrate may be used in patients who do not tolerate ACE inhibitors.

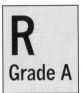

R

Grade A

DRUGS AFFECTING THE RENIN–ANGIOTENSIN SYSTEM

Angiotensin converting enzyme (ACE) inhibitors

ACE inhibitors have been introduced for the treatment of heart failure within the past decade. Their potential value was suggested by studies showing improved symptomatology,[86] hemodynamics[87,88] and survival.[89] It was hypothesized that ACE inhibitors might attenuate left ventricular remodeling after myocardial infarction[90,91] and thus possibly prevent the progression to symptomatic heart failure. Neuroendocrine activation has been shown to be of prognostic importance[92] and ACE inhibitors have the potential of modulating this activation.[93] Several studies have reported results on the effects of ACE inhibitors on survival in patients with clinical heart failure, following acute myocardial infarction generally and following myocardial infarction with left ventricular dysfunction or heart failure.

SURVIVAL TRIALS

In CONSENSUS I it was demonstrated that survival could be improved in severe heart failure by addition of an ACE inhibitor.[89] There were 253 patients in NYHA class IV randomized to placebo or enalapril. After a follow-up of 6 months (primary objective), the overall mortality was reduced by 27% ($P=0.003$). Number of days for hospital care was reduced and NYHA classification significantly improved with enalapril.

In the largest study, the Studies of Left Ventricular Treatment (SOLVD) trial, 2569 patients with symptomatic heart failure NYHA class II–III received placebo or enalapril besides conventional heart failure therapy.[94] The average follow-up was 41.4 months. Mortality was significantly reduced from 40% to 35% ($P=0.0036$). Hospitalizations for heart failure were also reduced. The largest reduction in mortality occurred among deaths attributed significantly to progressive heart failure. Symptoms and quality of life assessed by questionnaire were improved.[95]

In the Survival and Ventricular Enlargement (SAVE) trial, 2231 patients with ejection fraction of 40% or less, but without overt heart failure or symptoms of myocardial ischemia, were randomly assigned treatment with captopril or placebo.[96] Mortality from all causes was 20% in the captopril group and 25% in the placebo group (RR 19%; $P=0.019$).

In the TRACE study 1749 patients with left ventricular dysfunction were randomly assigned treatment with placebo or the ACE inhibitor trandolapril.[97] Treatment was initiated 3–7 days from the onset of myocardial infarction. All-cause mortality in the placebo group was 42.3% and 34.7% with trandolapril, a 22% relative reduction of mortality ($P=0.00065$).

In the AIRE study, 2006 patients with clinical evidence of heart failure any time after the index infarction, were randomly allocated to treatment with ramipril or placebo on the third to tenth day from the onset of infarction.[98] Clinical evidence of heart failure was defined as at least one of the following: signs of left ventricular failure on chest radiograph, bilateral auscultatory crackles extending at least one-third of the way up the lung fields in the absence of chronic pulmonary disease, or auscultatory evidence of a third heart sound with persistent tachycardia. The average follow-up was 15 months with a minimum of 6 months. Mortality from all causes at the end of the study was 17% in the ramipril group and 23% in the placebo group (RR 27%; $P=0.002$).

TRIALS ON EXERCISE CAPACITY

There are many trials that have focused on this objective. An extensive review of these trials has recently been published.[99] The key findings from this review were:

> Studies of ACE inhibitors confirm that these agents do improve the exercise capacity as well as symptoms in patients with chronic congestive heart failure. Study size, duration of follow-up and method of exercise testing appear to be three factors affecting the outcome of the studies. In the overall analysis, changes in exercise capacity are consistent with changes in symptoms.

TRIALS ON HEMODYNAMICS

ACE inhibitors were documented early to induce beneficial hemodynamic responses. These effects included a vasodilatory effect and an increased cardiac output, increased stroke volume and reduced pulmonary wedge pressure.[87,88]

TRIALS ON PREVENTION

A reduced incidence of heart failure by ACE inhibitors has been demonstrated in several trials. In the prevention arm of the SOLVD study,[94] the incidence of heart failure and the number of hospitalizations were reduced and similar findings were reported in

SAVE.[96] In an overview of ACE inhibitor trials[100] the preventive potential of ACE inhibitors is clearly demonstrated.

The potential antiatherosclerotic effect of ACE inhibitors, suggested from experimental animal studies, is supported by observations from the SOLVD[101] and SAVE[96] studies, in which the incidence of myocardial infarction and unstable angina were reduced. However, these findings need confirmation from ongoing prospective trials.

COST-EFFECTIVENESS

Enalapril therapy for patients with heart failure (SOLVD) was cost-effective and justified by added benefits compared to other vasodilator therapy.[102] In asymptomatic patients with left ventricular dysfunction after an acute myocardial infarction (SAVE), captopril was cost-effective in patients 50–80 years of age compared to other interventions.[103] Ramipril therapy for patients with clinical heart failure after acute myocardial infarction appears highly cost-effective when assessed using data from the AIRE study.[104] ACE inhibitor treatment was considered cost-effective in an evaluation of five independent economic analysis.[105]

Documented value of ACE inhibitors

Proven indication: always acceptable

- Symptomatic chronic heart failure and documented systolic myocardial dysfunction. Improved survival and reduced morbidity have been demonstrated. Symptoms will be attenuated and exercise capacity improved.
- Following acute myocardial infarction with clinical signs of heart failure or significant systolic dysfunction (ejection fraction<40%). Improved survival and reduced morbidity have been demonstrated.

Acceptable indication but of uncertain efficacy and may be controversial

- Heart failure due to diastolic dysfunction.

Not proven: potentially harmful (contraindicated)

- Treatment of patients with significant aortic or mitral stenosis.
- Treatment of patients with hypotension (systolic blood pressure <80 mmHg)
- Treatment of patients with pronounced renal dysfunction.

CLINICAL PERSPECTIVE

Chronic heart failure and left ventricular dysfunction

All patients with documented left ventricular systolic dysfunction by any method, in the order of ejection fraction <35–40%, should be considered for treatment with an ACE inhibitor. In symptomatic patients this should be considered first line therapy in addition to a diuretic agent. Treatment should be continued long term. Patients with clinical congestive heart failure should be maintained on ACE inhibitor treatment in combination with a diuretic.

Contraindications to ACE inhibitors include hypotension (in general systolic blood pressure <80 mmHg), pronounced renal dysfunction (serum creatinine >200 µmol/l), history of angioneurotic edema and important valve stenosis.

The dosage to be used should be titrated from a low dose and increased to the moderate high levels employed in clinical trials. If no hypotension or renal dysfunction develops, titration up to enalapril 10 mg b.i.d., captopril 50 mg b.i.d., ramipril 5 mg b.i.d., trandolapril 4 mg q.d. quinapril 10 mg b.i.d. will be most effective.

Angiotensin II receptor (AT$_1$) antagonists

As ACE inhibition does not provide complete blockade from the synthesis of angiotensin II, a more effective blockade has been postulated by a specific antagonism at the receptor (AT$_1$) level, speculating that such a blockade might offer better protection from sudden death in congestive heart failure. The first clinically available AT$_1$-receptor antagonist has been losartan. Hemodynamic effects of losartan have been similar to the effects of enalapril in comparative trial.[106] Recently, a pilot trial, ELITE, was published.[107] Patients >65 years with heart failure were randomized to losartan 50 mg q.d. or captopril 50 mg t.i.d. for 48 weeks. The primary endpoint was renal dysfunction. The effect on serum creatinine did not differ between the two groups. The secondary endpoint, death and/ or hospitalization for heart failure, was 9.4% in the losartan group and 13.2% in the captopril group ($P=0.075$). The difference was entirely due to a 46% decrease in total mortality among losartan-treated patients, 8.7% and 4.8% respectively ($P=0.035$). The effect of losartan is currently being evaluated in a survival study, ELITE II. Two other AT$_1$-receptor antagonists, valsartan and candesatril cilexitil, are also under evaluation in larger trials in heart failure.

In RESOLVD (Randomized Evaluation of Strategies of Left Ventricular Dysfunction), there were no differences between candesantan and enalapril in exercise tolerance, ventricular function and symptomatic status over 43 weeks. However, combined therapy with candesantan plus enalapril markedly reduced ventricular volumes and improved ejection fraction over 43 weeks compared to either candesantan or enalapril alone. There was greater inhibition of aldosterone levels with the combination at 20 weeks but this difference narrowed at 43 weeks. The study was too small to examine the impact of clinical outcomes.

In conclusion, AT$_1$ receptor antagonists are not clearly proven to be effective in reducing mortality or morbidity in patients with heart failure. There are promising observations that need confirmation in larger trials.

Documented value of AT$_1$-receptor antagonists

Acceptable indication but of uncertain efficacy and may be controversial
- Symptomatic treatment of patients with heart failure who do not tolerate ACE inhibitors.

NON-DIGITALIS INOTROPIC DRUGS

In congestive heart failure it is often apparent that the heart suffers from inotropic failure. It is therefore not surprising that vast effort has been invested in order to develop drugs that might increase contractility or the state of inotropy. Although several drugs with inotropic activity are available today, it has become increasingly evident that these drugs are associated with important negative effects.

There are inotropic agents in different classes according to their mode of action.[108] Cardiac glycosides affect sarcolemmal ions through the effects on ion channels or ion pumps. These drugs are covered in another section of this chapter. Other drugs increase the intracellular level of cyclic adenosine monophosphate (cAMP), either by receptor stimulation (beta-adrenergic agonists), or by decreasing cAMP breakdown (phosphodiesterase inhibitors). One class of agents affects intracellular calcium mechanisms by release of sarcoplasmic reticulum calcium, or by increasing the sensitivity of contractile proteins to calcium. Further, there are inotropic drugs with multiple mechanisms of action.

Beta-agonist drugs

DOBUTAMINE

Drugs with beta-receptor agonist properties induce an increase in intracellular cAMP activity by stimulation of cellular receptors. Already during the 1960s patients with cardiogenic shock were treated with beta-receptor agonists isoproterenol and norepinephrine.[109] It was realized that both drugs had potential negative effects, such as an increased risk for arrhythmias or – in the case of norepinephrine – an untoward vasoconstriction. The development of dobutamine, a drug which is a modification of the isoproterenol molecule, resulted in an agent with $beta_1$-, $beta_2$- and $alpha_1$-adrenergic activity.[110] Dobutamine induces vasodilation in combination with an increase in contractility, leading to an increase in stroke volume and cardiac output.[111–113] An enhancement of contractility is usually associated with an increase in myocardial oxygen consumption.[114] Side effects, such as arrhythmias or an unfavorable blood pressure response, are usually modest. Dobutamine can only be administered intravenously, in doses from 2 µg/kg/min up to 20–25 µg/kg/min.[115] It has been noticed that dobutamine may increase beta-receptor sensitivity.[116,117] However, prolonged infusion over 96 hours has been associated with a decrease in the hemodynamic effect by as much as 50%.[118] Beneficial short term action encouraged investigators to use the drug in patients with chronic heart failure on an outpatient basis. Intermittent therapy was found to increase quality of life and hemodynamics.[119] However, a clinical trial had to be stopped prematurely due to an increase in mortality in the dobutamine-treated group.[120]

DOPAMINE

Dopamine is an adrenergic agonist with predominantly $beta_1$-receptor activity.[121,122] This drug increases contractility with minor effects on heart rate or blood pressure. At low doses (0.5–2.0 µg/kg/min) dopamine acts on dopamine receptors, while at doses above 5.0 µg/kg/min it has effects through $beta_1$-receptors, and at higher doses also through alpha-receptors. Infusion at low doses causes dilation of smooth muscles in renal, mesenteric, and coronary arteries, leading to an increase in diuresis.[123,124]

IBOPAMINE

Ibopamine is an orally active dopaminergic agonist, with the active metabolite epinine N-methyldopamine acting on DA_1 and DA_2 receptors. This agent had positive hemodynamic effects in terms of an increase in cardiac output, a reduction in systemic vascular resistance, and no effect on heart rate.[125,126] In a study with digoxin and ibopamine in patients with mild to moderate chronic heart failure, it was observed that ibopamine had some positive effects in patients with less ventricular dysfunction, and no effects on mortality.[127] To evaluate the long-term effects of ibopamine a study (PRIME-II) was initiated in 1906 patients with NYHA class III–IV heart failure. However, the study was terminated prematurerly due to an increase in mortality in the ibopamine group: 25% in the ibopamine group died versus 20% in the placebo group ($P = 0.017$).[128]

XAMOTEROL

Xamoterol is a drug with beta-adrenergic blocking effects and high partial agonist activity. Long term effects are similar to other inotropic agents, and a multicenter trial had to be discontinued because of an increase in mortality in the active treatment group.[129]

Phosphodiesterase inhibitors

Through inhibition of cAMP breakdown, the phosphodiesterase inhibitors bypass the beta-receptor pathway. The first phosphodiesterase inhibitor was amrinone, a drug with inotropic and vasodilatory effects. During infusion, amrinone induced afterload reduction, a decrease in filling pressures, increase in cardiac index, and also an increased rate of contractility and relaxation.[130–132] The major side effect is thrombocytopenia. Similarly, the related agent milrinone has been found to enhance myocardial contractility, besides potent vasodilatory effects,[133–135] but without thrombocytopenia.[136] The short term effects of another agent – enoximone – have been similar to other phosphodiesterase inhibitors.[137–139] As phosphodiesterase inhibitors elicit intracellular effects through other pathways than beta-adrenergic drugs, it has been hypothesized that the combination of these two classes of drugs would enhance myocardial performance. Results from clinical trials have supported this concept.[140,141]

Whereas short term administration may improve myocardial performance and clinical condition in congestive heart failure,[135,142] the long term effects of phosphodiesterase inhibitors have been discouraging. Oral phosphodiesterase administration has been tested in several trials with chronic heart failure, all of which have demonstrated no beneficial effect or a substantial increase in mortality in patients receiving the investigated drug.[16,143–145]

Calcium-sensitizing drugs

Pimobendan is the most thoroughly studied drug in this class of inotropics. The effect is mediated by an increase in the affinity of troponin C for intracellular calcium.[146,147] Pimobendan inhibits phosphodiesterase and thereby has effects similar to milrinone.[146,148] In clinical trials pimobendan has been shown to exert improvement in cardiac index, exercise performance and quality of life.[149,150] However, treatment effects did not show congruity among different doses, and there was also a tendency toward increased mortality in a large 24 week trial.[151]

660

Levosimendan is a newer calcium-sensitizing agent with properties similar to pimobendan, but only limited data are available so far.[152,153]

Vesnarinone is a drug with muliple actions. It is a synthetic quinolinone derivative that in part inhibits phosphodiesterase, with simultaneous effects on transmembrane ion transports. This drug seemed to have effects on contractility without increasing the heart rate,[154,155] which made it an interesting candidate for long term therapy in heart failure. Furthermore, it was demonstrated that vesnarinone might inhibit the production of cytokines, including tumor necrosis factor (TNF-α).[156] A large trial with two doses of vesnarinone was started in 1989. Whereas the 120 mg treatment arm had to be stopped prematurely due to a significant increase in mortality in the active treatment group, the 60 mg group continued. Unexpectedly, by completion of the study it was shown that 60 mg of vesnarinone was associated with a marked 50% reduction in mortality risk ($P=0.003$).[157] This study was followed by a larger placebo-controlled trial (VEST), with 3800 patients. However, preliminary evaluation by the the Data Safety and Monitoring Committee has determined a 26% increase in mortality in patients treated with 60 mg of vesnarinone, and the study was terminated.[158]

Documented value of inotropic drugs

Proven indication: always acceptable

- Short term improvement of symptoms in patients with severe heart failure.
- Bridging towards more definitive surgical treatment, such as cardiac transplantation.

Acceptable indication but of uncertain efficacy and may be controversial

- Intermittent short term treatment in chronic heart failure.

Not proven: potentially harmful (contraindicated)

- Long term treatment in chronic heart failure. May increase mortality risk.

It should be obvious from the summary above that different inotropic drugs, with a wide variety of modes of action, may improve symptoms and cardiac function on a short term basis. However, inotropic drugs increase the risk of mortality. Whether these detrimental long term effects could be abolished in the development of any other compound is unclear.

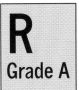

R
Grade A

BETA-ADRENERGIC BLOCKADE

Clinicians have generally been cautious in using beta-blockers in patients with congestive heart failure, even though investigators in the early 1970s were already proposing a possible beneficial effect of beta-blockers in such cases.[159,160] However, data have been gathered during recent years indicating that this class of drugs may have significant contribution to make in the heart failure treatment armamentarium of the near future.

Early case reports suggested that beta-blockers had a potential to elicit overt heart failure in some cases.[161,162] However, although the possibility of such an adverse reaction has been of concern, there are no placebo-controlled trials that have proved that beta-blockers are detrimental in congestive heart failure. On the contrary, analysis of several myocardial infarction studies has shown that patients with signs of congestive heart failure showed a similar or better response to beta-blockers than did patients without heart failure.[163–165]

Hemodynamic effects

The short term effects of beta-adrenergic blockade differs markedly from the long term effects, which might be one explanation for the difficulties in understanding the mode of action during long term therapy. After intravenous administration there is a rapid reduction in heart rate, contractility and blood pressure, with ensuing fall in cardiac output.[166–169] However, intraventricular volumes, stroke volume, and ejection fraction are unaffected.[167,168] Beta-blockers with vasodilating properties cause an acute reduction in afterload with reduction in filling pressures.[166,167] During 1–3 months of treatment, positive diastolic effects have been observed and these effects probably precede full effects on cardiac systolic function.[168,170]

During long term treatment (3–12 months), beta-blockers induce myocardial improvement, as expressed by an increase in ejection fraction, cardiac output, and exercise capacity.[171–175] Similar to the effects of ACE inhibitors, beta-blockers appear to attenuate left ventricular remodeling.[176–178]

Effects of neurohormones

Acute administration of metoprolol causes a reflex increase in peripheral catecholamines without alterations of the transmyocardial gradient.[168] Using radioactive labeling of norepinephrine, the non-selective beta-blocker propranolol was shown to reduce myocardial norepinephrine spillover as compared to the beta$_1$-selective blocker metoprolol.[179] There are sparse data on the long term effects of beta-adrenergic blockade on neurohormonal activation, but some studies suggest a beneficial reduction in peripheral norepinephrine level.[180–184]

Effects on quality of life and hospitalizations

A reduction of the need for hospitalizations has been demonstrated in studies with bisoprolol,[185] metoprolol,[186] and carvedilol.[187] Quality of life was improved in the Metoprolol in Dilated Cardiomyopathy (MDC) trial.[186] Whereas both patient and physician global assessments of heart failure symptoms improved, quality of life scores were not improved in the US carvedilol studies.[188,189] In the Australian–New Zealand study there was a tendency towards worse symptoms.[177] A health economic analysis has been performed on the MDC study data, suggesting an improved cost–benefit ratio for patients on metoprolol.[190] Further, carvedilol and metoprolol have been shown to reduce the progression towards overt heart failure.[177,186,188] In a substudy of RESOLVD, there was an early increase in heart failure hospitalizations with the use of metoprolol CR. However, over time, this difference decreased substantially. There was no difference in all causes of hospitalizations (S. Yusuf, personal communication).

Effects on survival

There is as yet no published study that has been specifically designed to test the effect of beta-adrenergic blockade on mortality in congestive heart failure. One of the first studies of beta-blockers in congestive heart failure showed a reduced mortality in patients treated by beta-blockade as compared to historical controls.[159] Not until 1993, when the MDC trial was published, did additional information on hard endpoints become available. This study showed a trend towards a 34% reduction in the combined endpoint deaths and need for heart transplantation ($P=0.058$), in 383 patients with idiopathic dilated cardiomyopathy, treated with placebo or metoprolol.[186] A late follow-up of this study has recently demonstrated that this trend was also maintained, or possibly reinforced, regarding all-cause mortality and actual cardiac transplantations 3 years after randomization.[191] In the CIBIS study, bisoprolol was used in a placebo-controlled trial in 641 patients. Overall there was a non-significant reduction in mortality (RR 0.80, 95% CI 0.56–1.15), whereas a subgroup of patients without a previous myocardial infarction had a more pronounced reduction in mortality (12% vs 22.5%, $P=0.01$).[185] Four combined studies in the United States, investigating different effects of carvedilol in a total of 1094 patients with varying degrees of heart failure, demonstrated a lower mortality ($P=0.0001$). In the recent RESOLVD substudy there was a favorable effect on mortality ($P=0.052$).[187] However, there was no statistically beneficial effect of carvedilol regarding survival in the ANZ trial in 415 patients with chronic heart failure of varying etiology.[192] None of the aforementioned trials were designed to specifically study mortality. Although a recent meta-analyses on collective available data support the view that beta-blockers are beneficial for long term survival in heart failure patients,[193,194] this requires confirmation in well-designed large trials. Presently, there are four ongoing trials testing the hypothesis that beta-blockers would improve survival in patients with chronic heart failure. Bisoprolol is tested in the CIBIS II study, bucindolol in the BEST study, metoprolol in the MERIT trial, and carvedilol vs metoprolol in the COMET trial. When all these four survival studies are concluded – comprising more than 12 000 patients – beta-blockers will be one of the most thoroughly investigated drugs in congestive heart failure.

Documented value of beta-blockers

Proven indication: always acceptable

- To improve cardiac function and symptoms in patients with symptomatic chronic heart failure, already on conventional treatment with ACE inhibitors, diuretics or digitalis.
- Patients with acute myocardial infarction and mild to moderate symptoms of congestive heart failure.

Acceptable indication but of uncertain efficacy and may be controversial

- Symptomatic heart failure due to diastolic dysfunction.
- To improve long term survival in patients with heart failure.

Not proven: potentially harmful (contraindicated)

- Acute decompensated heart failure.
- Congestive heart failure with pronounced hypotension and/or bradycardia.

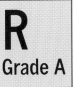

Clinical perspective

DRUG TITRATION AND INTOLERANCE

Due to initial negative inotropic effects, treatment with beta-blockers requires a slow titration procedure. Parallel to myocardial recovery beta-blocker dosages can usually safely be increased. It has been noticed that patients with simultaneous marked hypotension and tachycardia, expressing severe decompensation, may not tolerate beta-blockers. Nevertheless, figures of intolerance have been low in randomized trials, comparable to those of ACE inhibitors. Starting doses with different beta-blockers have been: bisoprolol 1.25 mg o.d.; carvedilol 3.125–6.25 mg b.d.; metoprolol 5 mg b.d. or 25 mg o.d. Doses are increased every 1–2 weeks, when doses are doubled, until maintenance doses of full conventional beta-blockade are achieved.

Although a reduction in heart rate probably is important, it has not been possible to adequately identify responders from non-responders to beta-blocker therapy. In cases with significant obstructive pulmonary disease, beta-blockers should be used with caution, and a selective beta-blocker would be preferred.

ANTIARRHYTHMIC DRUGS IN HEART FAILURE

Although progressive pump dysfunction is a common cause of death in heart failure, sudden death is probably the most common reason, and has been considered responsible in 25–50% of all deaths.[195–198] Besides a few cases of primary asystole, the majority of sudden deaths are due to ventricular arrhythmias.[199] The issue of antiarrhythmic therapy in heart failure patients has therefore been of major interest. Internal cardioversion defibrillators are now used for prevention of sudden death due to ventricular arrhythmias, and the use of these therapeutic devices is dealt with elsewhere in this book.

Most antiarrhythmics cause a depression of left ventricular function. Although frequent and complex ventricular arrhythmias may be predictive of sudden death, left ventricular dysfunction is a more powerful predictor.[200] Furthermore, these drugs may have a proarrhythmic effect, especially in cases of left ventricular dysfunction. In the CAST study the efficacy of antiarrhythmic drugs in patients with left ventricular dysfunction after myocardial infarction and with complex ventricular arrhythmias was evaluated. Patients who responded with attenuation of arrhythmias after drug testing were randomized to encainide, flecainide, or moricizine. The results showed an increase in mortality in patients treated with these agents.[201] Amiodarone is a class III antiarrhythmic drug with no or little negative inotropic effect. Previous promising smaller trials encouraged larger trials, such as the GESICA study. In this study, 516 patients with heart failure on conventional treatment were randomized to open label amiodarone treatment ($n = 260$) or conventional treatment ($n = 256$). Both sudden deaths and deaths due to heart failure were reduced, comprising in total 87 deaths in patients on amiadorone and 106 in the placebo group ($P = 0.02$).[202] However, these results were not reproduced in another study in patients with congestive heart failure and asymptomatic ventricular arrhythmias.[203] In this study 674 patients were investigated, but amiodarone treatment was not associated with reduction of overall mortality or mortality due to sudden death. Two other parallel studies have recently been finished, in which amiodarone was used in patients with a recent myocardial infarction and left ventricular dysfunction.[204,205] In addition, patients in the CAMIAT study had complex ventricular arrhythmias. Although all-cause mortality was not significantly lower in the treatment groups, both studies showed a reduction in arrhythmic deaths. A meta-analysis of all amiodarone trials demonstrated a significant reduction in mortality (Amiodarone Pooling Project – trial results to be published).

Sotalol, a beta-blocker with class III antiarrhythmic properties, has not been found to reduce deaths from ventricular arrhythmias. On the contrary, a study with the non beta-blocker isoform *d*-sotalol in post-MI patients had to be terminated in advance because of an increased mortality in the sotalol group.[206]

ACE inhibitors reduce the risk of progressive heart failure deaths. The possibility of ACE inhibitors to affect arrhythmias has been reviewed.[207] In some of the heart failure trials there has also been a reduction in the rate of sudden deaths.[74,208] However, these findings were not confirmed in the SOLVD trial.[209]

Documented value of antiarrhythmic therapy in heart failure

Proven indication: always acceptable

- No proven indication.

Acceptable indication but of uncertain efficacy and may be controversial

- The use of amiodarone in patients with ventricular arrhythmias after myocardial infarction.
- Beta-adrenergic blockade in patients with ischemic heart failure.
- Class I antiarrhythmic drugs in patients with symptomatic ventricular arrhythmias.

Not proven: potentially harmful (contraindicated)

- Class I antiarrhythmic drugs in patients with asymptomatic ventricular arrhythmias.
- Class III antiarrhythmic drugs, besides amiodarone.

Table 40.1 Key recommendations

Aim of treatment	Class of drug	Level of evidence
Symptomatic improvement of congestion, improvement of exercise capacity	Diuretics	Grade A
Improvement of symptoms, exercise capacity, and decreased hospitalization	Digitalis	Grade A
Improvement of survival, symptoms and exercise capacity, and reduced morbidity, in patients with asymptomatic and symptomatic left ventricular systolic dysfunction	Angiotensin converting enzyme inhibitors	Grade A
Symptomatic treatment of patients with heart failure who do not tolerate ACE inhibitors	Angiotensin II receptor antagonists	Grade A
Short-term improvement of symptoms in patients with severe congestive heart failure. Bridging towards more definitive surgical treatment, such as cardiac transplantation	Non-digitalis inotropic drugs	Grade A
Improvement of cardiac function and symptoms in patients with symptomatic chronic heart failure, already on conventional treatment	Beta-adrenergic blockers	Grade A
Improvement of survival	Beta-adrenergic blockers	Grade A
Prevention of arrhythmic deaths in patients with symptomatic ventricular arrhythmias	Amiodarone	Grade A

REFERENCES

1 Ribner B, Plucinski DA, Hsieh AM *et al.* Acute effects of digoxin on total systemic vascular resistance in congestive heart failure due to dilated cardiomyopathy. *Am J Cardiol* 1985;**56**: 896.

2 Gheorghiade M, St Clair J, St Clair C, Beller GA. Hemodynamic effects of intravenous digoxin in patients with severe heart failure initially treated with diuretics and vasodilators. *J Am Coll Cardiol* 1987;**9**:849.

3 Cohn K, Selzer A, Kersh ES *et al.* Variability of hemodynamic response to acute digitalization in chronic cardiac failure due to cardiomyopathy and coronary artery disease. *Am J Cardiol* 1975; **31**:461.

4 Braunwald E. Effects of digitalis on the normal and the failing heart. *J Am Coll Cardiol* 1985;**5**: 51A.

5 Ferguson DW, Berg WJ, Sanders JS *et al.* Sympathoinhibitory responses to digitalis glycosides in heart failure patients. *Circulation* 1989;**80**:65–77.

6 Ferguson DW. Baroreflex-mediated circulatory control in human heart failure. *Heart Failure* 1990;**6**:3.

7 Goldsmith SR, Simon AB, Miller E. Effect of digitalis on norepinephrine kinetics in congestive heart failure. *J Am Coll Cardiol* 1992;**20**:858–63.

8 Dobbs SN, Kenyon WI, Dobbs RJ. Maintenance digoxin after an episode of heart failure. Placebo controlled trial in outpatients. *Br Med J* 1977; **1**:749.

9 Fleg L, Gottlieb SH, Lakatta EG. Is digoxin really important in compensated heart failure? *Am J Med* 1982;**73**:244.

10 Taggart AJ, Johnston GD, McDevitt DG. Digoxin withdrawal after cardiac failure in patients with sinus rhythm. *J Cardiovasc Pharmacol* 1983;**5**: 229.

11 Lee DCS, Johnston RA, Bingham JB *et al.* Heart failure in outpatients. A randomized trial of digoxin versus placebo. *N Engl J Med* 1982;**306**: 699.

12 Guyatt GH, Sullivan MJJ, Fallen EL *et al.* A controlled trial of digoxin in congestive heart failure. *Am J Cardiol* 1988;**61**:371.

13 Haerer W, Bauer U, Hetzel M, Fehske J. Long-term effects of digoxin and diuretics in congestive heart failure. Results of a placebo-controlled randomized double-blind study. *Circulation* 1988;**78**:53.

14 The Captopril–Digoxin Multicenter Research Group. Comparative effects of therapy with captopril and digoxin in patients with mild moderate heart failure. *JAMA* 1988;**259**: 539–44.

15 German and Austrian Xamoterol Study Group. Double-blind placebo-controlled comparison of digoxin and xamoterol in chronic heart failure. *Lancet* 1988;**i**:489.

16 DiBianco R, Shabetai R, Kostuk W *et al.* A comparison of oral milrinone, digoxin, and their combination in the treatment of patients with chronic heart failure. *N Engl J Med* 1989;**320**: 677–83.

17 Uretsky BF, Young JB, Shahidi FE *et al.* Randomized study assessing the effect of digoxin withdrawal in patients with mild to moderate chronic congestive heart failure: results of the PROVED Trial. *J Am Coll Cardiol* 1993;**22**: 955–62.

18 Packer M, Gheorghiade M, Young JB *et al.* Withdrawal of digoxin from patients with chronic heart failure treated with angiotensin-converting enzyme inhibitors. *N Engl J Med* 1993;**329**:1–7.

19 Perry G, Brown E, Thornton R *et al.* The effect of digoxin on mortality and morbidity in patients with heart failure. *N Engl J Med* 1997;**336**: 525–33.

20 Stason WR, Cannon PJ, Heinemann HO, Laragh JH. Furosemide: a clinical evaluation of diuretic action. *Circulation* 1966;**34**:910–20.

21 Cody RJ, Ljungman S, Covit AB *et al.* Regulation of glomerular filtration rate in chronic congestive heart failure patients. *Kidney Int* 1988;**34**:361–7.

22 Francis GS, Goldsmith SR, Levine TB, Olivari MT, Cohn JN. The neurohumoral axis in congestive heart failure. *Ann Intern Med* 1984;**101**:370–7.

23 Lal S, Murtagw JG, Pollock AM, Fletcher E, Binnion PF. Acute hemodynamic effects of furosemide in patients with normal and raised left atrial pressures. *Br Heart J* 1969;**31**:711–17.

24 Stampfer M, Epstein SE, Beiser D, Braunwald E. Haemodynamic effects of diuresis at rest and during intense uprights exercise in patients with impaired cardiac function. *Circulation* 1968;**37**: 900–11.

25 Magrini F, Niarchos AP. Hemodynamic effects of massive peripheral edema. *Am Heart J* 1983; **105**:90–4.

26 Francis GS, Siegel RM, Goldsmith SR *et al.* Acute vasoconstrictor response to intravenous furosemide in patients with chronic congestive heart failure. *Ann Intern Med* 1985;**103**:1–6.

27 Dikshit K, Vyden JK, Forrester JS *et al.* Renal and extrarenal hemodynamic effects of furosemide in congestive heart failure after myocardial infarction. *N Engl J Med* 1973;**288**:1087–90.

28 Nelson GIC, Ahuja RC, Silke B, Taylor SH. Haemodynamic effects of furosemide and its influence on repetitive rapid volume loading in acute myocardial infarction. *Eur Heart J* 1983; **4**:706–11.

29 Verma SP, Silke B, Reynolds G *et al.* Immediate effects of bumetanide on systemic haemodynamics and left ventricular volume in acute and chronic heart failure. *Br J Clin Pharmacol* 1987;**24**:21–32.

30 Ramirez A, Abelman WH. Haemodynamic effects of diuresis by ethacrynic acid. *Ann Intern Med* 1968;**121**:320–7.

31 Valette H, Hebert JL, Apoil E. Acute haemodynamic effects of a single intravenous dose of piretanide in congestive heart failure. *Eur J Clin Pharmacol* 1983;**24**:163–7.

32 Fiehring H, Achhammer I. Influence of 10 mg torasemide iv and 20 mg furosemide iv on the intracardiac pressures in patients with heart failure at rest and during exercise. *Prog Pharmacol Clin Pharmacol* 1990;**8**:87–104.

33 Mackay IG, Muir AL, Watson ML. Contribution of prostaglandins to the systemic and renal vascular response to frusemide in normal man. *Br J Clin Pharmacol* 1984;**17**:513–19.

34 Ikram H, Chan W, Espiner EA, Nicholls ME. Haemodynamic and humoral responses to acute and chronic frusemide therapy in congestive heart failure. *Clin Sci* 1980;**59**:443–9.

35 Haerer W, Bauer U, Sultan N. Acute and chronic effects of a diuretic monotherapy with piretanide in congestive heart failure – a placebo controlled trial. *Cardiovasc Drugs Ther* 1990;**4**:515–22.

36 Podszus T, Piesche L. Effect of torasemide on pulmonary and cardiac haemodynamics after oral treatment of chronic heart failure. *Prog Pharmacol Clin Pharmacol* 1990;**8**:157–66.

37 Cheitlin MD, Byrd R, Benowitz N. Amiloride improves haemodynamics in patients with chronic congestive heart failure treated with chronic digoxin and diuretics. *Cardiovasc Drugs Ther* 1991;**5**:719–26.

38 Francis GS, Benedict C, Johnstone DE *et al.* Comparison of neuroendocrine activation in patients with left ventricular dysfunction with and without congestive heart failure. *Circulation* 1990;**82**:1724–9.

39 Bayliss J, Norell M, Canepa-Anson R, Sutton G, Poole-Wilson P. Untreated heart failure: clinical and neuroendocrine effects of introducing diuretics. *Br Heart J* 1987;**57**:17–22.

40 Achhammer I. Long-term efficacy and tolerance of torasemide in congestive heart failure. *Prog Pharmacol Clin Pharmacol* 1990;**8**:127–36.

41 Dusing R, Piesche L. Second-line therapy of congestive heart failure with torasemide. *Prog Pharmacol Clin Pharmacol* 1990;**8**:105–20.

42 Odemuyiwa O, Gilmartin J, Kenny D, Hall RJC. Captopril and the diuretic requirements in moderate and severe chronic heart failure. *Eur Heart J* 1989;**10**:586.

43 Anand IS, Kalra GS, Ferrari R *et al.* Enalapril as initial and sole treatment in severe chronic heart failure with sodium retention. *Int J Cardiol* 1990;**28**:341.

44 Richardson A, Bayliss J, Scriven AJ *et al.* Double-blind comparison of captopril alone against furosemide plus amiloride in mild heart failure. *Lancet* 1987;**ii**:709.

45 Cody RJ, Kubo SH, Pickworth KK. Diuretic treatment for the sodium retention of congestive heart failure. *Arch Intern Med* 1994;**154**:1905–14.

46 Pitt B. The randomized aldactone evaluation study (RALES). Parallel dose finding study. *J Am Coll Cardiol* 1995;**25**:45A.

47 Eichna LW, Sobel BJ, Kessler RH. Hemodynamic and renal effects produced in congestive heart failure by the intravenous administration of a ganglionic blocking agent. *Trans Assoc Am Phys* 1956;**69**:207–13.

48 Burch GE. Evidence for increased venous tone in chronic heart failure. *Arch Intern Med* 1956;**98**:750–66.

49 Zelis R, Mason DT, Braunwald E. A comparison of the effects of vasodilator stimuli on peripheral resistance vessels in normal subjects and in patients with congestive heart failure. *J Clin Invest* 1968;**47**:960–70.

50 Majid PA, Sharma B, Taylor SH. Phentolamine for vasodilator treatment of severe heart failure. *Lancet* 1971;**ii**:719–24.

51 Franciosa JA, Guiha NH, Limas CJ, Rodriguera E, Cohn JN. Improved left ventricular function during nitroprusside infusion in acute myocardial infarction. *Lancet* 1972;**i**:650–4.

52 Cohn JN, Franciosa JA. Vasodilator therapy of cardiac failure. *N Engl J Med* 1977;**297**:27–31.

53 Tsai SC, Adamik R, Manganiello VC, Moss J. Effects of nitroprusside and nitroglycerin on cGMP content and PGI#v2#v formation in aorta and vena cava. *Biochem Pharmacol* 1989;**38**:61–5.

54 Lavine SJ, Campbell CA, Held AC, Johnson V. Effect of nitroglycerin-induced reduction of left ventricular filling pressure on diastolic filling in acute dilated heart failure. *J Am Coll Cardiol* 1989;**14**:233–41.

55 Mason DT, Braunwald E. The effects of nitroglycerin and amyl nitrate on arteriolar and venous tone in the human forearm. *Circulation* 1965;**32**:755–65.

56 Armstrong PW, Armstrong JA, Marks GS. Pharmacokinetic-hemodynamic studies of intravenous nitroglycerin in congestive heart failure. *Circulation* 1980;**62**:160–6.

57 Leier CV, Bambach D, Thompson MJ *et al.* Central and regional hemodynamic effects of intravenous isosorbide dinitrate, nitroglycerin, and nitroprusside in patients with congestive heart failure. *Am J Cardiol* 1981;**48**:1115–23.

58 Flaherty JT, Reid PR, Kelly DT *et al*. Intravenous nitroglycerin in acute myocardial infarction. *Circulation* 1975;**51**:132–9.

59 Ludbrook PR, Byrne JD, Kurnik PB, McKnight RC. Influence of reduction of preload and afterload by nitroglycerin on left ventricular diastolic pressure-volume relation and relaxation in man. *Circulation* 1977;**56**:937–43.

60 DeMarco T, Chatterjee K, Rouleau JL, Parmley WW. Abnormal coronary hemodynamics and myocardial energetics in patients with chronic heart failure caused by ischemic heart disease and dilated cardiomyopathy. *Am Heart J* 1988; **115**:809–15.

61 Unverferth DV, Magorien RD, Lewis RP, Leier CV. The role of subendocardial ischemia in perpetuating myocardial failure in patients with nonischemic congestive cardiomyopathy. *Am Heart J* 1983;**105**:176–9.

62 Chiariello M, Gold HK, Leinbach RC, David MA, Maroko PR. Comparison between the effects of nitroprusside and nitroglycerin on ischemic injury during acute myocardial infarction. *Circulation* 1976;**54**:766–73.

63 Stevenson LW, Dracup KA, Tillisch JH. Efficacy of medical therapy tailored for severe congestive heart failure in patients transferred for urgent cardiac transplantation. *Am J Cardiol* 1989;**63**: 461–4.

64 Chatterjee K, Ports TA, Brundage BH *et al*. Oral hydralazine in chronic heart failure: sustained beneficial hemodynamic effects. *Ann Intern Med* 1980;**92**:600–4.

65 Franciosa JA, Nordstrom LA, Cohn JN. Nitrate therapy for congestive heart failure. *JAMA* 1978; **240**:443–6.

66 Miller RR, Awan NA, Maxwell KS, Mason DT. Sustained reduction of cardiac impedance and preload in congestive heart failure with the antihypertensive vasodilator prazosin. *N Engl J Med* 1977;**297**:303–7.

67 Franciosa JA, Jordan RA, Wilen MM, Leddy CL. Minoxidil in patients with chronic left heart failure: contrasting hemodynamic and clinical effects in a controlled trial. *Circulation* 1984;**70**: 63–8.

68 Leier CV, Desch CE, Magorien RD *et al*. Positive inotropic effects of hydralazine in human subjects. Comparison with prazosin in the setting of congestive heart failure. *Am J Cardiol* 1980; **46**:1039–44.

69 Rouleau JL, Chatterjee K, Benge W, Parmley WW, Hiramatsu B. Alterations in left ventricular function and coronary hemodynamics with captopril, hydralazine, and prazosin in chronic ischemic heart failure, a comparative study. *Circulation* 1982;**65**:671–8.

70 Daly P, Rouleau JL, Cousineau D, Burgess JH, Chatterjee K. Effects of captopril and a combination of hydralazine and isosorbide dinitrate on myocardial sympathetic tone in patients with severe congestive heart failure. *Br Heart J* 1986;**56**:152–7.

71 Magorien RD, Unverferth DV, Brown GP, Leier CV. Dobutamine and hydralazine. Comparative influences of positive inotropy and vasodilation on coronary blood flow and myocardial energetics in nonischemic congestive heart failure. *J Am Coll Cardiol* 1983;**1**:499–505.

72 Massie B, Chatterjee K, Werner J *et al*. Hemodynamic advantage of combined administration of hydralazine orally and nitrates nonparenterally in the vasodilator therapy of chronic heart failure. *Am J Cardiol* 1977;**40**: 794–801.

73 Packer M, Meller J, Medina N, Yushak M, Gorlin R. Provocation of myocardial ischemia events during initiation of vasodilator therapy for severe chronic heart failure. Clinical and hemodynamic evaluation of 52 consecutive patients with ischemic cardiomyopathy. *Am J Cardiol* 1981; **48**:939–46.

74 Cohn JN, Johnson G, Ziesche S *et al*. A comparison of enalapril with hydralazine-isosorbide dinitrate in the treatment of chronic congestive heart failure. *N Engl J Med* 1991; **325**:303–10.

75 Elkayam U, Amin J, Mehra A *et al*. A prospective, randomized, double-blind, crossover study to compare the efficacy and safety of chronic nifedipine therapy with that of isosorbide dinitrate and their combination in the treatment of chronic congestive heart failure. *Circulation* 1990;**82**:1954–61.

76 Danish Study Group on Verapamil in Myocardial Infarction. Secondary prevention with verapamil after myocardial infarction. *Am J Cardiol* 1990; **66**:331–401.

77 Iida K, Matsuda M, Ajisaka R *et al*. Effects of nifedipine on left ventricular systolic and diastolic function in patients with ischemic heart disease. *Jpn Heart J* 1987;**28**:495–506.

78 Barjon JN, Rouleau JL, Bichet D, Juneau C, De Champlain J. Chronic renal and neurohumoral effects of the calcium-entry blocker nisoldipine in patients with congestive heart failure. *J Am Coll Cardiol* 1987;**9**:622–30.

79 Gheorghiade M, Hall V, Goldberg D, Levine TB, Goldstein S. Long-term clinical and neurohormonal effects of nicardipine in patients with severe heart failure on maintenance therapy with angiotensin converting enzyme inhibitors. *J Am Coll Cardiol* 1991;**17**:274A.

80 Dunselman PHJM, Kuntze CEE, Van Bruggen A *et al*. Efficacy of felodipine in congestive heart failure. *Eur Heart J* 1989;**10**:354–64.

81 Cohn JN, Archibald DG, Ziesche S *et al*. Effect of vasodilator therapy on mortality in chronic

congestive heart failure. *N Engl J Med* 1986; **314**:1547–52.

82 Cohn JN, Ziesche SM, Loss LE *et al.* Effect of felodipine on short-term exercise and neurohormone and long-term mortality in heart failure. Results of V-HeFT III. *Circulation* (In press).

83 Packer M, O'Connor CM, Ghali JK *et al.* Effect of amlodipine on morbidity and mortality in severe chronic heart failure. *N Engl J Med* 1996;**335**:1107–14.

84 Packer M, Rouleau J, Swedberg K *et al.* Effect of flosequinan on survival in chronic heart failure. *Circulation* 1993;**88**:301.

85 McKenna WJ, Swedberg K, Zannad F *et al.* Experience of chronic intravenous epoprostenol infusion in end-stage cardiac failure: results of FIRST. *Eur Heart J* 1994;**15**:I-36.

86 Sharpe DN, Murphy J, Coxon R, Hannan SF. Enalapril in patients with chronic heart failure: a placebo-controlled, randomized, double-blind study. *Circulation* 1984;**70**:271–8.

87 DiCarlo L, Chatterjee K, Parmley WW *et al.* Enalapril A new angiotensin converting inhibitor in chronic heart failure: acute and chronic hemodynamic evaluations. *J Am Coll Cardiol* 1983;**2**:865–71.

88 Packer M, Medina N, Yushak M, Lee WH. Usefulness of plasma renin activity in predicting haemodynamic and clinical responses and survival during long term converting enzyme inhibition in severe chronic heart failure. Experience in 100 consecutive patients. *Br Heart J* 1985;**54**:298–304.

89 The Consensus Trial Study Group. Effects of enalapril on mortality in severe congestive heart failure. *N Engl J Med* 1987;**316**:1429–35.

90 Sharpe N, Murphy J, Heather S, Hannan S. Treatment of patients with symptomless left ventricular dysfunction after myocardial infarction. *Lancet* 1988;i:255–9.

91 Pfeffer JM, Pfeffer MA. Angiotensin converting enzyme inhibition and ventricular remodeling in heart failure. *Am J Med* 1988;**84**:37–44.

92 Swedberg K, Eneroth P, Kjekshus J, Wilhelmsen L, for the CONSENSUS Trial Study Group. Hormones regulating cardiovascular function in patients with severe congestive heart failure and their relation to mortality. *Circulation* 1990;**82**:1730–6.

93 Packer M. The neurohormonal hypothesis: a theory to explain the mechanism of disease progression in heart failure. *J Am Coll Cardiol* 1992;**20**:248–54.

94 The SOLVD Investigators. Effect of enalapril on mortality and the development of heart failure in asymptomatic patients with reduced left ventricular ejection fractions. *N Engl J Med* 1992;**327**:685–91.

95 Rogers WJ, Johnstone DE, Yusuf S *et al.* Quality of life among 5025 patients with left ventricular dysfunction randomized between placebo and enalapril: the studies of left ventricular dysfunction. *J Am Coll Cardiol* 1994;**23**:393–400.

96 Pfeffer MA, Braunwald E, Moyé LA *et al.* Effect of captopril on mortality and morbidity in patients with left ventricular dysfunction after myocardial infarction. *N Engl J Med* 1992;**327**:669–77.

97 Kober L, Torp-Pedersen C, Carlsen JE *et al.* A clinical trial of the angiotensin-converting-enzyme inhibitor trandolapril in patients with left ventricular dysfunction after myocardial infarction. *N Engl J Med* 1995;**333**:1670–6.

98 The Acute Infarction Ramipril Efficacy (AIRE) Study Investigators. Effect of ramipril on mortality and morbidity of survivors of acute myocardial infarction with clinical evidence of heart failure. *Lancet* 1993;**342**:821–8.

99 Narang R, Swedberg K, Cleland JG. What is the ideal study design for evaluation of treatment for heart failure? Insights from trials assessing the effect of ACE inhibitors on exercise capacity. *Eur Heart J* 1996;**17**:120–34.

100 Garg R, Yusuf S. Overview of randomized trials of angiotensin-converting enzyme inhibitors on mortality and morbidity in patients with heart failure. *JAMA* 1995;**273**:1450–6.

101 Yusuf S, Pepine CJ, Garces C *et al.* Effect of enalapril on myocardial infarction and unstable angina in patients with low ejection fractions. *Lancet* 1992;**340**:1173–8.

102 Paul SD, Kuntz KM, Eagle KA, Weinstein MC. Costs and effectiveness of angiotensin converting enzyme inhibition in patients with congestive heart failure. *Arch Intern Med* 1994;**154**:1143–9.

103 Tsevat J, Duke D, Goldman L *et al.* Cost effectiveness, of captopril therapy after myocardial infarction. *J Am Coll Cardiol* 1995;**26**:914–19.

104 Martinez C, Ball SG. Cost effectiveness of ramipril therapy for patients with clinical evidence of heart failure after acute myocardial infarction. *Br J Clin Pract* 1995;**78**(Suppl):26–32.

105 McMurray J, Davie A. The pharmacoeconomics of ACE inhibitors in chronic heart failure. *Pharmacoeconomics* 1996;**9**:188–97.

106 Dickstein K, Chang P, Willenheimer *et al.* Comparison of the effects of losartan and enalapril on clinical status and exercise performance in patients with moderate or severe chronic heart failure. *J Am Coll Cardiol* 1995;**26**:438–45.

107 Pitt B, Segal R, Martinez FA *et al.* Randomised trial of losartan versus captopril in patients over

65 with heart failure (Evaluation of losartan in the elderly study, ELITE). *Lancet* 1997;**349:** 747–52.

108 Feldman AM. Classification of positive inotropic agents. *J Am Coll Cardiol* 1993;**22:**1233–7.

109 Smith JH, Oriol A, Morch J *et al.* Hemodynamic studies in cardiogenic shock. Treatment with isoproterenol and metaraminol. *Circulation* 1967;**35:**1084–91.

110 Tuttle RR, Mills J. Dobutamine. Development of a new catecholamine to selectively increase cardiac contractility. *Circ Res* 1975;**36:**185–96.

111 Meyer SL, Curry GC, Donsky MS *et al.* Influence of dobutamine on hemodynamics and coronary blood flow in patients with and without coronary artery disease. *Am J Cardiol* 1976;**38:**103–8.

112 Akhtar N, Midulic E, Cohn JN, Chaudry MH. Hemodynamic effect of dobutamine in patients with severe heart failure. *Am J Cardiol* 1975;**36:** 202–5.

113 Leier CV, Webel J, Buch CA. The cardiovascular effects of the continuous infusion of dobutamine in patients with severe cardiac failure. *Circulation* 1977;**56:**468–72.

114 Pozen RG, DiBianco R, Katz RJ *et al.* Myocardial metabolic and hemodynamic effects of dobutamine in heart failure complicating coronary artery disease. *Circulation* 1981;**63:** 1279–85.

115 Leier CV, Unverferth DV, Kates RE. The relationship between plasma dobutamine concentrations and cardiovascular responses in cardiac failure. *Am J Med* 1979;**66:**238–42.

116 Colucci WS, Denniss AR, Leatherman GF. Intracoronary infusion of dobutamine to patients with and without severe congestive heart failure. *J Clin Invest* 1988;**81:**1103–10.

117 Bristow MR, Port JD, Hershberger RE, Gilbert EM, Feldman AM. The β-adrenergic receptor-adenylate cyclase complex as a target for therapeutic intervention in heart failure. *Eur Heart J* 1989;**10:**45–54.

118 Unverferth DV, Blanford M, Kates RE, Leier VI. Tolerance to dobutamine after a 72-hour continuous infusion. *Am J Med* 1980;**69:**262–6.

119 Applefeld MM, Newman KA, Grove WR *et al.* Intermittent continuous outpatient dobutamine infusion in the management of congestive heart failure. *Am J Cardiol* 1983;**51:**455–8.

120 Dies F, Krell MJ, Whitlow P *et al.* Intermittent dobutamine in ambulatory outpatients with chronic cardiac failure. *Circulation* 1986;**74:**II-38–II-38.

121 Goldberg LI. Cardiovascular and renal actions of dopamine. Potential clinical application. *Pharmacol Rev* 1972;**241:**1–29.

122 Goldberg LI, Volkman PH, Kohli JD. A comparison of the vascular dopamine receptor with other dopamine receptors. *Annu Rev Pharmacol Toxicol* 1978;**18:**57–79.

123 Rajfer SI, Goldberg LI. Dopamine in the treatment of heart failure. *Eur Heart J* 1982;**3:** 103–6.

124 Lockhandwala MF, Barrett RJ. Cardiovascular dopamine receptors. Physiological pharmaceutical and therapeutic implications. *J Auton Pharmacol* 1982;**2:**189–215.

125 Caponetto S, Terrachini V, Canale C *et al.* Long-term treatment of congestive heart failure with oral ibopamine: effects of rhythm disorders and neurohormonal alterations. *Cardiology* 1990;**77:** 43–8.

126 Itoh H, Taniguchi K, Tsajibayashi R, Koike A, Sato Y. Hemodynamic effects and pharmacokinetics of long-term therapy with ibopamine in patients with chronic heart failure. *Cardiology* 1992;**80:**356–60.

127 van Veldhuisen DJ, Man in 't Veld AJ, Dunselman PHJM *et al.* Double-blind placebo-controlled study of ibopamine and digoxin in patients with mild to moderate heart failure: results of the Dutch Ibopamine Multicenter Trial (DIMT). *J Am Coll Cardiol* 1993;**22:**1564–73.

128 Hampton JR, van Veldhuisen DJ, Kleber FX *et al.* Randomised study of effect of ibopamine on survival in patients with advanced severe heart failure. *Lancet* 1997;**349:**971–7.

129 The Xamoterol in Severe Heart Failure Study Group. Xamoterol in severe heart failure. *Lancet* 1990;**336:**1–6.

130 Alousi AA, Farah AE, Lesher GY, Opalka CJJ. Cardiotonic activity of amrinone-WIN 40680 [5-amino-3,4′bipyridin-6(1H)-one]. *Circ Res* 1979; **45:**666–77.

131 Millard RW, Dube G, Grupp G *et al.* Direct vasodilator and positive inotropic actions of amrinone. *J Mol Cell Cardiol* 1980;**12:**647–52.

132 Firth B, Ratner AV, Grassman ED *et al.* Assessment of the inotropic and vasodilator effects of amrinone versus isoproterenol. *Am J Cardiol* 1984;**54:**1331–6.

133 Rettig GF, Schieffer HJ. Acute effects of intravenous milrinone in heart failure. *Eur Heart J* 1989;**10:**39–43.

134 Baim DS, McDowell AV, Cherniles J *et al.* Evaluation of a new bipyridine inotropic agent-milrinone-in patients with severe congestive heart failure. *N Engl J Med* 1983;**309:**748–56.

135 Klocke RK, Mager G, Kux A *et al.* Effects of a twenty-four hour milrinone infusion in patients with severe heart failure and cardiogenic shock as a function of the hemodynamic initial condition. *Am Heart J* 1991;**121:**1965–73.

136 Kinney EL, Ballard JO, Carlin B, Zelis R. Amrinone-mediated thrombocytopenia. *Scand J Haematol* 1983;**31:**376–80.

137 Cowley AJ, Stainer K, Fullwood L, Muller AF, Hampton JR. Effects of enoximone in patients with heart failure uncontrolled by captopril and diuretics. *Int J Cardiol* 1990;**28**:S45–S53.

138 Bristow MR, Renlund DG, Gilbert EM, O'Connell JB. Enoximone in severe heart failure: clinical results and effects on β-adrenergic receptors. *Int J Cardiol* 1990;**28**:S21.

139 Herrmann HC, Ruddy TD, Dec GW *et al*. Diastolic function in patients with severe heart failure: comparison of the effects of enoximone and nitroprusside. *Circulation* 1987;**75**:1214–21.

140 Gage J, Rutman H, Lucido D, LeJemtel TH. Additive effects of dobutamine and amrinone on myocardial contractility and ventricular performance in patients with severe heart failure. *Circulation* 1986;**74**:367–73.

141 Uretsky BF, Lawless CE, Verbalis JG *et al*. Combined therapy with dobutamine and amrinone in severe heart failure. *Chest* 1987; **92**:657–62.

142 Anderson JL. Hemodynamic and clinical benefits with intravenous milrinone in severe chronic heart failure. Results of a multicenter study in the United States. *Am Heart J* 1991;**121**: 1956–64.

143 Packer M, Carver JR, Rodeheffer RJ *et al*. Effect of oral milrinone on mortality in severe chronic heart failure. *N Engl J Med* 1991;**325**:1468–75.

144 Uretsky BF, Jessup M, Konstam MA *et al*. Multicenter trial of oral enoximone in patients with moderate to moderately severe congestive heart failure. *Circulation* 1990;**82**:774–80.

145 DiBianco R, Shebetai R, Silverman BD *et al*. Oral amrinone for the treatment of chronic congestive heart failure. Results of a multicenter randomized double-blind and placebo-controlled withdrawal study. *J Am Coll Cardiol* 1984;**4**: 855–66.

146 Hagemeijer F. Calcium sensitization with pimobendan. Pharmacology, haemodynamic improvement, and sudden death in patients with chronic congestive heart failure. *Eur Heart J* 1993;**14**:551–66.

147 Fujino K, Sperelakis N, Solaro RJ. Sensitization of dog and guinea pig heart myofilaments to calcium activation and the inotropic effect of pimobendan. Comparison with milrinone. *Circ Res* 1988;**63**:911–22.

148 Böhm M, Morano I, Pieske B *et al*. Contribution of cAMP-phosphodiesterase inhibition and sensitization of the conctractile proteins for calcium to the inotropic effects of pimobendan in the failing human heart. *Circ Res* 1991;**68**: 689–701.

149 Katz SD, Kubo SH, Jessup M *et al*. A multicenter, randomized, double-blind, placebo-controlled trial of pimobendan, a new cardiotonic and vasodilator agent, in patients with severe congestive heart failure. *Am Heart J* 1992;**123**: 95–103.

150 Kubo SH, Gollub S, Bourge R *et al*. Beneficial effects of pimobendan on exercise tolerance and quality of life in patients with heart failure. *Circulation* 1992;**85**:942–9.

151 Just H, Hjalmarson Å, Remme WJ *et al*. pimobendan in congestive heart failure. Results of the PICO trial. *Circulation* 1995;**92**:722.

152 Pollesello P, Ovaska M, Kaivola J *et al*. Binding of a new Ca^2-sensitizer, levosimendan, to recombinant human cardiac troponin C. A molecular modelling, fluorescence probe and proton nuclear magnetic resonance study. *J Biol Chem* 1994;**269**:28584–9.

153 Sundberg S, Lilleberg J, Nieminen MS, Lehtonen L. Hemodynamic and neurohumoral effects of levosimendan, a new calcium sensitizer, at rest and during exercise in healthy men. *Am J Cardiol* 1995;**75**:1061–6.

154 Schwartz A, Wallick ET, Lee SW *et al*. Studies on the mechanism of action of 3,4-dihydro-6-[4-(3,4-dimethoxybenzoyl)-1-piperazinyl]-2(1H)-quinolinone (OPC-8212), a new positive inotropic drug. *Arzneimittelforschung* 1984;**34**: 384–9.

155 Yamashita S, Hosokawa T, Kojima M *et al*. In vitro and in vivo studies of 3,4-dihydro-6-[4-(3,4-dimethoxybenzoyl)-1-piperazinyl]-2(1H)-quinolinone on myocardial oxygen consumption in dogs with ischemic heart failure. *Jpn Circ J* 1986;**50**:659–66.

156 Matsumori A, Shioi T, Yamada T, Matsui S, Sasayama S. Vesnarinone, a new inotropic agent, inhibits cytokine production by stimulated human blood from patients with heart failure. *Circulation* 1994;**89**:955–8.

157 Feldman AM, Bristow MR, Parmley WW *et al*. Effects of vesnarinone on morbidity and mortality in patients with heart failure. *N Engl J Med* 1993;**329**:149–55.

158 Otsuka America, PNC. Letter to VEST Investigators, 29 July 1996.

159 Swedberg K, Waagstein F, Hjalmarson Å, Wallentin I. Prolongation of survival in congestive cardiomyopathy by beta-receptor blockade. *Lancet* 1979;**i**:1375–6.

160 Waagstein F, Hjalmarson Å, Varnauskas E, Wallentin I. Effect of chronic beta-adrenergic receptor blockade in congestive cardiomyopathy. *Br Heart J* 1975;**37**:1022–36.

161 Sloand EM, Thompson BT. Propranolol-induced pulmonary edema and shock in a patient with pheochromocytoma. *Arch Intern Med* 1984;**144**: 173–4.

162 Greenblatt DJ, Koch-Weser J. Adverse reactions to propranolol in hospitalized patients. *Am Heart J* 1973;**86**:478–84.

163 Herlitz J, Hjalmarson Å, Holmberg S *et al.* Development of congestive heart failure after treatment with metoprolol in acute myocardial infarction. *Br Heart J* 1984;**51**:539–44.

164 Chadda K, Goldstein S, Byington R, Curb JD. Effect of propranolol after acute myocardial infarction in patients with congestive heart failure. *Circulation* 1986;**73**:503–10.

165 Olsson G, Rehnqvist N. Effect of metoprolol in postinfarction patients with increased heart size. *Eur Heart J* 1986;**7**:468–74.

166 Gilbert EM, Anderson JL, Deitchman D *et al.* Long-term β-blocker vasodilator therapy improves cardiac function in idiopathic dilated cardiomyopathy: a double-blind, randomized study of bucindolol versus placebo. *Am J Med* 1990;**88**:223–9.

167 DasGupta P, Lahiri A. Can intravenous beta blockade predict long-term haemodynamic benefit in chronic congestive heart failure secondary to ischaemic heart disease? *Clin Invest* 1992;**70**:S98–S104.

168 Andersson B, Lomsky M, Waagstein F. The link between acute haemodynamic adrenergic beta-blockade and long-term effects in patients with heart failure. *Eur Heart J* 1993;**14**:1375–85.

169 Haber HL, Simek CL, Gimple LW *et al.* Why do patients with congestive heart failure tolerate the initiation of beta-blocker therapy. *Circulation* 1993;**88**:1610–19.

170 Andersson B, Caidahl K, Di Lenarda A, *et al.* Changes in early and late diastolic filling patterns induced by long-term adrenergic beta-blockade in patients with idiopathic dilated cardio-myopathy. *Circulation* 1996;**94**:673–82.

171 Woodley SL, Gilbert EM, Anderson JL *et al.* β-blockade with bucindolol in heart failure caused by ischemic versus idiopathic dilated cardiomyopathy. *Circulation* 1991;**84**:2426–41.

172 Eichhorn EJ, Bedotto JB, Malloy CR *et al.* Effect of β-adrenergic blockade on myocardial function and energetics in congestive heart failure. *Circulation* 1990;**82**:473–83.

173 Bristow MR, O'Connell JB, Gilbert EM *et al.* Dose-response of chronic β-blocker treatment in heart failure from either idiopathic dilated or ischemic cardiomyopathy. *Circulation* 1994;**89**:1632–42.

174 Eichhorn EJ, Heesch CM, Risser RC, Marcoux L, Hatfield B. Predictors of systolic and diastolic improvement in patients with dilated cardiomyopathy treated with metoprolol. *J Am Coll Cardiol* 1995;**25**:154–62.

175 Metra M, Nardi M, Giubbini R, Cas LC. Effects of short- and long-term carvedilol administration on rest and exercise hemodynamic vaiables, exercise capacity and clinical conditions in patients with idiopathic dilated cardiomyopathy. *J Am Coll Cardiol* 1995;**24**:1678–87.

176 Hall SA, Cigarroa CG, Marcoux L *et al.* Time course of improvement in left ventricular function, mass and geometry in patients with congestive heart failure treated with beta-adrenergic blockade. *J Am Coll Cardiol* 1995;**25**:1154–61.

177 Australia-New Zealand Heart Failure Research Collaborative Group. Effects of carvedilol, a vasodilator-β-blocker, in patients with congestive heart failure due to ischemic heart disease. *Circulation* 1995;**92**:212–18.

178 Waagstein F, for the Metoprolol in Mild to Moderate Heart Failure study group. Metoprolol in addition to ACE-inhibitors causes regression of left ventricular dilatation and increase exercise ejection fraction in ischemic cardiomyopathy. *J Am Coll Cardiol* 1997;**29**:206A.

179 Newton GE, Parker JD. Acute effects of β#v1#v-selective and nonselective β-adrenergic receptor blockade on cardiac sympathetic activity in congestive heart failure. *Circulation* 1996;**94**:353–8.

180 Andersson B, Blomström-Lundqvist C, Hedner T, Waagstein F. Exercise hemodynamics and myocardial metabolism during long-term beta-adrenergic blockade in severe heart failure. *J Am Coll Cardiol* 1991;**18**:1059–66.

181 Nemanich JW, Veith RC, Abrass IB, Stratton JR. Effects of metoprolol on rest and exercise cardiac function and plasma catecholamines in chronic congestive heart failure secondary to ischemic or idiopathic cardiomyopathy. *Am J Cardiol* 1990;**66**:843–8.

182 Eichhorn EJ, McGhie AI, Bedotto JB *et al.* Effects of bucindolol on neurohormonal activation in congestive heart failure. *Am J Cardiol* 1991;**67**:67–73.

183 Andersson B, Hamm C, Persson S *et al.* Improved exercise hemodynamic status in dilated cardiomyopathy after beta-adrenergic blockade treatment. *J Am Coll Cardiol* 1994;**23**:1397–404.

184 Yoshikawa T, Handa S, Anzai T *et al.* Early reduction of neurohumoral factors plays a key role in mediating the efficacy of beta-blocker therapy for congestive heart failure. *Am Heart J* 1996;**131**:329–36.

185 CIBIS Investigators and Committees. A randomized trial of β-blockade in heart failure. The Cardiac Insufficiency Bisoprolol Study (CIBIS). *Circulation* 1994;**90**:1765–73.

186 Waagstein F, Bristow MR, Swedberg K *et al.* Beneficial effects of metoprolol in idiopathic dilated cardiomyopathy. *Lancet* 1993;**342**:1441–6.

187 Packer M, Bristow MR, Cohn JN *et al.* The effect of carvedilol on morbidity and mortality in patients with chronic heart failure. *N Engl J Med* 1996;**334**:1349–55.

188 Colucci WS, Packer M, Bristow MR *et al.* Carvedilol inhibits clinical progression in patients with mild symptoms of heart failure. *Circulation* 1996;**94**:2800–6.

189 Packer M, Colucci WS, Sackner-Bernstein JD *et al.* Double-blind, placebo-controlled study of the effects of carvedilol in patients with moderate to severe heart failure. The PRECISE Trial. *Circulation* 1996;**94**:2793–9.

190 Waagstein F, for the MDC Study Group, Andersson F. Cost effectiveness of metoprolol in idiopathic dilated cardiomyopathy. *J Am Coll Cardiol* 1997;**29**:325A.

191 Andersson B, Waagstein F. Three-year follow-up of the metoprolol in dilated cardiomyopathy trial. *J Am Coll Cardiol* 1997;**29**:284A.

192 Australia/New Zealand Heart Failure Research Collaborative Group. Randomised, placebo-controlled trial of carvedilol in patients with congestive heart failure due to ischaemic heart disease. *Lancet* 1997;**349**:375–80.

193 Doughty RN, MacMahon S, Sharpe N. Beta-blockers in heart failure: promising or proved? *J Am Coll Cardiol* 1994;**23**:814–21.

194 Sharpe N. Beta-blockers in heart failure. Future directions. *Eur Heart J* 1996;**17**:39–42.

195 Kannel WB, Plehn JF, Cupples LA. Cardiac failure and sudden death in the Framingham study. *Am Heart J* 1988;**115**:869–75.

196 Kjekshus J. Arrhythmias and mortality in congestive heart failure. *Am J Cardiol* 1990;**64**:42I–48I.

197 Andersson B, Waagstein F. Spectrum and outcome of congestive heart failure in a hospitalized population. *Am Heart J* 1993;**126**:632–40.

198 Packer M. Sudden unexpected death in patients with congestive heart failure: a second frontier. *Circulation* 1985;**72**:681–5.

199 Stevenson WG, Stevenson LW, Middlekauff HR, Saxon LA. Sudden death prevention in patients with advanced ventricular dysfunction. *Circulation* 1993;**88**:2593–61.

200 Bigger TJJ, Fleiss JL, Kleiger R *et al.* The relationship between ventricular arrhythmias, left ventricular dysfunction and mortality in the two years after myocardial infarction. *Circulation* 1984;**69**:250–8.

201 Cardiac Arrhythmia Suppression Trial (CAST) Investigators. Preliminary report. Effect of encainide and flecainide on mortality in a randomized trial of arrhythmia suppression after myocardial infarction. *N Engl J Med* 1989;**321**:406–10.

202 Doval HC, Nul DR, Grancelli HO *et al.* Randomised trial of low-dose amiodarone in severe congestive heart failure. *Lancet* 1994;**344**:493–8.

203 Singh SN, Fletcher RD, Fisher SG *et al.* Amiodarone in patients with congestive heart failure and asymptomatic ventricular arrhythmia. *N Engl J Med* 1995;**333**:77–82.

204 Julian DG. Randomised trial of effect of amiodarone on mortality in patients with left-ventricular dysfunction after recent myocardial infarction: EMIAT. *Lancet* 1997;**349**:667–74.

205 Cairns JA. Randomised trial of outcome after myocardial infarction in patients with frequent or repetitive ventricular premature depolarisations: CAMIAT. *Lancet* 1997;**349**:675–82.

206 Waldo AL, Camm AJ, deRuyter H *et al.* Effect of D-sotalol on mortality in patients with left ventricular dysfunction after recent and remote myocardial infarction. *Lancet* 1996;**348**:7–12.

207 Pahor M, Gambassi G, Carbonin P. Antiarrhythmic effects of ACE inhibitors. A matter of faith or reality? *Cardiovasc Res* 1994;**28**:7–12.

208 Newman TJ, Maskin CS, Dennick LG *et al.* Effects of captopril on survival in patients with heart failure. *Am J Med* 1988;**84**:140–4.

209 The SOLVD investigators. Effect of enalapril on survival in patients with reduced left ventricular ejection fractions and congestive heart failure. *N Engl J Med* 1991;**325**:293–302.

41 Acute myocarditis and dilated cardiomyopathy

BARBARA A. PISANI,
JOHN F. CARLQUIST,
DAVID O. TAYLOR,
JEFFREY L. ANDERSON

DEFINITION OF MYOCARDITIS

"Myocarditis is an inflammatory disease of the myocardium which is diagnosed by established histological, immunological and immunochemical criteria." It is an inflammatory cardiomyopathy associated with cardiac dysfunction.[1] There are a variety of etiologic causes of myocarditis and the exact pathophysiologic mechanism remains to be elucidated.

IMMUNOPATHOGENESIS OF MYOCARDITIS

A broad spectrum of infectious and non-infectious agents have been associated with myocarditis (Tables 41.1–41.3). The application of virologic, serologic, and, most recently, molecular biological methods has substantiated epidemiologic observations of an infectious cause in many cases. While there are limited clinical data, there has been significant animal research into the etiology and pathophysiology of myocarditis. Coxsackie A and B viruses have been the most frequently implicated infectious agents in myocarditis. However, serologic studies suggestive of recent infection with Coxsackie virus are found in only about 40% of cases.[2] Similarly, it is uncommon to recover virus in culture from myocardial tissue obtained during or after acute myocarditis despite serologic evidence suggestive of viral infection.[3,4] Molecular genetic methods have continued to provide evidence for antecedent viral infection in some cases of myocarditis. Bowles et al.,[5] using Northern hybridization, identified Coxsackie B-specific RNA in nucleic acid extracts of myocardial tissue from nine of 17 patients with histologically proven myocarditis or inflammatory cardiomyopathy.

The use of the polymerase chain reaction (PCR) has produced variable results. Although some studies have found Coxsackie B or other enteroviral sequences in

Table 41.1 Common etiologies of myocarditis

Infectious	Systemic diseases
Adenovirus	Crohn's disease
Coxsackie virus	Kawasaki disease
Cytomegalovirus	Sarcoidosis
Epstein–Barr virus	Systemic lupus erythematosus
HIV-1	Ulcerative colitis
Borrelia (Lyme's disease)	Cardiac rejection
Toxoplasmosis	Giant cell myocarditis
	Peripartum myocarditis
Drug induced	
Amphetamines	**Hypersensitivity**
Anthracyclines (especially doxorubicin)	Hydrochlorothiazide
Catecholamines	Methyldopa
Cocaine	Penicillins
Cyclophosphamide	Sulfadiazine
Interleukin 2	Sulfamethoxazole

myocardial tissue from cases of cardiomyopathy or myocarditis by PCR,[6] others have failed to find any evidence of persistent Coxsackie B RNA in similar specimens[7] or have found a high frequency of enteroviral RNA in control specimens.[8] In a comparison of 34 children with myocarditis and 17 controls with congenital heart disease, 68% of 38 myocardial specimens had viral genome detected with PCR. There was a predominance of adenovirus when compared to adults. All control specimens and blood specimens were negative.[9] In a group of 40 postorthotopic heart transplant patients, 32% (41 samples) of 129 specimens obtained as a routine surveillance screen to rule out rejection had viral amplification with PCR. Of these, 16 were positive for CMV, 14 for adenovirus, six for enterovirus, three for parvovirus, and two for herpes simplex. In 13 of 21 patients with positive PCR, histologic scores also were consistent with moderate to severe rejection.[10] Matsumori[11] compared 36 patients with heart muscle disease and 40 consecutive patients who underwent cardiac catheterization. In six patients (16.7%) with dilated cardiomyopathy versus one patient (2.5%) with ischemic heart disease, hepatitis C was detected. Of these six patients, three had hepatitis C RNA identified on endomyocardial biopsy, utilizing the competitive nested PCR technique. The initial presentation in two patients was flu-like syndrome followed by heart failure (endomyocardial biopsy positive for myocarditis in one patient). The third patient presented with chronic heart failure. Thus, the accumulating evidence strongly implicates an antecedent or perhaps persistent or latent viral infection in the pathogenesis of myocarditis. However, the inability to convincingly establish one or a few etiologic agents in all cases suggests that other factors (e.g. immunologic and/or genetic) are contributory.

The difficulty in recovering infectious agents or even evidence of an ongoing infection in cases of lymphocytic myocarditis has prompted the speculation that this is at least partly autoimmune in etiology. Perhaps the best evidence for an autoimmune component in the progression of the disease comes from murine models of Coxsackie B3-induced myocarditis in susceptible animal strains. This experimental disease shows histologic resemblance to human disease[12–18] and has been useful in examining the immunologic and genetic elements of myocarditis. Original studies of this model showed a biphasic illness in which early (5–7 days postinfection) viral myocyte damage was supplanted

Table 41.2 Uncommon infectious etiologies of myocarditis

Viral
Arbovirus (dengue fever, yellow fever)
Arenavirus (Lassa fever)
Coronavirus
Echovirus
Encephalomyocarditis virus
Hepatitis B
Herpesvirus
Influenza virus
Junin virus
Mumps virus
Poliomyelitis virus
Rabies
Respiratory syncytial virus
Rubella virus
Rubeola virus
Vaccinia virus
Varicella virus
Variola virus

Bacterial
Brucellosis
Campylobacter jejuni
Chlamydia trachomatis
Clostridia
Diphtheria
Franciella (Tularemia)
Gonococcus
Hemophilus
Legionella
Listeria
Meningococcus
Mycobacteria (tuberculosis, avium-intercellulare, leprae)
Mycoplasma
Pneumococcus
Psittacosis

Salmonella
Staphylococcus
Streptococcus
Tropheryma whippelii (Whipple's disease)

Fungal
Aspergillus
Actinomycetes
Blastomyces
Candida
Coccidioides
Cryptococcus
Fusarium oxysporum
Histoplasma
Mucormycosis
Norcardia
Sporothrix

Rickettsial
Rickettsia rickettsii (Rocky Mountain spotted fever)
Coxiella burnetii (Q fever)
Scrub typhus
Typhus

Spirochetal
Leptospira
Syphilis

Helminthic
Cysticercus
Echinococcus
Schistosoma
Toxocara (visceral larva migrans)
Trichinella

Protozoal
Entamoeba
Leishmania

later (9–45 days) by mononuclear interstitial infiltration and chronic inflammation.[18,19] During the early phase, infectious virus was readily recovered from the myocardium; during the postinfectious phase, infectious virus was not recoverable. It is noteworthy that genetic factors dictated the susceptibility to the development of the late phase disease[18] as well as the susceptibility to the initial viral infection. This animal model closely resembles the currently held model for clinical disease in humans.

The nature of the antigen(s) that initiate and perpetuate the immune response in myocarditis is not known with certainty. The hypothesis of molecular mimicry is frequently invoked to explain the occurrence of autoimmune disease following an infection. Within the framework of this hypothesis, an immune response to a dominant epitope expressed by an infectious agent could induce disease following infection. In the

Table 41.3 Uncommon non-infectious causes of myocarditis

Drug induced

A. Toxic myocarditis
Amphetamines
Arsenic
Chloroquine
Emetine
5-Fluorouracil
Interferon alpha
Lithium
Paracetamol
Thyroid hormone

B. Hypersensitivity myocarditis
Acetazolamide
Allopurinol
Amphotericin B
Carbamazepine
Cephalothin
Chlorthalidone
Colchicine
Diclofenac
Diphenhydramine
Furosemide
Indomethacin
Isoniazid
Lidocaine
Methysergide
Oxphenbutazone
Para-aminosalicylic acid
Phenindione
Phenylbutazone
Phenytoin
Procainamide
Pyribenzamine
Ranitidine
Reserpine
Spironolactone
Streptomycin
Tetracycline
Trimethaprim

Toxins
Arsenic
Carbon monoxide
Copper
Iron
Lead
Mercury
Phosphorus
Scorpion stings
Snake venom
Spider bites
Wasp stings

Systemic diseases
Arteritis (giant cell, Takayasu)
Beta-thalassemia major
Churg–Strauss vasculitis
Cryoglobulinemia
Dermatomyositis
Diabetes mellitus
Hashimoto's thyroiditis
Mixed connective tissue disease
Myesthenia gravis
Periarteritis nodosa
Pernicious anemia
Pheochromocytoma
Polymyositis
Rheumatoid arthritis
Scleroderma
Sjögren's syndrome
Thymoma
Wegener's granulomatosis

Other
Eosinophilic myocarditis
Genetic
Granulomatous myocarditis
Head trauma
Hypothermia
Hyperpyrexia
Ionizing radiation
Mononuclear myocarditis

event that a similar or crossreacting epitope is also present on host cells, tissue damage might result.[20] Coxsackie B3 antibodies that crossreact with myosin have been described.[21] In addition, antibodies against myosin are frequently found in experimental myocarditis.[22,23] An alternative hypothesis is that immune reactivity to self antigens results from the aberrant expression of normally sequestered epitopes or upregulation of epitopes that are normally expressed at a density that favors tolerance.[24] Thus, an autoimmune component of disease pathology appears to be involved in the experimental model of the disease and, in all likelihood, is etiologic in clinical disease as well. However, the same etiologic pathway may not be followed in all cases of myocarditis. This may explain the failure to identify a consistent underlying immunopathologic picture in most cases of clinical myocarditis.

It appears, therefore, that the etiology of myocarditis is heterogeneous; likewise, a variety of immune effector mechanisms have been identified in myocarditis, further underscoring the heterogeneity of the disease. The earliest potential effector mechanism to be described in myocarditis was the production of autoantibodies to normal cellular antigens. A broad variety of tissue antigens have been identified as targets for autoantibodies. Among these are the beta-adrenergic receptor,[25] the adenine nucleotide translocator,[26] laminin,[27] branched chain ketoacid dehydrogenase,[28] heat shock protein-60 (HSP-60),[29] and sarcolemmal epitopes.[30] Although antibodies to these antigens are frequently identified in association with myocarditis, their significance is not known. They may function in the pathogenesis of the disease or they may be epiphenomena arising in conjunction with the principal pathogenic process. Perhaps these antibodies do not initiate myocyte damage/dysfunction, but contribute to pathology at later stages of the disease.

DILATED CARDIOMYOPATHY: BACKGROUND AND PATHOGENESIS

Idiopathic dilated cardiomyopathy (IDC) is characterized by dilation and impaired contraction of the left ventricle or both ventricles.[1] Dilated cardiomyopathy has been postulated to occur in some cases as a result of recognized or unrecognized myocarditis. Dec and colleagues[12] reported that endomyocardial biopsy examination revealed myocarditis in 66% of patients with acute dilated cardiomyopathy (of less then 6 months duration). However, in the Myocarditis Treatment Trial, only 10% of those screened with heart failure of less than 2 years duration had biopsy-proven myocarditis.[31] Nonetheless, in a substantial number of cases of IDC no identifiable etiologic process can be ascribed. Viral infections have been frequently implicated in IDC, as in myocarditis. Several serologic studies have found increased prevalence or levels of antibodies to Coxsackie B in cases of IDC.[32-34] Recent investigations have used the very sensitive PCR to search for persistent enteroviral RNA in IDC cases with equivocal results. Among the various studies, a wide percentage range of IDC cases with demonstrable enteroviral RNA has been reported (0–32%); in comparison, 0–38% of biopsies from non-IDC cases also have been reported positive for enteroviral RNA.[7,8,35] Thus, the finding of persistent virus or viral RNA in IDC does not appear to be specific for the disease although the overall consensus continues to favor an inciting infection in many cases.

A great deal of evidence is suggestive of autoimmune or autoimmune-like mechanisms in the pathogenesis of IDC. A spectrum of autoantibodies against similar cellular components as were identified for acute myocarditis has been found among cases of IDC. The principal cellular components reactive with antiheart antibodies associated with IDC are the adenine nucleotide translocator,[36] beta-adrenoceptors,[25] myosin,[37] laminin,[27] actin, tropomyosin, and heat shock protein-60 (HSP-60).[29] However, antibodies reactive with tissue antigens are often present in the circulation of asymptomatic individuals.[38] Thus, the source and significance of these antibodies relative to the pathology of IDC remain a mystery.

One of the most frequently examined aspects of IDC is the proposed linkage between disease frequency and the genes of the major histocompatibility complex (MHC). Such evidence would strengthen the argument for an immunologic component in IDC and establish a genetic component as well. The most frequently described linkage between IDC and MHC genes in Caucasian populations has been with class II alleles. Four of five independent studies identified a positive association of IDC with HLA DR4.[39] An association between HLA DR4 and anti-beta-receptor antibodies also has been noted.[23] Linkage with other class II alleles has been described in other ethnic groups,[40] underscoring possible ethnic differences. These studies strongly implicate genetically controlled immunologic factors with possible immune reactivity to tissue antigens in the pathogenesis of IDC. The specific predisposing HLA-related locus/loci, however, may depend on the genetic background (ethnicity) as well as the specific vector (viral strain) involved.

EPIDEMIOLOGY AND NATURAL HISTORY OF MYOCARDITIS AND IDC

The true incidence of myocarditis is unknown. In 12 747 autopsies performed in Sweden from 1975 to 1984, an incidence of 1.06% was found.[41] However, autopsies of children and young adults presenting with sudden death report an incidence as high as 17–21%.[2] In the Myocarditis Treatment Trial, 9.6% of 2333 patients with recent onset of heart failure (onset within 2 years of study enrollment) met pathologic criteria for myocarditis.[31] There is both a seasonal variation and a male predominance. Of 136 patients with biopsy-proven myocarditis, 63% presented between December and April.[42] A flu-like illness within 3 months of presentation was reported by 57%.[42] Only 41% reported a similar illness within 1 month of presentation.[42] Blacks and males were noted to have a 2.5-fold increased risk.[42] Patients with acute myocarditis tend to present at a somewhat younger age (43 ± 16 years) when compared to patients with IDC (50 ± 17 years).[42]

Of the more than three million people in the United States with heart failure, 25% of cases are secondary to IDC.[43] From 1975 to 1984, Codd and colleagues[44] detected 45 cases of dilated cardiomyopathy based on echocardiography, angiography, endomyocardial biopsy, and autopsy results. The median age at the time of diagnosis was 54 years, although presentation may be in childhood, adulthood or old age. Forty one cases (91%) were diagnosed during life. Of these, 36 patients (88%) were symptomatic prior to diagnosis, with dyspnea being the most common symptom (75% were New York Heart Association (NYHA) functional class III–IV). Five patients (14%) had a syncopal event. Twenty seven patients (75%) had clinical heart failure and nine (25%) had angina. Five of the 41 patients (12%) were identified during a routine medical evaluation and were asymptomatic. Four cases (9%) were diagnosed at autopsy although all had been symptomatic. The overall age- and sex-adjusted incidence was noted to increase from 3.9/100 000 person-years in 1975–1979 to 7.9/100 000 person-years in 1980–1984. The age- and sex-adjusted prevalence was 36.5/100 000 population. The prevalence of dilated cardiomyopathy in patients less than 55 years old was 17.9/100 000. Within this group, over one-third were NYHA functional class III or IV at the time of diagnosis. The annual incidence is 5–8 cases per 100 000.[43]

An increased incidence of IDC is noted in blacks.[45,46] The cumulative survival in blacks at 12 and 24 months is 71.5% and 63.6% respectively, compared to 92% and

86.3% among whites. One-year survival is adversely affected by an ejection fraction (EF) <25% or ventricular arrhythmias (<60% in both instances). Patients 60 years of age or greater had a three-fold increased risk of death among both blacks and whites.[46]

Males have an increased incidence of IDC.[45] The male:female ratio is 3.4:1. The incidence rate for men is greater than women within all age groups.[44] In a multicenter registry of IDC, DeMaria[47] et al. enrolled 65 women and 238 men (male:female ratio 3.66). Patients referred for cardiac transplant were excluded. Of the various clinical characteristics evaluated, 10 variables were significantly different between men and women. Men more frequently had a history of ethanol abuse and cigarette smoking. However, subgroup analysis revealed no influence of these variables on gender-related differences. Symptoms of heart failure were more frequently detected in women and were indicative of more advanced heart failure (NYHA class III–IV in 48%). Left bundle branch block (LBBB) was detected more frequently in women, while left anterior hemiblock (LAHB) was noted to be more common in men. There was more pronounced left ventricular dilation in women, with a slightly but not significantly higher mean myocardial thickness. Exercise tolerance was poorer in women. The median survival was 16 months for women and 19 months for men. Seven women (11%) and 17 men (7%) underwent cardiac transplantation, while 16% of women and 11% of men died due to cardiac causes.

Peripartum cardiomyopathy

Peripartum cardiomyopathy (PPCM) is the development of heart failure from the last month of pregnancy to within 5 months of delivery. There are no other determinable causes of heart failure or heart disease in the last month of pregnancy. Risk factors include age over 30, African descent, obesity, multiple pregnancies, twin gestation (7–10%), and long term (>4 weeks) tocolytic therapy.[48] The incidence varies from 1 in 15 000 to 1 in 100 live births.[49] Whether PPCM/peripartum myocarditis are distinct from IDC and myocarditis or are secondary to worsening subclinical IDC is unclear, but the natural history of the disease differs from IDC. Myocarditis has been reported in 8–78% of patients with PPCM.[48,50] Rizeq[51] et al. compared 34 women with PPCM and 30 age- and sex-matched IDC patients. The incidence of myocarditis was 8.8% (three of 34) in the PPCM group versus 9.1% (two of 22) in the control group. Mortality varies from 25% to 50%, with almost half of deaths secondary to heart failure, arrhythmias or thromboembolic events.[48] Almost half of the deaths occur within the first 3 months postpartum. Mortality secondary to thromboembolic events is as high as 30%. Approximately 50% of patients who regain normal cardiac function do so within 6 months of initial diagnosis. Witlin[52] noted that of 28 patients with PPCM, five died (18% mortality), three (11%) had cardiac transplant, 18 (64%) had continued functional impairment, and two (7%) had regression of their cardiomyopathy. Six subsequently became pregnant again. Of these, four deteriorated clinically, one remained well compensated on therapy, and one had no recurrence.

Therapy of PPCM consists of usual heart failure treatment measures, with the substitution of hydralazine for angiotensin converting enzyme inhibitors, cautious use of diuretics when sodium restriction fails, and the use of heparin in lieu of warfarin. Midei[50] reported on the use of immunosuppressants in 18 women with PPCM. Fourteen (78%) had biopsy evidence of myocarditis. Ten patients were treated with prednisone/

Table 41.4 Dallas Criteria classification of myocarditis[51]

Initial biopsy
Myocarditis: myocyte necrosis, degeneration or both in the absence of significant CAD with adjacent inflammatory infiltrate + / − fibrosis
Borderline myocarditis: inflammatory infiltrate too sparse or myocyte damage not apparent
No myocarditis

Subsequent biopsy
Ongoing (persistent) myocarditis + / −fibrosis
Resolving (healing) myocarditis + / −fibrosis
Resolved (healed) myocarditis + / −fibrosis

azathioprine and four were untreated. One patient died, despite treatment. Four patients with myocarditis improved clinically without treatment. Follow-up biopsy showed near complete resolution in two. Four patients without myocarditis were not treated. Two improved and two required transplantation. After completion of treatment, biopsy, LV stroke work index, and pulmonary capillary wedge pressure returned to normal in 12 (not repeated in two patients). Subsequent pregnancy in patients with persistent LV dysfunction should be discouraged as pregnancy may be associated with a high risk of complications and death.[48,52] Subsequent pregnancy in patients with recovery of LV function remains controversial. Patients who have recovered from PPCM have a lower contractile reserve upon dobutamine challenge when compared to normal controls, despite similar baseline ventricular size and function.[49] This may explain recurrent symptoms with subsequent pregnancies and may be helpful in determining which patients will tolerate future pregnancy.

CLINICAL PRESENTATIONS

Myocarditis

The presenting symptoms and physical examination are often non-specific in both myocarditis and IDC. A history of a flu-like syndrome may be present in up to 90% of patients with myocarditis, but only approximately 40% report a viral syndrome within the prior month.[2,41] The initial presentation may be one of acute or chronic heart failure or cardiogenic shock or may mimic an acute myocardial infarction.[53,54] Patients may experience life threatening arrhythmias or may remain asymptomatic. Lieberman *et al.*[55] proposed a clinicopathologic description of myocarditis, based on the initial manifestations, endomyocardial biopsy, and recovery (fulminant, acute, chronic active or chronic persistent myocarditis).

The Dallas Criteria[56] (Table 41.4) were developed in order to standardize histologic criteria for the diagnosis of myocarditis (Figure 41.1), facilitating a multicenter treatment study. However, a negative biopsy does not rule out myocarditis due to interobserver variability, sampling error, and the temporal evolution (transient presence) of pathologic features.

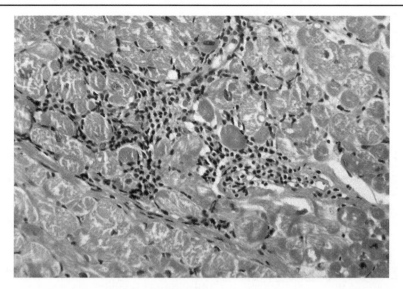

Figure 41.1   Acute myocarditis. Lymphocytic infiltrate of the myocardium with associated myocyte damage. (Hematoxylin and eosin; slide courtesy of Robert Yowell MD.)

IDC

IDC is initially manifest by heart failure in 75–85% of patients. Ninety percent of patients referred to a tertiary care center are NYHA functional class III–IV at presentation.[45] Other potential manifestations include asymptomatic cardiomegaly or LV dysfunction on routine evaluation, arrhythmias or even cardiogenic shock, as in myocarditis. Patients with LBBB have been noted to have a greater LV diastolic dimension normalized for body surface area. The presence of LBBB on electrocardiogram (ECG) may precede the development of cardiomyopathy in 40% of patients. LBBB may be noted on ECG for years prior to the onset of heart failure. At rest and when exercised, these patients may have a higher mean pulmonary artery pressure, although left ventricular end-diastolic volume remains normal, by comparison with normal patients.[57] Laboratory, X-ray, and other diagnostic tests are helpful but may be equally non-specific. Myocyte hypertrophy, degeneration of myocytes, interstitial fibrosis, and small clusters of lymphocytes (>5 per high power field) have been noted histologically (Figure 41.2).[45]

PROGNOSIS

Myocarditis

In patients with myocarditis, ECG abnormalities associated with a longer duration of illness (>1 month) include left ventricular hypertrophy (LVH), left atrial enlargement (LAE), left bundle branch block (LBBB), and atrial fibrillation (AF). The presence of an abnormal QRS complex on ECG correlates with severity of left ventricular damage and is an independent predictor of survival. LAE, AF, and LBBB also are associated with an increased mortality.[58] Higher baseline LVEF is positively associated with survival, while intensity of conventional therapy at baseline is negatively associated with survival.[31]

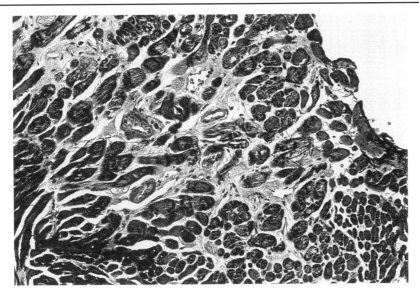

Figure 41.2 Idiopathic dilated cardiomyopathy. Myocyte hypertrophy with mild nuclear enlargement and increased interstitial collagen. (Trichrome stain; slide courtesy of Robert Yowell MD.)

The presence of right ventricular (RV) dysfunction, as evidenced by abnormal RV descent on echocardiogram, was shown to be the most important predictor of death or need for cardiac transplantation in a group of 23 patients with biopsy-proven myocarditis who were followed long term.[59] In addition, a net increase in LVEF (between initial and final EF) was associated with improved survival, whereas baseline EF was not predictive of outcome. The presence and degree of left ventricular regional wall motion abnormalities did not predict the clinical course.[59]

Light microscopic findings on biopsy have not been shown to predict outcome in myocarditis. Less than 10% of biopsies repeated at 28 weeks and 52 weeks continue to show evidence of ongoing or recurrent myocarditis, regardless of therapy. However, higher baseline serum antibodies to cardiac immune globulin (Ig) G by indirect immunofluoresence were associated with a better LVEF and a smaller left ventricular end-diastolic dimension.[31] Gagliardi *et al.*[60] followed 20 children with biopsy proven myocarditis who were treated with cyclosporin and steroids and found that 13 of 20 had persistent myocarditis at 6 months. At 1 year, 10 patients had persistent myocarditis by endomyocardial biopsy although ventricular size and function had improved on echocardiography. Echocardiography was unable to detect those patients with biopsy persistent versus resolved myocarditis. Despite histologic evidence of myocarditis, no patient died or required transplantation.

IDC

Spontaneous improvement in LVEF (over 10% points) occurs in 20–45% of patients with IDC. Improvement usually occurs within the first 6 months of presentation but may occur up to 4 years later. Outcome is adversely affected by progressive LV enlargement, RV enlargement, and markedly reduced LVEF. Both LVEF and RV enlargement are independent predictors of survival. Mortality rates of 25–30% at 1 year are noted. Overall, the annual mortality due to progression of disease is 4–10% but is greater in high risk subgroups. Twelve percent of patients with IDC die suddenly, which accounts for 28% of all deaths.[45] In a retrospective study of 104 patients with dilated cardiomyopathy, Fuster et al.[61] noted 77% of patients died. Two thirds of the deaths occurred within the first 2 years. Interestingly, the survival curve for the remaining patients was comparable to an age- and sex-matched control group. The 1- and 5- year mortality rates were 31% and 64%, respectively. Factors which were significantly associated with poorer survival were older age (97% mortality rate in patients 55 years and older), cardiothoracic ratio (86% mortality rate if the ratio was >0.55 vs 40% if <0.55), cardiac index (CI) (mortality rate 89% if CI <3.0 l/min vs 35% if CI >3.0 l/min) and left ventricular end-diastolic pressure (mortality rate 87% if ≥ 20 mmHg).

Referral bias and secular trends, new treatment modalities, and the prevalence of disease in the referral population should also be noted, as these may influence overall survival.[62] Patients with syncope, a third heart sound, RV dysfunction, hyponatremia, elevated plasma norepinephrine or atrial naturetic peptide or renin, a maximal systemic oxygen uptake (VO_2) of less than 10–12 ml/kg/min, CI of less than 2.5 l/min/m², systemic hypotension, pulmonary hypertension, increased central venous pressure or loss of cardiac myofilaments on high resolution microscopy show increased progression of disease and worse survival.[45] By comparison, when one assesses the natural history of asymptomatic IDC, patients have an excellent prognosis, with a 2-year survival of 100%, a 5-year survival of $78 \pm 8\%$, and a 7-year survival of $53 \pm 10\%$. However, there is no improvement in survival in these patients when compared to asymptomatic patients who have previously had symptoms of heart failure. The most common reason for cardiac evaluation in this group of patients is palpitations or an abnormal chest X-ray or ECG. When compared to patients with a prior history of congestive heart failure symptoms, these patients had a lower prevalence of cardiomegaly on chest X-ray (31% vs 57% of patients) and a smaller LV and better EF (33% vs 29% EF) on echocardiography.[63] Myocardial contractile reserve, as evaluated by change in LVEF with exercise, is an independent predictor of survival in patients with mildly symptomatic (NYHA class I or II) dilated cardiomyopathy. A change in LVEF >4% was associated with a 75% survival versus 25% survival for those whose EF changed <4% with exercise.[64] Coronary flow reserve is diminished in patients with dilated cardiomyopathy.

Treasure et al.[65] performed coronary angiography and Doppler flow studies of the left anterior descending (LAD) to estimate coronary artery flow velocities in seven normal controls and eight patients with dilated cardiomyopathy. The effect of acetylcholine and adenosine on epicardial vasoconstriction in patients with dilated cardiomyopathy was not significantly different from normal controls. However, infusion of intracoronary acetylcholine resulted in a dose-dependent increase in coronary blood flow in normal controls only, suggesting that endothelium-dependent coronary vasodilation is abnormal in dilated cardiomyopathy. There was a similar change in coronary blood flow with adenosine infusion in both groups.

In infants and children the outcome of IDC is more variable. A retrospective review of 24 patients under 20 years old with IDC revealed that in 92%, the initial manifestation was heart failure. Thirteen of the patients (54%) had onset of symptoms within 3 months of a viral syndrome although endomyocardial biopsy did not reveal active myocarditis in six. Sixty three percent had ECG evidence of LVH and 68% had ST-T wave abnormalities. The mean EF was 26% (5–51%). Fifteen patients died (63%). The cumulative survival was 63% at 1 year, 50% at 2 years, and 34% at 5 years of follow-up. Death was most frequently due to progressive heart failure. Of the nine patients who survived, the symptoms resolved in 3–24 months. Severe mitral regurgitation was a predictor of poor outcome. Survivors more frequently had viral symptoms within the preceding 3 months.[66] Five-year survival rates of 64–84% have been reported.[45] Sudden death is rare.[45]

Comparison of IDC and myocarditis

Grogan *et al.*[67] compared 27 patients with active (17) or borderline (10) myocarditis with 58 IDC patients. A viral illness was reported within the previous 3 months in 40% of patients with myocarditis versus 19% of the IDC patients. The EF was lower ($25 \pm 11\%$) in the group with IDC compared to the myocarditis group ($38 \pm 19\%$). Sixty three percent of the patients with IDC were NYHA functional class III–IV compared with only 30% of the patients with myocarditis. There was no difference in survival even when results were analyzed for the presence of active myocarditis, borderline myocarditis, or IDC (54% 5-year survival with IDC vs 56% with myocarditis).

Summary

While multiple causal factors have been implicated in both myocarditis and IDC, the precise etiology and pathophysiology remain unknown. Spontaneous improvement in left ventricular function may be noted with both myocarditis and IDC. Survival is similar (approximately 55% at 5 years) in both.

TREATMENT

Treatment of myocarditis: clinical and experimental

General supportive measures for patients with myocarditis include a low sodium diet, discontinuation of ethanol, and fluid restriction, especially in the presence of heart failure. Recommendations for the limitation of physical activity are based on the murine model of Coxsackie B3 myocarditis, in which forced exercise during the acute phase of illness was associated with increased inflammatory and necrotic lesions (although there was no effect on death rate).[68] The Task Force[69] on myopericardial diseases recommends a convalescent period of approximately 6 months after onset of clinical manifestations before a return to competitive sports.

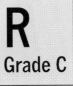

ANTIVIRAL THERAPY

The use of the antiviral ribaviron[70] in a murine (DBA/2) model of encephalomyocarditis (ECM) myocarditis improved survival and decreased myocardial viral titers when used in higher doses (200 or 400 mg/kg/day). Therapy resulted in fewer myocardial lesions, more pronounced inhibition of viral replication, a reduced inflammatory response, and less myocardial damage. However, treatment was started immediately after viral inoculation. There are no human studies of antiviral therapy to date and the ability to detect and begin therapy immediately upon onset is limited in the clinical setting.

CONVERTING ENZYME INHIBITION

Although there are multiple studies on the use of ACE inhibitors in heart failure (including patients with IDC), their utility in myocarditis has been studied only in the murine model. Studies of Coxsackie B3 myocarditis in CD1 mice reported that early treatment with captopril (starting on day 1 of infection) resulted in less inflammatory infiltrate, myocardial necrosis, and calcification. Heart weight, heart to body weight ratio, and liver congestion diminished. Even when therapy was begun later (10 days after inoculation), a beneficial effect – a reduction in left ventricular mass and liver congestion – was noted.[71]

A comparison of the ACE inhibitors captopril 7.5 g/kg/day and enalapril 1 mg/kg/day with the angiotensin II receptor blocker losartan 60 mg/kg/day in a murine model of ECM myocarditis revealed that only captopril and losartan, started 1 week after viral inoculation, resulted in decreased heart weight, body weight, heart weight to body ratio, and hypertrophy. Left ventricular cavity dimension decreased with the use of captopril and losartan 12 mg/kg/day or 60 mg/kg/day. These results are consistent with an improvement in heart failure and left ventricular hypertrophy. There was less necrosis with enalapril and captopril. However, the inflammatory score was reduced only by captopril.[72]

BETA-BLOCKERS

Similarly, beta-blockers have been studied in myocarditis only in murine models. Metoprolol was compared with saline in a murine model of acute Coxsackie B3 myocarditis, starting on the day of viral inoculation and continuing for 10 days. The result was an *increased* 30-day mortality (60% vs 0%) in metoprolol-treated mice associated with *increased* viral replication and myocyte necrosis.[73] The beta-blocker carteolol has been studied in a murine model (BALB/C and DBA/2 strains) of acute, subacute, and chronic ECM myocarditis. Metoprolol was compared with carteolol in the chronically infected group. There was no difference in survival between mice whose treatment was started on the day of viral inoculation, compared to therapy begun 14 days later. In chronically infected mice, carteolol resulted in a reduction in heart weight and heart weight to body ratio (not seen with metoprolol) and improved histopathologic scores (diminished wall thickness, cavity dimension, fiber diameter, cell necrosis, fibrosis, cellular infiltration, and calcification), suggesting that carteolol may prevent the development of lesions similar to those found in dilated cardiomyopathy.[74] The results suggest that early initiation of beta-blockers may be harmful, whereas in the chronic stages of illness beta-blockers improve manifestations of heart failure. In addition, non-cardioselective beta-blockers may be preferable.

CALCIUM-CHANNEL BLOCKERS

In a murine model of ECM induced myocarditis, verapamil pretreatment was associated with a reduction in microvascular necrosis, fibrosis, and calcification. Similar changes were noted if treatment was begun 4 days after viral inoculation. The development of microvascular constriction and microaneurysm formation was prevented when compared to controls. This suggests a possible role for calcium signaling and microvascular spasm in the pathogenesis of this form of viral myocarditis. Verapamil did not reduce mortality although the severity of illness and time to death were delayed.[75] There have been no human myocarditis trials with calcium-channel blockers to date.

NON-STEROIDAL ANTI-INFLAMMATORY AGENTS

The use of ibuprofen during the acute phase of murine Coxsackie B3 myocarditis resulted in significant exacerbation of myocardial inflammation, necrosis, and viral replication, when compared to control mice.[76,77]

VESNARINONE

Vesnarinone suppressed TNF-α, resulting in a reduction in myocardial necrosis, when given at a dose of 50 mg/kg, in a murine model of ECM myocarditis. At lower doses (10 mg/kg) the mortality rate was reduced in comparison to control mice, although both groups began to experience mortality on the fifth day after viral inoculation.[78]

IMMUNOSUPPRESSANTS

The data supporting an immunologic basis of myocarditis have resulted in multiple treatment trials using immunosuppressants. The largest of these trials, the Myocarditis Treatment Trial,[31] screened 2333 patients with heart failure of less than 2 years' duration. Two hundred and fourteen (10%) had endomyocardial biopsy evidence of myocarditis using the Dallas Criteria. One hundred and eleven patients had a qualifying LVEF of <45%. Patients were initially divided into three treatment groups: prednisone/ azathioprine, prednisone/cyclosporin, and no immunosuppressant treatment. The prednisone/azathioprine group was subsequently eliminated due to limited numbers of patients. Patients were treated for 24 weeks, during which time conventional heart failure therapy was continued. At both 28 and 52 weeks, no difference in pulmonary capillary wedge pressure or change in LVEF was observed (Figure 41.3). In addition, there was no significant change in LVEF in treated patients as compared with untreated (Figure 41.3). At 1 and 5 years, there was no difference in survival between groups or need for cardiac transplantation (Figure 41.4). On multivariate analysis, better baseline LVEF, less intensive conventional therapy, and shorter illness duration were independent predictors of improvement in LVEF during follow-up. Immunologic variables (cardiac IgG, circulating IgG, natural killer and macrophage activity, helper T cell level) were not associated with measures of cardiac function. A higher peripheral CD2$^+$T lymphocyte count was associated with a higher risk of death. At 5 years the combined endpoint of death or transplantation was 56%.

Gagliardi et al.[60] followed 20 children with biopsy-proven myocarditis who were treated with cyclosporin and prednisone. At 1 year, 10 of 20 patients still had histologic evidence of myocarditis. No patient died or required transplantation. However, there was no control group.

Certain subgroups might nonetheless benefit from immunosuppressant therapy, including those with giant cell myocarditis, hypersensitivity myocarditis or cardiac

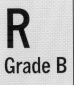

R

Grade B

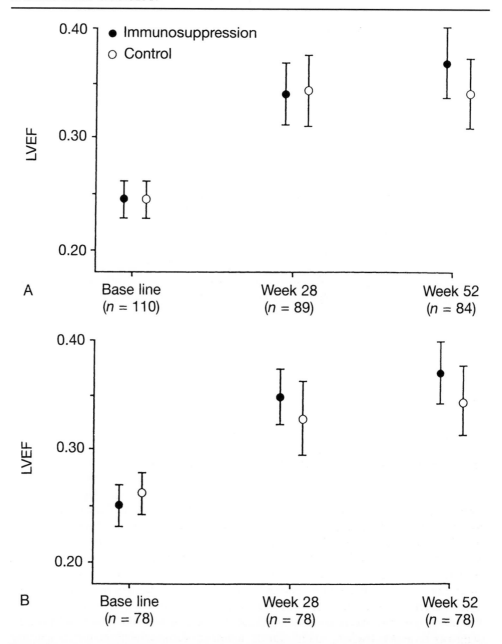

Figure 41.3 Mean (±SE) left ventricular ejection fraction (LVEF) in the immunosuppression and control groups at base line, week 28, and week 52. Panel A shows the mean values for all available studies at each time, with the numbers of patients indicated at the bottom of the panel. There was no difference between the two groups in the mean LVEF at base line, week 28 or week 52 (P=0.97, P=0.95, and P=0.45, respectively). Panel B shows the mean values for the 78 patients in whom data were available at all three times. Again, there was no significant difference between the groups (P=0.51, P=0.60, and P=0.50, respectively). (Adapted with permission from Mason *et al.*[31])

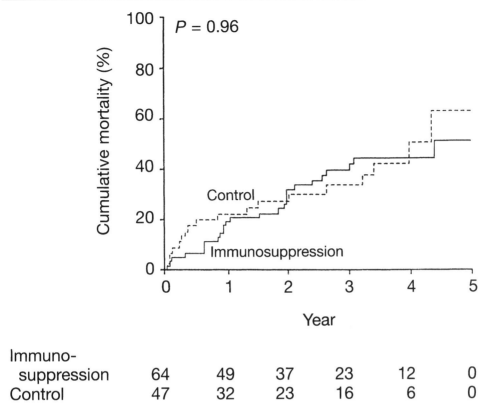

Figure 41.4 Actuarial mortality (defined as deaths and cardiac transplantations) in the immunosuppression and control groups. The numbers of patients at risk are shown at the bottom. There was no significant difference in mortality between the two groups. (Adapted with permission from Mason *et al.*[31])

sarcoidosis. Utilizing a multicenter database, Cooper[79] reviewed 63 patients with giant cell myocarditis. There was no difference in the number of men versus women or the age of men versus women. The mean age at onset was 42.6 ± 12.7 years. Eighty eight percent were white and 19% had an associated autoimmune disorder. Five patients (8%) had either Crohn's disease or ulcerative colitis, which preceded the onset of myocarditis. Seventy five percent presented with heart failure. Approximately half had sustained refractory ventricular tachycardia during the course of the illness. The rate of death or cardiac transplantation was 89%. Median survival was 5.5 months from symptom onset to death or transplantation. The median survival in patients treated with corticosteroids was 3.8 months versus 3.0 months in untreated patients. However, patients treated with corticosteroids and azathioprine had an average survival of 11.5 months. Cyclosporine in combination with corticosteroids, corticosteroids/azathioprine, or corticosteroids/azathioprine/OKT3 survived an average of 12.6 months. Survival was unaffected by sex, age or time to presentation. Cardiac transplantation was performed in 34 patients. Nine (26%) died during an average 3.7 years of follow-up. Five of these deaths occurred within 30 days of transplantation. Nine patients had recurrent giant cell myocarditis in the transplanted heart, after an average of 3 years post-transplantation. Comparison with 111 patients in the Myocarditis Treatment Trial revealed cumulative mortality was greater in patients with giant cell myocarditis (Figure 41.5).

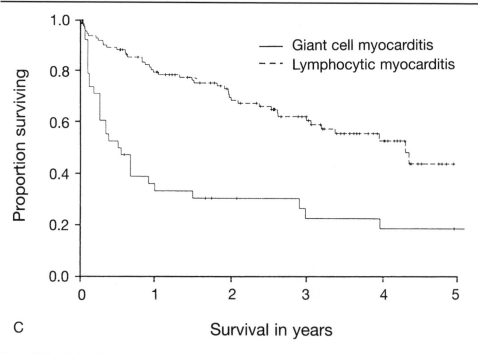

Figure 41.5 Kaplan–Meier survival curves for patients with giant cell myocarditis, showing the duration of survival among 38 patients in whom giant cell myocarditis was diagnosed by endomyocardial biopsy or by examination of a section of ventricular apex. Survival was significantly longer among patients with lymphocytic myocarditis (*P*<0.001 by the log rank test for each comparison). (Adapted with permission from Cooper *et al.*[79])

Other potential indications for a trial of immunosuppressant therapy include failure of myocarditis to resolve, progressive LV dysfunction despite conventional therapy, continued active myocarditis on biopsy or fulminant myocarditis that does not improve within 24–72 hours of full hemodynamic support, including mechanical assistance. Myocarditis associated with a known immune-mediated disease, such as systemic lupus erythematosus, may also benefit from immunosuppressive therapy.

These studies call into question the value of routine endomyocardial biopsy and immunosuppressant therapy in adults and children. Immunologic testing may be a more sensitive method of diagnosis and may reduce the sampling error noted with routine histology but awaits development and validation. Consideration of endomyocardial biopsy should be given whenever these specific immunosuppressant-responsive conditions are present or suspected. However, the low incidence of light microscopic evidence of histologic inflammatory disease, the fact that there is no specific therapy for most cases of myocarditis, and the fact that there are potential complications related to the procedure suggest that *routine* endomyocardial biopsy is not warranted.

Smaller studies have used differing immunosuppressant regimens. Kühl *et al.*[80] treated 31 patients with biopsies classified as immunohistologically positive (more than two cells per high power field and expression of adhesion molecules), negative Dallas Criteria, and LV dysfunction. Patients were treated with corticosteroids plus conventional therapy for 3 months followed by gradual tapering of methylprednisolone doses over 24 weeks (following biopsy and LVEF response). Therapy was associated with an improvement in

EF in 64% and improved NYHA functional class in 77%. Four patients (12%) had no change in EF despite improvement in inflammatory infiltrates. Three patients (9%) had no change in EF or inflammatory infiltrates. However, study conclusions are limited by the absence of a control group. These findings also reinforce the suggestion that light microscopy may not be the gold standard for the diagnosis of myocarditis or evaluation of therapy. Hopefully, new advances in immunohistochemistry will increase diagnostic and prognostic sensitivity and specificity.

Drucker et al.[81] retrospectively reviewed 46 children with congestive cardiomyopathy and Dallas Criteria of borderline or definite myocarditis. Twenty one patients were treated with intravenous IgG (2 g/kg over 24 hours) and were compared to 25 historical controls. Of the treated patients, four received a second dose of IgG and two were also treated with prednisone. Of the control patients, three received prednisone and two of these three patients also received cyclosporin. One died, one underwent heart transplantation, and one had persistent LV dysfunction. Overall survival was not improved although there was a trend toward improvement in 1-year survival in the treated group. In the IgG group, the mean LV end diastolic dimension was not significantly different from normal after 3 months. Fractional shortening improved in both groups but returned to normal only in the IgG group. Improvement in ventricular function persisted after adjustment for age, biopsy status, and use of ACE inhibitors and inotropes.

In a comparative study of interferon-alpha, thymomodulin, and conventional therapy in patients with biopsy-proven myocarditis or IDC, an improvement in the treatment groups was reported for EF (at rest and during exercise), maximum exercise time, functional class, and ECG abnormalities. Three of 12 conventionally treated patients died (one suddenly and two from heart failure), compared with one of 13 treated with interferon-alpha (sudden death in an IDC patient) and one of 13 treated with thymomodulin (of embolic cerebrovascular accident).[82] The use of intravenous immune globulin in 10 patients (NYHA III–IV) with symptoms of <6 months duration resulted in an improvement in LVEF (Figure 41.6) and functional improvement (NYHA I–II at 1 year of follow-up) in all nine patients who survived, regardless of biopsy results.[83]

Perhaps alternative immunosuppressant regimens and different diagnostic criteria may be more successful in demonstrating the utility of immunosuppressants. The European Study of Epidemiology and Treatment of Cardiac Inflammatory Disease (ESETCID)[84] is a prospective, multicenter, placebo-controlled, double-blind study intended to address the natural course of myocarditis, myopericarditis, pericarditis, and postmyocarditic muscle disease; the underlying processes which lead to progression of disease; and the benefit of immunosuppressant therapy based on etiology (autoimmune, enteroviral or cytomegalovirus induced). The primary endpoints are improvement in EF >5% points and improvement >10% in exercise tolerance time with bicycle ergometry. The secondary endpoints are reduction in LV end-diastolic dimension volume index, resolution of inflammatory infiltrates, lifestyle improvement, elimination of myocardial viral DNA and RNA, reduction of arrhythmias, and evaluation of mortality and need for cardiac transplantation. The treatment regimens will include conventional therapy with diuretics, ACE inhibitors, digoxin, and antiarrhythmics or defibrillators, and specific therapy for cytomegaloviral and enteroviral myocarditis, and prednisolone/azathioprine for myocarditis without detectable virus.

Other immunosuppressants have been studied in the murine model. The use of cyclophosphamide (CYA) in a murine model of Coxsackie B3 myocarditis revealed that therapy begun at the time of viral inoculation resulted in less severe cardiac lesions

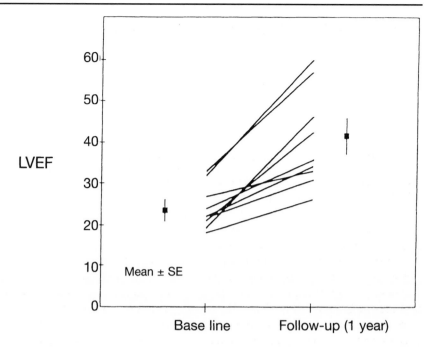

Change in LVEF

Figure 41.6   Change in LVEF ($P=0.003$) in patients treated with IV immune globulin. All patients demonstrated functional improvement and at 1-year follow-up were NYHA class I or II. No patient has been rehospitalized for congestive failure. (Adapted with permission from McNamara *et al*.[83])

compared to controls but no improvement in mortality. When therapy was begun later (8 days after viral inoculation), survival was worse in the CYA group despite improvement in cardiac lesions. When therapy was begun even later (day 21), there was no difference in survival or in cardiac infiltrates compared with controls.[85] In a murine model of EMC viral myocarditis, the use of tumor necrosis factor (TNF) resulted in greater myocardial viral content and more extensive myocardial necrosis and cellular infiltration. Anti-TNF-α monoclonal antibody did not alter mortality or prevent myocardial lesions unless given *before* viral infection.[86] There are no human studies with these agents. Preliminary data on the development of a enterovirus vaccine using chimeric Coxsackie virus B3 in a murine model of myocarditis suggest an attenuation of viral replication and diminished inflammatory infiltrates.[87]

CARDIAC TRANSPLANTATION

An analysis of outcome of 14 055 cardiac transplant recipients did not confirm the initial concern that there is a worse outcome if transplantation is performed during the acute stage of myocarditis. One-year actuarial survival in all groups transplanted (IDC, myocarditis, peripartum cardiomyopathy vs other diagnoses) was 80%.[88] Nonetheless, myocarditis may recur in the transplanted heart.[89]

Treatment of IDC: clinical and experimental

The same general supportive measures used in myocarditis are applicable in the management of IDC, except that moderate exercise is encouraged once heart failure symptoms have stabilized. Mild to moderate dynamic exercise is preferable to isometric exercise.[90]

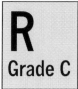

VASODILATORS, ACE INHIBITORS, AND ANGIOTENSIN RECEPTOR ANTAGONISTS

The beneficial effects of vasodilators (hydralazine and isosorbide dinitrate) and ACE inhibitors on symptomatic improvement and reduction in mortality have been shown in multiple large clinical trials.[91–95] Trials have included 15–18% of enrolled patients with a diagnosis of IDC.[91–95] These trials have documented a reduction in cardiac size, improvement in functional class, and a reduction in total and cardiovascular mortality. In addition, there is a reduction in the number of hospitalizations.[91–95].

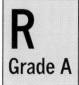

The use of enalapril in asymptomatic patients (EF <35%) resulted in a *non-significant* decrease in mortality. However, there was a reduction in the incidence of heart failure and related hospital admissions. The time to development of heart failure was shown to be prolonged from 8.3 months to 22.3 months.[93,94] The survival benefit of enalapril was found to be superior to the combination of hydralazine plus isosorbide dinitrate in the Second Vasodilator-Heart Failure Trial (V-HeFT-2).[95]

A short trial (8 weeks) comparing the angiotensin receptor II antagonist losartan with enalapril in 166 patients with NYHA class III–IV and an EF of <35% suggested comparable efficacy based on results of 6-minute walk test, dyspnea fatigue index, neurohumoral activation (norepinephrine and atrial naturetic factor levels), laboratory evaluation, and adverse events.[96] Larger trials of angiotensin receptor antagonists are currently underway. In a comparison of losartan (titrated to 50 mg/day) with captopril (50 mg three times a day) in 722 NYHA class II–IV patients over the age of 65, a 32% relative risk reduction of death and/or hospital admission was observed with the use of losartan (Evaluation of Losartan in the Elderly Study).[97] There was no difference in the number of hospital admissions for heart failure or improvement in functional class. This suggests that losartan may be used as an alternative to, if not preferred to, ACE inhibitors. A larger comparative study, powered to better address the issue of mortality, is underway.

DIGITALIS

Although the use of digitalis has long been a standard in the treatment of heart failure, only recently have large trials been conducted to adequately assess its safety and efficacy. Withdrawal trials of digitalis in patients with a depressed LVEF treated with diuretics and/or ACE inhibitors, in sinus rhythm, with mild to moderate heart failure, have shown a worsening of exercise performance and NYHA class, lower quality of life score, a need for additional drug therapy, more overall hospitalizations and hospitalizations for heart failure, and an increase in emergency room visits for heart failure compared with patients continued on digitalis. Patients who continued the use of digitalis had an increased time to treatment failure, higher LVEF, and lower heart rate and body weight. Its effect on mortality is neutral, with a balanced reduction in heart failure deaths and an increase in sudden arrhythmic deaths.[98–100] However, digoxin reduced hospitalization for heart failure.[100] Perhaps, unexpectedly, these results were similar in a group of patients with an EF ≥ 45%.[100] The symptomatic benefit of therapy was greatest in patients with an EF ≤ 25%, NYHA class III–IV, and in those with cardiomegaly. Idiopathic dilated cardiomyopathy was the etiology of heart failure in approximately 15–40% of patients enrolled in these trials.[98–100]

IMMUNOSUPPRESSANTS

The use of immunosuppressants is not as well studied in IDC as in myocarditis. Patients with IDC felt to be immune reactive, based on cellular infiltrate, Ig or complement deposition, elevated sedimentation rate or a positive gallium scan, were randomized to treatment with prednisone and compared to untreated controls by Parillo et al.[101] At 3 months, there was an improvement in EF, but this was not sustained at 9 months.[101] In another study, the use of interferon-alpha or thymomodulin in IDC appeared to improve EF (at rest and during exercise), maximum exercise time, functional class, and ECG abnormalities when compared with conventional therapy alone.[82] Ten patients with recent onset of heart failure and biopsy consistent with borderline myocarditis in one patient, non-specific inflammation in one patient, and six with no cellular infiltrate received intravenous immune globulin. There was an improvement in both LVEF (Figure 41.6), and functional classification (NYHA I–II at 1 year of follow-up) in all nine patients who survived.[83]

GROWTH HORMONE

Growth hormone has been suggested to be of therapeutic benefit in patients with IDC. In a recent pilot study, it resulted in improved quality of life, increased maximal exercise capacity, and increased LV mass and wall thickness, with resultant decreased wall stress, decreased chamber size, improved hemodynamics and systolic performance, and decreased myocardial oxygen consumption. Growth hormone therapy warrants further study.[102]

CALCIUM-CHANNEL BLOCKERS

The Prospective Randomized Amlodipine Survival Evaluation (PRAISE) trial[103] enrolled 1153 patients with NYHA class III–IV heart failure and an EF of <30%. Treatment with the calcium-channel blocker amlodipine was compared to placebo. On subgroup analysis, patients with dilated cardiomyopathy had a 31% reduction in fatal and non-fatal events and a 46% lower risk of death, although there was no significant reduction in overall mortality or fatal and non-fatal events. A follow-up study (PRAISE II) is prospectively testing the possibility that amlodipine is beneficial in IDC. The routine use of amlodipine in heart failure must await those results.

Cardiomyopathic Syrian hamsters are known to develop progressive focal myocardial necrosis, similar to lesions found in human cardiac diseases. In these hamsters, the process begins at 1 month of age, ultimately leading to heart failure. Using silicone rubber perfusion studies, Factor and colleagues[104] were able to document microvascular vasoconstriction, diffuse vessel narrowing, and lumenal irregularity associated with adjacent areas of myocytolytic necrosis. They were able to prevent the development of cellular necrosis by pretreatment of 30-day-old hamsters (the period when they normally develop these lesions) with verapamil. When treatment was begun at a later time (90 or 150 days), there was no alteration in scar or necrosis. However, verapamil had a positive effect on microvascular spasm, regardless of when treatment was begun, suggesting abnormal cellular calcium metabolism may be involved in the pathogenesis. Comparable human studies have not been done. These studies lend further support to the potential role of calcium and microvascular spasm.

BETA-BLOCKERS

Initial trials of the use of beta-blockers in IDC, while uncontrolled, suggested improved cardiac function and survival when added to digitalis and diuretics in patients with moderate to severe heart failure.[105] In addition, the withdrawal of such therapy appeared to result in the development of worsening heart failure.[105]

The long term effects of metoprolol were studied in an early double-blind, randomized study of limited size.[106] Patients also were frequently receiving treatment with digoxin, diuretics, and vasodilators. Patients had symptomatic heart failure with a baseline EF $\leq 49\%$. In the metoprolol-treated group, a significant improvement in functional class, exercise capacity, mean EF, and LV end-diastolic dimension was observed.[106] The subsequent larger Metoprolol in Dilated Cardiomyopathy (MDC) Trial[107] in symptomatic patients with an EF <40% showed a reduction in the composite endpoint of death or need for transplantation. However, all of the derived benefit was secondary to a reduction in cardiac transplantation, with no independent effect on all-cause mortality. Additional benefit was observed in several other measures; ejection fraction, pulmonary capillary wedge pressure, quality of life, exercise duration, and NYHA functional class improved significantly. The number of hospital readmissions for all patients and readmissions per patient were reduced with metoprolol. In a substudy of the Randomized Evaluation of Strategies of Left Ventricular Dysfunction (RESOLVD), of 450 patients with an EF<= 0.40, there was about a 50% risk reduction in mortality ($P=0.052$) and a significant improvement in ejection fraction with metoprolol CR compared to placebo over 20 weeks. There was no impact on cardiovascular or total hospitalizations[108] (personal communication, S. Yusuf).

The Cardiac Insufficiency Bisoprolol Study (CIBIS)[109] tested bisoprolol in heart failure and found no difference in sudden death or death due to documented venous thrombosis. On subgroup analysis, there was a reduction in mortality in IDC patients and those with NYHA class IV. There was also an improvement in functional status and fewer hospitalizations in patients treated with bisoprolol.

The alpha/beta-blocker carvedilol has been tested in patients with an EF of $\leq 35\%$ (NYHA classes II–IV), on digitalis, an ACE inhibitor, and diuretics, and was associated with a 65% reduction of all-cause mortality (not a prospective endpoint), a 27% reduction in hospitalization, and a 38% reduction in the combined endpoints of death and hospitalization (primary endpoint, progression of heart failure). The reduction in mortality was independent of age, sex, cause of heart failure, EF, exercise tolerance, systolic blood pressure, and heart rate.[110] The recent FDA approval of carvedilol for the treatment of heart failure represents a major advance in treatment options for heart failure, although the question of mortality effect is not completely resolved. Previously published randomized clinical trials of beta-blockers include over 1600 patients with heart failure. Taken together, these trials suggest a mortality risk reduction of approximately 20% but with wide confidence intervals.[110,111] Hence, the survival question requires additional study.

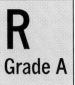

R

Grade A

Bucindolol is a non-selective beta-blocker with weak vasodilator properties that is well tolerated in compensated CHF. The use of bucindolol in IDC has resulted in a significant improvement in rest and exercise EF, hemodynamics, stroke work index, cardiac index, symptom score and functional class when compared to placebo controls.[112,113] There is also a decrease in central venous norepinephrine levels and maximum exercise heart rate with no change in maximal exercise time. The NHLBI/NIH supported Beta-blocker Evaluation of Survival Trial (BEST), which compares bucindolol in the placebo, is addressing the question of survival benefit: "Does addition of a beta-blocker to optimal therapy reduce total mortality in patients with moderate to severe heart failure?". Secondary objectives are to evaluate the effects of beta-blockade on total cardiovascular mortality, cardiovascular mortality due to worsening heart failure and sudden death, quality of life, hospitalization and costs, LVEF, incidence of myocardial infarction, combined transplant and mortality endpoints, and changes in the need for cotherapies.

INOTROPES

Multiple trials of different inotropes, both oral and intravenous, with various dose ranges have failed to result in an improvement in survival in patients with heart failure, although several agents may provide transient symptomatic improvement.[114–117] Thus, routine use of these agents cannot be recommended.

AMIODARONE

Over 40% of cardiac deaths occur suddenly, presumably due to arrhythmias. Both the Grupo de Estudio de la Sobrevida en la Insuficiencia Cardiaca en Argentina (GESICA)[118] and the Survival Trial of Antiarrhythmic Therapy in Congestive Heart Failure (CHF-STAT)[119] assessed the efficacy of amiodarone therapy in heart failure patients with asymptomatic ventricular arrhythmias.

GESICA[118] enrolled patients with NYHA class III–IV symptoms, an LVEF <35%, who were treated with routine heart failure therapy. The presence or absence of non-sustained ventricular tachycardia on Holter was noted. Patients were prospectively randomized to amiodarone 600 mg/day for 14 days, followed by 300 mg/day for 2 years. A total of 516 (260 in the amiodarone group) patients were enrolled. Within the amiodarone group, there was a 23% risk reduction (RR) in progressive heart failure. There was a 27% RR of sudden death, although there was no difference in non-cardiac deaths. There was also a 31% RR in death or heart failure admissions. On subgroup analysis, the effect of amiodarone was similar regardless of sex, functional class (NYHA class II–IV), and the presence or absence of non-sustained ventricular tachycardia. In addition, a larger proportion of amiodarone-treated patients were in the better functional classes.

CHF-STAT[119] enrolled 674 patients (336 amiodarone treated) with heart failure, >10 PVC/hour (unaccompanied by symptoms), with an EF <40% (PVC=premature ventricular complex). Patients were treated with amiodarone 800 mg/day for 2 weeks, then 400 mg/day for 50 weeks, followed by 300 mg/day until study completion. In contrast to the GESICA trial, there was no significant reduction in heart failure deaths, sudden deaths or non-cardiac deaths. Survival was unaffected by the suppression of PVCs or elimination of venous thrombosis. Amiodarone-treated patients had a significant improvement in LVEF at 6 months although this did not affect survival. When data were analyzed based on the etiology of heart failure, there was a trend toward improved mortality in non-ischemic patients ($P=0.07$). The difference between these two studies may be related to the different proportion of patients with coronary artery disease in the two trials and the fact that CHF-STAT but not GESICA was double-blind placebo-controlled.

Overview of treatment measures

While general supportive measures, with a period of no exercise, are recommended in the treatment of myocarditis, no specific therapies have been approved. ACE inhibitors, beta-blockers, and calcium-channel blockers have only been studied in animal models. The routine use of immunosuppressants is not supported by the Myocarditis Treatment Trial, although some subgroups may benefit, and other regimens may prove beneficial.

Supportive measures are also suggested in IDC and exercise is encouraged. Multiple trials support the use of vasodilators, ACE inhibitors and digoxin, when appropriate, in IDC. Preliminary data on the utility of beta-blockers are encouraging, but their routine use is not yet recommended. The potential for survival benefit of beta-blockers is being addressed by the ongoing BEST with bucindolol. There are insufficient data to support the use of immunosuppressants for the treatment of IDC. Further studies on the use of selected calcium-channel blockers are underway (PRAISE-II). The routine use of prophylactic antiarrhythmics is also unsupported. Transplantation is a valid treatment option for patients with endstage IDC and/or refractory myocarditis, although myocarditis may recur Grade B .

REFERENCES

1 Richardson P, McKenna W, Bristow M *et al.* Report of the 1995 World Health Organization/International Society and Federation of Cardiology Task Force on the Definition and Classification of Cardiomyopathies. *Circulation* 1996;**93**:841–2.

2 Taylor DO, Mason JW, Parmley WW. Myocarditis. In: Parmley W, Chatterjee K, Cheitlin MD *et al.* eds. *Cardiology.* Philadelphia: Lippincott-Raven, 1995, pp 1–26.

3 Daly K, Richardson PJ, Olsen EGJ *et al.* Acute myocarditis: role of histological and virological examination in the diagnosis and assessment of immunosuppressive treatment. *Br Heart J* 1984; **51**:30–5.

4 Parillo JE, Aretz HT, Palacios I, Fallon, Block PC. The results of transvenous endomyocardial biopsy can frequently be used to diagnose myocardial diseases in patients with idiopathic heart failure: endomyocardial biopsies in 100 consecutive patients revealed a substantial incidence of myocarditis. *Circulation* 1984;**69**: 93–101.

5 Bowles NE, Richardson PJ, Olsen EGJ, Archard LC. Detection of Coxsackie-B-virus-specific RNA sequences in myocardial biopsy samples from patients with myocarditis and dilated cardiomyopathy. *Lancet* 1986;**i**:1120–3.

6 Jin O, Sole MJ, Butany JW *et al.* Detection of enterovirus RNA in myocardial biopsies from patients with myocarditis and cardiomyopathy using gene amplification by polymerase chain reaction. *Circulation* 1990;**82**:8–16.

7 Grasso M, Arbustini E, Salini E *et al.* Search of Coxsackie B3 RNA in idiopathic dilated cardiomyopathy using gene amplification by polymerase chain reaction. *Am J Cardiol* 1992; **69**:658–64.

8 Weiss LM, Liu X-F, Chang KL, Billingham ME. Detection of enteroviral RNA in idiopathic dilated cardiomyopathy and other human cardiac tissues. *J Clin Invest* 1992;**90**:156–9.

9 Martin AB, Webber S, Fricker FJ *et al.* Acute myocarditis rapid diagnosis by PCR in children. *Circulation* 1994;**90**:330–9.

10 Schowengerdt KO, Jiyuan N, Denfield SW *et al.* Diagnosis, surveillance, and epidemiologic evaluation of viral infections in pediatric cardiac transplant recipients with the use of the polymerase chain reaction. *J Heart Lung Transplant* 1996;**15**:111–23.

11 Matsumori A, Matoba Y, Sasayama S. Dilated cardiomyopathy associated with hepatitis C virus infection. *Circulation* 1995;**92**:2519–25.

12 Dec GW Jr, Palacios IF, Fallon JT, *et al.* Active myocarditis in the spectrum of acute dilated cardiomyopathies. Clinical features, histologic correlates, and clinical outcome. *N Engl J Med* 1985;**312**:885–90.

13 Herskowitz A, Beisel KW, Wolfgram LJ, Rose NR. Coxsackievirus B3 murine myocarditis: wide pathologic spectrum in genetetically defined inbred strains. *Human Pathol* 1985;**16**:671–3.

14 Fenoglio JJ Jr, Ursell PC, Kellog CF, Drusin RE, Weiss MB. Diagnosis and classification of myocarditis by endomyocardial biopsy. *N Engl J Med* 1983;**310**:12–18.

15 Godman GC, Bunting H, Melnick JL. The histopathology of Coxsackie virus infection in mice. 1. Morphologic observations with four different viral types. *Am J Pathol* 1952;**28**: 223–45.

16 Woodruff JF. Viral myocarditis. *Am J Pathol* 1980; **101**:427–79.

17 Olsen EGJ. Endomyocardial biopsy. *Br Heart J* 1978;**40**:95–8.

18 Wolfgram LJ, Beisel KW, Herskowitz A, Rose NR. Variation in the susceptibility of congenic inbred mice to Coxsackie B3 induced myocarditis among different strains of mice. *J Immunol* 1986; **136**:1846–52.

19 Herskowitz A, Wolfgram LJ, Rose NR, Beisel KW. Coxsackie B3 myocarditis: a pathologic spectrum of myocarditis in genetically defined inbred strains. *J Am Coll Cardiol* 1987;**9**:1131–9.

20 Bhardwaj V, Kumar V, Geysen HM, Sercarz EE. Degenerate recognition of a dissimilar antigenic peptide by MBP-reactive T cells: implications for thymic education and autoimmunity. *J Immunol* 1993 **151**:5000–10.

21 Cunningham MW, Antone SM, Gulizia JM *et al.* Cytotoxic and viral neutralizing antibodies cross react with streptococcal M protein enteroviruses and human cardiac myosin. *Proc Natl Acad Sci USA* 1992;**89**:1320–24.

22 Alvarez FL, Neu N, Rose NR, Craig SW, Beisel KW. Heart-specific autoantibodies induced by Coxsackievirus B3: identification of heart autoantigens. *Clin Immunol Immunopathol* 1987; **43**:129–39.

23 Neu N, Beisel KW, Traystman MD, Rose NR, Craig SW. Autoantibodies specific for the cardiac myosin isoform are found in mice susceptible to Coxsackie B3-induced myocarditis. *J Immunol* 1987;**138**:2488–92.

24 Dahl AM, Beverley PCL, Stauss HJ. A synthetic peptide derived from the tumor-associated protein mdm2 can stimulate autoreactive, high avidity cytotoxic T lymphocytes that recognize naturally processed protein. *J Immunol* 1996; **157**:239–46.

25 Limas CJ, Goldenberg IF, Limas C. Autoantibodies against beta-adrenoreceptors in human dilated cardiomyopathy. *Circ Res* 1989;**64**:97–103.

26 Schultheiss HP, Schulze K, Huhl U, Ulrich G, Klingenberg M. The ADP/ATP carrier as a mitochondrial antigen – facts and perspectives. *Ann NY Acad Sci* 1986;**488**:44–64.

27 Wolff PG, Kuhl U, Schultheiss HP. Laminin distribution and autoantibodies to laminin in dilated cardiomyopathy and myocarditis. *Am Heart J* 1989;**117**:1303–9.

28 Ansari AA, Herskowitz A, Danner DJ. Identification of mitochondrial proteins that serve as targets for autoimmunity. *Circulation* 1988;**78**(Suppl):457 (Abstract).

29 Latif N, Baker CS, Dunn MJ *et al.* Frequency and specificity of antiheart antibodies in patients with dilated cardiomyopathy detected using SDS-PAGE and Western blotting. *J Am Coll Cardiol* 1993;**22**:1378–84.

30 Maisch B, Bauer E, Cirsi M, Kochsiek K. Cytolytic cross-reactive antibodies directed against the cardiac membrane and viral proteins in coxsackie B3 and B4 myocarditis. *Circulation* 1993;**87**(Suppl V):IV-49–IV-65.

31 Mason JW, O'Connell JB, Herskowitz A *et al.* A clinical trial of immunosuppressive therapy for myocarditis. *N Engl J Med* 1995;**333**:269–75.

32 Muir P, Tizley AJ, English TAH *et al.* Chronic relapsing pericarditis and dilated cardiomyopathy: serological evidence of persistent enterovirus infection. *Lancet* 1989;**1**: 804–7.

33 Cambridge G, MacArthur CG, Waterson AP, Goodwin JF, Oakley CM. Antibodies to Coxsackie B viruses in congestive cardiomyopathy. *Br Heart J* 1979;**41**:692–96.

34 Kawai C. Idiopathic cardiomyopathy: a study on the infection-immune theory as a cause of the disease. *Jpn Circ J* 1971;**35**:765–70.

35 Schwaiger A, Umlauft F, Weyrer K *et al.* Detection of enteroviral ribonucleic acid in myocardial biopsies from patients with idiopathic dilated cardiomyopathy by polymerase chain reaction. *Am Heart J* 1993;**126**:406–10.

36 Schultheiss HP, Bolte HD. Immunological analysis of auto-antibodies against the adenine nucleotide translocator in dilated cardiomyopathy. *J Mol Cell Cardiol* 1985;**17**: 603–17.

37 Caforio ALP, Grazzini M, Mann JM *et al.* Identification of a- and b-cardiac myosin heavy chain isoforms as major autoantigens in dilated cardiomyopathy. *Circulation* 1992;**85**:1734–42.

38 Herskowitz A, Neumann DA, Ansari AA. Concepts of autoimmunity applied to idiopathic

dilated cardiomyopathy. *J Am Coll Cardiol* 1993; **22**:1385–88.

39 Carlquist JF, Hibbs JB, Edelman LS, Watt RA, Anderson JL. Coxsackie B3 myocarditis in mice: viral clearance and post-infectious mortality are not associated with increased nitric oxide production. *Circulation* 1996;**94**(Suppl):I-468 (Abstract).

40 Nishi H, Kimura A, Koga Y, Toshima H, Sasazuki T. DNA typing of class II genes in Japanese patients with dilated cardiomyopathy. *J Mol Cell Cardiol* 1995;**27**:2385–92.

41 Gravanis M, Sternby N. Incidence of myocarditis: a 10-year autopsy study from Malmö, Sweden. *Arch Pathol Lab Med* 1991;**115**:390–2.

42 Herskowitz A, Campbell S, Deckers J *et al.* Demographic features and prevalence of idiopathic myocarditis in patients undergoing endomyocardial biopsy. *Am J Cardiol* 1993; **71**: 982–6.

43 Brown CA, O'Connell JB. Myocarditis and idiopathic dilated cardiomyopathy. *Am J Med* 1995;**99**:309–14.

44 Codd MB, Sugrue DD, Gersh BJ, Melton LJ. Epidemiology of idiopathic dilated and hypertrophic cardiomyopathy. *Circulation* 1989; **80**:564–72.

45 Dec GW, Fuster V. Medical progress: idiopathic dilated cardiomyopathy. *N Engl J Med* 1994; **331**:1564–75

46 Coughlin SS, Gottdiener JS, Baughman KL *et al.* Black-white differences in mortality in idiopathic dilated cardiomyopathy: the Washington DC Dilated Cardiomyopathy Study. *J Natl Med Assoc* 1994;**86**:583–91.

47 De Maria R, Gavazzi A, Recalcati F *et al.* Comparison of clinical findings in idiopathic dilated cardiomyopathy in women versus men. *Am J Cardiol* 1993;**72**:580–5.

48 Lampert MB, Lang RM. Peripartum cardiomyopathy. *Am Heart J* 1995;**130**:860–70.

49 Lampert MB, Weinert L, Hibbard J *et al.* Contractile reserve in patients with peripartum cardiomyopathy and recovered left ventricular function. *Am J Obstet Gynecol* 1997; **176**: 189–95.

50 Midei MG, DeMent SH, Feldman AM, Hutchins GM, Baughman KL. Peripartum myocarditis and cardiomyopathy. *Circulation* 1990;**81**:922–8.

51 Rizeq MN, Rickenbacher PR, Fowler MB, Billingham ME. Incidence of myocarditis in peripartum cardiomyopathy. *Am J Cardiol* 1994; **74**:474–7.

52 Witlin AG, Mabie WC, Sibai BM. Peripartum cardiomyopathy: an ominous diagnosis. *Am J Obstet Gynecol* 1997;**176**:182–8.

53 Dec GW, Waldman H, Southern J *et al.* Viral myocarditis mimicking acute myocardial infarction. *J Am Coll Cardiol* 1992;**20**: 85–9.

54 Costanzo-Nordin MR, O'Connell JB, Subramanian R, Robinson JA, Scanlon PJ. Myocarditis confirmed by biopsy presenting as acute myocardial infarction. *Br Heart J* 1985; **53**:25–9.

55 Lieberman EB, Herskowitz A, Rose NR, Baughman KL. A clinicopathologic description of myocarditis. *Clin Immunol Immunopathol* 1993;**68**:191–6.

56 Aretz HT. Myocarditis: the Dallas Criteria. *Human Pathol* 1987; **18**:619–24.

57 Kuhn H, Breithardt G, Knieriern HJ *et al.* Prognosis and possible presymptomatic manifestations of congestive cardiomyopathy (COCM). *Postgrad Med J* 1978;**54**:451–9.

58 Morgera T, Di Lenarda A, Dreas L *et al.* Electrocardiography of myocarditis revisited: clinical and prognostic significance of electrocardiographic changes. *Am Heart J* 1992; **124**:455–66.

59 Mendes LA, Dec GW, Picard MH *et al.* Right ventricular dysfunction: an independent predictor of adverse outcome in patients with myocarditis. *Am Heart J* 1994;**128**:301–7.

60 Gagliardi MG, Bevilacqua M, Squitieri C *et al.* Dilated cardiomyopathy caused by acute myocarditis in pediatric patients: evolution of myocardial damage in a group of potential heart transplant candidates. *J Heart Lung Transplant* 1993;**12**:S224-S229.

61 Fuster V, Gersh BJ, Giuliani ER *et al.* The natural history of idiopathic dilated cardiomyopathy. *Am J Cardiol* 1981;**47**:525–31.

62 Redfield MM, Gersh BJ, Bailey KR, Ballard DJ, Rodeheffer RJ. Natural history of idiopathic dilated cardiomyopathy: effect of referral bias and secular trend. *J Am Coll Cardiol* 1993;**22**: 1921–6.

63 Redfield MM, Gersh BJ, Bailey KR, Rodeheffer RJ. Natural history of incidentally discovered, asymptomatic idiopathic dilated cardio-myopathy. *Am J Cardiol* 1994; **74**:737–9.

64 Nagaoka H, Isobe N, Kubota S *et al.* Myocardial contractile reserve as prognostic determinant in patients with idiopathic dilated cardiomyopathy without overt heart failure. *Chest* 1997;**111**: 344–50.

65 Treasure CB, Vita JA, Cox DA *et al.* Endothelium-dependent dilation of the coronary microvasculature is impaired in dilated cardiomyopathy. *Circulation* 1990;**81**:772–9.

66 Taliercio CP, Seward JB, Driscoll DJ *et al.* Idiopathic dilated cardiomyopathy in the young: clinical profile and natural history. *J Am Coll Cardiol* 1985;**6**:1126–31.

67 Grogan M, Redfield MM, Bailey KR *et al.* Long-term outcome of patients with biopsy-proved myocarditis: comparison with idiopathic dilated

cardiomyopathy. *J Am Coll Cardiol* 1995;**26**: 80–84.

68 Ilbäck N-G, Fohlman J, Friman G. Exercise in coxsackie B3 myocarditis: effects on heart lymphocyte subpopulations and the inflammatory reaction. *Am Heart J* 1989;**117**: 1298–302.

69 Maron BJ, Isner JM, McKenna WJ. Task Force 3: hypertrophic cardiomyopathy, myocarditis and other myopericardial diseases and mitral valve prolapse. *J Am Coll Cardiol* 1994;**24**:845–99.

70 Matsumori A, Wang H, Abelmann WH, Crumpacker CS. Treatment of viral myocarditis with ribavirin in an animal preparation. *Circulation* 1985;**71**:834–9.

71 Rezkalla S, Kloner RA, Khatib G, Khatib R. Beneficial effects of captopril in acute coxsackie virus B₃ murine myocarditis. *Circulation* 1990; **81**:1039–46.

72 Araki M, Kanda T, Imai S *et al.* Comparative effects of losartan, captopril, and enalapril on murine acute myocarditis due to encephalomyocarditis virus. *J Cardiol Pharmacol* 1995;**26**:61–5.

73 Rezkalla S, Kloner RA, Khatib G, Smith FE, Khatib R. Effect of metoprolol in coxsackie virus B3 murine myocarditis. *J Am Coll Cardiol* 1988; **12**:412–14.

74 Tominaga M, Matsumori A, Okada I, Yamada T, Kawai C. β-Blocker treatment of dilated cardiomyopathy. Beneficial effects of carvedilol in mice. *Circulation* 1991;**83**:2021–8.

75 Dong R, Liu P, Wee L, Butany J, Sole MJ. Verapamil ameliorates the clinical and pathological course of murine myocarditis. *J Clin Invest* 1992;**90**:2022–30.

76 Costanzo-Nordin MR, Reap EA, O'Connell JB, Robinson JA, Scanlon PJ. A nonsteroid anti-inflammatory drug exacerbates coxsackie B₃ murine myocarditis. *J Am Coll Cardiol* 1985;**6**: 1078–82.

77 Rezkalla S, Khatib G, Khatib R. Coxsackie B₃ murine myocarditis: deleterious effects of nonsteroidal anti-inflammatory agents. *J Lab Clin Med* 1986;**107**:393–5.

78 Matsui S, Matsumori A, Matoba Y, Uchida A, Sasayama S. Treatment of virus-induced myocardial injury with a novel immunomodulating agent, vesnarinone. *J Clin Invest* 1994;**94**:1212–17.

79 Cooper LT, Berry GJ, Shabetai R, for the Multicenter Giant Cell Myocarditis Study Group Investigators. Idiopathic giant-cell myocarditis – natural history and treatment. *N Engl J Med* 1997;**336**:1860–6.

80 Kühl U, Schultheiss HP. Treatment of chronic myocarditis with corticosteroids. *Eur Heart J* 1995;**16**:168–72.

81 Drucker NA, Colan SD, Lewis AB *et al.* γ-Globulin treatment of acute myocarditis in the pediatric population. *Circulation* 1994;**89**:252–7.

82 Mirič M, Vasiljevič J, Bojič M *et al.* Long-term follow up of patients with dilated heart muscle disease treated with human leucocytic interferon alpha or thymic hormones. *Heart* 1996;**75**: 596–601.

83 McNamara DM, Rosenblum WD, Janosko KM *et al.* Intravenous immune globulin in the therapy of myocarditis and acute cardiomyopathy. *Circulation* 1997;**95**:2476–8.

84 Maisch B, Hufnagel G, Schönian U, Hengstenberg C. The European Study of Epidemiology and Treatment of Cardiac Inflammatory Disease (ESETCID). *Eur Heart J* 1995;**16**:173–5.

85 Kishimoto C, Thorp KA, Abelmann WH. Immunosuppression with high doses of cyclophosphamide reduces the severity of myocarditis but increases the mortality in murine coxsackievirus B₃ myocarditis. *Circulation* 1990;**82**:982–9.

86 Yamada T, Matsumori A, Sasayama S. Therapeutic effect of anti-tumor necrosis factor-alpha antibody on the murine model of viral myocarditis induced by encephalomyocarditis virus. *Circulation* 1994;**89**:846–51.

87 Chapman NM, Tracy S. Can recombinant DNA technology provide useful vaccines against viruses which induce heart disease? *Eur Heart J* 1995;**16**:144–6.

88 O'Connell JB, Breen TJ, Hosenpud JD. Heart transplantation in dilated heart muscle disease and myocarditits. *Eur Heart J* 1995;**16**(Suppl O): 137–9.

89 Loria K, Jessurun J, Shumway SJ, Kubo SH. Early recurrence of chronic active myocarditis after heart transplantation. *Human Pathol* 1994;**25**: 323–6.

90 Williams JF, Bristow MR, Fowler MB *et al.* Guidelines for the evaluation and management of heart failure. *Circulation* 1995;**92**:2764–84.

91 Cohn JN, Archibald DG, Ziesche S *et al.* Effect of vasodilator therapy on mortality in chronic congestive heart failure: results of a Veterans Administration Cooperative Study. *N Engl J Med* 1986;**314**:1547–52.

92 CONSENSUS Trial Study Group. Effects of enalapril on mortality in severe congestive heart failure: results of the Cooperative North Scandinavian Enalapril Survival Study (CONSENSUS). *N Engl J Med* 1987;**316**: 1429–35.

93 SOLVD Investigators. Effect of enalapril on survival in patients with reduced left ventricular ejection fractions and congestive heart failure. *N Engl J Med* 1991;**325**:293–302.

94 SOLVD Investigators. Effect of enalapril on mortality and the development of heart failure in asymptomatic patients with reduced left ventricular ejection fractions. *N Engl J Med* 1992; **327**:685–91.

95 Loeb HS, Johnson G, Henrick A *et al.* Effect of enalapril, hydralazine plus isosorbide dinitrate, and prazosin on hospitalization in patients with chronic congestive heart failure. The V-HeFT Cooperative Studies Group. *Circulation* 1993;**87** (Suppl 6): VI78–87.

96 Dickstein K, Chang P, Willenheimer R *et al.* Comparison of the effects of losartan and enalapril on clinical status and exercise performance in patients with moderate or severe chronic heart failure. *J Am Coll Cardiol* 1995; **26**:438–45.

97 Pitt B, Segal R, Martinez FA *et al.* Randomized trial of losartan versus captopril in patients over 65 with heart failure (Evaluation of Losartan in the Elderly Study, ELITE). *Lancet* 1997;**349**: 747–52.

98 Uretsky BF, Young JB, Shahidi FE *et al.* Randomized study assessing the effect of digoxin withdrawal in patients with mild to moderate chronic congestive heart failure: results of PROVED trial. *J Am Coll Cardiol* 1993;**22**: 955–62.

99 Packer M, Gheorghiade M, Young J *et al.* Withdrawal of digoxin from patients with chronic heart failure treated with angiotensin-converting-enzyme inhibitors. *N Engl J Med* 1993;**329**:1–7.

100 Digitalis Investigation Group. The effect of digoxin on mortality and morbidity in patients with heart failure. *N Engl J Med* 1997;**336**: 525–33.

101 Parillo JE, Cunnion RE, Epstein SE *et al.* A prospective, randomized, controlled trial of prednisone for dilated cardiomyopathy. *N Engl J Med* 1989;**321**:1061–8.

102 Fazio S, Sabatini D, Capaldo B *et al.* A preliminary study of growth hormone in the treatment of dilated cardiomyopathy. *N Engl J Med* 1996; **334**:809–14.

103 Packer M, O'Connor CM, Ghali JK *et al.* Effect of amlodipine on morbidity and mortality in severe chronic heart failure (PRAISE). *N Engl J Med* 1996;**335**: 1107–14.

104 Factor SM, Minase T, Cho S, Dominitz R, Sonnenblick EH. Microvascular spasm in the cardiomyopathic Syrian hamster: a preventable cause of focal myocardial necrosis. *Circulation* 1982;**66**:342–54.

105 Swedberg K, Hjalmarson A, Waagstein F, Wallentin I. Preliminary communications: prolongation of survival in congestive cardiomyopathy by beta receptor blockade. *Lancet* 1979; 1374–6.

106 Engelmeier RS, O'Connell JB, Walsh R *et al.* Improvement in symptoms and exercise tolerance by metoprolol in patients with dilated cardiomyopathy: double-blind, randomized, placebo-controlled trial. *Circulation* 1985;**72**: 536–46.

107 Waagstein F, Bristow MR, Swedberg K. Beneficial effects of metoprolol in idiopathic dilated cardiomyopathy. *Lancet* 1993;**342**:1441–6.

108 Tsuyuki RT, Yusuf S, Rouleau JL *et al.*, for the RESOLD Study Investigators. Combination of neurohormonal blockade with ACE inhibitors, angiotensin antagonists and beta-blockers in patients with congestive heart failure: design of the Random Evaluation of Strategies for Left Ventricular Dysfunction (RESOLVD) Pilot Study. *Can J Cardiol* 1997;**13** (in press).

109 CIBIS Investigators and Committees. A randomized trial of β-blockade in heart failure: the Cardiac Insufficiency Bisoprolol Study (CIBIS). *Circulation* 1994;**90**:1765–73.

110 Packer M, Bristow MR, Cohn JN *et al.* The effect of carvedilol on morbidity and mortality in patients with chronic heart failure. *N Engl J Med* 1996;**334**:1349–55.

111 Sharpe N. Beta-blockers in heart failure. Future directions. *Eur Heart J* 1996;**17**(Suppl B): 39–42.

112 Gilbert EM, Anderson JL, Deitchman D *et al.* Long term β-blocker vasodilator therapy improves cardiac function in idiopathic dilated cardiomyopathy: a double-blind, randomized study of bucindolol versus placebo. *Am J Med* 1990;**88**:223–9.

113 Woodley SL, Gilbert EM, Anderson JL *et al.* β-blockade with bucindolol in heart failure caused by ischemic versus idiopathic dilated cardiomyopathy. *Circulation* 1991;**84**:2426–41.

114 Simonton CA, Chatterjee K, Cody RJ *et al.* Milrinone in congestive failure: acute and chronic hemodynamic and clinical evaluation. *J Am Coll Cardiol* 1985;**6**:453–9.

115 DiBianco R, Shabetai R, Kostuk W *et al.* for the Milrinone Multicenter Trial Group. A comparision of oral milrinone, digoxin, and their combination in the treatment of patients with chronic heart failure. *N Engl J Med* 1989;**320**: 677–83.

116 Uretsky BF, Jessup M, Konstam MA *et al.* for the Enoximone Multicenter Trial Group. Multicenter trial of oral enoximone in patients with moderate to moderately severe congestive heart failure. *Circulation* 1990;**82**:774–80.

117 Feldman AM, Bristow MR, Parmley WW *et al.* for the vesnarinone study group. Effects of vesnarinone on morbidity and mortality in patients with heart failure. *N Engl J Med* 1993; **329**:149–55.

118 Doval HC, Nul DR, Grancelli HO *et al.* for Grupo de Estudio de la Sobrevida en la Insuficiencia Cardiaca en Argentina (GESICA). Randomised trial of low-dose amiodarone in severe congestive heart failure. *Lancet* 1994;**344**: 493–98.

119 Singh SN, Fletcher RD, Fisher SG *et al.* for the Survival Trial of Antiarrhythmic Therapy in Congestive Heart Failure. Amiodarone in patients with congestive heart failure and asymptomatic ventricular arrhythmia. *N Engl J Med* 1995;**333**:77–82.

Prevention of congestive heart failure and treatment of asymptomatic left ventricular dysfunction

42

R. S. McKelvie,
C. R. Benedict,
S. Yusuf

EPIDEMIOLOGY OF HEART FAILURE

Over the past three decades, epidemiological studies have been increasingly used to identify the cause of major chronic degenerative diseases such as systemic hypertension and atherosclerosis.[1] Early studies on the prevalence and incidence of heart failure were drawn from private practice, hospital wards, and admissions to hospitals.[1,2] Also, data from survey studies were used to determine the prevalence rate of heart failure.[3] The prevalence of heart failure shows some disparity among the published studies although generally the results are similar in demonstrating an increase with age.[4–7] Prevalence increases from approximately 0.7 cases/1000 persons in the younger age group (<50 years old) to approximately 27 cases/1000 persons in the older age (>65 years old) group. The incidence of heart failure is greater in men than in women and increases progressively with age.[6–10] The incidence in younger men (<50 years old) is approximately one case/1000 persons per year, increasing in the older age group (>65 years old) to 11 cases/1000 persons per year. In women the incidence increases in the younger group (<50 years old) from 0.4 cases/1000 persons per year to 5 cases/1000 persons per year in older individuals (>65 years old).

There are a number of reasons why some disparity has been observed among these studies examining incidence and prevalence in heart failure patients. The studies differ with regard to sampling methods (population-based vs cohort-based), geography and demographics, case finding methods (medical record review vs systematic questionnaires and examinations), and diagnostic criteria.[11] Even though these differences are

Table 42.1 Comparison of subjects with an ejection fraction ≥0.48 compared to those with an ejection fraction <0.48

	EF<0.48 (n=43)	EF≥0.48 (n=1523)
LV end-diastolic dimension (mm)	49.9*	47.8
LV end-systolic dimension (mm)	39.7*	30.6
LA dimension (mm)	40.2*	38.2
LV mass index (g/m²)	126.3*	111.4

LV, left ventricle; LA, left atrium.
* $P<0.05$ compared to EF≥0.48.
Adapted from Bröckel U *et al.* Prevalence of left ventricular dysfunction in the general population. *J. Am. Coll. Cardiol.* 1996; **27**(Suppl. A):25A, with permission.

responsible for the disparities among the studies, they also provide a more robust database and complementary information.

ASYMPTOMATIC LEFT VENTRICULAR DYSFUNCTION IN THE POPULATION

Studies assessing the epidemiology of heart failure have largely identified symptomatic individuals because identification of these patients is based on clinical criteria and does not require measuring left ventricular (LV) function.[11] Asymptomatic patients with LV dysfunction have therefore not been included in these studies. Consequently the available data on the prevalence of patients with asymptomatic LV dysfunction is limited, even though treatment of these patients may be expected to significantly improve their outcome.[12]

There have been at least two studies, both part of the WHO MONICA project, which screened the general population looking for the presence of asymptomatic LV dysfunction.[13-15] Bröckel *et al.*[13] used echocardiography to examine 1566 individuals in the general population in Augsburg, Germany. The overall prevalence of individuals with an ejection fraction (EF) less than 0.48 (2 SD below mean) was 2.8% (n=43), with a prevalence of 3.2% (n=24) in men, and 2.3% (n=19) in women. Of these 43 patients with an ejection fraction less than 0.48, there were 25 (58% of those with a low EF) who had a known history of cardiovascular disease while 18 (42% of those with a low EF) were without a history of cardiovascular disease. The 95th centile of 0.48 for EF in this study was high and only two of the individuals had an ejection fraction less than 0.35. Compared to individuals with an EF greater than 0.48, individuals with LV dysfunction had increases in LV dimensions and in LV mass (Table 42.1). The findings of this study demonstrated that moderate LV dysfunction is a relatively common finding in the general population, but that severe LV dysfunction in asymptomatic individuals was less frequent in this study. Therefore the authors suggested that echocardiographic screening cannot be recommended in the unselected, middle aged population to identify such patients.

McDonagh[14] performed a similar study in Glasgow, Scotland assessing 1617 men and women aged 25–74 years from the general population. Left ventricular dysfunction was defined as an ejection fraction less than 35%. The overall prevalence of LV

Table 42.2 Prevalence rate (%) of cardiovascular disease in patients with asymptomatic LV dysfunction (EF ≤0.35) compared to those with normal ventricular function (EF >0.35)

	EF ≤0.35 (n=135)	EF >0.35 (n=1482)
ECG evidence of previous MI	33	13
Previous MI reported	18	4
≥1 mm ST depression on exercise testing	25	14
Hypertension	37	23

Adapted from McDonagh TA *et al.* Global left ventricular systolic dysfunction in North Glasgow. *J. Am. Coll. Cardiol.* 1996; 27(Suppl. A);106A, with permission.

dysfunction was 8.4% (n=135 individuals), with the prevalence in women under 35 years of age being the lowest at 3.7% and increasing to 17.7% in men over age 66 years; men had the higher prevalence throughout the age groups. The prevalence for symptomatic LV dysfunction in this population was 2.9% and that of asymptomatic LV dysfunction was 4.8%. Compared to individuals with a normal ejection fraction, individuals with LV dysfunction more commonly had a previous history of cardiovascular disease (Table 42.2). Only 37% of those with symptomatic and 16% of those with asymptomatic LV dysfunction were receiving treatment with an ACE inhibitor and/or a diuretic and/or digoxin. The results of this study indicate asymptomatic LV dysfunction is common, underdiagnosed, and undertreated.

Individuals with asymptomatic LV dysfunction on average are younger than patients with heart failure documented in other studies.[11,13,16] The data from Bröckel et al.[13] and McDonagh et al.[14] indicate asymptomatic LV dysfunction is relatively common in the general population. However, they differ with regard to the prevalence of severe LV dysfunction, with Bröckel et al.[13] finding only two individuals (0.1%) with an ejection fraction less than 0.35 while McDonagh et al.[14] identified 135 individuals (8.4%). The main reason for the difference between the Augsberg and Glasgow studies may be the higher proportion of individuals with cardiovascular risk factors in the Scottish study. It may also have to do with age and method of echocardiographic measures. Both these studies demonstrated that there is frequently previous evidence of cardiovascular disease in these individuals.

Another factor which is gaining more recognition as a potentially important contributor to progression of LV systolic dysfunction and development of symptomatic heart failure is impaired LV diastolic function, whether by itself or in the presence of LV systolic dysfunction. The prevalence of normal ventricular systolic performance in patients with congestive heart failure (CHF) varies widely from 13% to 74%, with the majority of studies reporting a value of 40%.[17] Normal ventricular systolic function with CHF is more prevalent in patients >65 years of age than those ≤65 years old and among hypertensives with LV hypertrophy.[17] Studies report an annual mortality associated with diastolic heart failure of 3–9%, which is lower than that of patients with systolic heart failure.[17,18] A lack of consensus among physicians remains regarding what constitutes LV diastolic dysfunction measured by non-invasive techniques.[17] Therefore there is a need to develop a consensus for diagnostic criteria of diastolic heart failure which could then be used to provide a better estimate of its prevalence and prognosis. There is also a need for randomized clinical trials to determine the appropriate treatment for patients with established LV diastolic dysfunction.

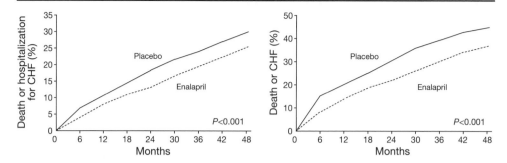

Figure 42.1 Death or hospitalization for congestive heart failure (CHF) and death or development of congestive heart failure in the Prevention Trial from SOLVD. (From SOLVD Investigators, *N Engl J Med* 1992;**327**:685–91, with permission.)

Although the presence of asymptomatic LV systolic dysfunction is a relatively common finding in the general population, a program of screening unselected middle aged individuals to identify such patients cannot be currently recommended. A more prudent approach would be to screen individuals who are at a greater risk of developing LV dysfunction such as those known to have ischemic heart disease or hypertension. Criteria which can be used to assess the risk of developing LV dysfunction will be outlined below in the subsequent sections.

FACTORS THAT LEAD TO THE DEVELOPMENT OF HEART FAILURE

Even though ACE inhibitors have recently been demonstrated to decrease morbidity and mortality, the event rate for heart failure remains very high. Obviously other measures are required to decrease the mortality and morbidity associated with heart failure. The results from the Survival and Ventricular Enlargement (SAVE) trial[19] and the Prevention trial of the Studies of Left Ventricular Dysfunction (SOLVD)[12] demonstrate the onset of heart failure can be prevented or delayed in patients with asymptomatic or minimally symptomatic LV systolic dysfunction with the use of ACE inhibitor (Figure 42.1). Therefore the most effective method to decrease mortality may be to identify patients who have asymptomatic LV dysfunction and treat them early to prevent the progression to symptomatic LV dysfunction. A number of factors have been identified which help predict whether an individual may have or develop LV dysfunction.

Hypertension

Hypertension for many years has been known to be an important risk factor for the development of heart failure.[6,8,10,20,21] In men and women, hypertension is associated with a three- to four-fold increase in the risk of heart failure for individuals between 35 and 64 years, and approximately two-fold increase for individuals over 65 years of age.[6,22] Although the relative risk is higher in the younger age group, the absolute excess risk is higher in the older age group, reflecting greater absolute risk differences.[22] Multivariate analyses have revealed that hypertension (defined as a systolic blood pressure of 140 mmHg or more or a diastolic blood pressure of 90 mmHg or more on the average of two physician measurements or current use of medications for treatment of high blood pressure) is associated with a high population-attributable risk for CHF accounting for 39% of cases in men and 59% in women.[21] Hypertension represents a continuous risk variable with no clear cut-off point below which CHF will not develop. Over four decades of observation there has been no significant change in the frequency of hypertension as an attributable cause of heart failure.[23] Therefore, hypertension remains an important risk factor for the development of heart failure.

Left ventricular hypertrophy

The presence of LV hypertrophy has been well documented as a risk factor for the development of heart failure, even after controlling for hypertension.[21–24] Electrocardiographic, chest radiographic, and echocardiographic criteria have all been used to document the presence of LV hypertrophy.[25] ECG evidence of LV hypertrophy criteria is associated with increased risk of CHF that is greater than the risk associated with cardiac enlargement on chest radiography. Data from Framingham demonstrate that the age-adjusted biennial rate of developing heart failure in men with ECG evidence of LV hypertrophy was 71/1000 patients aged 35–64 years and 102/1000 individuals aged 65–94 years, which was greater than that found when cardiac enlargement was present radiographically in men in the same age groups: 16/1000 individuals and 56/1000 individuals respectively.[25] This suggests that the ECG findings reflect ischemia in addition to anatomical hypertrophy.[25] LV hypertrophy is associated with a 15-fold increase in the incidence of heart failure in men less than or equal to 64 years of age and a five-fold increase in men greater than or equal to 65 years.[22] In women, LV hypertrophy is associated with a 13-fold increase in heart failure for the younger age group and a five-fold increase for the older age group.[22] Although the relative risk is higher in the younger age group, the absolute excess in risk is higher in the older age group, reflecting greater absolute risk differences.

Smoking

Cigarette smoking has been found in 42% of men and 24% of women who develop heart failure.[22] In men the relationship between cigarette smoking and development of heart failure is greater in the younger age group compared to the older age group.[6,22] Multivariate analyses have demonstrated smoking to be a strongly significant independent risk factor for the development of heart failure in men, even in the older age group.[6] The relationship between cigarette smoking and the risk of developing heart failure in women is inconsistent; although there has been a trend to an increase in relative risk in older women.[22] Therefore the data would suggest smoking is a risk factor for the development of heart failure and in fact the hazardous effects may be underestimated, as not all studies have taken into account changes in smoking habits over time and this could lead to an underestimation of smokers in the older age groups.[6]

Hyperlipidemia

Although a definite relationship between lipid abnormalities and the development of coronary artery disease has been demonstrated, the importance of lipid abnormalities has not been clearly demonstrated for heart failure. However, there is evidence to suggest a relationship between elevated triglyceride levels and the development of heart failure,[6] while a high ratio of total cholesterol to high density lipoprotein cholesterol is also associated with an increased incidence of heart failure.[22] The investigators in the Simvastatin Survival Study (4S) Group Trial found patients in the simvastatin group had a significantly lower incidence (6.2%) of heart failure compared to those in the placebo group (8.5%).[26] Interestingly, a higher triglyceride concentration and lower HDL concentration predicted the development of heart failure. These results further support the importance of lipid abnormalities as a factor responsible for the development of heart failure.

Diabetes mellitus

Diabetes mellitus is a well established risk factor for the development of coronary artery disease. Over the past 25 years, diabetes has been recognized as a factor responsible for the development of heart failure[6,8,9,21,23,27] working through an independent mechanism rather than simple acceleration of coronary atherosclerosis.[1,16,25,27] The presence of fibrosis in the hearts of diabetics has been described and it is thought to be due to diabetic microangiopathy.[28] The prevalence of diabetes in heart failure patients has been reported to be approximately 22%.[29] Recent data from the Randomized Evaluation of Strategies for Left Ventricular Dysfunction (RESOLVD) study has found in 568 CHF patients a 26% prevalence of documented diabetes, while 18% of additional patients were found to have abnormal fasting glucose levels but no diagnosis of diabetes.[30] Therefore approximately 44% of these patients had either known diabetes or abnormal fasting glucose levels. This suggests that most studies have underestimated the importance of glucose abnormalities in heart failure. Diabetes is more common in women than men with heart failure[16,22] and women with diabetes have a greater risk of developing heart failure than men with diabetes.[22,23,27] Following a myocardial infarction, patients with diabetes who develop heart failure have more severe symptoms than patients without diabetes who develop heart failure.[31] For any given level of infarct size, diabetic patients had a lower ejection fraction compared to non-diabetic patients (Yusuf et al., unpublished data). In the SOLVD trial in patients with asymptomatic LV dysfunction, diabetes is an independent predictor of development of heart failure and mortality.[32] Furthermore, the diabetic patients treated with enalapril had a greater mortality than the non-diabetic patients treated with enalapril, indicating that although ACE inhibitors benefit this subgroup of patients, diabetes still remains a significant predictor of outcome.

Therefore, the data would suggest abnormalities of glucose metabolism should be aggressively searched for and treated in CHF patients.

Microalbuminuria

In the ongoing Heart Outcomes Prevention Evaluation (HOPE) trial, microalbuminuria is a predictor of heart failure and other cardiovascular events in both diabetic and non-diabetic patients (Gerstein et al., unpublished observations). In this group of patients at high risk of a cardiovascular event, both the diabetic and non-diabetic patients with an albumin/creatinine ratio ≥ 2 mg/mmol were more likely to be hypertensive and smoking, and have a higher waist/hip ratio, lower ankle/arm systolic ratio, abnormal ECG and evidence of LV hypertrophy than normoalbuminuric patients ($P < 0.01$). After adjusting for these factors, 3.2% of all HOPE patients with elevated albumin/creatinine ratio were hospitalized for heart failure by one year compared to 0.9% of normoalbuminuric patients ($P<0.01$).

Vital capacity

A low or decrease in vital capacity over time has been found to be associated with an increased risk of developing heart failure.[25] The abnormality in vital capacity probably reflects the lungs being congested with blood due to LV dysfunction. However, the relationship between vital capacity and the development of heart failure has not been a consistent finding in all studies.[6]

Heart rate

In hypertensive patients, resting heart rate was a predictor of future development of heart failure.[33] Risk of heart failure increased with the heart rate in a continuous graded fashion from an age-adjusted biennial rate of 14.6/1000 patients at heart rates less than 64 beats per minute to a rate of 62.2/1000 patients at heart rates greater than 85 beats per minute. This may indicate asymptomatic LV dysfunction and subtle activation of the neuroendocrine system.

Obesity

Eriksson *et al.*[6] have reported that being overweight was an independent risk factor for the development of heart failure. This finding would support efforts directed at dietary modification which would promote weight loss and also help to correct lipid abnormalities.

PATHOPHYSIOLOGICAL ABNORMALITIES IN ASYMPTOMATIC LV DYSFUNCTION THAT PREDICT THE DEVELOPMENT OF CHF

Neuroendocrine activation

It has been well described that symptomatic heart failure is characterized by activation of several neuroendocrine systems.[34-38] The well documented finding that ACE inhibitor therapy improves survival in patients with heart failure further suggests neurohormones play a role in the pathogenesis of symptomatic heart failure.[39,40] Furthermore, the finding that ACE inhibitor therapy in asymptomatic patients with LV dysfunction reduces the rates of progression to symptomatic heart failure and hospitalization is consistent with neuroendocrine activation having a role in progression of early LV dysfunction to symptomatic heart failure.[12] A substudy of the SOLVD trial demonstrated that the

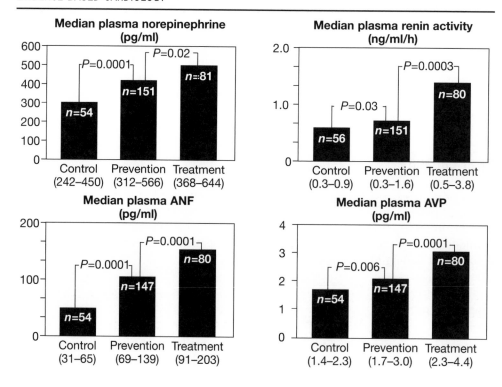

Figure 42.2 Comparison of norepinephrine, plasma renin activity, plasma atrial naturietic factor (ANF) and plasma arginine vasopressin (AVP) in healthy control subjects, patients with asymptomatic left ventricular dysfunction and patients with symptomatic congestive heart failure (From Francis GS *et al.*, *Circulation* 1990;82: 1724–9, with permission.)

median values for plasma norepinephrine, plasma atrial natriuretic factor (ANF), plasma arginine vasopressin (AVP), and plasma renin activity (PRA) were significantly higher in patients with asymptomatic LV dysfunction than in age and gender matched normal control individuals, with symptomatic patients having the highest neurohumoral values (Figure 42.2).[41] Plasma norepinephrine levels appear to increase early in the development of LV dysfunction, whereas the increase in PRA seems to occur only when the patients are taking diuretics. The degree of LV dysfunction is one of the mechanisms for activation of neurohormones as patients with an ejection fraction greater than 0.45 and pulmonary congestion on chest radiography were found to have only minimal neurohormonal activation with a modest increase in AVP and PRA.[42]

In the SOLVD Prevention trial, plasma norepinephrine level was the strongest predictor of the future development of heart failure.[43] This finding was independent of LV ejection fraction, NYHA class, age, sex, cause of heart failure, treatment assignment to placebo or enalapril, or pre-randomization ANF or PRA levels. Plasma norepinephrine levels above the median of 393 pg/ml were associated with a relative risk of 2.59 ($P = 0.002$) for all-cause mortality, 2.55 ($P = 0.005$) for hospitalization for heart failure, 1.88 ($P = 0.002$) for development of heart failure, 1.92 ($P = 0.001$) for ischemic events, and 2.59 ($P = 0.005$) for myocardial infarction (Figure 42.3). PRA and ANP were not as useful for predicting clinical outcome because although trends were observed for these hormones, they were not statistically significant. These data are very important because

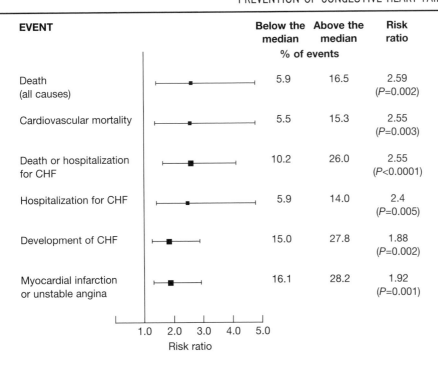

EVENT		Below the median	Above the median	Risk ratio
		% of events		
Death (all causes)		5.9	16.5	2.59 (P=0.002)
Cardiovascular mortality		5.5	15.3	2.55 (P=0.003)
Death or hospitalization for CHF		10.2	26.0	2.55 (P<0.0001)
Hospitalization for CHF		5.9	14.0	2.4 (P=0.005)
Development of CHF		15.0	27.8	1.88 (P=0.002)
Myocardial infarction or unstable angina		16.1	28.2	1.92 (P=0.001)

Figure 42.3 Effect of plasma norepinephrine level on all-cause mortality, cardiovascular mortality, development of CHF, hospitalization for CHF, and development of ischemic events. For each group, the increase in risk is shown as a percentage. Horizontal lines indicate the 95% CI. Size of each square is proportional to the number of events in that group. Vertical line corresponds to a finding of no effect. (From Benedict CR *et al.*, *Circulation* 1996;**94**:690–7, with permission.)

they suggest modulating the release or effect of plasma norepinephrine early in patients with asymptomatic left ventricular dysfunction may improve prognosis and prevent heart failure and perhaps ischemic events.

A recent study examines the location of adrenergic activity in patients with early heart failure.[44] In this study they found a selective increase in cardiac adrenergic drive in patients with early heart failure. This preceded the augmented sympathetic outflow to the kidneys and skeletal muscle found in advanced heart failure. These data collectively indicate that activation of the sympathetic system in early heart failure is causally related to the syndrome and drugs such as beta-blockers may be of value.

Cardiac dilation and remodeling

The process of LV remodeling in the setting of a prior myocardial infarction leading to ventricular dilation has been well described.[45–50] Even several years after the initial cardiac insult or remote from the precipitating cause of heart failure, this process continues progressively with continuing left ventricular dilation.[51–54] Among asymptomatic patients the rate of progression of ventricular dilation and systolic dysfunction is slower than in symptomatic patients.[51,52] It seems likely that asymptomatic and symptomatic patients represent a continuum of pathology, with the rate of ventricular

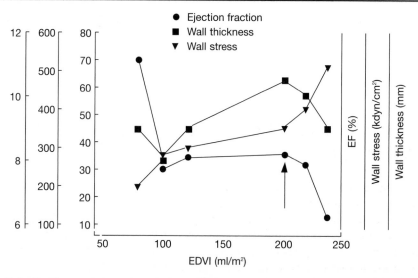

Figure 42.4 Hypothesis proposed to explain the changes in ejection fraction (EF), systolic wall stress, and wall thickness in relation to the progression of the left ventricular dilation (end-diastolic volume index, EDVI) after an acute myocardial insult. Under normal conditions, the EF is well above 50% and the wall stress is low. Immediately after the myocardial insult, EF and wall thickness decrease while wall stress increases. As the ventricle dilates, EF may recover slightly as a result of hypertrophy. The ventricle finally reaches a point that the rate and extent of dilation exceeds the capacity to hypertrophy, resulting in a rapid increase in wall stress (*arrow*). This would result in a decline in EF and a rapid deterioration of clinical status (From Pouleur HG *et al.*, *J Am Coll Cardiol* 1993;**22**(Suppl A):43A–48A 1993.)

dilation progression accelerating at later stages. Although the exact stimuli affecting these changes in myocardial structure remain unknown, increased myocardial wall stress has been postulated to represent an initiating factor. Activation of the renin–angiotensin system appears to play an important role in the pathogenesis of ventricular remodeling by contributing to the increase in wall stress and possibly by direct myocardial effects.[55–57]

The progression of LV dysfunction can be insidious in asymptomatic patients. When an initial insult causes the loss of large amounts of myocardium, the ejection fraction decreases and the end-diastolic volume increases (Figure 42.4). This increase in end-diastolic dimension is accompanied by relative thinning of the wall and an increase in wall stress.[58] As the compensatory remodeling process evolves, the ventricle dilates further, but as hypertrophy develops, wall thickness increases and the ejection fraction may recover slightly. The degree of hypertrophy is never sufficient to normalize left ventricular wall stress. The results from SOLVD support this hypothesis because in all patients studied the systolic and diastolic wall stresses were markedly augmented at baseline.[59] Neurohumoral systems are chronically activated in asymptomatic patients.[41] Because the mechanical and neurohumoral stimuli for hypertrophy continue to be activated, the remodeling process continues at a slow rate in asymptomatic patients with LV dysfunction. Furthermore, the ejection fraction may be maintained, probably because of new contractile units in the LV walls. Ventricular function is stable for a while until the rate of ventricular dilation increases and ejection fraction further declines. This is supported by data from the Treatment trial of SOLVD.[52] Hypertrophy is unable to keep pace with LV dilation, wall thickness decreases, wall stress increases rapidly resulting in a decrease in ejection fraction despite further LV dilation. Therefore, even when the asymptomatic patient with LV dysfunction appears stable, there are significant changes taking place in the heart which ultimately result in progression of LV dysfunction to symptomatic heart failure.

CLINICAL FACTORS PREDICTING PROGNOSIS IN ASYMPTOMATIC LV DYSFUNCTION

Although there are several studies that have examined the usefulness of clinical parameters, exercise tolerance, MVO_2 measurements, neurohormones, and echocardiographic parameters in predicting prognosis in patients with symptomatic heart failure, there are very little data available about prognostic markers in patients with asymptomatic LV dysfunction. The SOLVD Prevention trial was the first large study to examine the clinical outcome in patients with asymptomatic LV dysfunction. Specifically in this trial 2117 patients with EF $\leq 35\%$ were randomized to the placebo group (2111 to ACE inhibitors) and were followed for an average of 37.4 months (range 14.6–62 months). We examined this group of patients to determine the significant clinical, neurohormonal, and echocardiographic parameters that predicted prognosis in patients with asymptomatic LV dysfunction. Of these 2117 patients, 70% had an EF between 26 and 35% at the time of entry into the study while 26.1% had an EF between 16 and 25% and 3.9% had an EF $\leq 15\%$. By NYHA functional classification 67% of the patients were in class I while 33% were in class II. None was receiving treatment for heart failure. A more complete description of the clinical data in this group has been published elsewhere.[12]

During the follow-up period, there were 334 (15.8%) deaths and 640 (30.2%) developed congestive heart failure. There were also 273 (12.9%) first hospitalizations for heart failure in this population. Using the Cox multivariate model we examined the prognostic usefulness of several clinical, echocardiographic, and neurohormonal parameters in predicting the subsequent clinical outcome in these patients. The clinical parameters examined were age, sex, history of current smoking, etiology of LV dysfunction (ischemic heart disease, hypertension, diabetes mellitus or other), ejection fraction and cardiothoracic ratio (CT ratio). In the Cox multivariate model adjusted for age, ejection fraction, cardiothoracic ratio, NYHA functional class and etiology of heart failure, were found to be the important univariate predictors of one or more clinical outcomes. In a subset of these 2117 patients the prognostic usefulness of plasma neurohormones – plasma norepinephrine (PNE), ANF, AVP, and PRA – and echocardiographic parameters – end-diastolic volume (EDV) and end-systolic volume (ESV) – was also examined.

Age

Increasing age was a significant risk factor for mortality in patients with asymptomatic LV dysfunction. For every 10-year increase in age, the risk ratio for mortality was 1.2 (95% CI 1.08–1.32; $P<0.0014$), the risk ratio for hospitalization for CHF was 1.24 (95% CI 1.10–1.38; $P<0.0005$) and the risk ratio for development of CHF was 1.20 (95% CI 1.10–1.27; $P<0.0001$).

Sex

Unlike age, sex was not a prognostic variable for developing clinical endpoints. For example, the mortality rate in males was 16.06% while in females it was 13.5%, which was not significantly different. Similarly, hospitalization for CHF was 12.6% in males and 15.2% in females, and development of CHF was 28.9% in males and 30.4% in females, both of which were not significantly different. However, these results must be interpreted with caution because the SOLVD prevention trial predominantly consisted of males ($\approx 80\%$), which could have limited the ability to detect differences based on gender.

Ejection fraction

For a 5% reduction in EF, the risk ratio for mortality was 1.20 (95% CI 1.13–1.29; $P<0.0001$), the risk ratio for hospitalization for CHF was 1.28 (95% CI 1.18–1.38; $P<0.0001$) and the risk ratio for development of CHF was 1.20 (95% CI 1.13–1.26; $P<0.0001$).

NYHA functional class

The NYHA functional class was not a risk factor for mortality but was significant for risk of hospitalization for CHF (risk ratio 1.66; 95% CI 1.24–2.22; $P<0.0007$) and development of CHF symptoms (risk ratio 1.48; 95% CI 1.16–1.89; $P<0.0016$).

Etiology of heart failure

Patients were grouped by ischemic or non-ischemic causes. In this multivariate model patients with ischemic or non-ischemic etiology for asymptomatic LV dysfunction had similar outcomes with respect to mortality (15% vs 13.2%), hospitalization for heart failure (11.5% vs 13.9%) and development of heart failure (37% vs 40.3%). Then we examined the role of etiology by dividing the patients into hypertensive or non-hypertensive. Hypertension was not a significant contributor for development of clinical events. In contrast, presence or absence of diabetes was a major risk factor for mortality (risk ratio 1.89; 95% CI 1.27–2.24; $P=0.0003$), hospitalization for heart failure (risk ratio 1.98; 95% CI 1.46–2.69; $P=0.0001$) and for development of heart failure (risk ratio 2.06; 95% CI 1.58–2.59; $P<0.0001$). A current (but not past) history of smoking increased the risk of death (risk ratio 1.21; 95% CI 1.10–1.32; $P<0.001$) but only had a weak and non-significant impact on the development of heart failure.

Cardiothoracic ratio

Increased cardiothoracic ratio (>0.50) was a univariate risk factor for development of clinical endpoints but in the multivariate model it failed to reach statistical significance, most probably due to the impact of ejection fraction in this model.

Thus, in this cohort of 2117 patients followed for an average of 37.4 months, ejection fraction, age and diabetes emerged as the most powerful clinical predictors for development of subsequent clinical events. In contrast to the influence of diabetes, the lack of effect of ischemic heart disease or hypertension in contributing independently to the progression of LV dysfunction is surprising. A possible explanation could be that many of the individuals with ischemic and/or hypertensive etiology could have also had a greater depression in ejection fraction (large segmental wall motion abnormalities of the ventricle) when compared to those with diabetes, who have small vessel disease.

Neurohormonal predictors

Previous studies in patients with symptomatic LV dysfunction have indicated that several neurohormones, including PNE, PRA and ANF, are increased and both PNE and ANF may be useful for predicting clinical outcomes, including mortality, in these patients. However, it is important to note that these studies have not determined whether the neurohormonal activation present is a cause or consequence of heart failure in these patients. In contrast, examination of the prognostic usefulness of neurohormones in patients with asymptomatic LV dysfunction may help us to determine whether the neurohormonal system could possibly play a role in the progression of heart failure syndrome. In a subset of 514 patients with asymptomatic LV dysfunction, from the SOLVD Prevention trial, PNE, but not PRA, ANF and AVP, was found to be significantly associated with heart failure events and predicted the development of subsequent ischemic events (see Figure 41.3).[43] It is important to note that development of an interim ischemic event has been previously shown to worsen clinical outcome in this population.[60] Unlike PNE, the other neurohormones failed to predict the occurrence of subsequent clinical events in patients with asymptomatic LV dysfunction, which suggests that adrenergic activation in patients with LV dysfunction may be an early event.

Echocardiographic predictors

Greenberg et al.[53] have examined in a subset of patients from the SOLVD Prevention and Treatment trials the changes in echocardiographic parameters in patients with LV dysfunction, with 70% of the patients in this analysis from the SOLVD Prevention trial. In the placebo-treated group there was a significant increase in the end-diastolic volume from baseline after 4 months (200 ± 42 ml vs 208 ± 43 ml, $P = 0.025$) and after 1 year of follow-up (200 ± 42 ml vs 210 ± 46 ml, $P = 0.003$). The end-systolic volume increased significantly from baseline after 4 months (148 ± 38 ml vs 155 ± 43 ml, $P = 0.028$) and 1 year of follow-up (148 ± 38 ml vs 156 ± 42ml, $P = 0.014$). Recently, Vasan et al.[61] have reported from the Framingham study database that in asymptomatic individuals increases in LV internal dimension (both end-systolic and end-diastolic volumes) were important predictors for subsequent development of congestive heart failure.

Over 30 years ago Linzbach[62] described structural dilation of the LV as the morphological basis for the development of congestive heart failure. More recent studies on ventricular remodeling support this concept. Therefore it is not surprising that in patients with asymptomatic LV dysfunction, baseline ejection fraction and dilation of the LV emerged as important predictors for the development of subsequent clinical

715

Table 42.3 Effects of the treatment of hypertension on the development of congestive heart failure

Outcome drug regimen	Dose	No. of trials	Events: active treatment/control	RR (95% CI)
Diuretics	High	9	6/35	0.17 (0.07–0.41)
Diuretics	Low	3	81/134	0.58 (0.44–0.76)
Beta-blockers		2	41/175	0.58 (0.40–0.84)

RR, relative risk.
Adapted from Psaty BM *et al.* Health outcomes associated with antihypertensive therapies used as first-line agents. A systematic review and meta-analyses. *JAMA* 1997; **277**(9):739–45.

events. Since ventricular stretching is a powerful stimulus for adrenergic stimulation via the vagal afferents from the myocardium, it is not surprising that sympathetic activation as measured by PNE levels was also an important predictor of clinical events in these patients with asymptomatic LV dysfunction.

In summary, there is a paucity of data about the prognostic markers for development of CHF in patients with asymptomatic LV dysfunction. Data from the SOLVD Prevention trial provide important new information and confirm the importance of LV size, ejection fraction and increased PNE, as well as age and the etiology of LV dysfunction (diabetes), as important independent risk factors.

PREVENTION OF SYMPTOMATIC HEART FAILURE

Although a number of clinical trials have documented that pharmacological therapy reduces mortality in patients with symptomatic heart failure, the prognosis of this condition remains poor.[7,19,23,39,40,63,64] These results suggest that the greatest opportunity for reducing the incidence and excess mortality of heart failure is through preventive strategies.

Treatment of hypertension

The development of heart failure in the setting of hypertension could be due to a number of reasons, including activation of the renin–angiotensin–aldosterone system, acute or chronic subendocardial ischemia, inappropriately high wall stress, and alterations in the peripheral circulation.[65] A number of studies have demonstrated that the treatment of hypertension substantially reduces the risk for the development of heart failure.[10,66–70] A recent meta-analysis by Psaty *et al.*[71] demonstrated that CHF was effectively prevented (Table 42.3) with low dose diuretic therapy (relative risk 0.58; 95%; CI 0.44–0.76), high dose diuretic therapy (relative risk 0.17; 95% CI 0.07–0.41), and beta-blocker therapy (relative risk 0.58; 95% CI 0.40–0.84). The clinical trial evidence in terms of health outcomes is too meager to definitively state whether other drugs (calcium-channel blocks or ACE inhibitor therapy) for hypertension reduce the occurrence of CHF despite the finding that they effectively lower blood pressure. However, given the beneficial effects of ACE inhibitors in preventing worsening CHF in a variety of other circumstances (acute MI, post-MI, low EF), it is reasonable to expect that they

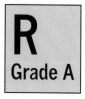

may also be effective in hypertension. Therefore, aggressive management of hypertension will help reduce the risk of developing heart failure.

Lipid lowering therapy to prevent congestive heart failure

It has been clearly demonstrated that lipid lowering therapy significantly reduces mortality in patients with coronary artery disease.[72] A recent report from the 4S Study Group suggests lipid lowering treatment with simvastatin ($n=2223$) compared to placebo ($n=2221$) prevents the onset of heart failure.[26] In this study, 189 patients (8.5%) in the placebo group were diagnosed with CHF during follow-up compared to 147 (6.2%) in the simvastatin group, resulting in a 27% ($P<0.003$) reduction in the incidence of CHF for the simvastatin group. Further studies are required to determine whether this reduction is related to the effect of lipid lowering on coronary artery disease or is exerted through another independent mechanism.

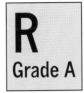

Prevention of myocardial ischemia

Treatment strategies should also be directed at preventing ischemia in patients with heart failure. In heart failure patients it has been demonstrated that the occurrence of a new myocardial infarction increases the risk of subsequent death by up to eight-fold and that one-third of all deaths are preceded by a major ischemic event.[60] Similar data have been reported by Rutherford *et al.*[73] from the SAVE trial. These data emphasize that reductions in ischemic events should be an integral part of the management of patients with LV dysfunction.

ACE inhibitors in asymptomatic LV dysfunction

There have been a number of trials demonstrating the effects of ACE inhibitors to reduce mortality and morbidity in patients with heart failure.[74] In fact, to date ACE inhibitors have been the only group of medications shown to consistently have these beneficial effects in heart failure patients. Therapy with ACE inhibitors in patients with asymptomatic LV dysfunction[12] has been shown to significantly reduce the total number of deaths or cases of CHF (risk reduction 29%; 95% CI 21–36%), and also reduce the total number of deaths or hospitalizations for CHF (risk reduction 20%; 95% CI 9–30%). Therefore an ACE inhibitor should be routinely administered to any patient with LV dysfunction (ejection fraction <0.40) who does not have a contraindication to this form of therapy.

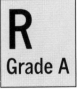

CONCLUSIONS

The incidence and prevalence of CHF is relatively high in the population. CHF is associated with significant mortality, morbidity, and poor quality of life for the patient. This is a progressive disorder and at present there are relatively few therapies that slow or prevent progression of the syndrome. There is recent evidence indicating that asymptomatic LV dysfunction occurs in 1–5% of the population depending on the prevalence of other cardiovascular risk factors. Although routine screening of the general population cannot be justified, screening high risk individuals may be of value. Risk factors for the development of CHF have been identified and these could be used to determine those who are at the greatest risk for the development of LV dysfunction and ultimately symptomatic CHF.

Suggested approach to identify and treat patients with asymptomatic left ventricular dysfunction

1. Determine those at greatest risk to develop left ventricular dysfunction:
   hypertension
   left ventricular hypertrophy
   diabetes mellitus and/or impaired glucose tolerance
   hyperlipidemia (hypertriglyceridemia and low HDL)
   previous extensive myocardial infarction
   age
   smoking
   obesity
2. Assess cardiac function using radionuclide ventriculography or quantitative echocardiography.
3. Ejection fraction <40% then start ACE inhibitors in all tolerant patients. Modify other risk factors (e.g. diabetes, hypertension, dyslipidemia) and treat symptoms of myocardial ischemia.
4. Ejection fraction ≥40% then counsel patients, modify risk factors (e.g. diabetes, hypertension, etc.), and treat symptoms of myocardial ischemia.

These individuals should receive appropriate counselling, lifestyle advice and therapy to alter risk factors for cardiovascular disease and CHF. The fact that the prognosis from CHF remains so poor makes it clear that the greatest opportunity for reducing the incidence and attendant high mortality of congestive heart failure is through strategies directed towards preventing its development.

REFERENCES

1 Smith WM. Epidemiology of congestive heart failure. *Am J Cardiol* 1985;**55**:3A–8A.

2 Klainer LM, Gibson TC, White KL. The epidemiology of cardiac failure. *J Chron Dis* 1965; **18**:797–814.

3 Gibson TC, White KL, Klainer LM. The prevalence of congestive heart failure in two rural communities. *J Chron Dis* 1966;**19**:141–52.

4 Parameshwar J, Shackell MM, Richardson A, Poole-Wilson PA, Sutton GC. Prevalence of heart failure in three general practices in north west London. *Br J Gen Pract* 1992;**42**:287–9.

5 Schocken DD, Arrieta MI, Leaverton PE, Ross EA. Prevalence and mortality rate of congestive heart failure in the United States. *J Am Coll Cardiol* 1992;**20**:301–6.

6 Eriksson H, Svärdsudd K, Larsson B *et al*. Risk factors for heart failure in the general population: the study of men born in 1913. *Eur Heart J* 1989; **10**:647–56.

7 Rodeheffer RJ, Jacobsen SJ, Gersh BJ *et al*. The incidence and prevalence of congestive heart failure in Rochester, Minnesota. *Mayo Clin Proc* 1993;**68**:1143–50.

8 McKee PA, Castelli WP, McNamara PM, Kannel WB. The natural history of congestive heart failure: the Framingham Study. *N Engl J Med* 1971;**285**:1441–6.

9 Remes J, Reunanen A, Aromaa A, Pyörälä K. Incidence of heart failure in eastern Finland: a population-based surveillance study. *Eur Heart J* 1992;**13**:588–93.

10 Yusuf S, Thom T, Abbott RD. Changes in hypertension treatment and in congestive heart failure mortality in the United States. *Hypertension* 1989;**13**(Suppl. I):I-74–I-79.

11 Yamani M, Massie BM. Congestive heart failure: insights from epidemiology, implications for treatment. *Mayo Clin Proc* 1993;**68**:1214–18.

12 The SOLVD Investigators. Effect of enalapril on mortality and the development of heart failure in asymptomatic patients with reduced left ventricular ejection fractions. *N Engl J Med* 1992;**327**:685–91.

13 Bröckel U, Hense HW, Muscholl M *et al*. Prevalence of left ventricular dysfunction in the general population. *J Am Coll Cardiol* 1996;**27**(Suppl. A): 25A.

14 McDonagh TA, Morrison CE, McMurray JJ *et al*. Global left ventricular systolic dysfunction in North Glasgow. *J Am Coll Cardiol* 1996;**27**(Suppl A):106A.

15 WHO MONICA Project. WHO MONICA project: objectives and design. *Int J Epidemiol* 1989;**18** (Suppl 1):S29–S37.

16 Johnstone D, Limacher M, Rousseau M *et al*. for the SOLVD Investigators. Clinical characteristics of patients in studies of left ventricular dysfunction (SOLVD). *Am J Cardiol* 1992;**70**:894–900.

17 Vasan RS, Benjamin EJ, Levy D. Prevalence, clinical features, and prognosis of diastolic heart failure: an epidemiologic perspective. *J Am Coll Cardiol* 1995;**26**:1565–74.

18 Gaasch WH. Diagnosis and treatment of heart failure based on left ventricular systolic or diastolic dysfunction. *JAMA* 1994;**271**:1276–80.

19 Pfeffer MA, Braunwald E, Moyé LA *et al*. Effect of captopril on mortality and morbidity in patients with left ventricular dysfunction after myocardial infarction: results of the Survival and Ventricular Enlargement trial. *N Engl J Med* 1992;**327**: 669–77.

20 Kannel WB, Castelli WP, McNamara PM, McKee PA, Feinleib M. Role of blood pressure in the development of congestive heart failure: the Framingham Study. *N Engl J Med* 1972;**287**: 781–7.

21 Levy D, Larson MG, Ramachandran S *et al*. The progression from hypertension to congestive heart failure. *JAMA* 1996;**275**:1557–62.

22 Ho KKL, Pinsky JL, Kannel WB, Levy D. The epidemiology of heart failure: the Framingham Study. *J Am Coll Cardiol* 1993;**22**(Suppl A): 6A–13A.

23 Ho KKL, Anderson KM, Kannel WB, Grossman W, Levy D. Survival after the onset of congestive heart failure in Framingham Heart Study subjects. *Circulation* 1993;**88**:107–15.

24 Kannel WB, Dannenberg AL, Levy D. Population implications of electrocardiographic left ventricular hypertrophy. *Am J Cardiol* 1987; **60**(Suppl I):85I–93I.

25 Kannel WB. Epidemiological aspects of heart failure. *Cardiol Clin* 1989;**7**:1–9.

26 Kjekshus J, Pedersen T, on behalf of the 4S Study Group. Lowering of cholesterol with simvastatin may prevent the development of heart failure in patients with coronary heart disease (abstract). *J Am Coll Cardiol* 1995;**25**:282A.

27 Kannel WB, Hjortland M, Castelli WP. Role of diabetes in congestive heart failure: the Framingham Study. *Am J Cardiol* 1974;**34**:29–34.

28 van Hoeven KH, Factor SM. A comparison of the pathological spectrum of hypertensive, diabetic, and hypertensive-diabetic heart disease. *Circulation* 1990;**82**:848–55.

29 Bangdiwala SI, Weiner DH, Bourassa MG *et al*. for the SOLVD Investigators. Studies of left ventricular dysfunction (SOLVD) registry: rationale, design, methods and description of baseline characteristics. *Am J Cardiol* 1992;**70**:347–53.

30 Suskin N, McKelvie RS, Wiecek E, Rouleau JL, Yusuf S. Insulin and glucose levels in heart failure (HF). Abstract to be presented at the Canadian Cardiovascular Society Meeting, Winnipeg, Manitoba, 1997.

31 Herlitz J, Malmberg K, Karlson BW, Rydén L, Hjalmarson Å. Mortality and morbidity during a five-year follow-up of diabetics with myocardial infarction. *Acta Med Scand* 1988;**224**:31–8.

32 Shindler DM, Kostis JB, Yusuf S *et al*. for the SOLVD Investigators. Diabetes mellitus, a predictor of morbidity and mortality in the Studies of Left Ventricular Dysfunction (SOLVD) Trials and Registry. *Am J Cardiol* 1996;**77**:1017–20.

33 Kannel WB. Epidemiology of heart failure in the United States. In: Poole-Wilson PA, Colucci WS, Massie BM, Chatterjee K, Coats AJS, eds. *Heart failure. Scientific principles and clinical practice.* New York: Churchill Livingstone, 1997, pp 279–88.

34 Francis GS, Goldsmith SR, Levine TB, Olivari MT, Cohn JN. The neurohumoral axis in congestive heart failure. *Ann Intern Med* 1984;**101**:370–7.

35 Cohn JN, Levine TB, Olivari MT *et al*. Plasma norepinephrine as a guide to prognosis in patients with chronic congestive heart failure. *N Engl J Med* 1984;**311**:819–23.

36 Gottlieb SS, Kukin ML, Ahern D, Packer M. Prognostic importance of atrial natriuretic peptide in patients with chronic heart failure. *J Am Coll Cardiol* 1989;**13**:1534–9.

37 Levine TB, Francis GS, Goldsmith SR, Simon A, Cohn JN. Activity of the sympathetic nervous system and renin–angiotensin system assessed by plasma hormone levels and their relationship to hemodynamic abnormalities. *Am J Cardiol* 1982; **49**:1659–66.

38 Curtiss C, Cohn JN, Vrobel T, Franciosa JA. Role of renin–angiotensin system in systemic vasoconstriction of chronic congestive heart failure. *Circulation* 1978;**58**:763–70.

39 The CONSENSUS Trial Study Group. Effect of enalapril on mortality in severe congestive heart failure. *N Engl J Med* 1987;**316**:1429–35.

40 The SOLVD Investigators. Effect of enalapril on survival in patients with reduced left ventricular ejection fractions and congestive heart failure. *N Engl J Med* 1991;**325**:293–302.

41 Francis GS, Benedict C, Johnstone DE *et al.* for the SOLVD Investigators. Comparison of neuroendocrine activation in patients with left ventricular dysfunction with and without congestive heart failure. A substudy of the Studies of Left Ventricular Dysfunction (SOLVD). *Circulation* 1990;**82**:1724–9.

42 Benedict CR, Weiner DH, Johnstone DE *et al.* for the SOLVD Investigators. Comparative neurohormonal responses in patients with preserved and impaired left ventricular ejection fraction: results of the Studies of Left Ventricular Dysfunction (SOLVD) Registry. *J Am Coll Cardiol* 1993;**22**(Suppl A):146A–153A.

43 Benedict CR, Shelton B, Johnstone DE *et al.* for the SOLVD Investigators. Prognostic significance of plasma norepinephrine in patients with asymptomatic left ventricular dysfunction. *Circulation* 1996;**94**:690–7.

44 Rundqvist R, Elam M, Bergmann-Sverrisdottir Y, Eisenhofer G, Friberg P. Increased cardiac adrenergic drive precedes generalized sympathetic activation in human heart failure. *Circulation* 1997;**95**:169–75.

45 Eaton LW, Weiss JL, Bulkley RH, Garrison JB, Weisfeldt ML. Regional cardiac dilatation after acute myocardial infarction: recognition by two-dimensional echocardiography. *N Engl J Med* 1979;**300**:57–62.

46 Fletcher PJ, Pfeffer JM, Pfeffer MA, Braunwald E. Left ventricular diastolic pressure-volume relations in rats with healed myocardial infarctions: effects on systolic function. *Circ Res* 1981;**49**:618–26.

47 Erlebacher JA, Weiss JL, Easton LW, Kallman C, Weisfeldt ML, Bulkley BH. Late effects of acute infarct dilatation on heart size: a two dimensional echocardiographic study. *Am J Cardiol* 1982;**49**:1120–6.

48 Roberts CS, MacLean D, Maroko P, Kloner RA. Early and late remodelling of the left ventricle after acute myocardial infarction. *Am J Cardiol* 1984;**54**:407–10.

49 McKay RG, Pfeffer MA, Pasternak RC *et al.* Left ventricular remodelling after myocardial infarction. A corollary to infarction expansion. *Circulation* 1986;**74**:693–702.

50 Sharpe N, Murphy J, Smith H, Hannan S. Treatment of patients with symptomless left ventricular dysfunction after myocardial infarction. *Lancet* 1988;**i**:255–9.

51 Konstam MA, Kronenberg MW, Rousseau MF *et al.* for the SOLVD Investigators. Effects of the angiotensin converting enzyme inhibitor enalapril on the long-term progression of left ventricular dilatation in patients with asymptomatic systolic dysfunction. *Circulation* 1993;**88**(I):2277–83.

52 Konstam MA, Rousseau MF, Kronenberg MW *et al.* for the SOLVD Investigators. Effects of the angiotensin converting enzyme inhibitor enalapril on the long-term progression of left ventricular dysfunction in patients with heart failure. *Circulation* 1992;**86**:431–8.

53 Greenberg B, Quiñones MA, Koilpillai C *et al.* for the SOLVD Investigators. Effects of long-term enalapril therapy on cardiac structure and function in patients with left ventricular dysfunction. Results of the SOLVD echocardiography substudy. *Circulation* 1995;**91**:2573–81.

54 Koilpillai C, Quiñones MA, Greenberg B *et al.* for the SOLVD Investigators. Relation of ventricular size and function to heart failure status and ventricular dysrhythmia in patients with severe left ventricular dysfunction. *Am J Cardiol* 1996;**77**:606–11.

55 Litwin SE, Litwin CM, Raya TE, Warner AL, Goldman S. Contractility and stiffness of non-infarcted myocardium after coronary ligation in rats: effects of chronic angiotensin converting enzyme inhibition. *Circulation* 1991;**83**:1028–37.

56 Pfeffer JM, Pfeffer MA, Braunwald E. Influence of chronic captopril therapy on the infarcted left ventricle of the rat. *Circ Res* 1985;**57**:84–95.

57 Jugdutt BI, Schwarz-Michorowski BL, Khan M. Effect of long-term captopril therapy on left ventricular remodelling and function during healing of canine myocardial infarction. *J Am Coll Cardiol* 1992;**19**:713–21.

58 Pouleur HG, Konstam MA, Udelson JE, Rousseau MF for the SOLVD Investigators. Changes in ventricular volume, wall thickness and wall stress during progression of left ventricular dysfunction. *J Am Coll Cardiol* 1993;**22**(Suppl A):43A–48A.

59 Pouleur H, Rousseau MF, van Eyll C *et al.* for the SOLVD Investigators. Cardiac mechanics during development of heart failure. *Circulation* 1993;**87**(Suppl IV):IV-14–IV-20.

60 Yusuf S, Pepine CJ, Garces C *et al.* Effect of enalapril on myocardial infarction and unstable angina in patients with low ejection fractions. *Lancet* 1992;**340**:1173–8.

61 Vasan RS, Larson MG, Benjamin, EJ, Evans JC, Levy D. Left ventricular dilation and the risk of congestive heart failure in people without myocardial infarction. *N Engl J Med* 1997;**336**:1350–5.

62 Linzbach AJ. Heart failure from the point of view of quantitative anatomy. *Am J Cardiol* 1960;**5**: 370–82.

63 Cohn JN, Archibald DG, Ziesche S *et al*. Effect of vasodilator therapy on mortality in chronic congestive heart failure: results of a Veterans Administration Cooperative Study. *N Engl J Med* 1986;**314**:1547–52.

64 Cohn JN, Johnson G, Ziesche S *et al*. A comparison of enalapril with hydralazine-isosorbide dinitrate in the treatment of chronic congestive heart failure. *N Engl J Med* 1991;**325**:303–10.

65 Litwin SE, Grossman W. Mechanisms leading to the development of heart failure in pressure-overload hypertrophy. *Heart Failure* 1992;April/May:48–54.

66 Veterans Administration Cooperative Study Group on Antihypertensive Agents. Effects of treatment on mortality in hypertension: results in patients with diastolic blood pressures averaging 115 through 129 mmHg. *JAMA* 1967;**202**:1028–34.

67 Veterans Administration Cooperative Study Group on Antihypertensive Agents. Effects of treatment on morbidity in hypertension, II: results in patients with diastolic blood pressure averaging 90 through 114 mmHg. *JAMA* 1970;**213**: 1143–51.

68 Furberg CD, Yusuf S. Effect of drug therapy on survival in chronic heart failure. *Adv Cardiol* 1986;**34**:124–30.

69 The Systolic Hypertension in the Elderly Research Group. Prevention of stroke by antihypertensive drug treatment in older persons with isolated systolic hypertension: final results of the Systolic Hypertension in the Elderly Program (SHEP). *JAMA* 1991;**265**:3255–64.

70 Cutler JA, Psaty BM, MacMahon S, Furberg CD. Public health issues in hypertension control: what has been learned from clinical trials. In: Laragh JH, Brenner BH, eds. *Hypertension: Pathophysiology, diagnosis and management*. New York, NY: Raven Press, 1995, pp 253–70.

71 Psaty BM, Smith NL, Siscovick DS *et al*. Health outcomes associated with antihypertensive therapies used as first-line agents. A systematic review and meta-analysis. *JAMA* 1997;**277**: 739–45.

72 Scandinavian Simvastatin Survival Study Group. Randomized trial of cholesterol lowering in 4444 patients with coronary heart disease: the Scandinavian Simvastatin Survival Study (4S). *Lancet* 1994;**344**:1383–9.

73 Rutherford JD, Pfeffer MA, Moyé LA *et al*. Effects of captopril on ischemic events after myocardial infarction. *Circulation* 1994;**90**:1731–8.

74 McKelvie RS, Yusuf S. Large trials and meta-analyses. In: Poole-Wilson PA, Colucci WS, Massie BM, Chatterjee K, Coats AJS, eds. *Heart failure. Scientific principles and clinical practice*. New York: Churchill Livingstone, 1997, pp 597–615.

43 Hypertrophic cardiomyopathy

PERRY M. ELLIOTT,
SANJAY SHARMA,
WILLIAM J. MCKENNA

INTRODUCTION

Hypertrophic cardiomyopathy (HCM) is defined by the presence of left and/or right ventricular hypertrophy in the absence of a cardiac or systemic cause. It is characterized by a predisposition to fatal cardiac arrhythmia and is an important cause of sudden death in individuals aged less than 35 years. The following chapter reviews current data on etiology, diagnosis, and treatment of the disease and briefly discusses areas of uncertainty.

GENETICS

In the majority of cases, HCM is an autosomal dominant inherited disease caused by mutations in genes encoding cardiac sarcomeric proteins; beta-myosin heavy chain on chromosome 14q11 (35%), cardiac troponin-T on chromosome 1q3 (15%), alpha-tropomyosin on chromosome 15q2 (<5%), and myosin binding protein C on chromosome 11p11.2 (15%).[1-4] Less than 1% of patients have mutations affecting the genes encoding the essential and regulatory myosin light chains (on chromosomes 3 and 12 respectively) that are associated with marked papillary muscle hypertrophy, midcavity obliteration, and skeletal muscle involvement.[5] A further as yet unidentified locus on chromosome 7q3 has been described in a large Irish family with HCM and Wolff–Parkinson–White syndrome.[6] Most recently, a mutation has been described in the cardiac troponin-I gene.[7] A causal association between sarcomeric protein gene abnormalities and HCM is supported by a number of observations: cosegregation of mutation and disease in adult patients, the presence of mutations in patients with familial HCM but not in unrelated unaffected individuals, and an association between *de novo* mutations and sporadic disease.[8] The manner in which specific mutations result in disease is still poorly understood, but it might be expected that point mutations occurring within critical domains of sarcomeric protein molecules would result in predictable cardiac phenotypes. Unfortunately, mutations affecting identical residues can result in very different clinical outcomes,[9] suggesting that other genetic and environmental factors influence disease expression. One such disease "modifier" may be angiotensin converting enzyme (ACE) gene polymorphism, with several papers suggesting that the DD genotype is associated with more severe hypertrophy than either ID or II genotypes.[10]

Recently, investigation of the functional consequences of sarcomeric protein mutations has been facilitated by the study of mutant beta-myosin within human skeletal muscle. The demonstration of selective type 1 fiber atrophy, reduced shortening velocity, and impaired isometric force contraction[11,12] suggests that the characteristic myocardial pathology of HCM is a compensatory response to impaired contractile function. A recently described mouse model, developed by introducing a [403]arginine to glutamine alpha-myosin mutation, has supported this hypothesis by demonstrating cardiac dysfunction before the development of disarray and myocyte hypertrophy.[13] This study also demonstrated that male mutant mice had more extensive disease than their female counterparts, indicating that gender may also modulate phenotype expression.

PATHOLOGY

Although any pattern of ventricular hypertrophy can be seen in HCM, it is usually asymmetrically distributed, affecting the interventricular septum more than the free or posterior walls of the left ventricle.[14] Isolated right ventricular hypertrophy is rare, but right involvement in association with left ventricular hypertrophy occurs in up to a third of patients. Microscopically, HCM is characterized by disturbance of myocyte-to-myocyte orientation, with cells forming whorls around foci of connective tissue ("disarray"). Individual cells vary in size and length and there is disruption of the normal intracellular myofibrillar architecture. Myocyte disarray is described in congenital heart disease, hypertension, and aortic stenosis, but it is more extensive in HCM, typically affecting more than 20% of ventricular tissue blocks at post-mortem and more than 5% of total myocardium. Other characteristic features include myocardial fibrosis and abnormal small intramural arteries.[15] The significance of the latter remains speculative, but the presence of extensive small vessel disease in areas of fibrosis suggests that they may cause myocardial ischemia.

PATHOPHYSIOLOGY

Hemodynamics

Systolic function is normal or hyperdynamic in most patients. Twenty five percent have a subaortic pressure gradient temporally associated with contact between the anterior mitral valve leaflet and the interventricular septum.[16] It is thought that the mitral valve leaflet is drawn anteriorly by Venturi forces generated as blood is rapidly ejected through a narrowed left ventricular outflow tract. More recently, the importance of abnormal anterior displacement of the papillary muscles during systole and other abnormalities of the mitral valve apparatus such as leaflet elongation have been recognized as additional contributory factors.[17,18] Although the magnitude of the outflow tract gradient is related to the time of onset and the duration of mitral valve–septal contact, its clinical significance is still debated. Several papers have shown that up to 80% of stroke volume may be ejected before a gradient develops, leading some authorities to suggest that "true" obstruction to flow does not occur.[19] In other patients, however, the presence of rapid deceleration in aortic flow at the time of septal–mitral contact, prolongation of left ventricular ejection time, and continued ventricular shortening after the onset of the outflow gradient in the absence of forward flow suggests that the gradient is of hemodynamic significance.[20] An analysis of published hemodynamic and echocardiographic data[16] has shown that the percentage of stroke volume ejected before mitral–septal contact is inversely related to the magnitude of the gradient. Using this model, the gradient only becomes hemodynamically "significant" when it exceeds 50 mmHg.

Diastolic function

Up to 80% of patients have a range of diastolic abnormalities that include slow and prolonged isovolumic relaxation, reduced rate of rapid filling, and increased left ventricular "stiffness".[21,22] The underlying cause of diastolic abnormalities is difficult to determine in the individual patient, but may include myocardial fibrosis, left ventricular hypertrophy, myocyte disarray, myocardial ischemia, and regional asynchrony. While diastolic abnormalities are undoubtedly the cause of symptoms in many patients, they are also observed in asymptomatic individuals.

Myocardial ischemia

Data accumulated over 30 years suggest that myocardial ischemia (despite normal coronary angiograms) is important in the natural history of HCM; ST segment changes are common during exercise and ambulatory electrocardiography,[23,24] reversible perfusion defects are described during single photon imaging and positron emission tomography,[23–26] and many patients have reduced coronary flow reserve and metabolic evidence for myocardial ischemia during pacing stress.[27] However, in routine clinical practice, the evaluation of chest pain remains difficult, as conventional electrocardiographic and scintigraphic markers of ischemia are difficult to interpret in the presence of left ventricular hypertrophy.

CLINICAL

Epidemiology

Five studies have examined the prevalence of HCM[28–32] and while comparison between them is difficult because of the different methodologies and selection criteria used (Table 43.1), most have suggested a figure of at least 0.2%. The exception[31] was based on an analysis of patient records from institutions in Olmsted County, Minnesota. Although the degree of surveillance of the resident population was admirably high, the fact that we now know that many patients with HCM have normal physical examinations and are asymptomatic makes it likely that some cases escaped detection during the initial

Table 43.1 Prevalence of hypertrophic cardiomyopathy

Author	n	Screening method	Prevalence (%)
Savage 1983[29]	3000	M-mode echo	0.3
Hada 1987[28]	12 841	ECG	0.17
Maron 1994[32]	714	2D-echo	0.5
Codd 1989[31]	3250	Echo/angio	0.02
Maron 1995[30]	4111	2D-echo	0.2

clinical screening process. Furthermore, the reliance in the early part of the study on M-mode echocardiography means that many patients with hypertrophy in those regions of the myocardium not within the "sight" of the M-mode beam may have been overlooked and would not have been allocated to one of the diagnostic codes used to select patients.

Natural history

It remains accepted wisdom that ventricular hypertrophy in patients with HCM usually develops during periods of rapid somatic growth, sometimes during the first year of life, but more typically during adolescence.[33–37] Very occasionally, HCM does not develop until the late teens or the early 20s (unpublished data) but most clinicians would still assert that the risk of a first degree relative of a patient with HCM developing ECG and/ or echocardiographic evidence of HCM after the age of 25 is extremely low (see Elderly HCM below). Patients may develop symptoms at any age or remain asymptomatic all their lives. While most patients with HCM experience an age-dependent decline in exercise capacity and left ventricular function, only 5–10% go on to develop rapid symptomatic deterioration in association with myocardial wall thinning and reduced systolic performance. Sudden death occurs throughout life, but the precise incidence varies in different series. Data from referral institutions suggest an overall annual mortality of 2%, with a maximum of 4–6% during childhood and adolescence,[33,34] whereas studies from several outpatient-based populations[35–37] suggest a lower figure of approximately 1% per annum. Data in infants with HCM are limited, but sudden death in the first decade is thought to be uncommon.[38]

Symptoms

In referral centers, exertional and atypical chest pain occur in approximately 30% of adult patients.[33,34] Dyspnea is also common in adults and is probably caused by elevated pulmonary venous pressure secondary to abnormal diastolic function. Paroxysmal nocturnal dyspnea may occur in patients with apparently mild hemodynamic abnormalities. Its mechanism is uncertain, but myocardial ischemia or arrhythmia may be responsible. Approximately 15–25% of patients experience syncope and 20% presyncope. In some this is caused by paroxysmal arrhythmia, conduction system disease or abnormal vascular responses during exercise, but in the majority no underlying cause is identified.

Examination

In most patients with HCM, physical examination is unremarkable. Patients may have a rapid upstroke to the arterial pulse, a forceful left ventricular impulse, and a palpable left atrial beat.[33] In approximately one-third of patients, there is a prominent "a" wave in the jugular venous pressure, caused by reduced right ventricular compliance. The first and second heart sounds are usually normal, but a fourth heart sound, reflecting atrial systolic flow into a "stiff" left ventricle, may be present. Up to one-third of patients have a systolic murmur caused by left ventricular outflow tract turbulence. Physiological and pharmacological maneuvers that decrease afterload or venous return (standing, Valsalva, amyl nitrate) increase the intensity of the murmur, whereas interventions that increase afterload and venous return (squatting and phenylephrine) reduce it. The majority of patients with left ventricular outflow murmurs also have mitral regurgitation. Rarely, right ventricular outflow obstruction causes a systolic murmur best heard in the pulmonary area.

Electrocardiogram

While the literature suggests that the ECG is abnormal in at least 80% of patients,[39] there are no specific changes diagnostic of HCM. Abnormal QRS morphology, repolarization abnormalities, and right and left atrial enlargement are common.[33,34,39] ST segment depression is frequent during exercise and daily life,[23,24] but is difficult to interpret in the presence of baseline ECG abnormalities. Abnormal Q-waves occur in 25–50% of patients,[39–41] most commonly in the inferolateral leads. Suggested causes include abnormal septal activation and myocardial ischemia. Giant negative T-waves in the mid-precordial leads may be more common in Japanese patients with apical hypertrophy,[42] but they are also seen in Western patients with involvement of other myocardial segments. Some patients have a short PR interval with a slurred QRS upstroke, but only a minority (approximately 5% of all patients with HCM[43]) have accessory atrioventricular pathways.

The incidence of arrhythmias detected during 48-hour ambulatory electrocardiographic monitoring is age dependent (Figure 43.1). Runs of non-sustained ventricular tachycardia (NSVT) occur in 25% of adults,[44,45] but most episodes are relatively slow, asymptomatic, and occur during periods of increased vagal tone (e.g. sleep). Sustained ventricular tachycardia is uncommon and is sometimes associated with apical aneurysms.[46] Paroxysmal supraventricular arrhythmias occur in 30–50% of patients,[47] with sustained atrial fibrillation present in 5% of patients at diagnosis. A further 10% of patients develop atrial fibrillation over the subsequent 5 years.[47]

Echocardiography

When echocardiographic diagnostic criteria for HCM were established using M-mode imaging, asymmetrical hypertrophy of the interventricular septum (ASH) was considered to be the *sine qua non* of the disease. However, subsequent two-dimensional echocardiography has shown that any pattern of hypertrophy is compatible with the diagnosis.[48] The proportion of patients with concentric versus asymmetric hypertrophy

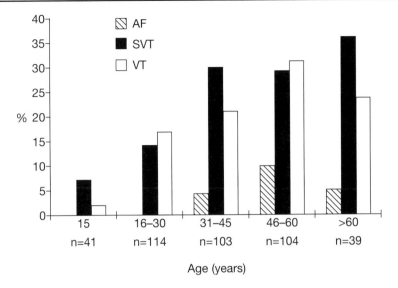

Figure 43.1 The frequency of supraventricular tachycardia (SVT), atrial fibrillation (AF), and non-sustained ventricular tachycardia (NSVT) at different ages in a consecutively referred population at St George's Hospital, London. (Unpublished data.)

depends on the definition employed. Thus, when a septal to posterior wall thickness ratio of 1.3:1 is used to define asymmetry, only 1–2% of patients have concentric left ventricular hypertrophy[48]. However, this proportion rises to approximately 30% when a ratio of 1.5:1 is used[49]. Criteria for abnormal wall thickness vary, but values exceeding two standard deviations from the mean corrected for age, sex, and height are generally accepted as diagnostic in the absence of any other cardiac or systemic cause. Doppler echocardiography is used to quantify the gradient across the left ventricular outflow tract using the modified Bernoulli equation; peak gradient $= 4V_{max}^2$, where V_{max} is the maximum velocity across the left ventricular outflow tract. When it is not possible to obtain accurate Doppler measurements, the gradient can be estimated using M-mode recordings of the mitral valve and the formula: peak gradient $= 25(X/Y) + 25$, where X is the duration of mitral–septal contact and Y the period from the onset of systolic anterior motion of the mitral valve to the onset of mitral–septal contact.[16]

Cardiac catheterization

In the modern era, cardiac catheterization is only performed in patients with refractory symptoms (particularly those with severe mitral regurgitation) and in order to exclude epicardial coronary artery disease in older patients with chest pain. In addition to an outflow gradient, a variety of hemodynamic abnormalities are described including elevated left ventricular end-diastolic and pulmonary capillary wedge pressures and a "spike and dome" appearance in the aortic waveform. Right atrial and right ventricular pressures are usually normal unless there is a substantial right ventricular outflow gradient or severe "restrictive" physiology. Resting cardiac output is typically normal or increased, except in patients with "end-stage" ventricular dilation.

In patients with hypertrophy confined to the distal left ventricle, ventriculography may show a characteristic "spade-shaped" appearance caused by the encroachment of hypertrophied papillary muscles. Coronary arteriography is usually normal, but systolic obliteration of epicardial vessels is described. Muscle bridges are also described but their relevance to individual patients' symptoms is often difficult to assess.

Radionuclide studies

Several studies have used stress radionuclide imaging to study myocardial perfusion in patients with HCM. So-called fixed thallium-201 perfusion defects are associated with increased left ventricular cavity dimensions, impaired systolic function, and reduced exercise capacity and are thought to represent myocardial scars.[25] Reversible regional thallium-201 defects are present in over 25% of patients, but correlate poorly with symptomatic status.[23,25] Recent suggestions that reversible defects relate to poor prognosis require further study.[50] "Apparent cavity dilation" is also described[23,25] and may represent subendocardial hypoperfusion. Radionuclide angiography has been used to investigate global and regional left ventricular function in HCM and has shown prolonged isovolumic relaxation, delayed peak filling, reduced relative volume during the rapid filling period, increased atrial contribution to filling and regional heterogeneity in the timing, rate and degree of left ventricular relaxation and diastolic filling.[51,52] A reduced peak filling rate has been shown to be associated with an increased disease-related mortality,[52] but its predictive value is not high and adds little to conventional risk stratification.

DIFFERENTIAL DIAGNOSIS

In adults, unexplained left ventricular hypertrophy exceeding two standard deviations from the normal (typically >1.5 cm) is usually sufficient to make a diagnosis of HCM. In children and adolescents the diagnosis can be more difficult as young "gene carriers" may not manifest the complete phenotype. A number of rare genetically determined disorders can present with a cardiac phenotype similar to HCM, but most are distinguished by the presence of other clinical features (Table 43.2). Rare exceptions include patients with Friedreich's ataxia who present with cardiac disease before the onset of obvious neurological deficit,[53] Noonan syndrome patients with only very mild somatic abnormalities,[54] and patients with primary mitochondrial disease who do not have clinical evidence for neuromuscular disease (unpublished data). In routine clinical practice the two most commonly encountered areas of difficulty are the differentiation of HCM from "secondary" left ventricular hypertrophy, as seen in hypertension and the "athlete's heart", and the more recently identified problem of incomplete penetrance in adults. A further as yet unresolved issue is the relation of so-called "elderly HCM" to early onset disease.

Hypertension

Left ventricular hypertrophy occurs in up to 50% of hypertensive patients. The hypertrophic response is determined by a number of factors including the degree of

Table 43.2 Other disorders characterized by left ventricular hypertrophy

Genetic disorders characterized by LVH and myocyte disarray
Noonan's syndrome
Friedreich's ataxia
Lentiginosis

Exaggerated "physiological" response
Renal and Afro–Caribbean hypertension
"Athlete's heart"
Obesity
? Elderly hypertensives

Metabolic disorders
Infants of diabetic mothers
Amyloid
Glycogen storage disease
Mitochondrial cytopathy
Pheochromocytoma
Fabry's disease
Disorders of fatty acid metabolism

Table 43.3 Relation of the pattern of left ventricular hypertrophy to underlying etiology (%)

	ASH[a]	Distal	Symmetrical	Wall thickness ≥ 2.0 cm
Sensitivity	56 (83)[b]	10	81	40 (40)
Specificity	81 (56)	100	66	93 (93)
Predictive value of positive test	83 (70)	100	58	81 (83)

[a] Defined by an interventricular septum to posterior wall thickness ratio of $\geq 1.5:1$.
[b] Values in parentheses from Keller *et al.*[57]

Sensitivity, specificity, and predictive value of asymmetric hypertrophy (ASH and distal) in diagnosing hypertrophic cardiomyopathy and symmetric hypertrophy in diagnosing secondary hypertrophy. The same parameters are shown for a maximal wall thickness or septal thickness of ≥ 2.0 cm in diagnosing HCM in patients with symmetric hypertrophy. Taken from Shapiro *et al.*[56] and Keller *et al.*[57]

hypertension, sex, and race.[55] In general, patients with HCM tend to have more severe hypertrophy than hypertensives and the presence of a maximal wall thickness of more than 2 cm in a Caucasian patient should always raise the suspicion of HCM (Table 43.3).[56,57] Concentric hypertrophy is more frequent in patients with hypertension and asymmetric septal hypertrophy more so in HCM, but the specificity of each pattern is not high. In contrast, isolated distal ventricular hypertrophy does seem to be highly predictive of HCM. Systolic anterior motion of the mitral valve (SAM) occurs in both diseases, but the combination of complete SAM with a substantial left ventricular outflow gradient and asymmetric septal hypertrophy is more indicative of HCM. A number of other echo-derived parameters such as left ventricular cross-sectional area and direction-dependent contraction have been suggested as discriminants but these require further study.[58]

Athlete's heart

While HCM is the commonest cause of unexpected sudden death in young athletes,[59,60] cardiovascular adaptation to regular training can make differentiation of the "athlete's heart" from HCM problematic. The ability to distinguish these two entities is of crucial importance as continued competitive activity in a young person with HCM may threaten that individual's life, whereas an incorrect diagnosis of HCM in a normal athlete may unnecessarily deprive them of their livelihood. The presence of symptoms and a family history of HCM and/or premature sudden death should always raise the level of suspicion for HCM. In general, athletic training is associated with only a modest increase in myocardial mass with less than 2% of elite athletes having a wall thickness greater than 13 mm.[61] A diagnosis of HCM in an elite athlete is very likely when an individual has a left ventricular wall thickness >16 mm in men or >=13 mm in females. Other echocardiographic features favoring a diagnosis of HCM include small left ventricular cavity dimensions (athletes tending to have increased left ventricular end-diastolic dimensions), left atrial enlargement, and the presence of a left ventricular outflow gradient.[62] Doppler evidence of diastolic impairment is also highly suggestive of HCM. The "athletic" ECG often displays voltage criteria for left ventricular hypertrophy, sinus bradycardia, and sinus arrhythmia, but Q waves, ST segment depression and/or deep T wave inversion are highly suggestive of HCM. The type of training may also be relevant to diagnosis as hypertrophy is greatest in specific sports such as rowing and cycling. Isometric activities do not appear to cause a substantial hypertrophic response. Very occasionally, a period of detraining over 3–6 months is required to distinguish HCM from the athlete's heart.

Incomplete penetrance in adults

It is increasingly recognized that some adults with sarcomeric protein mutations do not fulfill conventional echocardiographic criteria for HCM. New clinical diagnostic criteria for HCM, based on the assumption that the probability of disease in a first degree relative of a patient with HCM is 50%, have recently been proposed (Table 43.4).[63] It is important to realize that they are intended to apply only to *unexplained* ECG and echocardiographic abnormalities in first degree adult relatives of individuals with proven HCM and not to isolated cases of minor echocardiographic and electrocardiographic abnormalities.

HCM in the elderly

While there are no published reports of *de novo* HCM developing in middle age, idiopathic left ventricular hypertrophy has long been recognized in patients over the age of 65 years.[64-67] In comparison with their younger counterparts, patients with "elderly HCM" tend to have relatively mild hypertrophy localized to the anterior interventricular septum. The left ventricular cavity is said to be more commonly ovoid or ellipsoid in elderly

Table 43.4 Proposed diagnostic criteria for hypertrophic cardiomyopathy in first degree relatives of patients with definite diagnosis of hypertrophic cardiomyopathy

Major	Minor
Echocardiography	
Left ventricular wall thickness ≥ 13 mm in the anterior septum or posterior wall or ≥ 15 mm in the posterior septum or free wall	Left ventricular wall thickness of 12 mm in the anterior septum or posterior wall or 14 mm in the posterior septum or free wall
Severe SAM (septal leaflet contact)	Moderate SAM (no leaflet–septal contact)
	Redundant MV leaflets
Electrocardiography	
LVH + repolarization changes (Romhilt & Estes)	Complete BBB or (minor) interventricular conduction defects (in LV leads)
T-wave inversion in leads I and aVL (≥ 3 mm) (with QRS–T-wave axis difference ≥ 300), V3–V6 (≥ 3 mm) or II and III and aVF (≥ 5 mm)	Minor repolarization changes in LV leads
Abnormal Q-waves (>40 ms or >25% R wave) in at least 2 leads from II, III, aVF (in the absence of left anterior hemiblock), V1–V4; or I, aVL, V5–V6	Deep S in V2 (>25 mm)
	Unexplained syncope, chest pain, dyspnea

It is proposed that diagnosis of hypertrophic cardiomyopathy in first degree relatives of patients with the disease would be fulfilled in the presence of one major criterion or two minor echocardiographic criteria or one minor echocardiographic plus two minor electrocardiographic criteria. From McKenna et al.[63]

patients and crescentic in the young, but neither morphology is specific. Systolic anterior motion of the mitral valve and left ventricular outflow tract gradients occur at all ages, but the elderly tend to have more severe narrowing of the left ventricular outflow tract, anterior displacement of the mitral valve apparatus, restricted anterior excursion of the anterior mitral valve leaflet in systole, and a larger area of contact between the mitral valve leaflet and the septum. Mitral valve calcification is often seen in elderly patients, but it is not associated with a greater degree of left ventricular outflow tract obstruction. The frequency of moderate to severe symptoms is similar in young and elderly patients, but the limited published evidence indicates that the elderly respond well to pharmacological and surgical therapy and have a relatively good prognosis.[66]

The etiology of HCM in the elderly is still poorly understood. Hypertension is more frequent in the elderly population, but the failure to demonstrate any difference in left ventricular morphology in hypertensive and non-hypertensive HCM patients (with the possible exception of posterior wall thickness) has led some to suggest that it is not an important factor.[67] Other "hypertrophic" stimuli that may be present in older patients include increased angulation and decreased compliance of the aorta. Systematic pedigree analysis is not available in elderly patients, but the limited data from echocardiographic series indicate that only 11–13% of patients have a family history of HCM, suggesting that the underlying basis of the disease is different from early onset disease. Recent cross-sectional studies have suggested that the proportion of *proven* carriers of myosin binding protein C mutations with hypertrophy increases with age, raising the possibility that age-related penetrance continues beyond the second decade.[68] However, the number

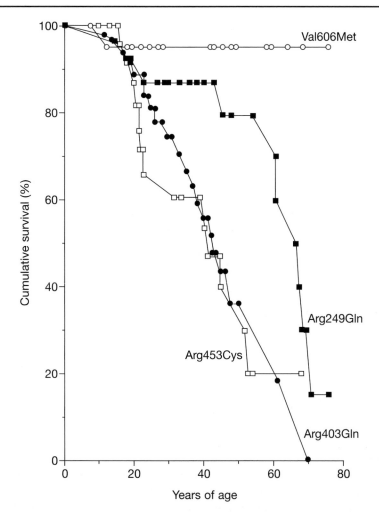

Figure 43.2 Kaplan–Meier survival curves for individuals with HCM and different beta-myosin gene mutations. Two beta-myosin points are reported to be associated with near normal survival: Val606→Met (○) and Leu908→Val. The mutations Arg403→Gln (●), Arg453Cys (□), and Arg249Gln (■) are associated with a poorer prognosis. (From Watkins *et al.*[9])

of patients studied to date is small and other factors such as referral bias may account for these findings.

RISK STRATIFICATION IN HYPERTROPHIC CARDIOMYOPATHY

Although sudden death in HCM is a relatively uncommon event, the fact that it frequently occurs in young asymptomatic individuals gives it a particular significance in families affected by HCM and for the wider community. Clinical risk stratification in patients with HCM is based on the premise that if sudden death can be prevented the

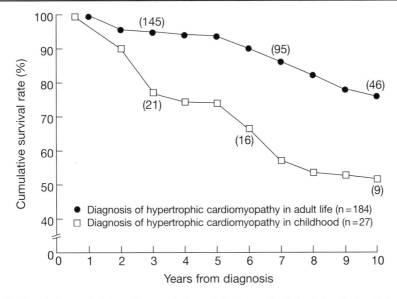

Figure 43.3 Cumulative survival from the year of diagnosis in 211 medically treated patients with HCM. (From McKenna and Deanfield.[81])

natural history of the disease for most patients is relatively benign. The absence of risk factors also facilitates reassurance of low risk individuals.

A number of studies have shown that individual sarcomeric protein gene mutations have different prognostic implications (Figure 43.2).[9] For example, all families with troponin-T mutations described to date have a poor prognosis with approximately 50% of individuals dying before middle age, whereas beta-myosin heavy chain mutations may have a benign or malignant course. Such data must, however, be considered preliminary as the number of families studied to date is relatively small and just as cardiac morphology varies between individuals with the same genotype, it is likely that the propensity for sudden death is also modulated by other genetic and environmental factors.

Clinically, a young age at diagnosis is associated with an increased risk of sudden death (Figure 43.3). Other recognized risk markers in this age group include a family history of multiple premature sudden deaths and recurrent unexplained syncopal episodes.[34] More recently abnormal blood pressure responses during exercise have been shown to be associated with a higher mortality in patients less than 40 years of age.[69] Abnormal responses are seen more frequently in patients with a family history of sudden death and small left ventricular cavity dimensions,[70] but the underlying mechanism for the abnormal response remains unknown. Some evidence suggests that inappropriate vasodilation in non-exercising muscles is responsible.[71]

Evidence published to date indicates that there is no direct correlation between severity of left ventricular hypertrophy and prognosis.[72] Symptomatic patients with particularly severe and diffuse hypertrophy may be at greater risk, but patients with very mild hypertrophy also die suddenly. Similarly, there is no conclusive evidence that left ventricular outflow gradients *per se* influence prognosis.

Two studies[44,45] have shown that NSVT in adults with HCM is associated with an increased risk of sudden death. In isolation, however, its clinical value is limited by a modest positive predictive accuracy of 22% and a low incidence in children. Recently, it has been suggested that NSVT is significant only when episodes are repetitive, prolonged, and/or associated with symptoms. A number of other non-invasive and invasive electrophysiological parameters have been evaluated in an attempt to further refine clinical risk stratification. QT and QTc intervals are often prolonged in patients with HCM, but no study has shown a convincing association with the risk of sudden death.[73–75] QT dispersion may be a more sensitive marker of the propensity to ventricular arrhythmia but further studies in large, well characterized populations are necessary. Abnormal signal averaged electrocardiograms (SAECG) are relatively common in patients with HCM and NSVT, the best predictor of NSVT being a reduced voltage (less than 150 µV) in the initial portion of the high gain QRS complex (sensitivity 95%, specificity 74%, postive predictive accuracy 64%).[76] Unfortunately, abnormal SAECGs are not associated with other clinical risk factors and do not identify patients who go on to develop sustained ventricular arrhythmia or sudden death. Similarly, while global and specific vagal components of heart rate variability (HRV) are reduced in patients with HCM and NSVT, abnormal HRV is not predictive of sudden catastrophic cardiac events.[77]

The role of programmed electrical stimulation in patients with HCM remains controversial. The largest series from a single center[43,78] report that programmed ventricular stimulation using up to three premature stimuli in the right and/or left ventricle produces sustained ventricular arrhythmia (i.e. lasting for more than 30 seconds or associated with hypotension) in 43% of patients selected on the basis of a history of previous cardiac arrest, syncope, palpitations or NSVT on Holter. Inducible sustained ventricular arrhythmia was associated with a history of cardiac arrest *or* syncope and, in a subsequent study, was associated with a reduced survival. The sensitivity, specificity, and predictive accuracy for predicting subsequent cardiac events were 82%, 68%, and 17% respectively. However, almost three-quarters of the patients with sustained ventricular arrhythmias required three premature stimuli for induction. The experience in other cardiac diseases has shown that while "aggressive" protocols using three or more stimuli are highly sensitive, their specificity is low. In addition, 76% of patients had polymorphic ventricular tachycardia (VT) or ventricular fibrillation (VF) rather than sustained monomorphic VT, which is generally thought to be a more sensitive and specific marker of sudden death risk. The interpretation of these published data in HCM and their translation into clinical practice is further complicated by the criteria used to select patients, as "low-risk" patients were underrepresented in the analysis. The general view at present is that programmed stimulation is of limited use in the assessment of risk in HCM.

Recently, the putative arrhythmogenic substrate in HCM has been investigated by analysing changes in individual paced electrocardiogram transitions ("fractionation") recorded at three sites in the right ventricle.[79] Compared with controls, patients with a history of VF have prolongation of the paced electrocardiogram at relatively long extrastimulus coupling intervals. Patients with a family history of premature sudden death or NSVT exhibit responses that span the range from "high risk" (VF) to "low risk" (no adverse prognostic features).

MANAGEMENT OF THE "HIGH RISK" PATIENT

In spite of over 20 years research and debate, the identification and management of patients at risk of sudden death are still determined by individual experience and local

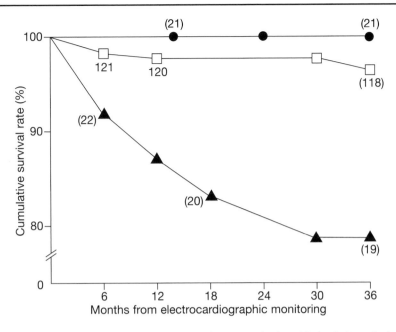

Figure 43.4 Cumulative survival curves for patients with non-sustained ventricular tachycardia treated with either conventional antiarrhythmic drugs (▲) or amiodarone (●), and for patients without non-sustained ventricular tachycardia (□). (From McKenna *et al.*[80])

resources, rather than by definitive prospective data. There is general agreement that low risk adult patients can be readily identified and in most populations these represent the majority of individuals with the disease. Patients who have survived out-of-hospital VF or have sustained VT are at particular risk and should be treated with antiarrhythmic drugs or implantable defibrillators (ICD). The treatment of patients without VT/VF is more controversial. Studies have shown that low dose amiodarone reduces the incidence of sudden death in adults with NSVT (Figure 43.4),[80] and in children considered to be at risk.[81] The principal limitations of the available data are the small size of the populations studied and their relatively low event rate in the context of a well controlled but non-randomized design. In addition, some physicians have expressed concern at the use of amiodarone in young children. Our own practice, based on retrospective analysis of a decade of experience at a single institution,[82] is to consider prophylactic amiodarone therapy in all patients with two or more clinical risk factors (i.e. NSVT, a family history of two or more sudden deaths below 40, recurrent unexplained syncope, and an abnormal exercise blood pressure response). However, as more data demonstrating the efficacy of ICD therapy in other cardiac diseases become available, it is likely that an increasing number of patients will receive an implantable device in preference to amiodarone. Several studies designed to test the predictive value of different clinical features and the effect of therapy on sudden death are in the planning stage and it is anticipated that more widely accepted treatment algorithms will become available.

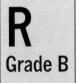

Table 43.5 Perioperative mortality and long term survival following surgical treatment of left ventricular outflow tract obstruction

Author	n	Early mortality (%)	LBBB (%) PPM (%)	5-year survival	10-year survival
Heric *et al.* 1975–1993[88]	178	6 4 SMM 8 (+other)	10	86 overall 93 (SMM) 51 (+MVR)	70 79 26
Robbins *et al.* 1972–1994[89]	158	3.2 2.3 SMM 7.4 (+other)	2.5	85	71
Schulte *et al.* 1963–1991[90]	364	4.9 2.9 SMM 10.9 (+other)	—	—	88
Williams *et al.* 1971–1986[87]	61	1.6	0 1.6	93	93
Maron *et al.* 1960–1975[86]	124	8	42 4	86	70
McCully *et al.*[91] 1986–1992	65	4.6 0 (SMM alone)	41 1.5	92	—
McIntosh *et al.*[92] 1983–1989	58 MVR only	8.6	— 5	86 (3 years)	—

LBBB, new left bundle branch block; MVR, mitral valve replacement; PPM, postoperative permanent pacemaker; SMM, septal myotomy-myectomy.

SYMPTOMATIC THERAPY

Obstructive hypertrophic cardiomyopathy

Most physicians still use beta-blockade as the first line drug therapy in patients with left ventricular outflow obstruction. While some studies have suggested that up to 70% of patients improve with beta-blockers, high doses are frequently required and side effects may be limiting. Disopyramide has been extensively used in some centers for symptomatic therapy in patients with significant outflow obstruction.[83,84] Reduction in SAM and left ventricular ejection time and improved exercise capacity and functional status are described but, in common with other therapies, the long term efficacy may not be maintained in some patients.[16] The anticholinergic effects of disopyramide (dry mouth, urinary retention, glaucoma) may also limit the drug's use, particularly in elderly patients. Some workers advocate the use of verapamil in patients with outflow gradients, but its effect is unpredictable and acute hemodynamic collapse is described in patients with substantial gradients or severe diastolic dysfunction.

When drug therapy fails or is only partially effective, surgery remains the "gold standard" treatment.[85–91] The most frequently performed operation is septal myotomy-myectomy in which a wedge of myocardium is excised from the upper interventricular septum via a transaortic approach. Operative mortality in experienced centers is now 1–2%, but may be higher in less experienced units. Most studies indicate that operative mortality is higher when myectomy is combined with other cardiac operations

R
Grade B

(Table 43.5). The incidence of non-fatal complications such as conduction system disease and ventricular septal defect has declined with modification of surgical practice and the use of intraoperative transesphageal echocardiography. Some data suggest that surgery reduces or abolishes resting gradients in 95% of cases and that 70% of patients show useful symptomatic and functional improvement. However, at least 10% continue to experience significant symptoms. Mitral valve replacement has been proposed as an alternative to myectomy, its attraction being that it avoids potential complications of ventricular septal defect and complete heart block. In a series of 58 patients, mitral valve replacement resulted in a substantial reduction in left ventricular outflow gradient, improved symptomatic class, and an actuarial survival at 3 years of 86%.[92] However, early operative mortality was 9% and only 68% of patients were free from thromboembolism, anticoagulant-related problems, congestive cardiac failure, and reoperation. Thus, mitral valve replacement, while successfully treating outflow obstruction, is usually only advocated when left ventricular outflow obstruction is associated with other primary or secondary abnormalities of the mitral valve.

R Grade B

There has been growing interest in the use of dual chamber pacing as a less invasive alternative to surgery. Several studies have described significant gradient reduction in patients treated with AV synchronous pacemakers programmed with a short AV delay to ensure constant capture of the right ventricle.[93–97] It was initially thought that pacing reduced the outflow gradient by causing paradoxical movement of the interventricular septum, but it is now realized that many aspects of ventricular activation are altered by right ventricular pacing and it is likely that reduced or delayed septal thickening, reduced contractility, and altered papillary muscle movement contribute to gradient reduction. In general, outflow gradients can be reduced by approximately 50%, but the translation of this benefit into useful clinical improvement is very variable and unpredictable. Some workers suggest that suboptimal responses to pacing may be caused by short native PR intervals that make it impossible to simultaneously achieve maximum pre-excitation and maintain normal atrial filling of the left ventricle. This can be overcome in some patients by pharmacologically increasing the PR interval with beta-blockers and/or calcium antagonists, but some groups controversially advocate radiofrequency ablation of the atrioventricular node in order to achieve "optimal" AV pacing. Other unresolved issues include the significance of the appreciable placebo effect of pacing demonstrated in at least two randomized studies, the effect of long term pacing on left ventricular wall thickness, and the role of pacing in the young. It is our view that, although effective in a minority of individuals, DDD pacing should still be considered experimental.

R Grade B

Several centers are now examining a novel approach to gradient reduction that uses injection of alcohol into the first septal perforator branch of the left anterior descending artery to produce a "chemical myectomy".[98–100] Preliminary data indicate that significant gradient reduction and improvement of symptoms can be achieved. However, as with dual chamber pacing, the actual mechanism of gradient reduction and symptomatic improvement is likely to be more complex than the creation of a "localized" scar in the interventricular septum. The most frequent complication reported to date is complete heart block, although the incidence varies between the small number of centers currently performing the procedure. There has been some concern regarding the short and long term consequences of deliberately producing a myocardial infarct and it is imperative that careful randomized trials are performed before this technique is more widely used.

Non-obstructive HCM

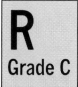

The treatment options in symptomatic patients without an outflow tract gradient are limited. Beta-blockers and calcium-channel antagonists can be used alone or in combination and in patients with symptoms suggestive of pulmonary venous congestion, diuretics may also be helpful. In a small number of patients with severe refractory chest pain, a variety of techniques such as transcutaneous nerve stimulation and cardiac denervation have been used with variable success.

MANAGEMENT OF SUPRAVENTRICULAR ARRHYTHMIA

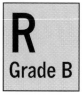

Established AF should be cardioverted but when restoration of sinus rhythm is not possible, control of the ventricular rate will improve symptoms in most patients.[47] Only rarely is it necessary to perform radiofrequency ablation of the AV node in order to achieve adequate rate control. AF in HCM is associated with a significant risk of thromboembolism and anticoagulation should be considered in all patients when AF is sustained or recurs frequently. Treatment for supraventricular arrhythmias is indicated only if they are sustained (>30 seconds) or associated with symptoms. Specific medical therapy with low dose amiodarone (1000–1400 mg weekly) or beta-blockers with Class III action (e.g. sotalol) is effective in maintaining sinus rhythm and in controlling the ventricular rate during breakthrough episodes. The role of other drugs such as Class I agents is uncertain.

CONCLUSION

HCM is a disorder of diverse etiology, pathology, and clinical presentation. While recent advances in molecular genetics and clinical characterization have led to greater understanding of the disease and its management, several clinical issues remain unresolved. Nevertheless, the pace of current research suggests that many of these controversies will be resolved over the next decade.

Key points

- The majority of cases of hypertrophic cardiomyopathy (HCM) are caused by mutations in genes encoding cardiac sarcomeric proteins.
- Although symptoms of chest pain, dyspnea, palpitation, and syncope are common, many patients are asymptomatic and may present for the first time with sudden death.
- Recurrent syncope, a family history of premature sudden death, non-sustained ventricular tachycardia during ambulatory electrocardiography, and abnormal exercise blood pressure responses are associated with an increased risk of sudden death.
- Symptomatic patients with left ventricular outflow gradients should be initially treated with beta-blockers or disopyramide. If drug therapy is ineffective patients should be considered for surgery or pacemaker therapy.
- All patients should undergo non-invasive risk stratification using ambulatory electrocardiography and exercise testing.
- Low risk adults can generally be reassured that their prognosis is good. High risk patients require further assessment and should be considered for amiodarone or ICD therapy.

REFERENCES

1 Jarcho JA, McKenna WJ, Pare JA *et al*. Mapping a gene for familial hypertrophic cardiomyopathy of chromosome 14q1. *N Engl J Med* 1989;**321**: 1372–8.

2 Thierfelder L, MacRae C, Watkins H *et al*. A familial hypertrophic cardiomyopathy locus maps to chromosome 15q2. *Proc Natl Acad Sci USA* 1993;**90**:6270–4.

3 Watkins H, MacRae C, Thierfelder L *et al*. A disease locus for familial hypertrophic cardiomyopathy maps to chromosome 1q3. *Nature Genet* 1993;**3**:333–7.

4 Bonne G, Carrier L, Bercovici J *et al*. Cardiac myosin binding protein C gene splice acceptor site mutation is associated with familial hypertrophic cardiomyopathy. *Nature Genet* 1995;**11**:438–40.

5 Poetter K, Jiang H, Hassanzadeh S *et al*. Mutations in either the essential or regulatory light chains of myosin are associated with a rare myopathy in human heart and skeletal muscle. *Nature Genet* 1996;**13**:63–9.

6 MacRae CA, Ghaisas N, Kass S *et al*. Familial hypertrophic cardiomyopathy with Wolff–Parkinson–White syndrome maps to a locus on chromosome 7q3. *J Clin Invest* 1995;**96**: 1216–20.

7 Kimura A, Harada H, Park J-E *et al*. Mutations in the cardiac troponin I gene associated with hypertrophic cardiomyopathy. *Nature Genet* 1997;**16**:379–82.

8 Watkins H, Thierfelder L, Hwang D *et al*. Sporadic hypertrophic cardiomyopathy due to de novo myosin mutations. *J Clin Invest* 1992;**90**: 1666–71.

9 Watkins H, Rozenzweig A, Hwang DS *et al*. Characteristics and prognostic implications of myosin missense mutations in familial hypertrophic cardiomyopathy. *N Engl J Med* 1992;**326**:1108–14.

10 Lechin M, Quinones MA, Omran A *et al*. Angiotensin converting enzyme genotypes and left ventricular hypertrophy in patients with hypertrophic cardiomyopathy. *Circulation* 1995; **92**:1808–12.

11 Rayment I, Holden HM, Sellers JR, Fananapazir L, Epstein ND. Structural interpretation of the mutations in the beta-cardiac myosin that have been implicated in familial hypertrophic cardiomyopathy. *Proc Natl Acad Sci USA* 1995; **92**:3864–8.

12 Lankford EB, Epstein ND, Fananapazir L, Sweeney HL. Abnormal contractile properties of muscle fibres expressing beta-myosin heavy chain gene mutations in patients with hypertrophic cardiomyopathy. *J Clin Invest* 1995;**95**:1409–14.

13 Geisterfer-Lowrance AA, Christe M, Conner DA *et al*. A mouse model of familial hypertrophic cardiomyopathy. *Science* 1996;**272**:731–4.

14 Davies MJ, McKenna WJ. Hypertrophic cardiomyopathy; pathology and pathogenesis. *Histopathology* 1995;**26**:493–500.

15 Maron BJ, Wolfson JK, Epstein SE, Roberts WC. Intramural ("small vessel") coronary artery disease in hypertrophic cardiomyopathy. *J Am Coll Cardiol* 1986;**8**:545.

16 Wigle ED, Sasson Z, Henderson MA *et al*. Hypertrophic cardiomyopathy: the importance of the site and extent of hypertrophy. A review. *Prog Cardiovasc Dis* 1985;**28**:1–83.

17 Levine RA, Vlahakes GJ, Lefebvre *et al*. Papillary muscle displacement causes systolic anterior motion of the mitral valve. Experimental validation and insights into the mechanism of subaortic obstruction. *Circulation* 1995;**91**: 1189–95.

18 Klues HG, Maron BJ, Dollar AL, Roberts WC. Diversity of structural mitral valve alterations in hypertrophic cardiomyopathy. *Circulation* 1992; **85**:1651–60.

19 Sugrue DD, McKenna WJ, Dickie S *et al*. Relation between left ventricular gradient and relative stroke volume ejected in early and late systole in hypertrophic cardiomyopathy. Assessment with radionuclide cineangiography. *Br Heart J* 1984; **52**:602–9.

20 Maron BJ, Epstein SE. Clinical significance and therapeutic implications of the left ventricular outflow tract pressure gradient in hypertrophic cardiomyopathy. *Am J Cardiol* 1986;**58**:1093–6.

21 Hanrath P, Mathey DG, Siegert R, Biefield W. Left ventricular and filling patterns in different forms of left ventricular relaxation and filling patterns in different forms of left ventricular hypertrophy. An echocardiographic study. *Am J Cardiol* 1980;**45**:15–23.

22 Maron BJ, Spirito P, Green KJ *et al*. Noninvasive assessment of left ventricular diastolic function by pulsed Doppler echocardiography in patients with hypertrophic cardiomyopathy. *J Am Coll Cardiol* 1987;**10**:733–42.

23 Cannon RO, Dilsizian V, O'Gara P *et al*. Myocardial metabolic, hemodynamic, and electrocardiographic significance of reversible thallium-201 abnormalities in hypertrophic cardiomyopathy. *Circulation* 1991;**83**:1660.

24 Elliott PM, Kaski JC, Prasad K *et al*. Chest pain during daily life in patients with hypertrophic cardiomyopathy: an ambulatory electro-cardiographic study. *Eur Heart J* 1996;**17**: 1056–64.

25 O'Gara PT, Bonow RO, Maron BJ *et al*. Myocardial perfusion abnormalities in patients

with hypertrophic cardiomyopathy: assessment with thallium-201 emission computed tomography. *Circulation* 1987;**76**:1214–23.

26 Camici P, Chiriatti G, Lorenzoni R *et al*. Coronary vasodilatation is impaired in both hypertrophied and non-hypertrophied myocardium of patients with hypertrophic cardiomyopathy: a study with nitrogen-13 ammonia and positron emission tomography. *J Am Coll Cardiol* 1991;**17**:879–86.

27 Cannon RO, Rosing DR, Maron BJ *et al*. Myocardial ischemia in patients with hypertrophic cardiomyopathy: contribution of inadequate vasodilator reserve and elevated left ventricular filling pressures. *Circulation* 1985;**71**:234–437.

28 Hada Y, Sakamoto T, Amano K *et al*. Prevalence of hypertrophy cardiomyopathy in a population of adult Japanese workers as detected by echocardiographic screening. *Am J Cardiol* 1987;**59**:183–4.

29 Savage DD, Castelli WP, Abbott RD *et al*. Hypertrophic cardiomyopathy and its markers in the general population: the great masquerader revisited. The Framingham Study. *J Cardiovasc Ultrason* 1983;**23**:41–7.

30 Maron BJ, Gardin JM, Flack JM *et al*. Prevalence of hypertrophic cardiomyopathy in a population of young adults. Echocardiographic analysis of 4111 subjects in the CARDIA study. Coronary Artery Risk Development in (Young) Adults. *Circulation* 1995;**92**:785–9.

31 Codd MB, Sugrue DD, Gersh BJ, Melton LJ. Epidemiology of idiopathic dilated and hypertrophic cardiomyopathy: a population based study in Olmsted County, Minnesota, 1975–1984. *Circulation* 1989;**80**:564–72.

32 Maron BJ, Peterson EE, Maron MS, Peterson JE. Prevalence of hypertrophic cardiomyopathy in an outpatient population referred for echocardiographic study. *Am J Cardiol* 1994;**73**:577–80.

33 Frank S, Braunwald E. Idiopathic hypertrophic subaortic stenosis: clinical analysis of 126 patients with emphasis on the natural history. *Circulation* 1968;**37**:759–88.

34 McKenna WJ, Deanfield J, Faruqui A *et al*. Prognosis in hypertrophic cardiomyopathy. Role of age and clinical, electrocardiographic and hemodynamic features. *Am J Cardiol* 1981;**47**:532–8.

35 Spirito P, Chiarella F, Carratino L *et al*. Clinical course and prognosis of hypertrophic cardiomyopathy in an outpatient population. *N Engl J Med* 1989;**320**:749–55.

36 Cecchi F, Olivotto I, Montereggi A *et al*. Hypertrophic cardiomyopathy in Tuscany: clinical course and outcome in an unselected regional population. *J Am Coll Cardiol* 1995;**26**:1529–36.

37 Cannan CR, Reeder GS, Bailey KR, Melton LJ III, Gersh BJ. Natural history of hypertrophic cardiomyopathy. A population based study, 1976 through 1990. *Circulation* 1995;**92**:2488–95.

38 Maron BJ, Tajik AJ, Ruttenberg HD *et al*. Hypertrophic cardiomyopathy in infants: clinical features and natural history. *Circulation* 1982;**65**:7–17.

39 Savage DD, Seides SF, Clark CE *et al*. Electrocardiographic findings in patients with obstructive and non-obstructive hypertrophic cardiomyopathy. *Circulation* 1978;**58**:402–9.

40 Lemery R, Kleinebenne A, Nihoyannopoulos P, Alfonso F, McKenna WJ. Q-waves in hypertrophic cardiomyopathy in relation to the distribution and severity of right and left ventricular hypertrophy. *J Am Coll Cardiol* 1990;**16**:368–74.

41 Cosio FG, Moro C, Alonso M, Saenz de la Calzada C, Llovet A. The Q-waves of hypertrophic cardiomyopathy. *N Engl J Med* 1980;**302**:96–9.

42 Yamaguchi H, Ishimura T, Nishiyama S *et al*. Hypertrophic nonobstructive cardiomyopathy with giant negative T-waves (apical hypertrophy): ventriculographic and echocardiographic features in 30 patients. *Am J Cardiol* 1979;**44**:401–12.

43 Fananapazir, L, Tracey CM, Leon MB *et al*. Electrophysiological abnormalities in patients with hypertrophic cardiomyopathy: a consecutive analysis in 155 patients. *Circulation* 1989;**80**:1259.

44 McKenna WJ, England D, Doi Y *et al*. Arrhythmia in hypertrophic cardiomyopathy. 1. Influence on prognosis. *Br Heart J* 1981;**46**:168–72.

45 Maron BJ, Savage DD, Wolfson JK, Epstein SE. Prognostic significance of 24 hour ambulatory electrocardiographic monitoring in patients with hypertrophic cardiomyopathy: a prospective study. *Am J Cardiol* 1981;**48**:252–7.

46 Alfonso F, Frenneaux MP, McKenna WJ. Clinical sustained uniform ventricular tachycardia in hypertrophic cardiomyopathy: association with left ventricular apical aneurysm. *Br Heart J* 1989;**61**:178–81.

47 Robinson K, Frenneaux MP, Stockins B *et al*. Atrial fibrillation in hypertrophic cardiomyopathy: a longitudinal study. *J Am Coll Cardiol* 1990;**15**:1279–85.

48 Maron BJ, Gottdiener JS, Epstein SE. Patterns and significance of the distribution of left ventricular hypertrophy in hypertrophic cardiomyopathy: a wide angle, two-dimensional echocardiographic study of 125 patients. *Am J Cardiol* 1981;**48**:418–28.

49 Shapiro LM, McKenna WJ. Distribution of left ventricular hypertrophy in hypertrophic cardiomyopathy: a two-dimensional echocardiographic study. *J Am Coll Cardiol* 1983; **2**:437–44.

50 Dilsizian V, Bonow RO, Epstein SE, Fananapazir L. Myocardial ischemia detected by thallium scintigraphy is frequently related to cardiac arrest and syncope in young patients with hypertrophic cardiomyopathy. *J Am Coll Cardiol* 1993;**22**:796–804.

51 Betocchi S, Bonow RO, Bacharach SL *et al.* Isovolumic relaxation period in hypertrophic cardiomyopathy: assessment by radionuclide angiography. *J Am Coll Cardiol* 1986;**7**: 74–81.

52 Chikamori T, Dickie S, Poloniecki JD *et al.* Prognostic significance of radionuclide-assessed diastolic dysfunction in hypertrophic cardiomyopathy. *Am J Cardiol* 1990;**65**: 478–82.

53 Child JS, Perloff JK, Bach PM *et al.* Cardiac involvement in Friedreich's ataxia. A clinical study of 75 patients. *J Am Coll Cardiol* 1986;**7**: 1370.

54 Burch M, Sharland M, Shinebourne E *et al.* Cardiologic abnormalities in Noonan syndrome: phenotypic diagnosis and echocardiographic assessment of 118 patients. *J Am Coll Cardiol* 1993;**22**:1189–92.

55 Devereux RB. Cardiac involvement in essential hypertension. Prevalence, pathophysiology and prognostic implications. *Med Clin North Am* 1987;**71**:813–26.

56 Shapiro LM, Kleinebenne A, McKenna WJ. The distribution of left ventricular hypertrophy in hypertrophic cardiomyopathy: comparison to athletes and hypertensives. *Eur Heart J* 1985;**6**: 967–74.

57 Keller H, Wanger K, Goepfrich M *et al.* Morphological quantification and differentiation of left ventricular hypertrophy in hypertrophic cardiomyopathy and hypertensive heart disease. *Eur Heart J* 1990;**11**:65–74.

58 Hattori M, Aoki T, Sekioka K. Differences in direction-dependent shortening of the left ventricular wall in hypertrophic cardiomyopathy and in systemic hypertension. *Am J Cardiol* 1992;**70**:1326–32.

59 Maron BJ, Roberts WC, McAllister HA, Rosing DR, Epstein SE. Sudden death in young athletes. *Circulation* 1980;**62**:218–29.

60 Burke AP, Farb A, Virmani R, Goodin J, Smialek JE. Sports-related and non-sports related sudden cardiac death in young adults. *Am Heart J* 1991; **121**:568–75.

61 Pelliccia A, Maron BJ, Spataro A, Proschan MA, Spirito P. The upper limit of physiologic cardiac hypertrophy in highly trained elite athletes. *N Engl J Med* 1991;**324**:295.

62 Maron BJ, Pellicia A, Spirito P. Cardiac disease in young trained athletes. Insights into methods for distinguishing athlete's heart from structural heart disease, with particular emphasis on hypertrophic cardiomyopathy. *Circulation* 1995; **91**:1569.

63 McKenna WJ, Spirito P, Desnos M, Dubourg O, Komajda M. Experience from clinical genetics in hypertrophic cardiomyopathy: proposal for new diagnostic criteria in adult members of affected families. *Heart* 1997;**77**:130–2.

64 Lewis JF, Maron BJ. Clinical and morphology expression of hypertrophic cardiomyopathy in patients 65 years of age. *Am J Cardiol* 1994;**73**: 1105–11.

65 Topol EJ, Traill TA, Fortuin NJ. Hypertensive hypertrophic cardiomyopathy of the elderly. *N Engl J Med* 1985;**312**:277–83.

66 Faye WP, Taliercio CP, Ilstrup DM, Tajik AJ, Gersh BJ. Natural history of hypertrophic cardiomyopathy in the elderly. *J Am Coll Cardiol* 1990;**16**:821–6.

67 Karam R, Lever HM, Healy BP. Hypertensive hypertrophic cardiomyopathy or hypertrophic cardiomyopathy with hypertension? A study of 78 patients. *J Am Coll Cardiol* 1989;**13**: 580–4.

68 Niimura H, Bachinski LL, Watkins H *et al.* Human cardiac myosin binding protein C mutations cause late-onset familial hypertrophic cardiomyopathy. *Proc Natl Acad Sci* 1997;**96**: 2987–91.

69 Sadoul N, Prasad K, Slade AKB, Elliott PM, McKenna WJ. Abnormal blood pressure response during exercise is an independent marker of sudden death in young patients with hypertrophic cardiomyopathy. *Circulation* 1997; **96**:2987–91.

70 Frenneaux MP, Counihan PJ, Caforio A, Chikamori T, McKenna WJ. Abnormal blood pressure response during exercise in hypertrophic cardiomyopathy. *Circulation* 1990; **82**:1995–2002.

71 Counihan PJ, Frenneaux MP, Webb DJ, McKenna WJ. Abnormal vascular responses to supine exercise in hypertrophic cardiomyopathy. *Circulation* 1991;**84**:686–96.

72 Spirito P, Maron BJ. Relation between extent of left ventricular hypertrophy and occurrence of sudden cardiac death in hypertrophic cardiomyopathy. *J Am Coll Cardiol* 1990;**15**: 1521–6.

73 Dritsas A, Sabarouni E, Gilligan D, Nihoyannopoulos P, Oakley CM. QT-interval abnormalities in hypertrophic cardiomyopathy. *Clin Cardiol* 1992;**15**:739–42.

74 Fei L, Slade AK, Grace AA *et al.* Ambulatory assessment of the QT interval in patients with hypertrophic cardiomyopathy: risk stratification and effect of low dose amiodarone. *Pacing Clin Electrophys* 1994;**17**:2222–7.

75 Buja G, Miorelli M, Turrini P, Melacini P, Nava A. Comparison of QT dispersion in hypertrophic cardiomyopathy between patients with and without ventricular arrhythmias and sudden death. *Am J Cardiol* 1993;**72**:973–6.

76 Kulakowski P, Counihan PJ, Camm AJ, McKenna WJ. The value of time and frequency domain, and spectral temporal mapping analysis of the signal-averaged electrocardiogram in identification of patients with hypertrophic cardiomyopathy at increased risk of sudden death. *Eur Heart J* 1993;**14**:941–50.

77 Counihan PJ, Fei L, Bashir Y *et al.* Assessment of heart rate variability in hypertrophic cardiomyopathy. Association with clinical and prognostic features. *Circulation* 1993;**88**: 1682–90.

78 Fananapazir L, Chang AC, Epstein SE, McAreavey D. Prognostic determinants in hypertrophic cardiomyopathy: prognostic evaluation of a therapeutic strategy based on clinical, Holter, hemodynamic and electrophysiological findings. *Circulation* 1992; **86**:730–40.

79 Saumarez RC, Slade AKB, Grace AA *et al.* The significance of paced electrocardiogram fractionation in hypertrophic cardiomyopathy. A prospective study. *Circulation* 1995;**91**: 2762–8.

80 McKenna WJ, Oakley CM, Krikler DM *et al.* Improved survival with amiodarone in patients with hypertrophic cardiomyopathy and ventricular tachycardia. *Br Heart J* 1985;**53**: 412–16.

81 McKenna WJ, Deanfield JE. Hypertrophic cardiomyopathy: an important cause of sudden death. *Arch Dis Childhood* 1984;**59**:971–5.

82 Elliott PM, Sharma S, Poloniecki J *et al.* Amiodarone and sudden death in hypertrophic cardiomyopathy. *Circulation* 1997;**96**:I-464.

83 Pollick C. Muscular subaortic stenosis: hemodynamic and clinical improvement after disopyramide. *N Engl Med* 1982;**307**:997–9.

84 Pollick C, Kimball B, Henderson M, Wigle ED. Disopyramide in hypertrophic cardiomyopathy I. Hemodynamic assessment after intravenous administration. *Am J Cardiol* 1988;**62**:1248–51.

85 Morrow AG, Reitz BA, Epstein SE *et al.* Operative treatment in hypertrophic subaortic stenosis: techniques, and the results of pre and postoperative assessments in 83 patients. *Circulation* 1975;**52**:88–102.

86 Maron BJ, Merrill WH, Freier PA *et al.* Long-term clinical course and symptomatic status of patients after operation for hypertrophic subaortic stenosis. *Circulation* 1978;**57**: 1205–13.

87 Williams WG, Wigle ED, Rakowski H *et al.* Results of surgery for hypertrophic obstructive cardiomyopathy. *Circulation* 1987;**76**(Suppl V): V104–8.

88 Heric B, Lytle BW, Miller DP *et al.* Surgical management of hypertrophic obstructive cardiomyopathy. Early and late results. *J Thorac Cardiovasc Surg* 1995;**110**:195–208.

89 Robbins RC, Stinson EB. Long-term results of left ventricular myotomy and myectomy for obstructive hypertrophic cardiomyopathy. *J Thorac Cardiovasc Surg* 1996;**111**:586–94.

90 Schulte HD, Bircks WH, Loesse B, Godehardt EAJ, Schwartzkopff B. Prognosis of patients with hypertrophic obstructive cardiomyopathy after transaortic myectomy. Late results up to 25 years. *J Thorac Cardiovasc Surg* 1993;**106**: 709–17.

91 McCully RB, Nishimura RA, Tajik J, Schaff HV, Danielson GK. Extent of clinical improvement after surgical treatment of hypertrophic obstructive cardiomyopathy. *Circulation* 1996; **94**:467–71.

92 McIntosh CL, Greenberg GJ, Maron BJ *et al.* Clinical and hemodynamic results after mitral valve replacement in patients with hypertrophic cardiomyopathy. *Ann Thorac Surg* 1989;**47**: 236–46.

93 Slade AKB, Sadoul N, Shapiro L *et al.* DDD pacing in hypertrophic cardiomyopathy: a multicentre clinical experience. *Heart* 1996;**75**:44–9.

94 Jeanrenaud X, Goy JJ, Kappenberger L. Effects of dual-chamber pacing in hypertrophic obstructive cardiomyopathy. *Lancet* 1992;**339**: 1318–23.

95 Fananapazir L, Epstein ND, Curiel RV *et al.* Long-term results of dual chamber (DDD) pacing in obstructive hypertrophic cardiomyopathy. Evidence for progressive symptomatic and hemodynamic improvement and reduction of left ventricular hypertrophy. *Circulation* 1994; **90**:2731–42.

96 Nishimura RA, Trusty JM, Hayes DL *et al.* Dual chamber pacing for hypertrophic cardiomyopathy: a randomised double-blind crossover trial. *J Am Coll Cardiol* 1997;**29**: 435–41.

97 Kappenberger L, Linde C, Daubert C *et al.* (PIC Study Group). Pacing in hypertrophic obstructive cardiomyopathy. A randomised crossover study. *Eur Heart J* 1997;**18**:1249–56.

98 Sigwart U. Non-surgical myocardial reduction for hypertrophic obstructive cardiomyopathy. *Lancet* 1995;**346**:211–14.

99 Gleichman U, Seggewiss H, Faber L *et al.* [Catheter treatment of hypertrophic cardio-myopathy]. (German) *Deutsche Medizinische Wochenschrift* 1996;**121**:679–85.

100 Knight C, Kurbaan AS, Seggewiss H *et al.* Non-surgical reduction for hypertrophic obstructive cardiomyopathy: outcome in the first series of patients. *Circulation* 1997;**95**:2075–81.

44 Other cardiomyopathies

José Antonio Marin-Neto,
Marcus Vinícius Simões,
Benedito Carlos Maciel

INTRODUCTION

From the vast array of clinical entities that comprise the cardiomyopathies, two conditions were selected for this chapter: Chagas' heart disease and endomyocardiofibrosis.

In neither disease have large randomized controlled trials been conducted to support recommendations for therapeutic options. Knowledge of natural history and pathophysiology is based almost entirely on observational studies, mostly of the case series kind. Most are flawed by heterogeneous criteria for patient selection and investigation. Thus, particularly in Chagas' heart disease, a large volume of incomplete and biased information has been obtained, so that even meta-analysis of available data is not feasible.

Despite this similarity in the status of evidence based knowledge, the diseases epitomize quite different but unique pathophysiological conditions. In essence, Chagas' heart disease is a myocarditis of parasitic origin, although the role of the etiologic agent in the chronic phase of the disease is still controversial. Endomyocardiofibrosis, on the other hand, has no defined etiology or pathogenesis. Reasonably good animal models exist for the study of Chagas' disease, but not for endomyocardiofibrosis.

There are many reasons for the lack of solid evidence based data in both diseases. However, while the apparently low prevalence of endomyocardiofibrosis is an obvious obstacle, the high prevalence of Chagas' heart disease in many countries has not helped to produce large randomized trials in therapeutic management.

CHAGAS' HEART DISEASE

Epidemiology

Chagas' disease is caused by *Trypanosoma cruzi* infection. Its transmission is mainly vectoral, through the feces of infected bloodsucking insects of the family *Reduviidae* (subfamily *Triatominae*). Many case series reports have also documented that the infection can occur by congenital and oral transmission, blood transfusion, laboratory contamination, and organ transplantation. Although virtually every organic system may be involved and megaesophagus and megacolon can produce florid clinical conditions, it is the cardiac involvement – the object of this chapter – that constitutes the most serious form of the disease.

The true prevalence of Chagas' heart disease is unknown because no large scale epidemiological screening has been carried out even in countries where the disease is endemic. Besides, the epidemiological information available from the different countries is strikingly varied. This reflects the diversity of public health programs, including the control of vectoral and transfusional transmission. Thus, a survey carried out from 1988 to 1990 in 850 municipalities of Brazil revealed that serological screening for Chagas' disease was performed in only two-thirds of all blood donors.[1] Also, a review of serological surveys for Chagas' infection among blood donors conducted over the last decade in several countries in the American continent disclosed a highly variable rate of prevalence, from 0% to 63%.[2]

Neither is case reporting reliable, even in areas of high endemicity. Recent rough estimates by the World Health Organization, based upon limited serological surveys, suggest that 15–20 million people are infected in extensive areas of the American continent.[3] Moreover, some 65 million are at risk.

Cross-sectional epidemiological studies have been carried out in scattered areas of Brazil and Venezuela to assess the prevalence of clinical manifestations and mortality due to Chagas' heart disease. However, probably because of marked variations in the genetic background, parasite strain, climate, socioeconomic and related hygienic alimentary conditions, and health care measures, the prevalence of both morbidity and mortality is extremely variable even within each country.[1]

Nevertheless, Chagas' heart disease is by far the most common form of cardiomyopathy in Latin-American countries. Further, because of modern migratory trends, it is likely to become ubiquitous. This tendency is exemplified by the recent information about the disease in the United States. Based on a prevalence of 4.5% of *T. cruzi* infection detected serologically in 205 Latin American immigrants to the United States and on rough estimates of the number of such legal and illegal immigrants, 400 000–500 000 infected people are believed to be living there now.[4] Also, rural–urban migration from endemic areas in Brazil is believed to have brought half a million infected people to cities such as São Paulo and Rio de Janeiro in the last three decades.

Chagas' heart disease has a very high social impact. It has been estimated that over 750 000 years of productive life are lost annually due to premature deaths in Latin American countries, at a cost of about US$1200 million/year.[5] These figures substantiate the need for the elimination of transmission – a goal which has already been achieved in some regions[6] and proved to be a highly cost effective public health policy.

Natural history and prognostic factors

There is sound experimental, pathological, and clinical evidence that Chagas' heart disease presents two different phases, acute and chronic. The long period – 10–30 years – between the acute condition and the appearance of clinically manifest chronic Chagas' heart disease is known as the indeterminate form of the disease and constitutes one of its most intriguing features.

Megaesophagus and megacolon are also frequently diagnosed in chagasic patients in Brazil, Argentina, and Chile, but not in Mexico or Venezuela. The hypothesis that different *T. cruzi* strains or environmental factors may cause this difference in morbidity has not, however, been evaluated by any appropriately designed studies.

The natural history of Chagas' heart disease is relatively well known from observational studies conducted mainly in endemic areas in Brazil, Argentina, and Venezuela since the early 1940s. There is also a wealth of case series reports dealing with acute Chagas' disease acquired through non-vector transmission. Most of these investigations consist of cross-sectional observations of infected people in rural areas. Very few studies have been conducted using case-control populations of chagasic and non-chagasic people.

There have also been some observational investigations focusing on the description and follow-up of hospital based cohorts of chagasic patients.

Both the rural and the hospital based studies have limitations. For example, usually there is no adequate identification of cardiac involvement provided in the rural based studies. Furthermore, because of the protracted course of heart involvement, from the acute phase to endstage heart failure, no prospective studies encompassing the whole span of the disease are available. Conversely, in hospital based studies the heart disease is usually well characterized, but their results could not be extended to the whole chagasic population.

PROGNOSIS IN THE ACUTE PHASE

This is not a simple matter. Case series using serological tests in endemic areas have shown that in no more than 10% of the acute cases were clinical manifestations sufficient to make a correct diagnosis.[7] This is a major deterrent for understanding the transition from the acute to the chronic stages of Chagas' disease.

For the minority in which the clinical diagnosis was possible, cardiac involvement occurred in around 90% of 313 successive cases; in 70–80%, cardiac enlargement was seen on X-rays, contrasting with only 50% of cases showing ECG abnormalities. The severity of myocarditis was inversely proportional to age; signs of heart failure were twice as intense in children aged up to 2 years than in those aged between 3 and 5 years.[7] Studies in experimental models of Chagas' disease are in general agreement with these findings.

Mortality in the acute phase, as seen in the 313 cases, was 8.3%. This was higher than the 3–5% reported in similar studies in other endemic areas in Brazil, Argentina, and Uruguay. The ECG was normal in 63.3% of the non-fatal cases and in only 14.3% of those who died in the acute phase. Seventy-five percent of all deaths were seen in children aged under 3 years. Heart failure was the constant finding in all fatal cases, with or without encephalitis and independent of age.[7]

Survival is characterized by disappearance of symptoms and signs of heart failure within 1–3 months and normalization of the ECG in over 90% of the cases after 1 year of the infection.

However, there is no evidence of spontaneous cure of the infection, as demonstrated by serial xenodiagnosis and serological tests in studies of several hundreds of chagasic patients.

Of 172 patients who were followed in Bambui (central Brazil) for up to 40 years after the acute infection, the development of cardiac involvement (based on clinical signs, ECG, and chest X-rays changes) occurred in 33.8%, 39.3%, and 58.1% for follow-up periods of 10–20 years, 21–30 years, and 31–40 years respectively.[7] In another review from the same area, for 268 patients whose acute phase of the disease had been diagnosed an average of 27 years before, the general mortality for the period was 13.8%.[7]

PROGNOSIS IN THE INDETERMINATE PHASE

The evolutive potential in the indeterminate phase, governed by still unknown factors, is shown by longitudinal cohort studies in endemic areas. A 1–3% per year rate of appearance of heart involvement has been observed in several studies. Of 400 young adults followed for 10 years, 91 (23%) showed clinical and/or ECG or chest X-ray markers of cardiac disease. Of note, eight deaths were recorded in that period, of which only one could be ascribed to reagudization of Chagas' heart disease.[8]

Another longitudinal study in Bambui, central Brazil, contrasted the evolution of 885 young chagasic patients in the indeterminate phase for 10 years with that of 911 chagasic patients with initially abnormal ECGs in the same period. Survival after 10 years was 97.4% and 61.3% respectively for the indeterminate group and the group with cardiac involvement.[9]

A third longitudinal study in a rural Venezuelan community, with 47% prevalence of positive serology for Chagas' disease, followed 364 patients for a mean period of 4 years. It revealed the appearance of heart disease at a rate of 1.1% per year in seropositive individuals. Mortality was 3% in the 4 years of follow-up and Chagas' heart disease was the cause of death in 69% of all fatal cases.[10]

In 1973 a longitudinal study was initiated in a rural community in north east Brazil. In the initial cross-sectional study, of 644 individuals aged >10 years, 53.7% were seropositive. The population initially described in 1973–1974 was re-examined in 1977, 1980, and 1983. The overall rate of development of abnormal ECG was 2.57% in seropositive (248) as compared to 1.25% per year in seronegative (332) individuals, a relative risk of 2 for the same geographical area. The age adjusted mortality rate was higher in seropositive (8.9/1000/year of 488 patients) than in seronegative individuals (7.8/1000/year of 509 individuals). However, mortality in this study was strongly associated with ventricular conduction defects and arrhythmias.[11]

It should be pointed out that these results were obtained in chagasic populations with more than 50% of the patients younger than 20 years and fewer indeterminate cases are found in the older age groups because of the evolutive nature of the disease.

Key points

- As long as the patients remain in the indeterminate phase, their prognosis is fine.
- After 10 years almost 80% of patients remain in the indeterminate phase of the disease and probably 50% of the entire population will have no signs of heart disease throughout their lives.
- There are no clues as to why some chagasic patients will evolve in this way, while others sooner or later will go through the chronic phase of heart involvement.

PROGNOSIS OF CHRONIC CHAGAS' HEART DISEASE

From the evidence provided by the studies mentioned above, it is apparent that the mere appearance of ECG changes suggests a bad prognosis. Also, a retrospective analysis of seropositive individuals followed over 18 years revealed that right bundle branch block was three times more common in fatal cases than in survivors.[12]

Another important negative prognostic factor once the heart disease is manifest is male gender. This is borne out by several studies carried out with long term follow-up of hospital based cohorts of chagasic patients.[7]

Only two case-control follow-up studies have been reported in Brazilian endemic areas. In central Brazil,[13] two cross-sectional clinical assessments (1974 and 1984) included 12-lead ECG and radiological evaluation of heart size. Serum positive patients and controls were matched by age and gender. In the first cross-sectional study 264 pairs of subjects were evaluated, of which 110 could be recomposed and re-examined after the 10-year follow-up period with the same clinical, ECG, and chest X-ray assessment. The incidence of heart disease in previously healthy but serologically positive individuals was 38.3% in the 10-year period. In those patients with previous heart involvement, a rate of 34.5% of deterioration was observed in the same period. In the chagasic population the overall mortality was 23%, compared to 10.3% in the controls. Moreover, cardiac mortality, including sudden death and death in heart failure, was 17% among chagasic patients and only 2.3% in the control population. Again, the overall mortality was much higher in chagasic males and largely predominated in the group aged 30–59 years.[13] The same group of investigators, applying similar methods in north eastern Brazil, showed that mortality rates were 1.6% and 0% for 125 matched pairs of respectively chagasic and non-chagasic patients followed for 4.5 years.[14] Progression of disease as assessed by ECG changes occurred in 10.4% of patients, as compared to 4.8% of controls. The hypothesis was that the different morbidity and mortality rates in the two regions were due to mean differences in the pathogenicity characteristics of *T. cruzi* strains, although there was no direct evidence to support this.[14]

There is also persuasive evidence to support the concept that the mortality associated with Chagas' disease is strongly associated with the severity of the myocardial dysfunction. For example, survival 2 years after the first episode of heart failure was only 33.4% in 160 cases.[15] Of note, 10% of deaths were sudden. In addition, 98 of deceased people were autopsied, revealing <20% prevalence of amastigote forms of *T. cruzi* in the cardiac tissue, but with a clear predominance of this finding in male patients.[15]

In a study of 107 chagasic patients followed for 10 years, a significant reduction in life expectancy, as compared to that of 22 non-chagasic patients, was detected only in those with ECG and/or clinical changes. A mortality rate of 82% over the 10-year follow-up period was seen in the group of 34 patients with signs of heart failure at the beginning of the study. In contrast, a 65% 10-year survival was associated with ECG abnormalities but in the absence of signs of heart failure.[16]

Another study of 104 male patients admitted to hospital with congestive heart failure revealed a mortality rate of 52% after 5 years. The strongest predictors of survival were LV ejection fraction and maximal oxygen uptake during exercise.[17]

In a series of 42 patients with Chagas' heart disease in the United States, 11 deaths occurred during a mean follow-up of nearly 5 years, always in association with global or regional LV dysfunction. Established or developing heart failure was a strong predictor of mortality but, surprisingly, not aborted sudden death or the presence of sustained ventricular tachycardia.[18] These results conflict with the evidence from 44 chagasic patients followed for a mean period of 2 years[19] that ventricular tachycardia detected during exercise testing is a marker of increased risk of sudden death. This discrepancy

Table 44.1 A clinical classification of Chagas' heart disease

| | Clinical phase | | | |
	Acute	Indeterminate	Overt heart disease	Heart failure
Symptoms	Fairly common	Absent	Minimal	Present
ECG changes	Common	Absent	RBBB, LAHB, AVB, PVCs	+ Q waves VT
Heart size (X-rays)	Usually abnormal	Normal	Normal	Enlarged
RV anatomy function	Usually abnormal	May be depressed	Usually abnormal	Abnormal
LV diastolic function	?	Mild abnormalities	Abnormal	Abnormal
LV systolic function	Abnormal	Mild regional dyssynergy	Segmental dyssynergy	Global depression
Perfusion defects	?	?	Common	Common
Autonomic function	?	May be abnormal	May be abnormal	Usually abnormal
RV biopsy	Abnormal	Usually abnormal	Abnormal	Abnormal

LV, left ventricle; RV, right ventricle; ECG, electrocardiogram; AVB, atrioventricular block; LAHB, left anterior hemiblock; RBBB, right bundle branch block; PVCs, premature ventricular complex; VT, ventricular tachycardia; ?, unknown.

probably reflects the limitations of small numbers and relatively short follow-up in both studies.

Key points

- There is substantial evidence that the most important prognostic factor in established Chagas' heart disease is the degree of myocardial dysfunction.
- Once overt cardiac failure is manifest, the prognosis is gloomily similar to that reported in the heart failure Framingham cohorts, with mortality rates approaching 50% in 4 years.
- It is possible – but by no means proven by good evidence – that sudden death and related ventricular dysrhythmia play a more prominent role in mortality due to Chagas' disease than in heart failure due to other etiologies.

Clinical features of Chagas' heart disease

Cardiac abnormalities are present in all stages of Chagas' disease, but their clinical expression is highly variable. The paucity of clinical indicators of the typical myocarditis of acute Chagas' disease has already been pointed out. There is also solid evidence – from necropsy studies as well as from *in vivo* investigations – that virtually all patients, even in the indeterminate phase of the disease, have some subtle degree of cardiac involvement.[4,20–24]

Patients with Chagas' heart disease are classified following the criteria shown in Table 44.1. All the anatomical and functional disturbances detected during life are consistent with the autopsy findings reported on several series of chagasic patients who died in the various stages of the disease.[20,25]

It is not uncommon for patients with ECG and marked LV regional abnormalities to be asymptomatic hard workers. When symptoms occur, they are usually in the form of fatigue and exertional dyspnea, palpitations, dizziness and syncope or chest pain. These are the expression of reduction of the cardiac reserve (including minor early signs of diastolic dysfunction), the presence of ventricular dysrhythmias, and atrioventricular block. The chest pain is usually atypical for myocardial ischemia but, in a subgroup of chagasic patients, may mimic an acute coronary syndrome.

Systemic and pulmonary embolism, arising from mural thrombi in the cardiac chambers, is a conspicuous complication of Chagas' heart disease, but post-mortem findings show they are often overlooked. The largest published series,[26] involving 1345 necropsies in patients with Chagas' heart disease, reported 595 cases (44%) with cardiac thrombi and/or visceral thromboembolism. The presence of cardiac thrombi was related to severity of ventricular enlargement. Embolism most frequently involved lungs (36%), kidneys (36%), spleen (14%), and brain (10%).

Congestive heart failure in Chagas' heart patients is more commonly expressed by prominent signs of systemic congestion and the symptoms and signs of left ventricular failure do not reach the severity seen in other cardiomyopathies.[27] There is evidence, from studies in a small number of patients, that this peculiar feature of Chagas' heart disease is due to early severe damage of the RV, a chamber frequently neglected in investigations that included evaluation of cardiac function.[28]

Finally, sudden unexpected death occurs with undefined but not negligible frequency even in patients previously asymptomatic. It is usually precipitated by physical exercise and associated with ventricular tachycardia and fibrillation or, more rarely, with complete AV block. From limited evidence from autopsy studies, it is apparent that such patients have constant but variable degrees of inflammatory abnormalities and neuronal cardiac depopulation.[21]

Patients with chronic Chagas' heart disease invariably have one or more positive serological tests. There is also recent and limited experience with a polymerase chain reaction method for detecting *T. cruzi* DNA sequences in the blood of chagasic patients. It is likely that this method will replace the standard cumbersome and unreliable method of direct demonstration of parasite infection by xenodiagnosis.

ECG abnormalities are present in most patients with chronic Chagas' heart disease, mainly in the form of conduction disturbances and ventricular arrhythmias. In more advanced stages pathological Q waves are found, compatible with extensive areas of myocardial fibrosis. The combination of right bundle branch block and left anterior hemiblock is very typical in chronic Chagas' heart disease. Nevertheless, no ECG changes can be considered specific to the disease.

Many case series reports have documented the typical feature of striking segmental wall motion abnormalities in several hundreds of chronic chagasic patients. The most characteristic lesion is the apical aneurysm, but it is the posterior basal dyssynergy that best correlates with the occurrence of malignant ventricular arrhythmia. A few small retrospective studies have evaluated the correlation between ventricular arrhythmia and symptoms in Chagas' heart disease. It is apparent that complex ventricular dysrhythmia may occur in asymptomatic patients, but it is usually a conspicuous manifestation associated with poor LV function. The aneurysms are also emboligenic sources in most thromboembolic events in chagasic patients, according to evidence from *post-mortem* studies.[26]

In spite of chest pain being a cardinal complaint in many chagasic patients, coronary angiography is usually normal. However, various types of myocardial perfusion defects have been detected in small groups of selected patients, possibly implying microvascular coronary disturbances.[4,23]

Cardiac autonomic dysfunction, mainly parasympathetic, has been shown in various studies, in groups of several hundreds of chagasic patients (including those with isolated digestive disease) whose response to various autonomic tests was compared to those of control subjects.[23,29,30] However, these abnormalities are neither correlated with any symptoms nor cause postural hypotension.

Pathophysiology and pathogenetic mechanisms

The clinical manifestations and organ damage arising during the acute phase are closely related to parasite presence in target organs such as the gastrointestinal tract, central nervous system and heart, coexisting with high grade parasitemia. Lymphadenopathy, liver and spleen enlargement are markers of widespread immunologic reaction.

As the parasitemia abates and the systemic inflammatory reaction subsides, it is believed that a silent relentless focal myocarditis ensues during the indeterminate phase. This causes cumulative destruction of cardiac fibers and marked reparative fibrosis. During this phase ventricular arrhythmias and sudden death may rarely occur as manifestations of the underlying focal inflammatory process. This is also eventually responsible for myocardial mass loss attaining critical degrees, thereby leading to cardiac dilation and setting the anatomic substrate for malignant ventricular dysrhythmia.

This hypothesis is based on several experimental animal models for Chagas' heart disease. Additional evidence has been provided by studies correlating clinical and pathological findings in autopsied humans dying in all phases of the disease. All studies were observational and usually included case series of dozens of chagasic patients for the acute and indeterminate phases and ranging from hundreds to thousands of cases for the chronic phase.

The most intriguing challenge for understanding the pathophysiology of Chagas' heart disease lies in the indeterminate phase. It remains to be explained why in many patients the myocardial aggression seems to have been controlled at low levels, whereas in others it leads to development of full blown chronic Chagas' cardiomyopathy.

Basically, four pathogenetic mechanisms have been identified and received substantial scientific focus.

NEUROGENIC MECHANISMS

Intense neuronal depopulation has been clearly demonstrated in a number of pathologic studies.[25,31] Also, as discussed above, abnormal autonomic cardiac regulation has been conclusively shown in many functional investigations.[23,29,30,32] However, various kinds of evidence militate against neurogenic derangements being a main pathogenetic mechanism. Thus, even in endemic areas where cardiac denervation is readily detectable in some patients, its prevalence and intensity are highly variable.[30,32] Also, no significant correlation has been shown between cardiac dysautonomia and the extent of myocardial dysfunction or the presence of dysrhythmia. Moreover, the typical chagasic cardiomyopathy is found in geographical regions where the disease is apparently caused by parasite strains devoid of neurotropism. Interestingly, in such regions, the typical chagasic digestive syndromes – considered to be causally related to parasympathetic denervation of the esophagus and colon – are rarely described.[30] Furthermore, no follow-up studies correlating autonomic regulation, myocardial function, and cardiac rhythm assessment have been reported in chagasic patients.

In conclusion, the role of dysautonomia remains to be determined. Furthermore, the attractive hypothesis implicating autonomic impairment in triggering sudden death has never been appropriately tested.

PARASITE-DEPENDENT INFLAMMATORY AGGRESSION

A direct cause–effect relationship between tissue parasitism and inflammatory findings in the chronic phase of Chagas' heart disease has until recently been discarded due to probably unreliable evidence from observational pathological studies. In essence, these studies found no regional association between the very scantly tissular nests of amastigotic *T. cruzi* and the diffuse focal inflammatory infiltrates. These findings seemed to be corroborated by the typical low grade parasitemia exhibited by chagasic patients examined with xenodiagnosis in the chronic phase of the disease. However, recent results from small groups of patients using a highly sensitive molecular biology detection method have shown that parasitemia may in fact be persistent in the chronic phase of Chagas' disease.[33] A similar kind of evidence concerning the presence of tissue parasitism in the chronic phase of Chagas' heart disease was obtained with a method for amplification of DNA sequences of *T. cruzi*.[34] These findings appear to be confirmed by recent studies applying immunofluorescent monoclonal antibodies for the detection of *T. cruzi* antigenic material in inflammatory foci seen in biopsy specimens obtained from Chagas' heart disease patients.[35] If confirmed by larger studies, this evidence would be persuasive in ascribing a direct role to parasitism in the pathogenesis of chronic Chagas' heart disease, with obviously relevant therapeutic implications.

MICROVASCULAR DISTURBANCES

Several independent studies focusing on histopathological changes, disturbances related to platelet activation, and the pharmacological regulation of endothelial function are compatible with the hypothesis that in Chagas' heart disease there are microvascular abnormalities. These findings have been reported in animal experimental models[36,37] and preliminary studies in humans.[38–40]

It is possible that such derangements are related to the ischemic-like symptoms and transient ECG changes often detected in chagasic patients. They might also constitute the mechanism responsible for the myocardial perfusion abnormalities described in chagasic patients with angiographically normal coronary arteries.[4,23]

On the basis of the evidence from these investigations, it has been postulated that microvascular derangements could represent a relevant mechanism for the amplification and perpetuation of myocardial damage triggered by the inflammatory process discussed above.[37] However, like autonomic impairment, it is more probable that microvascular disturbances are an ancillary rather than a main pathogenetic mechanism.

There is no information to date on the prognostic implications of these abnormalities.

IMMUNE MEDIATED CARDIAC DAMAGE

Studies in humans and in animal experiments provide evidence of the part played by the immunological mechanisms in chronic Chagas' heart disease. In particular, it is widely accepted that the mononuclear inflammatory infiltrates seen in chronic chagasic myocarditis are the expression of cell mediated aggression. Thus it has been shown, by ultrastructural microscopic studies in animal models, that immune effector cells cause lysis of non-parasitized myocardial cells.[41] Moreover, depletion of the TDC[4+] lymphocyte subpopulation annuls myocardial injury in the murine model of Chagas' heart disease.[42] Conversely, myocardial damage is induced in non-chagasic animals, by passive transfer of TDC[4+] lymphocytes from infected mice.[42] Furthermore, the identification of antigenic epitopes related to crossreactivity between *T. cruzi* and myocardial protein provides persuasive evidence that autoimmunity plays a relevant pathogenetic role.[43]

These findings support the theory that there is an organ-specific autoimmune aggression against self antigens modified since the acute phase. It is also possible that a dynamic damaging process is maintained through persistent presentation of crossreacting parasite antigens to the macrophage system, as a consequence of lifelong low grade tissular parasitism.

Key points

- The evidence gathered from pathophysiological studies in animal models and in humans is consistent with the hypothesis of immune mediated injury being a central pathogenetic mechanism in chronic Chagas' heart disease.
- The exacerbated immune responses are probably related to the presence of *T. cruzi* antigens in the cardiac tissue.
- Microvascular disturbances probably constitute important amplification mechanisms for the inflammatory myocardial injury.

Management of Chagas' heart disease

ETIOLOGIC TREATMENT

Two antitrypanosomal agents are available for clinical use: nifurtimox and benznidazole. These have been shown to be comparable both in efficacy and in having a high incidence of side effects including dermatitis, polyneuritis, leukopenia, and gastrointestinal intolerance – commonly resulting in discontinuation of treatment.

Acute phase

It is virtually consensual that in the acute phase etiologic treatment is mandatory to control symptoms and life threatening conditions such as myocarditis and encephalitis. However, in the absence of long term follow-up trials, there is no evidence for the prevention of chronic organ damage.

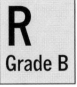

After adequate treatment parasitological evaluation shows negative xenodiagnosis in over 90% of cases and serological tests are negative in 80%. The impact on prognosis has not been established, again due to lack of appropriately designed follow-up studies.

Chronic phase

Evidence for potential benefits of chemotherapy in chronic Chagas' heart disease is extremely limited, due mainly to misleading criteria being employed in small trials. The parasitological criterion of persistent negativation of the xenodiagnosis is unreliable as this test is commonly negative in the chronic phase of Chagas' disease – approximately

60% – despite the presence of overt and progressive cardiac involvement. Moreover, large fluctuations of parasitemia occur over time. There was also bias in the trials caused by selection of patients with persistent parasitemia in the pretreatment period. Furthermore, results of experimental studies have shown that in the chronic phase the parasitemia is low or not detectable at all, while there is a predominant tissular parasitism by amastigotic forms of *T. cruzi*.

Conversely, because persistently positive serological tests may merely reflect mechanisms of immunological memory or be associated with crossreactivity to altered host antigens, results of any of the serological criteria used to assess etiological treatment are clearly inadequate. In fact, the observed rate of negativation of serological tests following treatment in the chronic phase is consistently low (4–8%) in trials suffering the same epidemiological restrictions as discussed above.

Thus, until an adequate laboratory method is available for assessment of cure, the only acceptable criteria for etiologic treatment must be based on the prevention of the appearance of the clinical form or the arrest of damage already detected. For this, a long follow-up period of large cohorts of patients would be required.

To date, only one prospective, non-randomized, controlled trial involving 131 patients treated with benznidazole (5 mg/kg/day for 30 days) and 70 untreated patients with a mean follow-up period of 8 years has been reported.[44] Progression of disease was assessed by ECG changes and deterioration of function. Treated patients presented fewer ECG changes than the control group (4.2% vs 30%) and less deterioration in the clinical condition (2.1% vs 17%). These results suggest that etiologic treatment may cause a favorable impact in the chronic phase. Nevertheless, the fact that the treated group also experienced some progression of disease indicates the relative inefficacy of available antitrypanosomal agents, so that development of new drugs would be warranted.

Clearly, no definitive recommendations are justifiable in this field until large randomized controlled studies encompassing patients in different stages of disease have been performed.

TREATMENT OF CONGESTIVE HEART FAILURE

R
Grade B

Hemodynamic derangements in chronic chagasic patients with heart failure are comparable to those reported in dilated cardiomyopathies of other etiologies. Similarly, the classic therapeutic interventions – sodium restriction, diuretics, digitalis, and vasodilation with nitrates and hydralazine – have been successful in relieving congestive symptoms. Small studies have documented short term hemodynamic beneficial effects of these agents and, to a lesser extent, improvement in exercise tolerance in chronic chagasic patients. However, no studies reported improvement in survival or even in long term outcome.

R
Grade B

Preliminary prospective studies on ACE inhibitors with small numbers of patients have shown promising results in heart failure complicating Chagas' disease. A multicenter, prospective, non-controlled trial assessed the impact of adding an ACE inhibitor to conventional therapy in 115 patients with heart failure (of whom 20 were chagasics). At the end of 12 weeks, irrespective of etiology, the NYHA functional class was significantly improved in most patients (85.2%).[45] A single-blind, crossover trial of ACE inhibitor and placebo for 6 weeks each, with a washout period of 2 weeks, was reported on 18 NYHA class IV chagasic patients.[46] Treatment with the ACE inhibitor was associated with significant reduction in neurohumoral activation and ventricular arrhythmias. These results indicate a potential beneficial role for this class of drugs in reducing active mechanisms related to sudden death. However, no long term controlled study has been reported assessing the impact on survival of chagasic patients treated with ACE inhibitors.

SURGICAL TREATMENT

Heart transplantation

Heart transplantation has been performed in small numbers of patients with refractory heart failure due to Chagas' disease. However, transplantation is limited by socioeconomic factors in the areas where the disease is endemic and by problems of immunosuppression.

Acute myocarditis with marked transitory LV systolic depression occurred in five of the first nine patients included in the largest series (22 patients) operated in a single surgical center.[47] Although the acute reactivation was usually responsive to antiparasite therapy, the possibility of chronic damage to the allograft could not be ruled out. The results reported on the latest 13 patients of this series, using a reduced regimen of immunosuppression with cyclosporin, are promising, with reactivation of disease occurring in only one patient. Also, a survival rate at 24 months post-transplantation of 80% in the latter group appears to compare favorably with those reported in clinical series. Nevertheless, the long term impact of heart transplantation in chagasic patients remains to be determined by adequately controlled studies in large cohorts.

Dynamic cardiomyoplasty

Reported experience with this procedure in chagasic patients is limited. While initial results in very few patients showed encouraging symptom and LV function improvement,[48] a recent survey of surgical centers in South America (112 patients of whom 96 had heart failure due to dilated cardiomyopathy and 13 due to Chagas' heart disease) was less optimistic.[49] Comparative analysis showed survival rates of 86.1% and 49.8% for patients with dilated cardiomyopathy and 40% and 9.5% for chagasic patients at 1 and 5 years follow-up respectively. There are no clues from these data to suggest why the prognosis for chagasic patients was worse.

Clearly large controlled randomized trials are needed to define the value of cardiomyoplasty as a temporary approach, before more radical interventions such as heart transplantation can be considered for wider application in refractory Chagas' heart disease.

PREVENTION OF THROMBOEMBOLIC EVENTS

There is very limited clinical information on the risk of embolism in patients with mural thrombus or apical aneurysm. In 65 selected patients with apical aneurysm, a follow-up study ranging from 19 to 176 months documented 17 episodes of thromboembolism in 14 patients (24.5%)[50] – seven to the brain, nine to the lung and one to the iliac artery. These patients also had congestive heart failure and 11 died in the observation period. In eight of those patients, the cause of death was related to heart failure and in three it was a consequence of cerebral embolism.

Another small study in an endemic region of South America addressed the contribution of Chagas' heart disease in 69 patients having embolic strokes.[51] Of 13 patients with non-ischemic dilated cardiomyopathy, Chagas' heart disease was detected in nine (13.0%). It was, the third most frequently identified cause of embolism after atrial fibrillation (29%) and rheumatic valvular heart disease (20.3%).

However, the real risk of thromboembolism in patients with Chagas' heart disease is unknown, as no specific studies have addressed this problem.

Furthermore, despite the preliminary evidence that thromboembolic events are relevant factors in the natural history of Chagas' disease, no clinical studies have been conducted to date on adequate treatment and prevention. Current recommendations for anticoagulant therapy are based on information derived from other dilated cardiomyopathies. Thus, chagasic patients presenting global LV dysfunction, atrial fibrillation, previous embolic episodes, and dyskinetic areas with detected mural thrombus are candidates for treatment with intravenous and/or oral anticoagulants. Social and economic factors limit the implementation of this treatment, however, even in chagasic patients with otherwise apparent clear indications for prevention of thromboembolism.

R Grade C

MANAGEMENT OF RHYTHM DISTURBANCES

A wide spectrum of rhythm disturbances is one of the main hallmarks of Chagas' heart disease. Sinus node dysfunction and other atrial dysrhythmias are common findings and usually at the early appearance of symptoms.

Management of rhythm disturbances does not differ from that recommended for other cardiomyopathies, although there is no sound evidence to support any specific treatment.

R Grade C

Complex ventricular dysrhythmia is the most important disturbance because of its implication for sudden death. It is believed that this is more common in chagasic patients than in other dilated cardiomyopathies, but no adequate comparative study has been reported to support this hypothesis. As may be expected, there is reasonable evidence that the more complex and frequent the ventricular dysrhythmia, the worse the ventricular function. However, there is convincing evidence that complex ventricular dysrhythmia may also occur in chagasic patients with preserved global LV function. This is more remarkable when dyskinesia in the posterior basal LV region seems to provide the electrophysiologic substrate for refractory ventricular tachycardia. Although no prospective controlled trial has been conducted, the scarce experience reported suggests that this subgroup may benefit from surgical excision of fibrotic tissue following careful electrophysiologic mapping of LV dyskinetic regions. Equally limited is the reported experience with implantable cardioverter defibrillators in chagasic patients surviving episodes of sudden death.[4]

Very scantly information has been published on the efficacy of pharmacological antiarrhythmic therapy in Chagas' heart disease. A prospective double-blind placebo-controlled randomized crossover study in a reduced number of patients reported similar effects of disopyramide and amiodarone for controlling ventricular dysrhythmia.[52] Another prospective open parallel randomized study in 81 chagasic patients with ventricular dysrhythmia compared the efficacy of flecainide and amiodarone.[53] The final evaluation by Holter monitoring after 60 days showed a significant and comparable reduction in the frequency of ventricular tachycardia achieved with both flecainide (96.5%) and amiodarone (92.6%). However, the follow-up was insufficient for conclusions to be drawn on the long term efficacy or the impact of arrhythmia control on the incidence of sudden death.

Two moderately large randomized trials included chagasics among patients treated with amiodarone. The GESICA (Grupo de Estudio de la Sobrevida en la Insuficiencia Cardiaca en Argentina) study concluded after 2 years of follow-up that low dose amiodarone was effective in reducing mortality and hospital admission in patients with severe heart failure, independent of the presence of complex ventricular dysrhythmia.[54] Unfortunately, the contingent of chagasic patients was very modest (48 of 516 patients) and subgroup analysis was not provided. Neither would it have been likely to be useful.

An ongoing prospective, multicenter, randomized, controlled study designed to evaluate the impact on survival of treatment of asymptomatic ventricular arrhythmia also included chagasic patients.[55] In its pilot phase, this trial enrolled 127 patients (24 with Chagas' heart disease) with LVEF <35%, presenting frequent ventricular premature complexes and/or repetitive forms of asymptomatic ventricular arrhythmia. The preliminary results after 12 months of follow-up showed a significant reduction in the incidence of sudden death in the amiodarone group (7.0% vs 20.4%). However, owing to a high dropout rate (16%), follow-up data were obtained in only 106 patients. Nevertheless, it is to be hoped that the final results, recruiting a larger number of chagasic patients, will provide some helpful evidence on treating ventricular dysrhythmia with amiodarone in Chagas' disease.

Complete atrioventricular block may also contribute to low cardiac output and cause syncope and sudden death in chagasic patients. In this situation pacemakers are used, as in other cardiac conditions. The evidence on the effects of pacemaker implantation comes from limited case series reports with historic control series of patients in whom this treatment was not possible.

The common association of atrioventricular disturbances and ventricular complex dysrhythmia in the same patient also requires pacemaker implantation associated with pharmacological antiarrhythmic therapy. This management is regarded as prophylactic, although it is not based on solid evidence.

> **Key points**
> Pharmacological, surgical, and device based strategies for the treatment of ventricular dysrhythmia in chagasic patients are empirical and not supported by any large randomized, controlled trials.

ENDOMYOCARDIAL FIBROSIS (EMF)

EMF is a restrictive cardiomyopathy with still unknown etiology occurring most frequently in tropical and subtropical countries. Major endocardial fibrotic involvement of the inflow portion of one or both ventricles, including the subvalvar region, leads to cavity obliteration, restriction of diastolic filling, and clinical manifestations of congestive heart failure and valvar regurgitation.[56]

A remarkably similar cardiac involvement occurring in non-tropical countries has been described as endomyocardial disease. This is commonly named Löffler endocarditis or hypereosinophilic syndrome.

Although a still disputed issue, it has been postulated that the two conditions represent different stages of the same disease.[57] Another controversial hypothesis is that eosinophil-derived factors have a toxic role in the pathogenesis of endomyocardial damage.[57]

Epidemiology and natural history

The low prevalence of EMF inhibits the study of the epidemiology and natural history. Even the larger published series have included only around 100 patients.

Symptoms and signs

Biventricular involvement has been documented in approximately half of the patients with EMF, while isolated right or left ventricular disease is variably described in 10–40% of cases in different published series. Depending upon predominant involvement of either chamber, symptoms and signs related to pulmonary congestion (leftsided) and systemic congestion (rightsided disease), and to mitral or tricuspid reflux, will tend to be more conspicuous.

Constrictive pericarditis is an important differential diagnosis in EMF, especially when the right ventricle is markedly involved.[58] Demonstration of ventricular obliteration by imaging techniques is essential for the diagnosis, but endomyocardial biopsy can be decisive in selected patients.

The magnitude of symptoms, the grade of ventricular obliteration (especially of the right ventricle), and the occurrence of valvar regurgitation are important prognostic determinants of mortality in this disease. These clinical markers are useful in selecting patients for surgery since a good long term prognosis has been reported for patients who have mild ventricular dysfunction and no valvar regurgitation.[59]

Surgical management

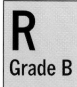

Extensive surgical excision of the fibrotic tissue, preserving or replacing the atrioventricular valves, can ameliorate symptoms and improve hemodynamics and has been suggested to improve the long term prognosis.[60] An operative mortality ranging from 4.6% to 25.0% has been reported in small case series studies.

It must be emphasized that no reports based on randomized controlled trials of treatment strategies are available.

> **Key points**
> - The etiology and pathogenesis of EMF are still to be determined.
> - The epidemiology, natural history, and pathophysiology are very incompletely understood, with available data based solely on retrospective evidence from small observational investigations.
> - Promising preliminary results obtained with surgical approaches await validation in large randomized, controlled studies before any general recommendation for improving quality of life and survival rates can be made.

REFERENCES

1 Wanderley DMV, Corrêa FMA. Epidemiology of Chagas' heart disease. *São Paulo Med J* 1995;**113**: 742–9.

2 Schmunis GA. *Trypanosoma cruzi*, the etiologic agent of Chagas disease: status in the blood supply in endemic and nonendemic countries. *Transfusion* 1991;**31**:547–57.

3 WHO. *Control of Chagas disease*. WHO Technical Report Series 811. Geneva: World Health Organization, 1991.

4 Hagar JM, Rahimtoola SH. Chagas' heart disease. *Curr Prob Cardiol* 1995;**10**:825–928.

5 Schofield CJ, Dias JCP. A cost benefit analysis of Chagas disease control. *Mem Inst Oswaldo Cruz* 1991;**86**:285–95.

6 Acquatella H, Catalioti F, Gomez-Mancebo JR, Davalos V, Villalobos L. Long-term control of Chagas disease in Venezuela: effects on serologic findings, electrocardiographic abnormalities, and clinical outcome. *Circulation* 1987;**76**:556–62.

7 Dias JCP. Cardiopatia chagásica: história natural. In: Cançado JR, Chuster M. eds. *Cardiopatia chagásica*. Belo Horizonte Fundação: Carlos Chagas de Pesquisa Médica, 1985, pp 99–113.

8 Macedo V. Forma indeterminada da doeņa de chagas. *J Bras Med* 1980;**38**:34–40.

9 Forichon E. *Contribution aux estimations de morbidité et de mortalité dans la maladie de Chagas*. Toulouse: Universite Paul-Sabatier, 1974.

10 Puigbó JJ, Rhode JRN, Barrios HG, Yépez CG. A 4-year follow-up study of a rural community with endemic Chagas' disease. *Bull World Health Organ* 1968;**39**:341–8.

11 Mota EA, Guimarães AC, Santana OO *et al.* A nine year prospective study of Chagas' disease in a defined rural population in northeast Brazil. *Am J Trop Med* 1990;**42**:429–40.

12 Dias JCP, Kloetzel K. The prognostic value of the electrocardiographic features of chronic Chagas' disease. *Rev Inst Med Trop São Paulo* 1968;**10**: 158–62.

13 Coura JR, Abreu LL, Pereira JB, Willcox HP. Morbidade da doença de chagas. IV. Estudo longitudinal de dez anos em Pains e Iguatama, Minas Gerais. *Mem Inst Oswaldo Cruz* 1985;**80**: 73–80.

14 Pereira JB, Cunha RV, Willcox HP, Coura JR. Development of chronic human Chagas' cardiopathy in the hinterland of Paraíba, Brazil, in a 4.5 year period. *Rev Soc Bras Med Trop* 1990; **23**:141–7.

15 Pugliese C, Lessa I, Santos Filho A. Estudo da sobrevida na miocardite crônica de chagas descompensada. *Rev Inst Med Trop São Paulo* 1976; **18**:191–201.

16 Espinosa R, Carrasco HA, Belandria F *et al.* Life expectancy analysis in patients with Chagas' disease: prognosis after one decade (1973–1983). *Int J Cardiol* 1985;**8**:45–56.

17 Mady C, Cardoso RHA, Barreto ACP *et al.* Survival and predictors of survival in congestive heart failure due to Chagas' cardiomyopathy. *Circulation* 1994;**90**:3098–102.

18 Hagar JM, Rahimtoola SH. Chagas' heart disease in the United States. *N Engl J Med* 1991;**325**: 763–8

19 de Paola AA, Gomes JA, Terzian AB *et al.* Ventricular tachycardia on exercise testing is significantly associated with sudden cardiac death in patients with chronic chagasic cardiomyopathy and ventricular arrhythmias. *Br Heart J* 1995; **74**:293–5.

20 Laranja FS, Dias E, Nobrega G, Miranda A. Chagas' disease: a clinical, epidemiologic, and pathologic study. *Circulation* 1956;**14**:1035–59.

21 Lopes ER, Chapadeiro E, Almeida HO, Rocha A, Rocha A. Contribuição ao estudo da anatomia patológica dos corações de Chagásicos falecidos subitamente. *Rev Soc Bras Med Trop* 1975;**9**: 269–82.

22 Barreto ACP, Arteaga-Fernandez E. RV endomyocardial biopsy in chronic Chagas' disease. *Am Heart J* 1986;**111**:307–12.

23 Marin-Neto JA, Marzullo P, Marcassa C. Myocardial perfusion defects in chronic Chagas' disease. Assessment with thallium-201 scintigraphy. *Am J Cardiol* 1992;**69**:780–4.

24 Barreto ACP, Ianni BM. The undetermined form of Chagas' heart disease: concept and forensic implications. *São Paulo Med J* 1995;**113**: 797–801.

25 Oliveira JSM. A natural human model of intrinsic heart nervous system denervation: Chagas' cardiopathy. *Am Heart J* 1985;**110**:1092–8

26 Oliveira JSM, Araújo RRC, Mucillo G. Cardiac thrombosis and thromboembolism in chronic Chagas' heart disease. *Am J Cardiol* 1983;**52**: 147–51.

27 Prata A, Andrade Z, Guimarães AC. Chagas' heart disease. In: Shaper AG, Hutt MSR, Fejfar Z. eds. *Cardiovascular disease in the tropics*. London: British Medical Association, 1974, pp 264–81.

28 Marin-Neto JA, Marzullo P, Sousa ACS *et al.* Radionuclide angiographic evidence for early predominant right ventricular involvement in patients with Chagas' disease. *Can J Cardiol* 1988; **4**:231–6.

29 Marin-Neto JA, Gallo L Jr, Manço JC, Rassi A, Amorin DS. Mechanisms of tachycardia on standing: studies in normal individuals and in chronic Chagas' heart patients. *Cardiovasc Res* 1980;**14**:541–50.

30 Amorim DS, Marin-Neto JA. Functional alterations of the autonomic nervous system in

Chages' heart disease. *São Paulo Med J* 1995;**113**: 772–83.

31 Köberle F. Chagas' heart disease and Chagas' syndromes: the pathology of American trypanosomiasis. *Adv Parasitol* 1968;**6**:63–116.

32 Amorim DS, Manço JC, Gallo L Jr, Marin-Neto JA. Chagas' heart disease as an experimental model for studies of cardiac autonomic function in man. *Mayo Clin Proc* 1982;**57**:48–60.

33 Avila HA, Sigman DS, Cohen LM, Millikan RC, Simpson L. Polymerase chain reaction amplification of *Trypanosoma cruzi* kinetoplast minicircle DNA isolated from whole blood lysates: diagnosis of chronic Chagas' disease. *Mol Biochem Parasitol* 1991;**48**:211–21.

34 Jones EM, Colley DG, Tostes S *et al.* A *Trypanosoma cruzi* DNA sequence amplified from inflammatory lesions in human chagasic cardiomyopathy. *Trans Assoc Am Physicians* 1992;**105**:182–9.

35 Bellotti G, Bocchi EA, Moraes AV *et al.* In vivo detection of *Trypanosoma cruzi* antigens in hearts of patients with chronic Chagas' disease. *Am Heart J* 1996;**131**:301–7.

36 Morris SA, Tanowitz HB, Wittner M, Bilezikian JP. Pathophysiological insights into the cardiomyopathy of Chagas' disease. *Circulation* 1990;**83**:1900–9.

37 Rossi MA. Microvascular changes as a cause of chronic cardiomyopathy in Chagas' disease. *Am Heart J* 1990;**120**:233–6.

38 Reis DD, Jones EM, Tostes S. Expression of major histocompatibility complex antigens and adhesion molecules in hearts of patients with chronic Chagas' disease. *Am J Trop Med Hyg* 1993; **49**:192–200.

39 Torres FW, Acquatella H, Condado J, Dinsmore R, Palacios I. Coronary vascular reactivity is abnormal in patients with Chagas' heart disease. *Am Heart J* 1995;**129**:995–1001.

40 Simões MV, Ayres-Neto EM, Attab-Santos JL, Maciel BC, Marin-Neto JA. Chagas' heart patients without cardiac enlargement have impaired epicardial coronary vasodilation but no vasotonic angina. *J Am Coll Cardiol* 1996;**27**:394–5A.

41 Andrade ZA, Andrade SG, Correa R, Sadigursky M, Ferrans VJ. Myocardial changes in acute *Trypanosoma cruzi* infection. *Am J Pathol* 1994; **144**:1403–11.

42 Santos RR, Rossi MA, Laus JL *et al.* Anti-CD4 abrogates rejection and reestablishes long-term tolerance to syngeneic newborn hearts grafted in mice chronically infected with *Trypanosoma cruzi*. *J Exp Med* 1992;**175**:29–39.

43 Cunha-Neto E, Duranti M, Gruber A *et al.* Autoimmunity in Chagas' disease cardiopathy: biological relevance of a cardiac myosin-specific epitope crossreactive to an immunodominant *Trypanosoma cruzi* antigen. *Proc Natl Acad Sci* 1995;**92**:3541–5.

44 Viotti R, Vigliano C, Armenti H, Segura E. Treatment of chronic Chagas' disease with benznidazole: clinical and serologic evolution of patients with long-term follow-up. *Am Heart J* 1994;**127**:151–62.

45 Batlouni M, Barretto AC, Armaganijan D *et al.* Treatment of mild and moderate cardiac failure with captopril. A multicenter trial. *Arq Bras Cardiol* 1992;**58**(5):417–21.

46 Roberti RR, Martinez EE, Andrade JL *et al.* Chagas cardiomyopathy and captopril. *Eur Heart J* 1992; **13**(7):966–70.

47 Bocchi EA, Bellotti G, Mocelin AO *et al.* Heart transplantation for chronic Chagas' heart disease. *Ann Thorac Surg* 1996;**61**(6):1727–33.

48 Jatene AD, Moreira LF, Stolf NA *et al.* Left ventricular function changes after cardiomyoplasty in patients with dilated cardiomyopathy. *J Thorac Cardiovasc Surg* 1991; **102**(1):132–8.

49 Moreira LF, Stolf NA, Braile DM, Jatene AD. Dynamic cardiomyoplasty in South America. *Ann Thorac Surg* 1996;**61**:408–12.

50 Albanesi-Filho FM, Gomes JB. O tromboembolismo em pacientes com lesão apical da cardiopatia chagásica crônica. *Rev Port Cardiol* 1991;**10**: 35–42.

51 Rey RC, Lepera SM, Kohler G, Monteverde DA, Sica RE. Cerebral embolism of cardiac origin. *Medicina (Buenos Aires)* 1992;**52**(3):206–16.

52 Carrasco HA, Vicuna AV, Molina C *et al.* Effect of low oral doses of disopyramide and amiodarone on ventricular and atrial arrhythmias of chagasic patients with advanced myocardial damage. *Int J Cardiol* 1985;**9**(4):425–38.

53 Rosembaum M, Posse R, Sgammini H *et al.* Comparative multicenter clinical study of flecainide and amiodarone in the treatment of ventricular arrhythmias associated to chronic Chagas cardiopathy. *Arch Inst Cardiol Mex* 1987; **57**:325–30.

54 Doval HC, Nul DR, Grancelli HD *et al.* Randomized trial of low-dose amiodarone in severe congestive heart failure. *Lancet* 1994;**344**:493–8.

55 Garguichevich JJ, Ramos JL, Gambarte A *et al.* Effect of amiodarone therapy on mortality in patients with left ventricular dysfunction and asymptomatic complex ventricular arrhythmias: Argentine pilot study of sudden death and amiodarone (EPAMSA). *Am Heart J* 1995;**130**: 494–500.

56 Wynne J, Baunwald E. Endomyocardiofibrosis. In: Baunwald E. ed. *The cardiomyopathies and myocarditides: A textbook of cardiovascular medicine*, 5th edn. Philadelphia: WB Saunders, 1997.

57 Olsen EGI, Spry CJF. Relationship between eosinophilia and endomyocardial disease. *Prog Cardiovasc Dis* 1985;**27**:241–54.

58 Somers K, Brenton DP, Sood NK. Clinical features of endomyocardial fibrosis of the right ventricle. *Br Heart J* 1968;**30**:309–21.

59 Barreto ACP, Luz PL, Mady C, Bellotti G, Pilleggi F. Determinants of survival in patients with endomyocardial fibrosis. *Circulation* 1988;**78**: 526–30.

60 Oliveira SA, Barreto ACP, Mady C, Bellotti G, Pilleggi F. Surgical treatment of endomyocardial fibrosis: a new surgical approach. *J Am Coll Cardiol* 1990;**5416**:1246–51.

Part III
Specific cardiovascular disorders
viii: Pericardial disease

BERNARD J GERSH, Editor

Grading of recommendations and levels of evidence used in *Evidence Based Cardiology*

GRADE A

Level 1a   Evidence from large randomized clinical trials (RCTs) or systematic reviews (including meta-analyses) of multiple randomized trials which collectively has at least as much data as one single well-defined trial.

Level 1b   Evidence from at least one "All or None" high quality cohort study; in which ALL patients died/failed with conventional therapy and some survived/succeeded with the new therapy (eg chemotherapy for tuberculosis, meningitis, or defibrillation for ventricular fibrillation); or in which many died/failed with conventional therapy and NONE died/failed with the new therapy (eg penicillin for pneumococcal infections).

Level 1c   Evidence from at least one moderate sized RCT or a meta-analysis of small trials which collectively only has a moderate number of patients.

Level 1d   Evidence from at least one RCT.

GRADE B

Level 2   Evidence from at least one high quality study of non-randomized cohorts who did and did not receive the new therapy.

Level 3   Evidence from at least one high quality case control study.

Level 4   Evidence from at least one high quality case series.

GRADE C

Level 5   Opinions from experts without reference or access to any of the foregoing (eg argument from physiology, bench research or first principles).

A comprehensive approach would incorporate many different types of evidence (eg RCTs, non-RCTs, epidemiologic studies, and experimental data), and examine the architecture of the information for consistency, coherence and clarity. Occasionally the evidence does not completely fit into neat compartments. For example, there may not be an RCT that demonstrates a reduction in mortality in individuals with stable angina with the use of beta-blockers, but there is overwhelming evidence that mortality is reduced following MI. In such cases, some may recommend use of beta-blockers in angina patients with the expectation that some extrapolation from post-MI trials is warranted. This could be expressed as Grade A/C. In other instances (e.g. smoking cessation or a pacemaker for complete heart block), the non-randomized data are so overwhelmingly clear and biologically plausible that it would be reasonable to consider these interventions as Grade A.

Recommendation grades appear either in a shaded margin box with an 'R' logo as shown, or within the text, for example Grade A.

Pericardial disease: an evidence based approach to diagnosis and treatment

45

Bongani M. Mayosi,
James A. Volmink,
Patrick J. Commerford

INTRODUCTION

Pericardial disease is a potentially curable cause of heart disease that accounts for about 7% of all patients who are hospitalized for cardiac failure in Africa.[1] Although there are no good epidemiologic data on the incidence or prevalence of pericarditis in different populations,[2] hospital based series indicate that the spectrum of pericardial disease is determined by the epidemiologic setting of the patient. In Western countries, most cases of primary pericarditis are of unknown cause, whereas tuberculosis accounts for the majority of patients in the developing world.[3,4] Thus, evidence based guidelines should be adapted according to the prevalence of certain diseases in particular geographic areas and patient populations.

A discussion of the large number of diseases that may affect the pericardium[5] (Table 45.1) cannot be covered in this short chapter. Consequently, this overview will focus on the diagnosis and treatment of idiopathic and tuberculous pericarditides. It will, in particular, aim to examine the extent to which existing treatments are supported by evidence from well designed prospective studies. The findings reported here are based on a comprehensive search of electronic databases and bibliographies of articles on pericarditis.

PRIMARY ACUTE PERICARDIAL DISEASE

Acute pericarditis may be caused by a variety of disorders (Table 45.1). Among the secondary forms of pericarditis, the underlying disorder is usually evident before pericardial involvement. The most challenging dilemma for the physician is the patient

Table 45.1 Causes of acute pericarditis[5]

Malignant tumor
Idiopathic pericarditis
Uremia
Bacterial infection
Anticoagulant therapy
Dissecting aortic aneurysm
Diagnostic procedures
Connective tissue disease
Postpericardiotomy syndrome
Trauma
Tuberculosis
Other
- radiation
- drugs inducing lupus-like syndrome
- myxedema
- postmyocardial infarction syndrome
- fungal infections
- AIDS-related pericarditis

Table 45.2 Etiology of primary acute pericarditis in the West

	Permanyer-Miralda *et al.* 1985[3] *n*=231	Zayas *et al.* 1995[5] *n*=100
Acute idiopathic pericarditis	199 (86%)	78 (78%)
Neoplastic pericarditis	13 (6%)	7 (7%)
Tuberculous pericarditis	9 (4%)	4 (4%)
Other infections	6 (3%)	3 (3%)
Collagen vascular disease	2 (0.5%)	3 (3%)
Other	2 (0.5%)	5 (5%)

with acute pericardial disease without apparent cause at the initial evaluation (primary acute pericardial disease). In Western series a specific etiology has been found in only 14–22% of these patients when they are subjected to a prospective diagnostic protocol (Table 45.2).[3,6]

DIAGNOSIS

Acute pericarditis is the occurrence of two or more of the following: characteristic chest pain, pericardial friction rub (pathognomonic of acute pericarditis), and an electrocardiogram showing characteristic ST segment elevation or typical serial changes.[7] The chest radiograph, echocardiogram, and radionuclide scans are of little diagnostic value in uncomplicated acute pericarditis.

The first step in the etiologic diagnosis of acute pericarditis consists of a search for an underlying disease that may require specific therapy. In most cases of suspected viral pericarditis, special studies for etiologic agents are not necessary because of the low diagnostic yield of viral studies and lack of specific therapy for viral disease.[7] However, a treatable condition such as *Mycoplasma*-associated pericarditis must be considered and

Table 45.3 Therapeutic strategies previously evaluated in recurrent pericarditis (after failure of non-steroidal anti-inflammatory drugs)

Study	Number of patients	Therapeutic strategy evaluated	Remission rate
Fowler[10]	9	Pericardiectomy	2/9 (22%)
Hatcher[11]	24	Pericardiectomy	20/24 (83%)
Asplen[12]	2	Azathioprine	2/2 (100%)
Melchior[13]	2	IV methylprednisolone as pulse therapy	2/2 (100%)
Marcolongo[14]	12	High dose prednisone with aspirin	11/12 (92%) Major side effects in 3
Guindo[15] and de la Serna[16]	9	Colchicine	9/9 (100%)
Spodick[17]	8	Colchicine	3/9 (33%)
Adler[18]	8	Colchicine	4/8 (50%)
Millaire[19]	19	Colchicine	14/19 (74%)

treated with antibiotics if the serological test is consistent with the diagnosis.[8] The Permanyer-Miralda *et al.* protocol[3] for the evaluation of acute pericardial disease is discussed under Pericardial Effusion below.

TREATMENT

Although there are no controlled trials, it is generally accepted that bedrest and oral non-steroidal anti-inflammatory drugs (NSAIDs) are effective in most patients with acute pericarditis.[7] The use of corticosteroids for acute idiopathic pericarditis when the disease does not subside rapidly is also untested in randomized trials, but it may be unnecessary and even dangerous in acute non-relapsing pericarditis in view of the availability of other agents, such as the parenteral NSAID ketorolac tromethamine.[9] Ketorolac is an extremely potent analgesic agent which appears to cause rapid resolution of symptomatic acute pericarditis. However, the limitation of this study of 20 patients with acute pericarditis was that there was no control group for comparison.[9]

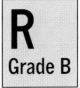

R
Grade B

Idiopathic relapsing pericarditis is the most troublesome complication of acute pericarditis, affecting about 20% of cases. There are no established therapeutic guidelines for patients who do not respond to NSAIDs.[7] Corticosteroids provide symptomatic relief in most of these patients, but symptoms recur in many when the prednisone dosage is reduced and severe complications are associated with prolonged steroid use.[10] Claims of effectiveness have been made in small uncontrolled studies for pericardiectomy, azathioprine, high dose oral and intravenous corticosteroids, and colchicine (Table 45.3).[10–15] The results of these studies are inconsistent and the effectiveness of these potentially harmful therapeutic modalities remains to be established in well designed randomized studies. Nevertheless, colchicine, used on the basis of its efficacy in the recurrent polyserositis seen in familial Mediterranean fever,[16] has aroused much interest following the dramatic effects which were initially reported with its use in recurrent pericarditis.[15] The accumulating experience with colchicine indicates that while its long term use is well tolerated, it is associated with a variable remission rate of 33–100%, and there is a tendency for a small proportion of patients to relapse after cessation of therapy.[16–19]

Table 45.4 Permanyer-Miralda *et al.* protocol for evaluation of primary acute pericardial disease[3]

Stage I	
General studies and echocardiogram	Electrocardiogram
	Chest radiograph
	Tuberculin skin test
	Serologic tests
Stage II	
Pericardiocentesis	Therapeutic pericardiocentesis: absolutely indicated for cardiac tamponade
	Diagnostic pericardiocentesis: clinical suspicion of purulent or tuberculous pericarditis
	Illness lasting for more than 1 week
Stage III	
Surgical biopsy of the pericardium	"Therapeutic" biopsy: as part of surgical drainage in patients with severe tamponade relapsing after pericardiocentesis
	Diagnostic biopsy: in patients with more than 3 weeks illness and without an etiologic diagnosis having been reached by previous procedures
Stage IV	
Empirical antitubercular treatment	Fever and pericardial effusion of unknown origin persisting for more than 5–6 weeks

Pericardial effusion

The spectrum of causes of pericardial effusion is similar to acute pericarditis (Table 45.1). However, prospective studies indicate that large pericardial effusions are more likely to be a result of serious underlying illnesses such as tuberculosis and cancer, where rapid diagnosis may lead to earlier therapy and improved survival.[3,20] The clinical features vary depending on the rate of accumulation of the fluid, the amount of fluid that accumulates, and the stage at which the patient is first seen.

DIAGNOSIS

The radiographic signs of pericardial effusion include an enlarged cardiac silhouette, a pericardial fat stripe, a predominant left-sided pleural effusion, and an increase in transverse cardiac diameter compared with previous chest radiographs. However, these signs cannot reliably confirm or exclude the presence of pericardial effusion, thus making radiography poorly diagnostic of pericardial effusion.[21] Similarly, electrocardiography is useful only in that it may suggest a cardiac abnormality. The QRS complexes are usually small, with generalized T-wave inversion. Electrical alternans, which suggests the presence of massive pericardial effusion, is uncommon. Even more uncommon is total electrical alternans (P-QRS-T alternation), which is pathognomonic of tamponade.[22]

Echocardiography, computed tomography, and magnetic resonance imaging can accurately detect and quantify pericardial effusion. Echocardiography, which is relatively

Table 45.5 Echocardiographic features of cardiac tamponade[26]

Echocardiographic/Doppler criteria	Comments
1. Right heart collapse: right atrial compression right ventricular diastolic collapse	Changes in blood volume may affect the sensitivity and specificity of right heart collapse as a sign of tamponade. False positives and false negatives may occur
2. Abnormal respiratory changes in ventricular dimensions	Inconstant finding
3. Abnormal respiratory changes in tricuspid and mitral flow velocities	May also be seen in obstructive airways disease, pulmonary embolism, and right ventricular infarction
4. Dilated inferior vena cava with lack of inspiratory collapse	Often seen with congestive heart failure and constrictive pericarditis
5. Left ventricular diastolic collapse	Frequent sign of regional cardiac tamponade and useful marker of tamponade in postoperative patients in a retrospective investigation[27]
6. Swinging heart	Not sensitive, specificity unknown

inexpensive, sensitive (capable of detecting as little as 17 ml pericardial fluid), harmless, and widely available, is the diagnostic method of choice for pericardial effusion.[5] Furthermore, it may also provide prognostic information. A large effusion with a circumferential echo-free space of >1cm in width at any point is reported to be a powerful predictor of tamponade[23] and intrapericardial echo images are associated with an increased likelihood of subsequent constriction.[24]

Permanyer-Miralda *et al.* have evolved a systematic approach for the evaluation of acute primary pericardial disease in developed countries with a low prevalence of tuberculosis (Table 45.4). It is based on a prospective study of 231 consecutive patients who were evaluated to determine the safest and most sensitive approach to the etiologic diagnosis of acute pericardial disease.[3] The findings were confirmed in a subsequent prospective study of a similar diagnostic protocol involving 100 patients with primary pericardial disease.[5] Firstly, these prospective studies indicate that a specific etiology is found in only 14–22% of patients with acute primary pericardial disease (Table 45.2). Secondly, while therapeutic pericardiocentesis is absolutely indicated for cardiac tamponade, it is not warranted as a routine investigation because of low diagnostic yield. The indications for diagnostic pericardiocentesis are the clinical suspicion of purulent or tuberculous pericarditis and those with an illness lasting longer than 1 week. Thirdly, the diagnostic yield of pericardiocentesis and pericardial biopsy is similar. Whereas biopsy is more invasive and may entail the need for general anesthesia, it is a safe procedure and direct histologic examination of the pericardium may allow immediate diagnosis in the case of tuberculosis. Furthermore, pericardial biopsy may allow a more direct visualization of the pericardium. However, even when detailed investigations are performed, including pericardioscopy and surgery, the etiology of pericardial effusion remains obscure in a significant number of patients.[25]

Cardiac tamponade

A pericardial effusion may result in the life threatening complication of cardiac tamponade, a condition caused by compression of the heart and impaired diastolic filling of the ventricles. It is an indication for pericardiocentesis.

Cardiac tamponade is a clinical diagnosis which is confirmed by echocardiography. The clinical examination shows elevated systemic venous pressure, tachycardia, dyspnea, and pulsus paradoxus.[26] Pulsus paradoxus may be absent in some instances such as left ventricular dysfunction, atrial septal defect, regional tamponade, and positive pressure breathing. Systemic blood pressure may be normal, decreased or even elevated. The diagnosis is usually confirmed by the echocardiographic demonstration of a large circumferential pericardial effusion and some of the features listed in Table 45.5. However, as a diagnostic test for tamponade, echocardiography may lack both sensitivity and specificity in certain clinical situations. For example, echocardiographic features of right heart collapse may be absent in the presence of loculated effusions causing regional left ventricular compression. This is particularly important after cardiac surgery when the absence of a circumferential effusion and right atrial collapse and right ventricular diastolic collapse may not exclude the presence of life threatening tamponade.[28] Furthermore, a dilated non-collapsing inferior vena cava and an abnormal respiratory pattern of diastolic flow are not specific signs of tamponade (Table 45.5).

CONSTRICTIVE PERICARDITIS

The etiology of constrictive pericarditis has changed over the past four decades.[29] Tuberculous constrictive pericarditis, which was a common cause of constriction worldwide before the 1960s, has since declined in incidence and is now rare in Western countries. In these countries the diminished importance of tuberculous pericarditis has been associated with a large contribution made by idiopathic cases. Postradiotherapy constriction, which was first recognized as an important disease in the 1960s, continues to feature prominently among the causes of constrictive pericarditis, while postsurgical constriction has emerged as an important cause.

Constrictive pericarditis is characterized anatomically by an abnormally thickened and non-compliant pericardium that limits ventricular filling in mid to late diastole. Consequently, nearly all ventricular filling occurs very rapidly in early diastole. This results in elevated cardiac filling pressures and the characteristic hemodynamic waveforms during which the diastolic pressures of the cardiac chambers equalize. The clinical manifestations of constrictive pericarditis, which are secondary to systemic venous congestion, mimic a variety of cardiopulmonary disorders, making the diagnosis of this condition difficult in some cases.

DIAGNOSIS

The chest radiograph and electrocardiogram are usually abnormal, drawing attention to the heart, but the abnormalities are largely non-specific. Chest radiography may reveal a small, normal or enlarged cardiac silhouette, and pleural effusions in 60%, and pericardial calcification in 5–50% of cases.[30,31] Calcification is not specific for constrictive pericarditis, as a calcified pericardium does not necessarily imply constriction. Non-specific but generalized T-wave changes are seen in most cases, while low voltage complexes occur in about 30%.

The ideal imaging technique for the accurate preoperative diagnosis of pericardial constriction would simultaneously provide both anatomic data describing the thickness of the pericardium and physiologic data describing the abnormal diastolic ventricular filling. Although echocardiography has proven useful in the diagnosis of pericardial effusion, its role in constrictive pericarditis is less certain. While constrictive wall motion abnormalities are suggestive, there is no single feature on M-mode echocardiography that is diagnostic of constrictive pericarditis[31] and two-dimensional echocardiography cannot accurately measure pericardial thickness.[32] Although Doppler echocardiography performed simultaneously with respiratory recording appears to be highly sensitive for diagnosing constrictive pericarditis and predictive of functional response to pericardiectomy, its specificity is unknown.[33]

Computed tomography and magnetic resonance imaging can demonstrate the extent and distribution of pericardial thickening. While this does not make the diagnosis of constriction, it is often very useful to know that the pericardium is abnormal in a patient in whom this diagnosis is suspected. In addition, computed tomographic or magnetic resonance imaging features of myocardial atrophy or fibrosis predict a poor outcome following pericardiectomy.[34] A promising new imaging technique is cine computed tomography which simultaneously provides both anatomic and physiologic data that may allow accurate preoperative diagnosis of pericardial constriction.[35] The validity of cine computed tomography as a non-invasive diagnostic test for constrictive pericarditis needs to be validated in larger studies.

Unless the diagnosis is very obvious, cardiac catheterization is usually performed. The characteristic finding is equal end-diastolic pressures in the two ventricles, persisting with respiration and fluid challenge. However, the diagnosis of constrictive pericarditis remains a challenge because it is often mimicked by restrictive cardiomyopathy. A number of studies, using different techniques, have attempted to distinguish the two conditions, including studies of left ventricular filling rate, mitral and tricuspid diastolic flow patterns, pulmonary venous flow velocity, hepatic flow velocity patterns, hemodynamic investigations, endomyocardial biopsy, and computed tomographic and magnetic resonance imaging studies.[36] Table 45.6 summarizes the important differences between the two conditions. No technique is totally reliable and in some patients, the only way of making the diagnosis is to perform a pericardiectomy.[37]

TREATMENT

The treatment for chronic constrictive pericarditis is complete resection of the pericardium. The average hospital mortality following pericardiectomy in several series ranges from about 5% to 16%.[38–40] Poor outcome is related mainly to preoperative disability, the degree of constriction, and myocardial involvement. The majority of early deaths are associated with low cardiac output, which has been attributed to myocardial atrophy. Thus, early pericardiectomy is recommended in patients with non-tuberculous constrictive pericarditis before severe constriction and myocardial atrophy occur.

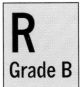

Among patients who survive the operation, symptomatic improvement can be expected in about 90% and complete relief of symptoms in about 50%. The 5-year survival rate ranges from 74% to 87%. Long term survival and symptomatic relief do not appear to be influenced by age, choice of median sternotomy or left thoracotomy or transient low

Table 45.6 The differentiation of constrictive pericarditis from restrictive cardiomyopathy[37]

Type of evaluation	Constrictive pericarditis	Restrictive cardiomyopathy
Physical examination	Regurgitant murmurs uncommon	Regurgitant murmurs common
Chest radiography	Pericardial calcification may be present	Pericardial calcification absent
Echocardiography	Normal wall thickness	Increased wall thickness, thickened cardiac valves and granular
	Pericardial thickness may be seen	sparkling texture (amyloid). Enlarged atria and low ejection fraction
	Prominent early diastolic filling with abrupt displacement of	favor restrictive cardiomyopathy
	interventricular septum	
Doppler studies	Early mitral flow is reduced with onset of inspiration and reciprocal	No respiratory variation in diastolic flow
	effect on tricuspid flow	Inspiratory increase of hepatic vein diastolic flow reversal
	Expiratory increase of hepatic vein diastolic flow reversal	Mitral and tricuspid regurgitation common
Cardiac	RVEDP and LVEDP usually equal	LVEDP often >5 mmHg greater than RVEDP, but may be identical
catheterization	RV systolic pressure <50 mmHg	
	RVEDP >one-third of RV systolic pressure	
Endomyocardial	May be normal or show non-specific myocyte hypertrophy or	May reveal specific cause of restrictive cardiomyopathy
biopsy	myocardial fibrosis	
CT/MRI	Pericardium may be thickened ≥3 mm	Pericardium usually normal

LV, left ventricular; RV, right ventricular; LVEDP, left ventricular end-diastolic pressure; RVEDP, right ventricular end-diastolic pressure; CT, computed tomography; MRI, magnetic resonance imaging.

output syndrome postoperatively. However, long term survival is unfavorably influenced by the presence of severe preoperative functional disability (NYHA class III or IV, diuretic use), renal insufficiency in the preoperative state, the presence of extensive non-resectable calcifications, incomplete pericardial resection, and the presence of radiation pericarditis, which is commonly complicated by myocardial fibrosis and restrictive myocardial disease.

TUBERCULOUS PERICARDITIS

The prevalence of tuberculous pericarditis follows the same pattern as that of tuberculosis in general. It is the most common cause of pericarditis in developing countries where tuberculosis remains a major public health problem, but accounts for only about 5% of cases in the West.[3,4,40] The incidence of tuberculous pericarditis is rising as a direct result of the human immunodeficiency virus epidemic in Africa[41] and this trend is likely to occur in other parts of the world where the acquired immnodeficiency syndrome epidemic is leading to the resurgence of tuberculosis. Tuberculosis caused by drug resistant *Mycobacterium tuberculosis* has emerged in the past few years as a serious threat to global public health, but its impact on pericardial tuberculosis has not been studied.

Tuberculous pericarditis appears to be more common in blacks than whites and males than females,[42,43] although the sex difference was reversed in the large prospective studies of Strang *et al.*[30,44] The disease can occur at any age.

Tuberculous pericardial effusion

Tuberculous pericarditis is usually detected clinically either in the effusive stage or after the development of constriction. Tuberculous pericarditis has a variable clinical presentation and it should be considered in the evaluation of all instances of pericarditis without a rapidly self-limited course.[43] While tuberculous pericarditis may cause effusions which do not produce cardiac compression, more commonly there is at least some degree of cardiac compression, which may be severe, causing tamponade.

Tuberculous pericardial effusion usually develops insidiously, presenting with non specific systemic symptoms such as fever, night sweats, fatigue, and loss of weight.[4,42,45] Chest pain, cough, and breathlessness are common.[45–47] Severe pericardial pain of acute onset characteristic of idiopathic pericarditis is unusual in tuberculous pericarditis.[42,45,48] Right upper abdominal aching due to liver congestion is also common in these patients.[4,42,49] In South African patients with tuberculous pericardial effusion, evidence of chronic cardiac compression that mimics heart failure is by far the most common presentation (Table 45.7).[4,47,49] While there is marked overlap between the physical signs of pericardial effusion and constrictive pericarditis, the presence of increased cardiac dullness extending to the right of the sternum favors a clinical diagnosis of pericardial effusion.

DIAGNOSIS

A definite diagnosis of tuberculous pericarditis is based on the demonstration of tubercle bacilli in pericardial fluid or on histologic section of the pericardium and a probable diagnosis is made when there is proof of tuberculosis elsewhere in a patient with

Table 45.7 Physical signs documented by a single observer in 88 patients with pericardial effusion and 67 patients with constrictive pericarditis in South Africa[4]

	Pericardial effusion (n = 88)	Constrictive pericarditis (n = 67)
Hepatomegaly	84 (95%)	67 (100%)
Increased cardiac dullness	83 (94%)	17 (25%)
Raised jugular venous pulse	74 (84%)	67 (100%)
Soft heart sounds	69 (78%)	51 (76%)
Sinus tachycardia	68 (77%) (Transient AF in 3)	47 (70%) (Persistent AF in 2)
Ascites	64 (73%)	60 (89%)
Apex palpable	53 (60%)	39 (58%)
Significant pulsus paradoxus	32 (36%)	32 (48%)
Edema	22 (25%)	63 (94%)
Pericardial friction rub	16 (18%)	—
Pericardial knock	—	14 (21%)
Third heart sound	—	30 (45%)
Sudden inspiratory splitting of the second heart sound	—	24 (36%)

AF, atrial fibrillation.

unexplained pericarditis. A definite or probable diagnosis is made in up to 73% of patients treated for tuberculous pericarditis.[44,50] The chest radiograph shows features of active pulmonary tuberculosis in only 30% and pleural effusion is present in 40–60% of cases.[43,44,46] The electrocardiogram is usually abnormal, drawing attention to the heart.[44,51] The ST segment elevations characteristic of acute pericarditis are usually absent. Echocardiographic findings are not specific for a tuberculous etiology.[50]

Pericardiocentesis is recommended in all patients in whom tuberculosis is suspected. The pericardial fluid is bloodstained in 80% of cases [4,52] and since malignant disease and the late effects of penetrating trauma cause bloody pericardial effusion, confirmation of tuberculosis as the cause is important. The difficulty in finding tubercle bacilli in the direct smear examination of pericardial fluid is well known. Culture of tubercle bacilli from pericardial effusions can be improved considerably by inoculation of the fluid into double strength liquid Kirchner culture medium at the bedside. A prospective study of the value of the double strength liquid Kirchner culture medium in patients considered to have tuberculosis reported a 75% yield compared to a 53% yield with conventional culture.[53] For *Mycobacterium tuberculosis*, the radiometric method (BACTEC) permits an average recovery and drug sensitivity testing time of 18 days, compared to 38.5 days for conventional methods, but the low yield of 54% is the major disadvantage of the former method.[53] Sputum with acid-fast bacilli will only be found in about 10% of patients.[4] Gastric washings from such patients may be studied and urine culture and lymph node biopsy may also demonstrate tubercle bacilli.

In developing countries tuberculin skin testing is of little value due to the high prevalence of primary tuberculosis, mass BCG immunizations and the likelihood of cross-sensitization from mycobacteria present in the environment.[54] Furthermore, the limited utility of the tuberculin skin test has also been documented in a prospective study performed in a non-endemic area.[43]

There is considerable urgency to establish the correct diagnosis of tuberculosis since early initiation of therapy is associated with a favorable outcome.[45] Since tubercle bacilli are often not found on stained smear of pericardial fluid[46,55] and their growth on culture requires 3–6 weeks, there is a need for other means of making an early diagnosis. Unfortunately, a rapid, simple, inexpensive, sensitive and specific diagnostic test for pericardial tuberculosis is not available.[54] Pericardial biopsy is an important option, but a normal result does not exclude the diagnosis.

Recently, the usefulness of measuring adenosine deaminase activity for the rapid diagnosis of pericardial tuberculosis has been reported in different study populations with consistent results showing a pericardial fluid activity of ≥ 40 u/l to have a sensitivity and specificity of more than 90%.[52,56,57] An analysis of the largest prospective study of the utility of the adenosine deaminase test for the diagnosis of pericardial tuberculosis,[58] which included a wide spectrum of patients with pericardial effusion, yielded a likelihood ratio of 3.8 and 0.05 for positive and negative tests respectively (Table 45.8). Fagan's nomogram (Figure 45.1) for interpreting diagnostic test results can be used to determine the usefulness of a positive (adenosine deaminase ≥ 40) or negative (adenosine deaminase <40) test result.[59,60] Although the likelihood ratio for a positive test is 3.8, a high pretest probability of 80% is associated with a post-test probability of 95% if the adenosine deaminase result is positive. The likelihood ratio of a negative adenosine deaminase test is 0.05, which should confer conclusive changes on pretest to post-test probabilities.

In addition to the adenosine deaminase test, the measurement of interferon gamma levels in pericardial fluid may offer another means of early diagnosis. A study involving 12 patients with definite tuberculous pericardial effusion and 19 controls indicated that

Table 45.8 Test properties of the adenosine deaminase (ADA) assay derived from Latouf *et al.*[56]

ADA level	Definite diagnosis of pericardial tuberculosis				Likelihood ratio
	Present		Absent		
	No.	Proportion	No.	Proportion	
ADA ≥ 40 u/l	77	77/80 = 0.963	26	26/103 = 0.253	3.8
ADA < 40 u/l	3	3/80 = 0.038	77	77/103 = 0.748	0.05
Total	80		103		

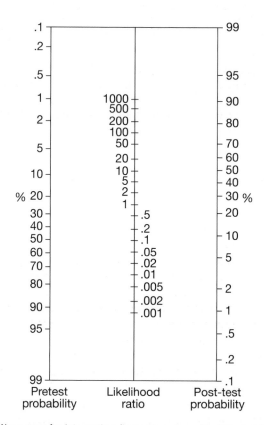

Figure 45.1 Nomogram for interpreting diagnostic test results. (Adapted from Fagan.[59,60])

elevated interferon gamma measured by radioimmunoassay in pericardial aspirate is a sensitive (92%) and highly specific (100%) marker of a tuberculous etiology in patients with a pericardial effusion.[61] This promising report needs confirmation in larger studies.

The polymerase chain reaction is useful in detecting *Mycobacterium tuberculosis* DNA in pericardial fluid,[62,63] but the technique involved is labor intensive and prone to contamination and false positive results and is thus not yet suitable for large numbers of specimens.[54] At present, serum antibody tests against specific tuberculoprotein epitopes have not offered a significant diagnostic advance over other methods.[54]

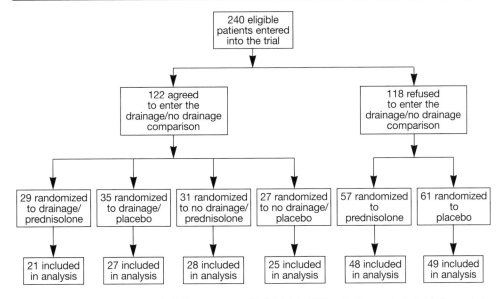

Figure 45.2 Tuberculous pericardial effusion trial profile.[44] A total of 198 patients were included in the analysis.

TREATMENT

In areas and communities with a high prevalence of tuberculosis, a pericardial effusion is often considered to be tuberculous unless an alternative cause is obvious and treatment often has to be commenced before a bacteriologic diagnosis is established.[53] A definite diagnosis is not made in about a third of patients treated for tuberculous pericarditis and an adequate response to antituberculous chemotherapy serves as confirmation. When systematic investigation fails to yield a diagnosis in patients living in non-endemic areas, good prospective data indicate that there is no justification for starting antituberculous treatment empirically.[7]

Antituberculous chemotherapy dramatically increases survival in tuberculous pericarditis. In the preantibiotic era, mortality was 80–90% and currently it ranges from 8% to 17%.[47,64,65] A regimen consisting of rifampicin, isoniazid and pyrazinamide in the initial phase of at least 2 months, followed by isoniazid and rifampicin for a total of 6 months of therapy has been shown to be highly effective in treating patients with extrapulmonary tuberculosis.[66,67] Treatment for 9 months or longer gives no better results and has the added disadvantages of increased costs and poor compliance.[67] Short course chemotherapy is also highly effective in curing tuberculosis in HIV infected patients,[68] although it has not been evaluated specifically in tuberculous pericarditis.

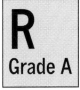

In 1988 Strang et al.[44] reported a prospective double-blind evaluation of patients with tuberculous pericardial effusion treated with antituberculous drugs who were randomly allocated to prednisolone or placebo during the first 11 weeks of therapy (Figure 45.2). Two hundred and forty patients entered the study and 198 were evaluated at 24 months; 42 patients (18%) were excluded from analysis mainly due to loss to follow-up and non-compliance with medication. In this trial, five of 97 patients given prednisolone compared with 11 of 101 given placebo died of pericarditis, seven and 17 needed repeat pericardiocentesis, three and seven open surgical drainage, and 91 and 88 had a favorable functional status at 24 months. Table 45.9 shows the outcomes for patients in the prednisolone and control groups together with the associated odds ratios (95%

Table 45.9 Pericardial effusion: prednisolone versus placebo[44]

Outcome	Group prednisolone (n=97)	Group placebo (n=101)	Peto's odds ratio (95% CI)	P value
1. Favorable status at 24 months[a]	91/97	88/101	2.15 (0.84, 5.53)	0.11
2. Repeat pericardiocentesis	7/97	17/101	0.41 (0.17, 0.95)	0.04
3. Subsequent open drainage	3/97	7/101	0.45 (0.13, 1.60)	0.22
4. Pericardiectomy	7/97	10/101	0.71 (0.26, 1.92)	0.50
5. Total with one or more adverse events[b]	21/97	35/101	0.53 (0.29, 0.98)	0.04
6. Death from pericarditis	5/97	11/101	0.46 (0.17, 1.29)	0.14

[a] Patients were classified as having a favorable status if the following criteria were fulfilled or if only one was still abnormal: pulse rate ≤100, jugular venous pulse ≤5 cm, arterial pulsus paradoxus ≤10mmHg, ascites and edema absent/just detectable, physical activity unrestricted, cardiothoracic ratio ≤55%, and electrocardiogram voltage ≥6 mm in V6 or ≥4 mm along the frontal axis.

[b] Includes outcomes numbered 2, 3, 4, and 6.

CI) and P values for the 198 patients who were analyzed in the trial. Patients treated with prednisolone were significantly less likely to require repeat pericardiocentesis and had fewer combined adverse events than the placebo group. Although there is a suggestion that prednisolone may have a beneficial effect with regard to other outcome events, including death from pericarditis, the 95% confidence intervals are consistent with a null effect.

It appears from these data that the adjuvant use of prednisolone in tuberculous pericarditis is associated with a reduced risk of reaccumulation of pericardial fluid and less morbidity during the treatment period, which may be clinically significant. It should, however, be noted that the exclusion of a high proportion of randomized patients from the analysis may be a source of substantial bias in the findings reported in this study. Further studies are indicated. Therefore, on the basis of the currently available data, prednisolone cannot be recommended for routine use in patients with tuberculous pericardial effusion. We concur with the recommendation that corticosteroids should be reserved for critically ill patients with recurrent large effusions who do not respond to pericardial drainage and antituberculous drugs alone.[31]

In the study by Strang et al.[44] which compared prednisolone and placebo, those who were willing were also randomized to open complete drainage by substernal pericardiotomy and biopsy under general anesthesia followed by suction drainage on admission or percutaneous pericardiocentesis as required to control symptoms and signs (Figure 45.2). One hundred and one patients participated in this comparison. Complete open drainage abolished the need for pericardiocentesis (odds ratio 0.12; 95% CI 0.04–0.39) but did not influence the need for pericardiectomy for subsequent constriction (odds ratio 0.45; 95% CI 0.10–2.06) or the risk of death from pericarditis (odds ratio 1.51; 95% CI 0.33–6.96).

Tuberculous pericardial constriction

Constrictive pericarditis is one of the most serious sequelae of tuberculous pericarditis and it occurs in 30–60% of patients despite prompt antituberculous treatment and the use of corticosteroids.[42–44] Tuberculosis is the most frequent cause of constrictive pericarditis in developing countries.[3,4] The presentation is highly variable, ranging from asymptomatic to severe constriction. The diagnosis is often missed on cursory clinical examination (Table 45.7). The diastolic lift (pericardial knock) which coincides with a high-pitched early diastolic sound and sudden inspiratory splitting of the second heart sound are subtle but specific physical signs, which are found in 21–45% of patients with constrictive pericarditis. These signs are often missed by the inexperienced observer unless specifically sought. Furthermore, if the investigation is not clinically guided, echocardiography has the potential to miss the signs that are suggestive of this diagnosis.

DIAGNOSIS

Most patients with constrictive pericarditis in South Africa have the subacute variety, in which a thick fibrinous exudate fills the pericardial sac, compressing the heart and causing a circulatory disturbance. As a result, calcification of the pericardium will be absent in the majority.[30] The chest radiograph findings are non-specific. In a study reported by Strang *et al.*, 70% of 143 patients had a cardiothoracic ratio greater than 55% and only 6% had a ratio greater than 75%.[30] It is uncommon to find concomitant pulmonary tuberculosis. Non-specific but generalized T-wave changes are seen in most cases, while low voltage complexes occur in about 30% of cases. Atrial fibrillation occurs in less than 5% of cases, is persistent, and usually occurs with a calcified pericardium. As with tuberculous pericardial effusion, the electrocardiogram is useful only in drawing attention to the presence of a cardiac abnormality.

Echocardiography is particularly valuable in confirming the diagnosis of subacute constrictive pericarditis. Typically, a thick fibrinous exudate is seen in the pericardial sac and is associated with diminished movements of the surface of the heart, normal sized chambers, absence of valvular heart disease, and absence of myocardial hypertrophy.[30] In time, the pericardial exudate condenses into a thick skin surrounding the heart, which usually, but not always, can be distinguished from myocardium.

TREATMENT

The treatment of tuberculous pericardial constriction involves the use of antituberculous drugs and pericardiectomy for persistent constriction in the face of drug therapy. In a double-blind, randomized, controlled trial in South Africa, 143 patients with tuberculous pericarditis and clinical signs of a constrictive physiology were allocated to receive prednisolone or placebo in addition to antituberculous drugs during the first 11 weeks of treatment (Figure 45.3).[30] One hundred and fourteen patients were available for evaluation at 24 months; 20% of patients were excluded from analysis mainly due to loss to follow up and non-compliance with medication. Although clinical improvement occurred more rapidly in the prednisolone group and there was a lower mortality from pericarditis at 24 months (4% vs 11%) and a lower requirement for pericardiectomy (21% vs 30%), these findings were not statistically significant (Table 45.10). The remarkable finding of this study is that constriction resolved on antituberculous chemotherapy within 6 months in most patients and only 29 (25%) of the 114 patients with constrictive pericarditis required pericardiectomy for persistent or worsening constriction.

No controlled studies have compared early pericardiectomy with late pericardiectomy in this condition. We recommend pericardiectomy if the patient's condition is static

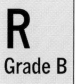

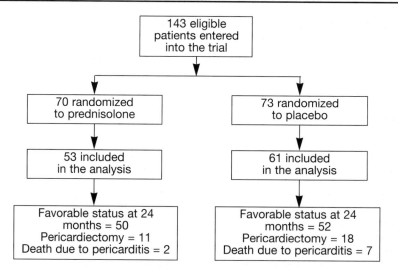

Figure 45.3 Tuberculous constrictive pericarditis trial profile.[30]

Table 45.10 Constrictive pericarditis: prednisolone versus placebo[30]

Outcome	Group prednisolone ($n=53$)	Group placebo ($n=61$)	Peto's odds ratio (95% CI)	P value
1. Favorable status at 24 months[a]	50/53	52/61	2.60 (0.79, 8.59)	0.116
2. Pericardiectomy	11/53	18/61	0.63 (0.27, 1.47)	0.29
3. Death from pericarditis	2/53	7/61	0.35 (0.09, 1.36)	0.13

[a] See note [a] in Table 45.9.

hemodynamically or deteriorating after 4–6 weeks of antituberculous therapy. However, if the disease is associated with pericardial calcification, which is a marker of chronic disease, surgery should be undertaken earlier under the antituberculous drug cover. The reported risks of death with pericardiectomy in patients with tuberculous constrictive pericarditis are variable, ranging from 3% to 16%.[40,69]

Effusive constrictive tuberculous pericarditis

This mixed form is a common presentation in Southern Africa. There is increased pericardial pressure due to effusion in the presence of visceral constriction and the venous pressure remains elevated after pericardial aspiration. In addition to physical signs of pericardial effusion, a diastolic knock may be detected on palpation and an early third heart sound on auscultation.

In patients with the effusive constrictive syndrome echocardiography may show a pericardial effusion between thickened pericardial membranes, with fibrinous pericardial bands apparently causing loculation of the effusion.

The treatment of effusive constrictive pericarditis is a problem because pericardiocentesis does not relieve the impaired filling of the heart and surgical removal of the fibrinous exudate coating the visceral pericardium is not possible. Antituberculous drugs should be given in the standard fashion and serial echocardiography performed to detect the development of a pericardial skin which is amenable to surgical stripping. The place of corticosteroids in such patients is unknown.

REFERENCES

1 Maharaj B. Causes of congestive heart failure in black patients at King Edward VIII Hospital, Durban. *Cardiovasc J S Afr* 1991;**2**:31–2.

2 Maisch B. Pericardial diseases, with a focus on etiology, pathogenesis, pathophysiology, new diagnostic imaging methods and treatment. *Curr Opin Cardiol* 1994;**9**:379–88.

3 Permanyer-Miralda G, Sagrista-Sauleda J, Soler-Soler J. Primary acute pericardial disease: a prospective series of 231 consecutive patients. *Am J Cardiol* 1985;**56**:623–9.

4 Strang JIG. Tuberculous pericarditis. *Clin Cardiol* 1984;**7**:667–70.

5 Fowler NO. Pericardial disease. *Heart Dis Stroke* 1992;**1**:85–94.

6 Zayas R, Anguita M, Torres F *et al.* Incidence of specific etiology and role of methods for specific etiologic diagnosis of primary acute pericarditis. *Am J Cardiol* 1995;**75**:378–82.

7 Permanyer-Miralda G, Sagrista-Sauleda J, Shebatai R *et al.* Acute pericardial disease: an approach to etiologic diagnosis and treatment. In: Soler-Soler J *et al.* Eds. *Pericardial disease: new insights and old dilemmas.* Dordrecht: Kluwer Academic Publishers, 1990.

8 Farraj RS, McCully RB, Oh JK, Smith TF. *Mycoplasma*-associated pericarditis. *Mayo Clin Proc* 1997;**72**:33–6.

9 Arunsalam S, Siegel RJ. Rapid resolution of symptomatic acute pericarditis with ketorolac tromethamine: a parenteral nonsteroidal antiinflammatory agent. *Am Heart J* 1993;**125**:1455–8.

10 Fowler NO, Harbin AD. Recurrent pericarditis: follow-up of 31 patients. *J Am Coll Cardiol* 1986;**7**:300–5.

11 Hatcher CR, Logue RB, Logan WD *et al.* Pericardiectomy for recurrent pericarditis. *J Thorac Cardiovasc Surg* 1971;**62**:371–8.

12 Asplen CH, Levine HD. Azathioprine therapy of steroid responsive pericarditis. *Am Heart J* 1970;**80**:109–11.

13 Melchior TM, Ringsdal V, Hildebrandt P, Torp-Pedersen C. Recurrent acute idiopathic pericarditis treated with intravenous methylprednisolone given as pulse therapy. *Am Heart J* 1992;**123**:1086–8.

14 Marcolongo R, Russo R, Lavender F, Noventa F, Agostini C. Immunosuppressive therapy prevents recurrent pericarditis. *J Am Coll Cardiol* 1995;**26**:1276–9.

15 Guindo J, Rodriguez de la Serna A, Ramio J *et al.* Recurrent pericarditis. Relief with colchicine. *Circulation* 1990;**82**:1117–20.

16 Rodriguez de la Serna A, Guindo Soldevila J, Marti Claramunt V, Bayes de Luna A. Colchicine for recurrent pericarditis. *Lancet* 1987;**ii**:1517.

17 Spodick DH. Colchicine therapy for recurrent pericarditis. *Circulation* 1991;**83**:1830.

18 Adler Y, Zandman-Goddard G, Ravid M *et al.* Usefulness of colchicine in preventing recurrences of pericarditis. *Am J Cardiol* 1994;**73**:916–17.

19 Millaire A, deGroote P, Decoulx E *et al.* Treatment of recurrent pericarditis with colchicine. *Eur Heart J* 1994;**15**:120–4.

20 Corey RG, Campbell PT, van Trigt P *et al.* Etiology of large pericardial effusions. *Am J Med* 1993;**95**:209–13.

21 Eisenberg MJ, Dunn MM, Kanth N, Gamsu G, Schiller NB. Diagnostic value of chest radiography for pericardial effusion. *J Am Coll Cardiol* 1993;**22**:588–92.

22 Spodick DH. Electrical alternation of the heart. Its relation to the kinetics and physiology of the heart during cardiac tamponade. *Am J Cardiol* 1962;**10**:155–65.

23 Eisenberg MJ, Oken K, Guerrero S, Saniei MA, Schiller NB. Prognostic value of echocardiography in hospitalized patients with pericardial effusion. *Am J Cardiol* 1992;**70**:934–9.

24 Sinha PR, Singh BP, Jaipuria N *et al.* Intrapericardial echogenic images and development of constrictive pericarditis in patients with pericardial effusion. *Am Heart J* 1996;**132**:1268–72.

25 Nugue O, Millaire A, Porte H *et al.* Pericardioscopy in the etiologic diagnosis of pericardial effusion in 141 consecutive patients. *Circulation* 1996;**94**:1635–41.

26 Fowler NO. Cardiac tamponade: a clinical or an echocardiographic diagnosis? *Circulation* 1993;**87**:1738–41.

27 Chuttani K, Pandian NG, Mohanty PK *et al.* Left ventricular diastolic collapse: an echocardiographic sign of regional cardiac tamponade. *Circulation* 1991;**83**:1999–2006.

28 Chuttani K, Tischler MD, Pandian MG, Lee RT, Mohanty PK. Diagnosis of cardiac tamponade after cardiac surgery: relative value of clinical, echocardiographic and hemodynamic signs. *Am Heart J* 1994;**127**:913–18.

29 Cameron J, Oesterle SN, Baldwin JC, Hancock EW. The etiologic spectrum of constrictive pericarditis. *Am Heart J* 1987;**113**:354–60.

30 Strang JIG, Kakaza HHS, Gibson DG *et al.* Controlled trial of prednisolone as adjuvant in treatment of tuberculous constrictive pericarditis in Transkei. *Lancet* 1987;**ii**:1418–22.

31 Lorell BH. Pericardial diseases. In: Braunwald E. Ed. *Heart disease: a textbook of cardiovascular medicine*. Philadelphia: WB Saunders, 1997.

32 Pandian NG, Skorton DJ, Kieso RA, Kerber RE. Diagnosis of constrictive pericarditis by two-dimensional echocardiography: studies in a new experimental model and in patients. *J Am Coll Cardiol* 1984;**4**:1164–73.

33 Oh JK, Hatle LK, Seward JB *et al.* Diagnostic role of Doppler echocardiography in constrictive pericarditis. *J Am Coll Cardiol* 1994;**23**:154–62.

34 Reinmuller R, Gurgan M, Erdmann E, *et al.* CT and MR evaluation of pericardial constriction: a new diagnostic and therapeutic concept. *J Thorac Imaging* 1993;**8**:108–21.

35 Oren RM, Grover-McKay M, Stanford W, Weiss RM. Accurate preoperative diagnosis of pericardial constriction using sine computed tomography. *J Am Coll Cardiol* 1993;**22**: 832–8.

36 Fowler NO. Constrictive pericarditis: its history and current status. *Clin Cardiol* 1995;**18**: 341–50.

37 Kushwaha SS, Fallon JT, Fuster V. Restrictive cardiomyopathy. *N Engl J Med* 1997;**336**: 267–76.

38 Tirilomis T, Unverdorben S, von der Emde J. Pericardiectomy for chronic constrictive pericarditis: risks and outcome. *Eur J Cardiothor Surg* 1994;**8**:487–92.

39 McCaughan BC, Schaff HV, Piehler JM *et al.* Early and late results of pericardiectomy for constrictive pericarditis. *J Thorac Cardiovasc Surg* 1985;**89**: 340–50.

40 Bashi VV, John S, Ravikumar E *et al.* Early and late results of pericardiectomy in 118 cases of constrictive pericarditis. *Thorax* 1988;**43**: 637–41.

41 Cegielski JP, Ramaiya K, Lallinger GJ, Mtulia IA, Mbaga IM. Pericardial disease and human immunodeficiency virus in Dar es Salaam, Tanzania. *Lancet* 1990;**335**:209–12.

42 Schrire V. Experience with pericarditis of Groote Schuur Hospital, Cape Town: an analysis of one hundred and sixty cases over a six-year period. *S Afr Med J* 1959;**33**:810–17.

43 Sagrista-Sauleda J, Permanyer-Miralda G, Soler-Soler J. Tuberculous pericarditis: ten-year experience with a prospective protocol for diagnosis and treatment. *J Am Coll Cardiol* 1988; **11**:724–8.

44 Strang JIG, Kakaza HHS, Gibson DG *et al.* Controlled clinical trial of complete open surgical drainage and of prednisolone in treatment of tuberculous pericardial effusion in Transkei. *Lancet* 1988;**ii**:759–64.

45 Hageman JH, d'Esopo ND, Glenn WWL. Tuberculosis of the pericardium: a long-term analysis of forty-four proved cases. *N Engl J Med* 1964;**270**:327–32.

46 Fowler NO, Manitsas GT. Infectious pericarditis. *Prog Cardiovasc Dis* 1973;**16**:323–36.

47 Desai HN. Tuberculous pericarditis: a review of 100 cases. *S Afr Med J* 1979;**55**:877–80.

48 Quale JM, Lipschik GY, Heurich AE. Management of tuberculous pericarditis. *Ann Thorac Surg* 1987; **43**:653–5.

49 Heimann HL, Binder S. Tuberculous pericarditis. *Br Heart J* 1940;**2**:165–76.

50 Fowler NO. Tuberculous pericarditis. *JAMA* 1991; **266**:99–103.

51 Schrire V. Pericarditis (with particular reference to tuberculous pericarditis). *Aust Ann Med* 1967; **16**:41–51.

52 Koh KK, Kim EJ, Cho CH *et al.* Adenosine deaminase and carcinoembryonic antigen in pericardial effusion diagnosis, especially in suspected tuberculous pericarditis. *Circulation* 1994;**89**:2728–35.

53 Strang G, Latouf S, Commerford P *et al.* Bedside culture to confirm tuberculous pericarditis. *Lancet* 1991;**338**:1600–1.

54 Ng TTC, Strang JIG, Wilkins EGL. Serodiagnosis of pericardial tuberculosis. *Quart J Med* 1995;**88**: 317–20.

55 Schepers GWH. Tuberculous pericarditis. *Am J Cardiol* 1962;**9**:248–76.

56 Martinez-Vasquez JM, Ribera E, Ocana I *et al.* Adenosine deaminase activity in tuberculous pericarditis. *Thorax* 1986;**41**:888–9.

57 Komsouglu B, Goldeli O, Kulan K, Komsouglu SS. The diagnostic and prognostic value of adenosine deaminase in tuberculous pericarditis. *Eur Heart J* 1995;**16**:1126–30.

58 Latouf SE, Levetan BN, Commerford PJ. Tuberculous pericardial effusion: analysis of commonly used diagnostic methods. *S Afr Med J* 1996;**86**(Suppl):15 (Abstract).

59 Fagan TJ. Nomogram for Bayes' theorem (C). *N Engl J Med* 1975;**293**:257.

60 Jaeschke R, Guyatt GH, Sackett III DL. How to use an article about a diagnostic test: B. What are the results and will they help me in caring for my patients? *JAMA* 1994;**271**:703–7.

61 Brisson-Noel A, Gicquel B, Lecossier D *et al.* Rapid diagnosis of tuberculosis by amplification of mycobacterial DNA in clinical samples. *Lancet* 1989;**ii**:1069–71.

62 Latouf SE, Ress SR, Lukey PT, Commerford PJ. Interferon-gamma in pericardial aspirates: a new,

sensitive and specific test for the diagnosis of tuberculous pericarditis. *Circulation* 1991; **84**(Suppl):II-149.

63 Godfrey-Faussett P, Wilkins EGL, Khoo S, Stoker N. Tuberculous pericarditis confirmed by DNA amplification. *Lancet* 1991;**337**:176–7.

64 Harvey AM, Whitehill MR. Tuberculous pericarditis. *Medicine* 1937;**16**:45–94.

65 Bhan GL. Tuberculous pericarditis. *J Infect* 1980; **2**:360–4.

66 Cohn DL, Catlin BJ, Peterson KL, Judson FN, Sbarbaro JA. A 62-dose, 6-month therapy for pulmonary and extrapulmonary tuberculosis. A twice-weekly directly-observed, cost-effective regimen. *Ann Intern Med* 1990;**112**: 407–15.

67 Combs DL, O'Brien RJ, Geiter LJ. USPHS Tuberculosis Short-Course Chemotherapy Trial 21: effectiveness, toxicity and acceptability. The report of final results. *Ann Intern Med* 1990;**112**: 397–406.

68 Perriens JH, St Louis M, Mukadi YB *et al.* Pulmonary tuberculosis in HIV-infected patients in Zaire: a controlled trial of treatment for either 6 months or 12 months. *N Engl J Med* 1995;**332**: 779–84.

69 Pitt Fennell WM. Surgical treatment of constrictive tuberculous pericarditis. *S Afr Med J* 1982;**62**:353–5.

Part III
Specific cardiovascular disorders
ix: Valvular heart disease

Bernard J Gersh, Editor

Grading of recommendations and levels of evidence used in *Evidence Based Cardiology*

GRADE A

Level 1a   Evidence from large randomized clinical trials (RCTs) or systematic reviews (including meta-analyses) of multiple randomized trials which collectively has at least as much data as one single well-defined trial.

Level 1b   Evidence from at least one "All or None" high quality cohort study; in which ALL patients died/failed with conventional therapy and some survived/succeeded with the new therapy (eg chemotherapy for tuberculosis, meningitis, or defibrillation for ventricular fibrillation); or in which many died/failed with conventional therapy and NONE died/failed with the new therapy (eg penicillin for pneumococcal infections).

Level 1c   Evidence from at least one moderate sized RCT or a meta-analysis of small trials which collectively only has a moderate number of patients.

Level 1d   Evidence from at least one RCT.

GRADE B

Level 2   Evidence from at least one high quality study of non-randomized cohorts who did and did not receive the new therapy.

Level 3   Evidence from at least one high quality case control study.

Level 4   Evidence from at least one high quality case series.

GRADE C

Level 5   Opinions from experts without reference or access to any of the foregoing (eg argument from physiology, bench research or first principles).

A comprehensive approach would incorporate many different types of evidence (eg RCTs, non-RCTs, epidemiologic studies, and experimental data), and examine the architecture of the information for consistency, coherence and clarity. Occasionally the evidence does not completely fit into neat compartments. For example, there may not be an RCT that demonstrates a reduction in mortality in individuals with stable angina with the use of beta-blockers, but there is overwhelming evidence that mortality is reduced following MI. In such cases, some may recommend use of beta-blockers in angina patients with the expectation that some extrapolation from post-MI trials is warranted. This could be expressed as Grade A/C. In other instances (e.g. smoking cessation or a pacemaker for complete heart block), the non-randomized data are so overwhelmingly clear and biologically plausible that it would be reasonable to consider these interventions as Grade A.

Recommendation grades appear either in a shaded margin box with an 'R' logo as shown, or within the text, for example Grade A .

Rheumatic heart disease: prevention and acute treatment

46

EDMUND A. W. BRICE,
PATRICK J. COMMERFORD

INTRODUCTION

Rheumatic fever is the most important cause of acquired heart disease in children and young adults worldwide. Initiated by an oropharyngeal infection with group A beta-hemolytic streptococci (GAS) and following a latent period of approximately 3 weeks, the illness is characterized by an inflammatory process primarily involving the heart, joints, and central nervous system. Pathologically, the inflammatory process causes damage to collagen fibrils and connective tissue ground substance (fibrinoid degeneration) and thus rheumatic fever is classified as a connective tissue or collagen vascular disease. It is the destructive effect on the heart valves that leads to the important effects of the disease, with serious hemodynamic disturbances causing cardiac failure or embolic phenomena resulting in significant morbidity and mortality at a young age.

There have been many publications concerning the primary and secondary prevention of rheumatic fever and the treatment of the acute attack. The evidence from randomized controlled clinical trials is strongest in the field of primary prevention or the treatment of pharyngitis caused by group A streptococci. There are few randomized trials concerning secondary prevention. In the treatment of the acute attack, most publications have been observational studies with only a small minority of randomized trials.

EPIDEMIOLOGY

In the developed countries of the world, the incidence of rheumatic fever has fallen markedly during this century. For example, in the USA the incidence per 100 000 was 100 at the start of this century, 45–65 between 1935 and 1960, and is currently estimated to be approximately two per 100 000. This decrease in rheumatic fever incidence preceded the introduction of antibiotics and is a reflection of improved socioeconomic standards, less overcrowded housing and improved access to medical care. The current prevalence of rheumatic fever in the USA and Japan, 0.6–0.7 per

1000 population, contrasts sharply with that in the developing countries of Africa, Asia, and South America where rates as high as 15–21 per 1000 have been reported. For example, in a study of 12 050 schoolchildren in Soweto, South Africa, a peak prevalence of rheumatic heart disease of 19.2/1000 children was reported.[1]

As GAS pharyngitis and rheumatic fever are causally related, both diseases share similar epidemiological features. The age of first infection is commonly between 6 and 15 years. Also, the risk for developing rheumatic fever is highest in situations where GAS is more common, for example where people live in crowded conditions.

PATHOGENESIS

Clinical, epidemiological, and immunological observations tend to strongly support the causative role of untreated GAS pharyngitis in rheumatic fever. Beyond this, however, the pathogenesis of acute rheumatic fever and clinical heart disease remains unclear and several important and unexplained observations render the management of this important disease extremely difficult.

These are:

1. individual variability of susceptibility to GAS pharyngitis;
2. individual variability of development of symptomatic GAS pharyngitis;
3. individual variability of development of acute rheumatic fever after an episode of GAS pharyngitis;
4. individual variation in the development of carditis and chronic rheumatic heart disease after an attack of acute rheumatic fever;
5. the development of chronic rheumatic heart disease in patients who have no definite history of acute rheumatic fever.

Streptococcal skin infection (impetigo) has not been shown to cause rheumatic fever. While effective antibiotic treatment virtually abolishes the risk of rheumatic fever, in situations of untreated epidemic GAS pharyngitis up to 3% of patients develop it.[2] Worryingly, as many as a third of patients who develop rheumatic fever do so after virtually asymptomatic GAS and in more recent outbreaks, 58% denied preceding symptoms.[3] This does not augur well for the primary prevention of rheumatic fever where prompt diagnosis of GAS pharyngitis and treatment are essential.

The virulence of the streptococcal infection is dependent on the organisms' M protein serotype which determines the antigenic epitopes which are shared with human heart tissue, especially sarcolemmal membrane proteins and cardiac myosin.[4] It is these variations in virulence, as a result of M protein variation, which are thought to explain the occasional outbreaks of rheumatic fever in areas of previously low incidence.[5] Other factors influencing the risk for rheumatic fever are the magnitude of the immune response and the persistence of the organism during the convalescent phase of the illness.[2]

Evidence suggests that host factors play a role in the risk for rheumatic fever. In patients who have suffered an attack of rheumatic fever, the incidence of a repeat attack is approximately 50%. A specific B-cell alloantigen has been found to be present in 99% of patients with rheumatic fever versus 14% of controls.[6] Certain HLA antigens appear to be associated with increased risk for rheumatic fever. Approximately 60–70% of patients worldwide are positive for HLA-DR3, DR4, DR7, DRW53 or DQW2.[7] Such genetic markers for rheumatic fever risk may be useful to identify those in need of GAS prophylaxis. However, in view of the frequency with which these markers occur, they are unlikely to be of practical benefit in the short term.

CLINICAL FEATURES

While there is no specific clinical, laboratory or other test to confirm conclusively a diagnosis of rheumatic fever, the diagnosis is usually made using the clinical criteria first formulated in 1944 by T. Duckett Jones[8] and subsequently modified by the Committee on Rheumatic Fever, Endocarditis and Kawasaki Disease of the Council on Cardiovascular Disease in the Young (American Heart Association).[9] The revised criteria emphasize the importance of diagnosing *initial* attacks of rheumatic fever. The criteria are often incorrectly applied to the diagnosis of recurrent attacks, for which they were not originally intended. The diagnosis is suggested if, in the presence of preceding GAS infection, two major criteria (carditis, chorea, polyarthritis, erythema marginatum, and subcutaneous nodules) or one major and two minor criteria (fever, arthralgia, elevated erythrocyte sedimentation rate, elevated C-reactive protein, or a prolonged PR interval on ECG) are present. Evidence of preceding GAS infection, essential for the diagnosis, may be obtained from throat swab culture (only positive in approximately 11% of patients at the time of diagnosis of acute rheumatic fever)[3] or by demonstrating a rising titer of antistreptococcal antibodies, either antistreptolysin O (ASO) or anti-deoxyribonuclease B (anti-DNase B).

PREVENTION

The most recent recommendations on the prevention of rheumatic fever have been published by by the Committee on Rheumatic Fever, Endocarditis and Kawasaki Disease of the Council on Cardiovascular Disease in the Young (American Heart Association).[10]

Prevention of rheumatic fever may be considered to be either prevention of the initial attack (primary prevention) or prevention of recurrent attacks (secondary prevention). *True primary prevention* of rheumatic fever depends more on socioeconomic than medical factors. Upgrading housing and other aspects of urban renewal will do more toward eradicating the disease than antibiotic prophylaxis.

Primary prevention

Prevention of the initial attack of rheumatic fever depends on the prompt recognition of GAS pharyngitis and its effective treatment. While it has been demonstrated that therapy initiated as long as 9 days after the onset of GAS pharyngitis can prevent an attack of rheumatic fever,[11] early treatment reduces both the morbidity and the period of infectivity.

The first report of the use of penicillin for the treatment of GAS pharyngitis and prevention of most attacks of rheumatic fever was published in 1950.[11] Over the following 40 years, attention focused on accurate diagnosis and treatment of GAS pharyngitis. A single dose of intramuscular benzathine penicillin G became the most

Table 46.1 Cure rates for various penicillin dosage schedules used in treatment of streptococcal pharyngitis

Reference	Agent/dose	Bacteriologic cure rate (%)
Gerber *et al.* (1985)[21]	Pen V 250 mg 2 × daily × 10 days	82
	Pen V 250 mg 3 × daily × 10 days	71.5
Gerber *et al.* (1989)[22]	Pen V 750 mg once daily × 10 days	78
	Pen V 250 mg 3 × daily × 10 days	92
Vann & Harris (1972)[19]	Potassium Pen G 80 000 u 2 × daily × 10 days	88
Spitzer & Harris (1977)[20]	Pen V 500 mg 2 × daily × 10 days	83
	Pen V 250 mg 3 × daily × 10 days	84

common mode of treatment and avoided problems of non-compliance. Subsequently, as a result of the pain and possibility of allergic reaction associated with benzathine penicillin G, oral penicillin became the treatment of choice[12] and remains so today.[13] In situations where compliance with a 10-day course of oral penicillin would be unreliable, a single dose of intramuscular benzathine penicillin G would be preferred (dosage 1.2 million u if >27 kg, otherwise 600 000 u).

Early studies established a 10-day course of oral penicillin as optimal[14,15] and this has been supported in more recent studies.[16,17] Shorter treatment periods are associated with significant decreases in bacteriological cure while longer courses of treatment do not increase cure rate.

Current recommendations[10] for penicillin therapy in children cite a dose of 250 mg two or three times daily. These recommendations are based on trials (Table 46.1) of 250 mg given two, three or four times daily resulting in equivalent cure rates.[18–21] A dose of 750 mg penicillin once a day yielded significantly worse results than 250 mg three times daily when compared in a randomized study.[22] There is no evidence available for optimal doses of penicillin in adults but 500 mg two to three times daily is currently recommended.[10]

Over the past decade, many trials have been published comparing penicillin VK to a variety of other antimicrobial agents, most commonly cephalosporins and macrolides. This has been prompted by the reported increase in treatment failures with penicillin. It has been suggested that treatment failure rates of up to 38% are possible. This contention, however, has been thoroughly investigated in a study by Markowitz *et al.*[23] in which treatment failure rates of penicillin were compared between two time periods, 1953–1979 and 1980–1993. Of the almost 2800 patients with GAS serotyping, treatment failures ranged between 10.5% and 17%, with no significant difference between each time period. It was thus concluded that the overreporting of treatment failures was due to problems with the design of the individual studies.

An increased bateriological cure rate for streptococcal pharyngitis by cephalosporins was demonstrated in a meta-analysis[24] of 19 randomized comparisons of a variety of cephalosporins with 10 days of oral penicillin therapy. Throat swab cultures were used to determine the presence of GAS and clearance after treatment. The results showed a statistically significant advantage of cephalosporins for which a bacteriological cure rate of 92% was reported versus 84% for penicillin. The corresponding clinical cure rates were 95% and 89% respectively. It is suggested that the resistance of cephalosporins to penicillinase-producing anaerobes and staphylococci present in the pharyngeal flora may explain these findings. This difference in efficacy would mean that 12–13 patients would require cephalosporin treatment to potentially prevent one penicillin bacteriological treatment failure.

More recently, a multicenter comparison of 10-day therapy with cefibuten oral suspension (9 mg/kg/d in one dose) and penicillin V (25 mg/kg/d in three divided doses)[25] revealed a bacteriological cure rate of 91% versus 80% respectively (corresponding clinical cure rates were 97% vs 89%). Shorter courses of selected cephalosporins[26] (4 or 5 days) have been shown to be effective but current recommendations[10] suggest that further study of these regimens is required before their adoption. The cephalosporins offer statistically significant advantages over penicillin in controlled clinical trials. It remains to be demonstrated, however, whether this statistical benefit can be translated into clinical or epidemiological benefit in regions where the disease is endemic. Given the financial constraints on health care resources of developing nations and the considerable cost difference, it would seem that this is unlikely in the foreseeable future. Greater benefit is likely to be achieved by concerted efforts to identify, treat, and ensure compliance in large numbers of patients with the established, albeit inferior, penicillin schedules.

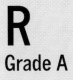

In patients allergic to penicillin, erythromycin has been shown to have an equivalent cure rate.[27] The recommended dosage for erythromycin estolate is 20–40 mg/kg/d in 2–4 divided doses and for erythromycin ethylsuccinate, it is 40 mg/kg/d in 2–4 divided doses, both for 10 days.[28] The efficacy of erythromycin estolate is superior to that of erythromycin ethylsuccinate and is associated with fewer gastrointestinal tract side effects.[29] GAS strains resistant to erythromycin have been reported in some parts of the world.[30]

Thus, penicillin V remains the treatment of choice in non-penicillin allergic patients as it has a long record of efficacy and is probably the most cost-effective option.

Appropriate antibiotic therapy in children with streptococcal pharyngitis should result in a clinical response within 24 hours – most children will become culture negative within the first or second day of treatment.[31] After completion of therapy, only patients who have persistent or recurring symptoms or those at an increased risk for recurrence, require repeat throat swab culture. If symptomatic patients are still harboring GAS in the oropharynx, a second course of antibiotics, preferably with another agent (amoxicillin clavulanate, cephalosporins, clindamycin or penicillin and rifampicin), is recommended.[10] Failure to eradicate GAS occurs more frequently following the administration of oral penicillin than intramuscular benzathine penicillin G.[32] Further treatment of asymptomatic patients, who are frequently chronic GAS carriers, is only indicated for those with previous rheumatic fever or their family members.

Secondary prevention

Following an initial attack of rheumatic fever, there is a high risk of recurrent attacks which increase the likelihood of cardiac damage and continuous antibiotic therapy is required. This is especially important as GAS infections need not be symptomatic to trigger a recurrence of rheumatic fever nor does optimal GAS treatment preclude a recurrence. It is recommended that patients who have suffered either proven attacks of rheumatic fever or Sydenham's chorea be given long term prophylaxis following the initial treatment to eradicate the pharyngeal GAS organisms. Recommendations regarding the duration of such prophylaxis are largely empiric and based on observational studies.

The duration of prophylaxis should be individualized and take into account the socioeconomic conditions and risk of exposure to GAS for that patient. Individuals who have suffered carditis, with or without valvular involvement, are at higher risk for recurrent attacks[33,34] and should receive prophylaxis well into adulthood and perhaps for life. If valvular heart disease persists then prophylaxis is indicated for at least 10 years after the last attack of rheumatic fever and at least until 40 years of age. Those patients who have not suffered rheumatic carditis can receive prophylaxis until 21 years of age or 5 years after the last attack.[35]

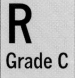

The choice of prophylactic agent has to be made with due regard for the likelihood of compliance with a regimen over a period of many years. Therefore, despite associated pain, intramuscular injection of benzathine penicillin G is the method of choice in most situations. The recommended dose is 1.2 million u every 3–4 weeks. A comparison of 3-weekly ($n=90$) versus 4-weekly ($n=63$) benzathine penicillin prophylaxis[36] demonstrated the superiority of the 3-weekly dosage. The only prophylaxis failure in the 3-weekly dosage group was due to partial compliance, versus five true failures in the 4-weekly dosage group. A long term follow-up study[37] for a mean period of 6.4 years (range 1–12 years) in 249 consecutively randomized patients to 3- or 4-weekly regimens further supported the former schedule (0.25% versus 1.29% prophylaxis failures respectively). Assays for penicillin levels in blood have also shown that 4-weekly dosage did not provide adequate drug levels throughout the intervening period between doses.[38] Therefore, only those considered at low risk should receive a 4-weekly dose.

Oral prophylaxis has been shown to be less effective than intramuscular penicillin G prophylaxis, even when compliance is optimal.[32] Penicillin V 250 mg twice daily for adults and children is the recommended dose. No published data exist on other penicillins, macrolides or cephalosporins for secondary prophylaxis of rheumatic fever. However erythromycin, at a dose of 250 mg twice daily, is usually recommended for those allergic to penicillin.

Patients who have either had prosthetic valves inserted and/or who are in atrial fibrillation require warfarin anticoagulation. This is a situation which may necessitate the use of an oral prophylaxis regimen. In such patients intramuscular injections of penicillin may carry the risk of hematoma formation, especially in patients rendered asthenic as a consequence of their underlying illness. This important circumstance is, as far as we are aware, not addressed in the literature.

ACUTE MANAGEMENT

The aim of the acute treatment of a proven attack of rheumatic fever is to suppress the inflammatory response and so minimize the effects on the heart and joints, to eradicate the GAS from the pharynx, and provide symptomatic relief.

The longstanding recommendation of bedrest would appear to be appropriate, mainly in order to lessen joint pain. The duration of bedrest should be individually determined but ambulation can usually be started once the fever has subsided and acute phase reactants are returning towards normal. Strenuous exertion should be avoided, especially for those with carditis.

Even though throat swabs taken during the acute attack of rheumatic fever are rarely positive for GAS, it is advisable for patients to receive a 10-day course of penicillin V (or erythromycin if penicillin allergic). Although conventional, this strategy is untested.

Table 46.2 Randomized trials of acute rheumatic fever treatment

Reference	Number of patients analyzed	Agent/dose	Apical murmur present at 1 year (%)
Combined Rheumatic Fever Study Group (1960)[40]	57	Prednisone 60 mg/d ×21 d than teper vs ASA 50 mg/lb/d ×9 wk, then taper	Steroids 57.1% vs ASA 37%
Combined Rheumatic Fever Study Group (1965)[41]	73	Prednisone 3 mg/lb/d ×7 d then taper vs ASA 50 mg/lb/d ×6 wk	Steroids 25.3% vs ASA 32.1%
Dorfman *et al.* (1961)[42]	129	Hydrocortisone 250 mg then taper and/or ASA to 20–30 mg%	Steroids 12.5% vs ASA 34.4%
Rheumatic Fever Working Party (1955)[43]	497	ACTH 80–120 u and taper vs cortisone 300 mg and taper vs ASA 60 mg/lb/d and taper	Steroids 48.6% vs ASA 44%
Stolzer *et al.* (1965)[44]	128	ASA 30–60 mg/lb/d ×6 wk vs cortisone 50–300 mg/d vs ACTH 20–120 mg/d	Steroids 26.3% vs ASA 34.6%

Thereafter, secondary prophylaxis should commence as described in the previous section.

The choice of anti-inflammatory agent is between salicylates and corticosteroids. Recently, a meta-analysis of trials comparing these two agents has been published.[39] In this review, a total of 130 publications from 1949 were assessed. While 11 studies had been randomized, only five (Table 46.2)[40–44] fulfilled the meta-analysis criteria of:

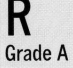

R

Grade A

- adequate case definition by the Jones criteria;
- proper randomization to either salicylates or some form of corticosteroid;
- non-overlap of subjects between studies;
- follow-up for at least a year for assessment of the presence of an apical systolic murmur suggesting structural cardiac damage as a result of carditis.

The trials varied in the use of steroid agent used – either cortisone, ACTH or prednisone.

The largest study of the five selected for the meta-analysis was that of the Rheumatic Fever Working Party where ACTH, cortisone, and aspirin were compared in a trial involving 505 children in the USA and United Kingdom.[43] This study found no long term advantage to be associated with either therapy. While apical systolic murmurs disappeared more rapidly in the steroid treated groups, the prevalence of a cardiac murmur at 1 year follow-up was the same as for the salicylate treated group. The erythrocyte sedimentation rate was found to normalize and nodules resolved faster in the steroid group.

When the five studies were examined in the meta-analysis, it was found that the advantage of corticosteroids over salicylates, in preventing the development of a pathological apical systolic murmur after 1 year of treatment, was not statistically significant (estimated odds ratio 0.88; 95% CI 0.53–1.46).

All these trials may be criticized on two important points. Firstly, the method used to assess cardiac involvement was clinical with the development or persistence of an apical systolic murmur the usual criterion. It could be argued that observer error and interobserver variability of clinical methodology could invalidate the results and that the question should be re-examined using modern non-invasive techniques. It has, however, been shown that, at least during the acute phase of the illness, transthoracic two-dimensional echocardiography with color flow imaging does not add significantly to the clinical evaluation of the degree of cardiac involvement.[45] The second point relates to the duration of follow-up. Lack of clinical evidence of cardiac involvement at 1 or 2 years following the initial attack of acute rheumatic fever is no guarantee that the important sequelae of valvular incompetence or stenosis will not develop in the ensuing decades.

Appropriate dosages of anti-inflammatory agents are aspirin 100 mg/kg/d in four or five divided doses or prednisone 1–2 mg/kg/d. Patients with severe cardiac involvement appear to respond more promptly to corticosteroids.[46]

The duration of therapy must be gauged from the severity of the attack, the presence of carditis, and the rate of response to treatment. Milder attacks with little or no carditis may be treated with salicylates for approximately a month or until inflammation has subsided, as assessed by clinical and laboratory evidence. More severe cases may require 2–3 months of steroid therapy before this can be gradually weaned. Up to 5% of patients may still have rheumatic activity despite treatment at 6 months. Occasionally a "rebound" of inflammatory activity can occur when anti-inflammatory therapy is reduced and may require salicylate treatment.

Alternative non-steroidal anti-inflammatory agents have not been adequately assessed in trials and would only be of benefit in individuals allergic to or intolerant of aspirin.

In patients whose initial attack of rheumatic fever is inadequately treated, there is a high risk that the rheumatic activity will continue and result in valvular incompetence, most commonly of the mitral valve. The end result of an ongoing rheumatic process with deteriorating valvular function is heart failure. Experience has shown that in such cases prompt surgical management[47] is the sole option and can result in the survival of up to 90% of patients.[48] It has been suggested that the reduction in cardiac workload following valve surgery results in a settling of the rheumatic process – akin to the beneficial effect observed for bedrest.

CONCLUSION

While questions regarding the pathogenesis of rheumatic fever remain, sufficient evidence is available to offer guidance on the appropriate prevention and acute treatment of this common illness (Table 46.3). It must be remembered that as most sufferers of this disease are in poor socioeconomic environments and in countries where resources are scarce, the regimens used must be cost-effective and chosen with a view to maximizing patient compliance. A recent study of the effect of a 10-year education program on the reduction of rheumatic fever incidence[49] demonstrated what can be achieved by a structured approach to patient identification, community education, and effective diagnosis and treatment. This intervention resulted in a 78% reduction in the incidence of rheumatic fever within 10 years. Much could be achieved through the establishment of similar programs where rheumatic fever is rife.

Table 46.3 Recommendations for prophylaxis and therapy

Primary prevention

Agent	Dose	Route	Duration
Benzathine penicillin G	600 000 u if ≤27 kg, 1200 000 u if >27 kg	Intramuscular injection	Once
Penicillin V	Children 250 mg, 2–3 × daily Adults 500 mg 2–3 × daily	Oral	10 days
Erythromycin estolate	20–40 mg/kg/d 2–4 × daily (max 1 g/d)	Oral	10 days

Secondary prevention (prevention of recurrent attacks)[a]

Agent	Dose	Route
Benzathine penicillin G	1200 000 u every 3 weeks (low risk, every 4 weeks)	Intramuscular injection
Penicillin V	250 mg 2 × daily	Oral
Erythromycin	250 mg 2 × daily	Oral

Treatment of the acute attack of rheumatic fever
- Bedrest
- Salicylates 100 mg/kg/d in 4–5 doses (in severe attacks with cardiac involvement, prednisone 1–2 mg/kg/d)
- Valve repair/replacement surgery for severe valve dysfunction

[a] Duration of secondary prophylaxis depends on history of carditis and if valvular involvement persists. For details see text.

REFERENCES

1 McLaren MJ, Hawkins DM, Koornhof HJ et al. Epidemiology of rheumatic heart disease in black schoolchildren of Soweto, Johannesburg. Br Med J 1975;3:474–8.

2 Siegel AC, Johnson EE, Stollerman GH. Controlled studies of streptococcal pharyngitis in a pediatric population. 1. Factors related to the attack rate of rheumatic fever. N Engl J Med 1961;265: 559–65.

3 Dajani AS. Current status of nonsuppurative complications of Group A streptococci. Pediatr Infect Dis J 1991;10:S25–7.

4 Dale JB, Beachey EH. Sequence of myosin cross-reactive epitopes of streptococcal M protein. J Exp Med 1986;164:1785–90.

5 Schwartz B, Facklam RR, Breiman RF. Changing epidemiology of group A streptococcal infection in the U.S.A. Lancet 1990;336:1167–71.

6 Khanna AK, Buskirk DR, Williams RC et al. Presence of non-HLA B cell antigen in rheumatic fever patients and their families as defined by a monoclonal antibody. J Clin Invest 1989;83: 1710–16.

7 Haffejee I. Rheumatic fever and rheumatic heart disease: the current state of its immunology, diagnostic criteria and prophylaxis. Quart J Med 1992;84:641–58.

8 Jones TD. Diagnosis of rheumatic fever. JAMA 1944;126:481–4.

9 Dajani AS, Ayoub EM, Bierman FZ et al. Guidelines for the diagnosis of rheumatic fever: Jones criteria, updated 1992. JAMA 1992;268:2069–73.

10 Dajani A, Taubert K, Ferrieri P et al. Treatment of acute streptococcal pharyngitis and prevention of rheumatic fever: a statement for health professionals. Paediatrics 1995;96:758–64.

11 Denny FW, Wannamaker LW, Brink WR, Rammelkamp CH Jr, Custer EA. Prevention of rheumatic fever: treatment of the preceding streptococci infection. JAMA 1950;143:151–3.

12 Gerber MA, Markowitz M. Management of streptococcal pharyngitis reconsidered. Pediatr Infect Dis 1984;4:518–26.

13 Nelson JD, McCracken GH Jr. Streptococcal infections (editorial). Pediatr Infect Dis J Newsletter 1993;12:12.

14 Wannamaker LW, Rammelkemp CR Jr, Denny FW et al. Prophylaxis of acute rheumatic fever by the treatment of the preceding streptococcal infection

with varying amounts of depot penicillin. *Am J Med* 1951;**10**:673–95.

15 Breese BB. Treatment of beta haemolytic streptococcal infections in the home: relative value of available methods. *JAMA* 1953;**152**: 10–14.

16 Schwartz RH, Wientzen RL, Pedreira F *et al.* Penicillin V for group A streptococcal pharyngotonsillitis: a randomised trial of seven vs. ten day therapy. *JAMA* 1981;**246**:1790–5.

17 Gerber MA, Randolf MF, Chanatry J *et al.* Five vs. ten days of penicillin V therapy for streptococcal pharyngitis. *Am J Dis Child* 1987;**141**:224–7.

18 Breese BB, Disney FA, Talpey WB. Penicillin in streptococcal infections: total dose and frequency of administration. *Am J Dis Child* 1965;**110**: 125–30.

19 Vann RL, Harris BA. Twice a day penicillin therapy for streptococcal upper respiratory infections. *South Med J* 1972;**65**:203–5.

20 Spitzer TG, Harris BA. Penicillin V therapy for streptococcal pharyngitis: comparison of dosage schedules. *South Med J* 1977;**70**:41–2.

21 Gerber MA, Spadaccini LJ, Wright LL, Deutsch L, Kaplan EL. Twice daily penicillin in the treatment of streptococcal pharyngitis. *Am J Dis Child* 1985; **139**:1145–8.

22 Gerber MA, Randolf MF, DeMeo K, Feder HM, Kaplan EL. Failure of once-daily penicillin therapy for streptococcal pharyngitis. *Am J Dis Child* 1989; **143**:153–5.

23 Markowitz M, Gerber MA, Kaplan EL. Treatment of streptococcal pharyngotonsillitis: reports of penicillin's demise are premature. *J Pediatr* 1993; **123**:679–85.

24 Pichichero ME, Margolis PA. A comparison of cephalosporins and penicillins in the treatment of group A beta-haemolytic streptococcal pharyngitis: a meta analysis supporting the concept of microbial copathogenicity. *Pediatr Infect Dis J* 1991;**10**:275–81.

25 Pichichero ME, McLinn SE, Gooch WM IIIrd *et al.* Cefibuten vs. penicillin V in group A beta-haemolytic streptococcal pharyngitis. Members of the Cefibuten Pharyngitis International Study Group. *Pediatr Infect Dis J* 1995;**14**:S102–7.

26 Aujard Y, Boucot I, Brahimi N, Chiche D, Bingen E. Comparative efficacy and safety of four-day cefuroxime axetil and ten day penicillin treatment of group A beta-haemolytic streptococcal pharyngitis in children. *Pediatr Infect Dis J* 1995; **14**:295–300.

27 Shapera RM, Hable KA, Matsen JM. Erythromycin therapy twice daily for streptococcal pharyngitis: a controlled comparison with erythromycin or penicillin phenoxymethyl four times daily or penicillin G benzathine. *JAMA* 1973;**226**:531–5.

28 Derrick CW, Dillon HC. Erythromycin therapy for streptococcal pharyngitis. *Am J Dis Child* 1976; **130**:175–8.

29 Ginsberg CM, McCracken GH Jr, Crow SD *et al.* Erythromycin therapy for group A streptococcal pharyngitis. Results of a comparative study of the estolate and ethylsuccinate formulations. *Am J Dis Child* 1984;**138**:536–9.

30 Seppala H, Missinen A, Jarvinen H *et al.* Resistance to erythromycin in group A streptococci. *N Engl J Med* 1992;**326**:292–7.

31 Krober MS, Bass JW, Michels GN. Streptococcal pharyngitis placebo controlled double-blind evaluation of clinical response to penicillin therapy. *JAMA* 1985;**253**:1271–4.

32 Feinstein AR, Wood HF, Epstein JA *et al.* A controlled study of three methods of prophylaxis against streptococcal infection in a population of rheumatic children. *N Engl J Med* 1959;**260**: 697–702.

33 Majeed HA, Yousof AM, Khuffash FA *et al.* The natural history of acute rheumatic fever in Kuwait: a prospective six year follow up report. *J Chronic Dis* 1986;**39**:361–9.

34 Kuttner AG, Mayer FE. Carditis during second attacks of rheumatic fever – its incidence in patients without clinical evidence of cardiac involvement in their initial rheumatic episode. *N Engl J Med* 1963;**268**:1259–61.

35 Berrios X, delCampo E, Guzman B, Bisno AL. Discontinuing rheumatic fever prophylaxis in selected adolescents and young adults. *Ann Intern Med* 1993;**118**:401–6.

36 Lue HC, Wu MH, Hseih KH *et al.* Rheumatic fever recurrences: controlled study of 3-week versus 4-week benzathine penicillin prevention programs. *J Pediatr* 1986;**108**:299–304.

37 Lue HC, Wu MH, Wang JK *et al.* Long-term outcome of patients with rheumatic fever receiving benzathine penicillin G prophylaxis every three weeks versus every four weeks. *J Pediatr* 1994;**125**:812–6.

38 Kaplan EL, Berrios X, Speth J *et al.* Pharmacokinetics of benzathine penicillin G: serum levels during the 28 days after intramuscular injection of 1 200 000 units. *J Pediatr* 1989;**115**:146–50.

39 Albert DA, Harel L, Karrison T. The treatment of rheumatic carditis: a review and meta-analysis. *Medicine (Baltimore)* 1995;**74**:1–12.

40 Combined Rheumatic Fever Study Group (RFSG). A comparison of the effect of prednisone and acetylsalicylic acid on the incidence of residual rheumatic carditis. *N Engl J Med* 1960;**262**: 895–902.

41 Combined Rheumatic Fever Study Group (RFSG). A comparison of short-term intensive prednisone and acetyl salicylic acid therapy in the treatment

of acute rheumatic fever. *N Engl J Med* 1965;
272:63–70.

42 Dorfman A, Gross JI, Lorincz AE. The treatment of acute rheumatic fever. *Pediatrics* 1961;**27**: 692–706.

43 Rheumatic Fever Working Party (RFWP) of the MRC, Great Britain, and the Subcommittee of Principal Investigators of the American Council on Rheumatic Fever and Congenital Heart Disease, American Heart Association. The treatment of acute rheumatic fever in children: a cooperative clinical trial of ACTH, cortisone and aspirin. *Circulation* 1955;**11**:343–71.

44 Stolzer BL, Houser HB, Clark EJ. Therapeutic agents in rheumatic carditis. *Arch Intern Med* 1955;**95**:677–88.

45 Vasan RS, Shrivastava S, Vijayakumar M *et al.* Echocardiographic evaluation of patients with acute rheumatic fever and rheumatic carditis. *Circulation* 1996;**94**:73–82.

46 Czoniczer G, Amezcua F, Pelargonio S, Massel BF. Therapy of severe rheumatic carditis: comparison of adrenocortical steroids and aspirin. *Circulation* 1964;**29**:813–19.

47 Lewis BS, Geft IL, Milo S, Gotsman MS. Echocardiography and valve replacement in the critically ill patient with acute rheumatic carditis. *Ann Thorac Surg* 1979;**27**:529–35.

48 Barlow JB, Kinsley RH, Pocock WA. Rheumatic fever and rheumatic heart disease. In: Barlow JB. Ed. *Perspectives on the mitral valve*. Philadelphia: FA Davis, 1987.

49 Bach JF, Chalons S, Forier E *et al.* 10-year educational programme aimed at rheumatic fever in two French Caribbean islands. *Lancet* 1996; **347**:644–8.

Indications for surgery

47 Mitral valve disease

BLASE A. CARABELLO

INTRODUCTION

In mitral valve disease, symptomatic status, ventricular functional status, and the kind of operation which will ultimately be performed all affect the indication for valve surgery. This chapter will integrate these aspects into a strategy for surgical correction. It should be noted that in surgery for valve disease there are few large controlled trials of therapy. Most knowledge of the response of valve disease to surgery accrues from reports of surgical outcome in both selected and unselected patients.

MITRAL REGURGITATION

Surgical objectives

Like all valvular lesions, mitral regurgitation imposes a hemodynamic overload on the heart. Ultimately, this overload can only be corrected by surgically restoring valve competence. For valve surgery in general, the timing of surgery has two opposing tenets. First, since surgery has an operative risk and, if a prosthesis is inserted, imposes the risks inherent to valve prosthesis, surgery should be delayed for as long as possible. Second, surgery which is delayed until the hemodynamic overload has caused irreversible left ventricular dysfunction will result in a suboptimal outcome. In some patients, far advanced left ventricular dysfunction may militate against operating at all.

The timing of valve surgery is made even more complex in mitral regurgitation since frequently valve repair rather than valve replacement can be effected. Because valve repair does not involve the use of a valvular prosthesis and because it also helps to preserve left ventricular function, it is applicable at the two ends of the spectrum of mitral regurgitation. Repair might be considered in asymptomatic patients with normal left ventricular function because the disease could be cured then without the need for intense follow-up and without the use of a valve prosthesis.[1] At the other end of the

798

spectrum, patients with severe impairment of left ventricular function who might not be candidates for mitral valve replacement with chordal disruption might have a good result from mitral valve repair.[2] However, for most patients, mitral valve surgery is performed for the relief of symptoms or for prevention of worsening of asymptomatic left ventricular dysfunction.

Etiology

The mitral valve apparatus consists of the mitral valve annulus, the valve leaflets, the chorda tendineae, and the papillary muscles. Abnormalities of any of these structures may cause mitral regurgitation. The common causes of mitral regurgitation include infective endocarditis, the mitral valve prolapse syndrome with myxomatous degeneration of the valve, spontaneous chordal rupture, rheumatic heart disease, collagen disease such as Marfan's syndrome and coronary artery disease leading to papillary muscle ischemia or necrosis. These etiologies of mitral regurgitation are important especially with regard to surgical correction. For instance, the spontaneous rupture of a posterior chorda tendineae leads to mitral valve repair in almost 100% of cases. On the other hand, severe rheumatic deformity of the valve which has led to mitral regurgitation may be irreparable, necessitating mitral valve replacement.

Pathophysiology

HEMODYNAMIC PHASES OF MITRAL REGURGITATION

Figure 47.1 depicts the pathophysiologic phases of mitral regurgitation.[3] In the acute phase, such as might occur with spontaneous chordal rupture, there is sudden volume, overload on both the left ventricle and left atrium. The regurgitant volume, together with the venous return from the pulmonary veins, distends both chambers. Distention of the left ventricle increases use of the Frank–Starling mechanism by which increased sarcomere stretch increases end-diastolic volume modestly and also increases left ventricular stroke work. The new orifice for left ventricular ejection (the regurgitant pathway) facilitates left ventricular emptying and end-systolic volume decreases. Acting in concert, these two effects increase ejection fraction and total stroke volume. However, as shown in Figure 47.1, panel A, if only 50% of the total stroke volume is ejected into the aorta there is a net loss of 30% of the initial forward stroke volume. At the same time, volume overload on the left atrium increases left atrial pressure. At this point in time, the patient suffers from low output and pulmonary congestion and appears to be in left ventricular failure although left ventricular muscle function is either normal or even augmented by sympathetic reflexes. Acute severe mitral regurgitation may lead to shock and pulmonary edema, requiring intra-aortic balloon counterpulsation and urgent mitral valve repair or replacement. However, if the patient can be maintained in a relatively stable condition, he or she may then enter the chronic compensated phase (Figure 47.1, panel B) within 3–6 months.

In the chronic compensated phase of mitral regurgitation, eccentric cardiac hypertrophy, in which sarcomeres are laid down in series, allows enlargement of the left ventricle, enhancing its total volume pumping capacity. Total stroke volume is increased, allowing

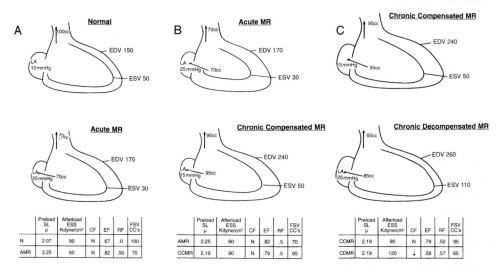

	Preload SL μ	Afterload ESS Kdyne/cm²	CF	EF	RF	FSV CC's
N	2.07	90	N	.67	.0	100
AMR	2.25	60	N	.82	.50	70

	Preload SL μ	Afterload ESS Kdyne/cm²	CF	EF	RF	FSV CC's
AMR	2.25	60	N	.82	.5	70
CCMR	2.19	90	N	.79	.5	95

	Preload SL μ	Afterload ESS Kdyne/cm²	CF	EF	RF	FSV CC's
CCMR	2.19	90	N	.79	.50	95
CDMR	2.19	120	↓	.58	.57	65

Figure 47.1 (Panel A) Normal hemodynamic state compared to acute mitral regurgitation (AMR). In AMR, total stroke volume and ejection performance increase as preload is increased and afterload is reduced. However, forward stroke volume is reduced and left atrial pressure is increased. (Panel B) AMR compared to chronic compensated mitral regurgitation (CCMR). In CCMR, increased end-diastolic volume permitted by eccentric hypertrophy increases both total and forward stroke volume. Enlargement of atrium and ventricle allows increased volume to be accommodated at lower filling pressure. Increase in afterload toward normal in this state of compensation reduces ejection performance slightly. (Panel C) Chronic decompensated mitral regurgitation (CDMR) compared with CCMR contractile function is reduced and afterload is increased in CDMR. Both reduce ejection performance and forward cardiac output. There is further cardiac dilation in CDMR, leading to worsening mitral regurgitation, further compromising pump function by reducing forward stroke volume and increasing filling pressure. CF, contractile function; EDV, end-diastolic volume; EF, ejection fraction; ESS, end-systolic stress; ESV, end-systolic volume; FSV, forward stroke volume; LA, left atrial pressure; N, normal hemodynamic state; RF, regurgitant fraction; SL, sarcomere length. (Reproduced with permission from Carabello.[3])

normalization of forward stroke volume. Enlargement of the left atrium accommodates the volume overload at a lower pressure, eliminating pulmonary congestion. In this phase the patient may be remarkably asymptomatic, able to perform normal daily activities, and can even engage in sporting events of modest physical demands.[4]

The patient may remain in the compensated phase for months or years. However, eventually the persistent volume overload leads to a decline in left ventricular function (Figure 47.1, panel C). A loss of myofibrils or an insensitivity to cyclic AMP may be responsible, at least in part, for loss of left ventricular contractility.[5,6] In this phase, left ventricular end-systolic volume increases because reduced force of contraction results in poor left ventricular emptying, forward stroke volume falls, and left ventricular dilation may worsen the mitral regurgitation. At this time there is re-elevation of the left atrial pressure, resulting again in pulmonary congestion. Of note, the still favorable loading conditions of mitral regurgitation (increased preload and normal afterload) permit a "normal" ejection fraction even though left ventricular dysfunction has developed.

IMPORTANCE OF THE MITRAL VALVE APPARATUS

Although the contribution of the mitral valve apparatus to left ventricular function was noted by Rushmer and Lillehei decades ago,[7,8] its physiologic significance and impact on patient care have only recently received widespread appreciation. It is quite clear that the mitral valve apparatus has a wider role than to simply prevent mitral regurgitation. Rather, the apparatus is an integral part of the left ventricular internal skeleton. In early systole, tugging on the apparatus by the chorda tendineae may shorten the major axis while lengthening the minor axis, in turn augmenting preload there during ejection systole. In addition, the apparatus helps to maintain the normal and efficient ellipsoid shape of the left ventricle.

Transsection of the chordae causes an immediate fall in left ventricular function.[9] Until the importance of chordal preservation during mitral valve surgery was recognized, ejection fraction almost always fell following surgery. This fall was attributed to increased afterload from surgical closure of the low impedance pathway which preoperatively had facilitated ejection into the left atrium. However, it is now clear that closure of the same low impedance pathway in which chordal integrity is maintained does not result in a fall in ejection fraction, suggesting that the increased postoperative load theory is not the sole mechanism for why ejection fraction falls.[2,10–13] In fact, chordal preservation can actually effect a lowering of systolic wall stress (afterload) instead of an increase as left ventricular radius decreases following surgery [stress = pressure × radius/2 × thickness].[10] Thus, chordal integrity should be maintained whenever possible. A recent randomized study demonstrated that maintenance of just the posterior apparatus lowers mortality and leads to superior postoperative function compared to posterior and anterior chordal transection.[14]

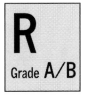

Apart from the benefits on left ventricular function, if mitral valve repair instead of a replacement can be performed, operative mortality is lower, postoperative survival is better and the need for anticoagulation is removed while thromboembolism remains low.[14–17] Even if the mitral valve is so badly damaged that a mitral valve prosthesis must be inserted, chordal preservation, especially of the posterior chords, can usually be performed resulting in better ventricular function than if all the chords were removed.[10,11]

Indications for surgery

SEVERITY OF MITRAL REGURGITATION

Under most circumstances only severe mitral regurgitation is corrected surgically. Mild to moderate regurgitation (regurgitant fraction <40%) under most circumstances neither causes symptoms nor leads to left ventricular dysfunction even over a protracted period of time. Severity is difficult to ascertain by physical examination alone, especially in acute mitral regurgitation. As noted above, in acute mitral regurgitation there has been no time for cardiac dilation to occur. Thus, palpation of the precordium does not reveal a hyperdynamic left ventricular impulse. Although the murmur of mitral regurgitation is present, severity cannot be gauged from its intensity. In most cases of severe mitral regurgitation an S3 should be present. This finding does not necessarily indicate heart failure but may simply be the result of a large regurgitant volume filling the left ventricle under a higher than usual left atrial pressure. In chronic mitral regurgitation there should be evidence on physical examination of an enlarged hyperdynamic left ventricle unless the patient's size or habitus makes physical examination difficult. Failure to find evidence of an enlarged heart suggests that the mitral regurgitation is not either severe enough or chronic enough to cause left ventricular enlargement.

In chronic severe mitral regurgitation, the chest radiograph should also show cardiac enlargement and the electrocardiogram is likely to demonstrate left atrial abnormality and left ventricular hypertrophy.

In most cases, quantitation of regurgitant severity is estimated during echocardiography with Doppler interrogation of the mitral valve. In acute mitral regurgitation, transthoracic echocardiography may underestimate regurgitant severity.[18] In such cases, transesophageal echocardiography is helpful. It should be noted that Doppler flow studies visually demonstrate blood flow velocity across the mitral valve and not true flow. Because of this, both under- and overestimation of regurgitant severity is possible. Flow mapping, which expresses the regurgitant jet in terms relative to left atrial size, has been used extensively. However, limitations of this method are well known and the technique is semiquantitative at best.[19,20] Other methods, such as the proximal isovelocity surface area, have been employed experimentally and in clinical investigation.[21–23] In using proximal isovelocity surface area to estimate regurgitation flow, the area of convergence of the regurgitant jet on the ventricular side of the mitral valve is measured at the point of aliasing. By multiplying proximal isovelocity surface area by the known aliasing velocity, actual flow is obtained, which should be a better indication of regurgitant severity. Unfortunately, the convergence pattern is often difficult to pinpoint clinically and is not applicable in many cases.

When regurgitation severity is in doubt because of discordance between left ventricular size and the regurgitant signal, i.e. a small left ventricle and left atrium suggesting mild disease and a Doppler signal suggesting severe disease, the issue should be resolved at cardiac catheterization. During cardiac catheterization, hemodynamics and a left ventriculogram give additional although also imperfect information about the degree of mitral regurgitation. The left ventriculogram, unlike the Doppler study, visualizes actual flow of contrast media from the left ventricle into the left atrium. Care must be taken to inject enough contrast agent (at least 60 ml) to opacify both the enlarged left ventricle and left atrium of mitral regurgitation. Coronary arteriography is also performed at cardiac catheterization if there is any suspicion of an ischemic etiology for mitral regurgitation or when risk factors for coronary disease coexist.

ACUTE MITRAL REGURGITATION

In almost all cases of severe acute mitral regurgitation, the patient is symptomatic. The acute hemodynamic changes noted above cause decreased forward output and sudden left atrial hypertension resulting in pulmonary congestion, reduced forward flow, and the symptoms of dyspnea, orthopnea, exercise intolerance, and fatigue. Vasodilator therapy may be successful in alleviating symptoms by preferentially increasing forward flow while simultaneously decreasing left ventricular size, partially restoring mitral valve competence.[24] If vasodilators fail or if the patient is so severely decompensated that hypotension contraindicates the use of vasodilators, intra-aortic balloon counterpulsation is necessary. In such cases surgery should follow soon after. This is especially true for the patient with ischemic mitral regurgitation. Such patients may have a volatile course with initially mild heart failure which progresses unpredictably in severity. These patients require close follow-up.[25,26] In milder cases where symptoms can be relieved by medical therapy, patients should be given a trial of medical therapy during which they may enter the compensated chronic phase. In such cases, patients may then become asymptomatic for months or years.

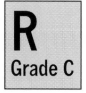

CHRONIC MITRAL REGURGITATION

Symptomatic disease

The onset of symptoms of congestive heart failure or a more subtle decrease in exercise tolerance is usually indicative of a change in physiologic status which usually has important clinical significance. The onset of new atrial fibrillation is also probably indicative of a significant change in disease status. Further, atrial fibrillation by itself leads to increased morbidity and decreased cardiac output. In most cases, the onset of symptoms or persistent atrial fibrillation is an indication for mitral valve surgery even when objective indicators of left ventricular function do not show advancement to dysfunction. Early surgery in the mildly symptomatic patient is especially indicated when there is a high probability that mitral valve repair can be effected. In this circumstance there is no need to delay longer, waiting for more severe symptoms or the onset of more apparent left ventricular dysfunction. A valve repair will allow improvement in lifestyle while at the same time avoiding the risks of a prosthesis. Early surgery may be especially important when mitral regurgitation is due to a flail leaflet because this condition may be associated with a modest increase in the risk of sudden death.[27] If preoperative evaluation indicates repair is unlikely, close follow-up of the patient is indicated. If symptoms continue to worsen or if left ventricular dysfunction develops, mitral competence should be restored.

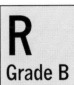

In the patient with mild symptoms and normal left ventricular function, transesophageal echocardiography to determine valve anatomy is crucial. This procedure is the best preoperative test to define whether or not repair can be performed or if replacement will be necessary.

Assessment of left ventricular function

A major goal in the management of the patient with mitral regurgitation is to correct the lesion prior to the development of irreversible left ventricular contractile dysfunction. Unfortunately, contractility is difficult to measure clinically. Standard ejection phase indices such as ejection fraction, which are used to gauge left ventricular function in most cardiac diseases, are confounded by the abnormal loading conditions present in mitral regurgitation, necessitating alterations in the way these indices are used.[28] Because ejection fraction is augmented by increased preload in mitral regurgitation,[29] the value for ejection fraction should be supernormal in the face of normal contractility. A "normal" ejection fraction for the patient with mitral regurgitation is probably 0.65 to 0.75. Indeed, Enriquez-Sarano and colleagues have demonstrated that once the ejection fraction falls to less than 0.60 in patients with mitral regurgitation, long term mortality is increased, suggesting that left ventricular dysfunction has already developed at that threshold for ejection fraction.[30]

End-systolic dimension, which is less dependent upon preload, has also been developed as an important indicator of left ventricular dysfunction in this disease. As demonstrated in Figure 47.2, when the end-systolic dimension exceeds 45 mm, the postoperative outcome is worsened.[31] This figure or its angiographic equivalent has been found to be predictive in other studies.[32,33] Careful evaluation of the patient with mitral regurgitation with history and physical examination augmented with serial echocardiograms should avoid the situation in which unrecognized left ventricular dysfunction develops. Yearly follow-up is probably adequate as long as the ejection fraction exceeds 0.65 and the

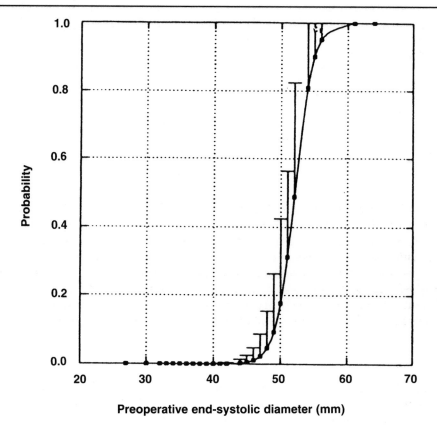

Figure 47.2 Plot of an S-shaped curve-related computed probability of postoperative death or severe heart failure to measured preoperative end-systolic diameter. Individual data coordinates are indicated by solid squares and bars represent upper 95% confidence intervals that were computed from the standard error (some points are overlapping; total $n=61$). (Reproduced with permission from Wisenbaugh *et al.*[29])

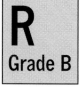

R

Grade B

end-systolic dimension is less than 40 mm. If the ejection fraction is lower or the end-systolic dimension is higher, more frequent follow-up is indicated. When the ejection fraction approaches 0.60 or when the end-systolic dimension approaches 45 mm, surgery should be contemplated.

INDICATIONS FOR SURGERY IN THE ASYMPTOMATIC PATIENT WITH MITRAL REGURGITATION

Patients with normal left ventricular function

At first glance, the asymptomatic patient with mitral regurgitation who has normal left ventricular function would not seem to require surgery. In this patient, surgery will neither improve lifestyle nor prevent reversible left ventricular dysfunction from developing imminently. However, patients with flail leaflet may become symptomatic within the next year[27] and may be at some increased risk for sudden death. In other cases where it is apparent that the severity of mitral regurgitation will eventually necessitate surgery, it could be argued that if mitral valve repair could be performed, little is to be gained by waiting. This circumstance is much like atrial septal defect

Table 47.1 Indications for mitral surgery in asymptomatic patients with severe non-ischemic mitral regurgitation

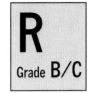

Grade **B/C**

Repair likely	Repair unlikely
Patients aged <75 yr with flail leaflet	—
Patient aged <75 yr with persistent atrial fibrillation	—
Patient aged <75 yr with EF <0.60 or ESD >45 mm	Patient aged <75 yr with EF <0.60 or ESD >45 mm

ESD, end-systolic minor axis dimension; EF, ejection fraction.

where at low operative mortality (less than 1%) the defect can be repaired without the use of a prosthesis before unwanted sequelae develop (in the case of atrial septal defect, persistent atrial arrhythmias and pulmonary hypertension; in the case of mitral regurgitation, left ventricular dysfunction). If this approach is taken it must be clear that repair rather than replacement can be effected. If the asymptomatic patient with normal left ventricular function is ultimately treated with a prosthesis when a repair had been anticipated, it should be considered a complication of surgery since the unwanted risks of a prosthesis could have been at least temporarily avoided.

Asymptomatic patients with left ventricular dysfunction

It is the asymptomatic patient with left ventricular dysfunction at whom serial follow-up is aimed. If left ventricular dysfunction has developed (ejection fraction <0.6, end-systolic dimension >45 mm), surgery should be performed to prevent further irreversible left ventricular dysfunction even if surgery entails a prosthetic valve. Since left ventricular dysfunction has already been indicated by non-invasive testing in such patients, every effort should be made to spare at least part of the mitral valve apparatus to prevent a further decline in left ventricular function postoperatively.

Grade **B**

Asymptomatic elderly patients

Patients with mitral regurgitation over the age of 75 are at increased risk for operative death and a poor outcome. This is especially true if mitral valve replacement instead of repair is performed or if concomitant coronary disease, a consequence of aging, is present.[12,34] Thus, elderly asymptomatic patients with mild left ventricular dysfunction should probably be managed medically. Only patients with severe symptoms in whom medical therapy is ineffective should undergo this relatively high risk procedure. A summary of indications for surgery is shown in Table 47.1.

Establishment of symptom status

Because of the insidious nature of mitral valve disease, patients may subtly alter their lifestyle to maintain their asymptomatic status. Thus, history alone may fail to identify this gradual decline in exercise tolerance. Therefore, in patients with mitral valve disease, formal exercise testing is useful to objectively quantify changes in exercise tolerance over the time of follow-up and to separate truly asymptomatic patients from those who avoid situations which produce symptoms.

FAR ADVANCED DISEASE

Occasionally patients reach the first attention of the physician in severe congestive heart failure with far advanced left ventricular dysfunction. Many patients in this category may benefit from surgery because correction of mitral regurgitation will lower left atrial pressure and perhaps increase forward output. However, in such cases postoperative left ventricular function will remain depressed and lifespan is likely to be shortened. It is often difficult to decide whether left ventricular dysfunction is so far advanced that surgery should not be performed. The answer to this question is predicated upon what kind of operation is contemplated. If repair with sparing of most chordal structures can be performed, patients with an ejection fraction as low as 30% can survive surgery with postoperative ejection performance maintained at this relatively low level.[2] However, for patients with an ejection fraction <40% in whom only mitral valve replacement can be performed, operative mortality might be prohibitive. Wisenbaugh has further suggested that if the end-systolic dimension exceeds 50 mm in patients with rheumatic mitral regurgitation, postoperative risk is extremely high whether repair can be effected or not.[31]

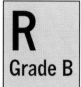

R

Grade B

Ischemic mitral regurgitation

The prognosis for ischemic mitral regurgitation remains substantially worse than for non-ischemic disease.[35,36] A worsened prognosis probably accrues from the automatic presence of a second potentially fatal and independently progressive cardiac disease and from the presence of ischemic myocardial dysfunction. Guidelines for surgery are not well developed. Common sense indicates that surgery should be performed when ischemic mitral regurgitation has caused shock or intractable pulmonary congestion.

Medical therapy

Apart from the use of prophylactic antibiotics against infective endocarditis, there is no proven medical therapy for chronic mitral regurgitation. While vasodilators are effective in treating the acute disease, no large long term trials have been performed to examine their effect in chronic disease. The trials which have been performed differ regarding benefit from this therapy.[37,38] Further, since afterload is not typically elevated in chronic mitral regurgitation, the physiologic underpinnings for vasodilators used for afterload reduction are less clear. In fact, vasodilators in this case might lead to cardiac atrophy, potentially putting the patient at a disadvantage when mitral valve replacement is finally performed.

Summary

Patients with acute mitral regurgitation with severe hemodynamic instability require surgical correction. In less severe situations, medical therapy may allow the patient to enter the chronic compensated phase in which surgery can be delayed.

When symptoms develop in chronic mitral regurgitation, they are usually an indication for valve surgery. This is especially true if left ventricular dysfunction is developing or if it is certain that a mitral valve repair can be performed. In asymptomatic patients with normal ventricular function, surgery should only be contemplated when there is certainty of repair. On the other hand, if left ventricular dysfunction is developing, surgery should be performed to prevent further deterioration whether or not a repair can be effected.

MITRAL STENOSIS

Etiology and pathophysiology

Most mitral stenosis in adults is acquired through rheumatic heart disease. In developed countries it typically appears in women in their fourth or fifth decades. In developing nations, where the rheumatic process appears to be more aggressive, stenosis may develop in adolescence or early adulthood.

As mitral stenosis worsens, a gradient develops between the left atrium and left ventricle during diastole. At the same time the stenotic valve impairs left ventricular filling, limiting cardiac output. The combination of pulmonary congestion caused by left atrial hypertension and diminished forward cardiac output caused by inflow obstruction mimics the hemodynamics of left ventricular failure even though the left ventricle itself is usually spared from the rheumatic process, especially in developed countries.[39] However, in approximately one-third of patients, left ventricular ejection performance is reduced despite no impairment in contractility.[40] Reduced ejection fraction is caused by reduced preload from the impairment of left ventricular filling and from increased left ventricular afterload secondary to reflex systemic vasoconstriction in the face of decreased cardiac output. Ejection performance may return to normal shortly after mitral stenosis is relieved.[41]

Although the left ventricle is usually spared from direct involvement in this disease, the right ventricle experiences pressure overload because it supplies the hemodynamic force propelling blood across the stenotic mitral valve. Thus, as left atrial pressure rises, pulmonary pressure and right ventricular pressure also must increase, placing a pressure overload on the right ventricle. For unclear reasons, as the disease progresses, reversible pulmonary vasoconstriction develops, leading to a worsening of pulmonary hypertension and eventually to right ventricular failure.

Indications for surgery

In most cases, mitral stenosis can be relieved by balloon valvotomy which offers results comparable to open commissurotomy, as shown in a randomized trial.[42] Surgery is reserved for those cases in which valve anatomy is unfavorable for balloon valvotomy or in which balloon valvotomy has been attempted and failed. Although in some instances open surgical commissurotomy can be successful even though balloon valvotomy was predicted to be unsuccessful, the unfavorable anatomy for balloon valvotomy will also be unfavorable for commissurotomy, necessitating valve replacement. Thus when surgery is anticipated, the risks and complications of a prosthesis should also be anticipated.

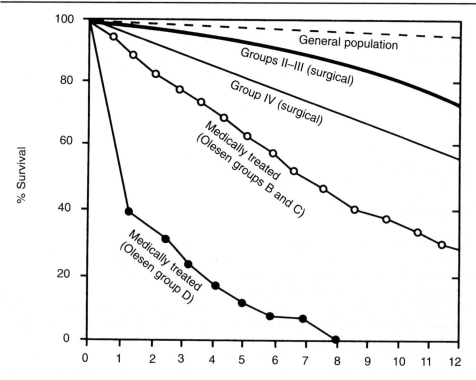

Figure 47.3 Comparison of surgically treated patients with medically treated patients with mitral stenosis. Groups II, III, and IV equivalent to NYHA classifications II, III, and IV are approximately similar to the groups represented by letters B, C, and D, respectively. Class IV patients had better improved survival when treated surgically than did class D patients who were treated medically. Class II and III patients also had better survival when treated surgically than did the patients in groups B and C, although the difference is not as dramatic. (Reproduced with permission from Roy & Gopinath N.[43])

The timing of surgery for mitral stenosis can largely be predicated on symptomatic status as shown in Figure 47.3.[43] Once more than New York Heart Association (NYHA) class II symptoms develop, mortality increases abruptly and surgery should be performed before class III symptoms appear. Additionally, some studies indicate that the presence of pulmonary hypertension substantially increases operative risk[33,44] and thus surgery should be contemplated in patients who develop asymptomatic pulmonary hypertension (pulmonary artery systolic pressure >50 mmHg). When surgery precedes severe pulmonary hypertension, operative mortality, even with the insertion of a prosthesis, is 1–3%.

The most difficult situation for timing surgery arises in the young woman who wishes to bear children. In such patients in whom balloon valvotomy has already been ruled out because of unfavorable valve anatomy, the choice of prosthetic valve becomes quite difficult. If a mechanical valve is placed, it will require anticoagulation which is problematic during pregnancy. Administration of warfarin causes a particularly high incidence of fetal malformation, especially when used during the first trimester. It can be substituted by daily injections of heparin but serious thrombotic complications have occurred in such circumstances, suggesting that this therapy is inadequate at least in some cases.[45] On the other hand, if a bioprosthesis is placed in a young woman it is likely to degenerate within a decade or sooner, forcing the patient to have a reoperation

R

Grade B

attended by increased surgical risk. There is no correct solution to this dilemma and the prosthesis which is eventually inserted is chosen after lengthy consultation between both the patient and surgeon.

Summary

In most cases, mitral stenosis can be treated successfully with balloon valvotomy. However, if this procedure is unfeasible, open commissurotomy or valve replacement is indicated for greater than NYHA class II symptoms or for the development of pulmonary hypertension.

R

Grade B

REFERENCES

1 Carabello BA. Timing surgery for mitral regurgitation in asymptomatic patients. *Choices Cardiol* 1991;**5**:137–8.

2 Goldman ME, Mora F, Guarino T, Fuster V, Mindich BP. Mitral valvuloplasty is superior to valve replacement for preservation of left ventricular function. An intraoperative two-dimensional echocardiographic study. *J Am Coll Cardiol* 1987;**10**:568–75.

3 Carabello BA. Mitral regurgitation, Part 1: basic pathophysiologic principles. *Mod Concepts Cardiovasc Dis* 1988;**57**:53–8.

4 Cheitlin MD, Douglas PS, Parmley WW. 26th Bethesda Conference: recommendations for determining eligibility for competition in athletes with cardiovascular abnormalities. Task Force 2: acquired valvular heart disease. *J Am Coll Cardiol* 1994;**24**:874–80.

5 Urabe Y, Mann DL, Kent RL *et al.* Cellular and ventricular contractile dysfunction in experimental canine mitral regurgitation. *Circ Res* 1992;**70**:131–47.

6 Mulieri LA, Leavitt BJ, Martin BJ, Haeberle JR, Alpert NR. Myocardial force-frequency defect in mitral regurgitation heart failure is reversed by forskolin. *Circulation* 1993;**88**:2700–4.

7 Rushmer RF. Initial phase of ventricular systole: asynchronous contraction. *Am J Physiol* 1956;**184**:188–94.

8 Lillehei CW, Levy MJ, Bonnabeau RC. Mitral valve replacement with preservation of papillary muscles and chordae tendineae. *J Thorac Cardiovasc Surg* 1964;**47**:532–43.

9 Hansen DE, Cahill PD, DeCampli WM *et al.* Valvular–ventricular interaction: importance of the mitral apparatus in canine left ventricular systolic performance. *Circulation* 1986;**73**:1310–20.

10 Rozich JD, Carabello BA, Usher BW *et al.* Mitral valve replacement with and without chordal preservation in patients with chronic mitral regurgitation. Mechanisms for differences in postoperative ejection performance. *Circulation* 1992;**86**:1718–26.

11 David TE, Burns RJ, Bacchus CM, Druck MN. Mitral valve replacement for mitral regurgitation with and without preservation of chordae tendineae. *J Thorac Cardiovasc Surg* 1984;**88**:718–25.

12 Enriquez-Sarano M, Schaff HV, Orszulak TA *et al.* Valve repair improves the outcome of surgery for mitral regurgitation. A multivariate analysis. *Circulation* 1995;**91**:1022–8.

13 Duran CG, Pomar JL, Revuelta JM *et al.* Conservative operation for mitral insufficiency: critical analysis supported by postoperative hemodynamic studies in 72 patients. *J Thorac Cardiovasc Surg* 1980;**79**:326–37.

14 Horskotte D, Schulte HD, Bircks W, Strauer BE. The effect of chordal preservation on late outcome after mitral valve replacement: a randomized study. *J Heart Valve Dis* 1993;**2**:150–8.

15 Cohn LH, Couper GS, Aranki SF *et al.* Long-term results of mitral valve reconstruction for regurgitation of the myxomatous mitral valve. *Cardiovasc Surg* 1994;**107**:143–51.

16 Cosgrove DM, Chavez AM, Lytle BW *et al.* Results of mitral valve reconstruction. *Circulation* 1986;**74** (suppl I):I-82–I-87.

17 Wells FC. Conservation and surgical repair of the mitral valve. In: Wells FC, Shapiro LM. Eds. *Mitral valve disease*, 2nd edn. London: Butterworths, 1996, pp 114–34.

18 Castello R, Fagan L Jr, Lenzen P, Pearson AC, Labovitz AJ. Comparison of transthoracic and transesophageal echocardiography for assessment of left-sided valve regurgitation. *Am J Cardiol* 1991;**68**:1677–80.

19 Smith MD, Kwan OL, Spain MG, DeMaria AN. Temporal variability of color Doppler jet areas in patients with aortic and mitral regurgitation. *Am Heart J* 1992;**123**:953–60.

20 Slater J, Gindea AJ, Freedberg RS *et al.* Comparison of cardiac catheterization and Doppler echocardiography in the decision to operate in aortic and mitral valve disease. *J Am Coll Cardiol* 1991;**17**:1026–36.

21 Recusani F, Bargiggia GS, Yoganathan AP *et al.* A new method for quantification of regurgitant flow rate using color Doppler flow imaging of the flow convergence region proximal to a discrete orifice: an in vitro study. *Circulation* 1991;**83**: 594–604.

22 Utsunomiya T, Ogawa T, Doshi R *et al.* Doppler color flow 'proximal isovelocity surface area' method for estimating volume flow rate: effects of orifice shape and machine factors. *J Am Coll Cardiol* 1991;**17**:1103–11.

23 Vandervoort PM, Rivera JM, Mele D *et al.* Application of color Doppler flow mapping to calculate effective regurgitant orifice area: an in vitro study and initial clinical observations. *Circulation* 1993;**88**:1150–6.

24 Yoran C, Yellin EL, Becker RM *et al.* Mechanisms of reduction of mitral regurgitation with vasodilator therapy. *Am J Cardiol* 1979;**43**:773–7.

25 Nishimura RA, Schaff HV, Shub C *et al.* Papillary muscle rupture complicating acute myocardial infarction: analysis of 17 patients. *Am J Cardiol* 1983;**51**:373–7.

26 Nishimura RA, Schaff HV, Gersh BJ, Holmes DR Jr, Tajik AJ. Early repair of mechanical complications after acute myocardial infarction. *JAMA* 1986; **256**:47–50.

27 Ling LH, Enriquez-Sarano M, Seward JB *et al.* Clinical outcome of mitral regurgitation due to flail leaflet. *N Engl J Med* 1996;**335**:1417–23.

28 Eckberg DL, Gault JH, Bouchard RL, Karliner JS, Ross J Jr. Mechanics of left ventricular contraction in chronic severe mitral regurgitation. *Circulation* 1973;**47**:1252–9.

29 Wisenbaugh T, Spann JF, Carabello BA. Differences in myocardial performance and load between patients with similar amounts of chronic aortic versus chronic mitral regurgitation. *J Am Coll Cardiol* 1984;**3**:916–23.

30 Enriquez-Sarano M, Tajik AJ, Schaff HV *et al.* Echocardiographic prediction of survival after surgical correction of organic mitral regurgitation. *Circulation* 1994;**90**:830–7.

31 Wisenbaugh T, Skudicky D, Sareli P. Prediction of outcome after valve replacement for rheumatic mitral regurgitation in the era of chordal preservation. *Circulation* 1994;**89**:191–7.

32 Zile MR, Gaasch WH, Carroll JD, Levine HF. Chronic mitral regurgitation: predictive value of preoperative echocardiographic indexes of left ventricular function and wall stress. *J Am Coll Cardiol* 1984;**3**:235–42.

33 Crawford MH, Souchek J, Oprian CA *et al.* Determinants of survival and left ventricular performance after mitral valve replacement. Department of Veterans Affairs Cooperative Study on Valvular Heart Disease. *Circulation* 1990;**81**: 1173–81.

34 Nair CK, Biddle WP, Kaneshige A *et al.* Ten-year experience with mitral valve replacement in the elderly. *Am Heart J* 1992;**124**:154–9.

35 Connolly MW, Gelbfish JS, Jacobowitz IJ *et al.* Surgical results for mitral regurgitation from coronary artery disease. *J Thorac Cardiovasc Surg* 1986;**91**:379–88.

36 Akins CW, Hilgenberg AD, Buckley MJ *et al.* Mitral valve reconstruction versus replacement for degenerative or ischemic mitral regurgitation. *Ann Thorac Surg* 1994;**58**:668–75.

37 Schon HR, Schroter G, Barthel P, Schomig A. Quinapril therapy in patients with chronic mitral regurgitation. *J Heart Valve Dis* 1994;**3**:303–12.

38 Wisenbaugh T, Sinovich V, Dullabh A, Sareli P. Six month pilot study of captopril for mildly symptomatic, severe isolated mitral and isolated aortic regurgitation. *J Heart Valve Dis* 1994;**3**: 197–204.

39 Hildner FJ, Javier RP, Cohen LS *et al.* Myocardial dysfunction associated with valvular heart disease. *Am J Cardiol* 1972;**30**:319–26.

40 Gash AK, Carabello BA, Cepin D, Spann JF. Left ventricular ejection performance and systolic muscle function in patients with mitral stenosis. *Circulation* 1983;**67**:148–54.

41 Liu C-P, Ting C-T, Yang T-M *et al.* Reduced left ventricular compliance in human mitral stenosis. Role of reversible internal constraint. *Circulation* 1992;**85**:1447–56.

42 Reyes VP, Raju BS, Wynne J *et al.* Percutaneous balloon valvuloplasty compared with open surgical commissurotomy for mitral stenosis. *N Engl J Med* 1994;**331**:961–7.

43 Roy SB, Gopinath N. Mitral stenosis. *Circulation* 1968;**38**(1, Suppl V):V68–76.

44 Ward C, Hancock BW. Extreme pulmonary hypertension caused by mitral valve disease. Natural history and results of surgery. *Br Heart J* 1975;**37**:74–8.

45 Sbarouni E, Oakley CM. Outcome of pregnancy in women with valve prostheses. *Br Heart J* 1994; **71**:196–201.

Indications for surgery in aortic valve disease

48

SHAHBUDIN H. RAHIMTOOLA

There are no prospective randomized trials of surgical procedures vs medical therapy in patients with aortic valve disease. One randomized trial in the early 1950s evaluated the role of antibiotic prophylaxis for prevention of recurrences of rheumatic carditis. Otherwise, there is only one prospective randomized trial evaluating patient outcome with use of a pharmacologic agent in patients with aortic valve disease.

This chapter reminds the reader of Sir William Broadbent's observation 100 years ago of the importance of age as a determinant of prognosis. Sir Thomas Lewis pointed out 80 years ago the inadequacy of knowledge of prognosis in patients with heart disease. He proposed a system for prospective follow-up of patients which we now call "databases" or "registries". The latter are, of course, the major evidence used in this chapter to delineate the indications for surgery.

AORTIC VALVE STENOSIS

Etiology

A wide variety of disorders may produce aortic valve obstruction;[1] however, those that result in severe stenosis in adults are:

- Congenital
- Acquired
  Rheumatic
  Calcific (degenerative/autoimmune)

The most common cause in younger adults is a congenitally bicuspid valve; rheumatic is still common in underdeveloped and poorer countries. In most patients aged ≥ 40 years, the severely stenotic valve is calcified. In patients aged ≥ 65 years, 90% of severely stenotic valves are tricuspid. Non-rheumatic calcified valves are thought to be "degenerative" but recent data suggest that it may be the result of an autoimmune reaction to antigens present in the valve.[2]

Natural history

To understand the natural history, one needs to know the normal aortic valve and the classification of severity of aortic stenosis. The aortic valve area is larger in larger individuals, probably because of the need of a larger stroke volume and cardiac output, therefore, valve area is related to the body size (m^2).

The normal aortic valve area ranges from 3 to 4 cm^2. It is reduced to half its size before a systolic gradient occurs.[3] In acute studies, the orifice area has to be reduced to one-third of its size before significant hemodynamic changes are seen,[4] gradients increase precipitously after that, and in *acute* experimental studies when it is reduced to one-fourth of its size or less the left ventricle fibrillates.[4] The obvious clinical problem is that in an individual patient with aortic stenosis one usually does not know the valve area prior to the onset of disease.

The natural history of aortic stenosis is variable depending on the degree of stenosis and the rate at which it progresses. Cardiac catheterization and echocardiographic–Doppler ultrasound studies indicate the systolic pressure gradient increases on an average by 10–15 mmHg per year. The 10–15 mmHg increase is a linearized value whereas the increase is not linear but a stepwise function with periods of steady state interspersed by an increase in gradient. The range is also wide, from minimal increases to as much as 19 mmHg per year. In all such studies, selected patients were evaluated, for example, patients who had repeat cardiac catheterizations probably had a clinical indication for the second catheterization. Moreover, the systolic gradient across the stenotic aortic value is dependent on the following.[5]

1. The stroke volume (not the cardiac output because the gradient and valve area are a per beat, and not a per minute, function).
2. The duration of the systolic ejection time per beat. Both the stroke volume and the systolic ejection time are dependent on the heart rate and determinants of ventricular function, that is, left ventricular pre- and afterload and myocardial contractility.
3. Systolic pressure in the ascending aorta. Furthermore, the stenotic valve area is inversely related not to the mean systolic gradient, but to the square root of the mean systolic gradient. Thus, measurement of valve area is more meaningful; the valve area may decrease by as much as 0.12 ± 0.19 cm^2 per year.[6]

To obtain these values by the echocardiography/Doppler ultrasound requires meticulous measurement of the left ventricular outflow tract with regard to its size and blood flow velocity, measurements that are often difficult in many patients. In a blinded study from a center with exceptional experience and skill in echocardiography/Doppler ultrasound and cardiac catheterization, simultaneously measured gradients in 100 consecutive patients showed the 95% confidence limit of the Doppler ultrasound measured mean systolic gradient when compared to catheter measured gradient was ± 20 mmHg.[7] To obtain the valve area by cardiac catheterization also requires meticulous measurements, particularly when the gradient is not large and flow is small. Ideally, one requires simultaneous measurement of left ventricular pressure, aortic pressure after pressure recovery has occurred, which is 2–3 cm beyond the aortic valve, cardiac output, and heart rate. However, the stenosis progresses more rapidly in patients with calcific/degenerative disease than with congential or rheumatic valve disease (-0.26 ± 0.25 vs -0.06 ± 0.15 cm^2, $P < 0.001$, determined over a 3-year time period).[8]

From the early days of modern cardiology, aortic stenosis has been classified as mild, moderate, or severe; for example, in 1956 Paul Wood used it in his classic textbook.[9] In 1951, Paul Dudley White classified it as slight, moderate, and marked.[10] A word that is used not uncommonly is "critical", but "critical" is not defined, and is usually a subjective description by the physician who feels the patient needs valve replacement.

Ross and Braunwald[11] reviewed seven autopsy studies published before 1955, and Horstkotte and Loogen[12] reported on 35 patients (10 of whom were asymptomatic) with aortic valve area of <0.8 cm^2 by cardiac catheterization and who refused surgery. The findings are shown in Table 48.1.

Table 48.1 Survival, according to symptoms, of patients with "severe" aortic stenosis

	Average survival	
	Autopsy data[a]	Post cardiac catheterization[b]
Overall	3 yr	23 mth
Angina[c]	5 yr	45 mth
Syncope	3 yr	27 mth
Heart failure	<2 yr	11 mth

[a] Data of Ross and Braunwald.[11]
[b] Data of Horstkotte and Loogen.[12]
[c] Angina in patients with aortic stenosis occurs even in those without associated obstructive coronary artery disease.

The mortality of symptomatic patients with "severe" aortic stenosis from eight studies[5] is given in Table 48.2.

Table 48.2 Mortality of symptomatic patients with "severe" aortic stenosis

Authors	Year of publication	Number of patients	Mortality follow-up time (years)					
			1	2	3	5	10	11
Frank et al.	1973	15			36%	52%	90%	
Rapaport	1975					62%	80%	
Chizner et al.	1980	23	26%	48%		64%		94%
Schwarz et al.	1982	19			79%			
O'Keefe et al.	1987	50	43%	63%	75%			
Turina et al.	1987	50	40%					
Kelly et al.	1988	39	38%					
Horstkotte et al.	1988	35			82%			

Mild aortic stenosis

In two studies, patients with aortic valve area >1.5 cm^2 by catheterization had no mortality on follow-up. At the end of 10 years, in one study 8% had severe stenosis and in the other, 15% had a cardiac event. At the end of 20 years, aortic stenosis had become severe in only 20% and continued to be mild in 63%.[5,12]

Moderate aortic stenosis

An aortic valve area of 1.1–1.5 cm^2 is characterized as moderate stenosis. It has a prognosis between mild and severe stenosis. In one study in which patients were followed after cardiac catheterization, the 1-year and 10-year mortality was 3% and 15%, respectively; and at 10 years 65% of patients had had a cardiac event.[5]

Severe aortic stenosis

Many different criteria have been used to define severe aortic stenosis, with aortic valve areas ranging from ≤0.5 cm^2 to ≤1.0 cm^2 and also from ≤0.4 cm^2/m^2 or 0.75 cm^2/m^2.[5]

Braunwald and Morrow defined severe aortic stenosis as an aortic valve area index ≤0.7 cm^2/m^2.[13] The subsequent natural history study of Frank et al.[14] from the same center used this criterion but all the patients in their study had an aortic valve area of ≤0.63 cm^2/m^2; thus, it is this criterion (≤0.63 to 0.7 cm^2/m^2) that now has the backing of a natural history study. Tobin et al.,[4] on the basis of left ventricular stroke work loss ≥30% and knowledge that an orifice must be reduced to ≤25% of its natural size before very serious consequences occur, showed that aortic stenosis was severe when the valve area was ≤1 cm^2 or ≤0.6 cm^2/m^2. The valve area values from these two studies are very close (≤0.63 and ≤0.6 cm^2/m^2); the value of ≤0.6 cm^2/m^2 is equal to ≤1 cm^2, assuming an average body size of 1.75 m^2.

Many clinicians frequently consider an aortic valve area ≤0.8, ≤0.75 or ≤0.7 cm^2 as severe aortic stenosis;[5] thus, they include patients with a valve area >0.8, >0.75, or >0.7 cm^2 up to 1 or 1.1 cm^2 as having moderate aortic stenosis. Chizner et al.[15] showed that 10 asymptomatic patients with an aortic valve area of 0.71 to 1.09 cm^2 had a very poor outcome – 60% died in an average time of 9 months (range 2 days to 22 months) and another 20% underwent aortic valve replacement. Data from a large multicenter database (492 patients) showed that the 1-year mortality of those with aortic valve areas after catheter balloon valvuloplasty for calcific aortic stenosis of ≤0.7 cm^2 vs that of those with valve areas >0.7 cm^2 was 37% vs 42%, respectively.[16] Kennedy and coworkers[17] reported on 66 patients with aortic valve areas of 0.7–1.2 cm^2 (0.92 cm^2±0.15 cm^2), normal left ventricular volumes and ejection fraction, whose average age was 67 years. In an average follow-up of 35 months, 21% died and 32% had valve replacement; at 4 years, the actuarial incidence of death or valve replacement was 41%.[17] Thus, these studies show that patients with aortic valve areas of 0.7–1.0 cm^2 have an outcome without valve replacement that is not benign, and is not consonant with moderate stenosis; these patients should be considered as having severe stenosis. In other words, in most patients, aortic stenosis should be considered to be severe when the aortic valve area is ≤1.0 cm^2.

Since gradients are frequently measured initially by Doppler ultrasound, a suggested conservative guideline for relating Doppler ultrasound gradient to severity of aortic stenosis (AS) in adults with normal cardiac output and normal average heart rate is shown in Table 48.3.

A suggested grading of the degree of aortic stenosis is given in Table 48.4.

The duration of the asymptomatic period after the development of severe aortic stenosis is uncertain. In a study of asymptomatic patients with varying grades of severity of aortic stenosis, 21% of 143 patients[18] with a mean age of 72 years required valve replacement within 3 months of evaluation at a referral center; and at 2 years the mortality was 10% and the event rate (death/valve replacement) in the remaining

Table 48.3 Doppler ultrasound gradient as an indicator of severe aortic stenosis (AS)

Peak gradient	Mean gradient	AS severe
≥ 80 mmHg	≥ 70 mmHg	High likely
60–79 mmHg	50–69 mmHg	Probable
<60 mmHg	<50 mmHg	Uncertain

From Rahimtoda,[5] with permission.

Table 48.4 Grading of stenosis by aortic valve area (AVA)

Aortic stenosis	AVA (cm^2)	AVA index (cm^2/m^2)
Mild	>1.5	>0.9
Moderate	1.1–1.5	>0.6–0.9
Severe[a]	$\leq$0.8–1.0	$\leq$0.4–0.6

[a] Patients with AVAs that are at borderline values between the moderate and severe grades (0.9–1.1 cm^2; 0.55–0.65 cm^2/m^2) should be individually considered.

From Rahimtoola,[5] with permission.

patients was 26%. Moreover, it is important to recognize that most patients in this study had only *moderate* aortic stenosis. In another study of 123 asymptomatic adults[6] also with varying grades of severity of aortic stenosis aged 63 ± 16 years, only the actuarial probability of death or aortic valve surgery is provided. It was $7 \pm 5\%$ at 1 year, $38 \pm 8\%$ at 3 years and $74 \pm 10\%$ 5 years. The event rate at 2 years for aortic jet velocity by Doppler ultrasound of >4.0 m/s (peak gradient by Doppler ultrasound >64 mmHg) was $79 \pm 18\%$, for a velocity of 3.0–4.0 m/s (peak gradient 36–64 mmHg) was $66 \pm 13\%$, and for a velocity of <3.0 m/s (peak gradient of <36 mmHg) was $16 \pm 16\%$.[6] Aortic jet velocity is also influenced by the same parameters as are gradients (see above). Thus, the duration of the asymptomatic period, particularly in those aged ≥ 60 years, is probably very short.

Sudden death

Paul Dudley White in 1951[10] credited the first recorded occurrence of sudden death to T. Bonet in 1679.[19] In the past 70 years the reported incidence of sudden death in eight series has ranged from 1 to 21%. Ross and Braunwald,[11] after reviewing seven autopsy series published before 1955, concluded the incidence was 3–5%. The incidence in asymptomatic adult patients has been 33% (1 in 3)[14] and 30% (3 of 10).[12] All of this information is difficult to utilize in clinical decision-making because they do not provide the important data, which is, the incidence by actuarial analysis of sudden death in a significant number of asymptomatic patients with severe stenosis. It is reasonable to conclude that the true incidence in adults is unknown and that most likely sudden death usually occurs after symptoms have occurred, however minor or minimal the symptoms may be. The incidence is believed to be higher in children.

Management

Patients with valvular heart disease need antibiotic prophylaxis against infective endocarditis; those with rheumatic valves need additional antibiotic prophylaxis against recurrences of rheumatic fever.[20] Grade A

Surgery is only recommended in those with severe valve stenosis and is the only specific and direct therapy for severe aortic stenosis, and unless the valve is suitable for repair, this means valve replacement.[20] Grade B

The operative mortality of valve replacement is $\leq 5\%$.[20,21] In those without associated coronary artery disease, heart failure or other co-morbid conditions, it is $\leq 2\%$ in experienced and skilled centers.[22] The operative mortality in those ≥ 70 years and in octogenarians is much higher, averaging 8% for valve replacement and 13% for those undergoing valve replacement and associated coronary bypass surgery;[20] however, operative mortality in these patients is also dependent on the associated factors listed above.[23]

Patients with associated coronary artery disease should have coronary bypass surgery at the same time as valve replacement, because it results in a lower operative mortality (4.0% vs 9.4%) and better 10-year survival (49% vs 36%).[22] This was in spite of the fact that those who underwent coronary bypass surgery had more coronary artery disease (34% had three-vessel disease, 11% had left main artery disease, and 38% had single-vessel disease) than those who did not undergo coronary bypass surgery (13% had three-vessel disease, 1% had left main disease, and 65% had single-vessel disease).[22] The presence of coronary artery disease, its site and severity can be estimated only by selective coronary angiography, which should be performed in all patients 35 years of age or older who are being considered for aortic valve surgery and in those aged <35 years if they have left ventricular dysfunction, symptoms or signs suggesting coronary artery disease or they have two or more risk factors for premature coronary artery disease (excluding gender).[20] The incidence of associated coronary artery disease will vary considerably depending on the prevalence of coronary artery disease in the population;[5,24] in general, in persons 50 years of age or older it is about 50%.[20]

In severe aortic stenosis, valve replacement results in an improvement of survival (Figure 48.1) even if they have normal left ventricular function preoperatively.[12,25]

Normal preoperative left ventricular function remains normal postoperatively if perioperative myocardial damage has not occurred.[26] Left ventricular hypertrophy regresses toward normal;[26,27] after 2 years, the regression continues at a slower rate up to 10 years after valve replacement.[27] In those with excessive ventricular hypertrophy preoperatively,[28] the hypertrophy may regress slowly or not at all. Preoperatively, these patients have a small left ventricular cavity, severe wall thickness, and "supernormal" ejection fraction; this occurs in 42% of women and 14% of men in those aged ≥ 60 years.[28] After valve replacement their clinical picture often resembles that of hypertrophic cardiomyopathy without outflow obstruction, which is a difficult clinical condition to treat, both in the early postoperative period and after hospital discharge;[20] therefore, surgery should be performed prior to development of excessive hypertrophy.

Surviving patients are functionally improved.[20]

After valve replacement, the 10-year survival is $\geq 60\%$, 15-year survival is $\geq 45\%$.[20,29] One-half or more of the late deaths are not related to the prosthesis but to associated cardiac abnormalities and other comorbid conditions.[29] Thus, the late survival will vary in different subgroups of patients. The older patients (≥ 60 years) have a 12-year

R
Grade B

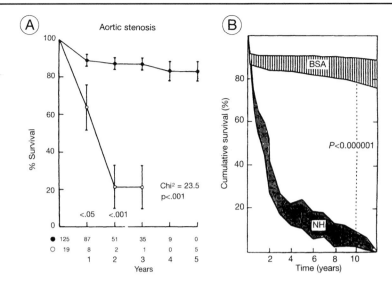

Figure 48.1   There are no prospective randomized trials of aortic valve replacement in severe aortic stenosis (AS), and there are unlikely to be any in the near future. Two studies have compared the results of aortic valve replacement with medical treatment in their own center during the same time period in symptomatic patients with normal left ventricular systolic pump function. *Panel A*: patients who had valve replacement (closed circles) had a much better survival than those treated medically (open circles). (From Schwarz *et al.*[25] with permission.) *Panel B*: patients who were treated with valve replacement (BSA) had a better survival than those treated medically (NH). (From Horstkotte and Loogen,[12] with permission.) These differences in survival between those treated medically and surgically are so large that there is a great deal of confidence that aortic valve replacement significantly improves the survival of those with severe aortic stenosis. Grade A

actuarial survival of 60% or greater.[30] Relative survival refers to survival of patients compared to age and gender matched people in the population. The relative 10-year survival after surgery is significantly better in those aged ≥65 than in those aged ≤65 years (94% vs 81% respectively, Figure 48.2);[31] the 94% relative survival is not significantly different from the 100% relative survival. Thus, surgery should not be denied to those ≥60–65 years old and should be performed early.[20,30–32]

Patients who present with heart failure should be hospitalized and treated with digitalis, diuretics, and ACE inhibitors and should undergo surgery as soon as possible. ACE inhibitors should be used with great caution in such patients, and in such a dosage that hypotension and significant fall of blood pressure is avoided. They should not be used if the patient is hypotensive. If heart failure does not respond satisfactorily and rapidly to medical therapy, surgery becomes a matter of considerable urgency.[20] Catheter balloon valvuloplasty can be an important bridge procedure in selected patients.[33] It usually improves patients' hemodynamics and makes them better candidates for valve replacement. In patients with heart failure, valve replacement that was performed 25 years ago had an operative mortality of <20%,[34] but in the current era it is ≤10%.[35] Although this is higher than in patients not in heart failure, the risk is justified, because late survival in those who survive the operation is excellent and is far superior to that which can be expected with medical therapy; the 7-year survival of patients who survive operation is 84%.[36] The 5-year survival in those without associated coronary artery disease is greater than in those with coronary artery disease (69% vs 39%, $P = 0.02$).[35] The impaired left ventricular function improves in all such patients provided there has

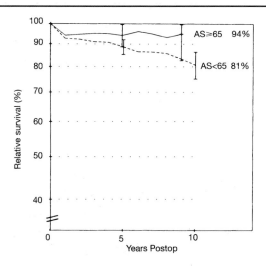

Figure 48.2 Data from the Karolinska Institute in Sweden has provided an interesting perspective on the long term survival after valve replacement in patients with aortic stenosis (AS) aged ≥65 years. They have examined the relative survival, that is, compared the survival of the patient who has undergone aortic valve replacement with another age and sex matched person in the same population. Actuarial survival ±95% confidence interval is shown. Patients under the age of 65 had a relative survival of 81% which is significantly lower than 100% and is also lower than that of those aged ≥65 years. On the other hand, patients who underwent valve replacement at age 65 or greater had a relative survival of 94% at the end of 10 years and this was not significantly different from 100%. These data indicate that survival following valve replacement for aortic stenosis in patients aged 65 and above is not significantly different from an age and sex matched individual in the population who does not have aortic stenosis; and the late relative survival of patients aged 65 years or greater is much better than that of patients aged under 65. (From Lindblom et al.[31] with permission.)

been no perioperative myocardial damage and becomes normal in two-thirds of the patients unless there was irreversible preoperative myocardial damage (Figure 48.3).[34] In one study, the left ventricular ejection fraction (LVEF) improved in only 76% of the patients;[35] however, in this study, the ejection fraction in the majority of patients was subjectively determined by visual inspection of the echocardiogram. In addition, the operative survivors are functionally much improved and are in NYHA classes I or II.[34] Left ventricular hypertrophy and dilation (if present preoperatively) regress toward normal.[34] Despite the excellent results of valve replacements in patients with severe aortic stenosis who are in heart failure, these results are not as good as for those who are not in heart failure; therefore, it is important to recognize that surgery should *not* be delayed until heart failure develops.

Six per cent of older patients present in cardiogenic shock.[33] The hospital mortality in such patients is very high, almost 50%. The subsequent mortality is also very high if the patients have not had their stenosis relieved.[33] Thus, these patients need to be managed aggressively by hemodynamic monitoring and intensive medical therapy; they need emergent surgery with or without catheter balloon valvuloplasty as a "bridge" procedure.[33]

The boxes on page 820 summarize the results of valve replacement in those with severe aortic stenosis and the factors predictive of a worse postoperative survival, less recovery of left ventricular function, and less improvement of symptoms in those with severe aortic stenosis and preoperative left ventricular systolic dysfunction.[5,20,23,25–27,29–31,34–36]

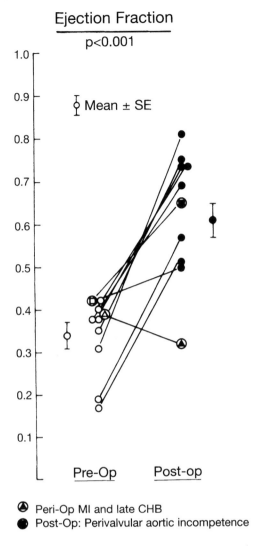

Ejection Fraction

p<0.001

Pre-Op   Post-op

◉ Peri-Op MI and late CHB
● Post-Op: Perivalvular aortic incompetence

Figure 48.3 Examination of changes in LVEF in each individual patient among those who had left ventricular systolic dysfunction and clinical heart failure. After valve replacement the LVEF improved from 0.34 to 0.63. All but one patient showed an improvement in LVEF; the only patient who showed a deterioration in ejection fraction suffered a perioperative myocardial infarction and had a complete heart block, and the only patient who showed only a small increase in ejection fraction had had a myocardial infarct prior to valve replacement. Note that ejection fraction normalized in two-thirds of the patients and in the two patients with the lowest ejection fraction (0.18 and 0.19), ejection fraction normalized in both. These data indicate that there is probably no lower limit of ejection fraction at which time these patients become inoperable. This also indicates that the lower the ejection fraction, the more urgent the need for valve replacement. (From Smith et al.,[34] with permission.)

In some patients, a small gradient across the valve may be associated with a small calculated aortic valve area that would be in a range which indicates severe aortic stenosis. There are at least two possible causes for this clinical circumstance. First, there is a small or reduced stroke volume and a normal or near normal systolic ejection time, thus, the gradient is small and the calculated aortic valve area correctly indicates severe aortic stenosis; or secondly, the stroke volume is reduced, the valve needs to open only

---

Results of valve replacement in patients with severe aortic valve stenosis

- Improved survival in symptomatic patients, especially so in those with left ventricular systolic dysfunction, in those in clinical heart failure, and in those aged ≤ 65 years.
- Improvement in left ventricular systolic dysfunction, which normalizes in two-thirds of the patients.
- Regression of left ventricular hypertrophy.
- Improvement in functional class, more marked in those with severe symptoms preoperatively.

Factors predictive of a less favorable outcome

- Extent and severity of associated comorbid condition.
- Presence and severity of clinical heart failure preoperatively.
- Severity of depression of preoperative LVEF.
- Duration of preoperative left ventricular systolic dysfunction.
- Extent of preoperative irreversible myocardial damage.
- Skill and experience of operating and other associated professional teams, for example, anesthetists, etc.
- Extent of perioperative myocardial damage.
- Complications of a prosthetic heart valve.

---

to a small extent to allow the left ventricle to eject the small stroke volume and the calculated aortic valve area accurately reflects the extent to which the valve has opened but overestimates the severity of aortic stenosis. Use of a provocative test using an inotropic agent, such as dobutamine,[37] may allow one to make the correct differentiation between the two. Dobutamine increases systolic flow per second due to increases in stroke volume or shortening of ejection time or both. In the first circumstance described above, dobutamine will result in an increase in gradient but the calculated valve area remains more or less unchanged. On the other hand, in the second circumstance described above, the gradient may or may not increase with dobutamine but the calculated valve area increases significantly, indicating the stenosis is not severe.

When performing the dobutamine test, it is important to measure meticulously cardiac output and simultaneous left ventricular and aortic pressures both before and during dobutamine infusion. Alternatively, the gradient and valve area may be assessed by echocardiography/Doppler during dobutamine infusion; however, one needs to be certain that cardiac output had increased significantly with dobutamine.

Operation should be advised for the symptomatic patient who has severe aortic stenosis. In young patients, if the valve is pliable and mobile, simple commissurotomy or valve repair may be feasible. Older patients and even young patients with calcified, rigid valves will need valve replacement.

In view of the dismal natural history of symptomatic patients with severe aortic stenosis, the excellent outcome after surgery – particularly in those without comorbid cardiac and non-cardiac conditions – and the uncertain natural history of the asymptomatic patient, which may be quite short and not as benign, it is reasonable to recommend surgery even to the asymptomatic patient in centers with the appropriate skill and experience. However, there is no consensus about valve replacement in the truly asymptomatic patient. Clearly, if the patient has left ventricular dysfunction, associated significantly obstructive coronary artery disease or other valve disease that needs surgery, then valve replacement should be performed. Some would recommend valve replacement in all asymptomatic patients with severe aortic stenosis, while others

---

Recommendations: Aortic valve replacement/repair in severe aortic stenosis

Indication	Class
• Symptomatic patients	I
• Asymptomatic patients with:	
Left ventricular dysfunction	I
Associated significantly obstructed CAD needing surgery	I
Other valve disease needing surgery	I
Aged $\geq$ 60–65 years	IIa
Severe left ventricular hypertrophy	IIa
Painless ischemia	IIb
Significant arrhythmias	IIb
Left ventricular dysfunction on exercise	IIb
• Prevention of sudden death in asymptomatic patients	III

CAD, coronary artery disease

Class I: Conditions for which there is evidence and/or general agreement that a given procedure or treatment is useful and effective.

Class II: Conditions for which there is conflicting evidence and/or a divergence of opinion about the usefulness/efficacy of a procedure or treatment.

   IIa: Weight of evidence or opinion is in favor of usefulness/efficacy.

   IIb: Usefulness/efficacy is less well established by evidence/opinion.

Class III: Conditions for which there is evidence and/or general agreement that the procedure/treatment is not useful, and in some cases, may be harmful.

---

would recommend it in all those with aortic valve area of $\leq 0.70\,\text{cm}^2$ and in only selected patients with aortic valve area of $0.71–1.0\,\text{cm}^2$.

CHRONIC AORTIC VALVE REGURGITATION

Etiology

The causes of chronic aortic regurgitation are:[38]

- Aortic root/annular dilation.
- Congenital bicuspid valve.
- Previous infective endocarditis.
- Rheumatic.
- In association with other diseases: surgery is rarely necessary in these cases.

In developed countries, aortic root/annular dilation and congenital bicuspid valve are the commonest causes of severe chronic aortic regurgitation.

Natural history

During the First World War, Sir Thomas Lewis and his colleagues[39] at Hampstead and Colchester Military Hospitals reported to the Medical Research Council highlighting the inadequacy of the knowledge of heart disease, especially from the standpoint of prognosis.

821

Sir Thomas Lewis proposed a system,[40] subsequently called "after histories",[40] which was a prospective follow-up of patients. All patients in R.T. Grant's "after histories"[40] had valvular heart disease – most had aortic regurgitation – in whom the patient characteristics were defined and described in detail, particularly by the degree of cardiac enlargement and the grade of cardiac failure. This probably was the start of databases or registries in cardiovascular medicine.

The natural history of aortic regurgitation can be considered by three different eras: the era of syphilis, the era of rheumatic fever/carditis, and the current era of non-invasive quantification of left ventricular function.

ERA OF SYPHILIS

The data are from the 1930s and 1940s, and thus, largely prior to availability of antibiotics.[41] The duration from syphilis infection to death was 20 years. The duration of the asymptomatic period after aortic regurgitation was 5 years in 60% of patients; and the 5-year survival was 95%. Once symptoms had developed, the 10-year survival ranged from 40 to 60%. Heart failure was associated with a 1-year survival of 30–50%, and 10-year survival of 6%. In a study of 161 patients reported in 1935, the 10-year survival after heart failure had developed was 34% but was 66% in those treated with arsenic.[41] Syphilis still occurs, but current therapy of syphilis is cheap and efficacious if diagnosed early. Syphilitic aortic regurgitation is not common, and the outcome in syphilitic aortic regurgitation may be more benign in the current era.

ERA OF RHEUMATIC FEVER/CARDITIS

Although the incidence of rheumatic valve disease is low in developed countries, rheumatic heart disease is a common form of heart disease in many parts of the world. Moreover, some people now domiciled in the developed world have had their initial attack(s) of acute rheumatic fever whilst living in less developed and poorer countries.

The detection of murmur after the episode of acute rheumatic fever averages 10 years.[41] The average interval from detection of murmur to development of symptoms is 10 years and the percentage of patients who are still symptom-free 10 years after detection of the murmur is 50%.[41]

In 1971, Spagnuolo and coworkers[42] reported on 15 year actuarial follow-up of 174 young people who had a median follow-up of 10 years. Patients were considered to be in a cumulative high risk group if they had systolic blood pressure >140 mmHg and/or diastolic blood pressure <40 mmHg, moderate or marked left ventricular enlargement on chest radiography, and two of three ECG abnormalities (S in V_2+R in V_5 ≥51 mm, ST segment depression or T wave inversion in left ventricular leads). The group's findings are summarized in Table 48.5.

In 1973, Goldschlager and coworkers[43] reported on the duration of the asymptomatic period in 126 patients with varied etiology (Table 48.6).

CURRENT ERA

In the current era, patients have been followed after non-invasive tests (echocardiography/Doppler ultrasound, radionuclide LVEF) or after invasive studies (cardiac catheterization or angiography). Reported outcomes are shown in Table 48.7.

Table 48.5 Reported outcome in 174 young people followed for a mean of 10 years after an episode of rheumatic fever

Symptoms/outcome	Outcome at:	%
Cumulative high risk group		
• Mortality	6 yr	30
• Angina	7 yr	60
• Heart failure	6 yr	60
• Mortality or angina or heart failure	6 yr	87
Cumulative low risk group		
• Mortality	6 yr	0
	15 yr	5[a]
• Angina	5 yr	2
• Heart failure	6 yr	2
	15 yr	5
• Mortality or angina or heart failure	15 yr	8

[a] The one patient (of the 72 patients) in this subgroup who died had developed two of the three risk factors.

Table 48.6 Asymptomatic period observed in 126 patients following an episode of rheumatic fever

Age group	Patients symptomatic at 10 years[a] (%)
11–20 yr	0
21–30 yr	24
31–40 yr	35
41–50 yr	71
51–60 yr	77
61–70 yr	89

[a] Symptoms were those of dyspnea and fatigue and less frequently chest pain and palpitations. Patients deteriorated from NYHA functional Class I to Classes II, III, or IV.

From Goldschlager *et al.*[43]

The limitations of some of the studies in the literature must be kept in mind. For example, data from the hydralazine trial which was reported as natural history[46] included some of the patients in the placebo arm, some who were dropouts from the hydralazine arm, and others who were patients outside the trial. The hydralizine trial is discussed later in this chapter. Moreover, 36% of the patients were in NYHA functional class II and were being treated with digoxin and diuretics, and thus, were not asymptomatic. Also, there is an apparent discrepancy in the rate of development of asymptomatic left ventricular dysfunction. In the Bonow study[47] of patients who developed symptoms and/or left ventricular dysfunction (4% per year), most (75%) had developed symptoms as well as left ventricular dysfunction, and only 25% developed isolated left ventricular dysfunction. The rate of development of asymptomatic left ventricular systolic dysfunction was 0.4% per year; however, most patients had follow-up at one-year intervals. In the digoxin arm of the nifedipine trial,[51] which is discussed later in this chapter, 47 patients developed symptoms and/or left ventricular systolic dysfunction at a rate of 6% per year, 75% developed left ventricular systolic dysfunction, 10% developed both symptoms

Table 48.7 Outcomes of patients with severe aortic regurgitation

	Incidence
Asymptomatic patients with normal left venticular systolic function[44–51]	
Progression to symptoms and/or left ventricular systolic dysfunction	2.4–5.7% per year (average 3.8% per year)
Progression to asymptomatic left ventricular dysfunction:	
Follow-up at 12 month intervals[a 47]	0.9% per year
Follow-up at 6 month intervals[a 51]	3.4% per year
Sudden death	0.1% per year
Asymptomatic patients with left ventricular systolic dysfunction[52–54]	
Progression to cardiac symptoms	>25% per year
Symptomatic patients[42,54–56]	
Mortality rate	average >10% per year
Angina	>10% per year
Heart failure	>20% per year

[a] See text for details.

Likelihood of symptoms or left ventricular dysfunction or death

- Left ventricular end-diastolic dimension
  - ≥ 70 mm — 10% per year
  - < 70 mm — 2% per year
- Left ventricular end-systolic dimension
  - ≥ 50 mm — 19% per year
  - 40–49 mm — 6% per year
  - < 40 mm — 0% per year

---

and left ventricular systolic dysfunction and 15% developed symptoms but had normal left ventricular systolic function. However, all patients in this randomized trial had follow-up at 6-monthly intervals. Thus, it seems plausible that if patients are evaluated more frequently, a larger percentage will be discovered to have left ventricular systolic dysfunction prior to onset of symptoms. Furthermore, even when follow-up is at annual intervals, at least 25% of patients who develop left ventricular systolic dysfunction do so before they have symptoms, thus emphasizing the need for quantitative assessment of left ventricular systolic function at follow-up in asymptomatic patients with severe aortic regurgitation and normal left ventricular systolic function. More recent studies indicate a poor outcome of symptomatic patients with medical therapy, even among those with preserved systolic function.[50,57]

Sir William Broadbent[58] stated 100 years ago that "The *age* of the patient at the time when the lesion is acquired is the most important consideration in prognosis ...". In asymptomatic patients with normal left ventricular systolic function, the independent predictors of symptoms, left ventricular systolic dysfunction, and death by multivariate analysis[47] were: older age, decreasing resting LVEF, and left ventricular dimension on M-mode echocardiography.[47]

However, in many of these patients, M-mode images were not obtained from two dimensionally directed echocardiograms. Very importantly, most of these dimensions were obtained in the United States, and US women have smaller left ventricular dimensions than men, even when they become symptomatic.[59] Thus, the above criteria most likely do not apply to women and almost certainly will not be applicable to populations of smaller body size, for example, Latin Americans, sub-Saharan Africans, Asians, and Orientals. Patients also develop symptoms and/or left ventricular systolic dysfunction at a faster rate if their initial left ventricular end-diastolic volume is $\geq 150 \, ml/m^2$ when compared to those with volumes $<150 \, ml/m^2$.[46]

Patients with severe ventricular dilation when exercised have shown mean pulmonary artery wedge pressure $\geq 20 \, mmHg$ and/or exercise ejection fraction <0.50, and such patients have demonstrated reduced exercise capacity, with reduced maximum VO_2.[60,61]

Patients who present with ventricular tachycardia, ventricular fibrillation or syncope and have inducible ventricular tachycardia on electrophysiologic studies have an 80% probability of a serious arrhythmic event up to 4 years of follow-up, versus 47% in those in whom ventricular tachycardia could not be induced ($P<0.005$).[62]

Management options

Angina is a result of a relative reduction of myocardial blood flow because of an increased need or associated obstructive coronary artery disease or both.[63] It does not respond to nitrates as well as in aortic stenosis. The options are to reduce the amount of aortic regurgitation and/or to revascularize the myocardium by coronary bypass surgery or by percutaneous catheter techniques.

Clinical heart failure is treated with the traditional first line triple therapy, that is, digitalis, diuretics, and ACE inhibitors. Parenteral inotropic and vasodilator therapy may be needed for those in severe heart failure.[64]

The only direct method(s) to reduce the amount of regurgitation is by arterial dilators[65] and valve surgery, that is, valve replacement or valve repair.

ARTERIAL DILATORS

In symptomatic patients with severe, chronic aortic regurgitation, an arteriolar dilator, hydralazine, resulted in reduction of resting pulmonary artery wedge pressure, increases of cardiac and stroke indices, and reduction of systemic vascular resistance.[65] On exercise, there was a reduction of mean arterial and mean pulmonary artery wedge pressures, increase of cardiac index and reduction of systemic vascular resistance. These beneficial effects were the result of reductions of regurgitant volume, regurgitant fraction, and left ventricular end-diastolic and end-systolic volumes, and a small increase of LVEF.[65] One dose of sublingual nifedipine produced similar changes in resting intracardiac pressures, cardiac index, and systemic vascular resistance.[65]

In symptomatic patients, an 11 month study of hydralazine did not produce any beneficial effects on left ventricular function.[5] In asymptomatic patients no beneficial effect was seen in a 6-month trial of hydralazine in 17 patients.[65] In a larger trial of 80 patients over 2 years[66] in which 36% of patients were symptomatic (NYHA class II) and were being treated with digitalis and diuretics, hydralazine produced very minor improvements of left ventricular size and function. Left ventricular end-diastolic and end-systolic volumes had decreased by $24 \pm 6 \, ml/m^2$ and $12 \pm 3 \, ml/m^2$, respectively; LVEF increased by only 0.02 ± 0.01.[66] Side effects associated with long term use of hydralazine seriously impaired compliance with therapy and only 46% of the patients completed

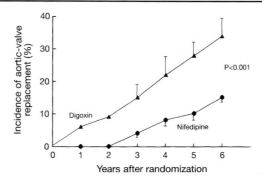

Figure 48.4 The role of long term, long acting nifedipine therapy in asymptomatic patients with severe aortic regurgitation and normal left ventricular systolic pump function was evaluated in 143 asymptomatic patients in a prospective randomized trial. By actuarial analysis, at 6 years, 34±6% of patients in the digoxin group underwent valve replacement versus 15±3% of those in the nifedipine group (P<0.001). This randomized trial demonstrates that long term arteriolar dilator therapy with long acting nifedipine reduces and/or delays the need for aortic valve replacement in asymptomatic patients with severe aortic regurgitation and normal left ventricular systolic pump function. (From Scognamiglio *et al*.[51] with permission.)

the trial. The major use of hydralazine is when an arteriolar dilator is needed for a short period of time to tide the patient over an acute reversible complication or in preparation for elective surgery in selected patients with left venticular dysfunction. On the other hand, a randomized trial of 72 patients for 12 months of long acting nifedipine showed major statistically significant reductions of left ventricular end-diastolic volume index and left ventricular mass and increase of LVEF.[51]

There is *only* one trial which has evaluated patient outcome.[51] The role of long acting nifedipine on *patient outcome* has been evaluated in a prospective, randomized trial of 143 asymptomatic patients with chronic, severe aortic regurgitation, and normal left ventricular systolic function; 69 patients were randomized to long acting nifedipine and 74 patients to digoxin. The patients were evaluated at 6-month intervals for medication complication and had a complete history, physical examination, ECG, chest radiograph, and echocardiographic/Doppler study. Each echocardiographic/Doppler study was read by two independent blinded observers. Criteria for valve replacement were established prior to the start of the study. If the patients developed left ventricular dysfunction, this had to be confirmed by a repeat echocardiographic/Doppler study at one month and by preoperative left ventricular angiographic study. At 6 years, the need for valve replacement was 34±6% in the digoxin treated group and 15±3% in the nifedipine group, P<0.001 (Figure 48.4).[51] Thus, for every 100 patients treated with nifedipine, 19 fewer valve replacements were needed at the end of 6 years; note that even after 6 years, the curves are not parallel and do not converge (see Figure 48.4). Compared to the digoxin group, the nifedipine treated group had reductions of left ventricular volumes and mass; ejection fraction increased in the digoxin arm of the trial, volumes and mass increased. After aortic valve replacement, 12 of 16 patients (75%) in the digoxin group and all 6 patients in the nifedipine group who had an abnormal LVEF before surgery had a normal ejection fraction. The study can be criticized because there was no "true" placebo group. However, it is to be noted that 85% of the patients in the digoxin group who needed valve replacement did so because of development of left ventricular systolic dysfunction, that is, left ventricular ejection fraction <0.50 (an objective blinded measurement) and there is no study anywhere showing that digitalis produces left

R

Grade A

ventricular dysfunction. Thus, digoxin was like a placebo. Long-acting nifedipine is the drug of choice and should be used in all asymptomatic patients with severe chronic aortic regurgitation and normal left ventricular systolic function unless there is a contraindication to its use.[63]

In an acute study in the catheterization laboratory, 20 patients were randomized to either oral nifedipine or oral captopril.[67] Nifedipine produced a reduction of regurgitant fraction but captopril did not. Nifedipine produced a greater increase of forward stroke volume and of cardiac output and a greater fall of systemic vascular resistance. This study showed that, acutely, nifedipine was superior to an ACE inhibitor. A short term 6 month randomized trial of a small number of patients showed that the results with captopril were similar to placebo, that is, there were no significant changes in M-mode echocardiographic left ventricular dimensions.[68] One study with quinapril involved 10 patients, many of whom had moderate aortic regurgitation.[63] In one randomized trial of enalapril versus hydralazine,[69] patients in the hydralazine arm showed no benefit. Patients in the enalapril arm were benefitted; however, 71% of the 38 enalapril-treated patients had mild to moderate aortic regurgitation and many had severe systemic hypertension with an average diastolic arterial blood pressure of 82 ± 13 mmHg and 47% of the patients had systolic blood pressure greater than 180 mmHg.[69] In these patients, ACE inhibitors would be beneficial for their systemic hypertension. Moreover, there is no published data to show that ACE inhibitor therapy reduces the need for valve surgery. In brief, ACE inhibitors are not of proven benefit in asymptomatic patients with severe chronic aortic regurgitation and normal left ventricular systolic function.

VALVE SURGERY (REPLACEMENT/REPAIR)

(See also section on Aortic Valve Stenosis above).

In a comparative study, survival at 5 years was identical in those treated surgically or "medically".[25] However, surgery was performed in those with two of three features, symptoms, abnormal left ventricular ejection fraction or progressive increase of left ventricular size on chest radiography. Thus, the two groups were not similar[25] and the operated patients would be expected to have a worse outcome without valve replacement. Survival in symptomatic patients is better after valve replacement in those with normal or mildly impaired left ventricular systolic function (ejection fraction ≥ 0.45) than in those with greater impairment of left ventricular systolic function (ejection fraction <0.45).[70] In one study, those with preoperative LVEF of ≥ 0.60 had a better survival than those with LVEF of <0.60;[71] however, in this study, the ejection fraction in the majority of patients was determined by visual inspection of the echocardiogram.

After valve replacement, patients with normal preoperative left ventricular systolic function have reductions of left ventricular volumes and hypertrophy.[72] There is an increase of ejection fraction even if the preoperative ejection fraction is in the normal range, presumably because of a reduction of myocardial stress.[26,73] Left ventricular hypertrophy continues to decline for up to 5–8 years in those with normal preoperative left ventricular systolic function but at a slower rate after 18–24 months.[26,73] Most patients are symptomatically improved and are in NYHA class I.[63]

After valve replacement in those with abnormal preoperative left ventricular systolic function (ejection fraction 0.25–0.49), there is a reduction of heart size and of left ventricular end-diastolic pressure, end-diastolic and end-systolic volumes and hypertrophy.[70] LVEF improves or normalizes only if the ejection fraction was abnormal

---

Results of valve replacement in patients with severe chronic aortic valve regurgitation

- Improved survival in those with mild to moderate impairment of left ventricular systolic function and in those with severe left ventricular enlargement irrespective of their symptomatic status.
- Improvement in left ventricular systolic dysfunction; function normalizes if the dysfunction is of ≤ 12 months' duration preoperatively.
- Regression of left ventricular hypertrophy.
- Improvement in functional class, particularly in those with preoperative mild to moderate impairment and in those with preoperative left ventricular diastolic dysfunction.

Factors predictive of a less favorable outcome

- Extent and severity of associated comorbid conditions.
- Presence and severity of clinical heart failure preoperatively.
- Severity of depression of preoperative LVEF.
- Duration of preoperative left ventricular systolic dysfunction.
- Extent of preoperative irreversible myocardial damage.
- Severity of increase in left ventricular end-diastolic and end-systolic size (left ventricular end-diastolic and end-systolic volumes of ≥ 210 and $\geq 110 \, ml/m^2$, respectively, or end-diastolic and end-systolic dimensions of $\geq 80 \, mm$ and $\geq 60 \, mm$).
- Skill and experience of operating and associated professional teams, for example, anesthetists.
- Extent of perioperative myocardial damage.
- Complications of a prosthetic heart valve.

---

for 12 months or less prior to surgery.[73] Moreover, unless there is a complication, most patients are symptomatically improved and are in NYHA class I or II.[63] In those with severe symptoms and severe reduction of ejection fraction or severe left ventricular dilation preoperatively, survival as well as the beneficial effects on left ventricular function and functional class are less marked.[72,74]

The boxes summarize the results of valve replacement in those with severe chronic aortic valve regurgitation and the factors predictive of a worse postoperative survival, less recovery of left ventricular function, and of less improvement in symptomatic state in those with severe regurgitation and preoperative left ventricular systolic dysfunction.

There are two questions that are very important in clinical decision-making in patients with severe aortic regurgitation. First, if and when does the symptomatic patient become inoperable? Secondly, when should one operate on asymptomatic patients with severe aortic regurgitation? In the discussion, I am assuming that associated comorbid conditions do not make the patient inoperable or at high risk for surgery.

The major reason that makes the patient inoperable is left ventricular systolic dysfunction. In the published study of left ventricular dysfunction in which the patient and left ventricular function improved, the patients had an ejection fraction of 0.25–0.49.[70,72] Personal experience indicates that with skilled and experienced surgery, patients with an ejection fraction of 0.18–0.24 are improved. Thus, unless there are extenuating or special circumstances, or until additional data become available, patients with an ejection fraction of ≤ 0.15–0.17 are probably inoperable.

In the asymptomatic patient, clinical decision-making about recommending valve surgery is much more difficult. If patients have developed left ventricular systolic dysfunction, then their outcome is poor without surgery and left ventricular dysfunction if present for 12 months or longer does not normalize after surgery;[73]

therefore, surgery is advisable. Patients who need surgery for associated conditions, for example, obstructive coronary artery disease, thoracic aortic disease such as an aortic aneurysm, or another valve lesion, should have surgery for the severe aortic regurgitation. Patients who have developed severe left ventricular dilation are on the edge of developing symptoms at a high rate. One could wait for symptoms to develop and follow these patients very carefully at frequent intervals. On the other hand, if one does a right heart catheterization (with a balloon flotation catheter) and on exercise the patient develops pulmonary artery wedge pressure ≥ 20 mmHg, then the patient is shown to have developed left ventricular dysfunction on exercise; it is thus appropriate to recommend valve surgery. If pulmonary artery wedge pressure on exercise is <20 mmHg, if the ejection fraction on exercise is <0.50, or if the patient has significant arrhythmias, then the patient is likely to be at higher risk and the benefits of surgery are unclear; therefore, recommending surgery in such patients is much more controversial. Patients who do not have severe left ventricular dilation and those who do not have left ventricular dysfunction at rest or exercise should not have surgery for chronic aortic valve regurgitation.

Recommendations: Aortic valve replacement/repair in severe chronic aortic regurgitation

Indication	Class
● Symptomatic patients with:	
Normal left ventricular systolic function	
LVEF ≥ 0.5	I
Left ventricular systolic dysfunction	
LVEF 0.25–0.49	I
LVEF 0.18–0.24	IIa
● Asymptomatic patients with:	
Left ventricular systolic dysfunction	
LVEF 0.25–0.49	I
LVEF 0.18–0.24	IIa
Normal left ventricular function and:	
Associated severe obstructive coronary artery disease needing surgery	IIa
Other valve or thoracic aortic disease needing surgery	IIa
Severe left ventricular dilatation	
EDD ≥ 70 mm *or* ESD ≥ 55 mm	
or LVEDVI >150 ml/m^2	
and pulmonary artery wedge pressure ≥ 20 mmHg on exercise	IIa
and pulmonary artery wedge pressure <20 mmHg on exercise	IIb
Ejection fraction <0.50 on exercise	IIb
Significant arrhythmias	IIb
Left ventricular dilation is not severe	III
Ejection fraction ≥ 0.50 on exercise	III

EDD, end-diastolic dimension; ESD, end-systolic dimension; LVEDVI, left ventricular end-diastolic volume index

For definition of classes, see p 821.

REFERENCES

1 Rahimtoola SH. Aortic valve stenosis. In: Rahimtoola SH, ed. *Valvular heart disease*, Vol II. St Louis: CV Mosby, 1997, pp 6.01–6.21.

2 Olsson N, Dalsgaaro C-J, Haegerstrand A *et al.* Accumulation of T lymphocytes and expression of interluken-2 receptors in nonrheumatic stenotic aortic valves. *J Am Coll Cardiol* 1994;**23**:1162–70.

3 Rahimtoola SH. The problem of valve prosthesis–patient mismatch. *Circulation* 1978; **58**:20–4.

4 Tobin Jr JR, Rahimtoola SH, Blundell PE, Swan HJC. Percentage of left ventricular stroke workloss: a simple hemodynamic concept for estimation of severity in valvular aortic stenosis. *Circulation* 1967;**35**:868–79.

5 Rahimtoola SH. Perspective on valvular heart disease: Update II. In: Knoebe S, Dacks S, eds. *Era in cardiovascular medicine.* New York: Elsevier, 1991, pp 45–70.

6 Otto CM, Burwask IG, Legget ME *et al.* Prospective study of asymptomatic valvular aortic stenosis: clinical, echocardiographic, and exercise predictors of outcome. *Circulation* 1997;**95**: 2262–70.

7 Currie PJ, Seward JB, Reeder GS *et al.* Continuous-wave Doppler echocardiographic assessment of severity of calcific aortic stenosis: a simultaneous Doppler-catheter correlative study in 100 adult patients. *Circulation* 1985;**71**:1162–9.

8 Wagner S, Selzer A. Patterns of progression of aortic stenosis: a longitudinal hemodynamic study. *Circulation* 1982;**65**:709–12.

9 Wood P. *Diseases of the heart and circulation*, 2nd edn. London: Eyre & Spottiswoode, 1956, p 581.

10 White PD. *Heart disease*, 4th edn. New York: Macmillan, 1951, pp 687–8.

11 Ross Jr J, Braunwald E. Aortic stenosis. *Circulation* 1968;**36**(Suppl IV):61–7.

12 Horstkotte D, Loogen F. The natural history of aortic valve stenosis. *Eur Heart J* 1988;**9**(Suppl E):57–64.

13 Braunwald E, Morrow AG. Obstruction to left ventricular outflow: current criteria for the selection of patients for operation. *Am J Cardiol* 1963;**12**:53–9.

14 Frank S, Johnson A, Ross Jr J. Natural history of valvular aortic stenosis. *Br Heart J* 1973;**35**:41–6.

15 Chizner MA, Pearle DL, deLeon AC. The natural history of aortic stenosis in adults. *Am Heart J* 1980;**99**:419–24.

16 O'Neill WW. Predictors of long-term survival after percutaneous aortic valvuloplasty: report of the Mansfield Scientific Balloon Aortic Valvuloplasty registry. *J Am Coll Cardiol* 1991;**17**:193–8.

17 Kennedy KD, Nishimura RA, Holmes Jr D, Bailey KR. Natural history of moderate aortic stenosis. *J Am Coll Cardiol* 1991;**17**:313–19.

18 Pellikka PA, Nishimura PA, Bailey KR, Tajik AJ. The natural history of adults with asymptomatic, hemodynamically significant aortic stenosis. *J Am Coll Cardiol* 1990;**15**:1012–27.

19 Bonet T. *Sepulchretum, sire Anatomia Practica.*, Geneva: Leonard Chouët, 167, Vol I, Book II, Section XI. Cited by White PD. *Heart Disease*, 4th edn. New York: Macmillan, 1951, p 692.

20 Rahimtoola SH. Aortic valve stenosis. In: Schlant R, Alexander RW, Fuster V, eds., *Hurst's The Heart*, 9th edn. New York: McGraw-Hill, 1998, pp 1759–69.

21 Sethi GK, Miller DC, Sonchek J *et al.* Clinical, hemodynamic and angiographic predictors of operative mortality in patients undergoing single valve replacement. *J Thorac Cardiovasc Surg* 1987; **93**:884–7.

22 Mullany CJ, Elveback ER, Frye RL *et al.* Coronary artery disease and its management: influence on survival in patients undergoing aortic valve replacement. *J Am Coll Cardiol* 1987;**10**:66–72.

23 Rahimtoola SH. Lessons learned about the determinants of the results of valve surgery. *Circulation* 1988;**78**:1503–7.

24 Enriquez-Sarano M, Klodas E, Garratt KN *et al.* Secular trends in coronary atherosclerosis – analysis in patients with valve regurgitation. *N Engl J Med* 1996;**335**:316–22.

25 Schwarz F, Banmann P, Manthey J *et al.* The effect of aortic valve replacement on survival. *Circulation* 1982;**66**:1105–10.

26 Pantely G, Morton M, Rahimtoola SH. Effects of successful uncomplicated valve replacement on ventricular hypertrophy, volume, and performance in aortic stenosis and aortic incompetence. *J Thorac Cardiovasc Surg* 1978;**75**: 383–91.

27 Monrad ES, Hess OM, Murakami T *et al.* Time course of regression of left ventricular hypertrophy after aortic valve replacement. *Circulation* 1988;**77**:1345–55.

28 Carroll JD, Carroll EP, Feldman T *et al.* Sex-associated differences in left ventricular function in aortic stenosis of the elderly. *Circulation* 1992; **86**:1099–107.

29 Hammermeister KL, Sethi GK, Henderson WG *et al.* A comparison of outcomes in men 11 years after heart-valve replacement with a mechanical valve or bioprosthesis. *N Engl J Med* 1993;**328**: 1289–96.

30 Murphy ES, Lawson RM, Starr A, Rahimtoola SH. Severe aortic stenosis in patients 60 years of age and older: left ventricular function and ten-year survival after valve replacement. *Circulation* 1981;**64**(Suppl II):184–8.

31 Lindblom D, Lindblom U, Qvist J, Lundström H. Long-term relative survival rates after heart valve replacement. *J Am Coll Cardiol* 1990;**15**:566–73.

32 Sprigings DC, Forfar JC. How should we manage symptomatic aortic stenosis in the patient who is 80 or older? *Br heart J* 1995;**74**:481–4.

33 Rahimtoola SH. Catheter balloon valvuloplasty for severe calcific aortic stenosis: a limited role. *J Am Coll Cardiol* 1994;**23**:1076–8.

34 Smith N, McAnulty JH, Rahimtoola SH. Severe aortic stenosis with impaired left ventricular function and clinical heart failure: results of valve replacement. *Circulation* 1978;**58**:255–64.

35 Connolly H, Oh JK, Orszulak TA *et al*. Aortic valve replacement for aortic stenosis with severe left ventricular dysfunction. Prognostic indicators. *Circulation* 1997;**95**:2395–400.

36 Rahimtoola SH, Starr A. Valvular surgery. In: Braunwald E, Mock MB, eds. *Congestive heart failure: current research and clinical applications*. New York: Grune and Stratton, 1982, pp 303–16.

37 deFilippi CR, Willett DL, Brickner ME *et al*. Usefulness of Doppler echocardiography is distinguishing severe from non-severe valvar aortic stenosis in patients with depressed left ventricular function and low transvalvular gradients. *Am J Cardiol* 1995;**75**:191–4.

38 Rahimtoola SH. Aortic valve regurgitation. In: Rahimtoola SH, ed. *Vavular heart disease*, Vol II. St Louis: CV Mosby, 1997, pp 7.01–7.26.

39 Lewis T (Sir). Special Report Series of the National Health Insurance Joint Committee, Medical Research Committee, London, No. 8, 1917.

40 Grant RT. After histories for 10 years of a thousand men suffering from heart disease. *Heart* 1933;**16**:275–334.

41 McKay CR, Rahimtoola SH. Natural history of aortic regurgitation. In: Gaasch WH, Levine HJ, eds. Chronic aortic regurgitation. New York: Kluwer, 1980, pp 1–17.

42 Spagnuolo M, Kloth H, Taranta A, Doyle E, Pasternack B. Natural history of rheumatic aortic regurgitation. Criteria predictive of death, congestive heart failure, and angina in young patients. *Circulation* 1971;**34**:368–80.

43 Goldschlager N, Pfeifer J, Cohn K, Popper R, Selze R. Natural history of aortic regurgitation: a clinical and hemodynamic study. *Am J Med* 1973;**54**:577–88.

44 Bonow RO, Rosing DR, McIntosh CL *et al*. The natural history of asymptomatic patients with aortic regurgitation and normal left ventricular function. *Circulation* 1983;**68**:509–17.

45 Scognamiglio R, Fasoli G, Dalla Volta S. Progression of myocardial dysfunction in asymptomatic patients with severe aortic insufficiency. *Clin Cardiol* 1986;**9**:151–6.

46 Siemienczuk D, Greenberg B, Morris C *et al*. Chronic aortic insufficiency: factors associated with progression to aortic valve replacement. *Ann Intern Med* 1989;**110**:587–92.

47 Bonow RO, Lakatos E, Maron BJ, Epstein SE. Serial long-term assessment of the natural history of asymptomatic patients with chronic aortic regurgitation and normal left ventricular systolic function. *Circulation* 1991;**84**:1625–35.

48 Scognamiglio R, Fasoli G, Ponchia A, Dalla Volta S. Long-term nifedipine unloading therapy in asymptomatic patients with chronic severe aortic regurgitation. *J Am Coll Cardiol* 1990;**16**:424–9.

49 Tornos MP, Olona M, Permanyer-Miralda G *et al*. Clinical outcome of severe asymptomatic chronic aortic regurgitation. A long-term prospective follow-up study. *Am Heart J* 1995;**130**:333–9.

50 Ishii K, Hirota Y, Suwa M *et al*. Natural history and left ventricular response in chronic regurgitation. *Am J Cardiol* 1996;**78**:357–61.

51 Scognamiglio R, Rahimtoola SH, Fasoli G, Nistri S, Dalla Volta S. Nifedipine in asymptomatic patients with severe aortic regurgitation and normal left ventricular function. *N Engl J Med* 1994;**331**:689–95.

52 Henry WL, Bonow RO, Rosing DR, Epstein SE. Observations on the optimum time for operative intervention for aortic regurgitation. II. Serial echocardiographic evaluation of asymptomatic patients. *Circulation* 1980;**61**:484–92.

53 McDonald IG, Jelinek VM. Serial M-mode echocardiography in severe chronic aortic regurgitation. *Circulation* 1980;**62**:1291–96.

54 Bonow RO. Radionuclide angiography in the management of asymptomatic aortic regurgitation. *Circulation* 1991;**84**:I.296–I.302.

55 Hegglin R, Scheu H, Rothlin M. Aortic insufficiency. *Circulation* 1968;**38**(Suppl 15):V77–V92.

56 Rapaport E. Natural history of aortic and mitral valve disease. *Am J Cardiol* 1975;**35**:221–7.

57 Aronow WS, Ahn C, Kronzon I, Nanna M. Prognosis of patients with heart failure and unoperated severe aortic valvular regurgitation and relation to ejection fraction. *Am J Cardiol* 1994;**74**:286–8.

58 Broadbent WH. In *Heart disease*: *with special reference to prognosis and treatment*. London: Baillière, Tindall & Cox, 1897.

59 Klodas E, Enriquez-Sarano M, Tajik AJ *et al*. Surgery for aortic regurgitation in women: contrasting indications and outcomes compared with men. *Circulation* 1996;**94**:2472–8.

60 Boucher CA, Wilson RA, Kanarek DJ *et al*. Exercise testing in asymptomatic or minimally symptomatic aortic regurgitation: relationship of left ventricular ejection fraction to left ventricular filling pressure during exercise. *Circulation* 1983;**67**:1091–100.

61 Kawanishi DT, McKay CR, Chandraratna PAN *et al*. Cardiovascular response to dynamic exercise

in patients with chronic symptomatic mild–moderate and severe aortic regurgitation. *Circulation* 1986;**73**:62–72.

62 Martinez-Rubio A, Schwammenthal Y, Schwammenthal E *et al*. Patients with valvular heart disease presenting with sustained ventricular tachyarrhythmias or syncope: results of programmed ventricular stimulation and long-term follow-up. *Circulation* 1997;**96**:500–8.

63 Rahimtoola SH. Aortic valve regurgitation. In: Schlant R, Alexander RW, Fuster V, eds. *Hurst's The Heart*, 9th edn. New York: McGraw-Hill, 1998, pp 1769–87.

64 Rahimtoola SH. Management of heart failure in valve regurgitation. *Clin Cardiol* 1992;**15**(Suppl I):22–27.

65 Rahimtoola SH. Vasodilator therapy in chronic, severe aortic regurgitation. *J Am Coll Cardiol* 1990;**16**:430–2.

66 Greenberg B, Massie B, Bristow JD *et al*. Long-term vasodilator therapy of chronic aortic insufficiency: a randomized double-blind, placebo-controlled clinical trial. *Circulation* 1988;**78**: 92–103.

67 Röthlisberger C, Sareli P, Wisenbaugh T. Comparison of single-dose nifedipine and captopril for chronic severe aortic regurgitation. *Am J Cardiol* 1993;**72**:799–804.

68 Wisenbaugh T *et al*. Six month pilot study of captopril for mildly symptomatic, severe isolated mitral and isolated aortic regurgitatiion. *J Heart Valve Dis* 1994;**3**:197.

69 Lin M, Chian H-T, Lin S-L *et al*. Vasodilator therapy in chronic asymptomatic aortic regurgitation: enalapril versus hydralazine. *J Am Coll Cardiol* 1994;**24**:1046–53.

70 Greves J, Rahimtoola SH, McAnulty JH *et al*. Preoperative criteria predictive of late survival following valve replacement for severe aortic regurgitation. *Am Heart J* 1981;**101**:300–8.

71 Cunha CL, Giuliani ER, Fuster V *et al*. Preoperative M-mode echocardiography as a predictor of surgical results in chronic aortic insufficiency. *J Thorac Cardiovasc Surg* 1980;**79**:256–65.

72 Clark DG, McAnulty JH, Rahimtoola SH. Valve replacement in aortic insufficiency with left ventricular dysfunction. *Circulation* 1980;**61**: 411–21.

73 Bonow RO, Dodd JT, Maron BJ *et al*. Long-term serial changes in left ventricular function and reversal of ventricular dilatation after valve replacement for chronic aortic regurgitation. *Circulation* 1988;**78**:1108–20.

74 Klodas E, Enriquez-Sarano M, Tajik AJ *et al*. Aortic regurgitation complicated by extreme left ventricular dilation: long-term outcome after surgical correction. *J Am Coll Cardiol* 1996;**27**: 670–7.

Balloon valvuloplasty: aortic valve

49

Daniel J. Diver,
Jeffrey A. Breall

AORTIC STENOSIS: NATURAL HISTORY AND PROGNOSIS

There are three major etiologies for valvular aortic stenosis in the adult patient: rheumatic aortic stenosis; congenital bicuspid aortic stenosis with secondary calcification; and senile-calcific or degenerative aortic stenosis. In rheumatic aortic stenosis, the major pathologic feature is commissural fusion, with associated thickening and fibrosis of the valve leaflets. Symptoms may not occur until ages 50–60, and are often accompanied by evidence of other valvular disease, usually mitral. Patients with congenital bicuspid aortic stenosis develop progressive narrowing and calcification of the aortic valve over time, with symptoms often present by ages 40–50. Degenerative calcific (senile) aortic stenosis appears to result from years of normal mechanical stress on the aortic valve, with progressive immobilization of cusps secondary to calcium accumulation in the pockets of the aortic cusps and eventual fibrosis. Degenerative calcific aortic stenosis is now the most common cause of aortic stenosis in patients presenting for aortic valve replacement.[1]

Most data regarding the natural history of aortic stenosis are derived from clinical experience during the presurgical era. The natural history of aortic stenosis is characterized by a long latent period marked by slowly increasing obstruction and adaptive myocardial hypertrophy. The majority of patients are free of cardiovascular symptoms until relatively late in the course of the disease. However, once patients with aortic stenosis develop symptoms of angina, syncope or heart failure, survival with medical therapy is dismal, with death occurring within 2–5 years in most patients following the development of symptoms (Figure 49.1). Average survival in patients with aortic stenosis and angina or syncope is 2–3 years, and may be as short as 1.5 years in patients with aortic stenosis who develop heart failure.[2] Concomitant atrial fibrillation decreases survival in all symptom groups.

Asymptomatic patients with aortic stenosis have an excellent prognosis, and rarely die without premonitory symptoms. A study by Pellikka et al. showed that mortality was slightly higher in asymptomatic patients treated with "prophylactic" valve

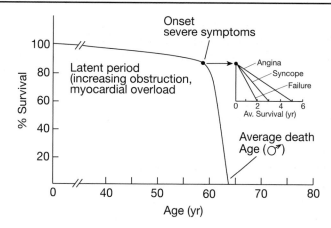

Figure 49.1 Natural history of aortic stenosis without operative treatment. (Reproduced with permission from Ross and Braunwald.[56])

replacement than in patients not operated on until symptoms develop.[3] A recent study by Otto and colleagues reported follow-up of 123 patients with asymptomatic aortic stenosis. During the follow-up period of 2.5 years, there were no sudden cardiac deaths. This study suggested that the rate of hemodynamic progression and clinical outcome in adults with asymptomatic aortic stenosis may be predicted by echocardiographic aortic jet velocity. Of those patients who entered the study with a peak aortic jet velocity greater than 4 meters per second, only 21% were alive and free of valve replacement at 2 years follow-up.[4]

The timing of aortic valve replacement in patients with aortic stenosis is predicated on development of symptoms or deterioration in left ventricular performance rather than severity of valve gradient or reduction in valve orifice area. Carabello has proposed a definition of "critical" aortic stenosis as that valve area small enough to cause the *symptoms* of aortic stenosis that often presage sudden death: a "critical" situation indicating the need for aortic valve replacement.[5] The aortic valve area associated with such symptom development varies significantly from patient to patient.

Aortic stenosis: natural history and prognosis

- Long latent period without symptoms.
- Poor prognosis following symptom development with death in 2–5 years.
- Prognosis significantly improved by valve replacement surgery.

SURGERY FOR AORTIC STENOSIS

The initial surgical approach to treatment of aortic stenosis involved surgical valvuloplasty. In contrast to the situation with pulmonary and mitral stenosis, the stenotic aortic valve did not respond favorably to surgical valvuloplasty techniques. Closed aortic commissurotomy was associated with a high incidence of acute aortic regurgitation and operative mortality, and was abandoned after the development of open aortic valve surgical techniques. Surgical valvuloplasty under direct vision for aortic stenosis was first described in 1956, but was limited by a high rate of restenosis leading to subsequent aortic valve replacement, as well as a significant incidence of complications including aortic regurgitation, infective endocarditis, and systemic embolization.[6] While ultrasonic decalcification and careful surgical sculpturing procedures carried out under direct vision are initially effective in some patients, restenosis remains a serious problem.[7] However, open surgical valvulotomy remains an important treatment for infants and children with critical aortic stenosis, a situation where initial prosthetic valve replacement is undesirable.

The development and refinement of surgical aortic valve replacement significantly improved morbidity and mortality in patients with symptomatic aortic stenosis. Although there is no prospective randomized controlled study comparing aortic valve replacement with medical therapy in such patients, long-term follow-up in high-quality case-series has convincingly demonstrated the long-term benefits of aortic valve replacement, including hemodynamic improvement, regression of left ventricular hypertrophy, improvement of left ventricular function, and improved survival.[8-10] Operative mortality for aortic valve replacement ranges from 2 to 8%, but may be as low as 1% in patients less than 70 years of age without significant comorbidity.

Aortic valve replacement, however, is associated with increased morbidity and mortality in certain subgroups.[9,11-13] Aortic valve replacement in the presence of left ventricular failure may be associated with perioperative mortality as high as 10–25%, and the need for emergency aortic valve replacement with operative mortality as high as 40%. Surgical risk is increased in the elderly patient, and may be increased several fold with the need for concomitant bypass or multiple valve surgery. While advanced age remains a strong predictor of operative death for aortic valve replacement even in recent studies, age alone is not a contraindication to aortic valve replacement in patients with aortic stenosis.[14] Fremes and colleagues at the University of Toronto described the result of valve surgery in 469 consecutive patients greater than 70 years of age, and found that the predicted probability of operative mortality ranged from 0.9 to 76%, depending on the presence of other risk factors, including urgent operation, double valve surgery, coronary artery disease, female gender, and left ventricular dysfunction.[15] The authors suggested that elderly patients in good risk categories should be offered surgical intervention for the correction of valvular lesions, while alternative therapy might be indicated in patients with multiple risk factors, in whom surgical mortality was prohibitively high. Levinson and colleagues at the Massachusetts General Hospital reported on aortic valve replacement for aortic stenosis in octogenarians.[16] In their cohort of 64 patients, serious comorbid non-cardiac conditions were infrequent. In-hospital mortality was 9.4%. An additional 10% of patients had permanent severe neurologic deficits, and an additional 38% had a "complicated" course, marked by temporary encephalopathy, discharge to a rehabilitation facility, or some combination thereof, albeit with ultimately good results. Although most survivors were ultimately free of cardiac symptoms, there was a high price to pay in terms of perioperative mortality and morbidity to achieve these results.

Therefore, while surgical aortic valve replacement has clearly improved the outcome in most patients with critical aortic stenosis, the higher risk in some patient subgroups, including elderly patients, often leads to physician or patient deferral of aortic valve replacement. In an attempt to define the natural history of such patients, O'Keefe and colleagues at the Mayo Clinic performed a case comparison study[17] of 50 patients with severe, symptomatic aortic stenosis, in whom surgery was declined by the patient ($n = 28$) or the physician ($n = 22$). The actuarial survival at 1, 2, and 3 years was 57, 37,

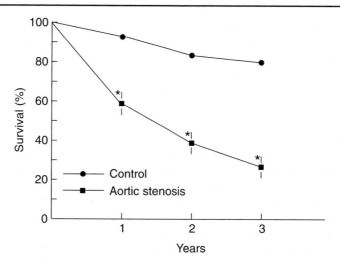

Figure 49.2 Survival among 50 patients with severe aortic stenosis who did not undergo surgical treatment in comparison with an age- and sex-matched control group from the US population. Asterisks denote significant difference (*P*<0.0001) between the two groups. Standard errors are shown as vertical lines. (Reproduced with permission from O'Keefe *et al.*[17])

and 25%, respectively. The survival of age- and sex-matched control subjects was 93, 85, and 77%, respectively (*P*<0.0001 at each 1-year interval) (Figure 49.2). This study suggested that the natural history of untreated aortic stenosis remains dismal and has not improved in the modern era, and confirmed the necessity of evaluating alternative non-surgical therapy, such as balloon aortic valvuloplasty, in patients likely to decline aortic valve replacement, or for whom surgery is not an option.

DEVELOPMENT OF BALLOON AORTIC VALVULOPLASTY

Children and adolescents with congenital aortic stenosis generally have non-calcified valves with commissural fusion. Since aortic valve replacement is not desirable in this age group, commissural incision under direct vision is the preferred surgical procedure, and has been shown to confer significant hemodynamic improvement at low risk.[18] The contribution of commissural fusion to the etiology of valvular stenosis and mechanism of surgical improvement in this patient group led to consideration of balloon aortic valvuloplasty as an alternative, non-surgical therapy.

In 1984 Lababidi and colleagues reported the first series of 23 children and young adults with congenital aortic stenosis treated with percutaneous balloon aortic valvuloplasty.[19] The patients ranged in age from 2 to 17 years. Balloon valvuloplasty was performed by the retrograde approach from the femoral artery, utilizing balloons of 10–20 mm in diameter. Percutaneous balloon dilation resulted in a decrease in the peak aortic valve gradient from 113 to 32 mmHg, with no change in cardiac output. The excellent initial results of percutaneous balloon valvuloplasty for aortic valve stenosis were confirmed by Rosenfeld and colleagues in young adults with congenital aortic stenosis. Long-term follow-up appeared to be excellent, with a 58% event-free rate at mean follow-up of 38 months.[20]

The excellent results of balloon valvuloplasty in pediatric patients with congenital aortic stenosis led to consideration of this technique in adult patients with acquired calcific aortic stenosis. Two reports in 1986 described the first successful balloon valvuloplasty procedures in adult patients. Cribier and colleagues in France performed percutaneous balloon dilation in three elderly patients with calcific aortic stenosis.[21] The peak aortic gradient decreased from 75 to 33 mmHg, with an increase in calculated aortic valve area from 0.5 to 0.8 cm². All patients had symptomatic improvement. McKay and colleagues at the Beth Israel Hospital in Boston described two elderly patients (aged 93 and 85 years) with calcific aortic stenosis treated with balloon valvuloplasty with 12–18-mm balloons.[22] This report likewise described substantial reduction in the transaortic pressure gradient and significant increase in aortic valve area, with symptomatic improvement in both patients, and significant improvement in left ventricular function in one. Despite initial concern regarding the possibility of valve disruption or embolization in the calcific valves present in adult patients, no patient in either report developed emboli or significant increase in aortic regurgitation.

MECHANISM OF BALLOON AORTIC VALVULOPLASTY

To assess the safety, efficacy, and mechanism of balloon aortic valvuloplasty, Safian and colleagues performed balloon dilation of stenotic aortic valves in 33 postmortem specimens and in six patients undergoing aortic valve replacement, prior to removal of the stenotic valve.[23] The cause of aortic stenosis was degenerative nodular calcification in 28 cases, calcific bicuspid aortic stenosis in eight cases, and rheumatic heart disease in three cases. The distribution of the etiology of aortic stenosis in this report is in concordance with the observation that degenerative calcific aortic stenosis is now the most common cause of aortic stenosis in adults presenting for aortic valve replacement.[1]

Safian and colleagues performed balloon dilation with 15–25-mm balloons in the postmortem specimens, and with 18–20-mm balloons in the surgical patients. Balloon dilation resulted in increased leaflet mobility and valve orifice dimensions in all patients. The mechanism of successful dilation included fracture of calcified nodules within the leaflets in 16 valves, separation of fused commissures in five valves, both in six valves, and "grossly inapparent microfractures" (or stretching) in 12 valves. Liberation of calcific debris, valve ring disruption, and mid-leaflet tears did not occur in any valve, although valve leaflet avulsion was produced in one postmortem specimen after inflation with a clearly oversized balloon. The authors concluded that there were several mechanisms for successful balloon aortic valvuloplasty, with the predominant mechanism in a given patient depending on the *etiology* of aortic stenosis. Furthermore, it appeared that embolic phenomena and acute regurgitation were not likely to be frequent complications following valvuloplasty.

The study of Safian and colleagues suggested that the most common etiology of aortic stenosis in the balloon aortic valvuloplasty population is degenerative nodular calcification, and that the predominant mechanism of valve dilation is fracture of calcified nodules within leaflets and leaflet stretching. Considered in conjunction with the disappointing surgical experience when stenotic aortic valves were dilated or cracked, the results of this mechanistic study predicted that there might be only mild improvement in aortic valve orifice area in patients treated with balloon aortic valvuloplasty, and that any such improvement might be short-lived. As will be seen, these implications were subsequently borne out in clinical trials.

Technical aspects

In the original reports by Cribier[21] and McKay,[22] balloon valvuloplasty was performed by the retrograde femoral approach. The most common balloon size used with the single-balloon retrograde approach is a 20-mm balloon, although smaller balloons can be used initially in small or frail patients. If no waist is produced in the inflated balloon or if the aortic valve gradient is not sufficiently decreased by a given balloon size, a larger balloon may produce a better result.

Several modifications of the percutaneous retrograde femoral approach have been described. Block and Palacios described an antegrade transseptal technique, which they advocated for patients with severe iliac occlusive disease, tortuous iliac vessels, or abdominal aortic aneurysm.[24] A retrograde brachial approach may also be useful in such situations, although care must be taken to avoid injury to the brachial artery by the large valvuloplasty balloon. Dorros and colleagues described a double-balloon technique, using both femoral arteries or a combined brachial and femoral approach.[25] The combined diameter of the balloons used in the double-balloon approach usually exceeds the diameter of the largest balloon used with single-balloon techniques. While initial results with double-balloon aortic valvuloplasty showed a greater enlargement of aortic valve area, follow-up studies showed no reduction in subsequent restenosis compared to single-balloon valvuloplasty.[26]

INITIAL RESULTS OF BALLOON AORTIC VALVULOPLASTY

Single center studies

Within several years of the initial reports of balloon valvuloplasty in adult patients with aortic stenosis, several centers reported large single center experiences with balloon aortic valvuloplasty.[27–30] Cribier *et al.* reported their initial experience with 92 adult patients with symptomatic aortic stenosis and a mean age of 75 years.[27] The aortic valve gradient was reduced from 75 to 30 mmHg, with an increase in calculated aortic valve area from 0.5 to 0.9 cm^2. The left ventricular ejection fraction rose from 48% at baseline to 51% immediately following the procedure. The majority of patients had marked symptomatic improvement. There were three in-hospital deaths and eight late deaths.

Safian *et al.* reported the initial experience with balloon aortic valvuloplasty in 170 consecutive patients treated at the Beth Israel Hospital in Boston.[28] The procedure was completed successfully in 168 patients and resulted in significant increases in the mean aortic valve area (0.6–0.9 cm^2) and cardiac output (4.6–4.8 liters per minute) and significant decrease in the aortic valve pressure gradient (71–36 mmHg) ($P<0.01$ for all comparisons). There were six in-hospital deaths, and five patients required early aortic valve replacement. The majority of patients had marked symptomatic improvement following the procedure. The most common complication was vascular complication involving the femoral access site; 40 patients required transfusion and 17 required surgical repair. Transient dysrhythmias, most commonly left bundle branch block, occurred in 28 patients. Left ventricular perforation and tamponade occurred in three patients, marked increase in aortic regurgitation in two patients, and a non-Q wave myocardial infarction in one patient. No patient suffered a stroke.

Table 49.1 Acute hemodynamic results of balloon aortic valvuloplasty

Author	Patients (no.)	Aortic valve gradient (mmHg)		Aortic valve area (cm^2)	
		Pre	Post	Pre	Post
Cribier[27]	92	75	30	0.5	0.9
Safian[28]	170	71	36	0.6	0.9
Block[29]	162	61	27	0.5	0.9
Lewin[30]	125	87	32	0.6	1.0

Table 49.2 Complications of balloon aortic valvuloplasty

Author	Patients (no.)	Complications (%)					
		Death	CVA	Perforation	MI	AI	Vascular
Safian[28]	170	3.5	0	1.8	0.6	1.2	10.0
Block[29]	162	7.0	2.0	0	0	0	7.0
Lewin[30]	125	10.4	3.2	0	1.6	1.6	9.6
Total	457	6.6	1.5	0.7	0.7	0.9	8.8

AI, aortic insufficiency; CVA, cerebrovascular accident; MI, myocardial infarction.

Hemodynamic results and complications of balloon aortic valvuloplasty in several large single center studies are summarized in Tables 49.1 and 49.2, respectively. The results are remarkable for their similarity across study sites. In general, balloon aortic valvuloplasty resulted in a 50–70% decrease in aortic valve gradient and a 50–70% increase in aortic valve area, resulting in early symptomatic improvement in most patients. The most common complication was vascular complication at the access site; there was a low incidence of life-threatening procedural complications. Death during the periprocedural period occurred in about 6% of patients.

Multicenter studies

Two large multicenter studies reported the initial results of balloon valvuloplasty in adult patients with symptomatic aortic stenosis.[31,32] The Mansfield Balloon Aortic Valvuloplasty Registry evaluated data from 27 clinical centers in the United States and included 492 patients treated with balloon aortic valvuloplasty between December 1986 and October 1987.[31] The mean age of patients was 79 years. All patients had severe symptoms, with 92% reporting congestive heart failure. Balloon aortic valvuloplasty was performed by the femoral approach in 92% of patients, by the brachial approach in 6%, and by the transseptal approach in 2%. A single-balloon technique was used in 72% of patients. The largest balloon size was 20 mm in over half of patients.

In the Mansfield Registry, balloon aortic valvuloplasty resulted in a decrease in mean aortic valve gradient from 60 to 30 mmHg, an increase in cardiac output from 3.9 to 4.0 liters per minute, and an increase in aortic valve area from 0.5 to 0.8 cm^2. Most patients had significant symptomatic improvement. Death occurred during the procedure in 4.9% of patients, and within 7 days of the procedure in an additional 2.6%. The most common complication (11%) was local vascular injury, requiring surgical repair in 5.7% of patients. Embolic complications, ventricular perforation resulting in tamponade, and significant increase in aortic insufficiency each occurred in 1–2% of patients, and significant arrhythmia or myocardial infarction in less than 1%. Emergency aortic valve replacement was required in 1% of patients following balloon valvuloplasty.

The National Heart Lung and Blood Institute (NHLBI) Balloon Valvuloplasty Registry enrolled 674 elderly (average age 78 years) patients at 24 centers between November 1987 and November 1989.[32] Heart failure was the most common presenting symptom, occurring in 92% of patients; 45% of patients had angina and 35% had syncope. A single-balloon retrograde valvuloplasty technique was used in 94% of patients; the largest balloon used was a 20-mm balloon in over half. The mean gradient decreased from 55 to 29 mmHg, and the aortic valve area increased from 0.5 to 0.8 cm^2, associated with symptomatic improvement in most patients. Procedural mortality was 3%; other major complications associated with the valvuloplasty procedure included cardiac arrest (5%), emergency aortic valve replacement (1%), left ventricular tamponade (2%), cerebral vascular accident (1%), systemic embolus (1%), emergency temporary pacing (5%), and ventricular arrhythmia requiring countershock (3%).

In summary, the initial results of the multicenter studies were similar to each other, and to the results of the previously described single center studies, and suggested that balloon aortic valvuloplasty resulted in modest hemodynamic improvement and significant symptomatic improvement in many patients considered to be at high risk for aortic valve surgery.

Left ventricular function

Aortic valve replacement has been shown to improve left ventricular function in many patients with aortic stenosis and left ventricular dysfunction.[8,9] Safian and colleagues at Beth Israel Hospital examined the effect of balloon aortic valvuloplasty on left ventricular performance in 28 patients with a low left ventricular ejection fraction (mean 37%), severe aortic stenosis, and a mean age of 79 years.[33] Balloon valvuloplasty resulted in significant increases in aortic valve area (0.5–0.9 cm^2), systolic pressure (120–135 mmHg), and cardiac output (4.2–4.8 liters per minute) ($P<0.01$ for all comparisons), and significant decreases in transaortic pressure gradient (69–35 mmHg) and pulmonary capillary wedge pressure (24–20 mmHg) ($P<0.01$ for both comparisons). All patients were symptomatically improved at the time of discharge.

Serial radionuclide ventriculography showed an increase in left ventricular ejection fraction from 37% prior to valvuloplasty to 44% 48 hours post-procedure and 49% at 3-month follow-up. However, there was substantial heterogeneity of response, with 13 patients showing progressive increases in left ventricular ejection fraction (34% to 49% to 58%, $P<0.001$), while 15 patients showed no significant change in ejection fraction (41% to 40% to 41%, $P=$NS) over 3 months. There was no difference between the groups with respect to age, extent of coronary disease, history of myocardial infarction, or baseline or postprocedure aortic valve area. However, peak systolic wall stress and left ventricular dimensions were higher in those patients who showed no improvement in ejection fraction. It may be that the failure to increase ejection fraction in this group is due to irreversible impairment in myocardial contractile function, secondary to previous infarction or longstanding aortic stenosis. Davidson and colleagues at Duke

University also found that fewer than half of patients with a baseline left ventricular ejection fraction less than 45% showed sustained improvement following percutaneous balloon aortic valvuloplasty, even at short-term follow-up.[34]

FOLLOW-UP

Despite the moderate hemodynamic improvement and significant symptomatic improvement initially achieved in most patients with aortic stenosis following percutaneous balloon valvuloplasty, this technique is severely limited by the high incidence of restenosis. The Beth Israel group reported follow-up results in 170 patients (mean age 77 years) with symptomatic aortic stenosis who underwent balloon aortic valvuloplasty between October 1985 and April 1988.[28] The procedure was completed successfully in 168 patients, with significant improvement in aortic valve area and gradient. There were six in-hospital deaths, and five patients required early aortic valve replacement. Follow-up averaging 9.1 months was available for all 157 patients discharged from the hospital after successful valvuloplasty. In 44 patients (28%), recurrent symptoms developed a mean of 7.5 months after the procedure; 16 were treated by repeat valvuloplasty, 17 by aortic valve replacement, and 11 with medical therapy. Two patients had a second restenosis, treated by aortic valve replacement in one patient and a third valvuloplasty procedure in the other. At latest follow-up, 103 patients (66%) were symptomatically improved, including 15 patients with restenosis who successfully underwent redilation. Twenty-five patients died after discharge, a mean of 6 months after balloon valvuloplasty. The most common cause of death was progressive congestive heart failure.

Repeat cardiac catheterization was performed in 35 patients in the Beth Israel follow-up cohort, including 21 with recurrent symptoms, a mean of 6 months after valvuloplasty. Significant aortic valve restenosis was found in all 21 patients with recurrent symptoms, and in eight of the 14 patients without symptoms. If restenosis was assumed to have occurred in all 25 patients who died, and in all 44 patients with recurrent symptoms, then the "clinical" rate of restenosis following valvuloplasty was 44% at only 9 months. The probability of survival at 1 year was 74% for the entire study population. However, if both recurrent symptoms and death were considered as events, the probability of event-free survival at 1 year was only 50%.

Similarly poor long-term results with high rates of early restenosis were reported by both of the multicenter studies of balloon aortic valvuloplasty. Among the 492 patients treated with balloon valvuloplasty in the Mansfield registry, the 1-year survival rate was 64%, with an event-free survival rate of only 43%.[35] Among the 674 patients reported in the National Heart, Lung and Blood Institute Balloon Valvuloplasty Registry, survival at 1, 2, and 3 years was 55, 35, and 23%, respectively.[36] Lieberman and colleagues from Duke reported long-term follow-up in 165 patients undergoing balloon aortic valvuloplasty.[37] The median duration of follow-up was 3.9 years, with follow-up achieved in 99% of patients. Ninety-three per cent of patients died or underwent aortic valve replacement, and 60% died of cardiac related causes. The probability of event-free survival, defined as freedom from death, aortic valve replacement, or repeat balloon aortic valvuloplasty, at 1, 2, and 3 years after balloon valvuloplasty was 40%, 19%, and 6%, respectively. By contrast, the probability of survival 3 years after balloon aortic valvuloplasty in a subset of 42 patients who underwent subsequent aortic valve replacement was 84%.

Mechanism of restenosis

Since the mechanism by which balloon aortic valvuloplasty increases aortic valve area appears to consist chiefly of fracture of calcified nodules within leaflets and leaflet stretching, and only rarely involves separation of commissural fusion,[23] it is not surprising that the initial improvement in aortic valve area is modest at best, and that significant and early restenosis occurs in most patients. Any element of improvement in the aortic valve area due to leaflet stretching is likely to be rapidly compromised by elastic recoil, and in fact postprocedure echocardiographic follow-up suggests early loss of initial valve area in many patients.[38] Histologic examination in patients who underwent balloon aortic valvuloplasty and had subsequent valve tissue examined at the time of aortic valve replacement or necropsy, showed evidence of closing of fractures in calcified nodules by granulation tissue that may lead to valvular scarring.[39,40] The more rapid time course of this type of inflammatory response, compared to the slowly developing valvular calcification initially leading to aortic stenosis, may explain the relatively rapid progression to symptomatic restenosis following initially successful balloon aortic valvuloplasty.

Results of balloon aortic valvuloplasty
- Initial hemodynamic and symptomatic improvement.
- Early restenosis, with recurrent symptoms.
- No improvement in long-term survival or event-free survival.

PREDICTORS OF OUTCOME FOLLOWING BALLOON AORTIC VALVULOPLASTY

Following recognition of the high incidence of restenosis after balloon aortic valvuloplasty, attempts were made to identify patient subsets more likely to derive long-term benefit. Kuntz and colleagues analyzed event-free survival in 205 patients who underwent balloon aortic valvuloplasty for symptomatic critical aortic stenosis.[41] They evaluated 40 demographic and hemodynamic variables as univariate predictors of event-free survival by Cox regression analysis, and attempted to identify independent predictors of event-free survival by stepwise multivariate analysis. The rate of event-free survival, defined as survival without recurrent symptoms, repeat balloon valvuloplasty, or subsequent aortic valve replacement, was 18% over a mean follow-up period of 24 months (Figure 49.3). Direct predictors of long-term event-free survival in the univariate analysis included female gender, left ventricular ejection fraction, and left ventricular and aortic systolic pressure. Inverse predictors of event-free survival included pulmonary capillary wedge and pulmonary artery pressure. While the prevalvuloplasty and postvalvuloplasty aortic valve area and aortic valve gradient were not associated with event-free survival, the percent reduction in the peak aortic valve gradient was a strong predictor of long-term event-free survival. For patients with a left ventricular ejection fraction of less than 40% at baseline, improvement in the ejection fraction was also directly associated with event-free survival. Of note, when patients 80 years of age or older were analyzed as a subgroup, univariate analysis indicated that the predictors of

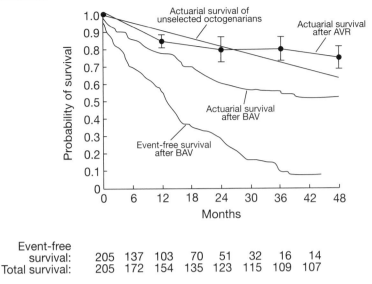

Event-free survival:	205	137	103	70	51	32	16	14
Total survival:	205	172	154	135	123	115	109	107

Figure 49.3 Actuarial total and event-free survival among 205 patients treated by balloon aortic valvuloplasty (BAV). Shown for comparison are the actuarial survival rates among unselected octogenarians in the United States and among octogenarians who undergo aortic-valve replacement (AVR). The numbers below the figure show how many patients were alive or alive without an event at each follow-up. (Reproduced with permission from Kuntz et al.[41])

long-term event-free survival were the same in elderly patients as in the entire patient cohort.

In the stepwise multivariate analysis, the only independent predictors of event-free survival following balloon aortic valvuloplasty were the baseline aortic systolic pressure, the baseline pulmonary capillary wedge pressure (inversely related), and the percent reduction in the peak aortic valve gradient. A baseline aortic systolic pressure less than 110 mmHg was associated with a relative risk of late events of 2.03, and a baseline pulmonary capillary wedge pressure greater than 25 mmHg was associated with a relative risk of 1.73, as compared with the risk in patients with a baseline aortic systolic pressure greater than or equal to 140 mmHg and a pulmonary capillary wedge pressure less than 18 mmHg, respectively. Furthermore, a reduction of less than 40% in the peak aortic valve gradient was associated with a relative risk of late events of 1.75, as compared with the risk in patients in whom valvuloplasty produced a reduction of 55% or more in the peak aortic valve gradient.

To facilitate prediction of outcome following aortic valvuloplasty, using only information available *prior* to the procedure, Kuntz and colleagues utilized the two independent baseline hemodynamic predictors in the Cox model, and estimated the probability of event-free survival at 6, 12, 18, and 24 months for all patients (Table 49.3). According to this two-variable predictive model, patients with baseline pulmonary capillary wedge pressure less than 18 mmHg and aortic systolic pressure greater than or equal to 140 mmHg (the most favorable patient subgroup) had event-free survival rates of 65% at 1 year and 41% at 2 years. On the other hand, patients with baseline pulmonary capillary wedge pressure greater than 25 mmHg and aortic systolic pressure less than 110 mmHg had event-free survival rates of only 23% at 1 year and 4% at 2 years.

Table 49.3 Estimated event-free survival according to baseline hemodynamic variables

Pre PCWP (mmHg)	Pre AOSP (mmHg)	Event-free survival (%)			
		6 mth	12 mth	18 mth	24 mth
<18	≥140	79	65	51	41
<18	110–139	73	58	42	31
<18	>110	64	46	30	19
18–25	≥140	74	59	43	32
18–25	110–139	68	50	34	23
18–25	>110	58	38	22	13
>25	≥140	63	44	28	18
>25	110–139	55	35	19	10
>25	>110	43	23	10	4

AOSP, aortic systolic pressure; PCWP, pulmonary capillary wedge pressure.
Reproduced with permission from Kuntz RE, Tosteson AN, Berman AD *et al.*[41]

In summary, Kuntz and colleagues found that the most important predictors of event-free survival following balloon aortic valvuloplasty were factors related to baseline left ventricular performance, a finding confirmed by analysis of long-term outcome in both large multicenter balloon aortic valvuloplasty registries.[35,36] The best long-term results following valvuloplasty were observed in patients who would also have been expected to have excellent long-term results after aortic valve replacement. In fact, comparison with the surgical data on aortic valve replacement in octogenarians suggests that patients with good hemodynamic performance have better survival after aortic valve replacement than after balloon aortic valvuloplasty.[16] Among patients with poor left ventricular performance or advanced heart failure, event-free survival following balloon aortic valvuloplasty was dismal, and did not appear to improve the natural history of untreated aortic stenosis.[17] Therefore, even in elderly patients with advanced heart failure and higher perioperative risk,[12] aortic valve replacement may increase the likelihood of long-term survival compared to balloon aortic valvuloplasty. In such high-risk patients, however, balloon aortic valvuloplasty may have a role in providing transient hemodynamic improvement, perhaps decreasing the risk of subsequent aortic valve replacement.

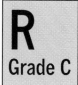

R
Grade C

REPEAT BALLOON AORTIC VALVULOPLASTY

In patients who are not candidates for surgery, development of restenosis following balloon aortic valvuloplasty can be managed with repeat balloon valvuloplasty. Studies of repeat valvuloplasty have shown that the absolute aortic valve areas tend to be slightly smaller both before and after the repeat valvuloplasty, even when larger balloons or balloon combinations are used.[42] The incidence of repeat restenosis remains high; follow-up of the 47 patients in the Mansfield registry who underwent repeat valvuloplasty showed that 66% of patients had died, undergone subsequent valve replacement, or required a third valvuloplasty at a mean follow-up of 5 months.[43] Histologic study of valves treated with balloon valvuloplasty, and excised prior to subsequent surgery or examined at autopsy, has shown active cellular proliferation within the splits in calcified nodules, as well as foci of ossification.[39] These findings suggest an active scarring process in response to balloon valvuloplasty, which may explain the failure to achieve better results with the use of larger balloons, and raises the possibility that balloon-induced injury to the aortic valve may accelerate the natural history of aortic stenosis.

AORTIC VALVE SURGERY AFTER BALLOON AORTIC VALVULOPLASTY

Most surviving patients who have undergone balloon aortic valvuloplasty develop clinically significant restenosis within 1–2 years following the procedure. Many of these patients are subsequently treated with aortic valve replacement. Johnson and colleagues at the Beth Israel Hospital reported 45 patients (25% of the initial balloon valvuloplasty cohort) subsequently treated with aortic valve replacement.[44] Three patients required emergency operation immediately after unsuccessful valvuloplasty, and the remaining 42 had an elective operation at a mean of 8 months following valvuloplasty, primarily for development of symptomatic restenosis. Despite the fact that the majority of these patients had initially undergone balloon valvuloplasty because they were considered to be at high risk for surgery, there were only four hospital deaths among the 45 patients. Three additional patients died a mean of 11 months following surgery. All surviving patients had persistent symptomatic improvement following surgery.

Lieberman and colleagues at Duke reported 40 patients (24% of the initial balloon valvuloplasty treatment group) who subsequently underwent aortic valve replacement.[45] Only one patient (2.5%) suffered a perioperative death. The probability of survival 3 years from the date of the last mechanical intervention was 75% for patients treated with balloon valvuloplasty and subsequent aortic valve replacement, as compared to only 20% for patients whose restenosis was treated with repeat balloon valvuloplasty, and 13% for patients who had no further mechanical intervention after developing restenosis. The majority of surgically treated patients remained asymptomatic at last follow-up. It is important to note that this study is not a randomized comparison of treatment strategies for restenosis, and the results must be interpreted in light of the probable selection bias with regard to choice of management strategy for aortic valve restenosis. Nevertheless, it appears that in this group of patients initially felt to be at high risk for aortic valve replacement, surgery could be performed with an acceptable operative risk. Furthermore, as opposed to balloon valvuloplasty, aortic valve replacement appears to offer a reasonable chance of long-term freedom from symptoms. Although these reports do not specifically address potential reduction in the risk of subsequent surgery by prior performance of balloon valvuloplasty, a beneficial effect cannot be excluded.

BALLOON AORTIC VALVULOPLASTY VS AORTIC VALVE SURGERY

There are no randomized trials comparing balloon aortic valvuloplasty with aortic valve replacement in adult patients with critical aortic stenosis. However, Bernard and colleagues in France compared two non-randomized matched series of patients with aortic stenosis treated with either balloon aortic valvuloplasty or aortic valve replacement at the same institution between January 1986 and March 1989.[46] Forty-six patients were treated with balloon aortic valvuloplasty and 23 patients with aortic valve replacement with a bioprosthesis. Baseline clinical and hemodynamic parameters were similar in both groups; all patients were at least 75 years old. Follow-up was 22 months for the aortic valvuloplasty patients and 28 months following surgery. Among patients treated with balloon aortic valvuloplasty, three patients (6.5%) died within 5 days after the procedure, and an additional 24 patients (42%) died during subsequent follow-up, with 16 deaths due to recurrent heart failure. Sixteen patients (35%) underwent subsequent aortic valve replacement at a mean of 16 months following balloon valvuloplasty. At last follow-up, only three valvuloplasty patients (6.5%) remained alive without subsequent aortic valve replacement. Of the patients treated with initial aortic valve replacement, two patients (8.7%) died in the perioperative period, and an additional three patients (13%) died during the follow-up period. All remaining patients (78%) were alive and in New York Heart Association functional class I or II at last follow-up. The overall survival rate following balloon valvuloplasty was 75% at 1 year, 47% at 2 years, and 33% at 5 years. By contrast, survival following surgery was 83% at 1 and 2 years and 75% at 3 and 4 years. Although selection bias cannot be excluded in this non-randomized case-comparison study, nevertheless the results strongly suggest that percutaneous balloon aortic valvuloplasty does not compare favorably with aortic valve surgery in elderly patients with aortic stenosis.

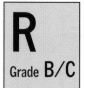

R

Grade B

SPECIFIC INDICATIONS FOR BALLOON VALVULOPLASTY

Aortic valvuloplasty prior to non-cardiac surgery

Patients with severe aortic stenosis are at increased risk for significant cardiac complications during non-cardiac surgery.[47] Three studies described the role of balloon aortic valvuloplasty in the management of patients with critical aortic stenosis requiring major non-cardiac surgery.[48–50] In these studies, 29 patients with critical aortic stenosis underwent balloon aortic valvuloplasty, complicated by procedural death due to ventricular perforation and tamponade in one patient. Valvuloplasty resulted in significant improvement in aortic valve gradient and aortic valve area. Twenty-eight of the 29 patients underwent the planned surgical procedure under general or epidural anesthesia. All but one patient had uncomplicated non-cardiac surgery, with no significant congestive heart failure, hypotension, myocardial infarction, arrhythmia, or conduction abnormality either during or immediately after surgery. One patient developed marked hypotension requiring transient intravenous pressor support during surgery for bowel carcinoma, resulting in interruption of surgery. This patient subsequently underwent aortic valve replacement and coronary artery bypass graft surgery, followed by repeat bowel resection. Procedures performed successfully following palliative balloon aortic valvuloplasty included aortic aneurysm repair, repair of hip fracture, exploratory laparotomy, and thoracotomy. While the cited reports are not randomized or case-control comparisons of preoperative balloon aortic valvuloplasty vs aortic valve replacement or medical therapy, nevertheless, they suggest that balloon valvuloplasty may reduce the risk of non-cardiac surgery in patients with critical aortic stenosis for whom preoperative aortic valve replacement is not possible or practical.

R

Grade B/C

Aortic valvuloplasty as a bridge to aortic valve replacement

As noted earlier, many patients treated with balloon aortic valvuloplasty subsequently undergo aortic valve replacement. Large series of patients undergoing subsequent aortic valve surgery after balloon valvuloplasty have demonstrated acceptable operative risk and excellent surgical outcome, with long-term freedom from symptoms in most surviving patients.[44,45] However, in most patients undergoing surgery in these studies, aortic valve replacement was performed because of failure of the initial balloon aortic valvuloplasty procedure, which was not specifically used to stabilize the patient for subsequent surgery.

Smedira and colleagues studied critically ill patients with aortic stenosis, in whom balloon aortic valvuloplasty was specifically used as a bridge to aortic valve replacement.[51] They reported five patients with severe aortic stenosis, multiple organ failure, and severe hemodynamic compromise, who were judged to be at excessive risk for aortic valve surgery. Balloon aortic valvuloplasty was used in these patients to provide transient hemodynamic improvement, improve organ function, and to decrease the risk of subsequent definitive surgical correction. Following successful balloon aortic valvuloplasty and clinical stabilization, subsequent elective aortic valve replacement was performed in all patients without complications. This report suggests that balloon aortic valvuloplasty may have a role as a bridge to subsequent aortic valve replacement for patients in whom heart failure or hypotension is so severe that the risk of primary aortic valve surgery is unacceptable.

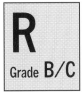

R
Grade B/C

Aortic valvuloplasty in cardiogenic shock

Of the 674 patients in the multicenter NHLBI Balloon Valvuloplasty Registry, 39 (6%) had cardiogenic shock. The largest reported series specifically describing the role of balloon aortic valvuloplasty in cardiogenic shock is that of Moreno and colleagues from the Massachusetts General Hospital.

Moreno studied 21 patients with critical aortic stenosis and cardiogenic shock treated with balloon aortic valvuloplasty.[52] All patients had major associated comorbid conditions precluding the use of emergent aortic valve replacement. The hemodynamic results were excellent, with an increase in systolic aortic pressure from 77 to 116 mmHg and an increase in aortic valve area from 0.5 to 0.8 cm^2 ($P=0.0001$ for both comparisons). Cardiac index increased from 1.84 to 2.24 liters/min/m^2 ($P=0.06$). Nine treated patients died in the hospital, two during the procedure and seven following successful balloon aortic valvuloplasty. Procedural complications were frequent, with five patients suffering vascular complications and one patient each developing stroke, cholesterol embolus, and aortic regurgitation requiring aortic valve replacement. Twelve patients (57%) survived and were discharged from the hospital. During follow-up of 15 months, five additional patients died. Actuarial survival was 38% at 27 months. The only predictor of improved survival was the postprocedure cardiac index.

In summary, the limited published data suggest that emergency percutaneous balloon aortic valvuloplasty can be successfully performed in patients with critical aortic stenosis and cardiogenic shock. Morbidity and mortality remain high even after hemodynamically successful procedures. Given the poor long-term outcome in patients treated with balloon

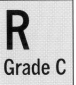

R
Grade C

aortic valvuloplasty, the use of aortic valvuloplasty in patients with cardiogenic shock should be considered a bridge to subsequent aortic valve replacement in those patients who improve sufficiently to undergo surgery at reasonable risk.

Aortic valvuloplasty in patients with low output, low gradient

Patients with left ventricular dysfunction and aortic stenosis in the presence of low cardiac output and low aortic valve gradient present a complex diagnostic and therapeutic challenge. Aortic valve surgery is associated with increased morbidity and mortality in such patients, a subset of whom have irreversible myocardial dysfunction.[9–11] Balloon aortic valvuloplasty has been proposed as a diagnostic tool in patients with aortic stenosis and low output, low gradient hemodynamics, to distinguish patients with reversible myocardial dysfunction due to abnormal loading conditions from those with irreversible myocardial dysfunction. It has been suggested that patients with low output, low gradient hemodynamics who have significant improvement in either ventricular function or symptoms following successful balloon aortic valvuloplasty are more likely to improve following aortic valve replacement than those patients in whom balloon aortic valvuloplasty produces no significant benefit.

Safian and colleagues studied 28 patients with a low left ventricular ejection fraction (mean 37%) and severe aortic stenosis who underwent balloon aortic valvuloplasty.[33] On the basis of response to balloon valvuloplasty, they were able to separate patients into a subset with progressive improvement in left ventricular ejection fraction, and a subset which showed no significant change in left ventricular function. Nishimura and colleagues, utilizing data from the multicenter Mansfield Aortic Valvuloplasty Registry, compared 67 patients with low output, low gradient hemodynamics versus 200 patients with a low cardiac index but *not* a low aortic valve gradient.[53] Patients with low output, low gradient hemodynamics had less of a decrease in aortic valve gradient after valvuloplasty, but a similar improvement in estimated aortic valve area. However, actuarial survival at 12 months was 46% for patients with low output, low gradient hemodynamics, compared to 64% in the comparison cohort ($P<0.05$). Furthermore, patients with low output, low gradient hemodynamics were less likely to show sustained symptomatic improvement. Therefore, since long-term outcome after balloon valvuloplasty is poor in patients with low output, low gradient hemodynamics, aortic valve replacement may be indicated in those patients in whom balloon aortic valvuloplasty produces an initial favorable response. While these reports suggest that it may be possible to identify a subset of patients with aortic stenosis and low output, low gradient hemodynamics likely to benefit from subsequent aortic valve replacement, the hypothesis that response to aortic valvuloplasty predicts subsequent outcome following surgery has not been tested.

Other indications

Case reports have described the use of balloon aortic valvuloplasty for the management of critical aortic stenosis in pregnancy, documenting safe performance of balloon valvuloplasty during pregnancy with subsequent normal births.[54] Given their age range, pregnant patients are more likely to have congenital or rheumatic aortic stenosis, and therefore to have valve stenosis due to commissural fusion, which responds more favorably to balloon dilation than the more frequently encountered degenerative calcific valvular disease. Use of balloon aortic valvuloplasty as a bridge to subsequent cardiac transplant in a patient with aortic stenosis and end-stage heart failure has also been described.[55]

Indications for balloon aortic valvuloplasty

- Symptomatic critical aortic stenosis in patients who are not candidates for aortic valve replacement.
- Bridge to aortic valve replacement in patients with severe hemodynamic compromise.
- Prior to urgent non-cardiac surgery.
- Aortic stenosis with low output, low gradient hemodynamics.

CONCLUSIONS

The development and analysis of balloon aortic valvuloplasty as a treatment strategy for adult patients with critical aortic stenosis offers a paradigm for investigation of new therapeutic techniques. The initial enthusiasm for new treatment modalities, often based on arguments of physiology, first principles, or small case series, is often replaced by sobering realization of limitations and complications, revealed by careful prospective multicenter clinical trials, ultimately resulting in the development of appropriate clinical indications for the new treatment strategy. The development and investigation of balloon aortic valvuloplasty for aortic stenosis followed just such a trajectory, and illustrates the impact of careful, early, prospective clinical trial data on the evolution and rapid development of appropriate indications for new therapeutic techniques.

Although aortic valve replacement clearly improves morbidity and mortality in patients with symptomatic aortic stenosis, concern regarding the higher morbidity in high-risk subgroups led to the investigation of balloon aortic valvuloplasty as an alternative therapy for aortic stenosis. Early evidence from both single center and multicenter series, showing hemodynamic and symptomatic improvement in most patients treated with balloon valvuloplasty, led to initial widespread enthusiasm for this new technique. However, this enthusiasm was quickly tempered as subsequent follow-up in these high-quality case series demonstrated a high rate of hemodynamic and clinical restenosis, and failure of balloon valvuloplasty to improve long-term survival or event-free survival.

Critical evaluation of the data from these large case series provided further understanding of the appropriate role of balloon aortic valvuloplasty in the management of patients with aortic stenosis. When patients were stratified by the independent predictors of event-free survival, it became clear that those patients who did best with balloon aortic valvuloplasty were acceptable candidates for aortic valve surgery, and had an even better event-free survival following surgery. On the other hand, patients with baseline profiles which indicated a high risk for surgery also did extremely poorly with balloon valvuloplasty, with event-free survival which did not appear to differ from the natural history of untreated aortic stenosis. The rapid accumulation and careful analysis of clinical trial data on patients treated with balloon valvuloplasty quickly established that the treatment of choice for adult patients with symptomatic aortic stenosis is aortic valve replacement, with balloon aortic valvuloplasty reserved for those patients in whom surgery is not possible or practical. Further refinement of the appropriate therapeutic niche for balloon aortic valvuloplasty has been aided by small case series targeted at specific indications for non-surgical therapy of aortic stenosis.

The following guidelines on appropriate utilization of balloon aortic valvuloplasty in adult patients with symptomatic critical aortic stenosis are based on case-series and case-control studies, and therefore should be considered as Level B Recommendations.

Based on the available evidence, balloon aortic valvuloplasty should be considered:

1. For patients with symptomatic aortic stenosis who are not operable, or who are poor candidates for aortic valve replacement, due to severe comorbid illness or advanced age in the presence of other significant predictors of surgical risk. It should be emphasized that advanced age alone in a patient without other significant surgical risk factors is not a contraindication to aortic valve replacement. It must be further stressed that the goal of balloon aortic valvuloplasty in this patient group is transient symptomatic relief, as there is no evidence that valvuloplasty improves survival or provides long-term freedom from symptoms. Grade B

2. As a bridge to subsequent aortic valve replacement in patients with advanced heart failure, hypotension or cardiogenic shock, when clinical presentation suggests excessive risk for an initial surgical strategy. The goal of balloon aortic valvuloplasty in this cohort is transient hemodynamic improvement, leading to stabilization of the patient for subsequent aortic valve replacement, the only treatment shown to ultimately improve long-term survival. Grade B

3. For patients with critical aortic stenosis and poor ventricular function, heart failure, or hypotension, who require urgent or emergent non-cardiac surgery. The goal of balloon aortic valvuloplasty in this patient subset is successful completion of the required non-cardiac surgical procedure, with subsequent aortic valve replacement for the underlying aortic stenosis. Grade B

4. For patients with aortic stenosis, diminished left ventricular function, and low output, low gradient hemodynamics, in whom the response to initial "diagnostic" balloon valvuloplasty may aid in identification of patients likely to benefit from subsequent aortic valve replacement. Grade B

Given the disparity in outcome between aortic valve replacement and balloon aortic valvuloplasty in large high-quality case series and non-randomized case-control studies, it is unreasonable to pursue randomized clinical trials comparing these treatment strategies. However, the high-quality case series rapidly performed and reported in patients treated with balloon aortic valvuloplasty not only established the appropriate role for balloon valvuloplasty in the treatment of aortic stenosis, but also confirmed the value of prompt clinical investigation in the rapid development of appropriate indications for new therapeutic techniques. When the *goal* of therapy is long-term survival or symptom-free survival, the available clinical trial data clearly support aortic valve replacement as the treatment of choice for aortic stenosis. However, in patients who are not candidates for surgery or refuse surgery, the trial data have demonstrated a role for balloon aortic valvuloplasty, albeit with the more limited goal of transient, palliative symptomatic relief, without improvement in survival or long-term symptomatic benefit.

REFERENCES

1 Passik CS, Ackermann DM, Pluth JR, Edwards WD. Temporal changes in the causes of aortic stenosis: a surgical pathologic study of 646 cases. *Mayo Clin Proc* 1987;**62**:119–23.

2 Frank S, Johnson A, Ross J. Natural history of valvular aortic stenosis. *Br Heart J* 1973;**35**:41–6.

3 Pellikka PA, Nishimura RA, Bailey KR, Tajik AJ. The natural history of adults with asymptomatic, hemodynamically significant aortic stenosis. *J Am Coll Cardiol* 1990;**15**:1012–17.

4 Otto CM, Burwash IG, Legget ME *et al.* Prospective study of asymptomatic valvular aortic stenosis. Clinical, echocardiographic, and exercise predictors of outcome. *Circulation* 1997;**95**:2262–70.

5 Carabello BA. Timing of valve replacement in aortic stenosis. Moving closer to perfection. *Circulation* 1997;**95**:2241–3.

6 Hsieh K, Keane JF, Nadas AS, Bernhard WF, Castaneda AR. Long-term follow-up of valvotomy before 1968 for congenital aortic stenosis. *Am J Cardiol* 1986;**58**:338–41.

7 McBride LR, Nannheim KS, Fiore AC *et al.* Aortic valve decalcification. *J Thorac Cardiovasc Surg* 1990;**100**:36–42.

8 Kennedy JW, Doces J, Stewart DK. Left ventricular function before and following aortic valve replacement. *Circulation* 1977;**56**:944–50.

9 Smith N, McAnulty JH, Rahimtoola SH. Severe aortic stenosis with impaired left ventricular function and clinical heart failure: results of valve replacement. *Circulation* 1978;**58**:255–64.

10 Lund O. Preoperative risk evaluation and stratification of long-term survival after valve replacement for aortic stenosis. *Circulation* 1990;**82**:124–39.

11 Magovern JA, Pennock JL, Campbell DB *et al.* Aortic valve replacement and combined aortic valve replacement and coronary artery bypass grafting: predicting high risk groups. *J Am Coll Cardiol* 1987;**9**:38–43.

12 Edmunds LH, Stephenson LW, Edie RN, Ratcliffe MB. Open-heart surgery in octogenarians. *N Engl J Med* 1988;**319**:131–6.

13 Verheul HA, Van Den Brink RBA, Bouma BJ *et al.* Analysis of risk factors for excess mortality after aortic valve replacement. *J Am Coll Cardiol* 1995;**26**:1280–6.

14 Asimakopoulos G, Edwards M, Taylor K. Aortic valve replacement in patients 80 years of age and older. Survival and cause of death based on 1100 cases: collective results from the UK Heart Valve Registry. *Circulation* 1997;**96**:3403–8.

15 Fremes SE, Goldman BS, Ivanou J, Weisel RD, David TE, Salerno T. Valvular surgery in the elderly. *Circulation* 1989;**80**(suppl I):177–90.

16 Levinson JR, Akins CW, Buckley MJ *et al.* Octogenarians with aortic stenosis. Outcome after aortic valve replacement. *Circulation* 1989;**80**(Suppl I):149–56.

17 O'Keefe JH, Vlietstra RE, Bailey KR, Holmes DR. Natural history of candidates for balloon aortic valvuloplasty. *Mayo Clin Proc* 1987;**62**:986–91.

18 Kirklin JW, Barratt-Boyes BG. Congenital aortic stenosis. In: *Cardiac Surgery*, 2nd edn. New York: Churchill-Livingstone, 1993, pp 1195–238.

19 Lababidi Z, Wu JR, Walls JT. Percutaneous balloon aortic valvuloplasty: results in 23 patients. *Am J Cardiol* 1984;**53**:194–7.

20 Rosenfeld HM, Landzberg MJ, Perry SB, Colan SD, Keane JF, Lock JE. Balloon aortic valvuloplasty in young adults with congenital aortic stenosis. *Am J Cardiol* 1994;**73**:1112–17.

21 Cribier A, Savin T, Saoudi N, Rocha P, Berland J, Letac B. Percutaneous transluminal valvuloplasty of acquired aortic stenosis in elderly patients: an alternative to valve replacement? *Lancet* 1986;**i**:63–7.

22 McKay RG, Safian RD, Lock JE *et al.* Balloon dilatation of calcific aortic stenosis in elderly patients: postmortem, intraoperative, and percutaneous valvuloplasty studies. *Circulation* 1986;**74**:119–25.

23 Safian RD, Mandell VS, Thurer RE *et al.* Postmortem and intraoperative balloon valvuloplasty of calcific aortic stenosis in elderly patients: mechanisms of successful dilation. *J Am Coll Cardiol* 1987;**9**:655–60.

24 Block PC, Palacios IF. Comparison of hemodynamic results of anterograde versus retrograde percutaneous balloon aortic valvuloplasty. *Am J Cardiol* 1987;**60**:659–62.

25 Dorros G, Lewin RF, King JF, Janke LM. Percutaneous transluminal valvuloplasty in calcific aortic stenosis: the double balloon technique. *Cathet Cardiovasc Diagn* 1987;**13**:151–6.

26 Fields CD, Lucas A, Desnoyers M *et al.* Dual balloon aortic valvuloplasty, despite augmenting acute hemodynamic improvement, fails to prevent post-valvuloplasty restenosis. *J Am Coll Cardiol* 1989;**13**:148A.

27 Cribier A, Savin T, Berland J *et al.* Percutaneous transluminal balloon valvuloplasty of adult aortic stenosis: report of 92 cases. *J Am Coll Cardiol* 1987;**9**:381–6.

28 Safian RD, Berman AD, Diver DJ *et al.* Balloon aortic valvuloplasty in 170 consecutive patients. *N Engl J Med* 1988;**319**:125–30.

29 Block PC, Palacios IF. Clinical and hemodynamic follow-up after percutaneous aortic valvuloplasty in the elderly. *Am J Cardiol* 1988;**62**:760–3.

30 Lewin RF, Dorros G, King JF, Mathiak L. Percutaneous transluminal aortic valvuloplasty:

acute outcome and follow-up of 125 patients. *J Am Coll Cardiol* 1989;**14**:1210–17.

31 McKay RG, for the Mansfield Scientific Aortic Valvuloplasty Registry. Balloon aortic valvuloplasty in 285 patients: initial results and complications. *Circulation* 1988;**78**(suppl II):II–594.

32 McKay RG, for the NHLBI Aortic Valvuloplasty Registry. Clinical outcome following balloon aortic valvuloplasty for severe aortic stenosis. *J Am Coll Cardiol* 1989;**13**:1218.

33 Safian RD, Warren SE, Berman AD *et al.* Improvement in symptoms and left ventricular performance after balloon aortic valvuloplasty in patients with aortic stenosis and depressed left ventricular ejection fraction. *Circulation* 1988;**78**:1181–91.

34 Davidson CJ, Harrison JK, Leithe ME, Kisslo KB, Bashore TM. Failure of balloon aortic valvuloplasty to result in sustained clinical improvement in patients with depressed left ventricular function. *Am J Cardiol* 1990;**65**:72–7.

35 O'Neill WW, for the Mansfield Scientific Aortic Valvuloplasty Registry Investigators. Predictors of long-term survival after percutaneous aortic valvuloplasty: report of the Mansfield Scientific Aortic Valvuloplasty Registry. *J Am Coll Cardiol* 1991;**17**:193–8.

36 Otto CM, Mickel MC, Kenedy JW *et al.* Three year outcome after balloon aortic valvuloplasty. Insights into prognosis of valvular aortic stenosis. *Circulation* 1994;**89**:642–50.

37 Lieberman EB, Bashore TM, Hermiller JB *et al.* Balloon aortic valvuloplasty in adults: failure of procedure to improve long-term survival. *J Am Coll Cardiol* 1995;**26**:1522–8.

38 Nishimura RA, Holmes DR, Reeder GS *et al.* Doppler evaluation of results of percutaneous aortic balloon valvuloplasty in calcific aortic stenosis. *Circulation* 1988;**78**:791–9.

39 Feldman T, Glagov S, Carroll JD. Restenosis following successful balloon valvuloplasty: bone formation in aortic valve leaflets. *Cathet Cardiovasc Diagn* 1993;**29**:1–7.

40 Isner JM. Aortic valvuloplasty: are balloon-dilated valves all they are "cracked" up to be? *Mayo Clin Proc* 1988;**63**:830–4.

41 Kuntz RE, Tosteson AN, Berman AD *et al.* Predictors of event-free survival after balloon aortic valvuloplasty. *N Engl J Med* 1991;**325**:17–23.

42 Kuntz RE, Tosteson AN, Maitland LA *et al.* Immediate results and long-term follow-up after repeat balloon aortic valvuloplasty. *Cathet Cardiovasc Diagn* 1992;**25**:4–9.

43 Ferguson JJ, Garza RA and the Mansfield Scientific Aortic Valvuloplasty Registry Investigators. Efficacy of multiple balloon aortic valvuloplasty procedures. *J Am Coll Cardiol* 1991;**17**:1430–5.

44 Johnson RG, Dhillon JS, Thurer RL, Safian RD, Wientraub RM. Aortic valve operation after percutaneous aortic balloon valvuloplasty. *Ann Thorac Surg* 1990;**49**:740–5.

45 Lieberman EB, Wilson JS, Harrison JK *et al.* Aortic valve replacement in adults after balloon aortic valvuloplasty. *Circulation* 1994;**90**(suppl II):II205–8.

46 Bernard Y, Etievent J, Mourand JL *et al.* Long-term results of percutaneous aortic valvuloplasty compared with aortic valve replacement in patients more than 75 years old. *J Am Coll Cardiol* 1992;**20**:796–801.

47 Goldman L, Caldera DL, Nussbaum SR. Multifactorial index of cardiac risk in noncardiac surgical procedures. *N Engl J Med* 1977;**297**:845–56.

48 Levine MJ, Berman AD, Safian RD, Diver DJ, McKay RG. Palliation of valvular aortic stenosis by balloon valvuloplasty as preoperative preparation for noncardiac surgery. *J Am Coll Cardiol* 1988;**62**:1309–10.

49 Roth RB, Palacios IF, Block PC. Percutaneous aortic balloon valvuloplasty: its role in the management of patients with aortic stenosis requiring major noncardiac surgery. *J Am Coll Cardiol* 1989;**13**:1039–41.

50 Hayes SN, Holmes DR, Nishimura RA, Reeder GS. Palliative percutaneous aortic balloon valvuloplasty before noncardiac operations and invasive diagnostic procedures. *Mayo Clin Proc* 1989;**64**:753–7.

51 Smedira NG, Ports TA, Merrick SH, Rankin JS. Balloon aortic valvuloplasty as a bridge to aortic valve replacement in critically ill patients. *Ann Thorac Surg* 1993;**55**:914–16.

52 Moreno PR, Ik-Kyung J, Block PC, Palacios IF. The role of percutaneous aortic balloon valvuloplasty in patients with cardiogenic shock and critical aortic stenosis. *J Am Coll Cardiol* 1994;**23**:1071–5.

53 Nishimura RA, Holmes DR, Michela ME *et al.* Follow-up of patients with low output, low gradient hemodynamics after percutaneous balloon aortic valvuloplasty: the Mansfield Scientific Aortic Valvuloplasty Registry. *J Am Coll Cardiol* 1991;**17**:828–33.

54 Banning AP, Pearson JF, Hall RJ. Role of balloon dilatation of the aortic valve in pregnant patients with severe aortic stenosis. *Br Heart J* 1993;**70**:544–5.

55 Vaitkus PT, Mancini D, Herrman HC. Percutaneous balloon aortic valvuloplasty as a bridge to heart transplantation. *J Heart Lung Transplant* 1993;**12**:1062–4.

56 Ross J, Braunwald E. Aortic stenosis. *Circulation* 1968;**38**(suppl V):61–7.

Balloon valvuloplasty: mitral valve

50

ZOLTAN G. TURI

INTRODUCTION

Percutaneous balloon mitral valvuloplasty is the latest technique in an evolution that began with Elliot Cutler advancing a knife retrograde through the apex of the left ventricle of a beating heart in 1923.[1] Neither he nor Henry Suttar, who performed a similar procedure in England two years later, received the expected accolades,[2] and there has been continuing dispute about the relative role of mitral obstruction in defining the spectrum of mitral stenosis. Sir Thomas Lewis' statement that valvotomy was based on an "erroneous idea, namely that the valve is the chief source of the trouble"[3] has few proponents in the modern era and relieving mitral obstruction is the de facto standard of care.

After a 20-year hiatus, the battlefield experience with closed heart procedures in the Second World War led to the application of these techniques outside the trauma arena. Although early results were confounded by significant morbidity and mortality, closed mitral valvotomy became a routine procedure for severe mitral stenosis, and is still the treatment of choice in many parts of the world where the disease is endemic and medical facilities limited. Large series[4,5] have claimed good long term results, but lack of systematic follow-up or comprehensive objective data obscure the actual restenosis rate and survival. In a Mayo Clinic retrospective analysis[6] there was a 79% 10-year and a 55% 20-year survival rate with re-operation in 34% by 10 years; however, nearly a quarter of patients were lost to follow-up and severity of disease at baseline could only be estimated. Open commissurotomy with the potential advantages of direct vision has supplanted closed procedures in industrialized nations. Controversy remains as to its superiority,[7–9] with the advantages of direct vision favoring cases where thrombus is present.

The percutaneous approach

A pediatric cardiac surgeon, Kanji Inoue, developed a double lumen atrial septostomy balloon catheter made of latex, with a mesh weave used to constrain the balloon during inflation into the classic wishbone shape depicted in Figure 50.1.[10] He then adapted the device for percutaneous balloon mitral valvuloplasty, demonstrated under direct vision in the operating room its ability to split fused mitral commissures,[11] and performed the first procedure in 1982.[12]

Mechanisms of valvuloplasty

The mechanisms responsible for the benefits of balloon mitral valvuloplasty[13] arise from the substantial radial force exerted by the enlarging balloon.[14] This stretches the mitral annulus, has the capacity to split fused commissures, and occasionally results in the cracking of calcifications. The stretching mechanism has been observed intraoperatively,[15] whereas the splitting of commissures[16] and cracking of calcifications have been demonstrated by direct observation in excised valves.[17] The largely successful nature of balloon mitral valvuloplasty is derived from commissural splitting; balloon dilation procedures where the other two mechanisms predominate, such as balloon valvuloplasty for calcific aortic stenosis, have less impressive short and long term results.

PRE-PROCEDURE EVALUATION

The most common reason for exclusion of patients is unsuitable valve anatomy. Specific relevant physical examination findings are diminution of the first heart sound (often indicative of extensive subvalvular disease) and a hyperdynamic ventricle, suggestive of volume loading secondary to mitral or aortic regurgitation, both of which are relative contraindications to the procedure.

Non-invasive methods

The echocardiographic findings of greatest predictive value have been debated at length. The standard,[18] the Wilkins–Weyman score, incorporates a scoring system for mitral valve leaflet thickening, mobility and calcification, and severity of subvalvular disease (Table 50.1), with a score of <8 described as an "ideal" patient population, and echo scores over 12 potentially predicting poorer results. The correlation between this echo score and initial as well as long term results is only fair, perhaps because it is a semiquantitative system based on partly subjective assessments and because other factors not included in the system have predictive value. Thus studies have alternately confirmed[19–21] or refuted[22–25] the predictive value of the Wilkins–Weyman score. One element of the score, leaflet mobility, correlates more strongly with outcome (r value $=0.67$) than the complete score,[26] while another element, severe calcification of the valve,[27] alone predicts a four-fold increase in cardiac complications and a 26% increase in 6-year mortality. In addition, important anatomic features that predict outcome, such as eccentricity of commissural fusion and a funnel-shaped subvalvular apparatus[28] (both negative predictors), are not included. Neither are the presence of moderate or severe mitral regurgitation or left atrial thrombus, both relative contraindications. In univariate analysis, the scoring system does predict long term results,[20] but so do age, presence of atrial fibrillation,[27] and severity of stenosis before and after the procedure.[29] Further, multivariate analyses that included the echo score *but not its individual components*, failed to

Table 50.1 Grading of mitral valve characteristics from the echocardiographic examination

Grade	Mobility	Subvalvar thickening	Thickening	Calcification
1	Highly mobile valve with only leaflet tips restricted	Minimal thickening just below the mitral leaflets	Leaflets near normal in thickness (4–5 mm)	A single area of increased echo brightness
2	Leaflet mid and base portions have normal mobility	Thickening of chordal structures extending up to one-third of the chordal length	Mid leaflets normal, considerable thickening of margins (5–8 mm)	Scattered areas of brightness confined to leaflet margins
3	Valve continues to move forward in diastole, mainly from the base	Thickening extending to the distal third of the chords	Thickening extending through the entire leaflet (5–8 mm)	Brightness extending into the mid portion of the leaflets
4	No or minimal forward movement of the leaflets in diastole	Extensive thickening and shortening of all chordal structures extending down to the papillary muscles	Considerable thickening of all leaflet tissue (>8–10 mm)	Extensive brightness throughout much of the leaflet tissue

Note. The total echocardiographic score was derived from an analysis of mitral leaflet mobility, valvar and subvalvar thickening, and calcification which were graded from 0 to 4 according to the above criteria. The total possible score ranges from 0 to 16. Reprinted with permission from Wilkins GT, Weyman AE, Abascal VM *et al.* Percutaneous balloon dilation of the mitral valve: an analysis of echocardiographic variables related to outcome and the mechanism of dilation. *British Heart Journal* **60**:299–309. Copyright ©1988 by the BMJ Publishing Group.[18]

demonstrate a single pre-procedure predictor of event-free survival.[30] Multivariate analysis that *includes* commissural calcification did reveal this to be a strong predictor of death, restenosis, and mitral valve replacement.[31] Perhaps the most compelling reason for routinely deriving the echo score is to allow for comparison with known data; most mitral valvuloplasty trials incorporate this or similar scoring systems. However, no absolute predictors of short and long term outcome have been developed.

Routine pre-procedure transesophageal echocardiography has been recommended because of its superiority for detection of left atrial thrombus,[32] as well as other structural abnormalities including vegetations or ruptured chordae. The case is most compelling in patients predisposed to clot formation such as those with spontaneous echo contrast ("smoke") on surface echocardiography and those with atrial fibrillation. The former was an independent predictor of left atrial thrombus in a prospective study of 100 patients.[33]

Cardiac catheterization

Cardiac catheterization prior to balloon commissurotomy is rarely necessary in young patients, but can be beneficial to exclude coronary artery disease in older subjects. The gradient alone is a poor proxy for assessment of severity of disease pre-valvuloplasty, since it can lead to overestimation of disease with poor heart rate control or underestimation in patients who have not had fluids for many hours prior to catheterization.

CONTRAINDICATIONS

While the usually cited contraindications are left atrial thrombus, greater than mild mitral regurgitation, severe calcification, or subvalvular disease, these were largely empirically derived and can be challenged.

Thrombus: Hung[34] and others have described at least three series involving a total of more than 70 patients with apparent organized left atrial appendage clot who underwent uncomplicated balloon commissurotomy. However, valvuloplasty should not be attempted when there is left atrial thrombus along the septum, free in the cavity, or on the surface of the valve.

Mitral regurgitation: The general presumption that valvuloplasty in patients with moderate or greater mitral regurgitation carried a high risk has not been prospectively tested; however, there have been two retrospective evaluations. A comparison of 25 patients with moderate mitral regurgitation and 25 age- and gender-matched patients with mild or no regurgitation did indeed demonstrate an increase in severe insufficiency post procedure; however, these patients had much higher echo scores and twice as frequently had severe calcification.[35] Further, while 20% of those with initially moderate mitral regurgitation developed severe regurgitation, hemodynamic improvement overall was similar, as was the incidence of post-procedure mitral valve replacement. Similarly, patients with mild mitral regurgitation also had less favorable anatomy at baseline and had lower event-free survival but a similar success rate.[36] Thus, the evidence suggests that balloon commissurotomy can still be considered for these patients if they are poor risks for heart surgery. Nevertheless, a theoretical disadvantage is additional volume loading of the left ventricle when antegrade flow is improved after balloon commissurotomy, a concern in the presence of aortic regurgitation as well.

Severe calcification: Patients with symmetric severe calcification may not respond at all to balloon commissurotomy;[22,37] those with asymmetric calcification are prone to leaflet tearing or rupture.[28] While high echo score alone does not predict the occurrence of severe mitral regurgitation,[38] one component, severe calcification, does.[39] Nevertheless, when the risk of surgery is prohibitive, growing experience with predominantly elderly patients with high echo scores and poor overall morphology has shown moderate improvement in hemodynamics and palliation of symptoms at the cost of high morbidity and mortality.[40]

PROCEDURE

Antegrade versus retrograde approaches

The predominant approach to percutaneous balloon mitral valvuloplasty is the antegrade transseptal approach. The techniques include single cylindrical balloon, Inoue, double and trefoil balloons, as well as monorail and metal valvulotomes. Inoue and the double cylindrical balloon methods account for virtually all mitral valvuloplasties performed.

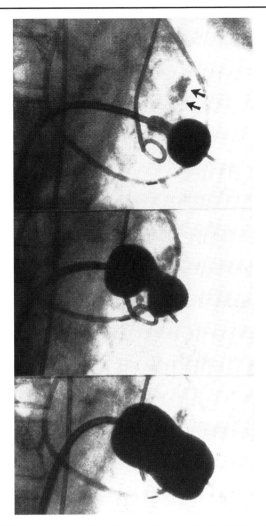

Figure 50.1 The Inoue balloon during staged deployment: (*top to bottom*) distal inflation with pullback against the valve; proximal inflation; full deployment. (Reprinted from Feldman *et al*.[38] with permission of the American Heart Association, Inc.)

The procedure has also been performed retrograde.[41–43] The advantages include avoidance of transseptal puncture; however, large devices are introduced into the femoral artery and balloons are passed across the submitral apparatus without balloon flotation (increasing the risk of catheter entrapment). There are no direct comparison studies between antegrade and retrograde techniques.

Inoue technique

The Inoue balloon's principal features are: a modifiable distal tip with reduced profile for transseptal passage, a nylon mesh covering that allows the balloon to straddle the mitral valve, and a compliance curve that allows the balloon to dilate over at least a 4 mm range of sizes (Figure 50.1). A stepwise approach involves evaluating the patient,

857

typically by echocardiography, between each balloon inflation to assess for improvement and detect presence of increasing mitral regurgitation. If improvement is suboptimal and regurgitation has not occurred/increased, the size is typically increased by one millimeter increments. In reviewing 19 series reporting results of Inoue valvuloplasty, a reported early success rate of 93% was noted in a total of 7091 patients.[44,45] Success was variably defined and in some reports overlapped with severe mitral regurgitation, atrial septal defect or embolic events, but included a doubling of the valve area in most studies.

Cylindrical balloon techniques

The cylindrical balloon technique, introduced in 1985,[46] did not uniformly result in adequate gradient reduction and gave way to a double balloon method.[47] A stepwise dilation technique is also used with progressively larger balloons placed side by side until adequate gradient reduction is obtained or an increase in mitral regurgitation is noted. The results of 12 studies incorporating 1864 patients reported a 90% overall success rate.

Long term follow-up

In an extraordinary series of 4832 patients across 120 centers in China, Chen and colleagues have claimed that 98.8% of patients were in NYHA functional Class I or II at a mean 32 months follow-up, with a 99.3% success rate, and virtually no complications.[48] Restenosis was reported as 5.2% over a mean 32 months follow-up. While there were likely problems with data gathering, the evidence from multiple studies of high success and low complication rates in patients with favorable anatomy is consistent.[20,49] Less favorable long term results were reported by Cohen et al.[50] for 145 patients followed for a mean of 3 years. Their 5-year event-free survival was only 51% (freedom from mitral valve replacement, redilation, or death); however, a high percentage of their patients had unfavorable anatomic features. In general, these descriptive series have suffered from incomplete follow-up, non-overlapping endpoints, and lack of serial hemodynamic measurements for assessing hemodynamics and restenosis.

Single vs double cylindrical balloons

The disadvantages of single balloons are related to the conundrum of a round balloon in an elliptical orifice – resulting in lower gradient reduction. Although no randomized comparisons were made, and much of the data are from sequential individual operator series, or sequential inflations with single followed by double balloons, the latter appears to be superior in retrospective comparisons (Figure 50.2)[52–54] as well as in an *in vitro* study.[55] The increased lateral force exerted by two balloons is one presumed mechanism for the superior splitting of the laterally directed commissures. However, a comparison of effective balloon dilating area to body surface area showed that a large single balloon could have similar hemodynamic benefits as two smaller balloons. Thus, geometry is not the sole determinant.

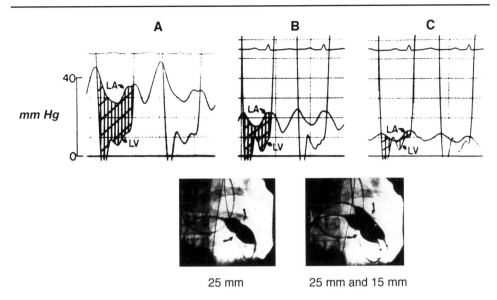

Figure 50.2 Single vs double balloon mitral valvotomy. Note the initial modest reduction of gradient from baseline (A) after single balloon commissurotomy (B), with near complete resolution of gradient after double balloon inflation (C). (Reprinted from Palacios *et al*.[51] with permission of the American Heart Association, Inc.)

Table 50.2 Comparative results of valvuloplasty techniques

	Inoue		Double balloon		Single balloon	
	MVA (mean ± SD)	*n*	MVA (mean ± SD)	*n*	MVA (mean ± SD)	*n*
Abdullah *et al*.[56]	1.9 ± 0.4	60	2.1 ± 0.5	60		
Arora *et al*.[57]	2.1 ± 0.4	310	2.2 ± 0.4	290		
Bassand *et al*.[58]	2.0 ± 0.5	71	2.0 ± 0.5	161		
Kasper *et al*.[59]	1.7 ± 0.7	23	2.2 ± 0.8	22		
Ortiz *et al*.[60]	1.8 ± 0.4	100	2.0 ± 0.5	36		
Park *et al*.[61 a]	1.9 ± 0.5	59	2.0 ± 0.5	61		
Rothlisberger *et al*.[62]	1.6 ± 0.6	145	1.8 ± 0.7	90		
Ruiz *et al*.[63]	1.9 ± 0.3	85	2.0 ± 0.6	322		
Sharma *et al*.[25]	2.2 ± 0.4	120	2.1 ± 0.5	230		
Trevino *et al*.[64]	2.0 ± 0.4	157	2.1 ± 0.5	56		
Zhang *et al*.[65]	1.8 ± 0.3	43	1.8 ± 0.4	43		
NHLBI *et al*.[66]			2.0 ± 0.8	591	1.7 ± 0.7	114

MVA, mitral valve area, in cm[2].
[a] This study was randomized.

Inoue vs double balloon (Table 50.2)

The Inoue technique's principal advantages are simplicity and short procedure times. The Inoue balloon differs from cylindrical single balloons because of the unique balloon design. The "slenderizing" feature that facilitates septal passage and the "dumbbell" shape of the inflated balloon have been reported by some to result in a lower incidence of atrial septal defect ($\leq 2.5\%$ vs up to 10% for the double balloon technique)[67] and a much lower likelihood of catastrophic apical perforation.

In a prospective randomized comparison between Inoue and double balloon valvotomy, no significant differences were noted in immediate results, including complications.[61] A trend toward fewer atrial septal defects with the Inoue balloon was not significant. Because of a lack of other prospective randomized comparisons by physicians equally experienced at both techniques, questions remain unanswered. It is likely that an easier procedure with lower complication rates (the Inoue technique) is a trade-off for slightly greater mitral regurgitation,[25,57] possibly because the distal portion of the balloon is oversized and may traumatize the subvalvular apparatus. There are also suggestive data that the double balloon technique, by virtue of the lateralization of forces, is advantageous in less favorable anatomy. One example is the result of dilation of asymmetrically fused commissures: where the Inoue technique has been used this led to significant risk of severe mitral regurgitation,[68] whereas with double balloon technique use this appeared to be less of a problem.[69] The disadvantages of the two balloon technique include longer procedure times, and higher risk of left ventricular apical perforation,[64,65,70,71] although the higher complication rates reported[58,64] may also reflect operator experience with this more complex procedure.

Intraprocedural transesophageal echocardiography

Use of transesophageal echocardiography "on-line" during balloon mitral valvuloplasty has been recommended for early detection of major complications (severe mitral regurgitation, tamponade, and large atrial septal defect).[72] In addition, transesophageal echo can confirm needle location during transseptal puncture.[73] Finally, decreased procedure time, mitral regurgitation, and residual atrial septal defects have been described in a randomized study of fluoroscopy plus transesophageal echo versus fluoroscopy without echo during balloon commissurotomy.[74] The evidence provided by these three studies is not compelling. The latter included a 60% rate of major complications in the non-echo group, suggesting limited experience. Surface two dimensional echocardiography is sensitive enough to detect increasing mitral regurgitation in most patients, and is an excellent tool for early appreciation of tamponade. Atrial septal defects are becoming substantially less common and are largely a post-procedure finding when they do occur. Finally, transseptal puncture in experienced hands has limited risk; arguably the procedure should not be performed by those who routinely need transesophageal echo guidance.

COMPLICATIONS

The learning curve is steep, which has had a major effect both on success and complication rates,[75] as well as skewing data in the literature.[67] The NHLBI Registry reported substantially lower rates of all major complications except acute mitral regurgitation at centers performing more than 25 cases and in the second year that sites enrolled patients; a willingness to attempt balloon commissurotomy in higher risk subsets in the second year may explain the mitral regurgitation. It is likely that the best interests of patients undergoing the procedure would be served by having relatively few centers perform a higher volume.

Overall mortality has been approximately 1%, most commonly related to tamponade not only from transseptal catheterization[76] but also from fenestration of the left ventricular apex, in particular by the cylindrical balloon technique. Tamponade has ranged from 2 to 4%, severe mitral regurgitation from 1 to 6%, and cerebral vascular accident and/or thromboembolism in up to 4%. Disturbingly, magnetic resonance imaging detected new hyperintensitivity foci suggestive of cerebral infarcts in 11 of 27 patients.[77] All had been evaluated before their procedure by transesophageal echocardiography without detection of clot. Thus, embolization may be common even if not clinically apparent. The probable sources are intracavitary clot, catheter-induced thrombus formation and showers of calcium.

Atrial septal defects were a significant source of early complications,[78] arising from transseptal tearing secondary to inadvertent proximal deployment of cylindrical balloons, withdrawal of winged balloons retrograde, or trauma to the septum from 5 or 8 mm balloons used to dilate the septum. Theoretically these problems should be avoidable by use of a dilator and a shorter balloon system, both features of the Inoue technique, and indeed this has been the finding.[79] It should be noted that decompression of the left atrium by a significant sized post-procedure atrial septal defect may have influenced the results of some balloon valvuloplasty series and may lead operators to overestimate the mitral valve area post procedure.[80]

Valvuloplasty for mild mitral stenosis

Several studies have looked retrospectively at the results of balloon valvuloplasty for patients with valve areas of $\geq 1.3–1.5\,cm^2$.[81,82] While historical comparisons suggest greater valve area increase than in patients with severe mitral stenosis, there is no evidence that the risk of occasional mortality, need for mitral valve replacement or other major morbidity warrants this approach. The possibility that early commissurotomy may affect the course of the disease, including progression to pulmonary hypertension, atrial fibrillation, and stroke, remains a hypothesis in need of prospective investigation.[83]

Pregnancy

There have been multiple reports of successful balloon commissurotomy during pregnancy.[84–86] The procedure has been performed with echo guidance and without fluoroscopy[87] to avoid radiation exposure to the fetus.

Dilation for restenosis

Reoperation for mitral valve stenosis has long been associated with increased morbidity and mortality.[88] Similarly several large balloon commissurotomy series have reported inferior overall results compared to de novo dilation. Davidson reported less symptomatic improvement[89] while Jang described a 20% lower success rate (only 51% having a valve area $>1.5\,cm^2$) and nearly 20% requiring mitral valve replacement by 4 years.[90] Cohen

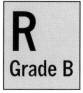

described twice the frequency[91] and Medina described a 10-fold increase in restenosis rates at 5 years for patients with prior commissurotomy[92] (both to approximately 20%). Most significant is the finding by Jang and colleagues that stratification by echo score resulted in nearly superimposable results for de novo and repeat commissurotomy procedures, suggesting that results are defined by valve morphology rather than history of prior commissurotomy.[90]

Bioprosthesis

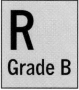

Several case reports have described successful balloon dilation of bioprosthetic mitral valves, although both the hemodynamic and longer term benefits were obscure in all but one.[93-95] However, bioprosthetic valves are typically similar histologically to those seen in calcific aortic stenosis: severe leaflet thickening, immobility and calcification, without commissural fusion.[96,97] Thus, a formal intraoperative study, examining the morphology of severely stenosed bioprosthetic valves before and after balloon dilation, revealed "completely ineffectual" dilation[98] with substantial leaflet tearing and cuspal perforation. Although the need for a percutaneous approach to the problem is great, the data do not support bioprosthetic mitral valve dilation.

Balloon vs closed surgical commissurotomy

Randomized trials comparing balloon and surgical commissurotomy were begun early in the development phase of the percutaneous technique. Because both are blind dilation of the valve with blunt instruments, and because closed commissurotomy was the predominant procedure in countries where mitral stenosis was prevalent, the early randomized trials compared balloon and closed commissurotomy. In these studies, surgeons were typically more experienced than the operators performing balloon valvuloplasty. In 1988 we randomized 40 patients with relatively ideal anatomy and severe mitral stenosis;[99] these patients have been followed with serial catheterization and echocardiography over a 7-year period. There were similar hemodynamic improvements in both groups, sustained through 7 years (Figure 50.3), with one late death in each group and need for repeat commissurotomy in 20%.[100] The actual restenosis rate (26% in the balloon group and 35% in the surgical group) as defined by a 50% loss of the gain and a valve area <1.5 cm², is significantly higher than the repeat commissurotomy rate because restenosis and functional class do not correlate strongly. Thus it is likely that restenosis rates in trials that have not done formal follow-up hemodynamics underestimated the true severity of disease during follow-up. Two other studies have compared balloon and closed commissurotomy with shorter, non-invasive follow-up only; these have demonstrated balloon results superior to[75] or similar to closed commissurotomy.[101] However, closed commissurotomy in the former study resulted in only a 1.3 cm² mean valve area, suggesting relatively unaggressive dilation. Finally, a randomized comparison by Ben Farhat and colleagues described superior acute results (2.2 ± 0.4 cm² vs 1.6 ± 0.4 cm²) for balloon valvuloplasty and a 4-year restenosis rate of 7% vs 37%.[102] Thus, balloon commissurotomy is at least equal and probably superior to closed surgical commissurotomy.

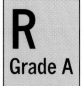

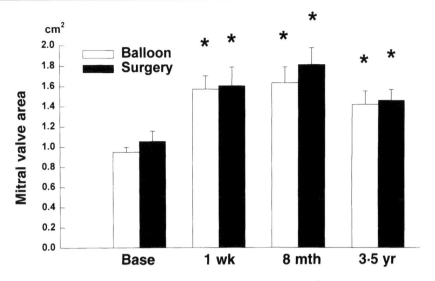

Figure 50.3 Mitral valve areas at baseline and each follow-up interval over $3\frac{1}{2}$ years in patients randomized to percutaneous balloon or surgical closed mitral commissurotomy.[100] Asterisk denotes $P<0.001$ compared with baseline.

Open commissurotomy vs balloon

The hypothesis that open commissurotomy would be superior to balloon valvuloplasty was based on the potential benefits of direct vision, including surgical splitting and remodeling of the subvalvular apparatus, neither of which is a feature of closed or balloon commissurotomy. A prospective series of 100 open commissurotomy patients had data gathering specifically for historical comparison to the then reported results of balloon valvuloplasty and concluded that open commissurotomy was distinctly superior.[103] The results of surgery – mean valve area 2.9 cm² – exceed expectations and may be related to technique of measurement[104] or patient selection, while mitral regurgitation was absent in all but 8 cases (where it was reported to be mild), results that are also testimony to great operator skill, but are in excess of prior reports.[8] On the contrary, the more compelling evidence from prospective randomized studies is for similar or superior results with balloon commissurotomy. In 1989 we randomized 60 patients to a prospective comparison of balloon vs open commissurotomy.[105] Patients had near identical baseline hemodynamics but those undergoing balloon commissurotomy had superior mitral valve areas at 3 years (Figure 50.4). A possible explanation for superior results in balloon commissurotomy patients is the direct and continuous feedback to the operator of hemodynamics during catheterization laboratory procedures, which even with the advent of transesophageal monitoring in the operating room is not available to the same degree to the surgeon.

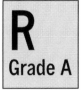

In the trial referred to earlier, Ben Farhat and colleagues[102] randomized 30 patients to balloon valvuloplasty as well as closed and open commissurotomy. In contrast to their findings with closed commissurotomy, the results for balloon and open commissurotomy were similar through 4 years.

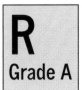

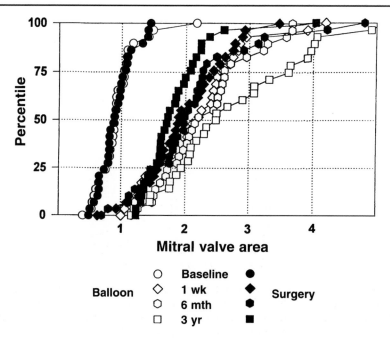

Figure 50.4 Mitral valve areas at baseline and at each follow-up interval in patients randomized to balloon or open surgical commissurotomy. The values represent the percentile of patients whose valve areas are ≤ the valve area on the abscissa. The baseline values overlap, but a shift to the right (representing higher valve areas) is seen for the balloon group at each time point. (Reprinted by permission of the *New England Journal of Medicine*. Copyright © 1994, Massachusetts Medical Society.[105])

Cost

Although formal cost comparison studies have not been reported, charges and costs at hospitals in India and in the United States have been estimated. Lau and Ruiz described cost to a United States hospital of $3000 for balloon valvuloplasty and $6000 for closed commissurotomy (assuming a hospital could be found that still performs this procedure). We published 1991 charges for balloon and closed commissurotomy in the United States and India (Figure 50.5) and demonstrated a potential six-fold greater expense for balloon valvuloplasty in India. However, our calculations did not include the extensive reuse of disposables in developing countries, where balloons can account for a much higher portion of the charges than physicians' fees or operating room billings.

The results of the randomized trials offer compelling evidence that balloon valvuloplasty is an effective alternative to surgery for patients with good valve anatomy. Even with a number of anatomic features predicting less favorable outcome, balloon commissurotomy, at the cost of higher risk in patients with unfavorable anatomy, still has the potential for palliation. The safety and efficacy of Inoue and double balloon valvuloplasty are not compellingly different in experienced hands and the selection of techniques should be based on operator preference, experience, and equipment availability. Low cost, avoidance of thoracotomy scar and discomfort, shorter hospitalization and excellent follow-up results to date mandate consideration of balloon valvuloplasty in most patients with rheumatic mitral valve stenosis without significant contraindications. Since balloon as well as surgical commissurotomy are largely palliative

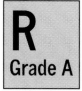

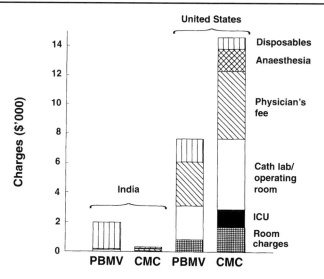

Figure 50.5 Charges for percutaneous balloon mitral valvuloplasty (PBMV) and closed surgical commissurotomy (CMC) at the Nizam's Institute of Medical Sciences in Hyderabad, India and at Harper Hospital in Detroit, MI in 1991. With the extensive reuse of disposables in developing countries, the cost of balloon valvuloplasty more closely approximates that for closed commissurotomy. (Copyright © 1993, F.A. Davis Co. Reprinted with permission.[106])

procedures, percutaneous balloon valvuloplasty has the added benefit of delaying the time until eventual thoracotomy.

In summary, percutaneous balloon mitral valvuloplasty is a superior alternative to surgical commissurotomy for a significant subset of patients with rheumatic mitral stenosis. Careful case selection and performance of the procedure by experienced teams will have a significant impact on outcome. Both clinical and financial considerations suggest that balloon valvuloplasty is the procedure of choice for rheumatic mitral stenosis in patients with suitable anatomy.

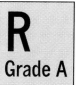

Key points

- Ideal patients have severe mitral stenosis without:
    > mild mitral regurgitation, severe subvalvular disease, or severe calcification;
    eccentric commissural fusion, clot in left atrium, volume loaded left ventricle.
- Procedure may be of benefit in:
    < critical mitral stenosis, but evidence for favorable long-term risk–benefit ratio is lacking;
    patients with unfavorable anatomy, including moderate mitral regurgitation, but with less favorable results and higher morbidity/mortality;
    patients with mitral restenosis, dependent on anatomic features;
    pregnant patients.
- Balloon valvuloplasty is superior to closed commissurotomy and is equivalent or superior to open commissurotomy in ideal patients.

REFERENCES

1 Cutler EC, Levine SA. Cardiotomy and valvulotomy for mitral stenosis. Experimental observations and clinical notes concerning an operated case with recovery. *Boston Med Surg J* 1923;**188**:1023–7.

2 Suttar HS. The surgical treatment of mitral stenosis. *Br Med J* 1925;**2**:603–6.

3 Lewis T. *Diseases of the heart*, 3rd edn. London: Macmillan, 1943.

4 John S, Bashi VV, Jairaj PS *et al.* Closed mitral valvotomy: early results and long-term follow-up of 3724 consecutive patients. *Circulation* 1983;**68**:891–6.

5 Toumbouras M, Panagopoulos F, Papakonstantinou C *et al.* Long-term surgical outcome of closed mitral commissurotomy. *J Heart Valve Dis* 1995;**4**(3):247–50.

6 Rihal CS, Schaff HV, Frye RL *et al.* Long-term follow-up of patients undergoing closed transventricular mitral commissurotomy: a useful surrogate for percutaneous balloon mitral valvuloplasty? *J Am Coll Cardiol* 1992;**20**:781–6.

7 Scalia D, Rizzoli G, Campanile F *et al.* Long-term results of mitral commissurotomy. *J Thorac Cardiovasc Surg* 1993;**105**:633–42.

8 Villanova C, Melacini P, Scognamiglio R *et al.* Long-term echocardiographic evaluation of closed and open mitral valvulotomy. *Int J Cardiol* 1993;**38**:315–21.

9 Hickey MS, Blackstone EH, Kirklin JW, Dean LS. Outcome probabilities and life history after surgical mitral commissurotomy: implications for balloon commissurotomy. *J Am Coll Cardiol* 1991;**17**:29–42.

10 Inoue K, Kitamura F, Chikusa H, Miyamoto N. Atrial septostomy by a new balloon catheter. *Jpn Circ J* 1981;**45**:730–8.

11 Inoue K, Nakamura T, Kitamura F. Nonoperative mitral commissurotomy by a new balloon catheter [abstract] *Jpn Circ J* 1982;**46**:877.

12 Inoue K, Owaki T, Nakamura T, Kitamura F, Miyamoto N. Clinical application of transvenous mitral commissurotomy by a new balloon catheter. *J Thorac Cardiovasc Surg* 1984;**87**:394–402.

13 Block PC, Palacios IF, Jacobs ML, Fallon JT. Mechanism of percutaneous mitral valvotomy. *Am J Cardiol* 1987;**59**:178–9.

14 Matsuura Y, Fukunaga S, Ishihara H *et al.* Mechanics of percutaneous balloon valvotomy for mitral valvular stenosis. *Heart Vessels* 1988;**4**:179–83.

15 Nabel E, Bergin PJ, Kirsh MM. Morphological analysis of balloon mitral valvuloplasty; intraoperative results. [abstract]. *J Am Coll Cardiol* 1990;**15**:97A.

16 Kaplan JD, Isner JM, Karas RH *et al. In vitro* analysis of mechanisms of balloon valvuloplasty of stenotic mitral valves. *Am J Cardiol* 1987;**59**:318–23.

17 McKay RG, Lock JE, Safian RD *et al.* Balloon dilation of mitral stenosis in adult patients: postmortem and percutaneous mitral valvuloplasty studies. *J Am Coll Cardiol* 1987;**9**:723–31.

18 Wilkins GT, Weyman AE, Abascal VM, Block PC, Palacios IF. Percutaneous balloon dilatation of the mitral valve: an analysis of echocardiographic variables related to outcome and the mechanism of dilatation. *Br Heart J* 1988;**60**:299–308.

19 Desideri A, Vanderperren O, Serra A *et al.* Long-term (9 to 33 months) echocardiographic follow-up after successful percutaneous mitral commissurotomy. *Am J Cardiol* 1992;**69**:1602–6.

20 Palacios IF, Tuzcu ME, Weyman AE, Newell JB, Block PC. Clinical follow-up of patients undergoing percutaneous mitral balloon valvotomy. *Circulation* 1995;**91**(3):671–6.

21 Abascal VM, Wilkins GT, O'Shea JP *et al.* Prediction of successful outcome in 130 patients undergoing percutaneous balloon mitral valvotomy. *Circulation* 1990;**82**:448–56.

22 Fatkin D, Roy P, Morgan JJ, Feneley MP. Percutaneous balloon mitral valvotomy with the Inoue single-balloon catheter: commissural morphology as a determinant of outcome. *J Am Coll Cardiol* 1993;**21**:390–7.

23 Levin TN, Feldman T, Bednarz J, Carroll JD, Lang RM. Transesophageal echocardiographic evaluation of mitral valve morphology to predict outcome after balloon mitral valvotomy. *Am J Cardiol* 1994;**73**(9):707–10.

24 Herrmann HC, Ramaswamy K, Isner JM *et al.* Factors influencing immediate results, complications, and short-term follow-up status after Inoue balloon mitral valvotomy: a North American multicenter study. *Am Heart J* 1992; **124**:160–6.

25 Sharma S, Loya YS, Desai DM, Pinto RJ. Percutaneous mitral valvotomy using Inoue and double balloon technique: comparison of clinical and hemodynamic short term results in 350 cases. *Cathet Cardiovasc Diagn* 1993;**29**:18–23.

26 Reid CL, Chandraratna PA, Kawanishi DT, Kotlewski A, Rahimtoola SH. Influence of mitral valve morphology on double-balloon catheter balloon valvuloplasty in patients with mitral stenosis. Analysis of factors predicting immediate and 3-month results. *Circulation* 1989;**80**: 515–24.

27 Zhang HP, Allen JW, Lau FY, Ruiz CE. Immediate and late outcome of percutaneous balloon mitral

valvotomy in patients with significantly calcified valves. *Am Heart J* 1995;**129**(3):501–6.

28 Miche E, Fassbender D, Minami K *et al.* Pathomorphological characteristics of resected mitral valves after unsuccessful valvuloplasty. *J Cardiovasc Surg* 1996;**37**:475–81.

29 Ruiz CE, Zhang HP, Gamra H, Allen JW, Lau FY. Late clinical and echocardiographic follow up after percutaneous balloon dilatation of the mitral valve. *Br Heart J* 1994;**71**(5):454–8.

30 Orrange SE, Kawanishi DT, Lopez BM, Curry SM, Rahimtoola SH. Actuarial outcome after catheter balloon commissurotomy in patients with mitral stenosis. *Circulation* 1997;**95**(2): 382–9.

31 Cannan CR, Nishimura RA, Reeder GS *et al.* Echocardiographic assessment of commissural calcium: a simple predictor of outcome after percutaneous mitral balloon valvotomy. *J Am Coll Cardiol* 1997;**29**(1):175–80.

32 Kronzon I, Tunick PA, Glassman E *et al.* Transesophageal echocardiography to detect atrial clots in candidates for percutaneous transseptal mitral balloon valvuloplasty. *J Am Coll Cardiol* 1990;**16**:1320–2.

33 Rittoo D, Sutherland GR, Currie P, Starkey IR, Shaw TR. A prospective study of left atrial spontaneous echo contrast and thrombus in 100 consecutive patients referred for balloon dilation of the mitral valve. *J Am Soc Echocardiogr* 1994; **7**(5):516–27.

34 Hung JS. Mitral stenosis with left atrial thrombi: Inoue balloon catheter technique. In: Cheng TO (ed) *Percutaneous balloon valvuloplasty.* New York: Igaku-Shoin, 1992, pp 280–3.

35 Zhang HP, Gamra H, Allen JW, Lau FY, Ruiz CE. Balloon valvotomy for mitral stenosis associated with moderate mitral regurgitation. *Am J Cardiol* 1995;**75**(14):960–3.

36 Alfonso F, Macaya C, Hernandez R *et al.* Early and late results of percutaneous mitral valvuloplasty for mitral stenosis associated with mild mitral regurgitation. *Am J Cardiol* 1993; **71**:1304–10.

37 Tuzcu EM, Block PC, Griffin B *et al.* Percutaneous mitral balloon valvotomy in patients with calcific mitral stenosis: immediate and long-term outcome. *J Am Coll Cardiol* 1994;**23**(7):1604–9.

38 Feldman T, Carroll JD, Isner JM *et al.* Effect of valve deformity on results and mitral regurgitation after Inoue balloon commissurotomy. *Circulation* 1992;**85**:180–7.

39 Herrmann HC, Lima JA, Feldman T *et al.* Mechanisms and outcome of severe mitral regurgitation after Inoue balloon valvuloplasty. North American Inoue Balloon Investigators. *J Am Coll Cardiol* 1993;**22**:783–9.

40 Tuzcu EM, Block PC, Griffin BP *et al.* Immediate and long-term outcome of percutaneous mitral

valvotomy in patients 65 years and older. *Circulation* 1992;**85**:963–71.

41 Bahl VK, Juneja R, Thatai D *et al.* Retrograde nontransseptal balloon mitral valvuloplasty for rheumatic mitral stenosis. *Cathet Cardiovasc Diagn* 1994;**33**(4):331–4.

42 Stefanadis C, Stratos C, Kallikazaros I *et al.* Retrograde nontransseptal balloon mitral valvuloplasty using a modified Inoue balloon catheter. *Cathet Cardiovasc Diagn* 1994;**33**(3): 224–33.

43 Stefanadis C, Stratos C, Pitsavos C *et al.* Retrograde nontransseptal balloon mitral valvuloplasty. Immediate results and long-term follow-up. *Circulation* 1992;**85**:1760–7.

44 Lau KW, Hung JS, Ding ZP, Johan A. Controversies in balloon mitral valvuloplasty: the when (timing for intervention), what (choice of valve), and how (selection of technique). *Cathet Cardiovasc Diagn* 1995;**35**(2):91–100.

45 Glazier JJ, Turi ZG. Percutaneous balloon mitral valvuloplasty. *Prog Cardiovasc Dis* 1997;**40**(1): 5–26.

46 Lock JE, Khalilullah M, Shrivastava S, Bahl V, Keane JF. Percutaneous catheter commissurotomy in rheumatic mitral stenosis. *N Engl J Med* 1985;**313**:1515–18.

47 al Zaibag M, Ribeiro PA, Al Kasab S, al Fagih MR. Percutaneous double-balloon mitral valvotomy for rheumatic mitral-valve stenosis. *Lancet* 1986; **i**:757–61.

48 Chen CR, Cheng TO. Percutaneous balloon mitral valvuloplasty by the Inoue technique: a multicenter study of 4832 patients in China. *Am Heart J* 1995;**129**(6):1197–203.

49 Iung B, Cormier B, Ducimetiere P *et al.* Functional results 5 years after successful percutaneous mitral commissurotomy in a series of 528 patients and analysis of predictive factors. *J Am Coll Cardiol* 1996;**27**(2):407–14.

50 Cohen DJ, Kuntz RE, Gordon SP *et al.* Predictors of long-term outcome after percutaneous balloon mitral valvuloplasty. *N Engl J Med* 1992;**327**: 1329–35.

51 Palacios I, Block PC, Brandi S *et al.* Percutaneous balloon valvotomy for patients with severe mitral stenosis. *Circulation* 1987;**75**:778–84.

52 Shrivastava S, Mathur A, Dev V *et al.* Comparison of immediate hemodynamic response to closed mitral commissurotomy, single-balloon, and double-balloon mitral valvuloplasty in rheumatic mitral stenosis. *J Thorac Cardiovasc Surg* 1992;**104**(5):1264–7.

53 Al Kasab S, Ribeiro PA, Sawyer W. Comparison of results of percutaneous balloon mitral valvotomy using consecutive single (25 mm) and double (25 mm and 12 mm) balloon techniques. *Am J Cardiol* 1989;**64**:1385–7.

54 Chen CG, Wang YP, Qing D, Lin YS, Lan YF. Percutaneous mitral balloon dilatation by a new sequential single- and double-balloon technique. *Am Heart J* 1988;**116**:1161–7.

55 Ribeiro PA, al Zaibag M, Rajendran V *et al.* Mechanism of mitral valve area increase by *in vitro* single and double balloon mitral valvotomy. *Am J Cardiol* 1988;**62**:264–9.

56 Abdullah M, Halim M, Rajendran V, Sawyer W, al Zaibag M. Comparison between single (Inoue) and double balloon mitral valvuloplasty: immediate and short-term results. *Am Heart J* 1992;**123**:1581–8.

57 Arora R, Kalra GS, Murty GS *et al.* Percutaneous transatrial mitral commissurotomy: immediate and intermediate results. *J Am Coll Cardiol* 1994;**23**(6):1327–32.

58 Bassand JP, Schiele F, Bernard Y *et al.* The double-balloon and Inoue techniques in percutaneous mitral valvuloplasty: comparative results in a series of 232 cases. *J Am Coll Cardiol* 1991;**18**:982–9.

59 Kasper W, Wollschlager H, Geibel A, Meinertz T, Just H. Percutaneous mitral balloon valvuloplasty – a comparative evaluation of two transatrial techniques. *Am Heart J* 1992;**124**(6):1562–6.

60 Ortiz FA, Macaya C, Alfonso F. Mono- versus double-balloon technique for commissural splitting after percutaneous mitral valvotomy. *Am J Cardiol* 1992;**69**:1100–1.

61 Park SJ, Kim JJ, Park SW *et al.* Immediate and one-year results of percutaneous mitral balloon valvuloplasty using Inoue and double-balloon techniques. *Am J Cardiol* 1993;**71**:938–43.

62 Rothlisberger C, Essop MR, Skudicky D *et al.* Results of percutaneous balloon mitral valvotomy in young adults. *Am J Cardiol* 1993;**72**:73–7.

63 Ruiz CE, Zhang HP, Macaya C *et al.* Comparison of Inoue single-balloon versus double-balloon technique for percutaneous mitral valvotomy. *Am Heart J* 1992;**123**:942–7.

64 Trevino AJ, Ibarra M, Garcia A *et al.* Immediate and long-term results of balloon mitral commissurotomy for rheumatic mitral stenosis: comparison between Inoue and double-balloon techniques. *Am Heart J* 1996;**131**(3):530–6.

65 Zhang HP, Gamra H, Allen JW, Lau FY, Ruiz CE. Comparison of late outcome between Inoue balloon and double-balloon techniques for percutaneous mitral valvotomy in a matched study. *Am Heart J* 1995;**130**(2):340–4.

66 Multicenter experience with balloon mitral commissurotomy. NHLBI Balloon Valvuloplasty Registry Report on immediate and 30-day follow-up results. The National Heart, Lung, and Blood Institute Balloon Valvuloplasty Registry participants. *Circulation* 1992;**85**:448–61.

67 Complications and mortality of percutaneous balloon mitral commissurotomy. A report from the National Heart, Lung, and Blood Institute Balloon Valvuloplasty Registry. *Circulation* 1992;**85**:2014–24.

68 Miche E, Bogunovic N, Fassbender D *et al.* Predictors of unsuccessful outcome after percutaneous mitral valvulotomy including a new echocardiographic scoring system. *J Heart Valve Dis* 1996;**5**:430–5.

69 Rodriguez L, Monterroso VH, Abascal VM *et al.* Does asymmetric mitral valve disease predict an adverse outcome after percutaneous balloon mitral valvotomy? An echocardiographic study. *Am Heart J* 1992;**123**:1678–82.

70 Fu XY, Zhang DD, Schiele F *et al.* Complications of percutaneous mitral valvuloplasty; comparison of the double balloon and the Inoue techniques. *Arch Mal Coeur Vaiss* 1994;**87**(11):1403–11.

71 Rihal CS, Nishimura RA, Reeder GS, Holmes DR Jr. Percutaneous balloon mitral valvuloplasty: comparison of double and single (Inoue) balloon techniques. *Cathet Cardiovasc Diagn* 1993;**29**:183–90.

72 Goldstein SA, Campbell A, Mintz GS *et al.* Feasibility of on-line transesophageal echocardiography during balloon mitral valvulotomy: experience with 93 patients. *J Heart Valve Dis* 1994;**3**(2):136–48.

73 Ballal RS, Mahan EF, Nanda NC, Dean LS. Utility of transesophageal echocardiography in interatrial septal puncture during percutaneous mitral balloon commissurotomy. *Am J Cardiol* 1990;**66**:230–2.

74 Ramondo A, Chirillo F, Dan M *et al.* Value and limitations of transesophageal echocardiographic monitoring during percutaneous balloon mitral valvotomy. *Int J Cardiol* 1991;**31**:223–33.

75 Rihal CS, Nishimura RA, Holmes DR Jr. Percutaneous balloon mitral valvuloplasty: the learning curve. *Am Heart J* 1991;**122**:1750–6.

76 Schoonmaker FW, Vijay NK, Jantz RD. Left atrial and ventricular transseptal catheterization review: losing skills. *Cathet Cardiovasc Diagn* 1987;**13**:233–8.

77 Rocha P, Mulot R, Lacombe P *et al.* Brain magnetic resonance imaging before and after percutaneous mitral balloon commissurotomy. *Am J Cardiol* 1994;**74**(9):955–7.

78 Yoshida K, Yoshikawa J, Akasaka T *et al.* Assessment of left-to-right atrial shunting after percutaneous mitral valvuloplasty by transesophageal color Doppler flow-mapping. *Circulation* 1989;**80**:1521–6.

79 Thomas MR, Monaghan MJ, Metcalfe JM, Jewitt DE. Residual atrial septal defects following

balloon mitral valvuloplasty using different techniques. A transthoracic and transoesophageal echocardiography study demonstrating an advantage of the Inoue balloon. *Eur Heart J* 1992;**13**:496–502.

80 Petrossian GA, Tuzcu EM, Ziskind AA, Block PC, Palacios I. Atrial septal occlusion improves the accuracy of mitral valve area determination following percutaneous mitral balloon valvotomy. *Cathet Cardiovasc Diagn* 1991;**22**: 21–4.

81 Pan M, Medina A, Suarez De Lezo J *et al*. Balloon valvuloplasty for mild mitral stenosis. *Cathet Cardiovasc Diagn* 1991;**24**:1–5.

82 Herrmann HC, Feldman T, Isner JM *et al*. Comparison of results of percutaneous balloon valvuloplasty in patients with mild and moderate mitral stenosis to those with severe mitral stenosis. The North American Inoue Balloon Investigators. *Am J Cardiol* 1993;**71**:1300–3.

83 Turi ZG. Mitral balloon valvuloplasty [Letter; comment]. *Cathet Cardiovasc Diagn* 1992;**25**: 343–4.

84 Glantz JC, Pomerantz RM, Cunningham MJ, Woods JR Jr. Percutaneous balloon valvuloplasty for severe mitral stenosis during pregnancy: a review of therapeutic options. *Obstet Gynecol Surv* 1993;**48**:503–8.

85 Patel JJ, Mitha AS, Hassen F *et al*. Percutaneous balloon mitral valvotomy in pregnant patients with tight pliable mitral stenosis. *Am Heart J* 1993;**125**:1106–9.

86 Ribeiro PA, Fawzy ME, Awad M, Dunn B, Duran CG. Balloon valvotomy for pregnant patients with severe pliable mitral stenosis using the Inoue technique with total abdominal and pelvic shielding. *Am Heart J* 1992;**124**:1558–62.

87 Kultursay H, Turkoglu C, Akin M *et al*. Mitral balloon valvuloplasty with transesophageal echocardiography without using fluoroscopy. *Cathet Cardiovasc Diagn* 1992;**27**:317–21.

88 Harken DE, Black H, Taylor WJ, Thrower WB, Ellis LB. Reoperation for mitral stenosis. A discussion of postoperative deterioration and methods of improving initial and secondary operation. *Circulation* 1961;**23**:7–12.

89 Davidson CJ, Bashore TM, Mickel M, Davis K. Balloon mitral commissurotomy after previous surgical commissurotomy. The National Heart, Lung, and Blood Institute Balloon Valvuloplasty Registry participants. *Circulation* 1992;**86**:91–9.

90 Jang IK, Block PC, Newell JB, Tuzcu EM, Palacios IF. Percutaneous mitral balloon valvotomy for recurrent mitral stenosis after surgical commissurotomy. *Am J Cardiol* 1995;**75**(8): 601–5.

91 Cohen JM, Glower DD, Harrison JK *et al*. Comparison of balloon valvuloplasty with operative treatment for mitral stenosis. *Ann Thorac Surg* 1993;**56**:1254–62.

92 Medina A, de Lezo JS, Hernandez E *et al*. Mitral restenosis: the Cordoba–Las Palmas experience. In: Cheng TO (ed) *Percutaneous balloon valvuloplasty*. New York: Igaku–Shoin, 1992, pp 294–304.

93 Calvo OL, Sobrino N, Gamallo C *et al*. Balloon percutaneous valvuloplasty for stenotic bioprosthetic valves in the mitral position. *Am J Cardiol* 1987;**60**:736–7.

94 Cox DA, Friedman PL, Selwyn AP, Lee RT, Bittl JA. Improved quality of life after successful balloon valvuloplasty of a stenosed mitral bioprosthesis. *Am Heart J* 1989;**118**:839–41.

95 Babic UU, Grujicic S, Vucinic M. Balloon valvoplasty of mitral bioprosthesis. *Int J Cardiol* 1991;**30**:230–2.

96 Waller BF, McKay C, VanTassel J, Allen M. Catheter balloon valvuloplasty of stenotic porcine bioprosthetic valves: Part II: mechanisms, complications, and recommendations for clinical use. *Clin Cardiol* 1991;**14**:764–72.

97 Waller BF, McKay C, Van Tassel J, Allen M. Catheter balloon valvuloplasty of stenotic porcine bioprosthetic valves: Part I: anatomic considerations. *Clin Cardiol* 1991;**14**: 686–91.

98 Lin PJ, Chang JP, Chu JJ, Chang CH, Hung JS. Balloon valvuloplasty is contraindicated in stenotic mitral bioprostheses. *Am Heart J* 1994; **127**(3):724–6.

99 Turi ZG, Reyes VP, Raju BS *et al*. Percutaneous balloon versus surgical closed commissurotomy for mitral stenosis. A prospective, randomized trial. *Circulation* 1991;**83**:1179–85.

100 Raju BS, Turi ZG, Raju R *et al*. Three and one-half year follow-up of a randomized trial comparing percutaneous balloon and surgical closed mitral commissurotomy. [abstract] *J Am Coll Cardiol* 1993;**21**:429A.

101 Arora R, Nair M, Kalra GS, Nigam M, Khalilullah M. Immediate and long-term results of balloon and surgical closed mitral valvotomy: a randomized comparative study. *Am Heart J* 1993;**125**:1091–4.

102 Ben Farhat M, Ayari M, Betbout F. Percutaneous balloon versus surgical closed and open mitral commissurotomy: short and long term results [abstract]. *J Am Coll Cardiol* 1993;**21**:428A.

103 Antunes MJ, Nascimento J, Andrade CM, Fernandes LE. Open mitral commissurotomy: a better procedure? *J Heart Valve Dis* 1994;**3**(1): 88–92.

104 Acar J. Open mitral commissurotomy or percutaneous mitral commissurotomy? [Editorial]. *J Heart Valve Dis* 1994;**3**(2): 133–5.

105 Reyes VP, Raju BS, Wynne J *et al.* Percutaneous balloon valvuloplasty compared with open surgical commissurotomy for mitral stenosis. *N Engl J Med* 1994;**331**:961–7.

106 Turi ZG, Valvuloplasty. In: Frankel W, Brest A (eds) *Valvular heart disease: comprehensive evaluation and treatment*, 2nd edn. Philadelphia: FA Davis, 1993, pp 293–326.

Valve repair and choice of valves

51

PAUL J. PEARSON,
HARTZELL V. SCHAFF

INTRODUCTION

Changes in treatment of mitral regurgitation provide a classic example of how advances in surgical technique influence the overall strategy of medical management of valvular heart disease, including both the indications for and timing of operation. In North America, degenerative diseases such as floppy valves and ruptured chordae tendineae are the most common causes of non-ischemic mitral valve regurgitation.[1–3]

Previously, clinicians observed patients with mitral regurgitation until symptoms developed or until there was evidence of left ventricular failure. Usually, operation resulted in replacement of the valve with a prosthesis. This left the patient with ventricular dysfunction, irreversible in some cases, and also the attendant prosthesis-related risks such as thromboembolism, hemorrhage cased by systemic anticoagulation, infection, and risks of mechanical failure. The advent of mitral valve repair, with its predictability and safety, lead to new criteria for intervention. Indeed, early operation for valve repair should be considered for all patients with severe mitral regurgitation.[4,5]

TIMING OF OPERATION FOR MITRAL VALVE REGURGITATION

Mitral valve regurgitation often progresses slowly and because of favorable loading conditions, left ventricular dysfunction can develop even though systolic indices of left ventricular performance are maintained. Indeed, with severe mitral valve regurgitation, normal ventricular function should result in a hyperdynamic left ventricle with a supranormal ejection fraction. When the ejection fraction falls below 60% in the presence of severe mitral regurgitation, the prognosis of patients after surgical correction worsens[4] (Figure 51.1). However, the relative insensitivity of ejection fraction in gauging ventricular performance in patients with mitral regurgitation has led to the development of indices of left ventricular function that are less dependent on preload, such as end

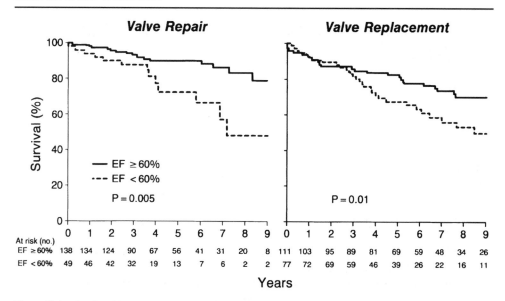

Figure 51.1 Graphs of late survival according to preoperative ejection fraction (EF) after valve repair (left) and valve replacement (right). (From Enriquez-Sarano *et al.*[4])

systolic dimension. Again, prognosis after valve repair or replacement is poor when preoperative left ventricular end systolic dimension exceeds 45 mm.[4] Thus, even in an asymptomatic patient with an ejection fraction greater than 60%, if left ventricular end systolic diameter approaches 45 mm, valve repair should be seriously considered.[4]

VALVE REPAIR VERSUS REPLACEMENT

There are no prospective, randomized studies comparing outcomes after mitral valve repair with replacement for mitral regurgitation. In addition, it is often difficult to compare these two modes of surgical treatment by review of the literature because of heterogeneous patient populations.[6] Patients with anatomy favorable to valve repair may have less advanced disease when compared to those patients in which valve replacement is necessary.[7]

However, even with these confounding factors, some generalizations can be made. First, analysis based upon adjustment for baseline differences in patient populations indicates that patients undergoing mitral valve repair have improved survival and better postoperative left ventricular function than patients undergoing mitral valve replacement[7,8] (Figure 51.2). In addition, patients undergoing valve repair have a lower operative mortality than their counterparts having prosthetic replacement[6,7] (Table 51.1). These good results following valvuloplasty are, at least in part, due to maintenance of normal left ventricular geometry and function through preservation of the valve–chordal–papillary muscle complex.[8–11]

Importantly, valve repair and replacement have similar low rates of reoperation. A recent study from our clinic comparing the outcomes of 195 patients undergoing valve repair with 214 who underwent valve replacement for organic mitral regurgitation demonstrated that freedom from reoperation was 90% and 93% (repair and replacement) at 5 years and 75% and 80% at 10 years respectively ($P=0.47$)[7] (Figure 51.3).

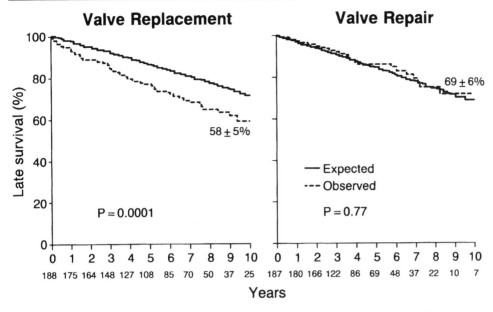

Figure 51.2 Plots of late survival (in operative survivors) of patients with valve replacement (left) and valve repair (right) compared with their expected survival. Note that in patients with valve repair, there is no difference in the expected survival, whereas in patients with valve replacement, the survival is significantly lower than expected. (From Enriquez-Sarano *et al.*[7])

Table 51.1 Operative mortality for mitral valve replacement versus repair

	Replacement	Repair	P
Overall	n=214 (10.3%)	n=195 (2.6%)	0.002
Age ≤75 years	n=39 (30.8%)	n=44 (6.8%)	0.0005
Age ≥75 years	n=175 (5.7%)	n=151 (1.3%)	0.036

From Enriquez-Sarano *et al.*[7]

Valve repair can even be undertaken in some patients with calcification of the leaflets and annulus. Although this presents a challenge to the surgeon, repair utilizing standard techniques after tissue decalcification and debridement does not adversely affect surgical outcome.[12,13] Mitral valve repair rather than replacement is also possible in the setting of native valve endocarditis, as this results in lower hospital mortality and improved long term outcome when compared to valve replacement.[14] Thus, valve repair for mitral regurgitation, whatever the etiology, should be the first choice of surgical correction.

Freedom from reoperation for structural valve-related degeneration has been reported as high as 90% at 10 years and 85% at 15 years following valve repair.[15] In patients who exhibit valve failure following repair, successful rerepair can be undertaken in 16–21% of patients.[16,17] Thus, the ultimate likelihood of requiring a mitral prosthesis following surgical repair of mitral regurgitation is very low.

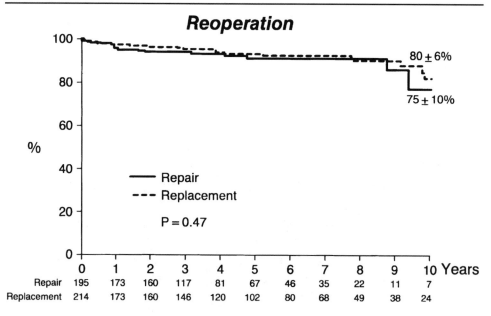

Figure 51.3 Plot of freedom from reoperation in valve repair and replacement groups. No significant difference is observed. (From Enriquez-Sarano *et al.*[7])

Basic concepts of repair

Prolapse of a segment of the posterior leaflet is treated by triangular or quadrangular resection of the unsupported portion or by plication of the redundant leaflet tissue.[18,19] In patients with anterior leaflet prolapse, with or without chordal rupture, we favor chordal replacement with Gore-Tex suture.[20]

Dilation of the valve annulus almost always accompanies mitral regurgitation.[21] Progressive annular enlargement worsens regurgitation by further decreasing the area of leaflet coaptation. The dilation tends to be asymmetrical, in that it affects the mural leaflet up to the commissures.[22] Dilation changes annular shape so that the anteroposterior diameter of the valve becomes greater than the transverse diameter. Because of this, an annuloplasty procedure is an integral part of mitral valve repair. The goals of an annuloplasty are four-fold:

1. decrease annulus diameter, thereby decreasing the area that the leaflets must seal;
2. prevent further dilation of the annulus;
3. allow coaptation of the leaflets along several millimeters from their free margins, thus decreasing the probability of tears in areas where segments of leaflets or chordae were repaired;
4. restoration of normal annulus shape.

Annuloplasty is typically performed with a prosthetic ring;[23,24] we favor a partial posterior ring[25] to reorient the anterior or posterior leaflets for adequate coaptation (Figure 51.4). Postoperative valve function as assessed by degree of regurgitation, transvalvular gradient, and valve area is comparable, irrespective of which technique is utilized.[25] It should be noted that the normal mitral annulus changes size and shape during the cardiac cycle.[26–29] This "sphincter-like" function results in a reduction in valve area by 26% during systole, which is associated with a change in shape from

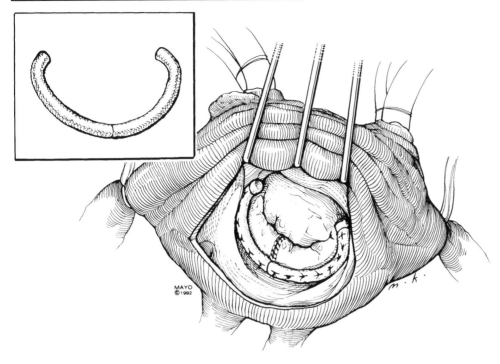

Figure 51.4 An annuloplasty ring.

circular to elliptical.[30] If a flexible annuloplasty is utilized for repair rather than a rigid ring, superior left ventricular systolic function can be demonstrated early and late following valve repair.[31,32]

VALVE REPLACEMENT

Choice of a valve prosthesis requires consideration of the qualities of the valve weighed against the patient's needs. Durability of the prosthesis is often the primary concern of the patient. Indeed, when discussing valve replacement with a patient, the most commonly asked question is "How long will it [the prosthesis] last?". For currently available mechanical valves in the United States, the answer is a qualified "forever", qualified in the sense that intrinsic material failure of mechanical valves is now extremely rare.[33] However, this does not mean that a valve might not need to be replaced because of extrinsic mechanical failure (for example, pannus ingrowth inhibiting proper function of the closure mechanism), and the patient should understand these differences. Durability of biologic valves is not so well defined for the individual patient. Indeed, as outlined below, by their very nature, tissue valves have a limited lifespan and their use must be matched to a patient's needs.

Anticoagulation and thrombogenicity are the other major issues with prosthetic valves. Mechanical valves offer excellent durability that clearly surpasses that of currently available tissue valves, but thrombus formation and thromboembolism are recognized hazards. Anticoagulation to prevent thromboembolism introduces an incremental risk

875

to a patient. Indeed, taken together, anticoagulant-related hemorrhage and thrombosis account for up to 75% of complications following mechanical valve replacement.[34]

Finally, when evaluating different types of cardiac valve prostheses, one must understand the concepts of valvular hemodynamics. These are directly related to valve design and determine the work the heart must expend to pump blood through the prosthesis. All currently approved prosthetic valves have a sewing ring which, with the housing of the valve, takes up a certain cross-sectional area in the path of blood flow. This "sewing ring area" is larger for the tissue valves than for the mechanical valves. The effective orifice area (EOA) of a valve is the actual area of the valve available for blood flow. If one divides the EOA by the sewing ring area, one can calculate the performance index (PI) of a given valve. The PI of currently available porcine valves ranges from 0.35 to 0.4, pericardial valves at 0.65, and tilting disc valves from 0.67 to 0.70, so that all stent mounted prosthetic valves are, by definition, stenotic compared to normal native valves. The potential for residual outflow obstruction when a small prosthetic valve is used in a large patient gives rise to the condition termed valve–prosthesis patient mismatch.[35,36] For most patients, the transvalvular gradient is small and of little clinical significance. It should be noted, however, that as the valve size decreases and the EOA concomitantly decreases, there can be a precipitous rise in the transvalvular gradient, which could cancel out the clinical improvement anticipated from valve replacement.

Two other aspects of valve function are often overlooked: dynamic and static prosthetic valve regurgitation. Dynamic regurgitant fraction is the amount of regurgitation that occurs through a valve before the occluder has a chance to close fully. This is lowest for the tilting disc valves, followed by the bileaflet prostheses; the greatest dynamic regurgitation is associated with the ball and cage prostheses.[37] Static regurgitation occurs through a valve after the valve has closed. Some static regurgitation is engineered into most valves to wash the valve components and eliminate microemboli. Bileaflet valves and Medtronic-Hall tilting disc valves have greater static regurgitation than ball and cage valves.[37] Although regurgitant volume through a normally functioning prosthesis is not important in a patient with adequate ventricular function, in the face of decreased ejection fraction, large regurgitant volumes may attenuate the hemodynamic improvement produced by valve replacement.

Mechanical valves

Currently in the United States, there are five categories of mechanical valves approved for implication by the Food and Drug Administration (FDA). These include the St Jude (St Jude Medical, Minneapolis, MN) bileaflet prosthesis, the Medtronic-Hall (Medtronic Inc, Minneapolis, MN) tilting disc valve, the CarboMedics (CarboMedics, Austin, TX) bileaflet prosthesis, the Starr-Edwards ball valve (Baxter Healthcare, Santa Ana, CA), and the Omnicarbon tilting disc valve, which evolved from the Omniscience valve. There are few prospective, randomized studies comparing outcomes between these categories of valves in the same patient populations.

Non-randomized studies and informal comparisons of published series show little difference in late patient outcome, either in morbidity or mortality, following implantation of currently approved mechanical prostheses (for review, see reference[37]). Several prospective, randomized studies comparing specific valves bear out this assertion. Schulte

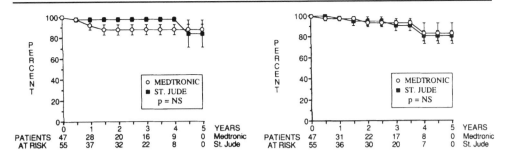

Figure 51.5 Actuarial freedom from thromboembolism (left) and hemorrhage (right) after mitral valve replacement with the St Jude and Medtronic-Hall valves (NS = not significant). (From Fiore *et al.*[39])

and associates randomized 150 consecutive patients to receive a tilting disc prosthesis or Starr-Edwards valve or mitral valve replacement; there was no significant difference in late patient survival (mean follow-up 14.8 years) between the two tilting disc valves (Bjork-Shiley, Lillehei-Kaster) and a ball and cage prosthesis (Starr-Edwards).[38]

In another randomized study of 102 patients, Fiore and colleagues found no significant difference in linearized rates of valve-related events and 3-year actuarial survival between a tilting disc (Medtronic-Hall) and bileaflet (St Jude) prosthesis[39] (Figure 51.5). Even when comparing an early model tilting disc prosthesis (Bjork-Shiley) with a bileaflet prosthesis (St Jude), no significant difference in early and late survival or major bleeding complications could be demonstrated in 178 patients in a prospectively randomized European study (mean follow-up of 52 months or 778 patient-years).[40] Thus, with regard to clinical performance and hemodynamic data, there are no large randomized studies that definitively demonstrate the superiority and thus preferential selection of one mechanical prosthesis over another.

Bioprosthetic valves

The three most commonly used bioprostheses are the Hancock porcine valve (Medtronic Inc) and the Carpentier-Edwards porcine and bovine pericardial valves (Baxter Healthcare). The main drawback of the bioprosthetic valves is structural deterioration which is not a simple linear function of time as the rate of structural dysfunction steadily accelerates after 5–6 years of implantation.[41–43] Regurgitation through cusp tears associated with calcific nodules is the most frequent form of bioprosthesis failure; pure stenosis due to calcified leaflets occurs infrequently. Structural dysfunction of bioprostheses is markedly accelerated in children, adolescents, and young adults, but is attenuated in very elderly patients. For aortic bioprostheses, patients younger than 39–44 years of age have structurally related event free estimates ranging from 58% to 70% at 10 years;[43–45] this drops to 33% at 15 years.[46] This is in contrast to patients over 70 years of age, who have event free estimates of 95% and 93% at 10 and 15 years following implantation.[46] Event free estimates for patients between 60 and 69 years of age 10 years following implantation range from 92% to 95%.[45–47]

Many investigators have compared the performance of the Hancock and the Carpentier-Edwards porcine bioprostheses. In general, no significant differences in the short and long term performance of these valves have been demonstrated.[48–51] Indeed, at 10-year follow-up of 174 patients undergoing mitral or aortic valve replacement who were prospectively randomized to receive either a Hancock or Carpentier-Edwards porcine bioprosthesis, there were no significant differences in patient survival, durability of the prosthesis or valve-related complications.[48] These findings were confirmed in another study of 147 patients randomized to receive either the Carpentier-Edwards or Hancock porcine bioprosthesis in the mitral position. At 10 years, no significant differences in survival or valve-related complications were apparent.[52]

Previously, all commercially available bioprostheses were mounted on a stent or frame to give the relatively flaccid tissue valve a fixed base to facilitate implantation. The stent and sewing ring, however, significantly decrease the EOA and make tissue valves relatively obstructive when compared with mechanical prostheses. There has been considerable interest recently in stentless bioprosthetic valves that are inserted in much the same fashion as homografts. Hemodynamic performance of stentless bioprostheses is good and like other tissue valves, no anticoagulation is required.[53-56] In one report, 254 patients with the Toronto SPV stentless valve (St Jude Medical) were followed for 3 years and the initially favorable EOAs and transvalvular gradients were said to improve with time.[53] In addition, left ventricular mass decreased by 14.3% in the study period.

The primary mode of failure of stentless valves, like all bioprostheses, is valvular regurgitation. Indeed, 27% of 200 patients were found to have aortic insufficiency 1 year following implantation of a stentless aortic valve (PRIMA Edwards; Baxter Healthcare); however, only one patient exhibited grade III insufficiency.[55] In addition, in a non-randomized study of 150 patients receiving either a stentless bioprosthesis (PRIMA Edwards), a traditional bioprosthesis or a homograft, no difference in morbidity or mortality was noted between the groups after 1 year.[57] While the initial data on stentless bioprostheses in the aortic position are encouraging, further long term studies will be needed to establish their ultimate role in the management of aortic valve disease.

Development of stentless valves for the mitral position has been difficult. Because the mitral valve annulus changes shape during the cardiac cycle, a stentless prosthesis in this location requires additional external support to maintain competence. This engineering challenge has been met by using artificial chordae to anchor the stentless valve to native papillary muscle.[58] Short term success has been reported, but a stentless prosthesis for the mitral position should be considered as experimental.

An additional category of tissue valves currently available for implantation are homografts. These are human tissue valves (either aortic or pulmonic) that have been harvested from cadavers, sterilized antibiotically, and cryopreserved.[59,60] Homografts have many attractive features including minimal gradients, low thrombogenicity without need for anticoagulation, and low risk of infection, even when used in patients with active endocarditis.[61,62] Implantation of a homograft is considered more difficult than implantation of a stent mounted bioprosthesis and both experience of the surgeon and surgical technique appear to influence late results.[63] Freedom from reoperation due to structural deterioration of homografts has been reported to range from 83% at 8 years[64] to 86% at 14 years.[60] When valve failure occurs, it is due to the gradual development of insufficiency.

The other homograft available for aortic valve replacement is the pulmonary valve autograft (termed the Ross procedure). The Ross procedure involves excision of a patient's normal pulmonic valve (autograft) and utilizing it to replace the diseased aortic valve.[65,66] A cryopreserved human pulmonary artery homograft (allograft) is then implanted to replace the native pulmonic valve. There are many positive aspects of the operation. First, as both of the valves are tissue valves, no anticoagulation is required.

Second, since the pulmonic valve autograft is not exposed to the antibiotic sterilization or cryopreservation process, it is viable and has potential for growth and long term durability.[67,68] In one series of 195 patients, the freedom from reoperation (autograft or allograft) was reported to be 89% at 5 years.[69] Compared to allograft replacement of the aortic valve, patients receiving the pulmonary autograft have comparable hemodynamics and early to medium term postoperative recovery.[70]

However, there are three potential drawbacks to the pulmonary autograft. First, the operation converts single valve disease to a double valve replacement. And even if the pulmonary autograft functions perfectly, there is potential for tissue degeneration and obstruction of the pulmonary allograft; in fact, the need for rightsided valve re-replacement may be underestimated. In the best of hands and in carefully selected patients, cumulative risk of reoperation for pulmonary valve substitute approaches 20% at 20 years postoperatively.[65,71] In addition, there is a 10–20% incidence of autograft aortic insufficiency, Grade 2 +, following operation.[72] Long term follow-up from multiple institutions is necessary to define the safety and durability of the pulmonary autograft for aortic valve replacement.

Comparative studies of mechanical versus bioprosthetic valves

In a prospective, randomized study in which 262 patients received either a mechanical (Bjork-Shiley) or porcine bioprosthesis (initially Hancock and subsequently Carpentier-Edwards) in the mitral position, actuarial survival and incidence of thromboembolism was comparable at 7 years follow-up.[73] Another prospective, randomized study also demonstrated comparable survival following valve replacement with either a mechanical valve or bioprosthesis.[74] Five hundred and seventy-five men, scheduled to undergo either aortic or mitral valve replacement, were randomized either to receive a mechanical valve (Bjork-Shiley) or porcine bioprosthesis (Hancock). After 11 years, survival rates and freedom from all valve-related complications were similar for both patient groups. However, the profile of valve-related complications was different in that structural failure was only observed with the bioprosthetic valves, whereas bleeding complications were more frequent in patients with mechanical valves. Thus, while the types of complications might differ between patients with either a bioprosthesis or mechanical valve, the actual incidence of the complications is comparable and survival is similar. As such, the choice between a bioprosthesis and a mechanical valve should be based on other factors.

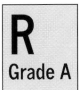

R
Grade A

MATCHING THE PATIENT TO THE PROSTHESIS: FACTORS IN SELECTING A VALVE FOR IMPLANTATION

Because patient survival following valve replacement is independent of the type of prosthesis used and dependent on other factors, one needs to focus on patient variables when selecting a valve. First, one must assess a patient's life expectancy after valve replacement. For patients aged 65–69 years undergoing aortic and/or mitral valve replacement, survival is approximately 53% at 10 years and 25% at 15 years; for patients 70 years of age or older, survival is 30–38% at 10 years and 25% at 15 years.[47]

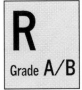

R
Grade A/B

Coronary artery disease requiring bypass grafting at the time of valve replacement further decreases long term survival.[75]

All other factors being equal, it has been our practice to suggest a mechanical valve to patients 70 years or younger and a bioprosthesis to those 75 years and older. In the "gray area" between 70 and 75 years, recommendations are made based upon a patient's general health and personal preference.

The other major issue related to the choice of a valve prosthesis is anticoagulation. Obviously, a mechanical valve, with its obligatory need for lifelong oral anticoagulation, would be contraindicated in a patient:

- who has bleeding tendencies;
- who, because of geography or psychosocial issues, would be unable to monitor the level of anticoagulation;
- who has an occupation with a high risk of trauma;
- who is a female of childbearing age who desires a future pregnancy.

In these situations, one of the tissue valves would be indicated. However, if a patient is likely to require anticoagulation for some other condition such as atrial fibrillation, a large left atrium, chronic deep venous thrombosis or a mechanical prosthesis in another location, then a mechanical valve is chosen for its durability. In addition, if for some reason a patient would be at great risk for reoperation and valve re-replacement, a mechanical valve is favored.

REFERENCES

1 Dare AJ, Harrity PJ, Tazelaar HD, Edwards WD, Mullany CJ. Evaluation of surgically excised mitral valves: revised recommendations based on changing operative procedures in the 1990s. *Hum Pathol* 1993;**24**(12):1286–93.

2 Olson LJ, Subramanian R, Ackermann DM, Orszulak TA, Edwards WD. Surgical pathology of the mitral valve: a study of 712 cases spanning 21 years. *Mayo Clin Proc* 1987;**62**:22–34.

3 Waller BF, Morrow AG, Maron BJ *et al.* Etiology of clinically isolated, severe, chronic, pure mitral regurgitation: an analysis of 97 patients over 30 years of age having mitral valve replacement. *Am Heart J* 1982;**104**:276–88.

4 Enriquez-Sarano M, Tajik AJ, Schaff HV *et al.* Echocardiographic prediction of survival after surgical correction of organic mitral regurgitation. *Circulation* 1994;**90**:830–7.

5 Ling LH, Enriquez-Sarano M, Sewrad JB *et al.* Clinical outcome of mitral regurgitation due to flail leaflet. *N Engl J Med* 1996;**355**:1417–23.

6 Perier P, Deloche A, Chauvaud S *et al.* Comparative evaluation of mitral valve repair and replacement with Starr, Bjork, and porcine valve prostheses. *Circulation* 1984;**70**:187–92.

7 Enriquez-Sarano M, Schaff HV, Orszulak TA *et al.* Valve repair improves the outcome of surgery for mitral regurgitation: a multivariate analysis. *Circulation* 1995;**91**:1022–8.

8 Goldman ME, Mora F, Guarino T, Fuster V, Mindich BP. Mitral valvuloplasty is superior to mitral valve replacement for preservation of left ventricular function: an intraoperative two-dimensional echocardiographic study. *JACC* 1987;**10**:568–75.

9 Rozich JD, Carabello BA, Usher BW *et al.* Mitral valve replacement with and without chordal preservation in patients with chronic mitral regurgitation. Mechanisms for differences in postoperative ejection performance. *Circulation* 1992;**86**:1718–26.

10 David TE, Uden DE, Strauss HD. The importance of the mitral apparatus in left ventricular function after correction of mitral regurgitation. *Circulation* 1983;**68**:1176–83.

11 David TE, Burns RJ, Bacchus CM, Druck MN. Mitral regurgitation with and without preservation of chordae tendineae. *J Thorac Cardiovasc Surg* 1984;**88**:718–25.

12 Grossi EA, Galloway AC, Steinberg BM *et al.* Severe calcification does not affect long-term outcome of mitral valve repair. *Ann Thorac Surg* 1994;**58**:685–8.

13 Carpentier AF, Pellerin M, Fuzellier JF, Relland JYM. Extensive calcification of the mitral valve annulus: pathology and surgical management. *J Thorac Cardiovasc Surg* 1996;**111**:718–30.

14 Muehrcke DD, Cosgrove DM, Lytle BW *et al.* Is there an advantage to repairing infected mitral valves? *Ann Thorac Surg* 1997;**63**:1718–24.

15 Alvarez JM, Deal CW, Loveridge K *et al.* Repairing the degenerative mitral valve: ten to fifteen year follow-up. *J Thorac Cardiovasc Surg* 1996;**112**: 238–47.

16 Cerfolio RJ, Orszulak TA, Pluth JR, Harmsen WS, Schaff HV. Reoperation after valve repair for mitral regurgitation: early and immediate results. *J Thorac Cardiovasc Surg* 1996;**111**:1177–84.

17 Gillinov AM, Cosgrove DM, Lytle BW *et al.* Reoperation for mitral valve repair. *J Thorac Cardiovasc Surg* 1997;**113**:467–75.

18 Carpentier A. Cardiac valve surgery: the French connection. *J Thorac Cardiovasc Surg* 1983;**86**: 323–37.

19 McGoon DC. Repair of mitral insufficiency due to ruptured chordae tendinae. *J Thorac Cardiovasc Surg* 1960;**39**:357–62.

20 David TE, Armstrong S, Sun Z. Replacement of chordae tendineae with Gore-Tex sutures: a ten-year experience. *J Heart Valve Dis* 1996;**5**(4): 352–5.

21 Ormiston JA, Shah PM, Tei C, Wong M. Size and motion of the mitral valve annulus in man. II. Abnormalities in mitral valve prolapse. *Circulation* 1982;**65**:713–19.

22 Carpentier A. Plastic and reconstructive mitral valve surgery. In Kalmanson D, ed. *The mitral valve, a pluridisciplinary approach.* London: Publishing Science Group, 1976, p 567.

23 Carpentier A, Deloche A, Dauptain J *et al.* A new reconstructive operation for correction of mitral and tricuspid insufficiency. *J Thorac Cardiovasc Surg* 1971;**61**:1–13.

24 Duran CMG, Umbago JL. Clinical and hemodynamic performance of a totally flexible prosthetic ring for atrioventricular valve reconstruction. *Ann Thorac Surg* 1976;**22**: 458–63.

25 Odell JA, Schaff HV, Orszulak TA. Early results of a simplified method of mitral valve anuloplasty. *Circulation* 1995;**92**(Suppl II):II–150–4.

26 David TE, Strauss HD, Mesher E *et al.* Is it important to preserve the chordae tendineae and papillary muscles during mitral valve replacement? *Can J Surg* 1981;**24**:236–9.

27 Hansen DE, Cahill PD, DeCampli WM *et al.* Valvular ventricular interactions: importance of the mitral apparatus in canine left ventricular systolic performance. *Circulation* 1986;**73**: 1310–20.

28 Hansen DE, Cahill PD, Derby GC, Miller DC. Relative contributions of the anterior and posterior mitral chordae tendineae to canine global left ventricular systolic performance. *J Thorac Cardiovasc Surg* 1987;**93**:45–55.

29 Sarris GE, Cahill PD, Hansen DE *et al.* Restoration of left ventricular systolic performance after reattachment of the mitral chordae tendineae.

The importance of the valvular-ventricular interaction. *J Thorac Cardiovasc Surg* 1988;**95**: 969–79.

30 Ormiston JA, Shah PM, Tei C, Wong M. Size and motion of the mitral annulus in man: a two-dimensional echocardiographic method and findings in normal subjects. *Circulation* 1981;**64**: 113–20.

31 David TE, Komeda M, Pollick C, Burns RJ. Mitral valve annuloplasty: the effect of the type on left ventricular function. *Ann Thorac Surg* 1989;**47**: 524–8.

32 Duran CG, Revuelta JM, Gaite L, Alonso C, Fleitas MG. Stability of mitral reconstructive surgery at 10–12 years for predominantly rheumatic valvular disease. *Circulation* 1988;**78**:191–6.

33 Grunkemeier GL, Rahimtoola SH. Artificial heart valves. *Annu Rev Med* 1990;**41**:251–63.

34 Edmonds LH. Thrombotic and bleeding complications of prosthetic heart valves. *Ann Thorac Surg* 1987;**44**:430–45.

35 Rahimtoola SH. The problem of valve prosthesis–patient mismatch. *Circulation* 1978; **58**:20–4.

36 Rahimtoola SH, Murphy E. Valve prosthesis–patient mismatch. A long-term sequela. *Br Heart J* 1981;**45**:331–5.

37 Akins CW. Results with mechanical cardiac valvular prostheses. *Ann Thorac Surg* 1995;**60**: 1836–44.

38 Schulte HD, Horstkotte D, Bircks W, Strauer BE. Results of a randomized mitral valve replacement with mechanical prostheses after 15 years. *Int J Artif Organs* 1992;**15**(10):611–16.

39 Fiore AC, Naunheim KS, d'Orazio S *et al.* Mitral valve replacement: randomized trial of St. Jude and Medtronic-Hall prostheses. *Ann Thorac Surg* 1992;**54**(1):68–73.

40 Vogt S, Hoffmann A, Roth J *et al.* Heart valve replacement with the Bjork-Shiley and St. Jude Medical prostheses: a randomized comparison in 178 patients. *Eur Heart J* 1990;**11**(7):583–91.

41 Jamieson WRE, Murno AI, Miyagishima RT *et al.* Carpentier-Edwards standard porcine bioprosthesis: clinical performance to seventeen years. *Ann Thorac Surg* 1995;**60**:999–1007.

42 Glower DD, White WD, Hatton AC *et al.* Determinants of reoperation after 960 valve replacements with Carpentier-Edwards prostheses. *J Thorac Cardiovasc Surg* 1994;**107**: 381–93.

43 Pelletier LC, Carrier M, Leclerc Y *et al.* Influence of age on late results of valve replacement with porcine bioprostheses. *J Cardiovasc Surg* 1992;**33**: 526–33.

44 Cohn LH, Collins JJ Jr, DiSesa V *et al.* Fifteen-year experience with 1,678 Hancock porcine bioprosthetic heart valve replacements. *Ann Surg* 1989;**210**:435–43.

45 Jones EL, Weintraub WS, Craver JM *et al.* Ten-year experience with the porcine bioprosthetic valves; interrelationship of valve survival and patient survival in 1,050 valve replacements. *Ann Thorac Surg* 1990;**49**:370–84.

46 Burdon TA, Miller DC, Oyer PE *et al.* Durability of porcine valves at fifteen years in a representative North American population. *J Thorac Cardiovasc Surg* 1992;**103**:238–52.

47 Burr LH, Jamieson WRE, Munro AI *et al.* Porcine bioprostheses in the elderly: clinical performance by age groups and valve positions. *Ann Thorac Surg* 1995;**60**:S264–9.

48 Sarris GE, Robbins RC, Miller DC *et al.* Randomized, prospective assessment of bioprosthetic valve durability: Hancock verses Carpentier-Edwards valves. *Circulation* 1993; **88**(pt 2):55–64.

49 Bolooki H, Kaiser GA, Mallon SM, Palatianos GM. Comparison of long-term results of Carpentier-Edwards and Hancock bioprosthetic valves. *Ann Thorac Surg* 1986;**42**:494–9.

50 Hartz RS, Fisher EB, Finkelmeier B *et al.* An eight-year experience with porcine bioprosthetic cardiac valves. *J Thorac Cardiovasc Surg* 1986;**91**: 910–17.

51 McDonald ML, Daley RC, Schaff HV *et al.* Hemodynamic performance of a small aortic valve bioprostheses: is there a difference? *Ann Thorac Surg* 1997;**63**:362–6.

52 Perier P, Deloche A, Chauvaud S *et al.* A ten-year comparison of mitral valve replacement with Carpentier-Edwards and Hancock porcine bioprostheses. *Ann Thorac Surg* 1989;**48**(1):54–9.

53 Del Rizzo DF, Goldman BS, Christakis GT, David TE. Hemodynamic benefits of the Toronto Stentless Valve. *J Thorac Cardiovasc Surg* 1996;**112**(6): 1431–45.

54 Sintek CF, Fletcher AD, Khonsari S. Small aortic root in the elderly: use of a stentless bioprosthesis. *J Heart Valve Dis* 1996;**5**(Suppl 3):S308–13.

55 Dossche K, Vanermen H, Daenen W, Pillai R, Konertz W. Hemodynamic performance of the PRIMA Edwards stentless aortic xenograft: early results of a multicenter clinical trial. *Thorac Cardiovasc Surg* 1996;**44**(1):11–14.

56 Wong K, Shad S, Waterworth PD *et al.* Early experience with the Toronto stentless porcine valve. *Ann Thorac Surg* 1995;**60**(Suppl 2):S402–5.

57 Dossche K, Vanermen H, Wellens F *et al.* Free-hand sewn allografts, stentless (Prima Edwards) and stented (CESA) porcine bioprostheses. A comparative hemodynamic study. *Eur J Cardiothorac Surg* 1995;**9**(1):562–6.

58 Deac RF, Simionescu D, Deac D. New evolution in mitral physiology and surgery: mitral stentless pericardial valve. *Ann Thorac Surg* 1995;**60**(Suppl 2):S433–8.

59 McGriffin DC, O"Brien MF, Stafford EG *et al.* Long-term results of the viable cryopreserved allograft valve: continuing evidence for superior valve durability. *J Cardiac Surg* 1988;**3**(Suppl): 289.

60 O'Brien MF, McGriffin DC, Stafford EG *et al.* Allograft aortic valve replacement: long-term comparative clinical analysis of the viable cryopreserved and antibiotic 4 C stored valves. *J Cardiac Surg* 1991;**6**(Suppl 4):534.

61 Tuna IC, Orszulak TA, Schaff HV, Danielson GK. Results of homograft aortic valve replacement for active endocarditis. *Ann Thorac Surg* 1990;**49**: 619–24.

62 Dearani JA, Orszulak TA, Schaff HV *et al.* Results of allograft aortic valve replacement for complex endocarditis. *J Thorac Cardiovasc Surg* 1997;**113**: 285–91.

63 Dearani JA, Orszulak TA, Daly RC *et al.* Comparison of techniques for implantation of aortic valve allografts. *Ann Thorac Surg* 1996;**62**: 1069–75.

64 Kirklin JK, Naftel DC, Novick W *et al.* Long-term function of cryopreserved aortic valve homografts: a ten year study. *J Thorac Cardiovasc Surg* 1993;**106**:154–66.

65 Ross D, Jackson M, Davies J. Pulmonary autograft aortic valve replacement: long-term results. *J Cardiac Surg* 1991;**6**(4):529–53.

66 Elkins RC, Santangelo K, Stelzer P, Randolph JD, Knott-Craig CJ. Pulmonary autograft replacement of the aortic valve: an evolution of technique. *J Cardiac Surg* 1992;**7**(2):108–16.

67 Gerosa G, McKay R, Ross DN. Replacement of the aortic valve or root with an autograft in children. *Ann Thorac Surg* 1991;**51**:424.

68 Walls JT, McDaniel WC, Pope ER *et al.* Documented growth of autogenous pulmonary valve translocated to the aortic valve position (letter). *J Thorac Cardiovasc Surg* 1994;**107**:1530.

69 Elkins RC, Lane MM, McCue C. Pulmonary autograft reoperation: incidence and management. *Ann Thorac Surg* 1996;**62**:450–5.

70 Santini F, Dyke C, Edwards S *et al.* Pulmonary autograft versus homograft replacement of the aortic valve: a prospective randomized trial. *J Thorac Cardiovasc Surg* 1997;**113**:894–900.

71 Ross D. Replacement of the aortic valve with a pulmonary autograft: the "switch" operation. *Ann Thorac Surg* 1991;**52**:1346.

72 Elkins RC. Editorial: pulmonary autograft – the optimal substitute for the aortic valve? *N Engl J Med* 1994;**330**:59.

73 Bloomfield P, Kitchin AH, Wheatley DJ *et al.* A prospective evaluation of the Bjork-Shiley, Hancock, and Carpentier-Edwards heart valve prostheses. *Circulation* 1993;**88**(5, pt 2): 1155–64.

74 Hammermeister KE, Sethi GK, Henderson WG *et al*. A comparison of outcomes in men 11 years after heart-valve replacement with a mechanical valve or bioprosthesis. *N Engl J Med* 1993;**328**:1289.

75 Jones EL, Weintraub WS, Craver JM *et al*. Interaction of age and coronary disease after valve replacement: implications for valve selection. *Ann Thorac Surg* 1994;**58**:378–85.

52 Diagnosis and management of infective endocarditis

DAVID T DURACK,
MICHAEL L TOWNS

The diagnosis and management of infective endocarditis (IE) present an ideal application for the principles of evidence based medicine. Many complex questions and decisions arise, most of which have not been formally asked or answered by means of controlled clinical studies. Current practice is based upon an extensive accumulation of uncontrolled clinical experience, rather than upon proven principles.

Here we will discuss common questions that arise during diagnosis and management of IE. Recommendations will be offered, along with an evidence based rating (on an A,B,C scale) of the basis for each recommendation.

BACKGROUND

Pathophysiology

Endocarditis refers to inflammation of the endocardial lining of the heart. The heart valves are most often involved, less commonly the lining of the heart chambers (mural endocarditis). When the lesions of endocarditis (vegetations) contain micro-organisms, the associated disease is termed infective endocarditis. This general term covers the various clinical subcategories of the disease (e.g. acute, subacute, prosthetic valve infection) and also the various etiologic agents (bacteria, yeasts or fungi).

The pathophysiology of this disease often begins with the formation of non-bacterial thrombotic endocarditis (NBTE). This lesion, which is sometimes called a "fibrin platelet plug", is a precursor site which may become infected by circulating organisms during the course of a bacteremia or fungemia.[1-3] NBTE is not normally found in healthy hearts, but it may develop on an endocardial lining which has been damaged by one of several mechanisms. One of the most common pathogenic mechanisms is that of a cardiac valvular lesion, such as scarring or stenosis, leading to high velocity turbulent flow across the valve, with resultant damage to the endothelial lining.[4,5] The damaged area may become a locus for deposition of fibrin and platelets, resulting in NBTE. The type of underlying cardiac valvular lesion determines where a vegetation is most likely to form on the endocardial surface. A bacteremia caused by organisms that have the capacity to adhere to this lesion may seed the NBTE and lead to development of an infected vegetation.[1,6]

Vegetations are the pathologic hallmark of IE.[2,6] They are composed of masses of organisms enmeshed with fibrin, platelets, and a variable (often scanty) inflammatory infiltrate. The vegetations may be of various sizes and may or may not progress to further valvular, perivalvular or extracardiac complications. Valvular complications may include valvular dysfunction, destruction or obstruction. Perivalvular complications include extension of infection into adjacent structures, which may result in the formation of a perivalvular abscess. Extracardiac complications most commonly result from embolic phenomena such as embolization into the coronary arteries or the systemic arterial tree, resulting in ischemia, infarcts or bleeding. Less commonly, abscesses or mycotic aneurysms may develop in various organs. Other extracardiac complications may include immune complex mediated disease such as glomerulonephritis.

Epidemiology

Infective endocarditis has been variously categorized in the past as acute, subacute, chronic, native valve, prosthetic valve, culture negative, and intravenous drug abuse-associated endocarditis. These terms have some value but may overlap. It is useful to specify the infecting organism because this allows prediction of the likely natural history, treatment requirements, and prognosis for an individual patient. Here we will briefly discuss the epidemiology of this disease in the context of three main categories: native valve, prosthetic valve, and culture negative endocarditis.[7,8]

Native valve endocarditis caused by virulent pathogens such as *Streptococcus pneumoniae* or *Staphylococcus aureus* may develop on previously normal valves. More often, native valve endocarditis develops in association with predisposing congenital or acquired valvular lesions, especially when caused by less virulent organisms such as the viridans streptococci. Table 52.1 shows the etiologic agents that are most commonly isolated in native valve infective endocarditis.

Prosthetic valve endocarditis can be subcategorized into early onset (less than 60 days postvalve replacement) or late onset (60 days or more). The observed spectrum of etiologic agents is different for the two categories, with the organisms causing late onset prosthetic valve endocarditis more closely resembling native valve subacute endocarditis, except that coagulase negative staphylococci remain important (Table 52.1).

Culture negative endocarditis has become less common in recent years, partly due to improvements in blood culture techniques and media. Organisms that previously were difficult to recover, such as nutritionally variant streptococci and the fastidious Gram-negative (HACEK: *Haemophilus* spp, *Actinobacillus actinomycetemcomitans*, *Cardiobacterium hominis*, *Eikenella* spp, and *Kingella kingae*) group, are now routinely isolated from optimized blood culture media, usually within 3–5 days. An exception to this is *Bartonella* spp. which have recently been found in association with endocarditis among homeless individuals and as a rare opportunistic infection in patients with AIDS.[9,10]

Table 52.1 Frequency of various organisms isolated in native valve infective endocarditis

Organism	NVE (%)	IV drug abusers (%)	Early PVE (%)	Late PVE (%)
Streptococci	65	15	5	35
Viridans, alpha-hemolytic	35	5	<5	25
Strep. bovis (group D)	15	<5	<5	<5
Strep. faecalis (group D)	10	8	<5	<5
Other streptococci	<5	<5	<5	<5
Staphylococci	25	50	50	30
Coagulase positive	23	50	20	10
Coagulase negative	<5	<5	30	20
Gram negative aerobic bacilli	<5	5	20	10
Fungi	<5	5	10	5
Miscellaneous bacteria	<5	5	5	5
Diphtheroids, propionibacteria	<1	<5	5	<5
Other anaerobes	<1	<1	<1	<1
Rickettsia	<1	<1	<1	<1
Chlamydia	<1	<1	<1	<1
Polymicrobial infection	<1	5	5	5
Culture negative endocarditis	5–10	<5	<5	<5

These are representative figures collated from the literature; wide local variations in frequency are to be expected. NVE, native valve endocarditis; PVE, prosthetic valve endocarditis.
(Reproduced, with permission, from Blanchard *et al.*[3])

DIAGNOSIS

Clinical manifestations

Patients with acute infective endocarditis typically present with an accelerated course typified by high fever, chills, and prostration, whereas those with subacute endocarditis present more insidiously. These patients often have a "flu-like" illness consisting of fever, chills, myalgias/arthralgias, and weakness, but there is great variability in the clinical presentation.[11]

Cardiac manifestations may dominate the clinical presentation in either acute or subacute disease with the presence of new or worsened murmurs or development of cardiac failure due to valvular damage. The patient may present with chest pain due to pleuritis, pericarditis or myocardial infarction resulting from coronary arterial embolism.

Extracardiac clinical manifestations consist of embolic as well as vascular phenomena. The patient may present with a headache without any definable neurologic abnormalities or may have focal abnormalities such as infarcts, areas of cerebritis, hemorrhages or mycotic aneurysms. Meningismus may also be present, although only a minority of patients have positive cerebrospinal fluid cultures. The patient may present with focal pain such as flank or leftsided upper quadrant pain due to embolic infarcts that may at times be complicated by the formation of an abscess, especially in the spleen. There are many other sites for potential embolization with clinical findings, although autopsy findings show that emboli often go undetected during life.

Various other vascular phenomena may occur including petechiae, splinter hemorrhages, Osler's nodes, Janeway lesions or clubbing of the fingernails.

Laboratory tests

Anemia is commonly present, usually of only mild to moderate severity with a normochromic, normocytic film typical of the anemia of chronic disease. Although many patients with acute or subacute endocarditis have some degree of leukocytosis, this is not a reliable laboratory finding. In approximately 90% of patients with IE the erythrocyte sedimentation rate (ESR) is elevated; the median value is about 65 mm/h, but the range is wide and about 10% are within the normal range. Urinalysis may show microscopic hematuria and/or mild proteinuria in approximately 50% of cases, with occasional red blood cell casts and heavy proteinuria in those patients who develop immune complex glomerulonephritis. Non-specific serologic abnormalities are common, especially positive rheumatoid factor which is seen in 30–40% of cases of the subacute form of the disease. A polyclonal increase in gammaglobulins is characteristic of active endocarditis.

MICROBIOLOGY

Blood cultures remain the definitive microbiologic procedure for diagnosis of IE.[12–14] The micro-organisms isolated from blood cultures may provide the clinician with clues to the diagnosis, given the clinical setting. For example, patients who present from the community with a fever of unknown origin and multiple positive blood cultures for the viridans group of streptococci, enterococci or the HACEK group should be considered to have IE until proven otherwise.[15,16] In addition, the temporal pattern of positive cultures may assist in the diagnosis. If three blood culture sets are drawn 1 hour apart and all are positive for the same micro-organism, this indicates that an endovascular infection is likely. Table 52.1 shows the leading organisms isolated from patients with acute, subacute, and prosthetic valve infective endocarditis.

OPTIMAL BLOOD CULTURE TECHNIQUES FOR DIAGNOSING INFECTIVE ENDOCARDITIS

Background

A positive blood culture is one of the two major criteria for diagnosis of IE.[12] Therefore, blood cultures should be obtained from every patient in whom this diagnosis is suspected. Optimal techniques are required in order to minimize the number of patients with IE that fall into the "culture negative" category and at the same time to limit the number of costly blood cultures obtained.[13,14]

Evidence

Typically, the bacteremia associated with endocarditis is continuous, with 10–200 colony-forming units per ml of blood.[17] If this were true in every case, it would only be necessary to draw one single blood sample of about 1 ml to make the diagnosis. In practice, however, some patients with IE have intermittent bacteremia and some have less than one organism per ml of blood. Therefore, the number of positive culture results is directly correlated with the number of blood samples drawn and the volume of blood in each individual sample.

Single samples should not be drawn because the most common contaminants of blood cultures, coagulase negative staphylococci from the skin, can cause IE.[18–20] Therefore, a single sample positive for a coagulase negative staphylococcus drawn from a patient who might have IE is uninterpretable.

Overall, about two-thirds of all samples drawn from patients with IE are positive. This figure represents the combined results from two patient populations. The first group includes the "classic" untreated IE patient with continuous bacteremia in whom all or nearly all cultures will be positive.[21] In such patients, more than 90% will be diagnosed by the first sample drawn, rising to more than 95% from three cultures.[18–21] The second population is a mixed group in whom the proportion of positive cultures is much lower. Many of these patients have received some antibiotic treatment, such as empirical oral ampicillin or cephalosporin, which has temporarily or permanently suppressed the bacteremia and turned the blood cultures negative without curing the underlying endocarditis. Others may have difficult to culture organisms, fungal infections or culture negative IE.[13]

The majority of clinical microbiology laboratories routinely hold their blood culture bottles for 5–7 days before issuing a negative report. In order to decrease the number of "culture negative" endocarditis episodes, investigators have tried to improve the yield by drawing blood during fever spikes or by culturing arterial instead of venous blood.[22] These practices are of marginal or no value. In addition, because some of the etiologic agents, e.g. HACEK group organisms,[23,24] have been traditionally regarded as slow growers, many laboratories have adopted the policy of prolonging incubation times for blood cultures to 14–21 days in cases of suspected IE. Recent data, however, suggest that with improvements in blood culture media, this practice may be unnecessary for all but a very few organisms such as *Bartonella* spp.[9,25,26] See Box 52.1.

SHOULD TRANSESOPHAGEAL ECHOCARDIOGRAPHY BE PERFORMED IN ALL PATIENTS WITH SUSPECTED INFECTIVE ENDOCARDITIS?

Background

Transthoracic M mode echocardiography (TTE) was first used for the detection of vegetations associated with endocarditis in 1973. Several years later a report describing 2D transthoracic echocardiographic findings of vegetations was published. Since then

Conclusions	Rating	References
Draw at least 2 sets (2 separate venepunctures, each sample divided between 2 bottles) for each blood culture ordered	A	This helps to identify contaminants and increases yield of positives[13,14,18]
Inoculate 8–10 ml blood into each bottle	B	This maximizes yield of positives[13,14,18]
Hold the culture bottles for 14–21 days before issuing the final negative report in order to minimize "culture negative" episodes	C	The yield is very low after 5 days[26]
Draw an arterial blood sample for culture if venous blood samples are negative but the diagnosis of IE still seems likely	C	The difference is none or very small[22,27]

Box 52.1

there have been many reports on the use of this technology to assist in the diagnosis of endocarditis, with the reported sensitivity of the procedure in the range of 60–75%.[28–31]

Transesophageal echocardiography (TEE) was initially described in the late 1980s and has proved especially valuable in evaluating patients with suspected endocarditis. TEE is more sensitive than TTE for detection of vegetations, abscesses, and valve perforations.[31–34] Because a TEE examination is more costly than a TTE examination, many comparative studies have been undertaken to determine which technology should be used in the initial diagnostic examination in a patient with suspected infective endocarditis.

Evidence

Multiple studies have demonstrated the superior sensitivity of TEE when compared to TTE. However, this fact does not resolve the question of which is the most appropriate and cost effective test for IE in patients with different pretest probabilities of having that disease.

TTE has an overall sensitivity for detection of intracardiac vegetations of 60–75%.[31] TEE has greater sensitivity – 95% or better overall, although the sensitivity in an individual case varies depending upon factors such as the location and size of the vegetations.[34–39]

TEE is far superior to TTE in detecting abscesses in patients with both native and prosthetic valve endocarditis (PVE), with a sensitivity of detection of 87%, compared to 28% with TTE in one study.[40] Because patients with PVE are more likely than those with native valve endocarditis (NVE) to have perivalvular abscesses, it is now accepted that TEE is the technique of choice in evaluating a patient with suspected PVE. TEE should also be applied in cases of NVE where there is a prolonged clinical course of infection, as well as those patients who do not respond to adequate medical therapy.

The need for TEE in the initial evaluation of patients with NVE, however, is not so clear. In a retrospective analysis of 180 patients referred for echocardiography for suspected infective endocarditis, in whom both TTE and TEE were done, the TTE was reported as technically inadequate in 46 patients (25%). In the remaining 134 patients, there was an almost equal distribution of patients who had a positive TTE (41 patients), a negative TTE (46 patients), and an abnormal but non-diagnostic TTE (47 patients).

All patients who had a positive TTE were subsequently found to have a positive TEE, while only two patients with a negative TTE were found to have a positive TEE, for a sensitivity of 100% and a specificity of 96% for TTE. The principal value of the TEE was in the non-diagnostic group, as well as those with a technically inadequate TTE. In the non-diagnostic group, nine patients (41%) were found to have positive TEE results for vegetations or abscesses. The study concluded that, for suspected native valve endocarditis, a TTE should be the initial echocardiographic study. If the TTE is technically inadequate, then a TEE should be performed. If the TTE is clearly positive or clearly negative, no additional echocardiographic study should be performed, as there was no incremental diagnostic value with TEE. A TEE, however, should be routinely performed if the TTE is abnormal but non-diagnostic.

Another study analyzed the diagnostic value of echocardiography in suspected infective endocarditis, based on the pretest probability of disease.[41] In this study, both TTE and TEE were performed on 105 consecutive patients with suspected endocarditis. On the basis of clinical criteria and (separately) echocardiography, patients were classified as having either low, intermediate or high probability of endocarditis. Echocardiography correctly classified the majority of patients with a low clinical probability of endocarditis, using either TTE (82%) or TEE (85%). The majority of patients (12/14) with an intermediate clinical probability of disease had technically adequate TTE; most of these (10/12) were classified as either high or low probability. Most of the patients with high clinical probability were placed in the low likelihood category by echocardiography – 15/24 by TTE and 12/24 by TEE. The authors concluded that echocardiography should not be used to make a diagnosis of IE in patients with a low clinical probability of disease. In addition, for those patients with an intermediate or high clinical probability of IE, TTE should be the initial echocardiographic procedure, reserving TEE for those patients with prosthetic valves and those with either a technically inadequate TTE or a TTE which indicates an intermediate probability of endocarditis.[41] See Box 52.2.

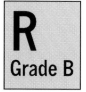

R

Grade B

HOW CAN THE DIAGNOSIS OF IE BE CONFIRMED?

Background

The vegetations of IE are located in an inaccessible site and can be directly seen only at surgery or autopsy. Therefore, for initial diagnosis of IE, they must be visualized indirectly, usually by means of echocardiography. Positive findings on echocardiography are a major criterion for diagnosis of IE, but they are not definitive because of possible false positive or false negative results.[42–44] Likewise, blood cultures, which constitute the second major criterion for diagnosis of IE, also can yield false positive or false negative results.

Evidence

In 1981, von Reyn and colleagues[45] published a paper on IE in which they proposed a set of diagnostic criteria in order to designate cases as definite, probable, possible, or rejected. These criteria, however, did not utilize echocardiography, which had only recently come into general use. In 1994, Durack and colleagues of the Duke Endocarditis

Conclusions	Rating	References
Echocardiography should not be used routinely as a screening test to "rule out endocarditis" in patients with fever and murmur	B	Not cost effective unless there is other evidence of IE, raising the pretest probability[31,41]
For suspected native valve infective endocarditis, TTE should be the initial echocardiographic study	A	[31,41]
If the TTE is technically inadequate in a patient with intermediate or high clinical probability of IE, then TEE should be performed	A	[31,41]
If the TTE is abnormal but non-diagnostic in a patient with intermediate or high pretest clinical probability of IE, then TEE should be performed	B	[31,41]
If the TTE is negative or abnormal but non-diagnostic in a patient with high pretest clinical probability of IE, then TEE should be performed	B	[31,41]
If the TTE is technically adequate and positive, no additional echocardiographic studies are warranted initially, i.e. it is not necessary to "confirm" a positive TTE with a TEE study	B	[31,41]
In patients with suspected prosthetic valve endocarditis, TEE should be performed	A	TEE is best for detection of abscesses[31,40,41]
Echocardiography should not be used routinely as a screening test to "rule out endocarditis" in patients with fever and murmur	B	Not cost effective unless there is other evidence of IE, raising the pretest probability[31,41]

Box 52.2

Service published a set of new criteria which differ from von Reyn's criteria, including echocardiographic findings and introducing the concept of major and minor diagnostic criteria[12] (Tables 52.2, 52.3). Subsequently, multiple studies have analyzed cases diagnosed by the gold standard of pathologic confirmation at surgery or autopsy, comparing both sets of criteria. In each of these studies the Duke criteria were found to be more sensitive than the von Reyn criteria (33–74%).[46–50] In most of these studies, it was felt that the inclusion of echocardiographic data was the primary factor resulting in the increased sensitivity, although even when compared with a modified von Reyn classification with addition of echocardiographic data, there was still an increase in sensitivity. Often increased sensitivity is associated with a concomitant decrease in specificity, but two studies indicate that the Duke criteria have good specificity.[51,52] These criteria should be useful to specify patient entry criteria for epidemiologic studies and clinical trials involving IE. See Box 52.3.

CAN IE BE CURED WITH BACTERIOSTATIC ANTIMICROBIALS?

Background

Antimicrobial agents are traditionally classified as bactericidal or bacteriostatic, according to whether they kill or inhibit growth, respectively. In fact, this classification

Table 52.2 Criteria for diagnosis of infective endocarditis

Definite infective endocarditis
Pathologic criteria
   Micro-organisms: demonstrated by culture or histology in a vegetation, or in a vegetation that has embolized, or in an intracardiac abscess, *or*
   Pathologic lesions: vegetation or intracardiac abscess present, confirmed by histology showing active endocarditis
Clinical criteria (use specific definitions listed in Table 52.3)
   2 major criteria, *or*
   1 major and 3 minor criteria, *or*
   5 minor criteria

Possible infective endocarditis
   Findings consistent with infective endocarditis that fall short of "definite", but not "rejected"

Rejected
   Firm alternate diagnosis for manifestations of endocarditis, *or*
   Resolution of manifestations of endocarditis, with antibiotic therapy for 4 days or less, *or*
   No pathologic evidence of infective endocarditis at surgery or autopsy, after antibiotic therapy for 4 days or less

(Adapted from Durack *et al.*,[12] with permission.)

is an oversimplification because an antimicrobial drug may be partially bactericidal or may be bacteriostatic for one species of bacteria and bactericidal for another. There is a widely quoted "general rule" that IE should be treated only with bactericidal drugs. The rationale often given to support this rule is that colonies of bacteria within a vegetation are protected from host defenses, especially neutrophils which in other sites would usually eliminate organisms which had been inhibited by bacteriostatic antibiotics.

Evidence

In the early days of antimicrobial therapy before penicillin was available, patients with IE were often treated with prolonged courses of sulfonamides. This nearly always failed. For example, in one study none of 42 patients with streptococcal IE treated with sulfonamides survived.[53] On the other hand, sulfonamide therapy occasionally cured a fortunate patient.[54] Sulfonamides were most likely to succeed in the small subgroup of cases of IE caused by *Haemophilus* species, which are especially susceptible to sulfonamides. In the special case of IE caused by *Coxiella burnetii* (the organism causing Q fever) bacteriostatic antibiotics such as tetracyclines are generally used for lack of better alternatives. In most cases they suppress but do not cure the endocardial infection; valve replacement surgery is required to increase the likelihood of cure. Similarly, few antibiotics are available to treat IE caused by resistant Gram negative bacilli such as *Pseudomonas cepacia* or *Stenotrophomonas maltophilia*; in these the combination of a (bacteriostatic) sulfonamide plus trimethoprim has been used with some success.[55] See Box 52.4.

Table 52.3   Definitions of terminology used in the diagnostic criteria for endocarditis

Major criteria

Positive blood culture for infective endocarditis

Typical micro-organism for infective endocarditis from two separate blood cultures:

Viridans streptococci, *Streptococcus bovis*, HACEK group or community acquired *Staphylococcus aureus* or enterococci, in the absence of a primary focus, *or*

Persistently positive blood culture, defined as recovery of a micro-organism consistent with infective endocarditis from:

  (i) blood cultures drawn more than 12 hours apart, *or*

  (ii) all of three or a majority of four or more separate blood cultures, with first and last drawn at least 1 hour apart

Evidence of endocardial involvement

Positive echocardiogram for infective endocarditis:

  (i) oscillating intracardiac mass, on valve or supporting structures, or in the path of regurgitant jet, or on implanted material, in the absence of an alternative anatomic explanation, *or*

  (ii) abscess, *or*

  (iii) new partial dehiscence of prosthetic valve, *or*

New valvular regurgitation (increase or change in pre-existing murmur not sufficient)

Minor criteria

- Predisposition: predisposing heart condition or injection drug use
- Fever: ≥38.0°C (100.4°F)
- Vascular phenomena: major arterial emboli, septic pulmonary infarcts, mycotic aneurysm, intracranial hemorrhage, conjunctival hemorrhages, Janeway lesions
- Immunologic phenomena: glomerulonephritis, Osler's nodes, Roth spots, rheumatoid factor
- Microbiologic evidence: positive blood culture, but not meeting major criterion as previously defined[a] or serologic evidence of active infection with organism consistent with infective endocarditis[b]
- Echocardiogram: consistent with infective endocarditis but not meeting major criterion as previously defined

HACEK = *Haemophilus* spp., *Actinobacillus actinomycetemcomitans*, *Cardiobacterium hominis*, *Eikenella* spp., and *Kingella kingae*.

[a] Excluding single positive cultures for coagulase negative staphylococci or organisms that do not cause endocarditis.

[b] Positive serology for *Coxiella burnetii* or *Bartonella* spp. may be used as a major criterion.

(Adapted from Durack *et al.*,[12] with permission.)

SHOULD COMBINATIONS OF ANTIMICROBIALS BE USED TO TREAT IE?

Background

IE is generally regarded as being difficult and/or slow to cure. Therefore, many attempts have been made to improve cure rates by using optimal antimicrobial regimens, even more so than in most other infections. In the course of this effort, many combinations of antibiotics have been tried and a general impression exists that combination therapy is appropriate for endocarditis. This is only partly true.

Conclusions	Rating	References
The diagnosis of IE is certain only if confirmed by suitable pathologic specimens and/or cultures obtained at surgery or autopsy	A	[12]
A "definite" diagnosis of IE (more than 95% confidence) can be made without surgical or autopsy specimens if defined major and minor criteria (the "Duke criteria") are applied	A	[12,46–49]
The diagnosis of IE can be rejected with high specificity if defined clinical criteria are applied, but this usually requires some delay to allow a period of observation	A	[51,52]
The decision as to whether or not to begin antibiotics should be made on the overall clinical assessment as to the likelihood of IE, not based solely upon the Duke criteria	B	Treatment decisions often need to be made before all diagnostic information is in[12,52]

Box 52.3

Conclusions	Rating	References
Bacteriostatic antibiotics often fail when used to treat IE	A	[53,54]
Bacteriostatic antibiotics may be used to treat IE in a few special cases, e.g. Q fever, resistant organisms like *Pseudomonas cepacia* or *Stenotrophomonas maltophilia*, or suppressive therapy for organisms not likely to be curable, such as *Pseudomonas* on a prosthetic valve	B	[55,56]

Box 52.4

Evidence

There is excellent documentation that enterococcal endocarditis is usually best treated with a combination of two antibiotics. The primary reason for this is that most strains of *Enterococcus faecalis* are relatively resistant to antibiotics, but are killed synergistically by a combination of a penicillin and an aminoglycoside.[57] This does not hold true, however, if the strain shows high level resistance to aminoglycosides (defined as resistance to 2000 µg/ml of streptomycin or 500 µg/ml of gentamicin). In the latter case, vancomycin should be substituted,[58] except for strains that are vancomycin resistant.[59] Ample documentation for the value of combination therapy has been published, based upon *in vitro* studies and *in vivo* treatment of both animals and humans.

Even when streptococci are fully sensitive to penicillin, combinations of a penicillin and an aminoglycoside or vancomycin act synergistically against them.[60] This has been convincingly demonstrated both *in vitro* and in experimental animals.[61,62] The human correlate is found in the fact that combination therapy cures more than 97% of cases within 2 weeks, whereas penicillin alone cures only 80–85% in the same interval and requires 4 weeks to reach 97% cure or better. This fact has been well proven.[54,63] See Box 52.5.

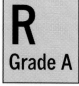

R
Grade A

894

Conclusions	Rating	References
Combination therapy should be used for IE caused by enterococci	A	59,64
A combination of at least two antibiotics (a beta-lactam plus an aminoglycoside) should be used for IE caused by coagulase negative staphylococci	A	65,66
A combination of three antibiotics (a beta-lactam plus an aminoglycoside plus rifampicin) should be used for IE caused by coagulase-negative staphylococci	C	Limited number of patients reported; no comparative trials[65,66]
An aminoglycoside should be added to a beta-lactam for the first few days of therapy for IE caused by *Staph. aureus*	C	A definitive outcome study has not been done[66,67]
Combination therapy should be used for rightsided IE caused by *Staph. aureus* if a short course (2 week) regimen is used	B	Only one major study available[68]
Addition of an aminoglycoside for IE caused by penicillin sensitive streptococci is beneficial and cost effective if a short course (2 week) regimen is used	A	69
Addition of an aminoglycoside for IE caused by penicillin sensitive streptococci is beneficial and cost effective if a standard (4 week) regimen is used	C	No modern cost effectiveness study has been done[69]

Box 52.5

OPTIMAL DURATION OF TREATMENT FOR IE

Background

Early experience established that endocarditis could not be cured by short courses of antibiotics which would have been adequate to cure other common infections such as pneumonia or gonorrhea. Trials of longer duration were more successful, eventually leading to the widely followed practice of treating IE for 6 weeks. This remains common practice today, despite the fact that more than half of all cases of IE could be reliably cured by 2–4 weeks of treatment.

Evidence

Before 1950 it was reported that IE could not be cured with 10 days of treatment, even when the organisms were highly susceptible to penicillin and/or high doses were given.[54,70,71] Subsequently, high cure rates were achieved by extending treatment to 4–6 weeks. For many years, 6 weeks of therapy was regarded as the standard duration for treatment of IE. In fact, this often led to overtreatment because 4 weeks would have been adequate for the majority of these cases.[54] Because of number preferencing for even numbers, 3 and 5 week regimens have not been studied, even though intuitively it seems likely that these durations would work as well as 4 and 6 week regimens.

Some cases of endocarditis can be cured with treatment for only 2 weeks. This is well supported by clinical experience for two important groups of patients: uncomplicated penicillin sensitive streptococcal native valve endocarditis[54,72] and intravenous drug addicts with rightsided *Staph. aureus* endocarditis.[68]

It should be noted that outpatient parenteral antibiotic therapy (OPAT) is appropriate for selected patients with IE.[73-75] In most cases, these will be patients without serious complications who have responded promptly to standard therapy begun in hospital. When OPAT is employed for treatment of IE, the total duration of therapy should normally be the same as if the patient had been hospitalized throughout the course of treatment.

The "B" ratings listed in the conclusions in Box 52.6 could be improved by publication of larger numbers of cases or by randomized controlled studies.

Conclusions	Rating	References
Penicillin sensitive IE can be cured in 2 weeks by combined penicillin plus aminoglycoside or in 4 weeks by penicillin alone	A	69,76
Enterococcal endocarditis should be treated for at least 4 weeks	B	58,69,77,78
Most cases of HACEK endocarditis can be cured in 3–4 weeks (*Haemophilus, Actinobacillus, Cardiobacterium, Eikenella, Kingella* species	B	Total number of reported cases is small[69,79,80]
Most cases of tricuspid valve *Staph. aureus* IE in intravenous drug users can be cured in 2 weeks	B	Only one major study done[68]
Most cases of leftsided native valve *Staph. aureus* IE can be cured in 4 weeks	B	Controlled study not done[69]

Box 52.6

MAIN INDICATIONS FOR SURGICAL INTERVENTION DURING MANAGEMENT OF IE

Background

The introduction of valve replacement, valve repair and other surgical procedures has revolutionized the management of IE, being second in importance only to the advent of antibiotic therapy for IE. Many studies have indicated that surgical intervention improves the prognosis of IE over medical therapy alone.[81-83] The benefits of early rather than late surgical intervention have been appropriately emphasized.[82-84] However, surgical placement of artificial cardiac valves is associated with high costs, significant morbidity, especially in the form of late complications, and some mortality. Furthermore, about two-thirds of all patients with IE can be cured without any surgical intervention. Therefore, correct selection of the subgroup of about one-third of patients who will benefit from surgery becomes of critical importance.

Evidence

Many hundreds of publications have reported on experience with surgery for IE, beginning in 1965[85] and continuing unabated today. The cumulative experience is based upon thousands of patients. However, this extensive experience does not include randomized studies of medical versus surgical therapy, primarily because selection bias (i.e. choosing more seriously ill patients for surgery) is virtually impossible to overcome. Therefore, the conclusions which have emerged, although often well supported by case studies, can only be rated "B" in terms of evidence based analyses. See Boxes 52.7, 52.8.

Conclusions I Strong indications for surgical intervention during IE	Rating	References
Heart failure unresponsive to medical therapy	B	7,8,83
Presence of a valve ring abscess	B	7,8,86,87
Early prosthetic valve infection (onset within 60 days of surgery)	B	7,8,88
Prosthetic valve infection caused by *Staph. aureus*	B	7,8,66,87,88
Prosthetic valve infection caused by Gram negative bacilli (not HACEK group)	B	7,8,88
Endocarditis caused by filamentous fungi (not yeasts)	B	89,90
Prosthetic valve infection caused by yeasts	B	88,91
Development of a sinus of Valsalva aneurysm	B	92
Occlusion of valves by very large vegetations	B	7,8,93

Box 52.7

Conclusions II Relative (less strong) indications for surgical intervention during IE	Rating	References
Recurrent arterial emboli	C	7,8,94
Native leftsided valve infection caused by *Staph. aureus*	C	7,8,66
Apparent failure of medical therapy (persistent bacteremia, persistent fever, increase in size of vegetation during treatment)	C	7,8
Native valve infection caused by Gram negative bacilli (not HACEK)	C	7,8
Large-sized leftsided vegetations by echo (greater than 15–20 mm)	C	7,8
Native valve infection caused by yeasts	C	90,91,95–97
Late onset prosthetic valve infection	C	7,8,88
Development of cardiac conduction abnormality during IE, but no abscess identified by TEE	C	7,8,86

Box 52.8

CORRECT TIMING FOR VALVE REPLACEMENT DURING MANAGEMENT OF IE

Background

In the past, it was often stated on empirical grounds that valve replacement surgery should be postponed until the patient had been cured by antibiotics. If the patient could not survive until cure, it was believed that surgery should be delayed as long as possible to allow suppression of the number of remaining bacteria to the lowest possible level to reduce the risk of relapse or infection of the new prosthetic valve. The available evidence does not support these widely held views.

Evidence

Actual experience showed that the frequency of relapse and/or infection of the prosthesis after surgery for IE was low, whether or not antibiotics had been given for long periods before operation. For patients with a good indication for valve replacement early in the course of active endocarditis, many authors have strongly advocated early surgery, before antibiotics have cured the patient, to avoid deaths and complications which might occur during antibiotic treatment.[81-84] See Box 52.9.

Conclusions	Rating	References
If there is no indication for early surgery, complete a standard course of antibiotic treatment before valve replacement	B	No randomized studies available
If there is an adequate indication for early surgery, proceed to valve replacement without regard to the duration of antibiotic treatment already given	A	Many uncontrolled reports support early surgery[81,84]

Box 52.9

CAN IE BE PREVENTED?

Background

IE sometimes develops as a complication of bacteremias associated with medical and dental procedures such as urinary catheterizations or tooth extractions. Although these represent only a small proportion – about 5% – of all cases of IE, much effort has been made to prevent them because IE carries high associated morbidity and mortality. Soon after antibiotics became available, various attempts were made to prevent bacteremias and/or IE by giving antibiotics before dental extractions or other procedures.[98-102] Subsequently, the American Heart Association[103] and many other groups[104-106] have issued recommendations for prevention of IE by this means.

Evidence

The evidence that bacteremias induced by medical and dental procedures can cause IE in patients with predisposing heart lesions consists of many uncontrolled case reports. There are enough of these to support the conclusion that there is a real risk after tooth extractions and procedures involving an infected genitourinary tract.[107-109] The evidence that lower risk procedures such as gastrointestinal endoscopy, procedures on the uninfected urinary tract, and biopsies and other minor surgical procedures cause a significant number of cases of IE is sketchy.[102,110-118]

Prophylaxis of IE has been unequivocally proven effective in experimental animal models of endocarditis by giving antibiotics before injecting bacteria intravenously.[119-126] However, there has been no definitive study to demonstrate the efficacy of antibiotic prophylaxis for infective endocarditis in humans.[110] One review of patients with prosthetic heart valves indicated that antibiotic prophylaxis before dental and urogenital procedures was effective,[127] but this study was retrospective, unrandomized, and unblinded. Analysis of prospectively collected cases in the Netherlands indicated that prophylaxis was either ineffective or, at best, only marginally effective.[128] Other analyses have indicated that even if prophylaxis is effective, it would probably not be cost effective as a general strategy.[129,130] Despite all this uncertainty, most authorities continue to recommend selective use of prophylaxis for patients with higher risk cardiac lesions undergoing higher risk procedures.[103,110] See Box 52.10.

Conclusions	Rating	References
Bacteremias following tooth extraction or surgical procedures involving an infected genitourinary tract can cause endocarditis	B	131
Bacteremias following gastrointestinal endoscopy or surgical procedures involving an uninfected genitourinary tract can cause endocarditis	C	118,131,132
Prevention of IE by giving antibiotics before medical and dental procedures that cause bacteremia is an empiric practice which has been proven effective in animal models but not in humans	A	110,123
Attempted prevention of IE in selected high risk groups undergoing high risk procedures such as tooth extraction is probably effective	C	127
Attempted prevention of IE in selected high risk groups undergoing high risk procedures such as tooth extraction is recommended	B	104–106
Extensive practice of attempted prophylaxis for IE is probably not cost effective	B	133,134

Box 52.10

REFERENCES

1 Durack DT, Beeson PB. Experimental bacterial endocarditis. I. Colonization of a sterile vegetation. *Br J Exp Pathol* 1972;**53**:44–9.

2 Angrist A, Oka M, Nakao K. Vegetative endocarditis. *Pathol Ann* 1967;**2**:155–212.

3 Blanchard DG, Ross RS, Dittrich HC. Nonbacterial thrombotic endocarditis. *Chest* 1993;**102**:954–6.

4 Rodbard S, Yamamoto C. Effect of stream velocity on bacterial deposition and growth. *Cardiovasc Res* 1969;**3**:68–74.

5 Grant RT, Wood JE Jr, Jones TD. Heart valve irregularities in relation to subacute bacterial endocarditis. *Am Heart J* 1928;**14**:247–61.

6 Livornese LL Jr, Korzeniowski O. Pathogenesis of infective endocarditis. In: Kaye D. ed. *Infective endocarditis*, 2nd edn. New York: Raven Press, 1992, pp 19–35.

7 Durack DT. Infective endocarditis. In: Schlant R, Hurst WJ. eds. *The heart*, 7th edition companion handbook. New York: McGraw-Hill, 1990, pp 153–67.

8 Scheld WM, Sande MA. Endocarditis and intravascular infections. In: Mandell GL, Douglas RG Jr, Dolin R. eds. *Principles and practice of infectious diseases*, 4th edn. New York: Churchill Livingstone, 1995, pp 740–83.

9 Raoult D, Fournier PE, Drancourt M *et al.* Diagnosis of 22 new cases of *Bartonella* endocarditis. *Ann Intern Med* 1996;**125**:646–52.

10 Schwartzman WA, Marchevsky A, Meyer RD. Epithelioid angiomatosis or cat scratch disease with splenic and hepatic abnormalities in AIDS: case report and review of the literature. *Scand J Infect Dis* 1990;**22**:121–33.

11 Durack DT. Infective and noninfective endocarditis. In: Hurst JW. ed. *The heart, arteries and veins*, 7th edn. New York: McGraw-Hill, 1990, pp 1230–55.

12 Durack DT, Bright DK, Lukes AS, Duke Endocarditis Service. New criteria for diagnosis of infective endocarditis: utilization of specific echocardiographic findings. *Am J Med* 1994;**96**: 200–9.

13 Washington JA II. The role of the microbiology laboratory in the diagnosis and antimicrobial treatment of infective endocarditis. *Mayo Clin Proc* 1982;**57**:22–32.

14 Washington JA II. The microbiological diagnosis of infective endocarditis. *J Antimicrob Chemother* 1987;**20**:29–39.

15 Maki DG, Agger WA. Enterococcal bacteremia: clinical features, the risk of endocarditis, and management. *Medicine* 1988;**67**:248–69.

16 Gullberg RM, Homann SR, Phair JP. Enterococcal bacteremia: analysis of 75 episodes. *Rev Infect Dis* 1989;**II**:74–85.

17 Beeson PB, Brannon ES, Warren JV. Observations of the sites of removal of bacteria from the blood in patients with bacterial endocarditis. *J Exp Med* 1945;**81**:9–23.

18 Weinstein M, Reller L, Murphy J, Lichtenstein K. Clinical significance of positive blood cultures: a comprehensive analysis of 500 episodes of bacteremia and fungemia in adults. I. Laboratory and epidemiologic observations. *Rev Infect Dis* 1983;**5**:35–53.

19 Towns M, Quartey S, Weinstein M *et al*. Clinical significance of positive blood cultures: a prospective, multicenter investigation. *ASM News* 1993; Abstract No. C232.

20 Weinstein M, Murphy J, Reller L, Lichtenstein K. Clinical significance of positive blood cultures: a comprehensive analysis of 500 episodes of bacteremia and fungemia in adults. II. Clinical observations, with special reference to factors influencing prognosis. *Rev Infect Dis* 1983;**5**: 54–70.

21 Belli J, Waisbren BA. The number of blood cultures necessary to diagnose most cases of bacterial endocarditis. *Am J Med Sci* 1956;**232**: 284–8.

22 Mallen MS, Hube EL, Brenes M. Comparative study of blood cultures made from artery, vein, and bone marrow in patients with subacute bacterial endocarditis. *Am Heart J* 1946;692–5.

23 Geraci JE, Wilson WR. Endocarditis due to gram-negative bacteria: report of 56 cases. *Mayo Clin Proc* 1982;**57**:145–8.

24 Chen YC, Chang SC, Luh KT, Hsieh WC. *Actinobacillus actinomycetemcomitans* endo-carditis: a report of four cases and review of the literature. *Q J Med* 1992;**81**:871–8.

25 Drancourt M, Birtles R, Chaumentin G *et al*. New serotype of *Bartonella henselae* in endocarditis and cat-scratch disease. *Lancet* 1996;**347**:441–3.

26 Doern GV, Davaro R, George M, Campognone P. Lack of requirement for prolonged incubation of Septi-Chek blood culture bottles in patients with bacteremia due to fastidious bacteria. *Diagn Microbiol Infect Dis* 1996;**24**:141–3.

27 Murray M, Moosnick F. Arterial vs venous blood cultures. *J Lab Clin Med* 1940;**26**:382–7.

28 Gilbert BW, Haney RS, Crawford F *et al*. Two-dimensional echocardiographic assessment of vegetative endocarditis. *Circulation* 1977;**55**: 346–53.

29 Plehn JF. The evolving role of echocardiography in management of bacterial endocarditis. *Chest* 1988;**94**:904–6.

30 Stewart JA, Silimperi D, Harris P *et al*. Echocardiographic documentation of vegetative lesions in infective endocarditis: clinical implications. *Circulation* 1980;**61**:374–80.

31 Irani WN, Grayburn PA, Afridi I. A negative transthoracic echocardiogram obviates the need for transesophageal echocardiography in patients with suspected native valve active infective endocarditis. *Am J Cardiol* 1996;**78**: 101–3.

32 Jaffe WM, Morgan DE, Pearlman AS, Otto CM. Infective endocarditis, 1983–1988: echo-cardiographic findings and factors influencing morbidity and mortality. *J Am Coll Cardiol* 1990; **15**:1227–33.

33 Martin RP. The diagnostic and prognostic role of cardiovascular ultrasound in endocarditis: bigger is not better. *J Am Coll Cardiol* 1990;**15**: 1234–7.

34 Taams MA, Gussenhoven EJ, Bos E *et al*. Enhanced morphological diagnosis in infective endocarditis by transesophageal echo-cardiography. *Br Heart J* 1990;**63**:109–13.

35 Rohmann S, Erbel R, Gorge G *et al*. Clinical relevance of vegetation localization by transoesophageal echocardiography in infective endocarditis. *Eur Heart J* 1992;**12**:446–52.

36 Shapiro SM, Bayer AS. Transesophageal and Doppler echocardiography in the diagnosis and management of infective endocarditis. *Chest* 1991;**100**:1125–30.

37 Pedersen WR, Walker M, Olson JD *et al*. Value of transesophageal echocardiography as an adjunct to transthoracic echocardiography in evaluation of native and prosthetic valve endocarditis. *Chest* 1991;**100**:351–6.

38 Morguet AJ, Werner GS, Andreas S, Kreuzer H. Diagnostic value of transesophageal compared with transthoracic echocardiography in suspected prosthetic value endocarditis. *Herz* 1995;**20**:390–8.

39 Anders K, Foley K, Stern WE, Brown WJ. Intracranial sparganosis: an uncommon infection. Case report. *J Neurosurg* 1984;**60**: 1282–6.

40 Daniel WG, Mugge A, Martin RP *et al.* Improvement in the diagnosis of abscesses associated with endocarditis by transesophageal echocardiography. *N Engl J Med* 1991;**324**: 795–800.

41 Lindner JR, Case RA, Dent JM *et al.* Diagnostic value of echocardiography in suspected endocarditis. An evaluation based on the pretest probability of disease. *Circulation* 1996;**93**: 730–6.

42 Hickey AJ, Wolfers J. False positive diagnosis of vegetations on a myxomatous mitral valve using two-dimensional echocardiography. *Aust NZ J Med* 1982;**12**:540–2.

43 Mintz GS, Kotler MN. Clinical value and limitations of echocardiography. Its use in the study of patients with infectious endocarditis. *Arch Intern Med* 1980;**140**:1022–7.

44 Sokil AB. Cardiac imaging in infective endocarditis. In: Kaye D. ed. *Infective endocarditis*, 2nd edn. New York: Raven Press, 1992, pp 125–50.

45 von Reyn CF, Levy BS, Arbeit RD, Friedland G, Crumpacker CS. Infective endocarditis: an analysis based on strict case definitions. *Ann Intern Med* 1981;**94**:505–17.

46 Bayer AS, Ward JI, Ginzton LE, Shapiro SM. Evaluation of new clinical criteria for the diagnosis of infective endocarditis. *Am J Med* 1994;**96**:211–19.

47 del Pont JM, de Cicco LT, Vartalitis C *et al.* Infective endocarditis in children: clinical analyses and evaluation of two diagnostic criteria. *Pediatr Infect Dis* 1995;**14**:1079–86.

48 Fournier PE, Casalta JP, Habib G, Messana T, Raoult D. Modification of the diagnostic criteria proposed by the Duke Endocarditis Service to permit improved diagnosis of Q fever endocarditis. *Am J Med* 1996;**100**:629–33.

49 Cecchi E, Parrini I, Chinaglia A *et al.* New diagnostic criteria for infective endocarditis. A study of sensitivity and specificity. *Eur Heart J* 1997;**18**:1149–56.

50 Olaison L, Hogevik H. Comparison of the von Reyn and Duke criteria for the diagnosis of infective endocarditis: a critical analysis of 161 episodes. *Scand J Infect Dis* 1996;**28**:399–406.

51 Hoen B, Beguinot I, Rabaud C *et al.* The Duke criteria for diagnosing infective endocarditis are specific: analysis of 100 patients with acute fever or fever of unknown origin. *Clin Infect Dis* 1996; **23**:298–302.

52 Dodds GA, Sexton DJ, Durack DT *et al.* Negative predictive value of the Duke criteria for infective endocarditis. *Am J Cardiol* 1996;**77**:403–7.

53 Galbreath WR, Hull E. Sulfonamide therapy of bacterial endocarditis: results in 42 cases. *Ann Intern Med* 1943;**18**:201–3.

54 Durack DT. Review of early experience in treatment of bacterial endocarditis, 1940–1955. In: Bisno AL. ed. *Treatment of infective endocarditis.* New York: Grune and Stratton, 1981, pp 1–14.

55 Speller DCE. *Pseudomonas cepacia* endocarditis treated with co-trimoxazole and kanamycin. *Br Heart J* 1972;**35**:47–8.

56 Street AC, Durack DT. Experience with trimethoprim-sulfamethoxazole in treatment of infective endocarditis. *Rev Infect Dis* 1988;**10**: 915–21.

57 Wilson WR, Wilkowske CJ, Wright AJ, Sande MA, Geraci JE. Treatment of streptomycin-susceptible and streptomycin-resistant enterococcal endocarditis. *Ann Intern Med* 1984; **100**:816–23.

58 Watanakunakorn C, Bakie C. Synergism of vancomycin–gentamicin and vancomycin–streptomycin against enterococci. *Antimicrob Agents Chemother* 1973;**4**:120–4.

59 Caron F, Lemeland JF, Humbert G, Klare I, Gutmann L. Triple combination penicillin–vancomycin–gentamicin for experimental endocarditis caused by a highly penicillin- and glycopeptide-resistant isolate of *Enterococcus faecium. J Infect Dis* 1993;**168**:681–6.

60 Watanakunakorn C, Glotzbecker C. Synergism with aminoglycosides of penicillin, ampicillin and vancomycin against non-enterococcal group-D streptococci and *Viridans streptococci. J Med Microbiol* 1976;**10**:133–8.

61 Sande MA, Irvin RG. Penicillin-aminoglycoside synergy in experimental *Streptococcus viridans* endocarditis. *J Infect Dis* 1974;**129**:572–6.

62 Fantin B, Carbon C. *In vivo* antibiotic synergism: contribution of animal models. *Antimicrob Agents Chemother* 1992;**36**:907–12.

63 Geraci JE. The antibiotic therapy of infective endocarditis: therapeutic data on 172 patient seen from 1951 through 1957: additional observations on short-term therapy (two weeks) for penicillin-sensitive streptococcal endocarditis. *Med Clin North Am* 1958;**42**: 1101–48.

64 Rice LB, Calderwood SB, Eliopoulos GM, Farber BF, Karchmer AW. Enterococcal endocarditis: a comparison of prosthetic and native valve disease. *Rev Infect Dis* 1991;**13**:1–7.

65 Karchmer AW, Archer GL, Dismukes WE. *Staphylococcus epidermidis* causing prosthetic valve endocarditis: microbiologic and clinical observations as guides to therapy. *Ann Intern Med* 1983;**98**:447–55.

66 Karchmer AW. Staphylococcal endocarditis. In: Kaye D. ed. *Infective endocarditis*, 2nd edn. New York: Raven Press, 1992, pp 225–49.

67 Sande MA, Courtney KB. Nafcillin–gentamicin synergism in experimental staphylococcal endocarditis. *J Lab Clin Med* 1976;**88**:118–24.

68 Chambers HF, Miller RT, Newman MD. Right-sided *Staphylococcus aureus* endocarditis in intravenous drug abusers: two-week combination therapy. *Ann Intern Med* 1988;**109**: 619–24.

69 Wilson WR, Karchmer A, Dajani A *et al*. Antibiotic treatment of adults with infective endocarditis due to viridans streptococci, enterococci, staphylococci and HACEK microorganisms. *JAMA* 1995;**274**:1706–13.

70 King FH, Schneierson SS, Sussman ML, Janowitz HD, Stollerman GH. Prolonged moderate dose therapy versus intensive short term therapy with penicillin and caronamide in subacute bacterial endocarditis. *J Mount Sinai Hosp* 1949;**16**: 35–46.

71 Bloomfield AL, Armstrong CD, Kirby WMM. The treatment of subacute bacterial endocarditis with penicillin. *J Clin Invest* 1945;**24**:251–67.

72 Kwon-Chung KJ, Hill WB. Studies on the pink, adenine-deficient strains of *Candida albicans*. I. Cultural and morphological characteristics. *Sabouraudia* 1970;**8**:48–59.

73 Francioli P, Etienne J, Hoigne R, Thys J, Gerber A. Treatment of streptococcal endocarditis with a single daily dose of ceftriaxone sodium for 4 weeks. Efficacy and outpatient treatment feasibility. *JAMA* 1992;**267**:264–7.

74 Francioli P, Ruch W, Stamboulian D, International Infective Endocarditis Study Group. Treatment of streptococcal endocarditis with a single daily dose of ceftriaxone and netilmicin for 14 days: a prospective multicenter study. *Clin Infect Dis* 1995;**21**:1406–10.

75 Stamboulian D, Bonvehi P, Arevalo C *et al*. Antibiotic management of outpatients with endocarditis due to penicillin-susceptible streptococci. *Rev Infect Dis* 1991;**13**:S160–S163.

76 Wilson WR, Geraci JE, Wilkowske CJ, Washington JA II. Short-term intramuscular therapy with procaine penicillin plus streptomycin for infective endocarditis due to viridans streptococci. *Circulation* 1978;**57**: 1158–61.

77 Geraci JE, Martin WJ. Antibiotic therapy of bacterial endocarditis. VI. Subacute enterococcal endocarditis: clinical, pathologic and therapeutic consideration of 33 cases. *Circulation* 1954;**10**: 173–94.

78 Moellering RC Jr, Wennersten C, Weinstein AJ. Penicillin–tobramycin synergism against enterococci: a comparison with penicillin and gentamicin. *Antimicrob Agents Chemother* 1973; **3**:526–9.

79 Shorrock PJ, Lambert PA, Aitchison EJ *et al*. Serological response in *Enterococcus faecalis* endocarditis determined by enzyme-linked immunosorbent assay. *J Clin Microbiol* 1990;**28**: 195–200.

80 Bieger RC, Brewer NS, Washington JA II. *Haemophilus aphrophilus*: a microbiologic and clinical review and report of 42 cases. *Medicine* 1978;**57**:345–55.

81 Bogers AJJC, van Vreeswijk H, Verbaan CJ *et al*. Early surgery for active infective endocarditis improves early and late results. *Thorac Cardiovasc Surg* 1991;**39**:284–7.

82 Aranki SF, Adams DH, Rizzo RJ *et al*. Determinants of early mortality and late survival in mitral valve endocarditis. *Circulation* 1995; **92**:143–9.

83 Middlemost S, Wisenbaugh T, Meyerowitz C *et al*. A case for early surgery in native left-sided endocarditis complicated by heart failure: results in 203 patients. *J Am Coll Cardiol* 1991;**18**: 663–7.

84 Jubair KA, Al Fagih MR, Ashmeg A, Belhaj M, Sawyer W. Cardiac operations during active endocarditis. *J Thorac Cardiovasc Surg* 1992;**104**: 487–90.

85 Wallace AG, Young G Jr, Osterhout S. Treatment of acute bacterial endocarditis by valve excision and replacement. *Circulation* 1965;**31**:450–3.

86 DiNubile MJ, Calderwood SB, Steinhaus DM, Karchmer AW. Cardiac conduction abnormalities complicating native valve active endocarditis. *Am J Cardiol* 1986;**58**:1213–17.

87 Tucker KJ, Johnson JA, Ong T, Mullen WL, Mailhot J. Medical management of prosthetic aortic valve endocarditis and aortic root abscess. *Am Heart J* 1993;**125**:1195–7.

88 Douglas JL, Cobbs CG. Prosthetic valve endocarditis. In: Kaye D. ed. *Infective endocarditis*, 2nd edn. New York: Raven Press, 1992, pp 375–96.

89 Woods GL, Wood P, Shaw BW Jr. *Aspergillus* endocarditis in patients without prior cardiovascular surgery: report of a case in a liver transplant recipient and review. *Rev Infect Dis* 1989;**II**:263–72.

90 Fowler VG, Durack DT. Infective endocarditis. *Curr Opin Cardiol* 1994;**9**:389–400.

91 Guzman F, Cartmill I, Holden MP, Freeman R. Candida endocarditis: report of four cases. *Int J Cardiol* 1987;**16**:131–6.

92 Scully RE, Mark EJ, McNeely WF, McNeely BU. Case records of the Massachusetts General Hospital. *N Engl J Med* 1996;**334**:105–11.

93 Khan SS, Gray RJ. Valvular emergencies. *Cardiol Clin* 1991;**9**:689–709.

94 Steckelberg JM, Murphy JG, Ballard D *et al*. Emboli in infective endocarditis: the prognostic value of echocardiography. *Ann Intern Med* 1991;**114**:635–40.

95 Kawamoto T, Nakano S, Matsuda H, Hirose H, Kawashima Y. Candida endocarditis with saddle embolism: a successful surgical intervention (abstract). *Ann Thorac Surg* 1989;**48**:723–4.

96 Tanka M, Toshio A, Hosokawa S, Suenaga Y, Hikosaka H. Tricuspid valve *Candida* endocarditis cured by valve-sparing debridement. *Ann Thorac Surg* 1989;**48**:857–8.

97 Isalska BJ, Stanbridge TN. Fluconazole in the treatment of candidal prosthetic valve endocarditis. *Br Med J* 1988;**297**:178–9.

98 Rhoads PS, Schram WR, Adair D. Bacteremia following tooth extraction: prevention with penicillin and N U 445. *J Am Dent Assoc* 1950; **41**:55–61.

99 Pressman RS, Bender IB. Antibiotic treatment of the gingival sulcus in the prevention of bacteremia. *Antibiotics Annual* 1954;92–104.

100 Northrop PM, Crowley MC. Further studies on the effect of the prophylactic use of sulfathiazole and sulfamerazine on bacteremia following extraction of teeth. *J Oral Surg* 1944;**2**:134.

101 Budnitz E, Nizel A, Berg L. Prophylactic use of sulfapyridine in patients susceptible to subacute bacterial endocarditis following dental surgical procedures. *J Am Dent Assoc* 1942;**29**:346.

102 Camara DS, Gruber M, Barde CJ *et al*. Transient bacteremia following endoscopic injection sclerotherapy of esophageal varices. *Arch Intern Med* 1983;**143**:1350–2.

103 Dajani AS, Taubert KA, Wilson WR *et al*. Prevention of bacterial endocarditis. Recommendations by the American Heart Association. *Circulation* 1997;**96**:358–66.

104 Delaye J, Etienne J, Feruglio A *et al*. Prophylaxis of infective endocarditis for dental procedures. Report of a working party of the European Society of Cardiology. *Eur Heart J* 1985;**6**:826–8.

105 Michel MF, Thompson J, Boering G, Hess J, van Putten PL. Revision of the guidelines of the Netherlands Heart Foundation for the prevention of endocarditis. *Geneesmiddelen-bull* 1986;**20**:53–6.

106 Shanson DC. Antibiotic prophylaxis of infective endocarditis in the United Kingdom and Europe. *J Antimicrob Chemother* 1987;**20**:119–31.

107 Meneely JK. Bacterial endocarditis following urethral manipulation. *N Engl J Med* 1948;**239**: 708–9.

108 Slade N. Bacteriaemia and septicaemia after urological operations. *Proc Roy Soc Med* 1958; **51**:331–4.

109 Sullivan NM, Sutter VL, Mims MM, Marsh VH, Finegold SM. Clinical aspects of bacteremia after manipulation of the genitourinary tract. *J Infect Dis* 1973;**127**:49–55.

110 Durack D. Prevention of infective endocarditis. *N Engl J Med* 1995;**332**:38–44.

111 Shorvon PJ, Eykyn SJ, Cotton PB. Gastrointestinal instrumentation, bacteraemia, and endocarditis. *Gut* 1983;**24**:1078–93.

112 Edson RS, van Scoy RE, Leary FJ. Gram-negative bacteremia after transrectal needle biopsy of the prostate. *Mayo Clin Proc* 1980;**55**:489–91.

113 Livengood CH III, Land MR, Addison WA. Endometrial biopsy, bacteremia, and endocarditis risk. *Obstet Gynecol* 1985;**65**: 678–81.

114 Mellow MH, Lewis RJ. Endoscopy-related bacteremia. Incidence of positive blood cultures after endoscopy of upper gastrointestinal tract. *Arch Intern Med* 1976;**136**:667–9.

115 Yin TP, Dellipiani AW. Bacterial endocarditis after Hurst bougienage in a patient with a benign oesophageal stricture. *Endoscopy* 1983;**15**:27–8.

116 Giglio JA, Rowland RW, Dalton HP, Laskin DM. Suture removal-induced bacteremia: a possible endocarditis risk. *J Am Dent Assoc* 1992;**123**: 65–70.

117 Ho H, Zuckerman MJ, Wassem C. A prospective controlled study of the risk of bacteremia in emergency sclerotherapy of esophageal varices. *Gastroenterology* 1991;**101**:1642–8.

118 Low DE, Shoenut JP, Kennedy JK *et al*. Prospective assessment of risk of bacteremia with colonoscopy and polypectomy. *Dig Dis Sci* 1987; **32**:1239–43.

119 Glauser MP, Bernard JP, Morceillon P, Francioli P. Successful single-dose amoxicillin prophylaxis against experimental streptococcal endocarditis: evidence for two mechanisms of protection. *J Infect Dis* 1983;**147**:568–75.

120 Bernard J, Francioli P, Glauser MP. Vancomycin prophylaxis of experimental *Streptococcus sanguis*; inhibition of bacterial adherence rather than bacterial killing. *J Clin Invest* 1981;**68**: 1113–16.

121 Moreillon P, Francioli P, Overholser P, Meylan P, Glauser MP. Mechanisms of successful amoxicillin prophylaxis of experimental endocarditis due to *Streptococcus intermedius*. *J Infect Dis* 1986;**154**:801–7.

122 Malinverni R, Overholser CD, Bille J, Glauser MP. Antibiotic prophylaxis of experimental endocarditis after dental extractions. *Lab Invest* 1988;**77**:182–7.

123 Glauser MP, Francioli P. Relevance of animal models to the prophylaxis of infective endocarditis. *J Antimicrob Chemother* 1987; **20**(Suppl A):87–93.

124 Durack DT, Petersdorf RG, Beeson PB. Penicillin prophylaxis of experimental *S. viridans* endocarditis. *Trans Assoc Am Physicians* 1972; **85**:222–30.

125 Durack DT, Petersdorf RG. Chemotherapy of experimental streptococcal endocarditis. I.

Comparison of commonly recommended prophylactic regimens. *J Clin Invest* 1973;**52**: 592–8.

126 Pelletier LL, Durack DT, Petersdorf RG. Chemotherapy of experimental streptococcal endocarditis. IV. Further observations on antimicrobial prophylaxis. *J Clin Invest* 1975; **56**:319–30.

127 Horstkotte D, Friedrichs W, Pippert H, Bircks W, Loogen F. Benefits of endocarditis prevention in patients with prosthetic heart valves (German). *Z Kardiol* 1986;**75**:8–11.

128 van der Meer JTM, van Wijk W, Thompson J *et al.* Efficacy of antibiotic prophylaxis for prevention of native-valve endocarditis. *Lancet* 1992;**339**:135–40.

129 Patton JP. Infective endocarditis: economic considerations. In: Kaye D. ed. *Infective endocarditis*, 2nd edn. New York: Raven Press, 1992, pp 413–22.

130 Imperiale TF, Horwitz RI. Does prophylaxis prevent postdental infective endocarditis? A controlled evaluation of protective efficacy. *Am J Med* 1990;**88**:131–6.

131 Everett ED, Hirschmann JV. Transient bacteremia and endocarditis prophylaxis. A review. *Medicine* 1977;**56**:61–77.

132 Biorn CL, Browning WH, Thompson L. Transient bacteremia immediately following transurethral prostatic resection. *J Urol* 1950;**63**: 155–61.

133 Clemens JD, Ransohoff DF. A quantitative assessment of pre-dental antibiotic prophylaxis for patients with mitral-valve prolapse. *J Chron Dis* 1984;**37**:531–44.

134 Bor DH, Himmelstein DU. Endocarditis prophylaxis for patients with mitral valve prolapse: a quantitative analysis. *Am J Med* 1984;**76**:711–17.

Antithrombotic therapy after heart valve replacement

53

ALEXANDER G. G. TURPIE

INTRODUCTION

Despite improvements in prosthetic materials and valve design, thromboembolism remains a serious complication in patients following heart valve replacement. It is generally agreed that lifelong oral anticoagulants are indicated in patients with mechanical prosthetic valves and in patients with tissue values, if they have atrial fibrillation or a history of thromboembolism.[1-3] In the absence of antithrombotic therapy, systemic embolism and stroke have been reported in between 5% and 50% of patients, depending upon the valve site, the type of valve replacement and the presence of comorbid conditions.[2,3] With the use of anticoagulants, the rate of systemic embolism has been reduced to 1–3% per year.[4] Antithrombotic therapy, however, carries an important risk of bleeding, which is related to the level of anticoagulation used.[5] Studies of long term oral anticoagulant therapy for deep vein thrombosis have shown that a less intense regimen (INR 2.0–3.0) is as effective but safer than the more intense regimen (INR 3.0–4.5) that was standard until recently.[6-8] Subsequently, studies in patients following either bioprosthetic or mechanical heart valve replacement have shown reduced bleeding with a lower intensity of anticoagulants without loss of efficacy,[9-11] and based on these studies there has been marked improvement in the safety of the long term anticoagulant regimens used following heart valve replacement.

BIOPROSTHETIC HEART VALVES

The risk of thromboembolism is less with uncomplicated bioprosthetic valves than with mechanical valves.[12-15] Oral anticoagulants, including warfarin, have been shown to be effective and safe when used at a targeted INR of 2.0–3.0 in such patients based on the results of one prospective clinical trial.[9] This study compared two intensities of anticoagulation to determine the safety and efficacy of a less intense anticoagulant regimen in patients following tissue valve replacement. One hundred and eight patients were randomized to standard anticoagulant control (INR 3.0–4.5), and 102 patients to

Table 53.1 Antithrombotic therapy in bioprosthetic heart valve replacement

	INR	Duration
Mitral	2.0–3.0	3 mth
Aortic	A/C optional	3 mth
Atrial fibrillation	2.0–3.0	Long term
Left atrial thrombosis	2.0–3.0	3 mth minimum Duration uncertain
Systemic embolism	2.0–3.0	3–12 mth Duration uncertain

(Aspirin optional long term in uncomplicated patients)

A/C, Anticoagulants.
From Stein *et al*.[4]

a less intensive regimen (INR 2.0–2.5). Treatment was continued for 3 months. In this study there was no difference in the frequency of major systemic emboli (1.8% vs 1.8%) between the two treatment groups, but there were significantly fewer major hemorrhagic complications (0.0% vs 4.5%; $P = 0.034$) and total hemorrhagic complications (5.4% vs 14.6%; $P = 0.042$) in the low intensity group (INR 2.0–3.0) compared to the high intensity group, respectively. This level of anticoagulation (INR 2.0–3.0) is now recommended by the American College of Chest Physicians (ACCP) for patients with tissue valve replacement.[4]

The risk of thromboembolism is limited mainly to the first 3 months postoperatively in uncomplicated patients with tissue valves, but is present indefinitely in patients with atrial fibrillation. Consequently, in uncomplicated patients with mitral bioprosthetic valves, anticoagulant therapy is recommended for 3 months while long term therapy is indicated in patients with atrial fibrillation, those with an atrial thrombus detected at echocardiography, and those who develop a systemic embolus.[4] Patients with uncomplicated bioprosthetic valves in the aortic position are at very low risk of systemic embolism and some authorities therefore suggest they do not require anticoagulant therapy, although this recommendation remains controversial.[4] The current recommendations by the ACCP for patients with tissue valves are shown in Table 53.1.

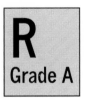

R
Grade A

MECHANICAL PROSTHETIC HEART VALVES

Patients with mechanical heart valve prostheses require lifelong anticoagulation therapy. The optimal level of anticoagulation in patients with mechanical heart valve replacements has been placed on a scientific footing based on the results of recent studies. Randomized trials have shown that oral anticoagulants are effective in reducing the risk of systemic embolism in patients with mechanical prosthetic valves when given at lower intensity than has been used in the past. In its 1995 guidelines the ACCP recommended long term oral anticoagulant therapy for patients with mechanical prostheses monitored to prolong the INR to 2.5–3.5.[4] This recommendation was based on two prospective studies that demonstrated that anticoagulant therapy maintained within this target INR range was as effective as a more intense level of anticoagulation, but with less bleeding. In the first study[10] there was no difference in the frequency of major embolic events in the patients treated with a high intensity regimen (INR 9.0) compared with patients treated with a less intense (INR 2.65) anticoagulant regimen (4.0 vs 3.7 embolic episodes per 100 patient years, respectively). However, there was significantly less bleeding in the less intense group (6.2 vs 12.1 hemorrhagic episodes per 100 patient years; P<0.02). The second study[11] compared low intensity (INR 2.0–2.99) with high intensity (INR 3.0–4.5) oral anticoagulants in patients with mechanical valves, all of whom were treated with aspirin (330 mg twice per day) in combination with dipyridamole (75 mg per day). In this study one transient ischemic attack occurred in the low intensity group and two in the high intensity group. There were significantly fewer bleeding events in the low intensity group, in which three episodes occurred compared with 12 in the high intensity group (P<0.02).

Although these studies form the basis for the recommendations for a less intense level of anticoagulation, they have a number of limitations. In the first study a very high intensity anticoagulant regimen was compared with a moderately high intensity anticoagulant regimen. The mean daily dose of warfarin in the high intensity group was 8.5 mg and in the low intensity group the mean daily dose of 5.9 mg was similar to the average daily dose of 5.4 mg used in the high intensity group in three venous thrombosis studies,[6–8] and in the randomized study in patients with tissue valves.[9] This suggests that the low intensity group in the first mechanical valve study[10] may have been equivalent to the standard intensity group in the venous thromboembolism studies.[8] The second study[11] was small, and therefore the claim that the two regimens were identical in efficacy is questionable. This latter study does, however, confirm the marked difference in bleeding between high intensity and low intensity anticoagulant regimens. A recent study from France[16] has confirmed the efficacy of a less intense level of anticoagulation following mechanical heart valve replacement. In this study 433 patients with mechanical prostheses were randomized to anticoagulant therapy monitored to achieve an INR of 2.0–3.0 or 3.0–4.5 and followed for 2.2 years. Thromboembolic outcome events, either clinical events or asymptomatic CNS abnormalities proven on CT scan, occurred in 10 of 185 (5.3%) patients in the low intensity group and 9 of 192 (4.7%) patients in the high intensity group (P=0.78). Importantly, there was a statistically significant difference in the rate of bleeding complications between the two groups. Bleeding events occurred in 34 patients (18.1%) in the lower intensity group compared with 56 patients (29.2%) in the high intensity group (P<0.01). The majority of patients in this trial, however, had aortic valve replacements and were in sinus rhythm, which limits the generalizability of the results. The ACCP recommendations for mechanical valves are shown in Table 53.2.

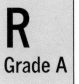

The ACCP recommendation of an INR target of 2.5–3.5 is lower than that reported in a study conducted in Europe which has recommended a target range of 3.0–4.0.[17] However, the European recommendation is based on retrospective data and largely on events that occurred in patients with older caged ball valve prostheses. Thus recommendations based on these data are unlikely to be applicable for use in patients with the modern bileaflet and tilting disc valves that are currently in use.

COMBINATION ANTITHROMBOTIC THERAPY

A major limitation to the current approach used to treat high risk patients with prosthetic heart valves is that systemic embolism, which may result in disabling stroke, still occurs

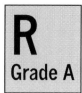

Grade A

Table 53.2 Antithrombotic therapy in mechanical heart valve replacement

	INR
Bileaflet	2.5–3.5
Tilting disc	2.5–3.5
Caged ball/disc	Consider higher INR
Systemic embolism	2.5–3.5 Plus aspirin 80 mg/day *or* Dipyridamole 400 mg/day

From Stein *et al*.[4]

Table 53.3 Dipyridamole plus anticoagulants following heart valve replacement

	Oral A/C alone	Oral A/C plus dipyridamole	% RR	2P
Thromboembolism	69/582 (11.9%)	31/559 (5.5%)	56	0.007
Non-fatal T/E	48/582 (8.2%)	24/559 (4.3%)	50	0.005
Fatal T/E	21/582 (3.6%)	7/559 (1.3%)	64	0.008
Death	67/582 (11.5%)	40/559 (7.2%)	40	0.013
Hemorrhage	87/539 (16.1%)	80/501 (16.0%)	−1	0.94

A/C, Anticoagulants; T/E, thromboembolism.
From Pouleur and Buyse.[20]

Grade A

at a rate of approximately 2–3% per year, despite the use of anticoagulants.[4] The addition of antiplatelet agents to oral anticoagulants has been advocated as an improved approach to the treatment of patients with mechanical valves, or high risk patients with tissue valves, to reduce further the risk of major systemic embolism. In an early study[18] the combination of dipyridamole and oral anticoagulants significantly reduced mortality in patients with early models of the Starr–Edwards prosthesis compared with anticoagulants alone. A subsequent study from the Mayo Clinic[19] reported that the addition of dipyridamole to oral anticoagulants significantly reduced the risk of thromboembolic events in patients with mechanical heart valve prostheses. A recent meta-analysis of the dipyridamole studies (Table 53.3) has confirmed improved outcomes with combined therapy compared with anticoagulants alone.[20] The routine use of dipyridamole in combination with oral anticoagulants is, however, not widely accepted for the treatment of patients with mechanical valves or high risk patients with tissue valves, because of the frequency of side effects, including intractable headache, dizziness, nausea, flushing, and syncope.

The combination of aspirin and oral anticoagulants has also been used in the treatment of patients with heart valve replacement with a significant reduction in embolic complications, but with an increased risk of bleeding complications.[21] In the early studies reported to date, aspirin was used in high doses (approximately 1 g/day), and in most cases the bleeding with the combination of high dose aspirin and high dose oral anticoagulants was gastrointestinal.[22] There is good evidence that gastrointestinal irritation and hemorrhage is dose-dependent over a range of 100 mg to 1000 mg of

Table 53.4 Effect of aspirin combined with antithrombotic therapy following heart valve replacement

	Aspirin + warfarin (n=186)	Placebo + warfarin (n=184)	RR % (95% CI)	2P
Systemic embolism	1.6	4.6	65.0 (1.8–37.5)	0.037
Vascular death	0.6	4.4	85.5 (36.0–96.7)	0.003
Death	2.8	7.4	61.7 (16.8–82.3)	0.009

Figures represent % annualized rates.
From Turpie et al.[23]

aspirin per day and that the antithrombotic effects of aspirin are independent of the dose over this range.

One completed study[23] compared low dose aspirin combined with warfarin in the treatment of patients with mechanical heart valve replacements to determine whether low dose aspirin would result in an improved antithrombotic effect, without the same high risk of bleeding that has been reported for the combination of oral anticoagulants with high dose aspirin. This was a double-blind, randomized trial to compare the relative efficacy and safety of aspirin (100 mg per day) with placebo in the prevention of systemic embolism or vascular death in patients with mechanical heart valve replacement or high risk patients with tissue valves who had atrial fibrillation or a history of thromboembolism. Three hundred and seventy patients were treated with oral anticoagulant therapy (warfarin: INR 3.0–4.5) and randomized to receive aspirin (186 patients) or placebo (184 patients) and followed for up to 4 years (average 2.5 years). The outcomes of the study were systemic embolism, valve thrombosis, vascular death, and hemorrhage. Systemic embolism or vascular death occurred in 6 (3.2%) of the aspirin-treated patients and 24 (13.0%) of the placebo-treated patients (risk reduction (RR) 77.2%; 90% confidence interval (CI) 51.7–89.2%; $P=0.0002$). The corresponding rates for systemic embolism or death from any cause were 13 (7.0%) and 33 (17.9%), respectively (RR 64.7%; 90% CI 39.6–79.5%; $P=0.0005$); for vascular death 2 (1.1%) and 13 (7.1%), respectively (RR 85.4%; 90% CI 49.8–95.9%; $P=0.0015$); and for death from any cause 9 (4.8%) and 22 (12.0%), respectively (RR 62.7%; 90% CI 44.5–80.5%; $P=0.0048$). Major bleeding events occurred in 24 (12%) of the aspirin-treated patients compared with 19 (10.3%) in the placebo-treated patients (absolute difference 2.6%; 90% CI 3.4 minus 8.3%; $P=0.2710$).

The results of this study, the annualized rates of which are summarized in Table 53.4, demonstrated that in patients with mechanical valve replacement or high risk patients with tissue valve replacement, the addition of aspirin (100 mg per day) to oral anticoagulation therapy (warfarin: INR 3.0–4.5) reduced mortality, vascular mortality, and systemic embolism, but with some increase in minor bleeding. In a recent study in patients with mechanical prostheses,[24] it was shown that low dose aspirin (100 mg/day) was as effective as high dose aspirin (650 mg/day) in combination with oral anticoagulants at a target INR of 2.0–3.0, but with a reduced risk of bleeding.

Ticlopidine may also be useful as an adjunct to oral anticoagulants, but the data are less solid since the one study in which it has been evaluated was not randomized.[25]

R
Grade A

SUMMARY

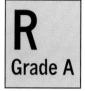

The demonstration that, for most indications for oral anticoagulant therapy, less intense anticoagulation (INR 2.0–3.0) is as efficacious as standard intensity anticoagulation (INR 3.0–4.5) but with significantly less bleeding is an important advance in antithrombotic therapy. It has greatly improved safety of long term oral anticoagulant therapy and has resulted in its more widespread use in the prevention and treatment of thromboembolism. It is the level of choice in uncomplicated patients with tissue prostheses. However, further evidence is required before this less intense regimen is routinely adopted for patients with mechanical valves and for high risk patients with tissue valves. The addition of low dose aspirin to anticoagulants may be more efficacious in the prevention of systemic embolism and vascular death in heart valve replacement patients than anticoagulants alone and may permit a lower intensity of anticoagulation to be used.

REFERENCES

1 Starr A. Late complications of aortic valve replacement with cloth-covered composite-seat prostheses. *Ann Thorac Surg* 1975;**19**:289.

2 Larsen GL, Alexander JA, Stanford W. Thromboembolic phenomena in patients with prosthetic aortic valves who did not receive anticoagulants. *Ann Thorac Surg* 1977;**12**:323.

3 Limet R, Lepage G, Grondin CM. Thromboembolic complications with the cloth-covered Starr–Edwards aortic prosthesis in patients not receiving anticogulants. *Ann Thorac Surg* 1977;**23**:529.

4 Stein PD, Alpert JS, Copeland JG, Dalen JE, Turpie AGG. Antithrombotic therapy in patients with mechanical and bioprosthetic heart valves. *Chest* 1995;**108**:371S–379S.

5 Levine MN, Hirsh J, Landefeld S *et al*. Hemorrhagic complications of anticoagulant treatment. *Chest* 1992;**102**(Suppl 4):352–63.

6 Hull R, Delmore T, Genton E *et al*. Warfarin sodium versus low-dose heparin in the long-term treatment of venous thrombosis. *N Engl J Med* 1979;**301**:855–8.

7 Hull R, Hirsh J, Jay R *et al*. Different intensities of oral anticoagulant therapy in the treatment of proximal vein thrombosis. *N Engl J Med* 1982;**307**:1676–81.

8 Hull R, Delmore T, Carter C *et al*. Adjusted subcutaneous heparin versus warfarin sodium in the long-term treatment of venous thrombosis. *N Engl J Med* 1982;**306**:189–94.

9 Turpie AGG, Gunstensen J, Hirsh J *et al*. A randomized trial comparing two intensities of oral anticoagulant therapy following tissue heart valve replacement. *Lancet* 1988;**i**:1242–5.

10 Saour JN, Sieck JO, Gallus AS. Trial of different intensities of anticoagulation in patients with prosthetic heart valves. *N Engl J Med* 1990;**332**:428–32.

11 Altman P, Rouvier J, Gurfinkel E *et al*. Comparison of two levels of anticoagulant therapy in patients with substitute heart valves. *J Thorac Cardiovasc Surg* 1991;**101**:427–31.

12 Cevese PG. Long-term results of 212 xenograft valve replacements. *J Cardiovasc Surg* 1975;**16**:639–42.

13 Pipkin RD, Buch WS, Fogarty TS. Evaluation of aortic valve replacement with a porcine xenograft without long-term anticoagulation. *J Thorac Cardiovasc Surg* 1976;**71**:179–86.

14 Stinson EB, Griepp RB, Oyer PE *et al*. Long-term experience with porcine aortic valve xenografts. *J Thorac Cardiovasc Surg* 1977;**73**:54–63.

15 Ionescu MI, Pakrashi BC, Mary DAS *et al*. Long-term evaluation of tissue valves. *J Thorac Cardiovasc Surg* 1974;**68**:361–79.

16 Acar J, Iung B, Boissel JP *et al*. AREVA: Multicenter randomized comparison of low-dose versus standard-dose anticoagulation in patients with mechanical prosthetic heart valves. *Circulation* 1996;**94**(9):2107–12.

17 Cannegieter SC, Rosendaal FR, Wintzen AR *et al*. Optimal oral anticoagulant therapy in patients with mechanical heart valves. *N Engl J Med* 1995;**333**(1):11–17.

18 Sullivan JM, Harken DE, Gorlin R. Pharmacologic control of thromboembolic complications of cardiac valve replacement. *N Engl J Med* 1971;**284**:1391–4.

19 Chesebro JG, Fuster V, Elveback LR *et al*. Trial of combined warfarin plus dipyridamole or aspirin therapy in prosthetic heart valve replacement: danger of aspirin compared with dipyridamole. *Am J Cardiol* 1983;**51**:1537–41.

20 Pouleur H, Buyse M. Effects of dipyridamole in combination with anticoagulant therapy on survival and thromboembolic events in patients

with prosthetic heart valves. A meta-analysis of the randomized trials. *J Thorac Cardiovasc Surg* 1995;**110**:463–6.

21 Dale J, Myhre E, Storstein O *et al*. Prevention of arterial thromboembolism with acetylsalicyl acid: a controlled clinical study in patients with aortic ball valves. *Am Heart J* 1977;**94**:101–11.

22 Hirsh J, Dalen JE, Fuster V *et al*. Aspirin and other platelet-active drugs: the relationship between dose, effectiveness and side effects. *Chest* 1995; **108**:247S–257S.

23 Turpie AGG, Gent M, Laupacis A *et al*. A double-blind randomized trial of acetylsalicylic acid (100 mg) versus placebo in patients treated with oral anticoagulants following heart valve replacement. *N Engl J Med* 1991;**329**:1365–9.

24 Altman R, Rouvier J, Gurfinkel E, Scazziota A, Turpie AGG. Comparison of high-dose with low-dose aspirin in patients with mechanical heart valve replacement treated with oral anticoagulant. *Circulation* 1996;**94**(9):2113–16.

25 Hayashi JI, Nakazawa S, Oguma F, Miyamura H, Eguchi S. Combined warfarin and antiplatelet therapy after St Jude mechanical valve replacement for mitral valve disease. *J Am Coll Cardiol* 1994;**23**:672–7.

Part III
Specific cardiovascular disorders
x: Other conditions

BERNARD J GERSH and SALIM YUSUF, Editors

Grading of recommendations and levels of evidence used in *Evidence Based Cardiology*

GRADE A

Level 1a   Evidence from large randomized clinical trials (RCTs) or systematic reviews (including meta-analyses) of multiple randomized trials which collectively has at least as much data as one single well-defined trial.

Level 1b   Evidence from at least one "All or None" high quality cohort study; in which ALL patients died/failed with conventional therapy and some survived/succeeded with the new therapy (eg chemotherapy for tuberculosis, meningitis, or defibrillation for ventricular fibrillation); or in which many died/failed with conventional therapy and NONE died/failed with the new therapy (eg penicillin for pneumococcal infections).

Level 1c   Evidence from at least one moderate sized RCT or a meta-analysis of small trials which collectively only has a moderate number of patients.

Level 1d   Evidence from at least one RCT.

GRADE B

Level 2   Evidence from at least one high quality study of non-randomized cohorts who did and did not receive the new therapy.

Level 3   Evidence from at least one high quality case control study.

Level 4   Evidence from at least one high quality case series.

GRADE C

Level 5   Opinions from experts without reference or access to any of the foregoing (eg argument from physiology, bench research or first principles).

A comprehensive approach would incorporate many different types of evidence (eg RCTs, non-RCTs, epidemiologic studies, and experimental data), and examine the architecture of the information for consistency, coherence and clarity. Occasionally the evidence does not completely fit into neat compartments. For example, there may not be an RCT that demonstrates a reduction in mortality in individuals with stable angina with the use of beta-blockers, but there is overwhelming evidence that mortality is  reduced following MI. In such cases, some may recommend use of beta-blockers in angina patients with the expectation that some extrapolation from post-MI trials is warranted. This could be expressed as Grade A/C. In other instances (e.g. smoking cessation or a pacemaker for complete heart block), the non-randomized data are so overwhelmingly clear and biologically plausible that it would be reasonable to consider these interventions as Grade A.

Recommendation grades appear either in a shaded margin box with an 'R' logo as shown, or within the text, for example Grade A.

Pregnancy and heart disease

54

CELIA M. OAKLEY

INTRODUCTION

Heart disease in pregnancy may be perceived as a rarity because most pregnant women have normal hearts and seek antenatal care from their general practitioner and local hospital rather than travel, so cardiologists, obstetricians, and anesthetists tend to see insufficient pregnant cardiac patients to feel confident. Yet heart disease is the third commonest non-obstetric cause of maternal death after hypertension and pulmonary embolism.[1] Rheumatic heart disease used to have a prevalence of up to 1% in young pregnant women but is now rare in the West. Congenital heart disease has become both relatively and absolutely more common in pregnancy as a result of the major improvement in survival of children with previously lethal congenital heart disease but with the separation of pediatric from adult cardiology, adult cardiologists are often inexperienced in their management.

The numerically small personal experience of most physicians and obstetricians explains a lack of randomized trials. These have been few even in the treatment of pregnancy-associated hypertension. The literature is largely composed of case reports, sometimes brought together into reviews of anecdotal experience. Even sizeable personal series are few. Most evidence is therefore level C, based on first principles, personal experience, small reported personal case series or published reviews of the anecdotal literature.

In general, heart disease tends to get worse over time. Women with any sort of heart disease who are ever going to have children should be advised to have them early. Advice about the safety and conduct of pregnancy follows a full diagnosis and appreciation of how the circulatory changes occurring during pregnancy will be handled. Most patients do well if they are in New York Heart Association (NYHA) symptomatic classes I or II before pregnancy, although there are exceptions (see Box at top of page 916).

915

Pre-existing heart disease

- Women with leftsided obstructive lesions or artificial heart valves need special care.
- Pulmonary hypertension carries the highest maternal mortality.
- Aortic dissection is a risk in the Marfan syndrome and in coarctation of the aorta.
- Cyanosed women get bluer and fetal growth is poor.

Cardiovascular disorders arising in pregnancy

- Hypertension is the main cause of maternal death followed by pulmonary embolism.
- Pulmonary embolism is commonest in the third trimester and postpartum, particularly after cesarean delivery.
- Peripartum cardiomyopathy may cause fatal heart failure (usually postpartum) but often with considerable recovery of function in survivors.
- Peripartum myocardial infarction is most often caused by spontaneous coronary artery dissection.

PHYSIOLOGICAL CHANGES DURING NORMAL PREGNANCY

Cardiac output increases between 30% and 50% during normal pregnancy. This starts at about the fifth week of gestation and most is achieved by a rise in stroke volume with only a small increase in heart rate of 10–20 beats/min at rest. At the same time circulating blood volume expands consequent upon prostaglandin-induced relaxation of smooth muscle, a greater increase in plasma volume than in red cell volume, giving rise to the physiological anemia of pregnancy.[2]

- Blood volume and cardiac output increase steadily by up to 50% (more in multiple pregnancies).
- Stroke volume rises more than heart rate.
- Diastolic blood pressure falls and pulse pressure widens.
- Coagulation factors, fibrinogen, and platelet turnover rise and fibrinolytic activity diminishes. The risk of thromboembolism increases.

Left ventricular mass and end diastolic volume increase, as do the contractile indices calculated by echocardiography which also often reveals mild physiological regurgitation through the tricuspid, pulmonary, and mitral valves.[3] The cardiac output nears its peak halfway through pregnancy with only a smaller increase thereafter. During the third trimester stroke volume is highly sensitive to changes in posture because the gravid uterus compresses the inferior vena cava (and to some extent the aorta) and reduces right atrial, pulmonary artery, and left atrial pressures in the supine position. This was used to good effect by obstetricians in the past who put their patients with mitral stenosis on bedrest which kept them out of pulmonary edema.

The magnitude of the circulatory changes correlates with the size and weight of the products of conception.[4] The hemodynamic load is therefore greater in multiple pregnancy, as is the risk of heart failure in heart disease.

The physiological changes in pregnancy, labor, and the puerperium have been measured by reliable means. High risk conditions (see Box at top of this page) are well recognized with concordance between published single center series, reviews, and personal experience. Preconceptual counseling, although desirable, is often impossible as most women are already pregnant when first seen but in girls with heart disease, future pregnancy should be discussed in the same way as future career and family planning advice should be given as they enter their reproductive years.

Preconceptual counseling

Preconceptual counseling in women with pre-existing heart disease considers:
- the effect of the hemodynamic changes on tolerance of the cardiac disorder;
- the effect of the cardiac disorder on fetal development (poor in women with cyanotic congenital heart disease);
- the effect of maternal drugs on the fetus;
- patient compliance, prognosis, and family support;
- the genetic risk to the fetus.

In addition to pre-existing heart disease, new cardiac disorders may arise in pregnancy and one may impinge on another. The coagulopathy of pregnancy increases the risk of both systemic and pulmonary thromboembolism in patients with valve disease and reduced collagen synthesis may lead to dissection of a previously normal aorta or increase the risk in a Marfan aorta.

Pre-existing disease	*Arising in or exacerbated by pregnancy*
Congenital	Pulmonary vascular disease
Valvular	Embolism
	pulmonary
	coronary
Marfan syndrome	Dissection
	aortic
	coronary
	pulmonary artery
Cardiomyopathy	Peripartum cardiomyopathy
Coronary disease	Myocardial infarction
Hypertension	Pre-eclampsia

CONGENITAL HEART DISEASE

Most common is atrial septal defect (ASD). Ventricular septal defect and patent arterial duct are less frequent as many have been closed in childhood and small ventricular defects often close spontaneously. Most of the simple acyanotic defects cause no trouble but pregnancy carries risks in women with severe left ventricular outflow tract obstruction, pulmonary hypertension, cyanosis or restricted cardiac output. Adults from medically unmonitored communities with previously unsuspected major cardiac defects may be seen in pregnancy for the first time (see Box at top of page 918).

Congenital heart disease and pregnancy

Well tolerated
Uncomplicated septal defects
Pulmonary stenosis
Hypertrophic cardiomyopathy (usually)
Acyanotic Ebstein's anomaly
Corrected transposition without other substantive defects

Moderate risk
Coarctation of the aorta
Cyanosed mother with pulmonary stenosis
Univentricular circulation after the Fontan procedure

High maternal (and fetal) risk
Pulmonary hypertension
Severe aortic stenosis

High fetal risk
Cyanosed mother with pulmonary stenosis or complex pulmonary atresia

---

Although only closure of a patent arterial duct can be regarded as a complete "cure", late problems are rare but arrhythmias may develop years after closure of secundum atrial septal defect and pulmonary vascular disease may progress after closure of a non-restrictive ventricular defect. Survivors of palliative surgery for complex congenital defects need to be assessed for cardiovascular reserve, ventricular function, pulmonary hypertension or stenosis, conduit stenosis, conduction defects, and arrhythmia.

Acyanotic congenital heart disease

While even severe pulmonary stenosis is well tolerated in pregnancy, leftsided obstruction carries risk. Hemorrhage, if it occurs postpartum, is poorly tolerated in ASD and can cause unexpected cardiac arrest, leading to massive left to right flow diversion with loss of left ventricular output and coronary flow.[5]

Both systemic and pulmonary artery dissections have an increased incidence in pregnancy either as a result of diminished collagen synthesis and wall thinning or due to increased uptake of water by connective tissue mucopolysaccharides. Dissection or rupture of the main pulmonary artery may develop when a duct is large and complicated by pulmonary hypertension. Aortic dissection may complicate coarctation of the aorta, sometimes even after surgical treatment, and arise either in the post-stenotic dilation distal to the coarctation or in the aortic root.[6]

Aortic stenosis

Aortic stenosis can be treacherous.[7] Women who were symptom free before pregnancy may develop angina, left ventricular failure, pulmonary edema or sudden death. The obstruction is usually valvular associated with some form of bicuspid valve. Subvalvar and supravalvar stenosis are much rarer. The increase in blood volume and stroke volume and decrease in systemic vascular resistance lead to an increase in left ventricular pressure and pressure drop across the obstruction. An increase in left ventricular work demands augmentation of coronary blood flow. Patients with mild or moderate stenosis do well but should plan to complete their families before the valve inevitably deteriorates. Assessment of fitness should occur before pregnancy is attempted.

Aortic stenosis and pregnancy

Fit for pregnancy
- Normal exercise tolerance
- Normal electrocardiogram or voltage increase only
- Negative exercise test with normal blood pressure rise, achievement of target heart rate, and absence of inducible ST-T wave changes
- Good left ventricular function on echo
- Peak aortic velocity on echocardiography <4.5 m/s.

Patients who have repolarization changes on the ECG, an impaired exercise test or left ventricular dysfunction should be advised against pregnancy until after the aortic stenosis has been relieved.

If all is well, serial Doppler velocities show an increase in the peak velocity of flow across the valve, indicating a normal rise in stroke volume. No change or a fall in stroke volume may be followed by dyspnea or angina. This may improve with rest and a beta-blocker to reduce demand and improve diastolic coronary blood flow. If intervention is needed and the fetus is not yet viable, balloon valvuloplasty may help to tide the patient through.[8] If the fetus is viable it should be delivered by cesarean section under general anesthesia *before* aortic valve replacement.

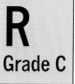

Children have an 18% risk of inheriting a bicuspid aortic valve from their mother (but only about 5% if the father has the condition).[9]

Coarctation of the aorta

Coarctation may be first recognized in pregnancy and most do well although there are risks of aortic dissection, rupture of an intracranial berry aneurysm, infective endocarditis or heart failure. These complications led to a mortality of 17% in early reports but to less than 3% in recent ones.[10,11]

Mild coarctations are uncommon and typically circulation to the distal segment is conducted almost entirely through collateral channels. Despite this, fetal development is normal and pre-eclampsia is rare, both suggesting that uteroplacental blood flow is well maintained. An associated bicuspid aortic valve increases the risk of endocarditis.

Drug treatment of the hypertension is unsatisfactory because surges in systolic pressure and pulse pressure occur with exercise and cannot be prevented pharmacologically. Overenthusiastic blood pressure reduction will diminish placental perfusion. Pregnant patients with uncorrected coarctations should therefore avoid strenuous exercise.

Corrected transposition

Corrected transposition (atrioventricular discordance with ventriculoarterial discordance) is usually accompanied by other defects, particularly ventricular septal defect, pulmonary stenosis, and malformation of the leftsided tricuspid valve. Sometimes other substantive defects are absent and the patient is referred because of a "mitral" regurgitant or ejection systolic murmur. A review of 18 patients without associated defects and first diagnosed between the ages of 16 and 61 years revealed that three of the nine women had had uneventful pregnancies producing seven children, none of whom had congenital heart disease.[12] Failure of the morphological right ventricle which supports the systemic circulation is the usual cause of death and its function should be observed closely during pregnancy, particularly in older women.

Cyanotic congenital heart disease

Cyanotic congenital heart disease is usually associated either with pulmonary hypertension (in the Eisenmenger syndrome) or with pulmonary stenosis (in the tetralogy of Fallot or with transposition or complex pulmonary atresia with extensive bronchial collateral supply to the lungs). Patients with Ebstein's anomaly of the tricuspid valve may be acyanotic or cyanosed. All are compatible with survival to adult life with or without previous palliative or radical surgery.

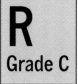

Cyanosis increases the risk for both the mother and the fetus. Patients with a low pulmonary artery pressure usually accomplish pregnancy without personal mishap but need bedrest to maximize arterial oxygen saturation and prophylactic subcutaneous heparin to reduce the risks of paradoxical embolism or closure of a systemic pulmonary shunt or stent. It has long been known (and exemplified by the late Helen Taussig's patients with the tetralogy and Blalock Taussig shunts)[13] that fetal growth is poor in cyanosed women. The chances of success are related to the arterial oxygen saturation and inversely to the hematocrit. Miscarriage is frequent and babies are almost always born prematurely and small for dates. Fetal growth needs careful monitoring and delivery should be accomplished as soon as it slows. Generous hydration is most important at all stages and the subcutaneous heparin should be exchanged for warfarin in the postpartum period until full mobilization has been achieved.

The Eisenmenger syndrome

Pulmonary hypertension in the Eisenmenger syndrome carries considerable dangers during pregnancy.[14-16] Firm advice should be given against it and early tubal ligation advised. Women with the Eisenmenger syndrome who become pregnant and refuse abortion should be admitted to hospital as soon as the hematocrit rises or oximetry shows a fall in resting arterial saturation or in any case by the middle of the second trimester. Prophylactic heparin, nasal oxygen, and continuous pulse oximetry are needed. Rest may enable some patients to achieve nearly normal arterial saturation and in that case fetal growth may continue at a normal rate.

In patients with persistently reduced arterial saturation, fetal growth will slow and cease before full term. As soon as this occurs the baby should be delivered by cesarean section. Although vaginal delivery under epidural anesthesia is often advised, this is associated with maternal exertion, systemic vasodilation and increased desaturation, causing greater risk to both baby and mother. General anesthesia gives the mother rest with maximal arterial saturation. Generous hydration should be maintained and any blood loss replaced promptly. After delivery mobilization of the mother should be slow and the patient returned to the ITU with oxygen, pulse oximetry, and subcutaneous heparin continued. Despite these precautions, many patients die suddenly, usually a week or so after delivery and at post-mortem there is no explanation. It is uncommon for these patients to die from pulmonary or paradoxical embolism if heparin has been given and the mechanism in monitored patients has been observed to be one of progressive increase in pulmonary vascular resistance with bradycardia, systemic vasodilation, a disastrous increase in right to left shunting, and ventricular fibrillation.

Pulmonary hypertension, either in the Eisenmenger syndrome or primary, is the single condition with the highest maternal mortality.[17] No effective pulmonary vasodilation can be achieved because changes in the resistance vessels are largely structural.

VALVULAR HEART DISEASE

The rarity of rheumatic valve disease in the indigenous community in the West has reduced clinical diagnostic skills. Five young women with previously undiagnosed mitral valve disease were described from Bradford, England.[18] Four were immigrant Asians and one was white with infective endocarditis. All had presented with sudden onset of pulmonary edema in pregnancy. Only one was in atrial fibrillation. Heart murmurs were heard in only two. There was mistaken reluctance to perform chest radiography and echocardiography was only performed after a cardiologist had finally seen them. Two of the patients died.

Previously asymptomatic or mildly dyspneic patients with mitral stenosis can develop rapidly progressive shortness of breath and pulmonary edema in pregnancy. Tachycardia causes the stroke volume to fall and the left atrial pressure to rise. A vicious circle of increasing reflex tachycardia, decreasing stroke volume, and rising left atrial pressure leads to pulmonary edema. Beta-adrenergic blocking drugs can be life saving by providing time for the left atrium to empty.[19] Digoxin does not slow the heart when it is in sinus rhythm because the minor vagotonic effect of digoxin is overcome by high circulating catecholamines. Side effects, feared by some, have not been seen in our patients with hypertrophic cardiomyopathy or mitral or aortic stenosis, given beta-blockers. (It is probable that reduction in uterine blood flow results from reducing perfusion pressure in hypertensives but if cardiac output increases with reduction in heart rate, the reverse may be true.)

Most young women with mitral stenosis have valves that are suitable for balloon valvuloplasty.[8,20] This should be carried out before pregnancy if the calculated mitral valve area is under 1.5 cm regardless of symptoms. It can also be successfully performed during pregnancy. Use of the Inoue ballon has reduced the time needed to about an hour and irradiation can be further minimized by utilizing transesophageal echocardiographic visualization. The optimal time is in the second trimester. Closed mitral valvotomy is still performed successfully and safely for both mother and fetus in parts of the world where the operation costs less than the balloon.

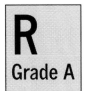

Valvular regurgitation is well tolerated, systemic vasodilation serving to reduce regurgitant flow.

Prosthetic valves

This is an area in which transatlantic controversy continues and in which good data from trials are much needed but would be very hard to obtain.

Women who are likely to need a future valve replacement should be encouraged to complete their families before a prosthesis becomes necessary because both bioprostheses and mechanical valves carry some hazards during pregnancy. Bioprostheses lack durability, particularly in the young and especially during pregnancy,[21-24] bringing the need for re-replacement at unpredictable risk when the children are still small. They are usually only recommended for elderly or sick patients whose prognosis is likely to be shorter than that of the prosthesis or for patients with an irremediable bleeding hazard, yet some cardiac surgeons still implant them in young women planning future pregnancy in order to avoid the perceived hazards of anticoagulant treatment. This planned obsolescence, chosen to provide time for one or more safe pregnancies, is often all too readily accepted by the potential parents but the dwindling numbers of such valves inserted into women under age 40 recorded by the UK Valve Registry suggests that the practice is becoming less common.[25]

The hypercoagulable state induced by pregnancy increases dependence on anticoagulant treatment in patients with mechanical valves and in some patients with bioprostheses. Because oral anticoagulants may cause fetal malformation during the first trimester, transfer to heparin has been advised without any evidence of its safety or efficacy in long term use. Randomized prospective trials to compare heparin with oral anticoagulation in pregnancy have not been carried out. They would be difficult to design and take years to complete given the relatively small numbers of patients, the need to have data on both dosage and anticoagulant effect throughout the pregnancies and the varying types, numbers, site, and sizes of valvular prostheses, all of which would have to be taken into account.

Despite this lack, heparin appears to offer inferior protection to the mother and does not reduce fetal wastage.

Patient numbers are small both in the US and in Europe because of the rarity of rheumatic carditis, the caution of many physicians and obstetricians in advising against pregnancy in women with valvular prostheses and the implantation of bioprostheses by some cardiac surgeons confident of their ability to replace these with mechanical valves later on.

Heparin does not reach the fetus but can cause early miscarriage and placental hemorrhage and its use is associated with an increased number of premature or stillbirths. Even in Hall's 1980 review, fetal wastage was as high with heparin as with oral anticoagulants.[26] Recommendations differ concerning heparin dosage, route, dose interval, and duration of heparin therapy. A much higher dose is needed to prevent prosthetic valve thrombosis or embolism than to prevent venous thromboembolism. Heparin treatment is arduous for the patient because of the need for twice-daily subcutaneous self-injection and stringent monitoring. Heparin's powerful antithrombin action, short duration of action, narrow therapeutic index, increasing dose requirement through pregnancy, and increasingly steep dose–response curve as the target is neared make it very difficult to maintain an antithrombotic effect without bleeding complications over the long term, even in the most compliant of patients.[27-30]

Salazar in Mexico City has studied pregnant patients under various regimens of heparin or oral anticoagulant treatment. His group have reported management of 370 pregnancies in 276 patients with various types of valve prostheses.[31] Fixed low dose heparin 5000 units b.d. resulted in prosthetic valve thrombosis.[32] Even with higher dose heparin, aiming to maintain the partial thromboplastin time (APTT) between 1.5 and 2.5 times the control in the first trimester, valve thrombosis was not prevented.[31] There was a 37.5% spontaneous miscarriage rate and Lee *et al.* had previously reported a 50% miscarriage rate when the heparin dose was adjusted to an APTT of 1.5.[33] Despite this, Ginsberg and Barron recently advised 12-hourly subcutaneous heparin with a target APTT a minimum of 2.0 times the control.[37] Elkayam suggests continuous intravenous heparin treatment in hospital at least between the sixth and 12th weeks for patients with older generation prosthetic valves, subcutaneous heparin for patients with older valves in the aortic position or newer generation valves in any position. He advises that the mid interval APTT be adjusted to between 2.0 and 3.0 with monitoring every 1 or 2 weeks and consideration of infusion via a programmable pump.[38] Such dosage is likely to lead to very high miscarriage rates as well as severe bleeding complications.

Heparin can cause thrombocytopenia which, being caused by platelet aggregation, brings a paradoxically increased risk of thrombosis and regular blood counts are required. It also causes osteopenia.[34,35] Low molecular weight fractionated heparins have not so far been studied for prevention of prosthetic valve thrombosis.

Oral anticoagulants provide effective protection against prosthetic valve thromboembolism but carry a risk of inducing embryopathy when taken between the sixth and 12th week of gestation and an increased risk of miscarriage. Salazar found the risk of major embryopathy to be 4.5% when coumarin compounds were used from the sixth to 12th weeks of gestation and he compared this favorably with the 7% risk of massive valve thrombosis which had occurred during carefully monitored heparin treatment.[31] His patients now remain on oral anticoagulation.

The fetal risk from oral anticoagulants is related to the maternal dose but the range of risks for different doses has never been computed. In a small series of 20 patients chosen because they required less than 5 mg warfarin daily, Cotrufo encountered no embryopathies.[36] Women taking a high warfarin dose also face a continuing higher risk of fetal hemorrhage. Both are caused by fetal vitamin K deficiency. The fetal overdose cannot be measured but it occurs because the immature fetal liver produces less procoagulant factors than the maternal liver and maternal procoagulant factors do not cross the placental barrier.

The newer mechanical prostheses carry a lower risk of thromboembolism. Sareli in South Africa found no thromboembolic complications in 39 patients with Medtronic–Hall prostheses or in seven women with St Jude Medical valves treated with warfarin throughout pregnancy, even though only 39% of international normalization ratios (INRs) were within the target range. There may be ethnic (genetic) differences in the propensity to thromboembolism.

Recommendations

- Oral anticoagulants should not be interrupted during pregnancy in women with native valvular disease or prostheses, who need anticoagulant treatment.[39,40]
- Elective cesarean section ensures a minimal time off warfarin and provides the safest delivery route for both baby and mother.[36,39,40]

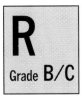

R

Grade **B/C**

- The risks should of course be fully discussed with both prospective parents before conception.
- Confusion still reigns in the US largely because both the manufacturers' guidelines and the Physicians' Desk Reference still state that coumarin is contraindicated in pregnancy regardless of the trimester.
- Anticoagulant control during pregnancy requires increased frequency of testing of INR. Self-testing and self-management using a home monitor allow the majority of patients to achieve better control than when advised by the anticoagulant clinic and it is more convenient.[41]
- An INR of 2.5 is sufficient for a patient with a third generation bileaflet prosthesis[39] in the aortic position and not more than 3.0 for patients with mitral prostheses. In non-pregnant patients these levels have been shown to diminish the risk of bleeding complications while not incurring an increase in thromboembolism.
- If low dose aspirin is added, this should be stopped at least 1 week before anticipated delivery because of possible premature closure of the arterial duct due to prostaglandin inhibition.
- Screening for known thrombotic risks such as the antiphospholipid syndrome and factor 7 Leiden should be considered a part of risk assessment.[42]

Reoperation may be required for dysfunctional bioprosthetic valves or thrombosed mechanical valves. The reoperation risk is highest if the need is emergent but even when performed electively, the mortality is still at least 5% and the patient must then again face the relatively high risk of the first postoperative year when paravalvular leaks, thromboembolism, and prosthetic valve endocarditis are most likely.

Thrombolytic treatment is the choice for thrombosis of tricuspid prostheses and has increasingly been shown to be practicable for leftsided valves.[43] Even though there is some risk of causing embolization, this risk may be less than that of reoperation. Thrombolytic treatment may cause loss of the fetus but this is not inevitable and has to be weighed against the very high risk to the fetus with reoperation in the emergency situation.

Fibrinolytic agents do not harm the fetus directly as they do not cross the placenta but, as with heparin, bleeding from the placental bed may cause loss of the fetus. There are anecdotal reports of a successful outcome to the pregnancy after maternal fibrinolytic treatment[43–46] (all were for treatment of pulmonary embolism rather than prosthetic valve thrombosis) which echo personal experience but such reports can give no indication of the size of the risk. Severe uterine bleeding should be anticipated if these drugs are given postpartum.

THE MARFAN SYNDROME

Fifty percent of aortic dissections in women under the age of 50 occur during pregnancy, most frequently during the third trimester or peripartum.[47] The majority are hypertensive but some have Marfan syndrome or aortic ectasia without Marfan phenotype. In the Marfan syndrome sudden rupture or dissection of the aorta is a risk which increases in pregnancy. If the aortic root is already widened (>4.5 cm) pregnancy is hazardous. The family history is important. In some families aortic dissection occurs at a low aortic root diameter (<4.0 cm).[48] Women deemed to be at high risk should be advised to defer pregnancy until after aortic root replacement, when their own valve can usually be resuspended. The risk of elective operation is <1% in experienced hands[49] and long term anticoagulants are not needed. It may soon be possible to assess individual risk with greater accuracy as different point mutations in the large gene on chromosome 15 involving the fibrillin protein are being correlated with different severities of the syndrome.

Recommendations

Patients should continue beta-blocker therapy. The aortic diameter should be measured by echocardiography at least every 2 months. Marfan women with any aortic root widening or a bad family history should be delivered by cesarean section under epidural anesthesia to minimize aortic wall stress. Women who show progressive increase in aortic root diameter should be rested in hospital and delivered by cesarean section at 32 weeks followed by elective surgery.

The risk of dissection is greatest in late pregnancy and increased risk persists for 6 months postpartum. The risk increases as age advances so Marfan women who desire children should complete their families early. All Marfan patients should avoid isometric stresses as far as possible and should not lift heavy children! A Marfan database for Europe is planned.

CARDIOMYOPATHY

Hypertrophic cardiomyopathy

Hypertrophic cardiomyopathy (HCM) may be first recognized after investigation of a murmur heard in the antenatal clinic followed by the finding of an abnormal ECG and echocardiogram.

The main hemodynamic abnormality is a small left ventricular cavity and restricted stroke volume. Outflow tract gradients are present in less than half of diagnosed cases and are labile, often present only with exertion, excitement or on pharmacological provocation. Diastolic stiffness increases with age, progressing from an increased active relaxation time to a restrictive pattern of rapid early filling with no later increment. Only a few young patients have seriously compromised diastolic function and most women with HCM do well in pregnancy, suggesting that left ventricular volume and compliance increase in response to the demands of pregnancy. Sudden death has been reported in two cases during pregnancy but the infrequency of such reports suggests that the risk is not increased and may indeed be diminished.[50] The presence of an outflow tract gradient is not prognostically significant.

Pharmacological treatment is only given for relief of symptoms. Shortness of breath and angina usually respond to a beta-blocker such as metoprolol. Verapamil is less suitable because of its vasodilator effect. Supraventricular arrhythmias are uncommon in this age group but because placental blood flow may become compromised, should be treated by DC reversion to safeguard the fetus. Women with ventricular arrhythmias or recurrent supraventricular tachycardias may need amiodarone. This drug is not teratogenic but can cause fetal hypothyroidism. Delivery should be planned to avoid vasodilation, maintain blood pressure and heart rate, avoiding excessive tachycardia, and blood lost should be promptly restored. Swan–Ganz pressure monitoring or cesarean

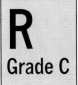

R
Grade C

section is only rarely indicated for the few women with advanced hemodynamic abnormality.

Prophylaxis against endocarditis is discretionary for normal delivery but patients with outflow tract obstruction are at risk from infective endocarditis.

Dilated and peripartum cardiomyopathy

Most women with diagnosed dilated cardiomyopathy are advised against pregnancy and there is little reported experience. Such women are probably at increased risk of developing a superimposed peripartum exacerbation so even if assessment suggests adequate cardiovascular reserve, pregnancy may bring an exacerbation and possibly permanent deterioration.

Peripartum cardiomyopathy is a term used to describe heart failure developing in temporal relationship to pregnancy and parturition. It usually develops during the last month of pregnancy or the first 3–6 months postpartum in women who have not previously been known to have heart disease. Severe heart failure may have an explosive onset within a few days of the birth.[51] Milder cases may be seen sometime later but most of them within days or weeks of delivery.

The true prevalence of the condition is unknown because mild cases may not be diagnosed and some may have had subclinical left ventricular dysfunction before the pregnancy. If cardiac biopsy is undertaken during the acute illness, it usually shows acute myocarditis.[52] A decrease in cell mediated immunity occurs during pregnancy. This prevents rejection of the foreign fetus but increases maternal susceptibility to some infections. However, evidence for a viral cause for the myocarditis is rarely found and other features of viral infection are absent.

Dilated cardiomyopathy is familial with other clinical or subclinical cases discovered during family screening in about 25% of family members. Patients with peripartum cardiomyopathy may have a genetic propensity to develop dilated cardiomyopathy which is now regarded as an immunologically based disease. In these predisposed subjects, pregnancy seems to be the trigger.

The postpartum heart failure reported among the Hausa women of northern Nigeria is different and attributable to traditional practices with fluid overload resulting from a high salt intake.[53]

Severe cases of peripartum cardiomyopathy present with biventricular failure. Echocardiography shows dilated, poorly contracting ventricles and serves to exclude other conditions which may cause heart failure at this time, such as pulmonary embolism, amniotic fluid embolism, and even previously undiagnosed valve disease.

The patients tend to be fluid overloaded with low blood pressure, tachycardia, and a third heart sound gallop. Ventricular tachycardia and sudden death may occur. Intraventricular thrombosis may lead to peripheral embolism.

The impact of acute myocarditis is sometimes focal and both the ECG and the echocardiogram may suggest acute myocardial infarction. Because myocardial infarction can also cause a peripartum emergency, cardiac catheterization with coronary angiography should be carried out with cardiac biopsy if the coronary arteries appear normal.

In the worst cases maximum cardiac support may be needed with intubation, ventilation, invasive monitoring, and intravenous inotropes. Cardiac transplantation has been performed but as in acute myocarditis outside pregnancy, there is a high chance of major improvement if the acute stage is survived. Treatment with ACE inhibitors, diuretics, and warfarin should continue while left ventricular function is subnormal. Ventricular arrhythmias may precipitate deterioration into cardiogenic shock and should be promptly treated by DC reversion or overdrive pacing. Amiodarone is the antiarrhythmic drug of choice should arrhythmias recur.

A strong case can be made for immunosuppression. Prednisolone 1.5 mg/kg plus azothiaprine 1 mg/kg daily should be started and continued for 4–6 weeks. Some guidance as to duration of therapy may be obtained from repeat biopsy but regional differences or sampling errors may only serve to confuse. There is no advantage in biopsying the left ventricle.

Heart failure does not necessarily recur but it is wise to advise against further pregnancy in patients with incomplete recovery. Since myocardial biopsy shows myocyte death, even patients who appear to show complete recovery have lost a measure of their cardiovascular reserve. The severity of left ventricular dysfunction does not necessarily predict outcome. A serial echocardiographic study of 10 women showed that despite improvement the ejection fraction became normal in only four, two of whom subsequently had normal pregnancies.[54]

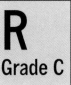

MYOCARDIAL INFARCTION

Atheromatous coronary artery disease is rare during pregnancy but is seen in patients with severe familial hypercholesterolemia and increasingly in older smokers or in diabetics.

When myocardial infarction complicates pregnancy it is usually caused by acute events in previously non-atheromatous coronary arteries and therefore usually develops without preceding angina. In reality, its prevalence is unknown but has been estimated to be about one in 10 000.[55,56] Now that more patients undergo early invasive investigation it has become appreciated that the most frequent underlying mechanism is coronary artery dissection[57] but numerous other contributory factors peculiar to or aggravated by pregnancy may be incriminated (see Box on page 928). It has been suggested that the dissection nearly always involves the left anterior descending artery but a higher proportion of anterior infarcts are likely to have been investigated or to have undergone autopsy. Spontaneous coronary artery dissection can be multiple and even involve all three arteries or cause angina without infarction.

Myocardial infarction is most often peripartum and may be precipitated by vasoactive drugs used for control of uterine hemorrhage or for termination of pregnancy. Infarction has been associated with the use of ergot derivatives, prostaglandin, and bromocriptine used to suppress lactation.[58,59] Acute chest pain may follow injection of vasoconstrictor agents causing coronary artery spasm and endothelial breaches which attract platelets, with subsequent clot formation.

Myocardial infarction is a well recognized complication of autoimmune disease, particularly in SLE and the antiphospholipid syndrome. It may occur in patients with old Kawasaki disease or in young drug abusers using crack cocaine. Other causes include coronary embolism. Because of its increasing prevalence, cocaine should be considered in any young patient with a sudden coronary event (see Box on page 928).

Myocardial infarction complicating pregnancy

Pregnancy-associated causes
Coronary artery dissection
    spasm
    thrombosis
Drug induced
    ergotamine
    prostaglandins
    bromocriptine
Pre-eclampsia
Embolism from placenta

Coexisting predisposing disorders
Coronary atheroma
    hypercholesterolemia
    smoking
    diabetes
Coronary arteritis
    systemic lupus erythematosus
    antiphospholipid syndrome
    old Kawasaki disease
Coronary embolism
    in mitral valve disease
    from prosthetic valve
    left atrial myxoma
    infective endocarditis
    paradoxical
Cocaine abuse

Myocardial infarction should be confirmed from ECG change and elevation of cardiac enzymes other than creatine kinase and its MB isoenzyme (which are released from the uterus postpartum).[60]

Coronary angiography should be undertaken without delay to confirm the diagnosis and the mechanism of coronary artery occlusion and if possible to reopen the vessel. Pregnancy is only a relative contraindication to the use of thrombolytic agents which are justified for large anterior infarcts associated with thrombus. If so, tPA can be delivered locally thereby minimizing the dose and maximizing efficacy. A small dissection may be sealed off by stenting but if a major dissection threatens the entire anterior descending artery territory, urgent coronary bypass is indicated. Both percutaneous angioplasty and coronary artery bypass grafting have been performed safely during pregnancy. Beta-blockers should be started as soon as possible. ACE inhibitors are contraindicated until after delivery. Every effort should be made to maintain the pregnancy until the infarct has healed and beta-blockers continued during delivery to reduce myocardial oxygen demand. Cesarean section is the safest mode of delivery if the left ventricle is compromised. If ventricular fibrillation occurs, the uterus should be displaced laterally during resuscitation as it causes significant aortocaval compression. If resuscitation fails, emergency cesarean section should be carried out within 15 minutes.

HYPERTENSION AND PRE-ECLAMPTIC TOXEMIA

Pre-eclampsia (gestational hypertension) is a multisystem vascular disorder characterized by a rise in blood pressure, peripheral edema, and proteinuria. In its most severe form, seizures may occur (eclampsia). It usually arises late in pregnancy and is most common in primagravidae with a family history of the condition. Women with pre-existing essential or renal hypertension are more likely to develop it than normotensive women and it is pre-eclampsia that makes hypertension the commonest cause of maternal death in the United Kingdom. The condition is a disorder of the endothelium and therefore a multisystem disease. Its treatment involves more than the management of hypertension alone.[61]

Hypertension in pregnancy

Chronic hypertension is >140/90 in first trimester (think essential, renal, coarctation, pheochromocytoma)

Gestational hypertension is an increase in
   systolic blood pressure >30 mmHg
   or diastolic blood pressure >15 mmHg
above the level in the first trimester.

Pre-eclampsia is
   blood pressure >140/90
   proteinuria >0.5 g in 24 hours
and edema usually after 24 weeks gestation.

Eclampsia – fits, disseminated intravascular coagulation, hypertensive crisis, and coma.

Chronic hypertension with superimposed pre-eclampsia is blood pressure rise >30/15 above the usual level, proteinuria and edema.

Blood pressure during pregnancy should be measured in the sitting position and the diastolic blood pressure should be taken to the fifth Korotkoff sound rather than the fourth.[62]

The Redman and Jeffries definition of pre-eclampsia is a diastolic blood pressure below 90 mmHg before 20 weeks, a rise in diastolic blood pressure after 20 weeks gestation to above 90 mmHg and by at least 25 mmHg above the first blood pressure recorded in pregnancy.[62] The definition is useful but not all patients with pre-eclampsia meet these blood pressure criteria and some who do will not have other features of pre-eclampsia (see Box above).

The onset is often heralded by rapid weight gain followed by edema. The face and hands appear puffy. The onset is usually after the 32nd week of pregnancy but is sometimes earlier, particularly in patients with pre-existing renal disease. Apart from the rise in blood pressure, the cardiovascular examination is usually normal but in severe cases left ventricular failure and pulmonary edema may occur. Pre-existing hypertension is usually noted during the first trimester although a fall in blood pressure at this time may render the patient temporarily normotensive. Pre-existing hypertension is usually associated with a gradual rather than a rapid gain in weight and the blood pressure, although higher, is better tolerated. Essential hypertension persists after delivery whereas the manifestations of pre-eclampsia usually resolve immediately the child is delivered and are only rarely observed during the postpartum period.

Pre-eclampsia is associated with a rapid increase in the peripheral vascular resistance resulting in reduced uteroplacental perfusion, fetal hypoxia, and intrauterine starvation.

Pre-eclampsia carries much greater risk than hypertension alone. Abnormalities on investigation include abnormal liver function tests, hyperuricemia, and increased packed cell volume.

Pre-eclampsia carries a major risk of eclampsia and of cerebral hemorrhage. Rapid lowering of blood pressure is necessary in order to avoid this, in contrast to the treatment

---

Diagnostic features on investigation of pre-eclampsia

Maternal
Thrombocytopenia
Abnormal liver function tests
Hyperuricemia
Raised packed cell volume
Proteinuria
Raised antithrombin III and von Willebrand factor

Fetal
Growth retardation
Hypoxemia
(Modified from de Swiet.[63])

Clinical features of pre-eclampsia which demand delivery

Central nervous system
Fits (eclampsia)
Cerebral hemorrhage
Cerebral infarction

Eyes
Retinal detachment
Retinal edema

Renal
Acute tubular necrosis
Acute cortical necrosis
Renal failure

Hepatic
Infarction or rupture
Jaundice
HELLP syndrome (hemolysis, elevated liver enzymes, low platelets)

Cardiorespiratory
Pulmonary edema
Adult respiratory distress syndrome

Coagulation
Thrombocytopenia
Microangiopathic hemolysis
Disseminated intravascular coagulation
HELLP syndrome
(Modified from de Swiet.[63])

---

of hypertension outside pregnancy when acute lowering of blood pressure may be hazardous and the main purpose of treatment is to prevent long term complications. Although the blood pressure can be lowered pharmacologically, the endothelial disorder progresses relentlessly. It is only stopped by delivery which is the ultimate therapeutic weapon, though responsible for premature and cesarean births carried out to save the lives of both mother and child. All patients with a rise in blood pressure above 150/ 100 and all patients who have proteinuria with a lower blood pressure should be managed in hospital in order to detect deterioration in either the maternal or the fetal condition which may demand rapid delivery (see Box on page 930). Treatment of maternal hypertension may allow the pregnancy to continue for long enough for dexamethasone to secure some maturation of the fetal lungs before delivery but once the blood pressure has risen to more than 170 systolic or 110 diastolic, it is unlikely to be possible to continue the pregnancy safely for more than a few days.[63]

A blood pressure of 170/110 is just below the level of blood pressure at which cerebral autoregulation fails and it needs to be reduced to about 140/90 to reduce the risk of cerebral hemorrhage. The Cochrane database meta-analysis of all trials of antihypertensive drugs for mild to moderate hypertension suggests that treatment of lesser degrees of blood pressure does not improve the fetal outcome[64] but in patients who were receiving antihypertensive medication before pregnancy, there is reason to believe that the use of methyldopa does improve fetal outcome. Most of the trials in the Cochrane database applied to patients without pre-existing hypertension. The earlier hypertension presents, the more likely that it already existed. In Redman's trial of methyldopa compared with placebo in women with hypertension noted before 30 weeks gestation, the perinatal loss rate was 1% in 106 women treated with methyldopa compared with 6% in 107 women given placebo.[65]

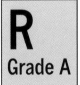

R
Grade A

In 1995 the Eclampsia Trial Collaborative Group reported the result of a multicenter international trial comparing magnesium and diazepam with magnesium and phenytoin in eclampsia.[66] The trial showed that magnesium was superior to either phenytoin or diazepam in preventing further seizures with insignificant trends also towards better maternal and fetal outcomes. Lucas et al. showed that magnesium was also considerably better than phenytoin for seizure prophylaxis.[67] Two thousand, three hundred and thirty-eight women with pre-eclampsia were randomized to receive phenytoin or magnesium and the trial was stopped prematurely when 10 of the women receiving phenytoin had seizures compared with none of those receiving magnesium. It has, however, been estimated that 5000 women would have to be treated prophylactically with magnesium in order to prevent one maternal death, the mortality of eclampsia being about 2%. It is not possible to predict which women with pre-eclampsia are at risk from seizures as some may have neither proteinuria nor significant hypertension at the time of the first fit and the study did not address the issue of blood pressure control in preventing seizures.

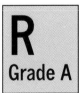

R
Grade A

Antihypertensive drugs used to lower blood pressure acutely in pre-eclampsia include hydralazine and labetalol (both of which are commonly given by intravenous infusion) and oral nifedipine.

Because of its record, methyldopa is the drug most commonly chosen for long term control of blood pressure in pregnancy but it may cause depression. Adequate clinical trials are lacking to support the use of other antihypertensives long term in pregnancy. One trial of atenolol compared with placebo found growth retardation in the atenolol treated group. Growth retardation may be a class effect of beta-blockers when used for

R
Grade B

the treatment of hypertension but not when used in normotensive patients in whom placental perfusion is less likely to be adversely affected.

Angiotensin converting enzyme inhibitors should not be used after the first trimester as they cause renal failure in the fetus which can be fatal. Grade A

ARRHYTHMIAS

Digoxin, beta-blockers, and verapamil are safe and have the usual indications. Intravenous adenosine for reversion of atrioventricular nodal re-entry tachycardia does not disturb the fetus nor does DC cardioversion when indicated. Amiodarone is not teratogenic but can cause fetal hypothyroidism.

CONDUCT OF LABOR AND DELIVERY IN THE HIGH RISK PATIENT

Normal labor involves intermittent surges in cardiac output and in blood pressure which may be dangerous for patients with an uncorrected coarctation, the Marfan syndrome or Takayasu aortitis.

Patients with a raised left atrial pressure will develop a further rise in pressure during the physical stresses of labor and also in the third stage when 500 ml or more of blood from the uterus and placenta is returned to the circulation. In such patients, frusemide 20 mg or 40 mg should be given intravenously at the commencement of labor and the patient sat up immediately after delivery. Swan–Ganz monitoring of the pulmonary artery and wedged pulmonary capillary pressures is only occasionally needed. If there is real concern a planned cesarean section is preferable in order to avoid maternal physical stress and expedite delivery.

Patients with cyanotic congenital heart disease have increased right to left shunting during normal labor which should be expedited in order to avoid fetal hypoxemia. Many need to be delivered prematurely on account of slowing fetal growth and this should be by cesarean section.

Epidural anesthesia is contraindicated in patients with limited stroke volume or congenital heart disease with right to left shunts. Patients with solitary pulmonary hypertension in whom neither pulmonary blood flow nor cardiac output can be increased are at greatest risk from systemic vasodilator agents.

HEART SURGERY IN PREGNANCY

Closed mitral valvotomy has been carried out for years with minimal risk to mother and baby. Balloon dilation can also be carried out successfully during pregnancy but should be avoided as far as possible during the first trimester.

Open heart surgery during pregnancy carries high risk because of the emergent nature of the situation which is the cause for this. It usually relates to failure of preconceptual diagnosis or advice, the development of infective endocarditis, aortic dissection or acute valvar regurgitation complicating a balloon aortic or mitral valvotomy. If the maternal cardiovascular state is critical the fetal state will also be precarious and continuous fetal monitoring is essential. Cardiopulmonary bypass should be carried out with high flow rates but fetal safety depends very much on the maternal condition at its conclusion. Full heparinization necessary during bypass may lead to retroplacental hemorrhage and separation.

ANTIBIOTIC PROPHYLAXIS

Antibiotic prophylaxis should be given to susceptible patients to cover prolonged or surgical deliveries and in patients with prosthetic valves or a history of infective endocarditis.

There is no evidence that it is either necessary or effective. Bacteremia with a range of bowel organisms occurs in only about 0.5% of normal deliveries and no proven case of endocarditis occurred among more than 2000 normal deliveries in unprotected women with susceptible heart disease in a study from Dublin.[68]

REFERENCES

1 Turnbull A *et al*. Report on confidential enquiries into maternal deaths in England and Wales 1982–1984. *Rep Health Soc Subj London* 1989; 34:1–166.

2 Robson SC, Hunter S, Boys RJ, Dunlop W. Serial study of factors influencing changes in cardiac output during human pregnancy. *Am J Physiol* 1989;**25b**:H1060–1050.

3 Campos O, Andrade JL, Bocanegra J *et al*. Physiological mutivalvular regurgitation during pregnancy: a longitudinal Doppler echocardiographic study. *Int J Cardiol* 1993;**40**:265–72.

4 Robson SC, Hunter S, Boys RJ, Dunlop W. Hemodynamic changes during twin pregnancy. A Doppler and M-mode echocardiographic study. *Am J Obstet Gynecol* 1989;**161**:1273–8.

5 Oakley C. Acyanotic congenital heart disease. In: Oakley C. ed. *Heart disease in pregnancy*. London: BMJ Books, 1997, pp 63–82.

6 Koller M, Rothlin M, Senning A. Coarctation of the aorta: reviewing 362 operated patients: long-term follow-up and assessment of prognostic variables. *Eur Heart J* 1987;**8**:670–9.

7 Arias F, Pineda J. Aortic stenosis and pregnancy. *J Reprod Med* 1978;**20**:229–32.

8 Presbitero P, Prever SB, Brusca A. Interventional cardiology in pregnancy. *Eur Heart J* 1996;**17**:182–8.

9 Nora JJ, Berg K, Nora AH. *Cardiovascular diseases. Genetics, epidemiology and prevention*. Oxford: Oxford University Press, 1991.

10 Deal K, Wooley CF. Coarctation of the aorta and pregnancy. *Ann Intern Med* 1973;**78**:706–10.

11 Clark SL. Cardiac disease in pregnancy. *Obstet Gynecol Clin North Am* 1991;**18**:237–56.

12 Presbitero P, Somerville J, Rabajoli F, Stone S, Conte MR. Corrected transposition of the great arteries without associated defects in adult patients. Clinical profile and follow-up. *Br Heart J* 1995;**74**:57–9.

13 Neill CA, Swanson S. Outcome of pregnancy in congenital heart disease. *Circulation* 1961;**24**:1003 (abstract).

14 Morgan-Jones A, Howitt G. Eisenmenger syndrome in pregnancy. *Br Med J* 1965;**1**:1627.

15 Gleicher N, Midwall J, Hochberger D, Jaffin H. Eisenmenger's syndrome and pregnancy. *Obstet Gynecol Surv* 1975;**34**:721–41.

16 Avila WS, Ginsberg M, Snitcowsky R *et al*. Maternal and fetal outcome in pregnant women with Eisenmenger's syndrome. *Eur Heart J* 1995;**16**:460–4.

17 de Swiet M. *Maternal mortality from heart disease in pregnancy*. DHSS Report on Confidential Enquiries into Maternal Deaths in England and Wales, 1985–1987. London: HMSO 1991.

18 Morley CA, Lim BA. The risks of delay in diagnosis of breathlessness in pregnancy. *Br Med J* 1995;**311**:1083–4.

19 Narasimhan C, Joseph G, Singh TC. Propranolol for pulmonary oedema in mitral stenosis. *Int J Cardiol* 1994;**44**:178–9.

20 Ben Farhat M, Betbout F, Gamra H *et al*. Results of percutaneous double-balloon mitral commissurotomy in one medical centre in Tunisia. *Am J Cardiol* 1995;**76**:1266–70.

21 Sbaroumi E, Oakley CM. Outcome of pregnancy in women with valve prostheses. *Br Heart J* 1994;**71**:198–201.

22 Bortolloti U, Milano A, Mazzucco A *et al*. Pregnancy in patients with porcine valve prosthesis. *Am J Cardiol* 1982;**50**:1051–4.

23 Salazar E, Zajarias A, Gutiarraz N, Iturbe I. The problem of cardiac valve prostheses:

anticoagulants and pregnancy. *Circulation* 1984; **70**:169–77.

24 Badduke ER, Jamieson RE, Miyashima RT *et al.* Pregnancy and childbearing in a population with biologic valvular prostheses. *J Thorac Cardiovasc Surg* 1991;**102**:179–86.

25 Taylor KM. *Report of the United Kingdom Heart Valve Registry 1993*. London: HMSO, 1995.

26 Hall JG, Pauli RM, Wilson KM. Maternal and fetal sequelae of anticoagulation during pregnancy. *Am J Med* 1980;**68**:122–40.

27 Oakley CM. Clinical perspectives: anticoagulation and pregnancy. *Eur Heart J* 1995;**16**:1317–19.

28 Oakley CM. Artificial heart valves. In: Oakley C. ed. *Heart disease in pregnancy*. London: BMJ, 1997.

29 Whitfield LR, Lele AS, Levy G. Effect of pregnancy on the relationship between concentration and anticoagulation action of heparin. *Clin Pharmacol Ther* 1983;**34**:23–8.

30 Barbour LA, Smith JM, Marler RA. Heparin levels to guide thromboembolism prophylaaxis during pregnancy. *Am J Obstet Gynecol* 1995;**173**: 1869–73.

31 Salazar E, Izaguirre R, Verdejo J, Mutchinick O. Failure of adjusted doses of subcutaneous heparin to prevent thromboembolic phenomena in pregnant patients with mechanical cardiac valve prosthesis. *J Am Coll Cardiol* 1996;**27**: 1698–1703.

32 Iturbe-Alessio I, Delcarmen Gonesca M, Mutchinik D *et al.* Risks of anticoagulant therapy in pregnancy: women with artificial heart valves. *N Engl J Med* 1986;**27**:1390–3.

33 Lee PK, Wang RYC, Cho JSF *et al.* Combined use of warfarin and adjusted heparin during pregnancy in patients with artificial valves. *J Am Coll Cardiol* 1986;**8**:221–4.

34 de Swiet M, Dorrington M, Fidler J. Prolonged heparin therapy in pregnancy causes bone demineralisation. *Br J Obstet Gynaecol* 1983;**90**: 1129.

35 Shefras J, Farquharson RG. Bone density studies in pregnant women receiving heparin. *Eur J Obstet Gynecol Reprod Biol* 1996;**65**:171–4.

36 Cotrufo M, de Luca TSL, Calabro R, Mastrogiovanni G, Lama D. Coumarin anticoagulation during pregnancy in patients with mechanical heart valve prostheses. *Eur J Cardiothorac Surg* 1991;**5**:300–5.

37 Ginsberg JS, Barron WM. Pregnancy and prosthetic heart valves. *Lancet* 1994;**344**: 1170–2.

38 Elkayam R. Anticoagulation in pregnant women with prosthetic heart valves. A double jeopardy. *J Am Coll Cardiol* 1996;**27**:1704–6.

39 Gohlke-Barwolf C, Acar J, Oakley C *et al.* Guidelines for prevention of thromboembolic events in valvular heart disease. *Eur Heart J* 1995; **16**:1320–30.

40 Gohlke-Barwolf C, Acar J, Oakley C *et al.*, for the Study Group of the Working Group on Valvular Heart Disease of the European Society of Cardiology. Guidelines for prevention of thromboembolic events in valvular heart disease. *Eur Heart J* 1995;**16**:1320–30.

41 Bernardo A, Halhuber C, Horstkotte D. Home prothrombin estimation. In: Butchart E, Bodnar E. eds. *Thrombosis, embolism and bleeding*. ICR Publishers, 1992.

42 Brenner B, Yulfsons SL, Lanir N, Nahir M. Co-existence of familial antiphospholipid syndrome and factor V Leiden: impact on thrombotic diathesis. *Br J Haematol* 1996;**94**:166–7.

43 Birdi I, Angelini GD, Bryan AJ. Thrombolytic therapy for left sided prosthetic heart valve thrombosis. *J Heart Valve Dis* 1995;**4**:154–9.

44 Delclos GL, Davila F. Thrombolytic therapy for pulmonary embolism in pregnancy: a case report. *Am J Obstet Gynecol* 1986;**155**:375–6.

45 Bando F, Caimi TM, Redaelli R *et al.* Emergency treatment with recombinant tissue plasminogen activator of pulmonary embolism in a pregnant woman with antithrombin III deficiency. *Am J Obstet Gynecol* 1990;**163**:1274–5.

46 Seifried E, Gabelmann A, Ellbruck D, Schmidt A. Thrombolytic therapy of pulmonary artery embolism in early pregnancy with recombinant tissue-type plasminogen activator. *Geburtshifte Frauenheilk* 1991;**51**:655–8.

47 Katz NM *et al.* Aortic dissections during pregnancy. *Am J Cardiol* 1984;**54**:699.

48 Child A. Management of pregnancy in Marfan syndrome, Ehlers-Danlos syndrome and the other heritable connective tissue disease. In: Oakley C. ed. *Heart disease in pregnancy*. London: BMJ, 1997.

49 Yacoub M, Gehle P, Chandrasekaran V *et al.* Late results of a valve preserving operation in patients with aneurysms of the ascending aorta and root. *J Thorac Cardiovasc Surg* (in press).

50 Oakley C. Hypertrophic cardiomyopathy. In: Oakley C. ed. *Heart disease in pregnancy*. London: BMJ, 1997, pp 201–9.

51 Julian DG, Szekely P. Peripartum cardiomyopathy. *Prog Cardiovasc Dis* 1985;**27**:223.

52 Midei MG, DeMent SH, Feldman AM *et al.* Peripartum myocarditis and cardiomyopathy. *Circulation* 1990;**81**:922–8.

53 Sanderson JE, Adesanya CO, Anjorin FI, Parry EHO. Postpartum cardiac failure: heart failure due to volume overload? *Am Heart J* 1979;**97**: 613.

54 Cole P, Cook F, Plappent T, Salzman D, Shilton M. Longitudinal changes in left ventricular architecture and function in peripartum cardiomyopathy. *Am J Cardiol* 1987;**60**:871–6.

55 Hankins GDV, Wendel GD Jr, Leveno KJ *et al.* Myocardial infarction during pregnancy. A review. *Obstet Gynecol* 1985;**65**:139.

56 Nolan TE, Hankins GD. Myocardial infarction in pregnancy. *Clin Obstet Gynecol* 1989;**32**:66–75.

57 Kearney P, Singh H, Hutter J *et al.* Spontaneous coronary artery dissection: a report of three cases and review of the literature. *Postgrad Med J* 1993; **69**:940–5.

58 Liao JK, Cockrill BA, Yurchak PM. Acute myocardial infarction after ergonovine administration for uterine bleeding. *Am J Cardiol* 1991; **68**:823–4.

59 Fjiwara Y, Yamanaka O, Nakamura T, Yokoi J, Yamaguchi H. Acute myocardial infarction induced by ergonovine administration for artifically induced abortion. *Jpn Heart J* 1993;**34**:803–8.

60 Leiserowitz GS, Evans AT, Samuels SJ, Oman K, Kost GJ. Creatine kinase and its MB isoenzyme in the third trimester and the peripartum period. *J Reprod Med* 1992;**37**:910–16.

61 Roberts JM, Taylor RN, Musci TJ *et al.* Pre-eclampsia: an endothelial cell disorder. *Am J Obstet Gynecol* 1989;**161**:1200–4.

62 Redman CWG, Jeffries M. Revised definition of pre-eclampsia. *Lancet* 1988;**2**:809–12.

63 de Swiet M. Hypertension and pre-eclamptic toxaemia. In: Oakley C. ed. *Heart disease in pregnancy.* London: BMJ, 1997, pp 293–306.

64 Collins R, Duley L. Any hypertensive therapy for pregnancy. The Cochrane Pregnancy and Childbirth Database, issue 1, 1995.

65 Redman CWG, Beilin LJ, Bonner J *et al.* Fetal outcome in trial of antihypertensive treatment in pregnancy. *Lancet* 1976;**ii**:753–6.

66 The Eclampsia Trial Collaborative Group. Which anticonvulsant for women with eclampsia? *Lancet* 1995;**345**:1455–63.

67 Lucas MJ, Leveno KJ, Cunningham FG. A comparison of magnesium sulphate with phenytoin for the prevention of eclampsia. *N Engl J Med* 1995;**333**:201–5.

68 Sugrue D, Blake S, Troy P, MacDonald D. Antibiotic prophylaxis against infective endocarditis after normal delivery – is it necessary? *Br Heart J* 1980;**44**:499–502.

55 Coronary intervention: angioplasty, stents, and atherectomy

Joseph P. Carrozza Jr,
David J. Cohen,
Donald S. Baim

INTRODUCTION

R
Grade B

From its humble beginnings 20 years ago, catheter intervention for the treatment of obstructive coronary artery disease has grown from a novelty into a mainstream therapy that has now surpassed coronary bypass in annual volume. In its first decade (through 1987), much of the growth of conventional balloon angioplasty – now referred to as plain old balloon angioplasty (POBA) – was due to progressive improvements in balloon technology and better understanding of the associated techniques for their use.[1] In its second decade, this growth has been further fueled by the introduction of new devices such as stents and atherectomy catheters, that are designed to overcome some of the inherent limitations of POBA (difficulty crossing or dilating certain lesion types, abrupt closure resulting from local dissection, restenosis due to unfavorable healing in the months after intervention). More so than in many other fields of medicine, these advances in interventional cardiology have been chronicled by a series of registries and randomized trials, which provide the evidential basis for clinical utilization and continued evolution in this area. One indirect benefit of these trials has been the demonstration that long term freedom from restenosis is related less to which *device* is used and more to how large a *final lumen diameter* is achieved – the so-called "bigger is better" hypothesis.[2] Data from each of the trials comparing a new device to balloon angioplasty have thus shown that once post-treatment lumen diameter is entered into a multivariable model of restenosis, the device used to obtain that result is no longer a significant determinant of restenosis (Figure 55.1). This recognition has focused the interventional strategy for each lesion towards using the device that is most likely to safely provide the largest lumen and then persisting with that device (or other secondary devices/ postdilation) until a near 0% residual stenosis has been achieved.

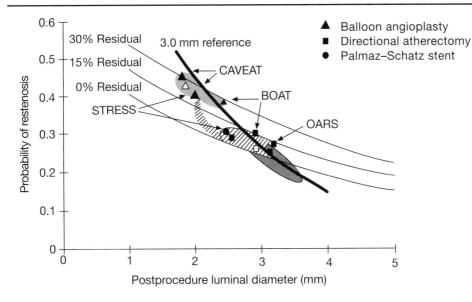

Figure 55.1   Device-independent relationship between post-treatment lumen diameter and the probability of subsequent angiographic restenosis. The acute results and late restenosis rates for several recent device trials (closed symbols) are superimposed on the generalized model derived from the Beth Israel experience with PTCA, directional coronary atherectomy (DCA), and the Palmaz–Schatz stent (open symbols; see reference[2]). Across all trials, the acute results for balloon angioplasty are tightly clustered (gray area) with minimal lumen diameter (MLD) 1.8–2.2 mm and late restenosis rates (defined as late stenosis >50%) of 40–50%. DCA results (crosshatched area) vary widely, with CAVEAT DCA results falling within the PTCA zone, but BOAT and OARS results falling in the range of larger acute MLD 2.8–3.1 mm and similarly low restenosis rates 25–30% to those reported in the original Beth Israel, Sequoia, and Washington Hospital experiences with this technique. Stent results (wavy line zone) also vary between the suboptimal results of STRESS and recent more optimal results showing post-treatment MLD 2.9–3.4 and angiographic restenosis rates of 20–25%. While results of other trials may differ slightly (based largely on use of different quantitative coronary angiographic techniques), multivariable modeling in all recent randomized trials has shown that post-treatment MLD is the most important single predictor of the probability of late angiographic restenosis and that once post-treatment MLD is included in the model there is no longer any additional effect of which particular device was used to obtain that result. This realization that restenosis is driven by the final acute result (and not the device used to obtain that result) has increased operator focus on using each device to the limits of its ability to safely enlarge the coronary lumen.

PLAIN OLD BALLOON ANGIOPLASTY

Although POBA was the initial progenitor of all percutaneous catheter coronary interventions, it has been subjected to relatively limited trials. Initial FDA approval was based on the first NHLBI PTCA Registry (1979–81) and increased use followed the demonstration in the second NHLBI PTCA Registry (1985–6) that improved catheter and guidewire design allowed treatment of more difficult lesion types with higher initial success and lower complication rates than seen in the first registry.[1] The main clinical trials focus on comparison of POBA to medical therapy in patients with single vessel disease and comparison to bypass surgery in patients with multivessel disease.

PERCUTANEOUS CORONARY REVASCULARIZATION vs MEDICAL THERAPY

Currently, approximately 50% of percutaneous coronary revascularization procedures are performed on patients with critical obstruction of only one major coronary artery.[1] Given the generally excellent prognosis for patients with single vessel coronary artery disease (CAD), it is not surprising that studies of coronary revascularization (either surgical or percutaneous) have failed to show an incremental survival benefit compared to the excellent prognosis on medical therapy. The decision to perform percutaneous coronary revascularization for such patients thus must be based on a clear understanding of the benefits (mostly improved symptomatic status) that may be expected from revascularization as compared with more conservative medical therapy.

Within the last 5 years, the first randomized trials have been performed comparing percutaneous revascularization with medical therapy. The VA-sponsored Angioplasty Compared with MEdicine (ACME) trial is the largest study to date to compare percutaneous transluminal coronary angioplasty (PTCA) with medical therapy for patients with single vessel CAD.[3] In this study, 212 patients with single vessel CAD and documented exercise-induced ischemia were randomized to a strategy of initial balloon angioplasty or intensive medical therapy. The primary study endpoint was the improvement in treadmill exercise time between baseline and 6-month follow-up. Although both study groups had improved exercise capacity at follow-up, the extent of improvement was significantly greater in patients randomized to PTCA compared with those assigned to medical therapy (2.1 vs 0.5 minutes, $P<0.001$). Moreover, patients randomized to PTCA reported less frequent angina at 6-month follow-up (36% vs 54%, $P<0.01$) and improved physical functioning and psychological well-being as well.[3,4]

The ACME trial also demonstrated that the symptomatic benefits of PTCA come with a price – to both the patient and society. From the patient's perspective, it appears that the choice of initial PTCA increases the likelihood of requiring bypass surgery – at least during the first year of follow-up. From a societal perspective, it is clear that medical care resource utilization and costs are greater with PTCA than with medical therapy. Nonetheless, formal cost-effectiveness analysis suggests that the benefits of PTCA are worth the cost for patients with single vessel disease, at least for those patients with moderate to severe angina.[5]

More recently, similar findings were reported in the Medicine, Angioplasty or Surgery Study (MASS) – a randomized clinical trial comparing medical therapy, balloon angioplasty, and coronary artery bypass surgery for patients with isolated stenosis of the proximal left anterior descending coronary artery (LAD).[6] Of patients assigned to initial PTCA, 82% were asymptomatic at the end of 3-year follow-up, as compared with only 32% of patients assigned to initial medical therapy ($P<0.01$). On the other hand, event-free survival (freedom from death, myocardial infarction, or refractory angina requiring surgical revascularization) was somewhat better for patients treated medically (83% vs 76%, $P=$NS). In this analysis, it should be noted that PTCA patients who required only an additional *percutaneous* revascularization were not considered to have experienced an endpoint.

Thus while the relative merits of PTCA over medical therapy for patients with mild to moderate angina due to a suitable lesion of a single vessel coronary disease for superior angina relief, increased exercise capacity, and improved overall quality of life are reasonably clear, PTCA has not been demonstrated to reduce infarction or death rates.

Table 55.1 Randomized clinical trials comparing angioplasty to bypass surgery for patients with multivessel coronary disease

Trial name	Country	Number of patients	Primary endpoint
CABRI[7]	Europe	1054	Death or non-fatal MI
RITA[8]	UK	1011[a]	Death or non-fatal MI
EAST[9]	USA	392	Death, MI or major thallium defect
GABI[10]	Germany	359	Angina-free survival
ERACI[11]	Argentina	127	Death, MI or recurrent angina
BARI[12]	USA	1829	All-cause mortality

[a] Includes 456 patients with single vessel disease.

Table 55.2 Mortality in randomized clinical trials comparing PTCA with CABG in patients with multivessel disease

Trial name	Follow-up	CABG deaths (%)	PTCA deaths (%)
CABRI[7]	1 year	14 (2.7)	21 (3.9)
RITA[8]	4.7 years	26 (5.2)	24 (4.7)
EAST[9]	3 years	12 (6.2)	14 (7.1)
GABI[10]	1 year	9 (5.1)	4 (2.2)
ERACHI[11]	3.8 years	3 (4.7)	6 (9.5)
BARI[12]	5 years	111 (10.7)	139 (13.7)
Overall	—	175 (7.4)	208 (8.6)

Comparison with bypass surgery in patients with multivessel coronary disease

In contrast to single vessel disease, there is an abundance of high quality data on the relative merits of percutaneous and surgical revascularization strategies in patients with multivessel coronary disease. Over the past 5 years, the results of six major randomized clinical trials involving more than 4300 patients with multivessel coronary disease have been published (Table 55.1).[7–12] Although each trial has somewhat different inclusion and exclusion criteria as well as varying revascularization strategies (complete anatomic, complete functional or culprit vessel revascularization), review of their results demonstrates a number of consistent findings.

First, and most importantly, there is no evidence that an initial strategy of percutaneous revascularization is associated with any worse long term survival than bypass surgery, for most patients with multivessel CAD (Table 55.2). A recent meta-analysis, combining data from all of the randomized trials, demonstrated that the relative risk for mortality with CABG as compared with PTCA was 0.89 with a 95% confidence interval of 0.74–1.08.[13,14] Although overall survival appears to be similar between PTCA and bypass surgery, there may be subgroups for whom initial bypass surgery is associated with improved survival. The BARI Trial reported a statistically significant survival benefit in diabetic patients randomized to bypass surgery (81% vs 66%; $P = 0.003$), for example.[12] This finding has not been confirmed by the other trials, however.

R
Grade A

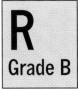
R
Grade B

Despite the lack of an overall survival advantage for PTCA or bypass surgery, there are important differences in long term outcome between these two strategies. Not surprisingly, patients undergoing initial PTCA require significantly more repeat revascularization procedures during the follow-up period.[14] In BARI, for example, 55% of patients treated with initial PTCA required one or more subsequent revascularization procedures during follow-up as compared with just 8% of CABG patients (P<0.001).[12] Nonetheless, nearly 70% of initial PTCA patients remained free from CABG after 5 years of follow-up. A second difference between PTCA and bypass surgery for such patients is in angina relief, at least in the short to intermediate term. Most of the randomized trials have shown that over the first 3 years of follow-up, patients treated with initial CABG have less frequent angina[8,15,16] and better physical functioning.[16] These differences likely reflect the less complete initial revascularization and frequent occurrence of restenosis with multivessel PTCA. Over time, however, these differences tend to diminish and by 5 years, angina and other quality of life outcomes tend to be similar.[16] Finally, medical care costs are clearly lower with multivessel PTCA than with bypass surgery during the initial hospitalization and the first 3 years of follow-up.[15,16] These differences tend to diminish with time, however, and by 5 years mean costs with initial PTCA are only 5% lower than with bypass surgery.[16]

STENTS

The increased lumen caliber seen following balloon angioplasty results from a combination of balloon-mediated vessel enlargement and plaque dissection. By serving as an endovascular scaffold, stents significantly reduce elastic recoil and seal dissection flaps, creating a larger, smoother vascular lumen than is possible with balloon dilation alone. Early experience with coronary stenting from registry and single-center experiences suggested that the Palmaz–Schatz coronary stent provided excellent acute results and low rates of angiographic restenosis.[17] The multicenter registry of the Gianturco–Roubin FlexStent also demonstrated that acute or threatened vessel closure following balloon angioplasty could be successfully treated with stenting.[18] However, data from the initial European experience with the Wallstent demonstrated an 18% incidence of thrombotic occlusion, necessitating aggressive anticoagulation and dampening the initial enthusiasm for stenting.[19]

Randomized trials of stenting vs balloon angioplasty

In August 1994, the randomized Stent Restenosis Study (STRESS) and Belgium Netherlands Stent (BENESTENT) trials compared elective Palmaz–Schatz coronary stenting with conventional balloon angioplasty for treatment of focal, *de novo* lesions in native coronary arteries 3–4 mm in diameter. Both trials demonstrated that stenting was associated with improved acute and long term clinical and angiographic outcome in patients randomized to stent placement[20,21] (Table 55.3). In both the STRESS and Benestent trials, the benefit seen with stenting was due to the fact that it provided a significantly larger postprocedure lumen which (despite greater late loss in lumen diameter), yielding a larger follow-up lumen diameter and lower incidence of angiographic restenosis compared to balloon angioplasty (31% vs 42%, P=0.046

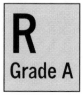

R

Grade A

Table 55.3 STRESS[20] and Benestent[21] Trials

	STRESS		Benestent	
	PTCA	Stent	PTCA	Stent
Clinical outcomes				
Procedural success (%)	85	92[a]	87	86
Inhospital events (%)	10	3[a]	10	7
Out-of-hospital events (%)	23	17	24	14[a]
Vascular surgery (%)	2	4	2	10[a]
Transfusion (%)	2	5	1	4[a]
Subacute thrombosis (%)	1	3	0.7	3
Target lesion revascularization (%)	22	14[a]	27	18[a]
Event-free survival (%)[b]	72	78[a]	60	70[a]
Angiographic outcomes				
Reference diameter (mm)	2.99	3.03	3.00	2.99
MLD preprocedure (mm)	0.75	0.77	1.08	1.07
MLD postprocedure (mm)	1.99	2.49[a]	2.05	2.48[a]
Stenosis postdevice (%)	35	19[a]	33	22[a]
MLD follow-up (%)	1.56	1.75[a]	1.73	1.82
Acute gain (mm)	1.23	1.72[a]	0.97	1.40[a]
Late loss (mm)	0.44	0.75[a]	0.32	0.65[a]
Restenosis rate (%)[c]	42	31[a]	32	22[a]

[a] $P<0.05$.
[b] Freedom from death, myocardial infarction or bailout stenting at 240 days (STRESS) and 210 days (BENESTENT).
[c] Defined as $\geq 50\%$ diameter stenosis.
MLD, minimum lumen diameter at follow-up.

[STRESS] and 22% vs 32%; $P=0.02$ [BENESTENT]). This improvement in late angiographic outcome with stenting was associated with better event-free survival (78% vs 72%, $P=0.03$ [STRESS] and 70% vs 60%, $P=0.03$ [BENESTENT]). The STRESS trial also confirmed that the strongest predictor of freedom from restenosis was a large post-treatment lumen diameter, with no independent effect attributable to the device itself. Other randomized trials comparing stenting to balloon angioplasty have shown similar benefits[22,23] (Table 55.4).

Since enrollment in the STRESS and BENESTENT trials was limited to elective stenting of *de novo* lesions in native coronary arteries, the favorable results reported in these trials cannot be directly extrapolated to the large cohort of patients in whom stents are placed in saphenous vein grafts, previously treated lesions, chronic total occlusions, or for unplanned indications (abrupt or threatened closure). Several smaller trials, however, have compared stenting to balloon angioplasty in these other subsets (Table 55.4). The randomized SAVED (Stent and balloon Angioplasty in saphenous VEin graft Disease) trial compared stenting to balloon angioplasty for treatment of *de novo* lesions in saphenous vein grafts, with stent placement resulting in greater procedural success (92% vs 69%, $P<0.001$) and lower incidence of adverse clinical events (death, myocardial infarction, or subsequent revascularization) (26% vs 38%; $P=0.05$).[24] The Stenting in Chronic Coronary Occlusion (SICCO) trial compared balloon angioplasty to Palmaz–Schatz stenting for the treatment of chronic total occlusion in native coronary arteries, showing that stenting was associated with a lower incidence of angiographic

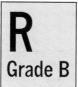

R
Grade A

R
Grade B

Table 55.4 Randomized trials of coronary stenting versus balloon angioplasty

Study	Lesion subset	Major findings	Stent (%)	PTCA (%)
STRESS[20]	*De novo* lesions in native vessels	Procedure success	92	85
		Restenosis	31	42
		TVR	14	22
Benestent[21]	*De novo* lesions in native vessels	Procedure success	87	86
		Restenosis	22	32
		TVR	18	27
		Vascular surgery	10	2
SAVED[24]	*De novo* lesions in saphenous vein grafts	Procedure success	92	69
		Restenosis	36	47
		MACE (6 months)	38	26
START[23]	*De novo* lesions in native vessels	Restenosis	22	37
		TVR	11	22
SICCO[25]	Chronic total occlusions in native vessels	Restenosis	32	74
		TVR	22	42
LAD[22]	*De novo* lesions in the left anterior descending artery	Procedure success	95	93
		Restenosis	19	40
		EFS (12 months)	87	70

TVR, target vessel revascularization; MACE, major cardiac events; EFS, event-free survival.

restenosis (32% vs 74%, $P<0.001$) and target vessel revascularization (22% vs 42%, $P=0.025$).[25]

Anticoagulation regimens for stenting

The enthusiasm for stenting based on the superior clinical and angiographic outcomes demonstrated in the STRESS and Benestent trials was tempered by the increased length of hospitalization and a higher incidence of hemorrhagic complications associated with the aggressive anticoagulation regimens than used to minimize the risk of stent thrombosis.[21] Colombo and others demonstrated that the incidence of stent thrombosis could be minimized by using "optimal" stenting techniques, under which circumstance only antiplatelet therapy (aspirin and ticlopidine) was required to reduce the risk of subacute stent thrombosis to ~1%.[26] This strategy was evaluated in the Intracoronary Stenting and Antithrombotic Regimen (ISAR) trial, comparing stenting with adjunctive anticoagulation (aspirin and warfarin) to antiplatelet agents (aspirin and ticlopidine) only. Patients treated with antiplatelet therapy only, had a significantly lower (1.6% vs 6.2%, $P<0.01$) incidence of major cardiac events (death, myocardial infarction, coronary artery bypass surgery or repeat balloon angioplasty) and subacute thrombosis (0.8% vs 5.4%, $P=0.004$).[27] In the larger Stent Antithrombotic Regimen Study (STARS), patients were randomized following optimal stenting to receive either aspirin alone, aspirin plus warfarin or aspirin plus ticlopidine. The incidence of ischemic cardiac events was significantly lower for patients treated with aspirin plus ticlopidine (0.6% [aspirin and ticlopidine] vs 2.6% [aspirin and warfarin] vs 2.9% [aspirin alone]), establishing the aspirin/ticlopidine regimen as the current "standard" for prophylaxis against occlusive stent thrombosis.[28]

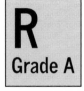

Future directions

While controlled trials have demonstrated that stenting is associated with improved clinical and angiographic outcome in a number of lesion subsets (native vessels, saphenous vein grafts, chronic total occlusions), ongoing trials are comparing stenting in a larger, expanding population of clinical indications (e.g. acute myocardial infarction) and lesion subsets (e.g. ostial location, long lesions, small vessels). In addition, several randomized trials comparing newer "second generation" stents with approved prototypes will address issues such as whether improvements in design are associated with greater ease of delivery and improved clinical outcome. Finally, ongoing evaluation of stent coatings (e.g. the heparin-coated Palmaz–Schatz coronary stent) and future evaluation of radioactive stents will provide valuable data regarding ability to further limit thrombosis and restenosis.

ATHERECTOMY

While conventional balloon angioplasty seeks to crack and displace outwardly the elements of an atherosclerotic obstruction, atherectomy quite literally seeks to enlarge the coronary lumen by removing portions of the atherosclerotic plaque. Doing so may overcome the tendency for local dissection and elastic recoil of the vessel wall inherent in POBA and potentially may leave behind a larger and smoother luminal surface.

Two main techniques have been popularized: directional atherectomy, in which a cutting blade within a windowed steel cylinder is used to resect and remove slivers of obstructing plaque, and rotational atherectomy, in which small diamond chips on the surface of a rapidly spinning brass burr are used to abrade the plaque into microscopic particles which are then washed away through the coronary microcirculation by normal arterial flow. These two mechanical techniques (which have been well studied and which together account for up to 15% of coronary intervention) will be emphasized in this discussion. The other techniques of extraction atherectomy (TEC) and laser atherectomy have much narrower niche applications, have generally not been subjected to high level clinical investigation and will thus not be discussed further.

Directional atherectomy

Directional atherectomy (DCA) was the first new (non-balloon) device approved by the Food and Drug Administration in 1990, based on a registry of 1000+ cases performed over the preceding 2 years.[29] Two randomized trials (CAVEAT (Coronary Angioplasty Versus Excisional Atherectomy Trial) and CCAT (Canadian Coronary Atherectomy Trial) were conducted in 1991–2 to evaluate the benefits of this device as compared to conventional balloon angioplasty.[30,31] Since the main benefits of this device were a smoother luminal surface with less proliferative response, and avoidance of balloon trauma, deep plaque resection or perforation, the technique for DCA utilized in these studies avoided attempts at complete plaque excision or maximal luminal enlargement through adjunctive balloon postdilation. Post-treatment lumen diameters and residual diameter stenoses were not significantly better than those obtained with POBA in the angioplasty arms of these trials (Table 55.5). Neither angiographic restenosis nor clinical

Table 55.5 Clinical trials of directional coronary atherectomy

	NACI Registry[39]	CAVEAT-DCA[30]	CAVEAT-PTCA[30]	BOAT-DCA[37]	BOAT-PTCA[37]
Number of pts	1196	512	500	497	492
Reference diameter (mm)	3.34	2.78	2.78	3.25	3.20
Post-treatment diameter (%)	2.72 (19%)	2.02 (29%)	1.80 (36%)	2.82 (14.7%)	2.33 (28)
% 7 Fr devices	43%	53%	N/A	95%	N/A
% postdilated	31%	<5%	N/A	81%	N/A
Major complications	2.8%	5.9%	3.7%	2.8%	3.3%
Angiographic restenosis	—	50%	57%	32%[a]	40%
Repeat revascularization	28.1%	33.7%	35%	25.4%	28.1%
TVR	22.6%[b]	24.4%	25.9%	17.1%	19.7%
1-year mortality	3.6%	2.2%	0.6%	0.6%	1.6%

[a] $P = 0.02$.
[b] Target vessel revascularization (TVR) was 13% for patients with acute residual stenosis <20%.
N/A, no DCA devices in PTCA arm.

Table 55.6 Excimer, Rotablator, Balloon Angioplasty in Complex lesions (ERBAC[41])

	PTCA	Excimer	Rotablator
Number of pts	215	210	195
Primary success	80%	76%	91%
Secondary success (after crossover)	82%	89%	92%
Post-treatment diameter stenosis	36%	32%	31%
Major complications (death/QMI/emCABG)	4.8%	6.2%	2.3%
Angiographic restenosis	51%	61%	56%
Repeat revascularization	35%	46%	46%
TVR	32%	42%	43%

restenosis (repeat revascularization by 6 months) was significantly reduced by DCA. While DCA did not increase the traditional major complications (death, Q-wave MI, emergency CABG), the incidence of non Q-wave MI defined as creatinine kinase (CK) >twice normal was doubled (14% vs 6%) and 1-year mortality was higher in the DCA arm (1.6% vs 0.6%). A similar lack of significant benefit was seen in the CAVEAT II trial comparing directional atherectomy to balloon angioplasty in the treatment of saphenous vein graft disease.[32] These data were taken to indicate that widespread use of directional atherectomy was unwarranted.[33]

Following the completion of these trials, there was a shift in understanding and technique for DCA in which the importance of maximizing the post-treatment lumen, the lack of increased restenosis when more complete resection of plaque and underlying media was undertaken, and the potential benefits of balloon postdilation to improve the results of successful (but suboptimal) atherectomy were appreciated.[34] Trials based on this "optimal" DCA technique included the OARS 200 patient registry,[35] the ABACAS 200 patient registry,[36] and the BOAT 1000 patient randomized comparison to balloon angioplasty[37] (Table 55.5). In contrast to the earlier studies, BOAT showed that optimal atherectomy could provide greater degrees of acute luminal enlargement, with a corresponding decrease in angiographic restenosis and a trend towards reduction in repeat revascularizations. Despite confirmation of the higher incidence of CK elevations after otherwise successful procedures (as observed in CAVEAT), there was no increase in major inhospital complications or in 1-year mortality (0.6% vs 1.6% for DCA and PTCA, respectively). This is at odds with findings from other retrospective series in which low order periprocedural CK elevation was associated with worsened longer term mortality.[38] This is a clear example of how important the technique of device use (and not just which device was used) is to the outcome of an interventional trial.

Rotational atherectomy

Rotational atherectomy was approved by the Food and Drug Administration in 1993, based on an extensive registry. That registry experience is included in the New Approaches to Coronary Intervention registry (NACI)[40] and suggests that the device had special utility in certain lesion types (ostial, calcified, diffuse) that are considered unfavorable for conventional balloon angioplasty. The ERBAC trial[41] randomized patients with such unfavorable lesions (AHA/ACC B2 or C) to excimer laser, rotational atherectomy or balloon angioplasty and found higher success and lower complication rates (although

Table 55.7 Trials of rotational atherectomy

	NACI Registry[40]	STRATAS aggressive[42]	STRATAS std- + PTCA	DART[43] Rota	DART-PTCA
Number of lesions	670	249	248	206	205
Reference diameter (mm)	2.77	2.41	2.37	2.45	2.47
Post-treatment diameter (% DS)	2.04 (26%)	1.78 (27.5%)	1.80 (26.5%)	1.75 (27.9%)	1.77 (29.8%)
Burr:artery ratio	0.71	0.90	0.80	—	—
Postdilation pressure atm (%)	— (88%)	1.7 (84%)	5.8 (98%)	—	—
Bailout stenting	—	7.2%	3.1%	6%	14%
Major complications	2.1%	2.0%	3.6%	1.3%	0
Death	0.8%	0.4%	2.0%	0.4%	0
QMI	1.1%	1.6%	0.8%	0	0
Em-CABG	0.4%	0.4%	2.0%	0.9%	0.9%
Angiographic rest	—	57.8%	51.7%	—	—
Repeat revascularization	34%				
TVR	26%	34.5%	28.6%	—	—
1-year mortality	5.0%	1.6%	4.0%	—	—

similar restenosis rates) with rotational atherectomy (Table 55.6). One criticism of this study is that the rotational atherectomy technique used a single (typically 1.75 mm) burr followed by standard balloon angioplasty. As with directional atherectomy, however, rotational atherectomy has undergone a progressive evolution in what is perceived as "optimal" technique. The STRATAS trial (Table 55.7)[42] compared two newer techniques: standard burring to a burr:artery ratio of 0.7 (2.15 mm burr in a 3 mm artery) followed by balloon angioplasty, versus aggressive burring to a burr:artery ratio of 0.8 or more followed by no or only low pressure (1–2 atm) balloon inflation. Relative to the technique in ERBAC, both rotablator arms in STRATAS used the serial burr technique (starting at 1.5 or 1.75 mm and then sizing up by 0.5 mm increments to a final burr size that was at least 70% of the reference diameter), lower rotational speeds (160–180 000 rpm), and careful burr advancement to avoid drops in rotational speed. Despite the theoretical benefits of maximal debulking with minimal balloon barotrauma, the aggressive burring strategy of STRATAS appeared to carry a higher incidence of non-Q-wave MI and bailout stenting, without reducing the incidence of late restenosis compared to the standard (0.7 burr:artery ratio, plus PTCA) strategy. To investigate whether rotational atherectomy offered any benefit over balloon angioplasty in simpler lesions, the DART trial[43] has randomized 400 patients to treatment with either conventional PTCA or rotational atherectomy using the standard STRATAS technique.

SUMMARY

The field of catheter coronary intervention represents a dynamic area where new devices are applied, with evolving techniques of use, to an ever broadening set of clinical and anatomic situations. The problem of accurately characterizing its performance across this broad front is further complicated by the fact that both alternative therapeutic techniques (medical therapy and surgical bypass) are undergoing progressive refinement as well (HMG-CoA reductase inhibitors, minimally invasive bypass, etc.). The "ultimate" answers to how each situation is best treated can thus never be obtained. This chapter has made clear, however, that the tradition of critically evaluating major issues (with careful registries and focused randomized trials) is now well established, making interventional cardiology one of the strong examples of evidenced based medicine.

REFERENCES

1 Detre K, Holubkov R, Kelsey S *et al.* Percutaneous transluminal coronary angioplasty in 1985–1986 and 1977–1981. The National Heart, Lung, and Blood Institute Registry. *N Engl J Med* 1988;**318**:265–70.

2 Kuntz RE, Baim DS. Defining coronary restenosis: newer clinical and angiographic paradigms. *Circulation* 1993;**88**:1310–1323.

3 Parisi AF, Folland ED, Hartigan P. A comparison of angioplasty with medical therapy in the treatment of single-vessel coronary artery disease. *N Engl J Med* 1992;**326**:10–16.

4 Strauss WE, Fortin T, Hartigan P, Folland ED, Parisi AF, on behalf of the Veterans Affairs Study of Angioplasty Compared to Medical Therapy Investigators. A comparison of quality of life scores in patients with angina pectoris after angioplasty compared with after medical therapy. Outcomes of a randomized clinical trial. *Circulation* 1995;**92**:1710–19.

5 Wong JB, Sonnenberg FA, Salem DN, Pauker SG. Myocardial revascularization for chronic stable angina. Analysis of the role of percutaneous transluminal coronary angioplasty based on data available in 1989. *Ann Intern Med* 1990;**113**: 852–71.

6 Hueb W, Bellotti G, Almedia de Oliveira S *et al.* The Medicine, Angioplasty, or Surgery Study (MASS): a prospective, randomized trial of medical therapy, balloon angioplasty, or bypass surgery

for single proximal left anterior descending artery stenoses. *J Am Coll Cardiol* 1995;**26**:1600–5.

7 CABRI Trial Participants. First-year results of CABRI (Coronary Angioplasty vs Bypass Revascularization Investigation). *Lancet* 1995; **346**:1179–84.

8 RITA Trial Participants. Coronary angioplasty versus coronary artery bypass surgery: the Randomized Intervention Treatment of Angina (RITA) trial. *Lancet* 1993;**343**:573–80.

9 King SB, Lembo NJ, Kosinski AS *et al.* A randomized trial comparing coronary angioplasty with coronary bypass surgery. *N Engl J Med* 1994; **331**:1044–50.

10 Hamm CW, Riemers J, Ischinger T *et al.* A randomized study of coronary angioplasty compared with bypass surgery in patients with symptomatic multi-vessel coronary disease. *N Engl J Med* 1994;**331**:1037–43.

11 Rodriguez A, Boullon F, Perez-Balino N *et al.* Argentine randomized trial of percutaneous transluminal coronary angioplasty versus coronary artery bypass surgery in multi-vessel disease (ERACI): in-hospital results and 1-year follow-up. *J Am Coll Cardiol* 1993;**22**:1060–7.

12 The Bypass Angioplasty Revascularization Investigation (BARI) Investigators. Comparison of coronary bypass surgery with angioplasty in patients with multivessel disease. *N Engl J Med* 1996;**335**:217–25.

13 Simoons ML. Myocardial revascularization – bypass surgery or angioplasty? *N Engl J Med* 1996;**335**:275–6.

14 Pocock SJ, Henderson RA, Rickards AF *et al.* Meta-analysis of randomized trials comparing coronary angioplasty with bypass surgery. *Lancet* 1995; **346**:1184–9.

15 Weintraub WS, Mauldin PD, Becker E, Kosiński AS, King SB. A comparison of the costs of and quality of life after coronary angioplasty or coronary surgery for multivessel coronary artery disease. Results from the Emory Angioplasty versus Surgery Trial (EAST). *Circulation* 1995;**92**:2831–40.

16 Hlatky MA, Rogers WJ, Johnstone I *et al.* Medical care costs and quality of life after randomization to coronary angioplasty or coronary bypass surgery. *N Engl J Med* 1997;**336**:92–9.

17 Carrozza JP Jr, Kuntz RE, Levine MJ *et al.* Angiographic and clinical outcome of intracoronary stenting: immediate and long-term results from a large single-center experience. *J Am Coll Cardiol* 1992;**20**:328.

18 George BS, Vorhees III WD, Roubin GS *et al.* Multicenter investigation of coronary stenting to treat acute or threatened closure after percutaneous transluminal coronary angioplasty: clinical and angiographic outcomes. *J Am Coll Cardiol* 1993;**22**:135.

19 Serruys PW, Strauss BH, Beatt KJ *et al.* Angiographic follow-up after placememt of a self-expanding coronary artery stent. *N Engl J Med* 1991;**324**:13.

20 Fischman DL, Leon MB, Baim DS *et al.* A randomized comparison of coronary-stent placement and balloon angioplasty in the treatment of coronary artery disease. *N Engl J Med* 1994;**331**:496.

21 Serruys PW, de Jaegere P, Kiemeneij F *et al.* A comparison of balloon-expandable stent implantation with balloon angioplasty in patients with coronary disease. *N Engl J Med* 1994;**331**:489.

22 Versaci F, Gaspardone A, Tomai F *et al.* A comparison of coronary-artery stenting with angioplasty for isolated stenosis of the proximal left anterior descending coronary artery. *N Engl J Med* 1997;**336**:817–822.

23 Serra A, Masotti M, Fernandez-Aviles F *et al.* Stent vs Angioplasty Restenosis Trial (START): influence of vessel size on angiographic restenosis. *Circulation* 1996;**94**:I–92a.

24 Savage MP, Douglas JS, Fishman DL *et al.* Stent placement compared with balloon angioplasty for obstructed coronary bypass grafts – saphenous vein de novo trial. *N Engl J Med* 1997;**337**:740–7.

25 Sirnes PA, Golf S, Myreng Y *et al.* Stenting in Chronic Coronary Occlusion (SICCO): a randomized, controlled trial of adding stent implantation after successful angioplasty. *J Am Coll Cardiol* 1996;**28**:1444–51.

26 Colombo A, Hall P, Nakamura S *et al.* Intracoronary stenting without anticoagulation accomplished with intravascular ultrasound guidance. *Circulation* 1995;**91**:1676–88.

27 Schomig A, Neumann FJ, Kastrati A *et al.* A randomized comparison of antiplatelet and anticoagulation therapy after the placement of coronary artery stents. *N Engl J Med* 1996;**334**:1084–9.

28 Leon MB, Baim DS, Gordon P *et al.* Clinical and angiographic results from the Stent Anticoagulation Regimen Study (STARS). *Circulation* 1996;**94**:I–685.

29 Baim DS, Hinohara T, Holmes D *et al.* Results of directional coronary atherectomy during multicenter preapproval testing. *Am J Cardiol.* 1993;**72**:6E–11E

30 Topol EJ, Leya F, Pinkerton CA *et al.* A comparison of directional atherectomy with coronary angioplasty in patients with coronary artery disease. *N Engl J Med.* 1993;**329**:221–227.

31 Adelman AG, Cohen EA, Kimball BP *et al.* A comparison of directional atherectomy with balloon angioplasty for lesions of the left anterior descending artery. *N Engl J Med* 1993;**329**:228–233

32 Holmes DR, Topol EJ, Califf RM *et al.* A multicenter randomized trial of coronary angioplasty versus directional atherectomy for patients with saphenous vein graft lesions. *Circulation* 1994; **91**:1966–74.

33 Holmes DR, Topol EJ, Adelman AG, Cohen EA, Califf RM. Randomized trials of directional atherectomy – implications for clinical practice and future investigation. *J Am Coll Cardiol* 1994; **24**:431–9

34 Gordon PC, Kugelmas AD, Cohen DJ *et al.* Balloon post-dilation can safely improve the results of successful (but sub-optimal) directional coronary atherectomy. *Am J Cardiol* 1993:**72**:71E–79E

35 Simonton CA, Leon MB, Kuntz RE *et al.* Acute and late clinical and angiographic results of directional atherectomy in the Optimal Atherectomy Restenosis Study (OARS). *Circulation.* 1995;**93**(suppl):2602

36 Hosokawa H, Suzuki T, Ueno K *et al.* Clinical and angiographic follow-up of Adjunctive Balloon Angioplasty following Coronary Atherectomy Study (ABACAS). *Circulation* 1996;**94**(suppl): I–318.

37 Baim DS, Cutlip DE, Popma JJ, Sharma SK *et al.* Final results in the Balloon vs Optimal Atherectomy Trial (BOAT) – 6 month angiographic and clinical follow-up. *Circulation* 1996;**94**:I–436 (abstract)

38 Abdelmequid AE, Topol EJ. The myth of the myocardial "infarctlet" during percutaneous coronary revascularization procedure. *Circulation* 1996;**94**:3369–75.

39 Waksman R, Popma JJ, Kennard ED. Directional coronary atherectomy–a report from the NACI Registry. *Am J Cardiol* 1997;**80**:50K–59K.

40 Brown DL, George CJ, Steenkiste AR *et al.* High speed rotational atherectomy in human coronary stenoses – acute and one year outcomes from the New Approaches to Coronary Intervention (NACI) Registry. *Am J Cardiol* (in press).

41 Reifart N, Vandormael M, Krajear M *et al.* Randomized comparison of angioplasty of complex coronary lesions at a single center – Excimer laser, Rotational atherectomy, and Balloon Angioplasty Comparison (ERBAC) study. *Circulation* 1997;**96**:91–8.

42 Whitlow PL, Cowley MJ, Kuntz RE *et al.* Study to determine Rotablator And Transluminal Angioplasty Strategy – acute results. *Circulation* 1996;**94**:I–434 (abstract).

43 Reisman M, Buchbinder M, Sharma SK. A multicenter randomized trial of rotational atherectomy vs PTCA–DART. *Circulation* 1997; **96**:I–467 (abstract).

56 Adjunctive therapy in PTCA

RONALD VAN DER WIEKEN,
MAARTEN SIMOONS

INTRODUCTION

The introduction of percutaneous transluminal coronary angioplasty has proven to be a major step forward in the treatment of coronary heart disease. Unfortunately, the gain has not come without a price: quite frequent and serious complications have been identified, acute as well as chronic. From the beginning in 1977, when Gruentzig introduced PTCA, it was clear that the technique cannot do without pharmacologic support. Since then, the development of adjunctive therapy has come a long way. Great progress has been made, but some major problems still wait to be resolved.

The goal of this chapter is to provide the reader with a general overview of adjunctive therapy directed against both acute and chronic complications as well as of the pathophysiologic principles involved.

Key points

Acute complications of PTCA
- Intimal dissection with or without thrombus
- Plaque rupture with thrombus
- Spasm

Acute complications

The complications in the key points box can each lead to abrupt vessel closure. This occurs in 6.8–8.3% of PTCA procedures and is responsible for a sizeable mortality (up to 1.7%), acute myocardial infarction (1.3–8.6%), emergency bypass surgery (1.3–3.6%), and emergency re-PTCA (4.5%).[1-5] Abrupt vessel closure usually happens in the catheterization laboratory, with the great majority taking place within 6 hours post-PTCA. If it is not possible to open the vessel rapidly, major problems can be expected: persisting anginal pain and myocardial infarction, hemodynamic instability and arrhythmias. Rather unexpectedly, these difficulties can also arise with the abrupt re-closure after opening a chronically occluded vessel. The incidence of abrupt vessel closure is more frequent in unstable coronary syndromes and in angiographically complicated lesions.

Intimal dissection is caused by intravascular maneuvering of guidewires, balloons or other devices. It occurs in a wide variety, from minor and acceptable to major and occlusive. It is usually but not always accompanied by thrombus formation. At present, the only feasible therapy for a significant dissection is mechanical. The most widely used therapy used to be prolonged balloon inflation at the site of the dissection, preferably with a perfusion catheter, but this has to a large extent been replaced by the application of stents.

Plaque rupture results from pressure applied to an atherosclerotic lesion. The fibrous cap of the plaque ruptures, uncovering highly thrombogenic plaque contents, in many ways resembling the events in the acute coronary syndromes. This probably happens in a large number of angioplastic maneuvers, often without deleterious consequence. It is only harmful if excessive thrombus formation takes place, leading to coronary occlusion or near occlusion.

Spasm can be caused by the mere touch of the intracoronary guidewire. Isolated spasm, without dissection or plaque rupture, can rarely lead to abrupt vessel closure. More often, spasm is associated with dissection and/or plaque rupture. Antispasmodic therapy consists of intracoronary nitroglycerin.[6,7] In refractory cases a calcium antagonist can be given.[8,9]

Chronic sequelae

Restenosis is an indirect sequel of the angioplastic trauma to the endovascular structures. Six months after successful conventional angioplasty, it is angiographically present in approximately 40% of cases.

Causal factors of chronic restenosis are shown in the key points box.

Key points

Events leading to chronic restenosis
- Elastic recoil
- Formation of mural thrombus
- Intimal proliferation and synthesis of intracellular matrix
- Pathological arterial remodeling

Many drugs have been named as potentially valuable in the prevention of chronic restenosis. A host of trials have been conducted but only a few reported a positive outcome. Very recently, it was shown in a double-blind, placebo-controlled, randomized trial that probucol, an antioxidant, was effective in reducing the restenosis rate.[10] One month before PTCA, 317 patients were randomly assigned to receive one of four treatments: placebo, probucol (500 mg b.d.d.), multivitamins (30 000 IU of betacarotene, 500 mg of vitamin C, and 700 IU of vitamin E, b.d.d.), or both probucol and multivitamins (b.d.d.). Patients were treated for 4 weeks before and 6 months after angioplasty. Follow-up angiography 6 months after PTCA showed restenosis in 20.7% in the probucol group, 28.9% in the combined treatment group, 40.3% in the multivitamin group, and

38.9% in the placebo group. The difference between the probucol and non-probucol groups is statistically highly significant ($P = 0.003$). These results need confirmation in other trials before probucol can be advocated as an indispensable adjunct to PTCA. Pharmacologic suppression of restenosis is, however, still under intense research. Trials with new pharmacologic agents, systemically or locally delivered, but also physical means such as intracoronary γ and β radiation will be conducted in the near future.

R

Grade A

In reduction of restenosis, stents have been successful, at least in large vessels.[11,12] Effects in smaller coronary arteries have to be awaited, but seem to be less promising. Stenting prevents recoil and pathological remodeling to a large extent, but leaves formation of mural thrombus and intimal proliferation unhampered. Stenting is thus at best a partial remedy to the problem of chronic restenosis, reducing the incidence of restenosis but not abolishing it.

THROMBUS, PLATELETS, AND THROMBIN

Thrombus formation

This plays a leading role in abrupt vessel closure and may be of importance in chronic restenosis. The composition of arterial thrombi ("white thrombi"), with their predominance of platelets, shows that thrombocytes are central in angioplasty-related thrombus formation and acute vessel occlusion. A second agent of great importance is thrombin.

Platelets, physiology, and pathophysiology

The properties of platelets relevant to the formation of thrombus are shown in the key points box and are discussed in some detail below. Platelets are produced by the megakaryocyte. Through processes yet unexplained, this cell fragments into many platelets, which are disk-shaped cells with a diameter of 2–3 μm derived from the cytoplasm of the megakaryocyte without a nucleus. They do contain platelet-specific granules and a dense tubular system as well as a skeleton consisting of actin. The surface has a host of receptors for a wide variety of agents all playing a role in the very complex processes of adhesion, aggregation, and release of granules.

Normally, platelets are in contact solely with the other blood components and the endothelial lining of the blood vessels. Any other contact is inducive to platelet adhesion, with the potential to escalate to aggregation. As long as the endothelial lining of the blood vessels is intact, platelets are not activated. This does not mean that they are inert. Platelets produce substances responsible for the maintenance of the integrity of the vessel walls.

Platelets are normally heterogeneous, both physically and functionally. Younger platelets seem to be larger and more responsive to thrombin than older ones.[13] The lifespan of the platelet is 7–10 days. They are not distributed evenly throughout the lumen; the arterial flow pattern is such that platelets tend to concentrate near the wall, while red blood cells are present predominantly in the central part of the vessel.

ADHESION

Platelets contacting surfaces other than erythrocytes, leukocytes or intact endothelium can adhere to them. They adhere to subendothelial structures, macrophages, activated leukocytes, and endothelial cells activated by inflammatory cytokines. They adhere through the expression of membrane integrins, a subset of the glycoprotein receptors situated on the platelet membrane. The main endothelial adhesive protein is the von Willebrand factor, but many others can play a role. Adhesion denotes the deposition of thrombocytes on a surface perceived as foreign, involving a monolayer of platelets and, at least theoretically, having the effect of providing a more natural environment for the other blood corpuscles. Often, however, aggregation ensues.

The most frequently encountered foreign structure is subendothelial tissue which is exposed when endothelium is damaged, for example during angioplasty. The level of platelet adherence is dependent on the nature of the foreign structure – deeper seated structures are a stronger stimulus than those just under the endothelial lining,[14] and on the presence of the von Willebrand factor. The von Willebrand factor can bind to certain types of collagen and form complexes that bind to the platelet membrane glycoprotein GPIb and thus cause adhesion.[15] Adhesion involves one single layer of thrombocytes only.

On adhesion, contact with subendothelial collagen can initiate the following physiologic events:

- intracellular platelet granules are released into the extracellular space;
- P-selectin, a platelet membrane glycoprotein, expresses itself on the platelet surface, mediating adhesion to white blood corpuscles;
- activation of the intraplatelet eicosanoid pathway, starting with the emanation of arachidonic acid;
- a profound change in the shape of the platelets, from a smooth disc to a spiculated structure.

These reactions together constitute the activation of the platelets which leads to platelet aggregation, a process that accelerates itself considerably in a short passage of time.

AGGREGATION

More extensive vessel damage induces platelets to aggregate. Activation and ensuing aggregation can be caused by many factors including adenosine diphosphate (ADP) and serotonin, which are produced (among many others) by the release of platelet granules, thromboxane A_2 (TXA_2), which is generated in the interior of the platelet as an end product of the eicosanoid pathway, and platelet activating factor, which is produced by injured endothelial cells. Adrenalin, noradrenalin and (most powerful) thrombin also activate platelets and, vice versa, platelet activation catalyzes the conversion of prothrombin to thrombin, thereby accelerating the process of activation and aggregation. Fibrillar collagen, which is exposed when the vessel is damaged, not only promotes adhesion but also induces aggregation.

After the specific agents have made contact with the platelet membrane, the platelet changes in shape from disc to spiculated sphere. This change in shape is regulated by a skeleton of actin situated interior to the plasmalemma. The filopodial projections that constitute the spiculae probably facilitate contact between GPIIb IIIa, the receptor on the platelet surface which is the final common pathway responsible for aggregation, and crucial proteins: fibrinogen and von Willebrand factor. In the next stage the GPIIb IIIa receptor changes in conformation, allowing fibrinogen and von Willebrand factor to bind simultaneously to the GPIIb IIIa receptors on the surface of two platelets, thus creating a link between them. This usually irreversible linkage is called aggregation. A plug of linked platelets constitutes a thrombus and may obstruct a vessel lumen.

SYNTHESIS AND RELEASE OF PROSTACYCLIN, THROMBOXANES, AND INTRACELLULAR GRANULES

The eicosanoid pathway exists in endothelial cells as well as in the interior of the platelet. Arachidonic acid is converted by cyclo-oxygenase to endoperoxides that form prostacyclin in the endothelial cells but generate TXA_2 in the platelet. TXA_2 enhances aggregation and is a vasoconstrictor; prostacyclin, on the other hand, has strong vasodilatory and antiaggregant properties. Platelets contain at least three different types of intracellular storage granules. These granules contain a host of substances that can be liberated from the activated platelets by an exocytotic mechanism.[16] The various materials are able to potentiate platelet aggregation and blood coagulation and increase vascular permeability.

Thrombin

Thrombin is the second major player in the pathogenesis of acute coronary thrombosis. It is at the center of reactions essential to thrombus formation. It can activate platelets strongly and independently.[17] Thrombin can cause the release of the von Willebrand factor from endothelium, facilitates the activation of factor V and VIII and the transition of fibrinogen to fibrin. It promotes the formation of a fibrin mesh around thrombi. Thrombin is abundantly generated during angioplasty.[18]

ANTIAGGREGATORY STRATEGIES

Four major classes of antiaggregatory agents can be discerned:

1. cyclo-oxygenase inhibitors, e.g. aspirin;
2. thienopyridines, e.g. ticlopidine;
3. glycoprotein IIb IIIa inhibitors, e.g. abciximab and integrilin;
4. thrombin inhibitors, e.g. heparin and hirudin.

Aspirin

Platelet aggregability can be inhibited to some extent by aspirin. In thrombocytes, aspirin irreversibly inhibits cyclo-oxygenase and thereby the generation of TXA_2 which is an aggregation promotor. Aspirin thus inhibits platelet aggregation and thrombus formation. However, also reduced is the production, in the endothelium, of antiaggregatory prostacyclin. Possibly this unfavorable side effect becomes more pronounced with higher doses of aspirin, rendering the lower doses relatively more effective.[19] Aspirin leaves other platelet activation pathways untouched. It is therefore a relatively weak antiaggregatory agent.

Aspirin has been used as premedication to angioplasty since its debut in 1977 and is a universally used adjunctive,[20] but with few prospective trials ever having proven the efficacy. In one, a daily dose of 990 mg aspirin combined with dipyridamole (225 mg daily) showed no effect on restenosis compared to placebo, but periprocedural infarctions were significantly less in the treatment group.[21] Among the 376 randomized patients, there were periprocedural Q wave infarctions in 6.9% in the placebo group and 1.6% in the active drug group, the difference reaching statistical significance ($P = 0.0113$). A retrospective angiographic study also showed a clear periprocedural advantage of aspirin and dipyridamole.[22] After doubts had been raised concerning the contribution of dipyridamole to the antithrombotic action of aspirin,[23] this drug disappeared from the adjunctive armamentarium.

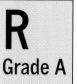

The optimal daily dosage of aspirin with a reliable effect in angioplasty is not known. In the US, 325 mg is usual, while in Europe 100 mg or 80 mg is accepted. The higher dosages (over 100 mg) are associated with more, predominantly gastrointestinal, side effects but not convincingly with greater efficacy. Aspirin is rapidly absorbed from the stomach and upper small intestine. Following ingestion, peak plasma levels are reached 20 minutes following ingestion.[24] Clinically relevant inhibition of platelet aggregation requires 80–90% blockade of TXA_2 synthesis.[25] With daily oral dosages of 80 mg it takes 48 hours to develop this effect on TXA_2 production and aggregation.[26] In higher dosages effective inhibition is reached earlier. It is therefore advisable to start oral aspirin at a low dose at least 48 hours before the angioplasty. Often time is lacking to prepare the patient along these lines. If an immediate procedure has to be performed and the patient is not on aspirin, chewing of enteric coated aspirin results in a sufficient antiplatelet effect after 30 minutes.[27] Intravenous injection of 250 or 500 mg aspirin results in an even more immediate platelet inhibition.[28]

Ticlopidine

Ticlopidine is metabolized to an as yet unknown substance, which inhibits ADP-induced platelet aggregation but has no effect on TXA_2-induced aggregation. It leads to a remarkable prolonging of the bleeding time. An effect on platelet aggregation is demonstrable only after 3–5 days of medication.

Ticlopidine has proven its usefulness in conjunction with aspirin in the prevention of acute and subacute stent thrombosis. This complication occurs after insertion of an intracoronary stent in 2–8% of cases, usually between days 2 and 14 with a peak between days 5 and 7 after stent placement. Very extensive regimens, consisting of vitamin K antagonists, dipyridamole, and dextran as well as aspirin and heparin, did not

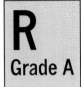

positively influence this complication and led to unacceptable bleeding complications.[11] However, the combination of aspirin and ticlopidine achieved a significant decrease of stent thrombosis as well as bleeding complications.[29] Simultaneously, significant improvement of stent delivery technique such as high pressure implantation also affected results.

Current practice is to administer ticlopidine daily, beginning 7 days before scheduled stent placement. If a stent is inserted as a bailout procedure or because of a suboptimal result, it is customary to start the drug immediately after the procedure. It is continued for 30 days in a regimen of 250 mg two times daily.

The main untoward but reversible effect is bone marrow depression, especially of the neutrophil granulocytes, occurring in less than 2% of patients.[30] In less than 1%, thrombocytopenia is encountered. Two weeks after starting ticlopidine, a white blood cell and thrombocyte count should be performed.

A newer drug, clopidogrel, while in many respects similar to ticlopidine, displays a lesser tendency to bone marrow depression.[31] It has not been tested as an adjunctive to PTCA.

IIb IIIa receptor blockers

Although there are many ways to activate the platelet, all converge into the same final common pathway, the IIb IIIa receptor. Blockade of this receptor impedes aggregation to a very large extent, if not completely, with all modes of platelet activation using the final common pathway.

Presently, IIb IIIa blockers are known in four forms:

1. a chimeric monoclonal antibody (derived from murine antibodies), abciximab, which is commercially available;
2. naturally occurring snake venom polypeptides. These non-enzymatic peptides have a low potency and short half-life, diminishing their therapeutic value;[32]
3. synthetic peptides, e.g. integrilin and tirofiban;
4. non-peptide IIb IIIa inhibitors, some with the interesting potential to be active orally, like lefradafibran.

Relevant large scale clinical investigation has been conducted with abciximab, integrilin, and tirofiban.

Abciximab was tested in the CAPTURE, EPILOG, and EPIC trials. All were prospective, multicenter, randomized, double-blind, placebo-controlled, phase III studies, with a grand total of 6156 patients. Table 56.1 shows the main results of these studies.

EPIC studied 2099 patients at increased risk for ischemic complications during or after PTCA:[33] unstable angina and/or recent non-Q wave infarction, acute Q wave infarction within 12 hours of symptom onset, and clinical and angiographic characteristics predictive of increased risk of ischemic complications according to AHA Medical/Scientific Statement Guidelines.[34] Patients were randomized to one of the following regimens:

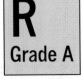

1. placebo bolus + infusion;
2. abciximab bolus 0.25 mg/kg IV + 12 hour infusion of placebo;
3. abciximab bolus 0.25 mg/kg IV + 12 hour infusion of abciximab 10 μg/min.

Table 56.1 Main results of CAPTURE, EPILOG and EPIC trials

	CAPTURE Refractory angina		EPIC High risk PTCA			EPILOG Elective PTCA		
	Placebo	Abcix-imab	Placebo	Bolus	Bolus + infusion	Placebo	Abcix. low hep.	Abcix. norm. hep.
No. pts	635	630	696	695	708	939	918	935
30 day MAE[a]	15.9	11.3	12.8	11.5	8.3	11.7	5.4	5.2
	$P=0.012$		$P=0.428$		$P=0.008$	$P<0.001$		$P<0.001$
Mortality	1.3	1.0	1.7	1.3	1.7	0.8	0.3	0.4
	n.s		n.s		n.s	$P=0.21$		$P=0.39$
Infarction	8.2	4.1	8.6	6.2	5.2	8.7	3.7	3.8
	$P=0.002$		$P=0.101$		$P=0.014$	$P<0.001$		$P<0.001$
Emerg. revasc.	10.9	7.8	7.8	6.4	4.0	5.2	2.3	1.6
	$P=0.054$				$P=0.003$	$P=0.001$		$P<0.001$
Major bleeding	1.9	3.8	6.6	11.1	14.0	3.1	2.0	3.5
	$P=0.043$		$P=0.003$		$P<0.001$	$P=0.19$		$P=0.7$
6 months MAE[a]	30.8	31.0	35.1	32.6	27.0	25.8	22.8	22.3
	n.s		$P=0.276$		$P=0.001$	$P=0.07$		$P=0.04$
3 year MAE[a]			47.2	41.1				
			$P=0.009$					

CAPTURE: C7E3 Anti Platelet Therapy in Unstable Refractory Angina.
EPIC: Evaluation of C7E3 to Prevent Ischemic Complications.
EPILOG: Evaluation in PTCA to Improve Long-term Outcome with abciximab GP IIb/IIIa blockade.
[a] MAE: major adverse events, comprising death, myocardial infarction, urgent revascularization of any sort, in percentages.

Treatment started at least 10 min before PTCA, all patients received 325 mg aspirin orally and 10 000–12 000 IU heparin intravenously.

Abciximab dosages were devised to reach a receptor blockade of at least 80%. Patients were followed for 30 days, 6 months and 3 years postprocedure. The 30-day composite endpoint, as in the other two studies, comprised death from any cause, acute infarction or the need for urgent coronary intervention and was statistically significantly reduced by 34.8% in the group treated with bolus and infusion of abciximab as compared to placebo bolus and infusion ($P=0.008$). Thirty days emergency repeat PTCA was necessary in 6% of the placebo group and in 1% of the bolus plus infusion group ($P=0.002$). At 6 months and after 3 years, the 30-day benefits were sustained.

Thrombocytopenia (<100 000/ml) was seen more often in the bolus plus infusion than in the placebo group (respectively 5.2% and 3.4%; $P=0.01$). Of the patients who received abciximab, 6.5% developed human antichimeric antibody, mostly in low titers; none showed allergic reactions.

Major hemorrhagic complications immediately after angioplasty, predominantly involving the access site, were higher in the abciximab treated patients. Hemorrhage was especially prominent in patients with a body weight under 75 kg receiving abciximab bolus plus infusion, suggesting that the fixed dose heparin was to blame.

This concept was tested in EPILOG.[35] A total of 2792 patients undergoing elective angioplasty were allocated among three regimens. In the EPIC trial an abciximab regimen was used almost similar to the bolus plus infusion in two of the three groups: one with standard dose heparin (100 IU/kg with a maximum of 10 000 IU) and one

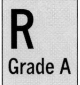

with low dose heparin (70 IU/kg, with a maximum of 7000 IU). A third cohort received placebo with standard dose heparin. In all groups additional heparin was administered to keep ACT above 300 s.

It was demonstrated that the efficacy of abciximab was preserved under the low dose regimen of heparin. It was also shown that the rate of major bleeding could be reduced to acceptable values: 2.0% in the low dose heparin group versus 3.1% and 3.5% in the heparin-only and the standard heparin with abciximab groups respectively ($P=$NS). Minor bleeding was 3.7% in the heparin-only group, 4.0% in the low dose heparin with abciximab and 7.4% in the standard heparin and abciximab group ($P=0.01$) In this study, too, the benefit of abciximab was preserved after 6 months: primary endpoints after 30 days were reached in 11.7% in the heparin-only group, 5.2% in the standard dose heparin with abciximab group, and 5.4% in the low dose heparin with abciximab group ($P<0.0001$).

In the recently concluded CAPTURE trial,[36] 1265 patients with refractory unstable angina were randomized to abciximab (bolus and infusion 18 hours preceding angioplasty) or placebo. Abciximab was given as a bolus and an infusion during 18–24 hours preceding the PTCA procedure. This infusion was stopped 1 hour after PTCA. Heparin was administered prior to randomization, until at least 1 hour after PTCA and adjusted to keep APTT between 2.0 and 2.5 times normal or an ACT of 300 s.

It should be noted that EPILOG and CAPTURE were terminated early, interim analyses demonstrating a significant reduction in endpoints in the abciximab treated groups.

The relative reduction of primary endpoints was of the same magnitude as in EPIC. The difference in primary endpoints between CAPTURE (placebo versus active drug: 15.9% versus 11.3%; $P=0.012$) and EPIC (12.8% versus 8.3%; $P=0.008$) can be explained by inclusion of more severely unstable patients in CAPTURE ("refractory" versus "high risk"). The significance of the difference in regimens – abciximab being administered before and during angioplasty in CAPTURE, and during and after in EPIC – is not yet clear.

Integrilin was tested in the IMPACT II study[37] which involved 4010 patients undergoing angioplasty or atherectomy. The incidence of major ischemic complications or emergency revascularization at 24 hours was lower in two groups treated with integrilin (0.5 μg/kg/min and 0.75 μg/kg/min, both for 20–24 hours) than in the placebo treated patients, but this was not statistically significant after 30 days (11.4% versus 9.2% versus 9.9% respectively for placebo, low dose, and high dose integrilin; $P=0.063$ placebo versus low dose integrilin). There was no difference in the occurrence of major bleeding.

Tirofiban was tested in the yet unpublished RESTORE (Randomized Efficacy of Tirofiban for Outcomes and Restenosis) study in 2139 patients with unstable angina or acute myocardial infarction, undergoing PTCA or atherectomy. Tirofiban (bolus of 10 μg/kg + 0.15 μg/kg/min for 36 hours) was compared with placebo, both groups receiving aspirin and heparin. At 30 days, the incidence of a composite endpoint of death, acute infarction, urgent or emergent PTCA or CABG was 10.5% in the placebo group and 8.0% in the tirofiban group ($P=0.052$). Here also, the incidence of major bleeding did not differ significantly.

Comparison of abciximab, integrilin, and tirofiban shows that abciximab is the most effective in reducing ischemic complications. This can be possibly explained by the tightness of the abciximab–IIb IIIa binding, while integrilin and tirofiban are loosely bound. Furthermore, it is probable that only abciximab also binds to the vitronectin receptor (which shares an epitope with IIb IIIa), extending its blocking capacities.

R

Grade A

Antithrombins

The most widely used thrombin antagonist is heparin. In its unfractionated form, it has been used in PTCA since its introduction. Its effect on periprocedural complications has never been demonstrated unequivocally.

Heparin is not a simple substance but consists of a combination of agents that all bind to antithrombin III (ATIII). Its molecular weight is 15 000. Through a reversible binding with ATIII, a naturally occurring inhibitor of activated blood coagulation factors,[38,39] heparin converts ATIII from a slow inhibitor to a rapid inhibitor of factors XIIa, XIa, IXa, Xa, and thrombin. Thrombin is more sensitive to the effects of heparin than is Xa and in keeping with this, unfractionated heparin exerts its action mainly through inhibition of thrombin-induced activation of factors V and VIII.[40] For thrombin inhibition it is necessary that both thrombin and ATIII bind to heparin. This requires a minimum chain length of 18 monosaccharides.

Heparin also comes in fractionated forms. These low molecular weight heparins (LMWH) have a molecular weight of 4000–5000 and a chain length <18 monosaccharides. These LMWH, when compared to the heavier components of unfractionated heparin, are more prone to bind to ATIII. They cannot bind to thrombin but they retain anti-Xa activity. The heavier components, on the other hand, are probably responsible for heparin associated thrombocytopenia and possibly for some platelet activation. LMWH can be administered subcutaneously once daily.

In accordance with the better binding to ATIII, LMWH are more effective than unfractionated heparin in the prevention of deep venous thrombosis.[41] Hopes for a better safety profile did not materialize: in a meta-analysis of 62 studies with a total of over 20 000 patients, it was shown that LMWH are associated with a higher bleeding risk than heparin.[42]

In the treatment of unstable angina, LMWH were proven valuable in various trials as compared to unfractionated heparin, without excessive bleeding.[43–45] LMWH inhibits *in vitro* smooth muscle cell migration and proliferation without affecting endothelial cell growth.[46] However, *in vivo*, one LMWH, enoxaparin, did not show any effect on the incidence of restenosis[47] nor did another, reviparin, compared to unfractionated heparin in patients undergoing PTCA.[48] Reviparin was not associated with a decrease in the incidence of bleeding complications nor did it show any advantage in the occurrence of acute complications during and after PTCA. Presently, there are no compelling evidence based arguments to replace unfractionated heparin with LMWH as an adjunctive to PTCA.

Heparin is a relatively weak antiplatelet agent, in part because it does not inhibit the other platelet activators that operate independently from thrombin. Also, it tends to bind to the platelet surface, thus increasing platelet activity.[49,50] Furthermore, thrombin is incorporated into a developing thrombus and binds to fibrin. This fibrin bound thrombin can generate activated factors V and VIII, producing additional thrombin and promoting thrombus growth.

The heparin–ATIII complex is a potent inhibitor of free thrombin but only weakly inhibits fibrin bound thrombin. Heparin therefore can only inhibit but not completely prevent the growth of thrombi.[51,52] Moreover, heparin can only exert its influence in the presence of adequate levels of antithrombin III.

Direct thrombin inhibitors have been developed to circumvent the need for antithrombin III. Hirudin is a natural antithrombin, produced by the salivary glands of the European leech. A recombinant form is equipotential. Both inhibit all known

959

functions of thrombin,[32] at least theoretically overcoming many of the disadvantages of heparin. However, in contrast to heparin, thrombin generation is left intact. In the HELVETICA (Hirudin in a European Trial versus Heparin in the Prevention of Restenosis after PTCA) trial hirudin was compared with heparin in patients with unstable angina undergoing PTCA.[53] This study in 1141 patients was designed to evaluate the effect of hirudin on chronic restenosis. In the occurrence of early cardiac events, a clear advantage could be attributed to hirudin: after 96 hours a combination of death, myocardial infarction, bypass surgery and second angioplasty occurred in 11% of the group treated with heparin, 7.9% in the intravenous hirudin group and 5.6% in the intravenous and subcutaneous hirudin group ($P=0.023$). There was a particular benefit in patients in Braunwald class III angina;[54] in patients who had angina at rest during the 48 hours before randomization, the event rate was 21.6% in the heparin group as compared with 5.3% in the patients receiving intravenous hirudin and 12.3% among the patients receiving intravenous and subcutaneous hirudin ($P=0.006$). After 7 months, however, there was no difference in major endpoints between the three cohorts, nor was there any difference in the angiographic degree of restenosis. Bleeding complications did not differ significantly. It was argued that the hirudin dosage was sufficient to limit acute thrombin mediated platelet aggregation and thus could affect acute complications, but insufficient to produce an adequate level of anticoagulation to influence restenosis.

In the GUSTO IIb study, in acute myocardial infarction, immediate angioplasty was performed in a subgroup. Patients were randomized to heparin and hirudin and to immediate angioplasty and thrombolysis. No beneficial effect of hirudin over heparin was found.[55]

Hirulog is a synthetic peptide designed on the structure of hirudin. Its effectiveness in angioplasty was studied in a prospective double-blind randomized trial. 4098 patients with unstable angina were treated with either heparin or bivalirudin (hirulog).[56] No difference was demonstrated in short and long term complications. Bivalirudin was associated with a lower incidence of major hemorrhage.

At present, neither a direct thrombin inhibitor nor LMWH can be advocated to take the place of heparin in PTCA.

RECOMMENDATIONS

Preventive

Aspirin is indispensable as an adjunct to PTCA. It is safe, cheap, and effective as well as easy to administer. It should be given in a single daily dose of 80 or 100 mg for at least 3 days before PTCA or 250–500 mg should be injected intravenously just before PTCA. It should be continued afterwards indefinitely.

If a stent is inserted, **ticlopidine** should be added to the regimen, in a dose of 250 mg b.i.d., preferably starting 7 days before and continuing 30 days after the procedure. In case of stenting as a bailout maneuver, the drug can be started immediately postprocedure. If the result of stent placement is considered suboptimal, it is advised (though randomized evidence is not available) to give heparin for 3–5 days as well, until ticlopidine can be expected to exert its influence.

Heparin is the thrombin inhibitor of choice in all PTCA procedures; dosage is a bolus of 70 IU/kg bodyweight or 5000 IU IV at the start of the procedure, with repeated injections of the same dose after every hour of the procedure. When a stent is implanted, another 5000 IU are administered. If deemed necessary, as in the case of a dissection, heparin can be given in an infusion, guided by APTT (around 70 s) or ACT (above 200 s), for 24 hours after angioplasty. It should be emphasized that heparin dosages are empirical and not evidence based.

In high risk procedures, as in unstable angina or angiographically complicated lesions (type B2, C), **abciximab** should be started, with a bolus of 0.25 mg/kg bodyweight 1 hour before the procedure, followed by a 12-hour infusion of 10 µg/min. Heparin should be rigorously weight adjusted.

It could be argued on the grounds of the EPILOG trial that abciximab should be administered before all coronary angioplasties. The cost factor would make that very hard to achieve at this moment.

Therapeutic

Spasm can be countered with nitroglycerin or nifedipine.

With modern antiplatelet strategies, thrombus formation can be prevented to a large extent. However, it may still occur and treatment often proves to be difficult. Though often used, thrombolysis in the form of intracoronary urokinase,[57] streptokinase or intravenous or intracoronary rTPA has not been proven to be effective in a randomized fashion. Furthermore, it may complicate an ensuing emergency bypass operation. It is likely that abciximab can be helpful in these often awkward situations and it is indeed frequently used for this indication, but its beneficial effect has not yet been demonstrated in a trial. Speculating that thrombus originates on and between the flaps of an intimal dissection (even if angiographically not visible), one could also defend the insertion of a stent, if the vessel diameter allows it.[58,59] Often vessel patency can be secured in this way.

References

1 Myler RK, Shaw RE, Stertzer SH *et al*. Lesion morphology and coronary angioplasty: current experience and analysis. *JACC* 1992;**9**:1641–52.

2 Detre KM, Holmes DR, Holubkov R *et al*. Incidences and consequences of periprocedural occlusion: the 1985–1986 National Heart, Lung, and Blood Institute Percutaneous Transluminal Coronary Angioplasty Registry. *Circulation* 1990; **82**:739–50.

3 De Feyter PJ, van den Brand M, Laarman GJ *et al*. Acute coronary artery occlusion during and after percutaneous transluminal coronary angioplasty: frequency, prediction, clinical course, management and follow up. *Circulation* 1991;**83**: 927–36.

4 Lincoff AM, Popma JJ, Ellis SG *et al*. Abrupt vessel closure complicating coronary angioplasty: clinical angiographic, and therapeutic profile. *JACC* 1992;**19**:926–35.

5 Ellis SG, Roubin GS, King SB III *et al*. Angiographic and clinical predictors of acute closure after native vessel coronary angioplasty. *Circulation* 1988;**77**: 372–9.

6 Margolis JR, Chen C. Coronary artery spasm complicating percutaneous transluminal angioplasty: role of intracoronary nitroglycerin. *Z Kardiol* 1989;**78**(Suppl 2):41–4.

7 Fischell TA, Derby G, Tse TM, Stadius ML. Coronary artery vasoconstriction routinely occurs after PTCA: a quantitative arteriographic analysis. *Circulation* 1988;**78**(6):323–34.

8 McIvor ME, Undemir C, Lawson J, Reddinger J. Clinical effects and utility of intracoronary diltiazem. *Cathet Cardiovasc Diagn* 1995;**35**(4): 287–91.

9 Pomerantz RM, Kuntz RE, Diver DJ, Safian RD, Baim DS. Intracoronary verapamil for the treatment of distal microvascular coronary artery spasm following PTCA. *Cathet Cardiovasc Diagn* 1991;**24**(4):283–5.

10 Tardif JC, Cote G, Lesperance J *et al*. Probucol and multivitamins in the prevention of restenosis after

coronary angioplasty. *N Engl J Med* 1997;**337**(6): 418–19.

11 Serruys PW, de Jaegere P, Kiemeney F *et al.* A comparison of balloon-expandable stent implantation with balloon angioplasty in patients with coronary artery disease (Benestent I). *N Engl J Med* 1994;**331**:489–95.

12 Fischman DL, Leon MB, Baim DS *et al.* A randomized comparison of coronary stent placement and balloon angioplasty in the treatment of coronary artery disease (STRESS). *N Engl J Med* 1994;**331**:496–501.

13 Peng JP, Friese P, Heilmann E, George JN, Burstein SA, Dale GL. Aged platelets have an impaired response to thrombin. *Blood* 1994;**83**:161–6.

14 Kehrel B. Platelet–collagen interactions. *Semin Thromb Hemost* 1995;**21**(2):123–9.

15 Stel HV, Sakariassen KS, de Groot PG *et al.* Von Willebrand factor in the vessel wall mediates platelet adherence. *Blood* 1985;**65**:85–90.

16 Heptinstall S, Hanley SP. Blood platelets and vessel walls. In: Walter Bowie EJ, Sharp AA, Eds. *Hemostasis and thrombosis.* London: Butterworths, 1985.

17 Coughlin SR, Vu TK, Hung DT, Wheaton VI. Characterization of a functional thrombin receptor: issues and opportunities. *J Clin Invest* 1992;**89**:351–5.

18 Marmur JD, Merlini PA, Sharma SK *et al.* Thrombin generation in human coronary arteries after percutaneous transluminal balloon angioplasty. *JACC* 1994;**24**:1484–91.

19 Verheugt FWA, van der Laarse A, Funke Kupper AJ *et al.* Effects of early intervention with low-dose aspirin (100 mg) on infarct-size, reinfarction and mortality in anterior wall acute myocardial infarction. *Am J Cardiol* 1990;**66**:267–70.

20 Antiplatelet Trialists' Collaboration. Collaborative overview of randomised trials of antiplatelet therapy. II. Maintenance of vascular graft or arterial patency by antiplatelet therapy. *Br Med J* 1994;**308**:159–68.

21 Schwartz L, Bourassa MG, Lesperance J *et al.* Aspirin and dipyridamole in the prevention of restenosis after percutaneous transluminal coronary angioplasty. *N Engl J Med* 1988;**318**: 1714–19.

22 Barnathan ES, Sanford Schwartz J, Taylor L *et al.* Aspirin and dipyridamole in the prevention of acute coronary thrombosis complicating coronary angioplasty. *Circulation* 1987;**76**: 125–34.

23 Fitzgerald GA. Dipyridamole. *N Engl J Med* 1987; **316**:1247–57.

24 Hirsh J, Dalen J, Fuster V, Harker LB, Salzman EW. Aspirin and other platelet-active drugs: the relationship between dose, effectiveness, and side effects. *Chest* 1992;**102**(suppl):327–36.

25 Reilly IAG, Fitzgerald GA. Aspirin in cardiovascular disease. *Drugs* 1988;**35**:154–76.

26 Ridker PM, Hebert PR, Fuster V *et al.* Are both aspirin and heparin justified as adjuncts to thrombolytic therapy for acute myocardial infarction? *Lancet* 1993;**341**:1574–7.

27 Jimenez AH, Stubbs ME, Tofler GH, Winther K, Williams GH, Muller JE. Rapidity and duration of platelet suppression by enteric coated aspirin in healthy young men. *Am J Cardiol* 1992;**69**: 258–62.

28 Husted SE, Kristensen SD, Vissinger H, Mann B, Schmidt EB, Nielsen HK. Intravenous acetyl-salicylic acid – dose related effects on platelet function and fibrinolysis in healthy males. *Thromb Haemost* 1992;**68**:226–9.

29 Schomig A, Neumann FJ, Kastrati A *et al.* A randomized comparison of platelet and anticoagulant therapy after the placement of coronary-artery stents. *N Engl J Med* 1996;**334**: 1084–9.

30 Bonita R. Epidemiology of stroke. *Lancet* 1992; **339**:342–4.

31 CAPRIE Steering Committee. A randomised, blinded, trial of clopidogrel versus aspirin in patients at risk of ischaemic events (CAPRIE). *Lancet* 1996;**348**:1329–39.

32 Verstraete M, Zoldhelyi P. Novel antithrombotic drugs in development. *Drugs* 1995;**49**(6): 856–84.

33 The EPIC Investigation. Use of a monoclonal antibody directed against the platelet glycoprotein IIb/IIIa receptor in high-risk coronary angioplasty. *N Engl J Med* 1994;**330**:956–61.

34 AHA Medical/Scientific Statement Guidelines for percutaneous transluminal coronary angioplasty. 1993;**88**:2987–3007.

35 The EPILOG Investigators. Effect of the platelet glycoprotein IIb/IIIa receptor inhibitor abciximab with lower heparin dosages on ischemic complications of percutaneous coronary revascularization. *N Engl J Med* 1997;**336**: 1689–96.

36 The CAPTURE Investigators. Refractory unstable angina; reduction of events by treatment with abciximab prior to coronary intervention. *Lancet* 1997;**349**:1429–35.

37 Tcheng JE, Lincoff AM, Sigmon KN, Califf RM, Topol EJ. Platelet glycoprotein IIbI IIa inhibition with Integrelin during percutaneous coronary intervention: the IMPACT II Trial (Integrilin to Manage Platelet Aggregation to Prevent Coronary Thrombosis II). *Circulation* 1995;**92**(Suppl I):543.

38 Rosenberg RD, Rosenberg JS. Natural anticoagulant mechanisms. *J Clin Invest* 1984; **74**:1–6.

39 Salzman EW, Rosenberg RD, Smith MH, Lindon JN, Favreau L. Effect of heparin and heparin

fractions on platelet aggregation. *J Clin Invest* 1980;**65**:64–73.

40 Ofusu FA, Hirsh J, Esmon CT *et al.* Unfractionated heparin inhibits thrombin-catalysed amplifications of coagulation more efficiently than those catalysed by Xa. *Biochem J* 1989;**257**:143–50.

41 Kakkar VV, Murray WJG. Efficacy and safety of low molecular weight heparin (CY216) in preventing postoperative venous thrombo-embolism: a cooperative study. *Br J Surg* 1985;**72**:786–91.

42 Rosendaal FR, Nurmohamed MT, Buller HR, Dekker E, Vandenbroucke JP. Low molecular weight heparins in the prophylaxis of venous thrombosis: a meta-analysis. *Haemost Thromb* 1991;**65**:927.

43 Gurfinkel EP, Manos EJ, Mejail RI *et al.* Low molecular weight heparin versus regular heparin or aspirin in the treatment of unstable angina and silent ischemia. *JACC* 1995;**26**(2):313–18.

44 Klein W, Buchwald A, Hillis SE *et al.* Comparison of low-molecular weight heparin with unfractionated heparin acutely and with placebo for 6 weeks in the management of unstable coronary artery disease (FRIC). *Circulation* 1997; **96**:61–8.

45 FRISC Study Group. Low-molecular weight heparin during instability in coronary artery disease. *Lancet* 1996;**347**:561–8.

46 Roth D, Betz E. Kultivierte Gefasswandzellen des Menschen. *Vasa* 1992;**35**(suppl):125–7.

47 Faxon DP, Spiro TE, Minor S *et al.* Low molecular weight heparin in prevention of restenosis after angioplasty. Results of the Enoxaparin Restenosis (ERA) trial. *Circulation* 1994;**90**(2):908–14.

48 Karsch KR, Preisack MB, Baildon R *et al.* Low molecular weight heparin (Reviparin) in PTCA: results of a randomized, double blind unfractionated heparin and placebo-controlled, multicenter trial (REDUCE trial). *JACC* 1996;**28**: 1437–43.

49 Coller BS. Antiplatelet agents in the prevention and therapy of thrombosis. *Annu Rev Med* 1992; **43**:171–80.

50 O'Reilly RA. Anticoagulant antithrombotic and thrombolytic drugs. In: Gilman AG, Goodman LS, Rall TW, Murad F. eds. *The pharmacological basis of therapeutics*, 7th edn. New York: Macmillan, 1985, ch 58.

51 Hirsh J, Fuster V. Guide to anticoagulant therapy. I. Heparin. *Circulation* 1994;**89**:1449–68.

52 Hull RD, Delamore T, Genton E *et al.* Warfarin sodium versus low dose heparin in the long term treatment of venous thromboembolism. *N Engl J Med* 1979;**301**:855–8.

53 Serruys PW, Herrman JR, Simon R *et al.* for the HELVETICA Investigators. A comparison of hirudin with heparin in the prevention of restenosis after coronary angioplasty. *N Engl J Med* 1995;**333**:757–63.

54 Braunwald E. Unstable angina: a classification. *Circulation* 1989;**80**:410.

55 Angioplasty Substudy Investigators. The global use of strategies to open occluded coronary arteries in acute coronary syndromes (GUSTO IIb). A clinical trial comparing primary coronary angioplasty with tissue plasminogen activator for acute myocardial infarction. *N Engl J Med* 1997; **336**:1621–8.

56 Bittl JA, Strony J, Brinker JA *et al.* Treatment with Bivalirudin (Hirulog) as compared with heparin during coronary angioplasty for unstable or postinfarction angina. *N Engl J Med* 1995;**333**: 764–9.

57 Schachinger V, Kasper W, Zeiker AM. Adjunctive intracoronary urokinase therapy during PTCA. *JACC* 1996;**77**(14):1174–8.

58 Roubin GS, Cannon AD, Agrawol SK *et al.* Intracoronary stenting for acute and threatened closure complicating PTCA. *Circulation* 1992; **85**(3):916–21.

59 Scott NA, Weintraub WS, Carlin SF *et al.* Recent changes in the management and outcome of acute closure after PTCA. *JACC* 1993;**71**(13): 1159–63.

57 Restenosis: etiologies and prevention

GIUSEPPE SANGIORGI,
DAVID R. HOLMES JR,
ROBERT S. SCHWARTZ

INTRODUCTION

Percutaneous coronary interventions have revolutionized the treatment of coronary atherosclerosis, creating an alternative strategy to medical and surgical therapy for myocardial ischemia and acute coronary events. The concept was that atherosclerotic plaque could be fractured, removed or ablated within the vessel by different device technologies. However, it was quickly understood that following the intervention, a healing response, known as restenosis, significantly reduced the long term success of the procedure.

Restenosis is a substantial medical problem not only because it occurs in 40–50% of patients undergoing coronary revascularization procedures, with increased patient morbidity, but also because of the significant burden of medical costs[1,2] which is estimated to be nearly $2.0 billion per year.[3] Restenosis may be effectively treated by repeat angioplasty. However, further interventional procedures entail additional cost and the redilated lesions are more prone to the development of restenosis than are the native lesions.

Because of this unacceptably high restenosis rate and the enormous health cost implications, it is not surprising that in the last decade there have been intense efforts to elucidate the pathophysiologic mechanisms of this process and, most importantly, extensive clinical trials aimed at a wide array of strategies to prevent restenosis. Today, while the cellular mechanisms and interactions involved in the pathobiology of restenosis are understood and powerful effects have been obtained in some animal models with the use of different drugs and devices, the search for successful therapies continues, because when transferred into the clinical practice, restenosis is still a shadow over the broad use of the interventional techniques.

Why does restenosis occur? A definitive answer does not yet exist, but major components in the evolution of the restenosis process have been identified.

Table 57.1 Angiographic definitions of restenosis

1. An increase of $\geq 30\%$ from immediate postangioplasty diameter stenosis to follow-up stenosis
2. An initial diameter stenosis $<50\%$ after angioplasty, increasing to $\geq 70\%$ at follow-up angiography
3. An increase in diameter stenosis at follow-up angiography to within 10% of the preangioplasty value
4. A loss of $>50\%$ of the initial diameter stenosis gain achieved by angioplasty, from immediate postangioplasty to follow-up angiography
5. A postangioplasty diameter stenosis $<50\%$ increasing to $>50\%$ at follow-up angiography
6. A decrease in the minimal lumen diameter at the lesion of >0.72 mm from immediate postangioplasty to follow-up angiography
7. Cumulative distribution of MLD

This chapter will review four aspects of the restenosis problem. First, it will highlight the mechanisms of restenosis including acute recoil, neointimal hyperplasia, and vascular remodeling. These, in turn, influence the response of the vessel wall to mechanical injury. Insights into the potential contribution of adventitia in the restenotic process will also be discussed. Second, key issues of stents and their clinical trials will be reviewed, with specific emphasis on restenosis. Included will be new technologies associated with stenting to limit the restenosis problem. Third, the issue of mural thrombus in restenosis will be addressed for both stenting and balloon angioplasty, since blood elements and factors produced by circulating cells play a key role in the initiation and propagation of neointima formation. The importance of antithrombotic agents such as GPIIb/IIIa receptor antagonists in reducing morbidity and mortality after PTCA and their potential in reducing the restenosis process will be reviewed. Finally, emerging concepts in restenosis treatment and potential solutions such as ionizing radiation and gene therapy will be addressed.

THE PROBLEM OF RESTENOSIS

Defining restenosis

Restenosis studies have suffered to various degrees from methodological problems. Since native coronary atherosclerotic and restenotic lesions are both identified and treated with the use of angiography, one would hope that a uniform angiographic definition of restenosis might exist. Unfortunately, such definitions are lacking, representing a major limitation in comparing different studies.

The numerous angiographic definitions used in clinical studies[4] and, more recently, definitions based on absolute changes in minimal lumen diameter at follow-up[5] have led to confusion and hampered investigations in this field[6] (Table 57.1).

Using clinical criteria, restenosis may be defined by evidence of recurrent myocardial ischemia after the revascularization procedure, discovered during clinical tests or indicated by the presence of symptoms (i.e. recurrence of angina, need for target vessel revascularization). Difficulties occur with a discordance between angiography and clinical status. A patient with a lesion fitting the angiographic criteria for restenosis but who is asymptomatic and/or has negative tests for ischemia will probably not be recatheterized on the basis of clinical criteria alone.

965

Restenosis has been previously characterized as an "all or none" phenomenon and, by subsequent studies, as a continuous variable that takes place to some extent in all treated lesions.[7] Many studies have been small and the timing and methods of follow-up have been variable,[1,8] introducing selection bias and misleading interpretations of the data. It is clear that a more uniform definition, that includes a combination of angiographic and clinical criteria, and studies with more uniform groups of patients may provide a more accurate picture of the restenosis phenomenon.[9]

Predicting restenosis

While many clinical studies have been performed to identify correlates of restenosis,[1,8,10–14] the ability to predict an excessive healing response after percutaneous interventions has remained particularly difficult.[15]

Three different categories of variables are related to an increased risk of restenosis. These include clinical patient-related factors, anatomic-related factors, and interventional procedure-related factors. Patient-related variables include older age, male gender, diabetes, hypertension, hyperlipidemia, unstable angina prior to angioplasty, vasospastic angina, and continued smoking after angioplasty. Anatomic and procedural factors include ostial lesions, longer lesions, total occlusions, multilesion and multivessel angioplasty procedures, saphenous vein graft location, left anterior descending location, presence of calcium, balloon to artery ratio, suboptimal results with significant residual stenosis, and extent of dissection. However, no variables have yet been found that predict restenosis with absolute certainty. Of all the factors, the most consistent in predicting a better long term outcome appears to be a large postprocedural lumen diameter.[16] This finding has lead to the current aphorism "bigger is better"[17] which has been widely applied as a therapeutic strategy of angioplasty and which may explain the improved long term outcome observed with coronary stents or directional atherectomy.[18,19]

Other factors that have not yet been fully evaluated may also predict restenosis. Angioscopic observations suggest that coronary thrombus is an important determinant of the late outcome.[20] Recent clinical studies using the glycoprotein IIb/IIIa receptor antagonist 7E3 have shown a significative reduction in the incidence of restenosis,[21] supporting the etiologic role of thrombotics. Experimental evidence suggests that oxidative stress may be important in the restenotic process and the results of the MVP Study[22] indicate that probucol is effective in reducing restenosis by means of LDL oxidation prevention, decreasing platelet aggregation, and modulation of prostaglandin and leukotriene synthesis.[23–25]

Studying restenosis

Traditionally, animal models are the cornerstone of test strategies aimed at developing treatments for pathologic conditions and understanding pathophysiologic mechanisms that may cause that particular condition. In this respect, restenosis is no exception and several animal models have been developed during the last decade in attempts to reproduce restenotic lesions and find a therapeutic strategy to reduce neointimal formation. Unfortunately, although several models of restenosis have been evaluated in the last 15 years, there is no perfect animal model for human restenosis. Common models include the rat carotid air desiccation or balloon endothelial denudation model,[26,27] the rabbit femoral or iliac artery balloon injury model with or without cholesterol supplementation,[28] and the porcine carotid and coronary artery model.[29]

The rat model, based on elastic arteries, does not develop severe stenotic neointimal lesions and is therefore very permissive in term of efficacy of pharmacological interventions. The cholesterol-fed rabbit model has been criticized for the high level of hyperlipidemia required for the development of lesions. They have a large macrophage foam cell component and resemble fatty streaks rather than human restenotic lesions. Conversely, the histopathologic features of neointima obtained in porcine models closely resemble the human neointima and the amount of neointimal thickening is proportional to severity of injury. This has allowed the creation of an injury–neointima relationship that can be used to evaluate the response to different therapies. However, the repair process in the pig coronary artery injury model using normal coronary arteries is certainly more rapid and may be different from the response to balloon angioplasty that characterizes human coronary atherosclerotic plaques.

The major limitation in the use of animal models of restenosis is that agents effective in reducing neointima in those models are ineffective when transferred into the clinical arena. Many explanations might be found for this, including different animal species, type of artery, degree of arterial injury, volume of neointima, drug dosage and timing regimen, and atherosclerotic substrate. We believe that before transferring the results obtained in animal models into clinical trials, a standardization of injury type, method of measurement, and dose and timing of drug among different animal models is necessary.

Other issues in the study of restenosis are the limitations in the design of clinical trials. Incomplete angiographic follow-up leading to the occurrence of selection and withdrawal biases and inadequate power due to small sample size leading to the potential of beta (type II) errors are the most common problems. Non-uniform definitions of angiographic restenosis and poor correlation between angiographic and clinical outcome are other problems that need to be resolved when comparing different trial results. Future restenosis studies should utilize composite clinical outcomes as primary endpoints, with multiple, simultaneous treatment approaches and careful choice of the appropriate regimen. These studies should also include an angiographic or intravascular ultrasound (IVUS) subset to allow assessment of mechanisms of action. Using these data can help limit the sample size necessary to detect efficacy in reducing neointima.

Understanding restenosis

To better understand the mechanisms of restenosis, it is useful to review briefly the potential mechanisms by which coronary interventional procedures increase lumen patency. Since the explanation given by Dotter and Judkins,[30] who ascribed the enlargement of a vessel lumen by balloon angioplasty to compression of atheromatous plaque against the arterial wall, several morphologic and histologic observations have been made in both human necropsy studies[31–33] and experimental models.[34] Different mechanisms of action have been identified. The original concept of plaque compression is unlikely to occur because the majority of atherosclerotic plaques are composed of dense fibrocollagenous tissue with hard calcium deposits and thus are difficult to compress. However, this mechanism can play a major role in the dilation of newly formed atherosclerotic plaques (i.e. soft plaques) or recently formed thrombus.

Subsequent data suggest that the major mechanisms of action of coronary angioplasty are breaking, cracking, and splitting of the intimal plaque with partial disruption of the media and vessel stretching of the plaque-free wall of the vessel.[35-37] In particular, intravascular ultrasound studies have shown that those mechanisms may vary depending on the histologic composition of the plaque, with more plaque dissection in calcified lesions and more vessel expansion in non-calcified plaques.[38]

Conversely, directional and rotational coronary atherectomy improve lumen caliber by tissue removal, with little disruption and expansion of the vessel wall. Finally, the mechanism of laser angioplasty is related to atherosclerotic tissue photoablation and dissection associated with vessel expansion.

Based on these clinical and experimental observations, the presumed healing and repair processes leading to arterial restenosis may be categorized as follows:

- exaggerated cell proliferation at the site of injury;
- incomplete plaque dissection by balloon angioplasty or incomplete tissue removal by DCA (directional coronary atherectomy), rotational atherectomy, and laser angioplasty;
- thrombus formation and organization at the site of injury;
- favorable or unfavorable arterial wall remodeling.

PATHOBIOLOGICAL EVENTS IN RESTENOSIS – FROM GROWTH REGULATORY FACTORS TO CELL CYCLE GENES

Essed *et al.* first documented intimal proliferation after PTCA as a cause of restenosis in 1983.[39] Since then, enormous progress has been made in defining the pathogenetic mechanisms of human restenotic lesions. At the same time, molecular techniques coupled with increasing understanding of the regulatory events at the level of nucleic acids have been applied to investigation of the restenotic process. Today, there is a general consensus that restenosis involves the interaction of cytokines, growth factors, vascular elements, blood cells, and the extent of injury.

Based on the experiences derived from experimental models, cell culture, human pathologic evidence, and angiographic, angioscopic, and intravascular ultrasound observations, the sequence of events that takes place in the artery and characterizes the restenotic process can be divided into three phases (Figures 57.1, 57.2):

1. a first phase of elastic recoil, usually occurring within 24 hours of the procedure;
2. a second phase of mural thrombus formation and organization in the subsequent 2 weeks;
3. a third phase of cell activation, proliferation, and extracellular matrix formation, which usually lasts from 2 to 3 months.[29,40]

Therefore, several factors may influence the production of excessive neointimal volume, including the amount of platelet-fibrin thrombus at the injury site, the total number of smooth muscle cells (SMC) within the neointima, and the amount of extracellular matrix elaborated by neointimal cells. Limiting one of those steps, either individually or in combination, might reduce the neointimal response following mechanical injury (Table 57.2).

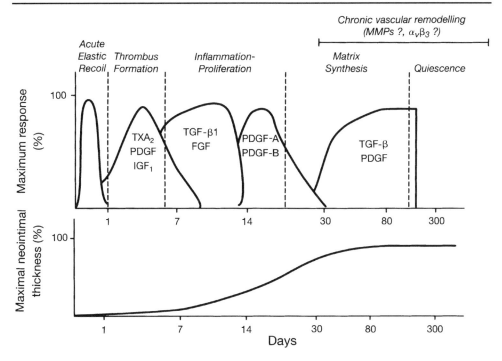

Figure 57.1 Different phases of the restenotic process. The lower panel shows the increase in neointimal thickening and the upper panel the associated expression of growth factors (for abbreviations see Table 57.3).

Phase I – elastic recoil

The vessel wall itself can participate in the acute lumen loss observed in some patients just after coronary interventions by a mechanism termed "recoil". Elastic recoil occurs within minutes to hours following balloon angioplasty and seems to be the consequence of the "spring-like" properties of the non-diseased vascular wall responding to its overstretching.[41–43] Other possible explanations are vasoconstriction due to vessel endothelial disruption[44] or platelet activation and thrombus formation with consequent release of vasoconstrictive substances.[45,46] Whenever the normal wall is significantly stretched, recoil may be the predominant mechanism of restenosis. Different studies have indeed shown that this very early vessel wall recoil increases the likelihood of subsequent restenosis, with a rate of 73.6% for the lesions that had lumen loss >10% but only 9.8% for lesions that diminished by <10%.[47,48] Early recoil may have a significant importance in restenosis when the vessel has not been severely injured and the lesion consists of SMC. When the vessel wall injury is more severe, thrombus formation with consequent activation of growth factors and release of cytokines may instead be the predominant mechanism of restenosis.

PREVENTION OF PHASE I – MECHANICAL VS PHARMACOLOGICAL APPROACHES

It is clear that the utilization of methods to minimize the angioplasty injury, reduce the elastic recoil, and enlarge the lumen size should result in a lower incidence of restenosis. Balloon angioplasty allows manipulation of some parameters that cause injury or recoil. Several studies have evaluated the number of balloon inflations,[49,50] duration of

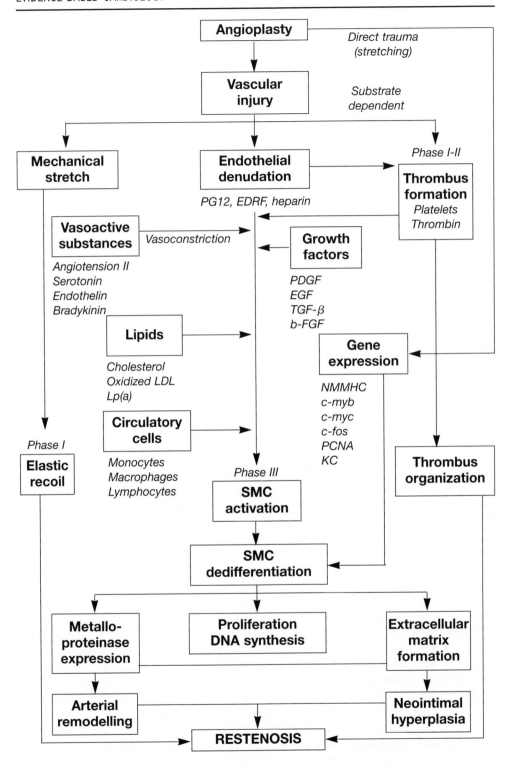

Figure 57.2 Sequence of events resulting in restenosis after vessel injury.

Table 57.2 Potential therapeutic approaches for the treatment of the different phases of the restenotic process

Response to vessel injury	Potential therapy
Early elastic recoil	Achievement of greater MLD by stents
Thrombus formation	Antithrombotic agents
	Antiplatelet agents
	Rapid re-endothelization
	Molecular therapies
Neointimal proliferation	
SMC activation	Molecular therapies
SMC migration	Rapid re-endothelization, MMP inhibitors
SMC proliferation	Antiproliferative agents, brachytherapy, rapid re-endothelization, molecular therapies
ECM formation	Antiproliferative agents, rapid re-endothelization, molecular therapies
Chronic vascular remodeling	Stents

MLD, minimal lumen diameter; MMP, metalloproteinases; SMC, smooth muscle cells; ECM, extracellular matrix.

inflation,[49,51–53] inflation pressure,[54–56] and balloon:artery ratio.[50,55,57,58] Although higher inflation pressures and larger balloon sizes have been related to reduced rates of restenosis, they also cause a substantial increase in acute complications such as rate of emergency surgery and myocardial infarction.[55,59]

One of the most important advantages of intracoronary stents is that these devices represent the "bigger is better" approach. Because of their rigid structure they address restenosis from the direction of greater luminal gain and a decrease in the elastic recoil. By this radial support, the technique results in increased residual lumen and expansion of the artery at long term follow-up.[17,60] Furthermore, coronary stents limit the exposure of deep vessel wall tissue to blood elements, diminishing the activation of unfavorable rheological factors and allowing a higher anterograde flow through a smooth-contoured lumen.

Randomized studies such as the Stent in Restenosis Study (STRESS)[61] and the European Belgian–Netherlands stent trial (BENESTENT)[18] have both shown a significant decrease in restenosis in the groups with stent placement compared with conventional balloon angioplasty.[18,62] The STRESS investigators reported a 10% decrease in restenosis rate with Palmaz–Schatz stent compared with balloon angioplasty (32% vs 42% respectively), and the Benestent trial also demonstrated a 10% decrease in restenosis (22% in the stent group vs 32% in the PTCA group), with better event-free survival and fewer revascularization procedures at 8-month follow-up. Stenting technique has continued to evolve and others trials have compared conventional balloon angioplasty with contemporary stenting techniques (high pressure deployment,[63] IVUS,[64] reduced anticoagulation,[64] ostial placement,[65] always demonstrating a reduction of restenosis rate in patients receiving coronary stents. The pilot phase of a new study, the Benestent-2 trial, has shown that the rate of restenosis was impressively reduced to less than 13% when heparin coated stents were placed with high pressure delivery.[66]

Other devices, such as directional atherectomy, rotational atherectomy, and TEC atherectomy, improve lumen patency by tissue removal and are associated with less vessel wall recoil and dissection.[67,68] The CAVEAT-1 and the C-CAT trials did not show

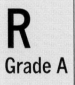

R
Grade A

a significant advantage of atherectomy over conventional balloon angioplasty.[69-71] This was a surprising finding since experimental and clinical studies have shown that a larger final lumen correlates with lower restenosis rates. However, it is important to note that in those trials the final lumen achieved with atherectomy did not differ from that obtained by balloon angioplasty. New trials, the Balloon versus Optimal Atherectomy Trial (BOAT) and the Optimal Atherectomy Restenosis Study (OARS), are at their final stage and the results are anxiously awaited since the lumen achieved in those trials was much bigger than that achieved with balloon angioplasty. OARS, a 200-patient multicenter registry, was designed to assess the impact of using IVUS-guided optimal atherectomy to achieve residual stenosis of less than 10%. Compared to CAVEAT, the initial results demonstrated a higher procedural success rate (88% vs 98%), lower residual stenosis (29% vs 7%), and fewer adverse outcomes in terms of composite events (death, myocardial infarction, and target lesion revascularization rates; 36.5% vs 23.7%).[72] Other trials involving rotational atherectomy (STRATAS, DART) are underway and the results are also awaited.

R

Grade B

Phase II – platelet aggregation and thrombus formation

As an integral part of the dilation mechanism, coronary angioplasty results in injury to the arterial wall, including endothelial damage with loss of antithrombotic properties (EDRF, PG12, tPA) and induction of procoagulant factors (thrombin, tissue factor). In addition, breaking of the internal elastic lamina and medial disruption, with exposure to the blood elements of wall constituents such as collagen, von Willebrand's factor, and extracellular matrix components, stimulates the interaction with platelet surface receptors (primarily glycoprotein Ib and IIb/IIIa integrins), resulting within minutes to hours after the intervention in platelet activation and deep mural thrombus formation[73-76] inaccessible to the action of heparin.[77,78] Experimental and clinical studies have also shown that platelets are activated by contrast media.[79,80] Activated platelets secrete several substances from their alpha granules that stimulate vasoconstriction, chemotaxis, and activation of neighboring platelets.[81,82] In addition, platelet aggregation releases or stimulates the production of numerous factors including thrombin, thromboxane A2, serotonin, plasminogen activator inhibitor (PAI-1), platelet-derived growth factor (PDGF), transforming growth factor-beta (TGF-β), basic fibroblast growth factor (b-FGF), epidermal growth factor (EGF), insulin-like growth factor (IGF-1), interleukin-1, and monocyte chemoattractant protein-1 (MCP-1)[83-85] (Table 57.3). These factors are believed to be responsible for neointimal growth by attracting and stimulating SMC migration and proliferation at the site of injury[86-89] (Figure 57.3). The severity of the thrombogenic response depends on the degree of vascular injury, the surface area of exposure, the type of substrate exposed in the underlying vessel wall, and the rheological conditions such as shear stress and time of exposure.

Platelet activation leads to the recruitment of glycoprotein IIb/IIIa integrin surface receptors, which mediate platelet aggregation and thrombus formation by binding fibrinogen molecules between adjacent receptors.[83,90,91] Aggregated platelets accelerate the conversion of prothrombin to thrombin, which in turn stimulates further platelet activation.[92] Thrombin is involved in thrombus formation, upregulation of E-selectin and P-selectin expression on endothelial cells, monocyte and neutrophil migration in the injured wall,[93] and stimulation of endothelin and tissue factor release from endothelial

Table 57.3 Extracellular factors involved in restenosis

Angiotensin-II
Collagen
Collagenase
Colony stimulating factors (CSFs)
Elastic fibers
Endothelins (ETs)
Epidermal growth factor/transforming growth factor alpha (EGF/TGF-α)
Fibroblast growth factors, acidic and basic (a-FGF, b-FGF)
Heparin
Heparin binding epidermal growth factor (HB-EGF)
Insulin-like growth factor-1 (IGF-1)
Interferon gamma (IFN-γ)
Interleukin-1 (IL-1)
Low density lipoprotein, oxidized (oxLDL)
Monocyte–macrophage colony stimulating factor (M-CSF)
Monocyte chemotatic protein 1 (MCP-1/MCAF-1)
Nitric oxide/endothelium-derived relaxing factor (NO/EDRF)
Plasmin
Plasminogen activator inhibitor (PAI-1)
Platelet-derived growth factor A (endothelium, PDGF-AA)
Platelet-derived growth factor B (smooth muscle cells, PDGF-BB)
Prostacyclin (PGI$_2$)
Prostaglandin E
Proteoglycans
Thrombin
Thromboxane A$_2$ (TXA$_2$)
Tissue plasminogen activator (tPA)
Transforming growth factor beta (TGF-β)
Tumor necrosis factor alpha (TNF-α)

cells with a mitotic effect on SMC.[94] Of interest, there is also evidence that monocyte–macrophage recruitment may contribute to thrombus myofibrotic organization.[95] Genes for the PDGF ligands and receptor components are expressed in normal and injured rat carotid arteries.[96] Basic FGF and FGF receptor type 1 are both expressed by endothelial and SMC after mechanical injury and inhibition of this growth factor reduces neointimal formation.[84,97,98] TGF-β seems to be the principal growth factor involved in the regulation and synthesis of proteoglycans, the major components of the extracellular matrix.[99–101] TGF-β induces both migration and proliferation of vascular cells and recent evidence suggests that it is an important factor in the vascular remodeling process associated with restenosis.[102,103]

In summary, the extent of vessel wall injury, amount of thrombus formation, and likelihood of neointimal proliferation are interrelated. Although the relationship of thrombus formation to restenosis remains to be elucidated, evidence suggests that thrombus contributes directly to restenosis by vessel occlusion[104] and indirectly by mediating the release of several factors, which in turn are also involved in the third phase of the restenotic process.[105]

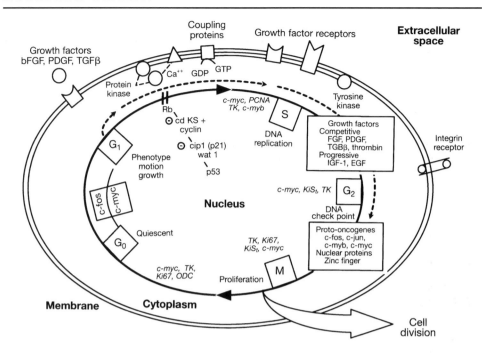

Figure 57.3 Cytoplasmic and nuclear control points for SMC division and proliferation. cdKS, cyclin-dependent kinases; TK, tyrosine kinase; ODC, ornithine decarboxylase gene; Rb, retinoblastoma protein (for other abbreviations, see text).

PREVENTION OF PHASE II – THE ROLE OF NEW ANTITHROMBOTIC DRUGS

Since platelet function and consequent thrombus formation are important in the vascular response to injury, they have been logical targets of several therapeutic strategies. In addition to existing antithrombotic and anticoagulant drugs (i.e. heparin and aspirin), antiplatelet therapies to prevent restenosis have recently been boosted by the development of newer agents that specifically inhibit critical steps in the coagulation cascade and proteins on the surface of platelets. These new drugs include inhibitors of thrombin generation (factor Xa inhibitors),[106,107] thrombin action (direct thrombin inhibitors)[108] or platelet aggregation (GP IIb/IIIa receptor antagonists).[109]

Although aspirin,[110] dypiridamole,[111] ticlopidine,[112] warfarin,[113–115] thromboxane antagonists,[116–118] and prostacyclin analogs[119,120] have been shown to be effective in animal models of restenosis, these drugs have failed to show any benefit in clinical practice. However, several factors may confound the interpretation of those studies. For example, differences in the lesion substrate, inappropriate drug doses or incomplete block of the target may explain the discrepancy between animal models and human studies. Moreover, while the magnitude of injury and thrombus formation correlates with the degree of neointimal formation in animals, the relationship in humans is by no means established. In addition, specific anticoagulant agents such as heparin,[121–124] low molecular weight heparin,[125–127] hirudin, and hirulog[128–131] did not show any favorable effect either on angiographic or clinical outcome related to restenosis.

Both animal models of restenosis and clinical trials demonstrated a significant reduction of neointimal proliferation by blocking the platelet GP IIb/IIIa ($\alpha_{IIb}\beta_3$) or the vitronectin receptors ($\alpha_v\beta_3$).[21,132–135] By using a chimeric 7E3 antibody directed against the platelet membrane IIb/IIIa receptor complex, the EPIC trial demonstrated a significant reduction in the onset of acute complications and clinical restenosis in high risk angioplasty.[21] Since this trial was published other studies have evaluated the effect of IIb/IIIa antagonists versus placebo at 6-month follow-up. Unfortunately, IMPACT,[136] IMPACT-2,[135] RESTORE,[137] EPILOG and CAPTURE trials,[138,139] that studied the efficacy of integrilin, tirofiban, and abciximab, respectively, did not demonstrate a reduction in target vessel revascularization compared to placebo treatment.

Phase III – smooth muscle cell activation and synthesis of extracellular matrix

This final phase of vascular healing is predominantly characterized by neointimal formation due to SMC proliferation and extracellular matrix accumulation produced by the neointimal cells at the injury site.[41,140-143] The healing response is a normal process which is essential in maintaining vascular integrity after an injury to the vessel wall, but varies in the degree to which it occurs. One pathogenetic explanation of restenosis is indeed an exaggeration of this healing response.

Phase III could be further divided into three different waves.[40] In the *first wave* (days 1–4 after vessel injury), medial SMC from the site of injury and possibly from adjacent areas are activated and stimulated by the triggering factors mentioned earlier. In addition to mitogenic factors released by endothelial cells, stretching of the arterial wall is a potent stimulus for SMC activation and growth.[144] Once activated, SMC undergo characteristic phenotypic transformation, from a "contractile" to a "synthetic" form,[141] which is responsible for the production of extracellular matrix rich in chondroitin sulfate and dermatan sulfate seen in the first 6 months after injury. The *second wave* (3–14 days after vessel injury) and the *third wave* (14 days to months after vessel injury) are respectively characterized by the migration of SMC through breaks in the internal elastic lamina into the intima, the local thrombus,[145] and SMC proliferation followed by extracellular matrix formation.[105,146-149] Those events are characterized by complex interactions between growth factors, second messengers, and gene regulatory proteins resulting in phenotypic change from a quiescent to a proliferative state.[86]

The peak of proliferation is observed 4–5 days after balloon injury but the duration of migration is not known, nor is it known whether a phase of cellular replication is required before SMC migration. Few studies have been done to identify the matrix molecules involved in the migration into the intima. Osteopontin is expressed in sites of marked remodeling[150] and antibodies to osteopontin inhibit SMC migration into the intima after balloon angioplasty.[151] Proteoglycans may also be important for the formation of neointima. CD44, a receptor for hyaluronic acid, seems to play a role in the migration of cells into fibrin or osteopontin.[152,153] SMC migration presumably requires degradation of the basement membrane surrounding the cells. Several metalloproteinases, including tissue plasminogen activator, plasmin, MMP-2, and MMP-9, may be responsible for this process[154,155] and the administration of a protease inhibitor reduces SMC migration into the intima.[156] Cell migration is probably initiated by recognition of extracellular matrix proteins by a family of cell surface adhesion receptors known as integrins.[157,158] *In vitro* and *in vivo* studies have demonstrated that the selective blockage of the $\alpha_v\beta_3$ integrin inhibits SMC migration and reduces neointimal formation.[133,159]

Experimental studies have suggested that endothelin-1 and endothelin receptors may also be indirectly implicated in the SMC migration and matrix synthesis.[160-162] Immunohistochemical studies demonstrate a time-dependent increase in endothelin immunoreactivity after balloon angioplasty in the rat model.[163] The administration of endothelin receptor antagonists in different animal models of balloon injury has been effective in reducing neointimal formation.[160,164,165]

Several *in vitro* studies have suggested that different growth factors, such as PDGF-AA, PDGF-BB, b-FGF, IGF, EGF, FGF, TGF-β, and angiotensin II, may also play a major role in this process.[86,148,166-170] Control of SMC proliferation is regulated by the actions of mitogens (i.e. PDGF) and the opposing effect of inhibitors (i.e. TGF-β). The growth factors bind to cell surface receptors and initiate a cascade of events which leads to cell migration and division. Components of the cascade include different tyrosine kinases, coupling proteins, and membrane-associated and cytoplasmic protein kinases (Figure 57.3). On stimulation by growth factors, proto-oncogenes are transiently activated and, together with other cell cycle-dependent proteins such as zinc finger proteins, mediate effects within the nucleus. Several studies have demonstrated that stimulation of SMC *in vitro* is associated with an increase of the proto-oncogenes c-myc, c-myb, and c-fos.[171-173] The ornithine decarboxylase gene and the thymidine kinase messenger RNA are both expressed in stimulated cells and in continuously cycling cells.[173] SMC proliferation may also result from a reduction in inhibitory factors which normally prevent cell division. Proteins such as p21 are inhibitors of the cyclin-dependent kinases which regulate the entry of the cell in the cycle (Figure 57.3). Stimulation of these proteins inhibits SMC proliferation and neointima formation after balloon injury.[174]

As smooth muscle cells decrease their proliferation rate, they begin to synthesize large quantities of proteoglycan matrix. The extracellular matrix production continues for up to 20-25 weeks and over time it is gradually replaced by collagen and elastin, while the SMC turn into quiescent mesenchymal cells. The resulting neointima is composed of a fibrotic extracellular matrix with few cellular constituents. The endothelial cells proliferate and cover the denuded area, resulting in a re-endothelization process, and the new endothelium begins to produce large quantities of heparan sulfate and nitric oxide, both of which inhibit SMC proliferation.[76] However, whether SMC proliferation and extracellular matrix production cease after re-endothelization is still unknown at this time.

PREVENTION OF PHASE III – THE PAST AND THE FUTURE

Multiple experimental and clinical trials[175,176] have been carried out to specifically target what seemed the key in the restenosis process: smooth muscle cell proliferation. To date, with only a few exceptions, no pharmacologic or mechanical agent has been conclusively shown to reduce restenosis.

Antiproliferative approaches

Several antiproliferative agents targeting SMC migration and proliferation have been evaluated, including glucocorticoids, colchicine, somatostatin, hypolipidemic drugs, antineoplastic agents, and angiotensin converting enzyme (ACE) inhibitors.

Both natural and synthetic corticosteroids are potent inhibitors of SMC proliferation, leukocyte migration and degranulation, PDGF and macrophage-derived growth factor

Table 57.4 Local drug delivery systems

Double balloon system
Iontophoretic porous balloon
Balloon with hydrophilic polyacrylic polymer (hydrogel)
Channel catheter
Transport porous catheter
Dispatch catheter
Rheolytic system
Ultrasonic energy and radiofrequency
Balloon over a stent
Biodegradeable drug releasing polymer stents
Dacron stent
Silicone stent
High molecular weight polyacetic acid stent
Nitinol stent with polyurethane coating
Fibrin coated stent
Stent with cell layer
Stent with radioactive substance

release, and matrix production.[177] While experimental and preclinical studies[178–180] have reduced SMC proliferation with the use of local glucocorticoid delivery, three different human trials using oral steroid dosage have failed to shown any reduction in restenosis rate.[110,181,182]

Contradictory results have also been obtained with antineoplastic agents such as methotrexate, cytarabine, azathioprine, etoposide, vincristine, taxol, and doxorubicin, with some *in vitro* and *in vivo* studies showing an attenuation of vascular SMC proliferation.[183,184] Other studies show no efficacy in reducing the incidence of restenosis after PTCA.[185–187] Colchicine, which has an antimitotic and anti-inflammatory action in addition to an inhibitory effect on platelet aggregation and release of secretory products, has been shown to reduce restenosis in animals.[188] However, no clinical benefit has been seen with colchicine in two randomized placebo-controlled clinical trials.[189,190] As with other chemotherapeutics, the narrow therapeutic index of these drugs may be of concern. The problem of systemic toxicity may be overcome by the use of different local drug delivery devices currently under investigation[191–196] (Table 57.4). Local therapy offers the combined advantages of high local concentrations at the injury site and diminished systemic levels, with decreased risk of side effects. However, despite the appeal of local delivery systems, there are still concerns on many unresolved and confounding issues.[197]

After verification of an inhibitory effect on neointimal hyperplasia in animal models,[198–200] ACE inhibitors have been extensively studied to assess the clinical effect on restenosis. Two large clinical studies (MERCATOR and MARCATOR), with over 2129 patients enrolled, failed to show any impact on clinical or angiographic restenosis.[201,202] Intensive treatment with cholesterol lowering agents, such as the HMG-CoA reductase inhibitors lovastatin, pravastatin, simvastatin, and fluvastatin, reduces intimal hyperplasia in the rat and rabbit models,[187,203,204] probably via serum lipid reduction and decreased platelet aggregation. Despite this promising preliminary data, chronic high dose lovastatin treatment does not attenuate the incidence of clinical restenosis.[205] Antioxidant agents such as probucol, ascorbic acid and alpha-tocopherol may be useful in limiting restenosis by reducing platelet aggregation and modulating prostaglandin and leukotriene synthesis. Both animal[206,207] and clinical[22,208] studies have recently shown a reduction in restenosis with the use of such agents.

Recent excitement has developed in the scientific community about the use of external or intravascular radiation (brachytherapy) in the form of low dose beta and gamma radiation for the inhibition of neointimal formation.[209–215] Ionizing radiation affects dividing cells by damaging the nucleus, causing single or double strand breaks of the DNA bases,[216] and may reduce neointima proliferation by increasing the rate of apoptosis within the intima.[217] External beam radiotherapy involves the generation of a beam of radiation from a source external to the patient, for example a linear accelerator or ^{60}Co unit. Brachytherapy is a method of delivering radiation to a target organ by placing radioactive sources, for example ^{90}Yt or ^{192}Ir sources, close to or within an organ. This method (as opposed to external beam radiation) is well suited to delivering high doses of radiation to a small defined region. In addition, gamma emitters deliver more uniform dose to the arterial wall than beta emitters, but at the cost of increased radiation risk. Encouraging results from small human clinical studies utilizing both gamma and beta emitters[218–221] have set the stage for human clinical trials. A double-blind, randomized trial (SCRIPPS study), in which 56 patients were enrolled, evaluated gamma emitter seeds on a guidewire following stent placement in restenosis patients.[222] A 6-month follow-up restenosis rate of less than 11% suggests this therapy is promising for restenosis prevention after coronary percutaneous revascularization procedures.

Growth factor approaches

Because several growth factors have been implicated in the pathogenesis of restenosis, interfering with the cellular processes that control cellular migration, replication, and matrix deposition they have attracted much interest in the continuous search for pharmacologic agents to reduce the incidence of restenosis.

Angiopeptin, an analog of somatostatin, prevents the mitotic effect of several growth factors including somatomedin-C, epidermal growth factor, insulin-like growth factor, and PDGF. It inhibits SMC proliferation and reduces neointimal hyperplasia in different experimental models.[223–225] A multicenter trial in which 1246 patients were randomized to receive placebo or three different doses of angiopeptin showed no reduction in clinical events and restenosis rates between the different groups.[226] On the other hand, in a smaller randomized study, angiopeptin treatment reduced restenosis after PTCA (7.5% vs 37.8% in the placebo group).[227] However, using the same drug regimen, this promising finding was not confirmed by another multicenter European study.[228] Questions remain on whether a more prolonged dosing of this agent is needed to affect neointimal growth.

Trapidil is a potent thromboxane-A2 and PDGF antagonist which significantly reduces neointimal formation in animal models of restenosis.[229] The STARC trial randomized 305 patients to receive trapidil or aspirin and showed a reduction in restenosis rate by 40%, and reduction in clinical symptoms at 6-month follow-up in the trapidil treatment group.[230]

Molecular approaches

With the growing understanding that the failure of several antiproliferative agents to reduce neointimal hyperplasia may be related to the amplification and redundancy present in membrane and nuclear protein signaling, several attempts have been made to control and transform gene expression at the molecular level.[231] The mechanisms by which genetic material transfers into the target tissue include:

1. *in vivo* gene transfer by infusion of naked DNA or antisense oligonucleotides;[232]
2. transport by hybrid liposomes containing viral coat particles;[233]
3. transport by cationic liposomes containing the DNA;[234]
4. via viral vectors using retro- or adenoviruses.[235,236]

Besides the potential safety concerns of gene therapy, there are also problems of transfection efficiency and which gene should be delivered. Previously, in agreement with the restenosis hypothesis, SMC were the preferential target. In more recent years, however, with improved knowledge of the pathogenetic mechanisms involved in the restenosis phenomenon, other targets have been selected, including endothelial cells, thrombus formation, growth factors, matrix production, and vascular remodeling.[237–241] In addition, increased extracellular growth inhibitors of SMC proliferation might be another potential approach.[174,242,243] Other future approaches may include enhancement of re-endothelization and repair by cell seeding[244–247] and photodynamic therapy with light which shows cytotoxic properties on SMC and cell membranes through the production of activated singlet oxygen species.[248–251]

NEW ETIOLOGIES IN RESTENOSIS – THE ROLE OF CHRONIC VASCULAR REMODELING AND ADVENTITIA

Vascular remodeling, first described in relation to atherosclerosis,[252,253] has assumed great importance in the last few years as a cause of coronary restenosis in non-stented patients. In atherosclerotic vessels a chronic focal enlargement of the artery occurs in response to plaque increase, in order to preserve blood flow.[254–258] Artery size changes also occur following coronary angioplasty.[259] The artery may exhibit three different remodeling responses: compensatory enlargement,[260] absence of compensation[261] or vascular constriction.[262,263] Intravascular ultrasound has become an important way to understand the concept of remodeling. IVUS imaging has shown that after PTCA there is an axial plaque redistribution and that failure to cause dissection is one cause of early lumen loss by elastic recoil.[35,38] More recently, serial IVUS studies indicated that the restenotic lesion led to contraction of the artery and late lumen narrowing.[264–267] While the mechanisms of chronic remodeling are poorly understood, several explanations have been postulated to explain the late lumen narrowing after PTCA: fibrosis of the vessel wall underlying the lesion, rearrangement of extracellular matrix composition and structure, and response to increased shear stress.[268–271] A recent paper suggests that $\alpha_v\beta_3$ may regulate contraction of the vessel wall.[272] The integrins may therefore play a role in active contraction as well as migration of SMC. Animal studies indicate that after PTCA, stretching of the adventitia may result in the proliferation and synthesis of extracellular matrix by myofibroblasts within the adventitia itself with consequent scarlike contraction and compression of the underlying vascular wall.[273–275] This mechanism, however, does not seem relevant for late lumen narrowing in human coronary arteries subjected to balloon angioplasty.[276]

The potential impact of neointimal hyperplasia and geometric remodeling on restenosis requires further studies. Methods to prevent constrictive remodeling or to promote compensatory enlargement should be investigated. The metallic stent or drugs like cytokalasin B, which seems to function as a biologic stent, may fulfill this function.[277]

CONCLUSIONS – IS THE PREVENTION OF RESTENOSIS POSSIBLE?

The failure to effectively circumvent the problem of restenosis after 15 years of research underscores the complexity of this biological process which, to date, has not been fully understood. The elimination of the intimal healing response to injury is probably not achievable, nor is it desirable considering that this physiologic response to preserve vascular integrity has been maintained across millions of years in different species. The more we delve into it, the more complex and redundant this process appears.

Although SMC proliferation and neointima formation undoubtedly play a central role in restenosis, it is more likely that multifactorial mechanisms, involving different stimuli interacting in a synergistic manner with each other, are responsible for the restenosis phenomenon. Given the multimechanistic nature of restenosis, it is too simplistic to expect that a single drug or mechanical device will solve this problem completely. The solution will most likely be multifactorial, possibly involving the use of drug therapy in conjunction with second generation mechanical devices. Of these devices, coronary stents are the most promising, especially for their ability to achieve the best post-treatment luminal size.

In the history of medicine, human attempts to interfere with the natural course of a disease have often lead to undesired consequences. Restenosis is a new disease, one of the many that medicine has encountered in trying to solve an old disease. Enormous progress has been made in the last few years in the understanding of the pathogenetic mechanisms of restenosis. However, much work still needs to be done. A combination of present and future strategies will probably represent the "magic bullet" to solve the problem of restenosis. If those therapies reduce the need for repeat intervention and decrease the incidence of subsequent coronary events, the future of interventional cardiology and vascular biology is indeed exciting.

REFERENCES

1 Califf RM, Fortin DF, Frid DJ et al. Restenosis after coronary angioplasty: an overview. *J Am Coll Cardiol* 1991;**17**:2B–13B.

2 Franklin SM, Faxon DP. Pharmacologic prevention of restenosis after coronary angioplasty: review of the randomized clinical trials. *Coronary Artery Dis* 1993;**4**:232–42.

3 Topol EJ, Ellis SG, Cosgrove DM et al. Analysis of coronary angioplasty: practice in the United States with an insurance-claims database. *Circulation* 1993;**87**:1489–97.

4 Holmes DR, Vlietstra RE, Smith HC et al. Restenosis after percutaneous transluminal coronary angioplasty (PTCA): a report from the PTCA registry of the National Heart, Lung, and Blood Institute. *Am J Cardiol* 1984;**53**: 77C–81C.

5 Serruys PW, Luijten HE, Beatt KJ et al. Incidence of restenosis after successful coronary angioplasty: a time-related phenomenon. A quantitative angiographic study in 342 consecutive patients at 1, 2, 3, and 4 months. *Circulation* 1988;**77**:361–71.

6 Serruys PW, Rensing BJ, Hermans WRM, Beatt KJ. Definition of restenosis after percutaneous transluminal coronary angioplasty: a quickly evolving concept. *J Interv Cardiol* 1991;**4**: 256–76.

7 Beatt KJ, Luijten HE, de Feyter PJ et al. Change in diameter of coronary artery segments adjacent to stenosis after percutaneous transluminal coronary angioplasty: failure of percent diameter stenosis measurement to reflect morphologic

changes induced by balloon dilation. *J Am Coll Cardiol* 1988;**12**:315–23.

8 Kuntz RE, Keaney KM, Senerchia C, Baim DS. A predictive method for estimating the late angiographic results of coronary intervention despite incomplete ascertainment. *Circulation* 1993;**87**:815–30.

9 Kuntz RE, Baim DS. Defining coronary restenosis: newer clinical and angiographic paradigms. *Circulation* 1993;**88**:1310–23.

10 Renkin J, Melin J, Robert A *et al*. Detection of restenosis after successful coronary angioplasty: improved clinical decision making with use of a logistic model combining procedural and follow-up variables. *J Am Coll Cardiol* 1990;**16**: 1333–40.

11 Weintraub W, Ghazzal Z, Liberman H, Cohen C, Morris D. Long term clinical follow-up in patients with angiographic restudy after successful angioplasty. *Circulation* 1991;**84**:II-364.

12 Weintraub WS, Kosinski AS, Brown CL, King SB. Can restenosis after coronary angioplasty be predicted from clinical variable? *J Am Coll Cardiol* 1993;**21**:6–14.

13 Mick MJ, Piedmonte MR, Arnold AM, Simpfendorfer C. Risk stratification for long-term outcome after elective coronary angioplasty: a multivariate analysis of 5000 patients. *J Am Coll Cardiol* 1994;**24**:74–84.

14 Melkert R, Violaris AG, Serruys PW. Luminal narrowing after percutaneous transluminal coronary angioplasty: a multivariate analysis of clinical, procedural and lesion related factors, affecting long-term angiographic outcome in the PARK study. *J Invas Cardiol* 1994;**6**:160–71.

15 Peters RJC, Wouter EM, Kok MD *et al*. for the PICTURE Study Group. Prediction of restenosis after coronary balloon angioplasty: results of PICTURE (post-intracoronary treatment ultrasound result evaluation), a prospective multicenter intracoronary ultrasound imaging study. *Circulation* 1997;**95**:2254–61.

16 Farb A, Virmani R, Atkinson JB, Anderson PG. Long-term histologic patency after percutaneous transluminal coronary angioplasty is predicted by the creation of a greater lumen area. *J Am Coll Cardiol* 1994;**24**:1229–35.

17 Kuntz RE, Gibson CM, Nobuyoshi M, Baim DS. Generalized model of restenosis after conventional balloon angioplasty, stenting and directional atherectomy. *J Am Coll Cardiol* 1993; **21**:15–25.

18 Serruys PW, de Jaegere P, Kiemeneij F *et al*., for the BENESTENT Study Group. A comparison of balloon expandable-stent implantation with balloon angioplasty in patients with coronary artery disease. *N Engl J Med* 1994;**331**:489–95.

19 Fischman DL, Leon MB, Baim DS *et al*., for the Stent Restenosis Study Investigators. A randomized comparison of coronary-stent placement and balloon angioplasty in the treatment of coronary artery disease. *N Engl J Med* 1994;**331**:496–501.

20 Feld S, Ganim M, Carrel ES *et al*. Comparison of angioscopy, intravascular ultrasound imaging and quantitative coronary angiography in predicting clinical outcome after coronary interventions in high risk patients. *J Am Coll Cardiol* 1996;**28**:97–105.

21 Topol EJ, Califf RM, Weisman HF *et al*. Randomised trial of coronary intervention with antibody against platelet IIb/IIIa integrin for reduction of clinical restenosis: results at six months. The EPIC Investigators. *Lancet* 1994; **343**:881–6.

22 Tardif JC, Cote G, Lesperance J *et al*. Prevention of restenosis by pre- and post-PTCA probucol therapy: a randomized clinical trial. *Circulation* 1996;**94**(Suppl I):I-91 (abstract).

23 Godfried SL, Deckelbaum LI. Natural antioxidants and restenosis after percutaneous transluminal coronary angioplasty. *Am Heart J* 1995;**129**:203–10.

24 Chisolm GR. Antioxidants and atherosclerosis: a current assessment. *Clin Cardiol* 1991;**14**: I25–30.

25 Schneider J, Berk B, Santoian E *et al*. Oxidative stress is important in restenosis: reduction of neointimal formation by the antioxidant probucol in a swine model of restenosis. *Circulation* 1992;**86**:I-186.

26 Clowes AV, Karnovsky MJ. Suppression by heparin of smooth muscle cell proliferation in injured arteries. *Nature* 1977;**265**:625–6.

27 Olson IV, Clowes AW, Reidy MA. Inhibition of smooth muscle cell proliferation in injured rat arteries. *J Clin Invest* 1992;**90**:2044–9.

28 Faxon DP, Weber VJ, Haudenschild C *et al*. Acute effect of transluminal angioplasty in three experimental models of atherosclerosis. *Arteriosclerosis* 1982;**2**:125–33.

29 Schwartz RS, Edwards WD, Huber KC *et al*. Coronary restenosis: prospects for solution and new perspectives from a porcine model. *Mayo Clin Proc* 1993;**68**:54–62.

30 Dotter CT, Judkins MP. Transluminal treatment of atherosclerotic obstruction: description of new technique and a preliminary report of its application. *Circulation* 1964;**30**:654–70.

31 Baughman KL, Pasternak RC, Fallon JT, Block PC. Transluminal coronary angioplasty of post mortem human hearts. *Am J Cardiol* 1981;**48**: 1044–7.

32 Block PC, Myler RK, Stertzer S, Fallon JT. Morphology after transluminal angioplasty in humans. *N Engl J Med* 19;**305**:382.

33 Waller BF. Pathology of transluminal balloon angioplasty used in the treatment of heart disease. *Human Pathol* 1987;**18**:476–84.

34 Sanborn TA, Faxon DP, Haudenschild C, Gottsman SB, Ryan TJ. The mechanism of coronary angioplasty: evidence for formation of aneurysms in experimental atheroslerosis. *Circulation* 1983;**68**:1136–40.

35 Potkin BN, Roberts WC. Effects of coronary angioplasty on atherosclerotic plaque composition and arterial size to outcome. *Am J Cardiol* 1988;**62**:41–50.

36 Kohchi K, Takebayashi S, Block PC *et al*. Arterial changes after percutaneous coronary angioplasty: results at autopsy. *J Am Coll Cardiol* 1987;**10**:592–9.

37 Mizuno K, Kurita A, Imazeki N. Pathologic findings after percutaneous transluminal coronary angioplasty. *Br Heart J* 1984;**52**:588–90.

38 Potkin BN, Keren GN, Mintz GS *et al*. Arterial responses to balloon coronary angioplasty: an intravascular ultrasound study. *J Am Coll Cardiol* 1992;**20**:942–51.

39 Essed CE, van der Brand M, Becker AE. Transluminal coronary angioplasty and early restenosis: fibrocellular occlusion after wall laceration. *Br Heart J* 1983;**49**:393–6.

40 Fuster V, Erling F, Fallon JT *et al*. The three processes leading to post PTCA restenosis: dependence on the lesion substrate. *Thromb Haemost* 1995;**74**:552–9.

41 Nobuyoshi M, Kimura T, Nosaka H *et al*. Restenosis after successful percutaneous transluminal coronary angioplasty: serial angiographic follow-up of 229 patients. *J Am Coll Cardiol* 1988;**12**:616–23.

42 Sanders M. Angiographic changes thirty minutes following percutaneous transluminal coronary angioplasty: serial angiographic follow-up of 229 patients. *Angiology* 1985;**36**:419–24.

43 Daniel WC, Pirwitz MJ, Willard JE *et al*. Incidence and treatment of elastic recoil occurring in the 15 minutes following successful percutaneous transluminal coronary angioplasty. *Am J Cardiol* 1996;**78**:253–9.

44 Fischell TA, Derby G, Tse TM, Stadius ML. Coronary artery vasoconstriction routinely occurs after percutaneous transluminal angioplasty. *Circulation* 1988;**78**:1323–34.

45 Mabin TA, Holmes DR, Smith HC *et al*. Intracoronary thrombus: role in coronary occlusion complicating percutaneous transluminal coronary angioplasty. *J Am Coll Cardiol* 1985;**5**:198–202.

46 Arora RR, Platko WP, Bhadwar K, Simpfendorfer C. Role of intracoronary thrombus in acute complications during percutaneous transluminal coronary angioplasty. *Cath Cardiovasc Diagn* 1989;**16**:226–9.

47 Rodriguez AE, Santaera O, Larribeau M, Sosa MI, Palacios IF. Early decrease in minimal luminal diameter after successful percutaneous transluminal angioplasty predicts late restenosis. *Am J Cardiol* 1993;**71**:1391–5.

48 Rodriguez AE, Santaera O, Larribeau M *et al*. Coronary stenting decreases restenosis in lesions with early loss in luminal diameter 24 hours after successful PTCA. *Circulation* 1995;**91**:1397–402.

49 Rupprecht HJ, Brennecke R, Bernhard G *et al*. Analysis of risk factors for restenosis after PTCA. *Cardiovasc Diagn* 1990;**19**:151–9.

50 Guiteras V, Bourassa MG, David PR *et al*. Restenosis after percutaneous transluminal coronary angioplasty: the Montreal Heart Institute experience. *Am J Cardiol* 1987;**60**:50B.

51 Staudacher RA, Hess KR, Harris SL, Abu-Khalil J, Heibig J. Percutaneous transluminal coronary angioplasty utilizing prolonged balloon inflations: initial results and six-month follow-up. *Cath Cardiovasc Diagn* 1991;**23**:239–44.

52 Kaltenbach M, Beyer J, Walter S *et al*. Prolonged application of pressure in transluminal coronry angioplasty. *Cath Cardiovasc Diagn* 1984;**10**:213–19.

53 Douglas GS, King SBI, Roubin GS. Influence of methodology of percutaneous transluminal coronary angioplasty on restenosis. *Am J Cardiol* 1987;**60**:29B.

54 Rensing BJ, Hermans WR, Deckers JW *et al*. Lumen narrowing after percutaneous transluminal coronary balloon angioplasty follows a near gaussian distribution: a quantitative angiographic study in 1,445 successfully dilated lesions. *J Am Coll Cardiol* 1992;**19**:939–45.

55 Meier B, Gruntzig AR, King SBI *et al*. Higher balloon dilatation pressure in coronary angioplasty. *Am Heart J* 1984;**107**:619–22.

56 Shaw RE, Myler RK, Fishman-Rosen J *et al*. Clinical and morphologic factors in prediction of restenosis after multiple vessel angioplasty. *J Am Coll Cardiol* 1986;**7**:63A.

57 Detre K, Holubkov R, Kelsey S *et al*. Percutaneous transluminal coronary angioplasty in 1985–1986 and 1977–1981; the NHLBI registry. *N Engl J Med* 1988;**318**:265.

58 Mata LA, Bosch X, David PR *et al*. Clinical and angiographic assessment 6 months after double vessel percutaneous coronary angioplasty. *J Am Coll Cardiol* 1985;**6**:1239–44.

59 Roubin GS, Douglas JSJ, King SBI *et al*. Influence of balloon size on initial success, acute complications and restenosis after percutaneous

coronary angioplasty: a prospective randomized study. *Circulation* 1988;**78**:557–65.

60 Sangiorgi G, Nunez BD, Keelan E *et al*. Detailed restenosis angiographic analysis after "crackers, stretchers, drillers, shavers and burners". *J Inv Cardiol* 1995;**7**(Suppl C): (abstract).

61 Schatz RA, Penn IM, Baim DS *et al*. for the STRESS Investigators. Stent Restenosis Study (STRESS): analysis of in-hospital results. *Circulation* 1993;**88**:I-594.

62 Serruys P, Macaya, C, de Jaegere P *et al*. Interim analysis of the BENESTENT trial. *Circulation* 1993;**88**:594.

63 Colombo A, Maiello L, Almagor Y *et al*. Coronary stenting: single institution experience with the initial 100 cases using the Palmaz–Schatz stent. *Cath Cardiovasc Diagn* 1992;**26**:171–6.

64 Colombo A, Hall P, Nakamura S. Intracoronary stenting without anti-coagulation accomplished with intravascular ultrasound guidance. *Circulation* 1995;**91**:1676–88.

65 Versaci F, Gaspardone A, Tomai F *et al*. A comparison of coronary stenting with angioplasty for isolated stenosis of the proximal left anterior descending coronary artery. *N Engl J Med* 1997;**336**:817–22.

66 Serruys PW, Emanuellsson H, van der Giessen W *et al*. Heparin-coated Palmaz–Schatz stents in human coronary arteries: early outcome of the Benestent-II Pilot Study. *Circulation* 1996;**93**: 412–22.

67 Tanaglia AN, Buller CE, Kisslo KB *et al*. Mechanisms of balloon angioplasty and directional atherectomy as assessed by intracoronary ultrasound. *J Am Coll Cardiol* 1992;**20**:685–91.

68 Kimball BP, Bui S, Cohen EA. Comparison of acute elastic recoil after directional coronary atherectomy vs standard balloon angioplasty. *Am Heart J* 1992;**124**:1459–66.

69 Elliot JM, Berdan LG, Homes DR *et al*. One year follow-up in the coronary angioplasty versus excisional atherectomy trial (CAVEAT I). *Circulation* 1995;**91**:2158–66.

70 Topol EJ, Leya F, Pinkerton CA *et al*. A comparison of patients with coronary artery disease. *N Engl J Med* 1993;**329**:221–7.

71 Adelman AG, Cohen EA, Kimball BP *et al*. A comparison of directional atherectomy with balloon angioplasty in the treatment of coronary artery disease for lesions of the left anterior descending arteries. *N Engl J Med* 1993;**329**: 228–33.

72 Simonton CA, Leon MB, Kuntz RE *et al*. Acute and late clinical and angiographic results of directional atherectomy in the Optimal Atherectomy Restenosis Study (OARS). *Circulation* 1995;**92**:I-545 (abstracts).

73 Uchida Y, Hasegawa K, Kawamura K, Shibuya I. Angioscopic observation of the coronary luminal changes induced by percutaneous transluminal coronary angioplasty. *Am Heart J* 1989;**117**: 769–76.

74 Miller DD, Boulet AJ, Tio FO *et al*. In vivo technetium-99m S12 antibody imaging of platelet alpha granules in rabbit endothelial neointimal proliferation after angioplasty. *Circulation* 1991;**83**:224–36.

75 den Heijer P, van Dijk RB, Hillege HL *et al*. Serial angioscopic and angiographic observations during the first hour after successful coronary angioplasty: a preamble to a multicenter trial addressing angioscopic markers for restenosis. *Am Heart J* 1994;**128**:656–63.

76 Ip JH, Fuster V, Israel D *et al*. The role of platelets, thrombin and hyperplasia in restenosis after coronary angioplasty. *J Am Coll Cardiol* 1991; **17**:77B–88B.

77 Weitz JI, Huboda M, Massel D, Maraganore J, Hirsh J. Clot-bound thrombin is protected from inhibition by heparin-antithrombin III but is susceptible to inactivation by antithrombin III-independent inhibitors. *J Clin Invest* 1990;**86**: 385–91.

78 Bar-Shavit R, Eldor A, Vlodavsky I. Binding of thrombin to subendothelial extracellular matrix: protection and expression of functional properties. *J Clin Invest* 1989;**84**:1096–104.

79 Chronos NAF, Goodall AH, Wilson DJ, Sigwart U, Buller NP. Profound platelet degranulation is an important side effect of some types of contrast media used in interventional cardiology. *Circulation* 1993;**88**(Part I):2035–44.

80 Kolarov P, Tschoepe D, Nieuwenhuis HK *et al*. PTCA: periprocedal platelet activation. Part II of the Dusseldorf PTCA Platelet Study (DPPS). *Eur Heart J* 1996;**17**:1216–22.

81 Fukami MH, Salganicoff L. Human platelet storage organelles. *Thromb Haemostat* 1977;**38**: 963–70.

82 Holmsen H. Secretable storage pools in platelets. *Ann Rev Med* 1979;**30**:119–34.

83 Le Breton H, Plow EF, Topol EJ. Role of platelets in restenosis after percutaneous coronary revascularization. *J Am Coll Cardiol* 1996;**28**: 1643–51.

84 Lindner V, Reidy MA. Expression of basic fibroblast growth factor and its receptor by smooth muscle cells and endothelium in injured rat arteries: an enface study. *Circ Res* 1993;**73**: 589–95.

85 Shimokawa H, Ito A, Fukumoto Y *et al*. Chronic treatment with interleukin-1 induces coronary intimal lesions and vasospastic responses in pigs in vivo. *J Clin Invest* 1996;**97**:769–76.

86 Casscells W. Migration of smooth muscle and endothelial cells. Critical events in restenosis. *Circulation* 1992;**86**:723–29.

87 Rekhter MD, O'Brien E, Shah N *et al.* The importance of thrombus organization and stellate cell phenotype in collagen I gene expression in human coronary atherosclerosis and restenotic lesions. *Cardiovasc Res* 1996;**32**: 496–502.

88 Poole JCF, Cromwell SP, Benditt EP. Behavior of smooth muscle cells and formation of extracellular structures in the reaction of the arterial walls to injury. *Am J Pathol* 1971;**62**: 391–413.

89 Jeong MH, Owen WG, Staab ME *et al.* Porcine model of stent thrombosis: platelets are the primary component of acute stent closure. *Cath Cardiovasc Diagn* 1996;**38**:38–43.

90 Plow EF, McEver RP, Coller SW *et al.* Related binding mechanisms for fibrinogen, fibronectin, von Willebrand factor and thrombospondin on thrombin-stimulated human platelets. *Blood* 1985;**66**:724–7.

91 Weiss HG, Hawiger J, Ruggeri ZW *et al.* Fibrinogen-independent platelet adhesion and thrombus formation on subendothelium mediated by glycoprotein IIb/IIIa complex at high share rate. *J Clin Invest* 1989;**83**:288–97.

92 Unterberg C, Sandrock D, Nebendhal K, Buchwald AB. Reduced acute thrombus formation results in decreased neointimal proliferation after coronary angioplasty. *J Am Coll Cardiol* 1995;**26**:1747–54.

93 Sugama Y, Malik A. Thrombin receptor 14-aminoacid peptide mediates endothelial hyperadhesivity and neutrophil adhesion by P-selectin-dependent mechanism. *Circ Res* 1992; **71**:1015–19.

94 Shi Y, Hutchinson HG, Hall DG, Zalewsky A. Downregulation of c-myc expression by antisense oligonucleotides inhibits proliferation of human smooth muscle cells. *Circulation* 1993; **88**:1190–5.

95 Moreno P, Falk E, Palacios I *et al.* Macrophage infiltration in acute coronary syndromes: implications for plaque rupture. *Circulation* 1994;**90**:775–8.

96 Majesky MW, Reidy MA, Bowen-Pope DF *et al.* PDGF ligand and receptor genes expression during repair of arterial injury. *J Cell Biol* 1990; **111**:2149–58.

97 Nabel EG, Yang ZY, Plautz G *et al.* Recombinant fibroblast growth factor-1 promotes intimal hyperplasia and angiogenesis in arteries in vivo. *Nature* 1993;**362**:844–6.

98 Lindner V, Reidy MA. Proliferation of smooth muscle cells after vascular injury is inhibited by an antibody against basic fibroblast growth factor. *Proc Natl Acad Sci USA* 1991;**88**: 3739–43.

99 Chen JK, Hoshi H, McKeehan WL. Transforming growth factor type beta specifically stimulates synthesis of proteoglycan in human adult arterial smooth muscle cells. *Proc Natl Acad Sci USA* 1987;**84**:5287–91.

100 Nikol S, Weir L, Sullivan A *et al.* Persistently increased expression of the transforming growth factor beta 1 gene in human vascular restenosis: analysis of 62 patients with one or more episodes of restenosis. *Cardiovasc Pathol* 1992;**3**:57–62.

101 Nabel EG, Shum L, Pompili VJ *et al.* Direct transfer of transforming growth factor beta 1 into arteries stimulates fibrocellular hyperplasia. *Proc Natl Acad Sci USA* 1993;**90**:10759–63.

102 Shi Y, O'Brien J, Fard A, Zalewski A. Adventitial myofibroblasts contribute to neointimal formation following coronary arterial injury. *Circulation* 1995;**92**:I-34 (abstract).

103 Shi Y, Pieniek M, Fard A *et al.* Adventitial remodeling after coronary arterial injury. *Circulation* 1996;**93**:340–8.

104 Violaris AG, Melkert R, Hermann JPR, Serruys PW. Role of angiographically identifiable thrombus on long-term luminal renarrowing after coronary angioplasty: a quantitative angiographic analysis. *Circulation* 1996;**93**: 889–97.

105 Schwartz RS, Holmes DRJ, Topol EJ. The restenosis paradigm revisited: an alternative proposal for cellular mechanisms. *J Am Coll Cardiol* 1992;**20**:1284–93.

106 Yamazaki M. Factor Xa inhibitors. *Drugs of the Future* 1995;**20**:911–18.

107 Schwartz RS, Holder DJ, Holmes DRJ *et al.* Neointimal thickening after severe coronary artery injury is limited by short-term administration of a factor Xa inhibitor: results in a porcine model. *Circulation* 1996;**94**: 2998–3001.

108 Deutsch E, Rao AK, Colman RW. Selective thrombin inhibitors: the next generation of anticoagulants. *J Am Coll Cardiol* 1993;**22**: 1089–92.

109 Fitzgerald GA, Meagher EA. Antiplatelets drugs. *Eur J Clin Invest* 1994;**24**:46–9.

110 Hillegas WB, Ohman EM, Califf RM. Restenosis: the clinical issues. In: Topol EJ. Ed. *Textbook of interventional cardiology*, 2nd edn. Philadelphia: WB Saunders, 1994, pp 415–35.

111 Schwartz L, Bourassa MG, Lesperance J *et al.* Aspirin and dipyridamole in the prevention of restenosis after percutaneous transluminal coronary angioplasty. *N Engl J Med* 1988;**318**: 1714–19.

112 White C, Knudson M, Schmidt D. Neither ticlopidine nor aspirin-dipyridamole prevents

restenosis post PTCA: results from a randomized placebo-controlled multicenter trial. *Circulation* 1987;**76**:IV–213 (abstract).

113 Thomton MA, Gruentzig AR, Hollman J *et al.* Coumadin and aspirin in prevention of restenosis after transluminal coronary angioplasty: a randomized study. *Circulation* 1984;**69**:721–7.

114 Urban P, Buller N, Kox K *et al.* Lack of effect of warfarin on the restenosis rate or on clinical outcome after balloon coronary angioplasty. *Br Heart J* 1988;**60**:485–8.

115 Bertrandt ME, Allain H, Lablanche JM. Results of a randomized trial of ticlopidine vs placebo for the prevention of acute closure and restenosis after coronary angioplasty: the TACT study. *Circulation* 1990;**82**:190 (abstract).

116 Serruys PW, Rutsch W, Heyndrickx GR *et al.* Prevention of restenosis after percutaneous transluminal coronary angioplasty with thromboxane A2-receptor blockade. A randomized, double-blind, placebo-controlled trial. Coronary Artery Restenosis Prevention on Repeated Thromboxane-Antagonism Study (CARPORT). *Circulation* 1991;**84**:1568–80.

117 Feldman RL, Bengston JR, Pryor DB, Zimmerman MB, for the GRASP Study Group. Use of a thromboxane A_2 receptor blocker to reduce adverse clinical events after coronary angioplasty. *J Am Coll Cardiol* 1992;**19**:259A.

118 Bove A, Savage M, Deutsch E *et al.* Effects of selective and non-selective thromboxane A2 blockade on restenosis after PTCA: M-Heart II. *J Am Coll Cardiol* 1992;**19**:259A (abstract).

119 Knudtson ML, Flintoft VF, Roth DL, Hansen JL, Duff HJ. Effect of short-term prostacyclin administration on restenosis after percutaneous transluminal coronary angioplasty. *J Am Coll Cardiol* 1990;**15**:691–7.

120 Raitzner AE, Holman J, Abukhalil J, Demke D. Ciprostene for restenosis revisited: quantitative analysis of angiograms. *J Am Coll Cardiol* 1993; **21**:321A (abstract).

121 Ellis SG, Roubin GS, Wilentz J, Douglas JSJ, King SB. Effect of 18- to 24-hour heparin administration for prevention of restenosis after uncomplicated coronary angioplasty. *Am Heart J* 1989;**117**:777–82.

122 Ellis S, Roubin G, Wilentz J *et al.* Results of a randomized trial of heparin and aspirin vs. aspirin alone for prevention of acute closure (AC) and restenosis (R) after angioplasty (PTCA). *Circulation* 1987;**76**:IV–213 (abstract).

123 Dryski M, Mikat E, Bjornsson TD. Inhibition of intimal hyperplasia after arterial injury by heparins and heparinoids. *J Vasc Surg* 1988;**8**: 623–33.

124 Lehmann KG, Doria RJ, Feuer JM *et al.* Paradoxical increase in restenosis rate with chronic heparin use, final results of randomized trials. *J Am Coll Cardiol* 1991;**17**:181A (abstract).

125 Cairns JA, Gill J, Morton B *et al.*, for the EMPAR collaborators. Fish oils and low-molecular-weight heparin for the reduction of restenosis after percutaneous transluminal coronary angioplasty. The EMPAR study. *Circulation* 1996; **94**:1553–60.

126 Currier JW, Pow TK, Haudenschild CC, Minihan AC, Faxon DP. Low molecular weight heparin (Enoxaparin) reduces restenosis after iliac angioplasty in the hypercholesterolemic rabbit. *J Am Coll Cardiol* 1991;**17**:118B–125B.

127 Faxon D, Spiro T, Minor S *et al.* Low molecular weight heparin in the prevention of restenosis after angioplasty: results of enoxaparin restenosis (ERA) trial. *Circulation* 1994;**90**: 908–14.

128 Topol EJ, Bonar R, Jewitt D *et al.* Use of a direct antithrombin, hirulog, in place of heparin during coronary angioplasty. *Circulation* 1993;**87**: 1622–9.

129 Serruys PW, Herrman JR, Simon R *et al.*, Investigators for the HELVETICA. A comparison of hirudin with heparin in the prevention of restenosis after coronary angioplasty. *N Engl J Med* 1995;**333**:757–63.

130 Heras M, Chesebro JH, Penny WJ *et al.* Effects of thrombin inhibition on the development of acute platelet-thrombus deposition during angioplasty in pigs. Heparin versus recombinant hirudin, a specific thrombin inhibitor. *Circulation* 1989;**79**:657–65.

131 van den Boss AA, Deckers JW, Heyndrickx GR *et al.* Safety and efficacy of recombinant hirudin (CGP 39393) vs heparin in patients with stable angina undergoing coronary angioplasty. *Circulation* 1993;**88**:2058–66.

132 Matsuno H, Stassen JM, Vermylen J, Deckmyn H. Inhibition of integrin function by a cyclic RGD-containing peptide prevents neointimal formation. *Circulation* 1994;**90**:2203–6.

133 Choi ET, Engel L, Callow AD *et al.* Inhibition of neointimal hyperplasia by blocking $\alpha_v\beta_3$ integrin with a small peptide antagonist GpenGRGDSPCA. *J Vasc Surg* 1994;**19**:125–34.

134 The EPIC Investigators. Use of monoclonal antibody direct against the platelet glycoprotein IIa/IIIb receptor in high risk coronary angioplasty. *N Engl J Med* 1994;**14**:956–61.

135 Lincoff AM, Tcheng JE, Ellis SG *et al.*, for the IMPACT-II Investigators. Randomized trials of platelet glycoprotein IIb/IIIa inhibition with Integrelin for prevention of restenosis following coronary interventions: the IMPACT-II angiographic substudy. *Circulation* 1995;**92**:I-607.

136 Tcheng JE, Harrington RA, Kottke-Marchant K et al. Multicenter, randomized, double-blind placebo-controlled trial of the platelet integrin glycoprotein IIb/IIIa inhibition blocker integrelin in elective coronary intervention. *Circulation* 1995;**91**:2151–7.

137 Tcheng JE. Glycoprotein IIb/IIIa receptor inhibitors: putting the EPIC, IMPACT II, RESTORE and EPILOG trials into perspective. *Am J Cardiol* 1996;**78**:35–40.

138 van der Werf F. More evidence for a beneficial effect of platelet glycoprotein IIb/IIIa- blockade during coronary interventions: latest results from the EPILOG and CAPTURE trials. *Eur Heart J* 1996;**17**:325–6 (editorial).

139 Ferguson J Jr. EPILOG and CAPTURE trials halted because of positive interim results. *Circulation* 1996;**93**:637 (news).

140 Ueda M, Becker AE, Tsukada T, Numano F, Fujimoto T. Fibrocellular tissue response after percutaneous transluminal coronary angioplasty. An immunocytochemical analysis of the cellular composition. *Circulation* 1991;**83**: 1327–32.

141 Nobuyoshi M, Kimura T, Ohishi H et al. Morphologic studies: restenosis after percutaneous transluminal coronary angioplasty: pathologic observations in 20 patients. *J Am Coll Cardiol* 1991;**17**:433–9.

142 Garratt KN, Edwards WD, Kaufmann UP, Vlietstra RE, Holmes DR. Differential histopathology of primary atherosclerotic and restenotic lesion in coronary arteries and saphenous vein bypass grafts: analysis of tissue obtained from 73 patients by directional atherectomy. *J Am Coll Cardiol* 1991;**17**:442–8.

143 van Beusekom H, van der Giessen W, van Suylen R et al. Histology after stenting of human saphenous vein bypass grafts: observations from surgically excised grafts 3 to 320 days after stent implantation. *J Am Coll Cardiol* 1993;**21**:45–54.

144 Clowes A, Clowes M, Fingerle J, Reidy M. Kinetics of cellular proliferation after arterial injury V. Role of acute distension in the induction of smooth muscle proliferation. *Lab Invest* 1989; **49**:360–4.

145 Clowes AW, Schwartz SN. Significance of quiescent smooth muscle cell migration in the injured rat carotid artery. *Circ Res* 1985;**56**: 139–45.

146 Forrester JS, Fishbein M, Helfant R, Fagin J. A paradigm of restenosis based on cell biology: clues for the development of new preventive therapies. *J Am Coll Cardiol* 1991;**17**:758–69.

147 Clowes AW, Reidy MA, Clowes MM. Kinetics of cellular proliferation after arterial injury, I. Smooth muscle growth in the absence of endothelium. *Lab Invest* 1983;**49**:327–33.

148 Clowes AW, Reidy MA, Clowes MM. Kinetics of cellular proliferation after arterial injury. *Lab Invest* 1987;**49**:327–33.

149 Clowes A, Clowes M, Reidy M. Kinetics of cellular proliferation after arterial injury: endothelial and smooth muscle growth in chronically denuded vessels. *Lab Invest* 1986;**54**:295–303.

150 Thayer JM, Giachelli PM, Mirkes PE, Schartz SM. Expression of osteopontin in the head process late in gastrulation in the rat. *J Exp Zool* 1995; **272**:240–4.

151 Liaw L, Lombardi DM, Almeida MM, Schwartz SM. Neutralizing antibodies direct against osteopontin inhibit rat carotid neointimal thickening following endothelial denudation. *Arterioscler Thromb Vasc Biol* 1997;**17**:188–93.

152 Weber GF, Ashkar S, Glimcher MJ, Cantor H. Receptor–ligand interaction between CD44 and osteopontin (Eta-1). *Science* 1996;**271**:509–12.

153 Jain M, He Q, Lee WS et al. Role of CD44 in the reaction of vascular smooth muscle cells to arterial wall injury. *J Clin Invest* 1996;**97**: 596–603.

154 Bendeck M, Zempo N, Clowes A, Galardy R, Reidy M. Smooth muscle cell migration and matrix metalloproteinase expression after injury in the rat. *Circ Res* 1994;**75**:539–45.

155 Schwartz SM. Smooth muscle migration in atherosclerosis and restenosis. *J Clin Invest* 1997; **99**:2814–17.

156 Bendeck MP, Irvin C, Reidy MA. Inhibition of matrix metalloproteinase activity inhibits smooth muscle cell migration but not neointimal thickening after arterial injury. *Circ Res* 1996; **78**:38–43.

157 Ruoslahti E. Integrins. *J Clin Invest* 1991;**87**: 1–5.

158 Hynes RO. Integrins: versatility, modulation, and signalling in cell adhesion. *Cell* 1992;**69**:11–25.

159 Samanen J, Ali FE, Romoff T et al. Development of a small RGD-peptide fibrinogen receptor antagonist with potent antiaggregatory activity in vitro. *J Med Chem* 1991;**34**:3114–25.

160 Douglas S, Ohlstein E. Endothelin-1 promotes neointima formation after balloon angioplasty in the rat. *J Cardiovasc Pharmacol* 1993;**22** (**Suppl** **8**):S371-3.

161 Helset E, Sildnes T, Seljelid R, Konoski ZS. Endothelin-1 stimulates human monocytes in vitro to release TNFα, IL-1β and IL-6. *Mediat Inflamm* 1993;**2**:417.

162 Scott-Burden T, Resink TJ, Hahn AWA, Vanhoutte PM. Induction of endothelin secretion by angiotensin II: effects on growth and synthetic activity of vascular smooth muscle cells. *J Cardiovasc Pharmacol* 1991;**17**:S96.

163 Wang X, Douglas SA, Louden C et al. Expression of endothelin-1, endothelin-3, endothelin-

converting-enzyme-1, endothelin-A and endothelin-B receptor mRNA following angioplasty-induced neointima formation in the rat. *Circ Res* 1996;**78**:322–8.

164 Tsjuno M, Hirata Y, Eguchi S *et al.* Nonselective ETA/ETB receptor antagonist blocks proliferation of rat vascular smooth muscle cells after balloon angioplasty. *Life Sci* 1995;**56**:PL449.

165 Wessale J, Adler A, Novosad E *et al.* Endothelin antagonism reduces neointima formed following balloon injury in rabbit. Fourth International Conference on Endothelin, London, UK, 1995.

166 Ferns GA, Raines EW, Sprugel KH *et al.* Inhibition of neointimal smooth muscle accumulation after angioplasty by an antibody to PDGF. *Science* 1991;**253**:1129–32.

167 Clowes AW, Clowes MM, Fingerle J, Reidy MA. Regulation of smooth muscle cell growth in injured artery. *J Cardiovasc Pharmacol* 1989;**14**: S12–S15.

168 Nabel EG, Yang Z, Plautz G *et al.* rFGF-1 gene expression in porcine arteries induces intimal hyperplasia and angiogenesis in vivo. *Nature* 1993;**362**:844–6.

169 Nabel EG, Liptay S, Yang Z *et al.* r-PDGF gene expression in porcine arteries induces intimal hyperplasia in vivo. *J Clin Invest* 1993;**91**: 1822–9.

170 Scott-Burden T, Vanhoutte PM. Regulation of smooth muscle cell growth by endothelium-derived growth factors. *Tex Heart Inst J* 1993; **21**:91–7.

171 Kindy MS, Sonenshein GE. Regulation of oncogene expression in cultured aortic smooth muscle cells: post-transcriptional control of c-myc m-RNA. *J Biol Chem* 1986;**261**:12865–8.

172 Simons M, Edelman ER, DeKeyser JL, Langer R, Rosenberg RD. Antisense c-myb oligonucleotides inhibit intimal arterial smooth muscle cell accumulation in vivo. *Nature* 1992;**359**:67–70.

173 Campan M, Desgranges C, Gadeau AP, Millet D, Belloc F. Cell cycle dependent gene expression in quiescent stimulated and asynchronously cycling arterial smooth muscle cells in culture. *J Cell Physiol* 1992;**150**:493.

174 Chang MW, Barr E, Lu MM, Barton K, Leiden JM. Adenovirus-mediated over-expression of the cyclin/cyclin-dependent kinase inhibitor p21 inhibits vascular smooth muscle cell proliferation and neointima formation in the rat carotid artery model of balloon angioplasty. *J Clin Invest* 1995;**96**:2260–8.

175 Paranandi SN, Topol EJ. Contemporary clinical trials of restenosis. *J Invest Cardiol* 1994;**6**: 109–24.

176 Dangas G, Fuster V. Management of restenosis after clinical intervention. *Am Heart J* 1996;**132**: 428–36.

177 Berk BC, Gordon JB, Alexander RW. Pharmacologic roles of heparin and glucocorticoids to prevent restenosis after coronary angioplasty. *J Am Coll Cardiol* 1991; **17**:111B–117B.

178 Longenecker JP, Kilty LA, Johnson LK. Glucocorticoid inhibition of vascular smooth muscle cells proliferation: influence of homologous extracellular matrix and serum mitogens. *J Cell Biol* 1984;**98**:534–40.

179 Longeneker JP, Kilty LA, Johnson LK. Glucocorticoid influence on growth of vascular cells in culture. *J Cell Physiol* 1982;**113**: 197–202.

180 Stone GW, Rutherford BD, McConahay DR *et al.* A randomized trial of corticosteroids for the prevention of restenosis in 102 patients undergoing repeat coronary angioplasty. *Cath Cardiovasc Diagn* 1989;**18**:227–31.

181 Pepine CJ, Hirshfield JW, MacDonald RG *et al.* A controlled trial of corticosteroids to prevent restenosis after coronary angioplasty. M-HEART Group. *Circulation* 1990;**81**:1753–61.

182 Villa AE, Guzman LA, Chen W *et al.* Local delivery of dexamethasone for prevention of neointimal proliferation in a rat model of balloon angioplasty. *J Clin Invest* 1994;**93**:1243–9.

183 Voisard R, Dartsch PC, Seitzer U *et al.* The in-vitro effect of antineoplastic agents on proliferative activity and cytoskeletal components of plaque-derived smooth muscle cells from human coronary arteries. *Coronary Artery Dis* 1993;**4**: 935–42.

184 Sollott SJ, Cheng L, Pauly RR *et al.* Taxol inhibits neointimal smooth muscle cell accumulation after angioplasty in the rat. *J Clin Invest* 1995; **95**:1869–76.

185 Murphy JG, Schwartz RS, Edwards WD *et al.* Methotrexate and azathioprine fail to inhibit porcine coronary restenosis. *Circulation* 1990; **82**:III-429.

186 Cox DA, Anderson PG, Roubin GS *et al.* Effect of local delivery of heparin and methotrexate on neointimal proliferation in stented porcine coronary arteries. *Coronary Artery Dis* 1992;**3**: 237–48.

187 Mullett DW, Topol EJ, Abrams GD, Gallagher KP, Ellis SG. Intramural methotrexate therapy for the prevention of the neointimal thickening after balloon angioplasty. *J Am Coll Cardiol* 1992;**20**: 460–6.

188 Muller D, Ellis S, Topol E. Colchicine and antineoplastic therapy for the prevention of restenosis after percutaneous coronary interventions. *J Am Coll Cardiol* 1991;**17**: 126B–131B.

189 O'Keefe J, McCallister B, Bateman T *et al.* Colchicine for the prevention of restenosis after

coronary angioplasty. *J Am Coll Cardiol* 1991; **17**:181A (abstract).

190 Grines CL, Rizik D, Levine A *et al*. Colchicine angioplasty restenosis trial (CART). *Circulation* 1991;**84**:II-365 (abstract).

191 Wolinsky H, Thung SN. Use of perforated balloon catheter to deliver concentrated heparin into the wall of the normal canine artery. *J Am Coll Cardiol* 1990;**15**:475–81.

192 Santoian EC, Gravanis MB, Schneider JE *et al*. Use of the porous balloon in porcine coronary arteries: rationale for low pressure and volume delivery. *Cath Cardiovasc Diagn* 1993;**31**:240–5.

193 Murphy JG, Schwartz RS, Edwards WD *et al*. Percutaneous polymeric stents in porcine coronary arteries. Initial experience with polyethylene terephthalate stents. *Circulation* 1992;**86**:1596–604.

194 van der Giessen WJ, Slager CJ, van Beusekom HMM *et al*. Development of a polymer endovascular prosthesis and its implantation in porcine arteries. *J Interv Cardiol* 1992;**5**:175–85.

195 Bier JD, Zalesky P, Li ST *et al*. A new bioabsorbable intravascular stent: in vitro assessment of hemodynamic and morphometric characteristics. *J Interv Cardiol* 1992;**5**:187–94.

196 Riessen R, Isner JM. Prospects for site-specific delivery of pharmacologic and molecular therapies. *J Am Coll Cardiol* 1994;**23**:1234–44.

197 Wolinsky H. Local delivery: let's keep our eyes on the wall. *J Am Coll Cardiol* 1994;**24**:825–7.

198 Powell JS, Clozel JP, Muller RK *et al*. Inhibitors of angiotensin-converting enzyme prevent myointimal proliferation after vascular injury. *Science* 1989;**245**:186–8.

199 Huber KC, Schwartz RS, Edwards WD, Camrud AR, Bailey K. Effects of angiotensin converting enzyme inhibition on neointimal hyperplasia in a porcine coronary injury model. *Am Heart J* 1993;**125**:695–701.

200 Janiak P, Libert O, Vilaine JP. The role of the renin-angiotensin system in neointima formation after injury in rabbits. *Hypertension* 1994;**24**:671–8.

201 The Multicenter European Research Trial with Cilazapril After Angioplasty to Prevent Transluminal Coronary Obstruction and Restenosis (MERCATOR) Study Group. Does the new angiotensin converting enzyme inhibitor cilazapril prevent restenosis after percutaneous transluminal coronary angioplasty? Results of the MERCATOR Study. *Circulation* 1992;**86**: 100–10.

202 Faxon D, on behalf of the MARCATOR Investigators. Angiotensin converting enzyme inhibition and restenosis: the final results of the MARCATOR trial. *Circulation* 1992;**88**:506 (abstract).

203 Rogler G, Lacknet KJ, Schmitz G. Effects of fluvastatin on growth of porcine and human vascular smooth muscle cells in vitro. *Am J Cardiol* 1995;**76**:114A–116A.

204 Gellman J, Ezekowitz MD, Sarembock IJ *et al*. Effect of lovastatin on intimal hyperplasia after balloon angioplasty: a study in an atherosclerotic hypercholesterolemic rabbit. *J Am Coll Cardiol* 1991;**17**:251–9.

205 Weintraub WS, Boccuzzi SJ, Klein JL *et al*. Lack of effect of lovastatin on restenosis after coronary angioplasty: Lovastatin Restenosis Trial study group. *N Engl J Med* 1994;**331**:1331–7.

206 Lafont AM, Chai Y-C, Cornhill JF *et al*. Effect of alpha-tocopherol on restenosis after angioplasty in a model of experimental atherosclerosis. *J Clin Invest* 1995;**95**:1108–25.

207 Schneider JE, Berk BC, Gravanis MB *et al*. Probucol decreases neointimal formation in a swine model of coronary artery balloon injury. *Circulation* 1993;**88**:628–37.

208 Watanabe K, Sekiya S, Miyagawa M, Hashida K. Preventive effects of probucol on restenosis after percutaneous transluminal coronary angioplasty. *Am Heart J* 1996;**23**:23–9.

209 Schwartz RS, Koval TM, Edwards WD *et al*. Effect of external beam irradiation on neointimal hyperplasia after experimental coronary artery injury. *J Am Coll Cardiol* 1992;**19**:1106–13.

210 Waksman R, Robinson KA, Crocker IR *et al*. Intracoronary low-dose beta-irradiation inhibits neointima formation after coronary artery balloon injury in the swine restenosis model. *Circulation* 1995;**92**:3025–31.

211 Wiedermann JG, Marboe C, Amols H, Schwartz A, Weinberger J. Intracoronary irradiation markedly reduces restenosis after balloon angioplasty in a porcine model. *J Am Coll Cardiol* 1994;**23**:1491–8.

212 Wiedermann JG, Marboe C, Amols H, Schwartz A, Weinberger J. Intracoronary irradiation markedly reduces neointimal proliferation after balloon angioplasty in swine: persistent benefit at 6-month follow-up. *J Am Coll Cardiol* 1995; **25**:1451–6.

213 Waksman R, Robinson KA, Crocker IR *et al*. Endovascular low-dose irradiation inhibits neointima formation after coronary artery balloon injury in swine. A possible role for radiation therapy in restenosis prevention. *Circulation* 1995;**91**:1533–9.

214 Verin V, Popowski Y, Urban P *et al*. Intra-arterial beta irradiation prevents neointimal hyperplasia in a hypercholesterolemic rabbit restenosis model. *Circulation* 1995;**92**:2284–90.

215 Liermann D, Boettcher HD, Schopohl B *et al*. Is there a method to prevent intimal hyperplasia after stent implantation in peripheral vessels? *Angiology* 1992;**92**:269–70.

216 Hall EJ. Cell-survival curves. In: Hall EJ (ed) *Radiobiology for the radiologist*, 3rd edn Philadelphia: Lippincott 1988, pp 18–38.

217 Sangiorgi G, Kline RW, Bonner JA *et al.* 17 kilovolt beta-radiation induces apoptosis following experimental balloon angioplasty: results in a tissue culture model. Restenosis Summit IX, 1997.

218 Popowski Y, Verin V, Papirov I *et al.* High dose rate brachytherapy for prevention of restenosis after percutaneous transluminal coronary angioplasty: preliminary dosimetric tests of a new source presentation. *Int J Radiation Oncol Biol Phys* 1995;**33**:211–5.

219 Condado JA, Gurdiel O, Espinoza R *et al.* Percutaneous transluminal coronary angioplasty (PTCA) and intracoronary radiation therphy (IRT): a possible new modality for treatment of coronary restenosis. A preliminary report of the first 10 patients treated with intracoronary radiation therapy. *J Am Coll Cardiol* 1995;**38**:228A (abstract).

220 Liermann D, Bottcher HD, Kollath J *et al.* Prophylactic endovascular radiotherapy to prevent intimal hyperplasia after stent implantation in femoropopliteal arteries. *Cardiovasc Interv Radiol* 1994;**17**:12–16.

221 Bottcher HD, Schopohl B, Liermann D, Kollath J, Adamietz IA. Endovascular irradiation – a new method to avoid recurrent stenosis after stent implantation in peripheral arteries: technique and preliminary results. *Int J Radiation Oncol Biol Phys* 1994;**29**:183–6.

222 Massullo V, Teirstein PS, Jani S *et al.* Endovascular brachytherapy to inhibit coronary artery restenosis: an introduction to the SCRIPPS Coronary Radiation to Inhibit Proliferation Post Stenting Trial. *Int J Radiation Oncol* 1996;**36**: 973–5.

223 Grant MB, Wargovich TJ, Ellis EA *et al.* Localization of insulin growth factor I and inhibition of coronary smooth muscle cell growth by somatostatin analogues in human coronary smooth muscle cells: a potential treatment for restenosis? *Circulation* 1994;**89**: 1511–17.

224 Lundergan CF, Foegh ML, Ramwell PW. Peptide inhibition of myointimal proliferation by angiopeptin, a somatostatin analogue. *J Am Coll Cardiol* 1991;**17**:132B–136B.

225 Santoian EC, Schneider JE, Gravanis MB *et al.* Angiopeptin inhibits intimal hyperplasia after angioplasty in porcine coronary arteries. *Circulation* 1993;**88**:11–14.

226 Kent KM, Williams DO, Cassagneau B *et al.* Double blind, controlled trial of the effect of angiopeptin on coronary restenosis following balloon angioplasty. *Circulation* 1993;**88**:506 (abstract).

227 Eriksen UH, Amtorp, Bagger JP *et al.*, for the Angiopeptin Study Group. Continuous angiopeptin infusion reduces coronary restenosis following coronary angioplasty. *Circulation* 1993;**88**:594 (abstract).

228 Emanuelsson H, Beatt KJ, Bagger JP *et al.* Long-term effect of angiopeptin treatment in coronary angioplasty: reduction of clinical events but not angiographic restenosis. *Circulation* 1995;**91**: 1689–96.

229 Liu MW, Roubin GS, Robinson KA *et al.* Trapidil in preventing restenosis after balloon angioplasty in the atherosclerotic rabbit. *Circulation* 1990;**81**:1089–93.

230 Maresta A, Balducelli M, Cantini L *et al.* Trapidil (triazolopyrimidine), a platelet-derived growth factor antagonist, reduces restenosis after percutaneous transluminal coronary angioplasty: results of the randomized, double-blind STARC study. *Circulation* 1994;**90**: 2710–15.

231 Ohno T, Gordon D, San H *et al.* Gene therapy for vascular smooth muscle cell proliferation after arterial injury. *Science* 1994;**265**:781–4.

232 Chapman G, Lim CS, Gammon RS *et al.* Gene transfer into coronary arteries of intact animals with a percutaneous balloon catheter. *Circ Res* 1992;**71**:27–33.

233 Morishita R, Gibbons GH, Kaneda Y, Ogihara T, Dzau VJ. Novel in vitro gene transfer method for study of local modulators in vascular smooth muscle cells. *Hypertension*1993;**21**:894–9.

234 Mazur W, Ali NM, Geske RS *et al.* Lipofectin-mediated versus adenovirus-mediated gene transfer in vitro and in vivo: comparison of canine and porcine models systems. *Coronary Artery Dis* 1994;**5**:779–86.

235 Kahn ML, Lee SW, Dichek D. Optimization of retroviral vector-mediated gene transfer into endothelial cells in vitro. *Circ Res* 1992;**71**: 1508–17.

236 French BA, Mazur W, Ali NM *et al.* Percutaneous transluminal in vivo gene transfer by recombinant adenovirus in normal porcine coronary arteries, atherosclerotic arteries, and two models of coronary restenosis. *Circulation* 1994;**90**:2402–13.

237 Epstein S, Siegall C, Biro S *et al.* Cytotoxic effects of a recombinant chimeric toxin on rapidly proliferating vascular smooth muscle cells. *Circulation* 1991;**84**:778–87.

238 Pickering G, Weir L, Jekanowski J, Isner J. Inhibition of proliferation of human vascular smooth muscle cells using antisense oligonucleotides to PCNA. *J Am Coll Cardiol* 1992;**19**:165A (abstract).

239 Pickering JC, Bacha P, Weir L *et al.* Prevention of smooth muscle cells outgrowth from human

989

atherosclerotic plaque by a recombinant cytotoxin specific for epidermal growth factor receptor. *J Clin Invest* 1993;**91**:724–9.

240 Biro S, Siegall CB, Fu YM *et al*. In vitro effects of a recombinant toxin targeted to the fibroblast growth factor receptor on rat vascular smooth muscle and endothelial cells. *Circ Res* 1992;**71**: 640–5.

241 Casscells W, Lappi DA, Olwin BB *et al*. Elimination of smooth muscle cells in experimental restenosis: targeting of fibroblast growth factor receptors. *Proc Natl Acad Sci USA* 1992;**89**:7159–63.

242 Chang MW, Barr E, Seltzer J *et al*. Cytostatic gene therapy for vascular proliferative disorders with a constitutively active form of the retinoblastoma gene product. *Science* 1995;**267**: 518–22.

243 von der Leyen H, Gibbons G, Morishita R *et al*. Gene therapy inhibiting neointimal vascular lesion: in vivo transfer of endothelial cell nitric oxide synthase gene. *Proc Natl Acad Sci USA* 1995;**92**:1137–41.

244 Nabel EG, Plautz G, Boyce FM, Stanley JC, Nabel GJ. Recombinant gene expression in vivo within endothelial cells on the arterial wall. *Science* 1989;**244**:1342–4.

245 Thompson MM, Budd JS, Eady SL *et al*. Endothelial cell seeding of damaged native vascular surfaces: prostacycline production. *Eur J Vasc Surg* 1992;**6**:487–93.

246 Thompson MM, Budd JS, Eady SL, James RFL, Bell PRF. A method to seed transluminal angioplasty sites with endothelial cells using a double balloon catheter. *Eur J Vasc Surg* 1993; **7**:113–21.

247 Baker JE, Nikolaychick V, Sahota H *et al*. Reconstruction of balloon injured artery with fibrin glue/endothelial cell matrix. *Circulation* 1994;**90–4**:1–492.

248 Ortu P, LaMuraglia GM, Roberts G, Flotte TJ, Hasan T. Photodynamic therapy of arteries. A novel approach for treatment of experimental intimal hyperplasia. *Circulation* 1992;**85**: 1189–96.

249 Eton D, Borhani M, Spero K *et al*. Photodynamic therapy. Cytotoxicity of aluminium phthalocyanin on intimal hyperplasia: acute and chronic. *J Vasc Surg* 1995;**19**:321–9.

250 LaMuraglia GM, Chandrasekar NR, Flotte TJ *et al*. Photodynamic therapy inhibition of experimental intimal hyperplasia: acute and chronic effects. *J Vasc Surg* 1994;**19**:321–9.

251 Tang G, Hyman S, Schneider JH, Giannotta SL. Application of photodynamic therapy to the treatment of atherosclerotic plaques. *Neurosurgery* 1993;**32**:438–43.

252 Mann GV, Spoerry A, Gray M, Jarashow D. Atherosclerosis in the Masai. *Am J Epidemiol* 1972;**95**:26–37.

253 Glagov S, Weisenberg E, Zarins CK, Stankunavicius R, Kolettis GJ. Compensatory enlargement of human atherosclerotic coronary arteries. *N Engl J Med* 1987;**316**:1371–5.

254 Kamiya A, Togawa T. Adaptative regulation of wall shear stress to flow change in the canine carotid artery. *Am J Physiol* 1980;**239**: H14–H21.

255 Zarins CK, Weisenberg E, Kolettis G, Stankunavicius R, Glagov S. Differential enlargement of artery segments in response to enlarging atherosclerosis plaques. *J Vasc Surg* 1988;**7**:386–94.

256 Langille BL, Bendeck MP, Keeley FW. Adaptations of carotid arteries of young and mature rabbits to reduced carotid blood flow. *Am J Physiol* 1989;**256**:H931–H939.

257 Langille BL. Remodeling of developing and mature arteries: endothelium, smooth muscle, and matrix. *J Cardiovasc Pharmacol* 1993;**21**: S11–S17.

258 Clarkson TB, Prichard RS, Morgan TM, Petrick GS, Klein KP. Remodeling of coronary arteries in human and nonhuman primates. *JAMA* 1994; **271**:289–94.

259 Zarins CK, Lu CT, Gewertz BL *et al*. Arterial disruption and remodeling following balloon dilatation. *Surgery* 1982;**92**:1086–95.

260 Kakuta T, Currier JW, Haudenschild CC, Ryan TJ, Faxon DP. Differences in compensatory vessel enlargement, not intimal formation, account for restenosis after angioplasty in the hypercholesterolemic rabbit model. *Circulation* 1994;**89**:2809–15.

261 Kakuta T, Currier JW, Horten K, Faxon DP. Failure of compensatory enlargement, not neointimal formation, accounts for lumen narrowing after angioplasty in the atherosclerotic rabbit. *Circulation* 1993;**88**:I-619 (abstract).

262 Pasterkamp G, Wensing PJW, Post MJ *et al*. Paradoxal arterial wall shrinkage may contribute to luminal narrowing of human atheroslerotic femoral arteries. *Circulation* 1995; **91**:1444–9.

263 Pasterkamp G, Borst C, Gussenhoven EJ *et al*. Remodeling of de novo atherosclerotic lesions in femoral arteries: impact on mechanism of balloon angioplasty. *J Am Coll Cardiol* 1995;**26**: 422–8.

264 Kovach JA, Mintz GS, Kent KM *et al*. Serial intravascular ultrasound studies indicate that chronic recoil is an important mechanism of restenosis following transcatheter therapy. *J Am Coll Cardiol* 1993;**21**:484A (abstract).

265 Mintz GS, Popma JJ, Pichard AD *et al.* Arterial remodeling after coronary angioplasty: a serial intravascular ultrasound study. *Circulation* 1996;**94**:35–43.

266 Mintz GS, Kenneth MK, Pichard AD *et al.* Contribution of inadequate arterial remodeling to the development of focal coronary artery stenoses: an intravascular ultrasound study. *Circulation* 1997;**95**:1791–8.

267 Kimura T, Kaburagi S, Tashima Y *et al.* Geometric remodeling and intimal regrowth as mechanisms of restenosis: observations from serial ultrasound analysis of restenosis (SURE) trial. *Circulation* 1995;**92**:I-76 (abstract).

268 Libby P, Schwartz D, Brogi E, Tanaka H, Clinton SK. A cascade model for restenosis. A special case of atherosclerosis progression. *Circulation* 1992;**86**(Suppl III):III-47–III-52.

269 Gibbons GH, Dzau VJ. The emerging concept of vascular remodeling. *N Engl J Med* 1994;**330**: 1431–8.

270 Glagov S. Intimal hyperplasia, vascular remodeling, and the restenosis problem. *Circulation* 1994;**89**:2888–91.

271 Isner JM. Vascular remodeling: honey, I think I shrunk the artery. *Circulation* 1994;**89**:2937–41 (editorial).

272 Mogford JE, Davies GE, Platts SH, Meininger GA. Vascular smooth muscle alpha(v)beta(3) integrin mediates arteriolar vasodilatation in response to RGD peptides. *Circ Res* 1996;**79**: 821–6.

273 Lafont A, Guzman LA, Whitlow PL *et al.* Restenosis after experimental angioplasty. Intimal, medial, and adventitial changes associated with constrictive remodeling. *Circ Res* 1995;**76**:996–1002.

274 Staab ME, Srivatsa SS, Lerman A *et al.* Arterial remodeling after percutaneous injury is highly dependent on adventitial injury histopathology. *Int J Cardiol* 1997;**58**:31–40.

275 Shi Y, Pieniek M, Fard A *et al.* Adventitial remodeling after coronary arterial injury. *Circulation* 1996;**93**:340–8.

276 Sangiorgi G, Farb A, Carter CJ *et al.* Contribution of neointima and adventitia to the creation of final lumen area in human coronary arteries treated by balloon angioplasty. *J Am Coll Cardiol* 1997;**29**:742 (abstract).

277 Kuntz LL, Anderson PG, Schroff RW, Roubin GS. Sustained dilatation and inhibition of restenosis in pig femoral artery injury model. *Circulation* 1994;**90**:I-197 (abstract).

58 The prevention of ischemic stroke

H. J. M. BARNETT,
H. E. MELDRUM,
M. ELIASZIW

THE DECLINE OF STROKE AND THE RECOGNITION OF RISK FACTORS

Stroke prevention has emerged as a major obligation for all who engage in the practice of medicine. The evidence that it is an effective pursuit is found in the statistics which reveal that in all developed countries the mortality from stroke has declined and in many, although not in all, the incidence also continues to decline.[1] Where the information is available, the number of useful years of life lost to stroke indicates a dramatic change. Stroke has dropped in Canada from third to sixth place in the disorders depriving patients of years of useful life. There is evidence that this decline is the result of stroke occurring later in life, in men but particularly in women.

The reasons for this decline are less well understood than in other disorders where dramatic decline has been identified. No single agent or change in lifestyle can be credited with this decrease. The possibility is strong that the recognition of risk factors followed by improving strategies to manage them effectively has brought about some but not all of this decline. This decline is not seen in the Eastern European countries where, in contrast to the developed countries, both stroke and heart disease mortality continue to increase. It has been assumed that this difference relates to neglect of manageable risk factors.

THE MANAGEABLE RISK FACTORS

It is beyond the scope of this chapter to detail all the risks which add to the likelihood of stroke. The paramount factors have been dubbed the Four Horsemen of the Stroke Apocalypse, displaying the recognized banners of hypertension, cigarette smoking, diabetes mellitus, and hyperlipidemia.[2] Evidence is now available from grade A trials to affirm that all but diabetes mellitus, when scrupulously managed, will result in a significant decline of ischemic stroke. The new cholesterol lowering compounds, the 3-hydroxy-3-methylglutaryl coenzyme A (HMG-CoA) reductase inhibitors (statins), have been shown to have a beneficial effect on cardiovascular events and stroke. Two meta-analyses of pravastatin tested against placebo have identified benefit within 12 months of beginning of therapy for middle aged subjects.[3,4] In older subjects, trials are needed to evaluate benefit. Stroke and myocardial infarction are reduced when subjects surviving a myocardial infarction receive vigorous anticholesterol therapy and middle to high normal levels are brought into lower ranges of normal.[5] Cigarette smoking studied in grade B observations ⟨Grade B⟩ and hypertension in grade A trials ⟨Grade A⟩ separately are recognized as risk factors.[6,7] Combined, they cause a 20-fold increase in stroke risk. At no age and in neither sex is a systolic blood pressure above 160 and diastolic pressure above 90 acceptable.[8] Substantial reduction of stroke incidence has been noted following cigarette smoking cessation even in elderly subjects and in those who had been heavy smokers for years.[9]

In the case of insulin-dependent diabetes mellitus (IDDM) the target organs which suffer from microvascular obliterative disease (the kidney, retina, and peripheral nerves) can be significantly spared by scrupulous compared to more casual control of hyperglycemia.[10] The large arteries are commonly affected in both IDDM and maturity onset diabetes and both strokes and heart attacks are more prone to occur than in non-diabetics. It has yet to be shown that rigid control of the glucose abnormality will lessen this tendency. Uncontrolled hyperglycemia existing at the time of an ischemic stroke will result in a greater functional loss than in normoglycemic individuals. Thus, all four of the most common culprits demand attention to reduce the risk of stroke.

The Four Horsemen bring about premature and advanced arteriosclerosis. Two other particularly important risk indicators can be added to the manageable conditions: clinical evidence of cerebral and coronary artery arteriosclerosis. Cerebral ischemic events (transient ischemic attacks (TIA) and non-disabling stroke events) as well as angina and other evidence of heart disease are both strong risk factors for stroke; so too is non-valvular atrial fibrillation, which is the most common cardiac lesion resulting in cerebral thromboembolism.

Familial tendencies to ischemic phenomena, especially in the years before age 45, require attention directed to the Four Horsemen. In addition, inflammatory small vessel disease, disorders associated with coagulation abnormalities, and familial forms of non-rheumatic and non-arteriosclerotic varieties of heart disease are to be considered. The widespread occurrence of homocysteinemia, which both brings about premature atheroma and provokes thrombogenesis, suggests that it be sought for in young patients with stroke, with and without a known family history.

Families with histories of premature stroke and heart disease commonly have predisposing risks which can be identified and increasingly can be managed. Extra attention must be given to these factors. A fatalistic attitude is not warranted. Although genetics deals the cards, the playing of them is determined by the environment and this can be altered substantially between the patient and his/her physician. In older patients the risk of stroke is increased and so too is the impact of the vascular risk factors. The older patient should be given more scrupulous rather than less scrupulous care of manageable risk factors.

The type of stroke which threatens is of consequence in deciding upon the therapeutic and preventive strategies. Intracerebral hemorrhage and subarachnoid hemorrhage should be excluded by CT or MR imaging. Further discussion of these entities is beyond the scope of this chapter. Large artery atherothrombotic stroke, cardioembolic stroke, and lacunar stroke are the three common varieties of ischemic stroke. In evaluating their diagnostic features, three considerations are worthy of comment. First, there may be difficulty in assigning the specific cause in a particular individual. The diagnostic prerequisites for two or even three of these causes may be coexistent. Second, each variety is equally likely to present with TIA. Third, diagnostic capabilities keep changing with advancing technology. This adds to diagnostic precision and the ability to define new entities. A good example of this is the compelling evidence from transesophageal echocardiography that atheroma in the arch of the aorta is a major cause of ischemic stroke. The pioneers in this work have claimed recently that 14% of cerebral ischemic events have their origin in this lesion.[11]

Whatever the cause of stroke, all physicians and health care personnel who can influence management are obliged to be alert to risk factors and to encourage their amelioration on an ongoing basis. Attention to them has been a major element in producing chinks in the armor of one of our most disabling disorders and leading causes of death.

ANTITHROMBOTIC STRATEGIES

Anticoagulants and platelet inhibitors have been studied in enough disciplined grade A clinical trials to allow their firm indications and the areas of uncertainty in their application to be spelled out.

Platelet inhibitors

In the late 1950s and mid-1960s two research paths converged. The first involved the identification of platelet fibrin thrombogenesis in producing transient retinal ischemic events. Visible retinal lesions were described and soon were confirmed as platelet fibrin material. By analogy, transient hemisphere attacks were identified as having this pathogenesis and in time the proof of platelet activity in at least some of the hemisphere TIA of arterial thromboembolic origin was apparent. Coincident with these events, investigators in Toronto and presently in New York and Oxford determined that there were safe drugs, sulfinpyrazone, aspirin, and dipyridamole, which altered platelet responsiveness both in the test tube and in experimentally injured arteries.[12-14] Trials of platelet inhibitors in stroke prevention preceded any use of them in other vascular beds. Launched first was a small trial of dipyridamole involving only 169 patients, which showed no benefit.[15] Aspirin was tested next in a factorial study design in which patients received either aspirin 1300 mg daily, sulfinpyrazone 800 mg, both together or double placebo.[16] Patients were randomized if they had recognizable arterial origin for their TIA or non-disabling stroke and did not have recognizable sources for cardioembolism. When 585 patients, two-thirds male and one-third female, had been followed for an average of 28 months, the investigators reported that patients in the two arms of the trial containing aspirin compared with those not on aspirin had a risk reduction of 31% for the combined outcome events of stroke and death. No benefit was detected in the sulfinpyrazone arm. A subgroup analysis reported no benefit for the 200 women in the trial and when the results for men alone were analyzed in a data generated

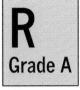

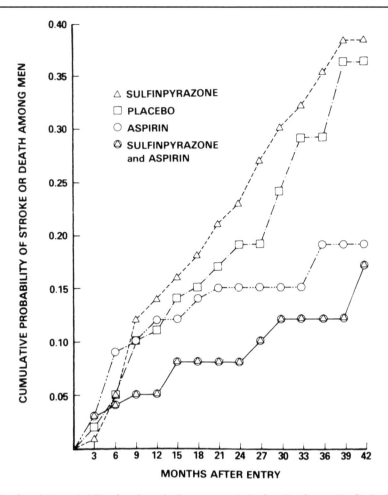

Figure 58.1 Cumulative probability of stroke or death among men in the Canadian Cooperative Study. (Reproduced with permission from CCSG.[16])

subgroup, a 48% benefit in stroke and death was observed in the aspirin containing groups (Figure 58.1).

Since the publication of the Canadian Cooperative Study there has been a flurry of activity. Most importantly, the mode of action of platelet inhibitors has become known. Aspirin has been shown to interfere with the cyclo-oxygenase enzyme responsible for releasing the platelet aggregating substance thromboxane A_2 from the platelet and simultaneously to be responsible for releasing prostacylin produced by the endothelial cell, a powerful antiaggregant.

New platelet inhibitors have been studied. Ticlopidine exhibited modest benefit over aspirin or placebo[17,18] and even more modest benefit was detected for clopidogrel over aspirin.[19]

Omitting from consideration the patients recently involved in the very large clopidogrel study (Clopidogrel versus Aspirin in Patients at Risk of Ischaemic Events – CAPRIE), 14 400 patients with symptoms of TIA and non-disabling stroke of non-cardiac origin have been studied in 15 randomized studies evaluating the above mentioned drugs. In

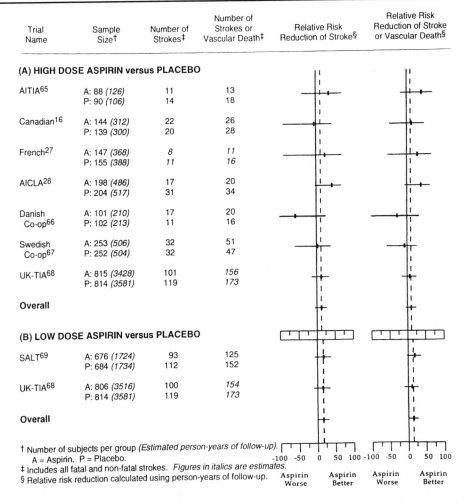

Trial Name	Sample Size†	Number of Strokes‡	Number of Strokes or Vascular Death‡	Relative Risk Reduction of Stroke§	Relative Risk Reduction of Stroke or Vascular Death§
(A) HIGH DOSE ASPIRIN versus PLACEBO					
AITIA[65]	A: 88 *(126)*	11	13		
	P: 90 *(106)*	14	18		
Canadian[16]	A: 144 *(312)*	22	26		
	P: 139 *(300)*	20	28		
French[27]	A: 147 *(368)*	*8*	*11*		
	P: 155 *(388)*	*11*	*16*		
AICLA[28]	A: 198 *(486)*	17	20		
	P: 204 *(517)*	31	34		
Danish Co-op[66]	A: 101 *(210)*	17	20		
	P: 102 *(213)*	11	16		
Swedish Co-op[67]	A: 253 *(506)*	32	51		
	P: 252 *(504)*	32	47		
UK-TIA[68]	A: 815 *(3428)*	101	*156*		
	P: 814 *(3581)*	119	*173*		
Overall					
(B) LOW DOSE ASPIRIN versus PLACEBO					
SALT[69]	A: 676 *(1724)*	93	125		
	P: 684 *(1734)*	112	152		
UK-TIA[68]	A: 806 *(3516)*	100	*154*		
	P: 814 *(3581)*	119	*173*		
Overall					

† Number of subjects per group *(Estimated person-years of follow-up)*.
   A = Aspirin. P = Placebo.
‡ Includes all fatal and non-fatal strokes. *Figures in italics are estimates.*
§ Relative risk reduction calculated using person-years of follow-up.

Figure 58.2 Meta-analyses showing the relative risk reduction of stroke and vascular death among patients with transient ischemic attack or stroke of non-cardiac origin receiving (A) high dose aspirin as compared with placebo and (B) low dose aspirin as compared with placebo. The trials administered high dose aspirin in the range of 900–1300 mg daily and low dose aspirin in the range of 75–300 mg daily. The relative risk reduction is indicated by a solid rectangle, with its corresponding 95% confidence interval (CI) as a horizontal line. The overall relative risk reduction is represented by the broken vertical line. (A) Stroke: 11%; 95% CI, −7 to 26%; P=0.205. Stroke and vascular death: 9%; 95% CI, −6 to 22%; P=0.230. (B) Stroke: 15%; 95% CI, −2 to 30%; P=0.079. Stroke and vascular death: 13%; 95% CI, −1 to 26%; P=0.076. A negative number indicates an increase in risk. All P values are two-tailed. Test for heterogeneity among relative risk reductions in each analysis was statistically non-significant. (Reproduced with permission from Barnett *et al.*[20])

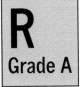

a meta-analysis the odds reduction was 22% for all major vascular events (CV death, MI or strokes) and 23% for non-fatal stroke alone.

Although no single trial in patients presenting with cerebral ischemic events has demonstrated that either aspirin in high or low dose, dipyridamole, ticlopidine or clopidogrel significantly prevents stroke, several showed a trend and the overall results significantly favored treatment.[20] The combined outcome events of stroke and vascular death, in all trials except one, show benefit. The results were similar for high or low aspirin dosage (Figure 58.2).

Ticlopidine does not act on the cyclo-oxygenase enzyme but reduces platelet aggregation by inhibiting the platelet fibrinogen binding mechanisms. Two trials have shown it to be effective in stroke prevention. In 3069 randomized patients with TIA and non-disabling stroke, 1300 mg of aspirin was tested against 500 mg of ticlopidine.[17] At 3 years the relative risk reduction marginally favored ticlopidine. Non-fatal stroke or death had occurred in 19% of the aspirin and 17% of the ticlopidine group for an absolute reduction of 2% ($P=0.048$). Stroke alone, whether fatal or non-fatal, was seen in 10% of the ticlopidine and 13% of the aspirin group, an absolute reduction of 3% ($P=0.024$).

The second trial did not enter patients with TIA, only those who had experienced ischemic stroke.[18] It tested ticlopidine against placebo. Combining three outcome events – stroke, myocardial infarction, and vascular death – the relative risk reduction favoring ticlopidine was 30% ($P=0.006$); the placebo event rate was 15% per year versus 11% with ticlopidine.

Ticlopidine has been heavily promoted as the first choice of antiplatelet agent for stroke-threatening patients, especially those occurring in women, after stroke, and in the posterior circulation. The following must be considered.

1. Its acceptance as superior to aspirin rests upon one study, the differences were modest and occurred mostly in the first 4 weeks.
2. Women benefited in the aspirin and the ticlopidine trials. The exception to this benefit was in the Canadian Cooperative Study. In retrospect, this lack of benefit was likely due to small numbers. It was not known at that time that after TIA or sentinel stroke women have a better prognosis than men and the 200 women in the Canadian study were insufficient to avoid a type II error.[21] The claim that ticlopidine is better for women than aspirin rests on dubious grounds.[22]
3. The fact that the Canadian American Ticlopidine Study (CATS) was for stroke victims alone does not support the claim that after a developed stroke there is superiority of ticlopidine over aspirin in preventing recurrence. The major aspirin trials included stroke as well as TIA. In both the aspirin trials and the ticlopidine CATS, patients with totally disabling strokes were not included for reasons of practicality in follow-up.
4. The claim that ticlopidine is better than aspirin in posterior circulation ischemic events is based on post-hoc analysis and small numbers.[23]
5. Diarrhea occurs in 20% of patients taking ticlopidine and at least 5% must abandon the drug.
6. Bone marrow suppression occurred in about 2% of those who took ticlopidine in the Ticlopidine Aspirin Stroke Study (TASS) and CATS. It was reversible but this reversibility is not a certainty.[24,25] Of the 645 instances of bone marrow suppression known to the manufacturers, 16% have been fatal,[26] some despite monitoring. No patients should receive ticlopidine without clearcut symptoms of cerebral ischemic events or if they are unable to tolerate enteric coated aspirin or continue to have ischemic events despite aspirin. Ticlopidine is the platelet inhibitor of second choice in stroke prevention.

The CAPRIE trial reported on 19 185 patients who had recently experienced either myocardial infarction, ischemic stroke or symptoms of peripheral vascular disease.[19] Clopidogrel, a close chemical relative of ticlopidine, was compared to 325 mg of aspirin, as opposed to the 1300 mg of aspirin against which ticlopidine had been tested. A non-significant benefit for stroke reduction (relative risk reduction 7.3%) favored clopidogrel.

R

Grade A

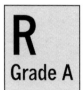

997

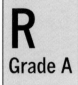

R

Grade A

The combined outcome events of MI, ischemic stroke, and vascular death yielded a relative risk reduction of 8.7% ($P = 0.04$). The absolute risk reduction comparing clopidogrel to aspirin was only 0.5% in favor of clopidogrel. This does not mean that it is of no value in practice. It had fewer side effects than ticlopidine, less diarrhea and skin rash, and the number of patients with non-fatal bone marrow suppression was only 10% of the number with ticlopidine. It is hoped, therefore, that the drug may continue to enjoy this record, replace ticlopidine and become the platelet inhibiting drug of second choice in stroke prevention. For the foreseeable future, blood counts will be required.

Dipyridamole was the first platelet inhibitor to be studied in a small randomized trial against placebo of 169 patients.[15] It was not effective. In three trials, 1575 patients were randomized to receive either aspirin with dipyridamole or aspirin alone.[27–29] In none of these trials was benefit found from the combination of dipyridamole with aspirin in doses of aspirin ranging from 900 to 1300 mg. A new study, the European Stroke Prevention Study 2 (ESPS-2), was published in 1996 wherein 6602 patients were studied in a factorial design.[30] One-quarter of the patients were denied platelet inhibitor, one-quarter received 50 mg of aspirin alone, one-quarter received 400 mg of dipyridamole, and one-quarter received the two active treatments. A benefit for the combined therapy over either single active agent was claimed.

This study must be repeated before it will be given widespread acceptance as evidence of rehabilitation of dipyridamole (in conjunction with ASA) as a stroke preventing drug. The investigators used a dose of aspirin (25 mg b.i.d.) which has never been studied nor proven of value in direct stroke prevention studies. They did not justify why they ignored previous trials with the 20-fold greater dose of aspirin when it might have been expected that two different doses could have been tried. They failed to supervise the conduct of the trial closely enough to observe that one of the major contributors had entered sufficiently dubious data that his 438 patients were eliminated from the sample analyzed for the results.[31] There is no evidence that this affected the results but there is lurking concern that other discrepancies may have been overlooked. The investigators excused the use of a placebo by stating that institutional review boards said it was acceptable despite the evidence from the meta-analyses presented in 1988 by the Anti-Platelet Trialists that there was a 23–25% reduction in stroke with platelet inhibitors. Dipyridamole is not acceptable until the details of closer scrutiny are available pertaining to this trial. To prove its usefulness as an adjunct to aspirin will require another trial using a two-level dose of aspirin. Hopefully, the second dose will be 650–1300 mg daily.

The optimum dose of aspirin in stroke prevention is not known. No adequate trials have been conducted with direct does comparisons. Using meta-analyses in which all platelet inhibitors, all doses, variable endpoints and a variety of target organs are involved is an unsatisfactory way to come to a decision about the dose. There is a serious difference of opinion on this subject.[32–34] Two compelling reasons existed at one point in time to consider the lowest dose. First, it was hypothesized that a larger dose (650–1300 mg) daily would lead to more thrombotic events. It can now be stated that within the range of dosage used in vascular disorders, outcomes have not been shown to be dose dependent.[35] Second, the evidence that serious gastrointestinal, intracranial or wound site bleeding is dose dependent has not been confirmed.[35,36]

The major reasons for avoiding a higher dose have been found to be of little consequence but three other observations must be kept in focus. In the Physicians

Health Study, in which 22 000 male doctors in the United States took either one tablet (325 mg) of aspirin every other day or a placebo, the risk of myocardial infarction (MI) was reduced by 44% and the stroke risk was unaffected by this regimen.[37] Similarly in 87 678 nurses who regularly took modest doses of aspirin, 32% fewer MIs occurred compared with those not taking aspirin. No change in stroke rate was observed.[38] Secondly, the stroke relative risk reductions were in the 25–42% range in the TIA and stroke trials where 900–1300 mg of aspirin daily were employed, compared with the 7–18% range in the trials with lesser dose. Finally, in the North American Symptomatic Carotid Endarterectomy Trial (NASCET) severe stenosis phase, an analysis done post-hoc, and therefore needing confirmation, found a five-fold increase in postoperative strokes in patients who were given 325 mg or less of aspirin daily compared to those taking 650–1300 mg daily. The Aspirin and Carotid Endarterectomy Study (ACE) is randomizing patients to one of four doses, 81 mg to 1300 mg, in whom therapy is begun 24 hours prior to endarterectomy. This trial has entered over 2000 patients and results will be available in 1998.[39]

Until a direct dose comparison study of TIA and stroke patients is conducted, the optimal dose of aspirin remains unknown. It may be more than required for patients with coronary artery disease. Without knowing the optimum dose, using from 50 to 325 mg of aspirin as the "standard" dose against which to judge other therapeutic agents may lead to misleading conclusions.

Our recommendation, based on imperfect data, is that patients with evidence of cerebral or retinal ischemic events of non-cardiac origin take 325 mg enteric-coated aspirin two to three times daily.

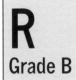

Anticoagulants in stroke prevention

Despite 50 years of empirical use of anticoagulants, it is only in the last decade that heparin and warfarin have been studied in good randomized grade A trials to evaluate their place in stroke prevention. What has been learned may be summarized as follows.

- Patients with non-valvular atrial fibrillation (NVAF) are obligatory subjects for consideration of long term warfarin. Six randomized trials have established this without equivocation.[40–45] Two other trials have compared warfarin with aspirin.[46,47] From a meta-analysis, there is a 64% relative risk reduction of stroke favoring warfarin over placebo and 48% relative risk reduction favoring warfarin over aspirin (Figure 58.3).

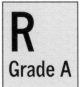

- Patients who are under age 60 and are free of the additional risk factors imposed by a history of systemic embolization, of hypertension with left ventricular hypertrophy, or who have had recent evidence of congestive heart failure should be considered for long term aspirin therapy rather than being put through the enduring risk of complications from long term anticoagulant therapy. Patients over age 75 must be carefully monitored when anticoagulants are used for NVAF and the international normalization ratio (INR) must not exceed 3.0.[33]
- Patients who have had a recent cerebral ischemic event in conjunction with a recent MI should be given heparin therapy followed by 3–6 months of warfarin therapy.[48]

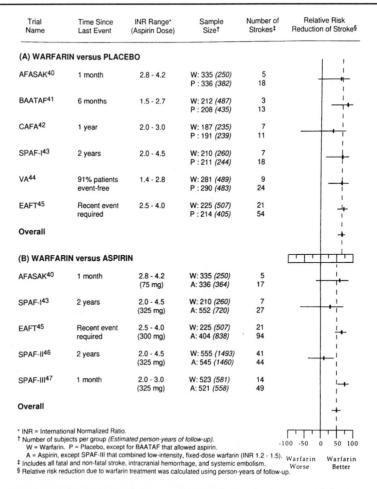

Trial Name	Time Since Last Event	INR Range* (Aspirin Dose)	Sample Size†	Number of Strokes‡	Relative Risk Reduction of Stroke§
(A) WARFARIN versus PLACEBO					
AFASAK[40]	1 month	2.8 - 4.2	W: 335 *(250)* P : 336 *(382)*	5 18	
BAATAF[41]	6 months	1.5 - 2.7	W: 212 *(487)* P : 208 *(435)*	3 13	
CAFA[42]	1 year	2.0 - 3.0	W: 187 *(235)* P : 191 *(239)*	7 11	
SPAF-I[43]	2 years	2.0 - 4.5	W: 210 *(260)* P : 211 *(244)*	7 18	
VA[44]	91% patients event-free	1.4 - 2.8	W: 281 *(489)* P : 290 *(483)*	9 24	
EAFT[45]	Recent event required	2.5 - 4.0	W: 225 *(507)* P : 214 *(405)*	21 54	
Overall					
(B) WARFARIN versus ASPIRIN					
AFASAK[40]	1 month	2.8 - 4.2 (75 mg)	W: 335 *(250)* A: 336 *(364)*	5 17	
SPAF-I[43]	2 years	2.0 - 4.5 (325 mg)	W: 210 *(260)* A: 552 *(720)*	7 27	
EAFT[45]	Recent event required	2.5 - 4.0 (300 mg)	W: 225 *(507)* A: 404 *(838)*	21 94	
SPAF-II[46]	2 years	2.0 - 4.5 (325 mg)	W: 555 *(1493)* A: 545 *(1460)*	41 44	
SPAF-III[47]	1 month	2.0 - 3.0 (325 mg)	W: 523 *(581)* A: 521 *(558)*	14 49	
Overall					

* INR = International Normalized Ratio.
† Number of subjects per group *(Estimated person-years of follow-up)*.
 W = Warfarin. P = Placebo, except for BAATAF that allowed aspirin.
 A = Aspirin, except SPAF-III that combined low-intensity, fixed-dose warfarin (INR 1.2 - 1.5).
‡ Includes all fatal and non-fatal stroke, intracranial hemorrhage, and systemic embolism.
§ Relative risk reduction due to warfarin treatment was calculated using person-years of follow-up.

Figure 58.3 Meta-analyses showing the relative risk reduction of stroke among patients with non-valvular atrial fibrillation receiving (A) warfarin as compared with placebo and (B) warfarin as compared with aspirin. The relative risk reduction is indicated by a solid rectangle, with its corresponding 95% confidence interval (CI) as a horizontal line. The overall relative risk reduction is represented by the broken vertical line. (A) 64%; 95% CI, 51 to 74%; *P*<0.001. (B) 48%; 95% CI, 33 to 60%, *P*<0.001. All *P* values are two-tailed. Test for heterogeneity among relative risk reductions in each analysis was statistically non-significant. (Reproduced with permission from Barnett *et al.*[20])

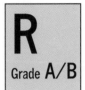

- Based on small studies only, patients will have a reduced incidence of stroke after recent anterior MI if warfarin or heparin is administered.[48,49] When heparin is used at the onset it should be followed for 3 months by warfarin with an INR ranging from 2.0 to 3.5.
- It is not known whether patients with TIA or non-disabling stroke of arterial origin should be given warfarin when platelet inhibitors are not tolerated or events continue despite their administration.
- There is no good evidence that heparin or warfarin is of benefit in the patient whose stroke is progressing.

CLINICAL TRIALS EVALUATING SURGICAL THERAPY IN CAROTID ARTERY DISEASE

Symptomatic disease

The introduction of carotid artery surgery in 1954 by Eastcott, Pickering and Rob heralded a new era in stroke prevention. In 1967 a randomized trial was launched to evaluate this exciting prospect of endarterectomy and the results were published in 1970.[50] The trial, despite being grade A, was not supportive of the procedure. Many problems can be identified. The trial was too small, only 316 patients were randomized. There was a perioperative complication rate of 11%. Almost half of the patients had symptoms only in the vertebral basilar territory. Too many patients were lost to follow-up: 12% in the surgical and 1.3% in the medical group. A second small trial, grade A, conducted at the same time but reported much later, was overwhelmingly negative due to a high perioperative complication rate.[51]

These negative trials did not reduce the enthusiasm for the procedure. By 1985 a total of 107 000 endarterectomies had been carried out annually in the United States and it has been estimated that by 1985 a cumulative total of one million endarterectomies had been conducted for symptomatic and asymptomatic disease. The appropriateness of patient selection and the awareness that in many centers a forbiddingly high level of operative morbidity and mortality existed lead to a requirement for disciplined clinical trials. Three have been conducted for patients with symptomatic disease and four for asymptomatic patients. These will be discussed separately.

Carotid endarterectomy for symptomatic disease

Two grade A trials, the NASCET and the European Carotid Surgery Trial (ECST), have between them randomized close to 6000 patients.[52,53] A third smaller trial, when stopped, had a trend towards the same result but involved only 189 patients.[54] NASCET and ECST required angiography for entry and demanded focal hemisphere or retinal events within 180 days. Both stopped randomization of patients with severe stenosis because of compelling evidence on interim analyses demonstrating a clear reduction in ipsilateral strokes with endarterectomy. In ECST, there was no benefit with surgery for patients with moderate and minor stenosis. NASCET has closed entry but will not analyze the results for patients with moderate stenosis until January 1998.

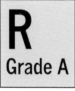

NASCET and ECST used measurement of the narrowest diameter of the stenosed segment as the numerator. The results from NASCET demonstrated a 2-year 65% relative and a 17% absolute risk reduction favoring endarterectomy (Table 58.1). When the ECST angiograms were remeasured by the NASCET method and the results calculated for the reduced number of patients who would be "severe" by NASCET criteria, the favorable results in the survival curves for surgery are very similar.[55] The results from ECST's moderate phase have been published and there is no benefit detected for endarterectomy.[56] Because of the differences in measurement, the patients reported by ECST who did not benefit would be in the low–moderate range of stenosis, <50%, by NASCET criteria. The results from 50–70% from NASCET will be of particular interest.

The compelling results favoring endarterectomy for severe stenosis in NASCET and ECST are dependent on two important facts. First, the surgical complication rate was

Table 58.1 Risk of ipsilateral stroke or any perioperative stroke or perioperative death–NASCET. (Reproduced with permission from *Neurology* 1996;**46**:605)

Study time	Risk (%) medical	Risk (%) surgical	Risk (%) difference	RRR (%)	NNT
30 days	3.3	5.8	−2.5	—	—
1 year	17.3	7.5	9.8	57	10
2 years	26.0	9.0	17.0	65	6

From the North American Symptomatic Carotid Endarterectomy Trial (NASCET), the risk of stroke for 331 medically treated and 328 surgically treated patients with symptoms appropriate to severe stenosis are given at 30 days, 1 and 2 years. To prevent one stroke in 2 years, six patients need to have endarterectomy.
RRR, relative risk reduction; NNT, number needed to treat by endarterectomy to prevent one stroke within the specified study time.

low. In NASCET the occurrence of any stroke, disabling or mild, lasting more than 24 hours or death in the 30-day period was 5.8%. For disabling stroke and perioperative death, the complication rate was 2.1%. A perioperative complication rate of 10% negates benefit. Surgeons must have above-average skill. Second, the results relate to a measurement of the degree of stenosis from conventional carotid angiograms.

Enthusiasts for ultrasonography have been recommending that ultrasound alone is adequate.[57] Unhappily, some patients known to benefit from endarterectomy will be erroneously considered by ultrasound to be in the moderate range.[58] Conversely, an overreading of the ultrasound commonly leads to endarterectomy where benefit is not known to exist. Ultrasound will not identify important lesions. The condition of the intracranial arteries is not studied. Intracranial stenosing or occluding lesions exist in about 5% of patients symptomatic with extracranial stenosis. If intracranial stenosis is as severe as the extracranial disease, the rationale for endarterectomy is not only questionable but the operative risk is doubled, making benefit dubious. Ultrasound does not identify intracranial aneurysm present in about 2% of the NASCET angiograms. It overlooks soft thrombi in the carotid arteries, visualized in 2% of all angiograms from NASCET and 4.3% in the angiograms with ≥ 70% of stenosis. This dangerous lesion carries an operative risk of about 20% and is one of the few vascular risk factors not eliminated by endarterectomy. Medically treated patients have an equally high 30-day stroke risk, thereby presenting a major therapeutic dilemma. One month on anticoagulant therapy is the current empirically based recommendation, with endarterectomy recommended when and if the intraluminal thrombus disappears.

Conventional angiography carries a risk. A worldwide literature review reported a 1% stroke complication rate; one stroke in five was disabling.[59] In NASCET, from 2929 angiograms performed in 100 centers, the minor and non-disabling stroke rate was 0.6%, the disabling stroke rate 0.1%. This is too high but is only one-tenth of the risk of stroke from endarterectomy: 5.8% for any stroke or death and 2.1% for disabling stroke or death. Patients should not face these odds until endarterectomy is indicated. To date this requires conventional angiography.

Studies from the NASCET database include five particularly interesting observations.

1. A high vascular risk profile compared to a low profile adds to the risk for patients given only medical therapy for symptomatic and asymptomatic carotid lesions

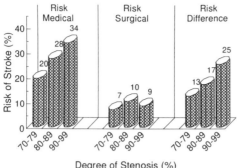

Figure 58.4 Kaplan–Meier estimates of the risk of any ipsilateral stroke at 2 years by degree of angiographically defined stenosis in the symptomatic carotid artery of patients in NASCET. For medically treated patients, the risk of stroke increases with increasing degrees of stenosis, whereas the risk remains similar across all degrees of stenosis for surgically treated patients. The net result, in absolute terms, is that patients with the most severe stenosis receive the greatest benefit from carotid endarterectomy. (Reproduced with permission from Barnett HJM, Meldrum HE, Eliasziw M. Lessons from the symptomatic trials for the management of asymptomatic disease. In: Caplan LR, Shifrin EG, Nicolaides AN, Moore WS. Eds. *Cerebrovascular ischaemia investigation and management.* Med-Orion 1996, p 385.)

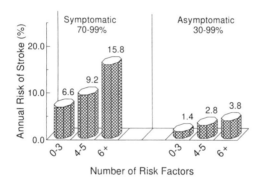

Figure 58.5 Kaplan–Meier estimates of the average annual risk of ipsilateral stroke related to the number of risk factors present. The list of 16 risk factors that comprise the risk profile has been previously published.[52] In the medically treated patients of NASCET with 70–99% stenosis of the randomized carotid artery, the risk of stroke rises with an increasing number of risk factors for both the symptomatic artery and the asymptomatic contralateral artery. (Reproduced with permission from *Neurology* 1996;**46**:606.)

(Figure 58.4). Endarterectomy for symptomatic patients is equally beneficial for high and low vascular risk patients.

2. The prognosis is worst for patients with the most severe degrees of stenosis. Conversely, the surgical benefit is greatest for those with the most severe stenosis (Figure 58.5).

3. The benefit of the operative procedure is durable over an 8-year follow-up (Figure 58.6).

4. Readily identifiable ulcerative lesions carry a three-fold increase in stroke risk compared to medically treated patients without this lesion. Surgical therapy eliminates this without extra risk.

5. Hemisphere TIA have three times the risk of stroke in medically treated patients at 2 years as compared to patients experiencing only retinal TIA.

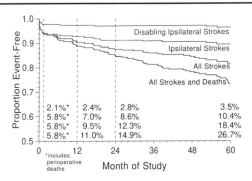

Figure 58.6 Kaplan–Meier curves showing event-free survival after carotid endarterectomy in symptomatic NASCET patients with 70–99% stenosis. The percentages at the bottom are the Kaplan–Meier risk estimates at 30 days, 12, 24, and 60 months respectively for three types of stroke and death. (Reproduced with permission from Barnett HJM, Meldrum HE, Eliasziw M. In: Barnett HJM, Mohr JP, Stein BM, Yatsu FM. Eds. *Stroke*, 3rd edn. New York: Churchill Livingstone (in press).)

Carotid endarterectomy for asymptomatic disease

Four grade A randomized trials have addressed the problem of benefit from endarterectomy in patients with asymptomatic carotid stenosis. A fifth trial has been initiated because of the failure of the first four trials to answer this question satisfactorily. Design flaws prevented conclusive evidence being gained from the Carotid Artery Stenosis with Asymptomatic Narrowing: Operation Versus Aspirin (CASANOVA) and Mayo Asymptomatic Carotid Endarterectomy (MACE) trials. In the CASANOVA trial, patients with ≥ 90% stenosis were excluded and crossovers were commonly allowed from medical to surgical therapy. In the MACE trial the baseline of medical care, particularly of aspirin, was not extended to the surgical arm. The United States VA trial was small, with only 444 patients, and reported a perioperative complication rate of 4.4%.[60] Immediate and long term stroke-free survival curves were similar in patients receiving endarterectomy and those given best medical care alone.

The fourth trial, the Asymptomatic Carotid Atherosclerosis Study (ACAS), randomized 1662 patients and after 2.7 years of average follow-up, claimed a statistically significant benefit favoring endarterectomy with a relative risk reduction of 53%.[61] Table 58.2

Table 58.2 Risk of ipsilateral stroke or any perioperative stroke or perioperative death (based upon 825 patients randomized to CEA) — ACAS. (Reproduced with permission from *Neurology* 1996;**46**:605)

Study time	Risk (%) medical	Risk (%) surgical	Risk (%) difference	RRR (%)	NNT
30 days	0.4	2.3	−1.9	—	—
1 year	2.4	3.0	−0.6	—	—
2 years	5.0	3.5	1.5	30	67
5 years	11.0	5.1	5.9	53	17

From the Asymptomatic Carotid Atherosclerosis Study (ACAS), the risk of stroke is compared between the medically and surgically treated patients. To prevent one stroke in 2 years, 67 patients need to have endarterectomy. Adjusting the surgical arm to include only the patients who had endarterectomy, the 30-day surgical risk becomes 2.6% and the 1-, 2- and 5-year risks rise to 3.3%, 3.8% and 5.4% respectively. The number needed to treat to prevent one stroke in 2 years becomes 83. RRR, relative risk reduction; NNT, number needed to treat by endarterectomy to prevent one stroke within the specified study time.

demonstrates reservations about the clinical significance of this result. The absolute risk reduction is only 1% per year. Sixty seven patients must undergo endarterectomy to prevent one stroke in 2 years. This is in contrast to the six required in symptomatic patients with similarly severe disease. When the perioperative complication rate exceeds 3% the benefits are negated. A higher figure is known to be common. For example, in the ongoing ACE trial, in which 45% of 2000 patients have received endarterectomy for asymptomatic disease, the perioperative stroke and death rate is 4.6%.[39]

All of the symptomatic trials and major observational case-series studies have observed a worsening of prognosis with increasing degrees of stenosis.[62,63] The reduction in strokes after endarterectomy was found to be greatest in those with the most severe stenosis. The ACAS was unable to distinguish between results in the higher or lower range of stenosis, partly because of small numbers of outcome events in a relatively benign disorder and partly because the trial depended upon Doppler ultrasound to characterize the lesion.

A high risk subgroup with benefit from endarterectomy for asymptomatic disease may emerge from ongoing studies. They will possibly be patients with 85–99% stenosis by angiogram measurement and include especially those with a high vascular risk profile. Meanwhile, selected patients who fit this description may reasonably be candidates for endarterectomy conducted by the most expert of surgeons.

Hopefully, the fifth and largest trial being conducted in Europe, the Asymptomatic Carotid Surgery Trial (ACST), will give more information in this direction.[64]

CONCLUSION

Three decades of clinical observation and random trials in stroke prevention have given very positive and promising results.

Key points

- The vascular risk profile which identifies individuals at greatest risk of stroke has been identified. The Four Horsemen of the Stroke Apocalypse are hypertension, diabetes mellitus, high blood cholesterol, and cigarette smoking. All are manageable.
- Aspirin has emerged as the platelet inhibiting drug of first choice for patients threatening further ischemic events of arterial origin. The optimal dose of aspirin is unknown. The authors favor 650–975 mg daily of enteric coated aspirin.
- Ticlopidine is the platelet inhibiting drug of second choice and may be replaced in time by the closely related compound clopidogrel.
- Warfarin is indicated in patients with NVAF. Low risk NVAF patients below age 60 should receive aspirin therapy. In high risk patients over the age of 75, warfarin should be used with caution.
- Warfarin is indicated in patients with or likely to have a left ventricular thrombus as a potential or known source of cerebral ischemic events.
- Heparin appears to be of benefit in preventing stroke in patients with recent anterior myocardial infarction but more studies are required.
- Carotid endarterectomy is indicated for patients with focal hemisphere or retinal symptoms appropriate to a 70–99% carotid stenosis.
- The place of endarterectomy for symptomatic patients with 50–69% stenosis is not yet clarified.
- Despite the clinical trials, there is uncertainty about the place of endarterectomy in patients with carotid stenosis without symptoms.
- Patients with 80–99% asymptomatic stenosis with a high vascular risk profile will probably benefit from endarterectomy if done by surgeons with exceptional skill.

REFERENCES

1 Gale CR, Martyn CN. The conundrum of time trends in stroke. *J Roy Soc Med* 1997;**90**:138–43.

2 Barnett HJMB, Meldrum HE. *Stroke prevention – a medical obligation*. Jacksonville: Florida Medical Association, 1997 (in press).

3 Byington RP, Jukema JW, Salonen JT *et al.* Reduction in cardiovascular events during pravastatin therapy. Pooled analysis of clinical events of the pravastatin atherosclerosis intervention program. *Circulation* 1995;**92**:2419–25.

4 Blauw GJ, Lagaay AM, Smelt AHM, Westendorp RGJ. Stroke, statins, and cholesterol. A meta-analysis of randomized, placebo-controlled, double-blind trials with HMG-CoA reductase inhibitors. *Stroke* 1997;**28**:946–50.

5 Sacks FM, Pfeffer MA, Moye LA, *et al.*, for the Cholesterol and Recurrent Events Trial Investigators. The effect of pravastatin on coronary events after myocardial infarction in patients with average cholesterol levels. *N Engl J Med* 1996;**335**:1001–9.

6 Kawachi I, Colditz GA, Stampfer MJ *et al.* Smoking cessation and decreased risk of stroke in women. *JAMA* 1993;**269(2)**:232–6.

7 MacMahon S, Rodgers A. The epidemiological association between blood pressure and stroke: implications for primary and secondary prevention. *Hypertens Res* 1994;**17**(Suppl):S23–S32.

8 SHEP Cooperative Research Group. Prevention of stroke by antihypertensive drug treatment in older persons with isolated systolic hypertension. Final results of the Systolic Hypertension in the Elderly Program (SHEP). *JAMA* 1991;**265**:3255–64.

9 Wolf PA. Epidemiology and risk factor management. In: Welch KMA, Caplan LR, Reis DJ, Siesjö BK, Weir B. Eds. *Primer on cerebrovascular diseases*. San Diego: Academic Press, 1997, pp 751–7.

10 The Diabetes Control and Complications Trial Research Group. The effect of intensive treatment of diabetes on the development and progression of long-term complications in insulin-dependent diabetes mellitus. *N Engl J Med* 1993;**329**:977–86.

11 Amarenco P, Cohen A, Tzourio C *et al.* Atherosclerotic disease of the aortic arch and the risk of ischemic stroke. *N Engl J Med* 1994;**331**:1474–9.

12 Mustard JF, Rowsell HC, Smythe HA, Senyi A, Murphy EA. The effect of sulfinpyrazone on platelet economy and thrombus formation in rabbits. *Blood* 1967;**29**:859–66.

13 Weiss HJ, Aledort LM. Impaired platelet/connective-tissue reaction in man after aspirin ingestion. *Lancet* 1967;**ii**:495–7.

14 Emmons PR, Harrison MJ, Honour AJ, Mitchell JR. Effect of a pyrimido pyrimidine derivative on thrombus formation in the rabbit. *Nature* 1965;**208**:255.

15 Acheson J, Danta G, Hutchinson EC. Controlled trial of dipyridamole in cerebral vascular disease. *Br Med J* 1969;**1**:614–15.

16 The Canadian Cooperative Study Group. A randomized trial of aspirin and sulfinpyrazone in threatened stroke. *N Engl J Med* 1978;**299**:53–9.

17 Hass WK, Easton JD, Adams HP Jr *et al.* A randomized trial comparing ticlopidine hydrochloride with aspirin for the prevention of stroke in high-risk patients. *N Engl J Med* 1989;**321**:501–7.

18 Gent M, Blakely JA, Easton JD *et al.* The Canadian American Ticlopidine Study (CATS) in thromboembolic stroke. *Lancet* 1989;**i**:1215–20.

19 CAPRIE Steering Committee. A randomised, blinded, trial of clopidogrel versus aspirin in patients at risk of ischaemic events (CAPRIE). *Lancet* 1996;**348**:1329–39.

20 Barnett HJM, Eliasziw M, Meldrum HE. Drugs and surgery in the prevention of ischemic stroke. *N Engl J Med* 1995;**332**:238–48.

21 Dyken ML. Antiplatelet aggregating agents in transient ischemic attacks and the relationship of risk factors. In: Breddin K, Loew D, Uberla K *et al.* Eds. *Prophylaxis of venous, peripheral, cardiac and cerebral vascular diseases with acetylsalicylic acid*. Stuttgart: Schattauer Verlag, 1981, pp 141–8.

22 Hershey LA. Stroke prevention in women: role of aspirin versus ticlopidine. *Am J Med* 1991;**91**:288–92.

23 Grotta JC, Norris JW, Kamm B, TASS Baseline and Angiographic Data Subgroup. Prevention of stroke with ticlopidine: who benefits most? *Neurology* 1992;**42**:111–15.

24 Oh PI, Lanctôt KL, Naranjo CA, Shear NH. Fatal aplastic anemia associated with ticlopidine therapy – approaches to an adverse drug reaction. *Can J Clin Pharmacol* 1995;**2**:19–22.

25 Shear NH. Prevention of ischemic stroke (letter). *N Engl J Med* 1995;**333**:460.

26 Barnett HJM, Eliasziw M, Meldrum HE. Prevention of ischemic stroke (reply). *N Engl J Med* 1995;**333**:460.

27 Guiraud-Chaumeil B, Rascol A, David JL *et al.* Prévention des récidives des accidents vasculaires cérébraux ischémiques par les anti-agrégants plaquettaires: résultats d'un essai thérapeutique contrôlé de 3 ans. *Rev Neurol (Paris)* 1982;**138**:367–85.

28 Bousser MG, Eschwege E, Haguenau M *et al.* "AICLA" controlled trial of aspirin and

dipyridamole in the secondary prevention of athero-thrombotic cerebral ischemia. *Stroke* 1983;**14**:5–14.

29 The American-Canadian Co-operative Study Group. Persantine. Aspirin trial in cerebral ischemia: endpoint results. *Stroke* 1985;**16**: 406–15.

30 Diener HC, Cunha L, Forbes C *et al.* European Stroke Prevention Study 2. Dipyridamole and acetylsalicylic acid in the secondary prevention of stroke. *J Neurol Sci* 1996;**143**:1–13.

31 Enserink M. Fraud and ethics charges hit stroke drug trial. *Science* 1996;**274**:2004–5.

32 Barnett HJM, Kaste M, Meldrum HE, Eliasziw M. Aspirin dose in stroke prevention: beautiful hypotheses slain by ugly facts. *Stroke* 1996;**27**: 588.

33 Hart RG, Harrison MJG. Aspirin wars: the optimal dose of aspirin to prevent stroke. *Stroke* 1996;**27**: 585–7.

34 Patrono C, Roth GJ. Aspirin in ischemic cerebrovascular disease: how strong is the case for a different dosing regimen? *Stroke* 1996;**27**: 756–60.

35 Cappelleri JC, Lau J, Kupelnick B, Chalmers TC. Efficacy and safety of different aspirin dosages on vascular diseases in high-risk patients: a metaregression analysis. *Online J Curr Clin Trials* 1995;Mar 14:doc no 174.

36 Munson RJ, Sharpe BL, Finan JW *et al.*, for the North American Symptomatic Carotid Endarterectomy Trial (NASCET) Group. The NASCET experience of bleeding complications of patients on aspirin. Abstract presented at the 22nd International Joint Conference on Stroke and Cerebral Circulation, February 6–8, 1997.

37 The Steering Committee of the Physicians Health Study Research Group. Special report. Preliminary report: findings from the aspirin component of the ongoing Physicians Health Study. *N Engl J Med* 1988;**318**:262.

38 Manson JE, Stampfer MJ, Colditz GA *et al.* A prospective study of aspirin use and primary prevention of cardiovascular disease in women. *JAMA* 1991;**266**:521–7.

39 Thorpe KE, Taylor DW, for the North American Symptomatic Carotid Endarterectomy Trial Collaborators. ASA and carotid endarterectomy. Abstract presented at the 22nd International Joint Conference on Stroke and Cerebral Circulation, February 6–8, 1997.

40 Petersen P, Godtfredsen J, Boysen G. Placebo-controlled, randomized trial of warfarin and aspirin for prevention of thromboembolic complications in chronic atrial fibrillation. The Copenhagen AFASAK study. *Lancet* 1989;**i**:175.

41 The Boston Area Anticoagulation Trial for Atrial Fibrillation Investigators. The effect of low-dose warfarin on the risk of stroke in patients with nonrheumatic atrial fibrillation. *N Engl J Med* 1990;**323**:1505.

42 Connolly SJ, Laupacis A, Gent M *et al.* Canadian atrial fibrillation anticoagulation (CAFA) study. *J Am Coll Cardiol* 1991;**18**:349–55.

43 Stroke Prevention in Atrial Fibrillation Investigators. Stroke Prevention in Atrial Fibrillation Study: final results. *Circulation* 1991; **84**:527–39.

44 Ezekowitz MD, Bridgers SL, James KE *et al.* Warfarin in the prevention of stroke associated with nonrheumatic atrial fibrillation. *N Engl J Med* 1992;**327**:1406–12. [Erratum, *N Engl J Med* 1993;**328**:148.]

45 EAFT (European Atrial Fibrillation Trial) Study Group. Secondary prevention in non-rheumatic atrial fibrillation after transient ischaemic attack or minor stroke. *Lancet* 1993;**342**:1255–62.

46 Stroke Prevention in Atrial Fibrillation Investigators. Warfarin versus aspirin for prevention of thromboembolism in atrial fibrillation: Stroke Prevention in Atrial Fibrillation II Study. *Lancet* 1994;**343**:687–91.

47 Stroke Prevention in Atrial Fibrillation Investigators. Adjusted-dose warfarin versus low-intensity, fixed-dose warfarin plus aspirin for high-risk patients with atrial fibrillation: Stroke Prevention in Atrial Fibrillation III randomised clinical trial. *Lancet* 1996;**348**:633–8.

48 Cerebral Embolism Task Force. Cardiogenic brain embolism: the second report of the Cerebral Embolism Task Force. *Arch Neurol* 1989;**86**:727.

49 Turpie AGG, Robinson JG, Doyle DJ *et al.* Comparison of high-dose with low-dose subcutaneous heparin to prevent left ventricular mural thrombosis in patients with acute transmural anterior myocardial infarction. *N Engl J Med* 1989;**320**:352.

50 Fields WS, Maslenikov V, Meyer JS *et al.* Joint study of extracranial arterial occlusion. V. Progress report of prognosis following surgery or nonsurgical treatment for transient cerebral ischemic attacks and cervical carotid artery lesions. *JAMA* 1970;**211**:1993–2003.

51 Shaw DA, Venables GS, Cartlidge NEF, Bates D, Dickinson PH. Carotid endarterectomy in patients with transient cerebral ischaemia. *J Neurol Sci* 1984;**64**:45–53.

52 North American Symptomatic Carotid Endarterectomy Trial Collaborators. Beneficial effect of carotid endarterectomy in symptomatic patients with high-grade carotid stenosis. *N Engl J Med* 1991;**325**:445–53.

53 European Carotid Surgery Trialists' Collaborative Group. MRC European Carotid Surgery Trial: interim results for symptomatic patients with severe (70–99%) or with mild (0–29%) carotid stenosis. *Lancet* 1991;**337**:1235–43.

54 Mayberg MR, Wilson SE, Yatsu F *et al.* Carotid endarterectomy and prevention of cerebral ischemia in symptomatic carotid stenosis. *JAMA* 1991;**266**:3289–94.

55 Barnett HJM, Warlow CP. Carotid endarterectomy and the measurement of stenosis. *Stroke* 1993; **24**:1281–4.

56 European Carotid Surgery Trialists' Collaborative Group. Endarterectomy for moderate symptomatic carotid stenosis: interim results from the MRC European Carotid Surgery Trial. *Lancet* 1996;**347**:1591–3.

57 Chervu A, Moore WS. Carotid endarterectomy without arteriography. *Ann Vasc Surg* 1994;**8**: 296–302.

58 Eliasziw M, Rankin RN, Fox AJ, Haynes RB, Barnett HJM, for the North American Symptomatic Carotid Endarterectomy Trial (NASCET) Group. Accuracy and prognostic consequences of ultrasonography in identifying severe carotid artery stenosis. *Stroke* 1995;**26**: 1747–52.

59 Hankey GJ, Warlow CP, Molyneuz AJ. Complications of cerebral angiography for patients with mild carotid territory ischaemia being considered for carotid endarterectomy. *J Neurol Neurosurg Psychiatr* 1990;**53**:542–8.

60 Hobson RW II, Weiss DG, Fields WS *et al.* Efficacy of carotid endarterectomy for asymptomatic carotid stenosis. *N Engl J Med* 1993;**328**:221–7.

61 Executive Committee for the Asymptomatic Carotid Atherosclerosis Study. Endarterectomy for asymptomatic carotid artery stenosis. *JAMA* 1995;**273**:1421–28.

62 Hennerici M, Hulsbomer HB, Hefter H, Lemmerts D, Rautenberg W. Natural history of asymptomatic extracranial arterial disease: results of a long-term prospective study. *Brain* 1987;**110**:777–91.

63 Norris JW, Zhu CZ, Bornstein NM, Chambers BR. Vascular risks of asymptomatic carotid stenosis. *Stroke* 1991;**22**:1485–90.

64 Halliday AW, Thomas D, Mansfield A. The Asymptomatic Carotid Surgery Trial (ACST) rationale and design. *Eur J Vasc Surg* 1994;**8**: 703–10.

65 Fields WS, Lemak NA, Frankowski RF, Hardy RJ. Controlled trial of aspirin in cerebral ischemia. *Stroke* 1977;**8**:301–16.

66 Sorensen PS, Pedersen H, Marquardsen J *et al.* Acetylsalicylic acid in the prevention of stroke in patients with reversible cerebral ischemic attacks: a Danish Cooperative Study. *Stroke* 1983;**14**: 15–22.

67 The Swedish Cooperative Study. High-dose acetylsalicylic acid after cerebral infarction. *Stroke* 1987;**18**:325–34.

68 UK-TIA Study Group. The United Kingdom transient ischemic attack (UK-TIA) aspirin trial: final results. *J Neurol Neurosurg Psychiatr* 1991; **54**:1044–54.

69 The SALT Collaborative Group. Swedish Aspirin Low-dose Trial (SALT) of 75 mg aspirin as secondary prophylaxis after cerebrovascular ischaemic events. *Lancet* 1991;**338**:1345–9.

Venous thromboembolic disease 59

Clive Kearon,
Jeffrey S. Ginsberg,
Jack Hirsh

INTRODUCTION

There are three main aspects to the management of venous thromboembolism (VTE): diagnosis, prevention, and treatment. Before focusing on each of these areas, those aspects of pathogenesis and natural history of VTE which are most relevant to clinical practice will be reviewed.

PATHOGENESIS OF VTE

Virchow is credited with identifying stasis, vessel wall injury, and hypercoagulability as the pathogenic triad responsible for thrombosis. This classification of risk factors for VTE remains valuable.

Venous stasis

The importance of venous stasis as a risk factor for VTE is demonstrated by the fact that most deep vein thrombi (DVT) associated with stroke affect the paralyzed leg,[1] and most DVT associated with pregnancy affect the left leg,[2] the iliac veins of which are prone to extrinsic compression by the pregnant uterus and the right common iliac artery.

Vessel damage

Venous damage, usually as a consequence of accidental injury or manipulation during surgery (e.g. hip replacement), is an important risk factor for VTE. Hence, three-quarters

1009

of proximal DVT which complicate hip surgery occur in the operated leg.[3] Similarly, indwelling venous catheters predispose to thrombosis.[4]

Hypercoagulability

A complex balance of naturally occurring coagulation and fibrinolytic factors and inhibitors serve to maintain blood fluidity and hemostasis. Congenital, or acquired, changes in this balance may predispose to thrombosis. The most important inherited biochemical disorders associated with VTE are due to defects in the naturally occurring inhibitors of coagulation: deficiencies of antithrombin III, protein C or protein S, resistance to activated protein C caused by a single amino acid substitution in factor V (factor V Leiden).[5] The first three of these disorders are rare in the normal population (combined prevalence of ~1%), and have a combined prevalence of ~5% in patients with a first episode of VTE.[6] Activated protein C resistance is comparatively common, occurring in ~5% of the normal population and ~20% in patients with a first episode of VTE.[7] Hyperhomocysteinemia is also a risk factor for VTE.[5] Prothrombotic abnormalities of the fibrinolytic system occur but are rare.[6]

Acquired hypercoagulable states include antiphospholipid antibody syndromes, systemic lupus erythematosus, malignancy, combination chemotherapy, and surgery.[5] Patients who develop immunologically related heparin-induced thrombocytopenia also have a high risk of developing arterial and venous thromboembolism.[8] Unlike the congenital abnormalities, acquired risk factors may be transient, which has important implications for the duration of anticoagulation if they are associated with VTE.

Combinations of risk factors

The risk of developing VTE depends on the prevalence and severity of risk factors. Based on an assessment of these factors (Table 59.1), patients (particularly surgical) can be categorized as having a low, moderate or high risk of VTE (Table 59.2). Probably because it is associated with other risk factors, advancing age is also an important risk factor. Even in the face of multiple risk factors, VTE is very rare before the age of 16 years. However, the risk of VTE increases exponentially with advancing age (i.e. 1.9-fold per decade), rising from an annual incidence of approximately 30/100 000 at 40 years to 90/100 000 at 60 years, and 260/100 000 at 80 years.[9]

NATURAL HISTORY OF VTE

DVT usually starts in the calf[10] (Table 59.3). When DVT causes symptoms, over 80% involve the popliteal or more proximal veins (proximal DVT).[11–13] However, if venography is used to diagnose DVT in asymptomatic high risk patients (e.g. following orthopedic surgery) only about one third of venous thrombi are proximal[3] (Table 59.2). Of patients with isolated calf DVT, about 20% subsequently extend to involve the proximal veins, usually within a week of presentation. Non-extending calf DVT rarely causes pulmonary embolism (PE), whereas proximal DVT often does.[14]

Table 59.1 Risk factors for venous thromboembolism

Patient factors
Previous VTE[a]
Age over 40
Pregnancy, puerperium
Varicose veins
Marked obesity

Underlying condition
Malignancy[a]
Cancer chemotherapy
Paralysis[a]
Prolonged immobility
Major trauma[a]
Lower limb injuries[a]
Familial hypercoagulable state
Heparin-induced thrombocytopenia

Type of surgery
Lower limb orthopedic surgery[a]
General anesthesia >30 min

[a] Common major risk factors for VTE.
Combinations of factors have at least an additive effect on the risk of VTE.

It is estimated that ~10% of symptomatic PE cause death within an hour of onset,[15] and that, left untreated, about one-third of patients with initially non-fatal PE will have a fatal recurrence.[10,16] Untreated, symptomatic, proximal DVT progresses to symptomatic PE in about 50% of cases, and in general, the risk of recurrent VTE is highest within days or weeks of an acute event.[17] The risk of recurrent VTE remains elevated in patients with persistent risk factors (e.g. malignancy, congenital hypercoagulable states) compared to those in whom VTE was associated with a transient risk factor (e.g. surgery).[18-21]

DIAGNOSIS OF VTE

Objective testing for DVT and PE is important because clinical assessment alone is unreliable, failure to diagnose VTE is associated with a high mortality and, although anticoagulation is effective, its inappropriate use needs to be avoided.

DIAGNOSIS OF DVT

Venography is the criterion standard for the diagnosis of DVT.[22,23] However, because of its invasive nature, technical demands, costs, and the risks associated with contrast media, non-invasive tests have been developed, of which venous ultrasound imaging (VUI) and impedance plethysmography (IPG) are most widely used. VUI has a sensitivity for proximal DVT of approximately 95% and a specificity of about 98%[12,13] in symptomatic patients. Coupled with a prevalence of proximal DVT of about 20% in patients who undergo investigation, this translates into a positive predictive value of 92% and a

Table 59.2 Risk stratification for postoperative VTE, frequency of VTE without prophylaxis, and recommended methods of prophylaxis

	Venographic DVT[a]		Pulmonary embolism		Recommended prophylaxis
	Calf	Proximal	Symptomatic	Fatal	
Low risk Less than 40 years and uncomplicated surgery and no additional risk factors	2%	0.4%	0.2%	<0.01%	Early mobilization
Moderate risk More than 40 years or prolonged/complicated surgery or additional "minor" risk factors	20%	5%	2%	0.5%	Low-dose UFH LMWH (~3000 u daily) GC stockings
High risk Major surgery for malignancy or previous VTE or knee/hip surgery or heparin-induced thrombocytopenia	50%	15%	5%	2%	LMWH (>3000 u per day) Warfarin (INR 2–3) Adjusted dose UFH IPC devices

[a] Asymptomatic DVT detected by surveillance bilateral venography.

Low dose UFH: 5000 u of subcutaneous unfractionated heparin preoperatively and twice or three times daily postoperatively.

LMWH: Subcutaneous low molecular weight heparin; higher doses (e.g. ~4000 u once daily with a preoperative start (Europe) or ~3000 u twice daily with a postoperative start (North America)) are used in high risk patients than in moderate risk patients (~3000 u daily with a preoperative start).

GC stockings: Graduated compression stockings, alone or in combination with pharmacological methods.

IPC devices: Intermittent pneumatic compression devices, alone or in combination with graduated compression stockings and/or pharmacological methods.

Warfarin: Usually started postoperatively and adjusted to achieve an INR of 2.0–3.0.

Adjusted dose UFH: Preoperative start with an adjusted, three times daily dose to raise the activated partial thromboplastin time to the upper limit of the normal range.

Table 59.3 Natural history of venous thromboembolism

- Clinical factors can identify high risk patients
- VTE usually starts in the calf veins
- Over 80% of symptomatic DVTs are proximal
- About 20% of symptomatic isolated calf DVTs subsequently extend to the proximal veins, usually within a week of presentation
- PE usually arises from proximal DVT
- The majority ($\sim$70%) of patients with symptomatic proximal DVT have asymptomatic PE and vice versa
- Only one-quarter of patients with symptomatic PE have symptoms or signs of DVT
- About 50% of untreated proximal DVTs are expected to cause symptomatic PE
- The risk of recurrent VTE after anticoagulants are stopped is much higher if there are persistent risk factors for VTE

negative predictive value of 99% for proximal DVT. Isolated calf DVT is more difficult to detect, with sensitivities of approximately 75%. The essential component of VUI is assessment of venous compressibility of the common femoral vein and popliteal vein with the application of gentle ultrasound probe pressure.[12]

IPG has a sensitivity for proximal DVT of about 85% and a specificity of about 95% in symptomatic patients, but generally does not detect isolated calf DVT.[24,25] This translates into a positive predictive value for DVT of about 85% and a negative predictive value for proximal DVT of about 97%. VUI has superior accuracy to IPG for proximal DVT.[25]

Isolated calf DVT cannot be excluded in symptomatic patients with a normal initial VUI and IPG and, since 20% of these are expected to extend into the proximal veins, follow-up testing is required. Two additional tests, over 7–10 days, are generally performed,[26] although one test after 7 days is probably adequate with VUI.[27] Of the tests which are initially normal, approximately 5% of IPG results and 2% of VUI results become positive during serial testing.[26] Serial testing with VUI or IPG has been shown to be a safe management approach in symptomatic patients, with rates of thromboembolism of less than 2% during the 6 months after serial negative testing.[26–30]

The accuracy of VUI or IPG in asymptomatic postoperative patients who have a high risk for DVT is poor; sensitivity for proximal DVT is approximately 60% for VUI[31] and 20% for IPG.[3] Venography is the only accurate test for diagnosing DVT in asymptomatic postoperative patients, but the clinical utility of routine venography in such patients is not known.

A structured clinical evaluation of patients with a suspected first DVT which includes an assessment of symptoms and signs, the presence of an alternative diagnosis to account for the patient's presentation, and risk factors for VTE allows stratification of the pretest probability of DVT into low (prevalence $\sim$5%), moderate (prevalence $\sim$33%), and high (prevalence $\sim$85%) categories.[13] Findings of clinical assessment and non-invasive tests are complementary and can be interpreted as shown in Figure 59.1. Tests for DVT based on measurement of D-dimer molecules, which are formed when crosslinked fibrin is lysed, are being introduced. Some such tests have been shown to have a high negative predictive value for DVT, although their specificity is generally too low for diagnosing thrombosis.[32]

Pregnant patients with suspected DVT can generally be managed with serial non-invasive testing.[29,30] In pregnant patients with normal non-invasive tests that have a

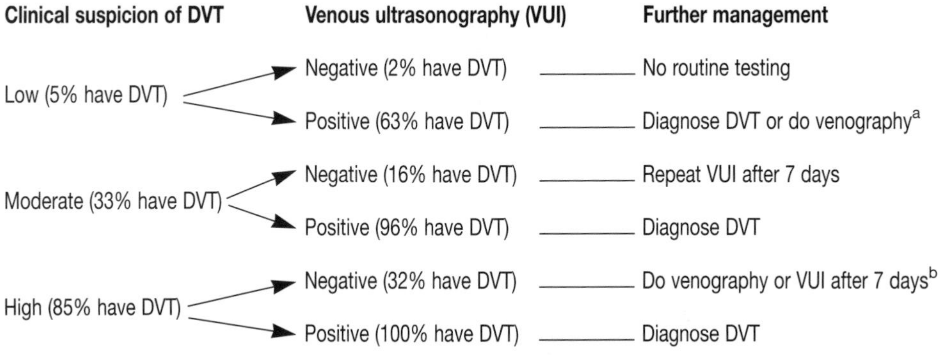

Clinical suspicion of DVT	Venous ultrasonography (VUI)	Further management
Low (5% have DVT)	Negative (2% have DVT)	No routine testing
	Positive (63% have DVT)	Diagnose DVT or do venography[a]
Moderate (33% have DVT)	Negative (16% have DVT)	Repeat VUI after 7 days
	Positive (96% have DVT)	Diagnose DVT
High (85% have DVT)	Negative (32% have DVT)	Do venography or VUI after 7 days[b]
	Positive (100% have DVT)	Diagnose DVT

[a] If VUI shows extensive non-compressibility and there is no suspicion of previous DVT, venography is not necessary.

[b] If symptoms and signs are severe and confined to the calf, venography should be considered.

Figure 59.1   Diagnosis of a first DVT using venous ultrasound. (Data from Wells *et al*.[13])

high clinical suspicion of either isolated iliac or calf DVT, venography (a complete study or a limited study using abdominal shielding, respectively) should be considered.

DIAGNOSIS OF RECURRENT DVT

Persistent abnormalities of the deep veins are common following DVT. Therefore, diagnosis of recurrent DVT requires evidence of new clot formation. A new non-compressible common femoral or popliteal venous segment using VUI, conversion of a normal IPG to abnormal or an intraluminal filling defect on venography are considered to be diagnostic for recurrent VTE. If initial IPG or the VUI is normal, anticoagulation can be withheld and serial testing performed.[33,34]

DIAGNOSIS OF PULMONARY EMBOLISM

Pulmonary angiography is the criterion standard for the diagnosis of PE, but it has similar limitations to venography.[35] The usual initial investigation in patients with suspected PE is a ventilation perfusion scan (Figure 59.2). A normal perfusion scan excludes PE[36] but is found in a minority (10–40%) of patients.[37,38] Perfusion defects are non-specific; only about one-third of patients with defects have PE.[37,39] The probability that a perfusion defect is due to PE increases with size and number and the presence of normal ventilation, as assessed by a ventilation scan ("mismatched" defect).[37,39] Mismatched perfusion defects which are segmental in size or larger are termed "high-probability" defects.[39] A single such defect is associated with a PE prevalence of ~80%.[40] Three or more mismatched defects are associated with a PE prevalence of $\geq 90\%$.[40] The clinical assessment of PE is complementary to ventilation perfusion lung scanning; a moderate or high clinical suspicion in a patient with a high probability lung scan provides grounds for treatment (prevalence of PE of $\geq 90\%$), but a low clinical suspicion

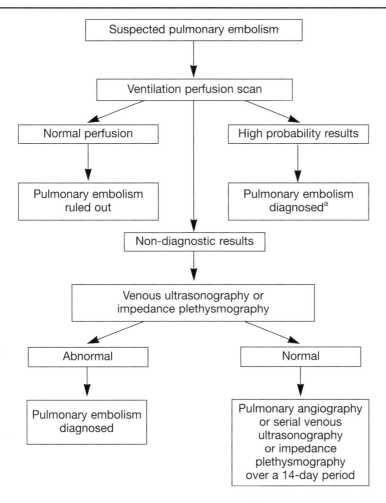

All abnormal perfusion scans which are not high probability for pulmonary embolism when combined with a ventilation scan are non-diagnostic.

[a] Further testing should be performed (i.e. pulmonary angiography) if the clinical suspicion is low for pulmonary embolism.

Figure 59.2 Diagnosis of pulmonary embolism.

with a high probability defect requires further investigation because the prevalence of PE with these findings is only ~50%.[37,39]

Patients with non-diagnostic combinations of clinical assessment and ventilation perfusion lung scan results have, on average, a prevalence of PE of ~20%.[37] Objective tests for DVT, with IPG, VUI or venography, can be performed in these patients. If DVT is diagnosed, it can be concluded that the patient's symptoms are due to PE.[38,39] However, if these tests are negative, further testing is required. Two management approaches are reasonable in patients who have non-diagnostic lung scans and negative tests for DVT. The first is to perform pulmonary angiography, which is usually definitive. The second is to withhold anticoagulants and perform serial non-invasive testing to detect evolving proximal DVT, the forerunner of the recurrent PE. If serial non-invasive testing for DVT (two to three tests) is negative after 2 weeks, the subsequent risk of recurrent VTE during the next 3 months is less than 2%[41] (Figure 59.2). Because the prevalence of PE is expected to be 5% or less in patients with subsegmental, matched, perfusion defects ("low probability"), a low clinical suspicion, and a normal initial non-invasive test for DVT, it is reasonable to withhold anticoagulants without further testing in such patients.

There is the potential for the high negative predictive value of some D-dimer tests to simplify the diagnosis of PE in patients with non-diagnostic lung scans. Similarly, spiral computer tomography may be accurate for the diagnosis of PE. However, there is inadequate evidence to advocate these approaches for clinical management at present.

Pregnant patients with suspected PE can be managed similarly to non-pregnant patients, with the following modifications:

- VUI or IPG can be performed first and lung scanning only performed if there is no DVT; patients with unequivocal evidence of DVT are treated.
- The amount of radioisotope used for the perfusion scan can be halved and the duration of scanning extended.
- If pulmonary angiography is performed, the brachial approach with abdominal screening is preferable.

These recommendations are based on a belief that the risk of inaccurate diagnosis of suspected PE during pregnancy is greater than the risk of radioactivity to the fetus.[42]

PREVENTION OF VTE

In a non-randomized trial, oral anticoagulation was shown to prevent PE in patients with fractured hips, without causing an unacceptable increase in bleeding[43] (Table 59.4). Subsequently, low dose unfractionated heparin was shown to reduce fatal postoperative PE[44] (Table 59.4). Meta-analysis confirmed that low dose heparin reduced the risk of postoperative DVT and fatal PE by ~66%.[45] Further studies have demonstrated that the efficacy of low dose unfractionated heparin can be improved by increasing the dose so as to minimally prolong the activated partial thromboplastin time (aPTT)[46] or by combining its use with graduated compression stockings[47] or intermittent pneumatic compression devices.[48]

Based on laboratory evidence that the low molecular weight fraction of heparin had higher bioavailability and less hemorrhagic potential than the parent compound, clinical evaluation of these agents commenced in the mid-1980s. Meta-analysis supports the belief that low molecular weight heparins (LMWH) are more effective than low dose unfractionated heparin or dextran for the prevention of postoperative VTE[49] and that this difference is of a clinically important magnitude in patients who have the highest risk (e.g. orthopedic surgery, major trauma). There is evidence that aspirin reduces the risk of postoperative VTE but the magnitude of this effect is uncertain.[50-53] Currently, the use of aspirin, as sole agent, is not recommended for the prevention of postoperative VTE.[53] This position may need to be revised when the results of a large ongoing trial (~10 000 patients) evaluating aspirin therapy in patients with hip fractures become available.[54] There is also preliminary evidence that the direct antithrombins (hirulog[55] and hirudin[56]) can prevent postoperative VTE. The evidence that short term prophylaxis (e.g. low dose unfractionated heparin) prevents clinically important VTE in immobilized medical patients is less convincing, partly because it has been less extensively studied

Table 59.4 Landmark trials in the prevention and treatment of VTE

Study	Population studied	Intervention		Outcome	Efficacy		Relative risk	95% CI
		Active	Control		Active	Control		
Prevention								
Sevitt & Gallagher[43]	Hip fracture	OA	Untreated	DVT/PE	4/150 (2.7%)	43/150 (29%)	0.09	0.02–0.25
Kakkar et al.[44]	Surgical	LD heparin	Untreated	Fatal PE	2/2045 (0.10%)	16/2076 (0.77%)	0.13	0.01–0.5
Acute treatment								
Barritt & Jordan[16]	PE	Heparin, OA	Untreated	PE	10/19 (53%)	0/16 (0%)	∞	2.20–∞
UPET I[78 a]	PE	Urokinase	No urokinase	Death	6/82 (7.3%)	7/78 (9.0%)	0.82	0.24–2.7
Gallus et al.[65]	DVT/PE	~4d Heparin	~10d Heparin	DVT/PE	5/139 (3.6%)	6/127 (4.7%)	0.76	0.19–2.9
Hull et al.[66]	DVT	5d Heparin	10d Heparin	DVT/PE	7/99 (7.1%)	7/10 (7.0%)	1.01	0.31–3.2
Brandjes et al.[67]	DVT	Heparin IV	No heparin	DVT/PE	4/60 (6.7%)	12/60 (20%)	0.33	0.08–1.0
Prandoni et al.[69]	DVT	LMWH	Heparin	DVT/PE	6/85 (7.1%)	12/85 (14.1%)	0.50	0.16–1.4
Hull et al.[70]	DVT	LMWH	Heparin	DVT/PE	6/213 (2.8%)	15/219 (6.8%)	0.41	0.13–1.1
de Vaik et al.[73]	DVT/PE	Danaparoid	Heparin	DVT/PE	25/127 (20%)	17/59 (29%)	0.68	0.39–1.2
Levine et al.[71]	DVT	Outpatient LMWH	Heparin	DVT/PE	13/247 (5.3%)	17/253 (6.7%)	0.78	0.36–1.7
Koopman et al.[72]	DVT	Outpatient LMWH	Heparin	DVT/PE	14/202 (6.9%)	17/198 (8.6%)	0.81	0.38–1.7
Oral anticoagulation								
Hull et al.[17]	DVT	OA	LD heparin	DVT/PE	0/33 (0%)	9/35 (26%)	0.0	0.0–0.5
Hull et al.[75]	DVT	INR ~2.1	INR ~3.2	DVT/PE	1/47 (2.1%)	1/49 (2.0%)	1.04	0.01–80
British Thoracic Society[19]	DVT/PE	4 weeks	3 months	DVT/PE	28/358 (7.8%)	14/354 (4.0%)	1.78	1.03–4.0
Schulman et al.[21]	DVT	6 weeks	6 months	DVT/PE	80/443 (18.1)	43/454 (9.5%)	1.91	1.33–2.8
Schulman et al.[77]	2nd DVT/PE	Indefinite	6 months	DVT/PE	3/116 (2.6%)	23/111 (21%)	0.12	0.02–0.40

95% CI, 95% confidence interval of relative risk; OA, oral anticoagulants; LD heparin, low dose subcutaneous heparin.
[a] Urokinase Pulmonary Embolism Trial (Phase 1).

in this population and because there is concern that medical patients remain at high risk of recurrence after prophylaxis is stopped.[57]

In addition to augmenting the efficacy of pharmacologic methods of prophylaxis, mechanical methods can be effective on their own. Graduated compression stockings prevent postoperative VTE in moderate risk patients (risk reduction of 68%),[58] and intermittent pneumatic compression devices prevent postoperative VTE in high risk orthopedic patients.[59,60] The relative efficacy of graduated compression stockings and intermittent pneumatic compression devices is uncertain. No difference in efficacy was evident in neurosurgical patients[61] but pneumatic compression devices are expected to be superior to graduated compression stockings in high risk patients.[53] Mechanical methods of prophylaxis should be used in patients who have a moderate or high risk of VTE and in whom anticoagulants are contraindicated (e.g. neurosurgical patients).[53]

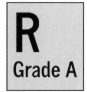

Because postoperative fatal PE is rarely preceded by symptomatic DVT,[44] prophylaxis is the only effective way to prevent it. Use of primary prophylaxis is strongly supported by cost-effectiveness analyses, which indicate that it reduces overall costs in addition to reducing morbidity.[62]

TREATMENT OF VTE

In 1960, Barritt and Jordan established that heparin (1.5 days) and oral anticoagulants (2 weeks) reduced the risk of recurrent PE and associated death[16] (Table 59.4). Based on expert opinion, 10–14 days of heparin therapy and 3 months of oral anticoagulation became widely adopted in clinical practice.

Heparin therapy

Studies in animals suggested that adjusting heparin dose in response to the results of a coagulation test might optimize the efficacy and safety of heparin therapy. This approach was supported by a prospective study which found a three-fold increase in the risk of recurrent VTE in patients who were initially treated with a heparin infusion of 1000 u/hour and who had an aPTT result of less than 1.5 times control for 3 or more days.[63] However, the importance of achieving "therapeutic" aPTT results is uncertain if patients are treated with adequate doses of heparin (i.e. 30 000 u per day by continuous intravenous infusion).[64]

Two studies have shown that 4 or 5 days of intravenous heparin is as effective as 10 days of therapy for the initial treatment of VTE[65,66] (Table 59.4). The assumption, based on indirect evidence, that effective anticoagulation requires an initial course of heparin therapy was verified in a recent randomized controlled trial[67] (Table 59.4). A large number of smaller studies and, in 1992, two larger randomized trials, which primarily evaluated clinical outcomes, established that weight adjusted LMWH (without laboratory monitoring) was as safe and effective as adjusted dose unfractionated heparin for the treatment of acute VTE[68–70] (Table 59.4). Outpatient treatment of acute VTE with fixed doses of subcutaneous LMWH was subsequently shown to be as effective and safe as inpatient treatment with adjusted dose unfractionated heparin[71,72] (Table 59.4) and results in major cost savings. The heparinoid danaparoid also appears to be as effective and safe as unfractionated heparin for the treatment of DVT[73] (Table 59.4) and as it has little immunologic crossreactivity with heparin preparations, it is a good treatment option for patients with heparin-induced thrombocytopenia.

Oral anticoagulation

A randomized trial of patients with DVT which compared 3 months of warfarin (international normalization ratio (INR) ~3.0–4.0) with low dose heparin after initial treatment with full dose intravenous heparin established the necessity for prolonged oral anticoagulation after initial heparin therapy[17] (Table 59.4). Prolonged high dose subcutaneous heparin was subsequently shown to be an equally effective alternative.[74] In the 1970s it was recognized that, because of differences in the responsiveness of thromboplastins to oral anticoagulants, a prothrombin time ratio of 2.0 reflected a much more intense level of anticoagulation in North America than in Europe. This prompted a comparison of two intensities of warfarin therapy (corresponding to mean INRs of ~2.1 and ~3.2) for the treatment of DVT[75] (Table 59.4). This study found that the lower intensity of oral anticoagulation was as effective as the higher intensity but caused much less bleeding (4% vs 22%).

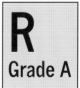

In the 1970s and 1980s, a number of small studies evaluated the optimal duration of oral anticoagulation in patients with VTE, but their results were inconclusive. Subsequently, a large study performed by the British Thoracic Society found that rates of recurrent VTE doubled if the duration of anticoagulation was reduced from 3 months to 4 weeks[19] (Table 59.4). This has been confirmed by two further studies,[20,21] the largest of which, compared 6 weeks and 6 months of oral anticoagulation[21] (Table 59.4). Subgroup analysis of these three studies indicates that patients who develop VTE secondary to a transient risk factor have a lower than average risk of recurrence, and suggest that four or six weeks of anticoagulation may be adequate treatment for these patients. Conversely, patients with idiopathic VTE, or continuous risk factors for VTE (e.g. malignancy, paralysis) had a higher than average risk of recurrence. Based on these observations, a subsequent study randomized patients with a first episode of idiopathic VTE who had been treated for 3 months to either stopping anticoagulants, or remaining on them for a further 2 years. This study was stopped early when clear benefit was shown for remaining on warfarin, despite an associated increase of major bleeding.[76]

Following a second episode of VTE, indefinite anticoagulation greatly reduces the risk of further episodes of recurrent VTE[77] (Table 59.4). However, this is achieved at the cost of an increase in major bleeding (8.6% vs 2.7% over 4 years). It is probable that the optimal duration of anticoagulation following VTE depends on individual risk of recurrent VTE and bleeding and that a previous episode of VTE, although important, is only one of the factors which needs to be considered.

Thrombolytic therapy

Thrombolytic therapy has an unproven benefit in patients with DVT and because of the risk of bleeding, is not recommended. Current evidence indicates that thrombolytic therapy accelerates the resolution of PE, but it has not been shown to achieve long term benefits.[78–80] Until there is evidence of improvement in clinically important outcomes, thrombolytic therapy should be restricted to patients who have hemodynamic instability due to PE.

Inferior vena caval filters

Inferior vena caval filters are used to prevent PE from DVT. A recent randomized trial demonstrated that a filter, as an adjunct to at least 3 months of anticoagulation, reduced the rate of PE from 5.6% to 1.6% during the year following insertion.[81] However, in the second year of follow-up, patients with a filter had a significantly higher rate of recurrent DVT (25% vs 17%), and no statistically significant difference in the rate of PE. This study supports the use of vena caval filters to prevent PE in patients with acute DVT who cannot be anticoagulated (i.e. bleeding), but does not support more liberal use of filters.

Key points

- Primary prophylaxis with pharmacologic and/or mechanical methods should be used in patients who have a moderate or high risk of VTE Grade A.
- Acute VTE (DVT and/or PE) should be anticoagulated with heparin and oral anticoagulants:
  - Heparin (unfractionated or LMWH) should be for a minimum of 4–5 days Grade A.
    If unfractionated heparin is used, a dose of at least (i) 30 000 u/d or 18 u/kg/h by intravenous infusion; or (ii) 33 000 u/d, by twice-daily, subcutaneous injection, should be administered Grade A. Dose of unfractionated heparin should be adjusted to achieve "therapeutic" APTT results Grade C.
  - Oral anticoagulation should be for 3–6 months Grade A, with a dose adjusted to achieve an INR of 2.0–3.0 Grade A. Prolonged therapeutic doses of heparin (unfractionated heparin or LMWH) is a satisfactory alternative Grade A. Anticoagulation should be continued for longer than 3 months in patients with a first episode of idiopathic VTE Grade A and when VTE is associated with a risk factor, for as long as such factors are active Grade C.

TREATMENT OF VTE DURING PREGNANCY

Unfractionated heparin and LMWH do not cross the placenta and are safe for the fetus, whereas oral anticoagulants cross the placenta and can cause fetal bleeding and malformations.[82] Therefore, pregnant women with VTE should be treated with therapeutic doses of subcutaneous heparin (unfractionated heparin or LMWH) throughout pregnancy. Care should be taken to avoid delivery while therapeutically anticoagulated, one management approach being to change from subcutaneous to intravenous heparin at 38 weeks gestation and then to induce labor. After delivery, warfarin, which is safe for infants of nursing mothers, should be given (with initial heparin overlap) for 4–6 weeks.

THE FUTURE

The results of basic research, in conjunction with randomized trials, have greatly improved the safety, efficacy, and cost-effectiveness of management of VTE. However, there are many questions relating to currently available antithrombotic agents which need to be answered and many new antithrombotic agents under development which will require clinical evaluation. Studies are expected to focus on subgroups of patients with different therapeutic requirements, different doses or durations of treatment, and improved methods of anticoagulant monitoring. In addition, the role of thrombolytic therapy for the treatment of PE requires further evaluation; broadening of indications may be appropriate.[80] In order to provide clear directions for clinical management, studies should evaluate clinically important outcomes (i.e. symptomatic VTE, major bleeding).

REFERENCES

1 Turpie AGG, Levine MN, Hirsh J *et al*. Double blind randomised trial of Org 10172 low-molecular-weight heparinoid in the prevention of deep vein thrombosis in thrombotic stoke. *Lancet* 1987;**i**: 523–26.

2 Ginsberg J, Brill-Edwards P, Burrows RF *et al*. Venous thrombosis during pregnancy: leg and trimester of presentation. *Thromb Hemost* 1992; **67**(5):519–20.

3 Cruickshank MK, Levine MN, Hirsh J *et al*. An evaluation of impedance plethysmography and ^{125}I-fibrinogen leg scanning in patients following hip surgery. *Thromb Hemost* 1989;**62**:830–4.

4 Bern MM, Lokich JJ, Wallach SR *et al*. Very low doses of warfarin can prevent thrombosis in central venous catheters. *Ann Intern Med* 1990; **112**(6):423–8.

5 Schafer AI. Hypercoagulable states: molecular genetics to clinical practice. *Lancet* 1994;**344**: 1739–42.

6 Heijboer H, Brandjes PM, Buller HR, Sturk A, ten Cate JW. Deficiencies of coagulation-inhibiting and fibrinolytic proteins in outpatients with deep-vein thrombosis. *N Engl J Med* 1990;**323**: 1512–16.

7 Koster T, Rosendaal FR, de Ronde H *et al*. Venous thrombosis due to poor anticoagulant response to activated protein C: Leiden thrombophilia study. *Lancet* 1993;**342**:1503–6.

8 Warkentin TE, Levine MN, Hirsh J *et al*. Heparin-induced thrombocytopenia in patients treated with low-molecular-weight heparin or unfractionated heparin. *N Engl J Med* 1995;**332**: 1330–5.

9 Anderson FA, Wheeler HB, Goldberg RJ *et al*. A population-based perspective of the hospital incidence and case-fatality rates of deep vein thrombosis and pulmonary embolism. *Arch Intern Med* 1991;**151**:933–8.

10 Alpert JS, Dalen JE. Epidemiology and natural history of venous thromboembolism. *Prog Cardiovasc Dis* 1994;**XXXVI**:417–22.

11 Heijboer H, Cogo A, Buller HR, Prandoni P, ten Cate JW. Detection of deep vein thrombosis with impedance plethysmography and real-time compression ultrasonography in hospitalized patients. *Arch Intern Med* 1992;**152**:1901–3.

12 Lensing AWA, Prandoni P, Brandjes D *et al*. Detection of deep-vein thrombosis by real-time B-mode ultrasonography. *N Engl J Med* 1989; **320**(6):342–5.

13 Wells P, Hirsh J, Anderson DR *et al*. Accuracy of clinical assessment of deep-vein thrombosis. *Lancet* 1995;**345**:1326–30.

14 Kakkar VV, Howe CT, Flanc C, Clarke MB. Natural history of postoperative deep-vein thrombosis. *Lancet* 1969;**ii**:230–2.

15 Stein PD, Henry JW. Prevalence of acute pulmonary embolism among patients in a general hospital and at autopsy. *Chest* 1995;**108**:978–81.

16 Barritt DW, Jordan SC. Anticoagulant drugs in the treatment of pulmonary embolism: a controlled trial. *Lancet* 1960;**i**:1309–12.

17 Hull R, Delmore T, Genton E *et al*. Warfarin sodium versus low dose heparin in the long-term treatment of venous thrombosis. *N Engl J Med* 1979;**301**:855–8.

18 Prandoni P, Lensing AWA, Cogo A *et al*. The long-term clinical course of acute deep venous thrombosis. *Ann Intern Med* 1996;**125**:1–7.

19 Research Committee of the British Thoracic Society. Optimum duration of anticoagulation for deep-vein thrombosis and pulmonary embolism. *Lancet* 1992;**340**:873–6.

20 Levine MN, Hirsh J, Gent M *et al*. Optimal duration of oral anticoagulant therapy: a randomized trial comparing four weeks with three months of

warfarin in patients with proximal deep vein thrombosis. *Thromb Hemost* 1995;**74**:606–11.

21 Schulman S, Rhedin A-S, Lindmarker P *et al.* A comparison of six weeks with six months of oral anticoagulant therapy after a first episode of venous thromboembolism. *N Engl J Med* 1995; **332**:1661–5.

22 Hull R, Hirsh J, Sackett DL *et al.* Clinical validity of a negative venogram in patients with clinically suspected venous thrombosis. *Circulation* 1981; **64**(3):622–5.

23 Agnelli G, Ranucci V, Veschi F *et al.* Clinical outcome of orthopaedic patients with negative lower limb venography at discharge. *Thromb Hemost* 1995;**74 (4)**:1042–4.

24 Hull R, Hirsh J, Sackett DL *et al.* Combined use of leg scanning and impedance plethysmography in suspected venous thrombosis. An alternative to venography. *N Engl J Med* 1977;**296**: 1497–1500.

25 Wells PS, Hirsh J, Anderson DR *et al.* Comparison of the accuracy of impedance plethysmography and compression ultrasonography in outpatients with clinically suspected deep vein thrombosis. *Thromb Hemost* 1995;**74 (6)**:1423–7.

26 Heijboer H, Buller HR, Lensing AWA *et al.* A comparison of real-time compression ultra-sonography with impedance plethysmography for the diagnosis of deep-vein thrombosis in symptomatic outpatients. *N Engl J Med* 1993; **329**:1365–9.

27 Cogo A, Lensing AWA, Koopman MMW *et al.* Compression ultrasound for the diagnostic management of clinically suspected deep-vein thrombosis. *Br Med J* (in press).

28 Hull RD, Hirsh J, Carter CJ *et al.* Diagnostic efficacy of impedance plethysmography for clinically-suspected deep-vein thrombosis. *Ann Intern Med* 1985;**102**:21–8.

29 Hull RD, Raskob GE, Carter CJ. Serial impedance plethysmography in pregnant patients with clinically suspected deep-vein thrombosis. *Ann Intern Med* 1990;**112**:663–7.

30 de Boer K, Buller HR, ten Cate JW, Levi M. Deep vein thrombosis in obstetric patients: diagnosis and risk factors. *Thromb Hemost* 1992;**67**(1): 4–7.

31 Wells PS, Lensing AWA, Davidson BL, Prins MH, Hirsh J. Accuracy of ultrasound for the diagnosis of deep venous thrombosis in asymptomatic patients after orthopedic surgery. *Ann Intern Med* 1995;**122**:47–53.

32 Wells PS, Brill-Edwards P, Stevens P *et al.* A novel and rapid whole-blood assay for d-dimer in patients with clinically suspected deep vein thrombosis. *Circulation* 1995;**91**:2184–7.

33 Hull RD, Carter CJ, Jay RM *et al.* The diagnosis of acute recurrent deep vein thrombosis: a diagnostic challenge. *Circulation* 1983;**67**(4): 901–6.

34 Huisman MV, Buller HR, ten Cate JW. Utility of impedance plethysmography in the diagnosis of recurrent deep-vein thrombosis. *Arch Intern Med* 1988;**148**:519–681.

35 Stein PD, Athanasoulis C, Alavi A *et al.* Complications and validity of pulmonary angiography in acute pulmonary embolism. *Circulation* 1992;**85**:462–8.

36 Hull RD, Raskob GE, Coates G, Panju AA. Clinical validity of a normal perfusion lung scan in patients with suspected pulmonary embolism. *Chest* 1990;**97**:23–6.

37 The PIOPED investigators. Value of the ventilation perfusion scan in acute pulmonary embolism. *JAMA* 1990;**263**:2753–9.

38 Hull RD, Hirsh J, Carter CJ *et al.* Pulmonary angiography, ventilation lung scanning, and venography for clinically suspected pulmonary embolism with abnormal perfusion lung scan. *Ann Intern Med* 1983;**98**:891–9.

39 Hull RD, Hirsh J, Carter CJ *et al.* Diagnostic value of ventilation-perfusion lung scanning in patients with suspected pulmonary embolism. *Chest* 1985; **88**:819–28.

40 Stein PD, Henry JW, Gottschalk A. Mismatched vascular defects. An easy alternative to mismatched segmental equivalent defects for the interpretation of ventilation/perfusion lung scans in pulmonary embolism. *Chest* 1993;**104**: 468–72.

41 Hull RD, Raskob GE, Ginsberg JS *et al.* A noninvasive strategy for the treatment of patients with suspected pulmonary embolism. *Arch Intern Med* 1994;**154**:289–97.

42 Ginsberg JS, Hirsh J, Rainbow AJ, Coates G. Risks to the fetus of radiologic procedures used in the diagnosis of maternal venous thromboembolic disease. *Thromb Hemost* 1989;**61**:189–96.

43 Sevitt S, Gallagher NG. Prevention of venous thrombosis and pulmonary embolism in injured patients. *Lancet* 1959;**ii**:981–9.

44 Kakkar VV, Corrigan TP, Fossard DP. Prevention of fatal postoperative pulmonary embolism by low doses of heparin. An international multicentre trial. *Lancet* 1975;**ii**:45–51.

45 Collins R, Scrimgeour A, Yusuf S, Peto R. Reduction in fatal pulmonary embolism and venous thrombosis by perioperative administration of subcutaneous heparin. *N Engl J Med* 1988;**318**:1162–73.

46 Leyvraz PF, Richard J, Bachmann F. Adjusted versus fixed dose subcutaneous heparin in the prevention of deep vein thrombosis after total hip replacement. *N Engl J Med* 1983;**309**:954–8.

47 Wille-Jorgensen P, Thorup J, Fischer A, Holst-Christensen J, Flamsholt R. Heparin with and

without graded compression stockings in the prevention of thromboembolic complications of major abdominal surgery: a randomized trial. *Br J Surg* 1985;**72**:579–81.

48 Ramos R, Salem BI, de Pawlikowski MP *et al.* The efficacy of pneumatic compression stockings in the prevention of pulmonary embolism after cardiac surgery. *Chest* 1996;**109**:82–5.

49 Leizorovicz A, Haugh MC, Chapuis F-R, Samama MM, Boissel JP. Low molecular weight heparin in prevention of perioperative thrombosis. *Br Med J* 1992;**305**:913–20.

50 Imperiale TF, Speroff T. A meta-analysis of methods to prevent venous thromboembolism following total hip replacement. *JAMA* 1994;**271**(**22**):1780–5.

51 Mohr DN, Silverstein MD, Murtaugh PA, Harrison JM. Prophylactic agents for venous thrombosis in elective hip surgery. *Arch Intern Med* 1993;**153**:2221–8.

52 Antiplatelet trialists' collaboration. Collaborative overview of randomised trials of antiplatelet therapy. III:reduction in venous thrombosis and pulmonary embolism by antiplatelet prophylaxis among surgical and medical patients. *Br Med J* 1994;**308**:235–46.

53 Clagett GP, Anderson FA, Heit J, Levine MN, Wheeler HB. Prevention of venous thromboembolism. *Chest* 1995;**108**(Suppl):312S-334S.

54 MacMahon S, Rodgers A, Collins R, Farrell B. Antiplatelet therapy to prevent thrombosis after hip fracture. *J Bone Joint Surg* 1996;**76B**:521–24.

55 Ginsberg JS, Nurmohamed MT, Gent M *et al.* Use of hirulog in the prevention of venous thrombosis after major hip or knee surgery. *Circulation* 1994;**90**:2385–9.

56 Eriksson BI, Ekman S, Kälebo P *et al.* Prevention of deep-vein thrombosis after total hip replacement: direct thrombin inhibition with recombinant hirudin, CGP 39393. *Lancet* 1996;**347**:635–9.

57 Gårdlund B. Randomised, controlled trial of low dose heparin for prevention of fatal pulmonary embolism in patients with infectious diseases. *Lancet* 1996;**347**:1357–61.

58 Wells PS, Lensing AWA, Hirsh J. Graduated compression stockings in the prevention of postoperative venous thromboembolism: a meta-analysis. *Arch Intern Med* 1994;**154**:67–72.

59 Hull R, Delmore T, Hirsh J *et al.* Effectiveness of an intermittent pulsatile elastic stocking for the prevention of calf and thigh vein thrombosis in patients undergoing elective knee surgery. *Thromb Res* 1979;**16**(1/2):37–45.

60 Hull RD, Raskob GE, Gent M *et al.* Effectiveness of intermittent pneumatic leg compression for preventing deep vein thrombosis after total hip replacement. *JAMA* 1990;**263**(17):2313–17.

61 Turpie AGG, Hirsh J, Gent M, Julian DH, Johnson J. Prevention of deep vein thrombosis in potential neurosurgical patients: a randomized trial comparing graduated compression stockings alone or graduated compression stockings plus intermittent pneumatic compression with control. *Arch Intern Med* 1989;**149**(4):679–81.

62 Salzman EW, Davies GC. Prophylaxis of venous thromboembolism: analysis of cost effectiveness. *Ann Surg* 1980;**191**:207–18.

63 Basu D, Gallus AS, Hirsh J, Cade J. A prospective study of the value of monitoring heparin treatment with the activated partial thromboplastin time. *N Engl J Med* 1972;**287**(7):324–7.

64 Anand S, Ginsberg JS, Kearon C, Gent M, Hirsh J. The relation between the activated partial thromboplastin time response and recurrence in patients with venous thrombosis treated with continuous intravenous heparin. *Arch Intern Med* 1996;**156**:1677–81.

65 Gallus AS, Jackaman J, Tillett J, Mills W, Sycherley A. Safety and efficacy of warfarin started early after submassive venous thrombosis or pulmonary embolism. *Lancet* 1986;**ii**:1293–6.

66 Hull RD, Raskob GE, Rosenbloom D *et al.* Heparin for 5 days as compared with 10 days in the initial treatment of proximal venous thrombosis. *N Engl J Med* 1990;**322**:1260–4.

67 Brandjes DPM, Heijboer H, Buller HR *et al.* Acenocoumarol and heparin compared with acenocoumarol alone in the initial treatment of proximal-vein thrombosis. *N Engl J Med* 1992;**327**:1485–9.

68 Leizorovicz A, Simonneau G, Decousus H, Boissel JP. Comparison of efficacy and safety of low molecular weight heparins and unfractionated heparin in initial treatment of deep venous thrombosis: meta-analysis. *Br Med J* 1994;**309**:299–304.

69 Prandoni P, Lensing AWA, Buller HR *et al.* Comparison of subcutaneous low-molecular-weight heparin with intravenous standard heparin in proximal deep-vein thrombosis. *Lancet* 1992;**339**(8791):441–5(abstract).

70 Hull RD, Raskob GE, Pineo GF *et al.* Subcutaneous low-molecular-weight heparin compared with continuous intravenous heparin in the treatment of proximal-vein thrombosis. *N Engl J Med* 1992;**326**:975–82.

71 Levine M, Gent M, Hirsh J *et al.* A comparison of low-molecular-weight heparin administered primarily at home with unfractionated heparin administered in the hospital for proximal deep-vein thrombosis. *N Engl J Med* 1996;**334**:677–81.

72 Koopman MMW, Prandoni P, Piovella F *et al.* Treatment of venous thrombosis with intravenous

unfractionated heparin administered in the hospital as compared with subcutaneous low-molecular-weight heparin administered at home. *N Engl J Med* 1996;**334**:682–7.

73 De Valk HW, Banga JD, Wester JWJ *et al.* Comparing subcutaneous danaparoid with intravenous unfractionated heparin for the treatment of venous thromboembolism. A randomized controlled trial. *Ann Intern Med* 1995; **123**:1–9.

74 Hull R, Delmore T, Carter C *et al.* Adjusted subcutaneous heparin versus warfarin sodium in the long-term treatment of venous thrombosis. *N Engl J Med* 1982;**306**:189–94.

75 Hull R, Hirsh J, Jay R *et al.* Different intensities of oral anticoagulant therapy in the treatment of proximal-vein thrombosis. *N Engl J Med* 1982; **307**:1676–81.

76 Kearon C, for the LAFIT Investigators. Two years of warfarin versus placebo following three months of anticoagulation for a first episode of idiopathic venous thromboembolism (VTE). *VIX International Congress on Thrombosis and Haemostasis*, 1997.

77 Schulman S, Granqvist S, Holmstrom M *et al.* and the Duration of Anticoagulation Trial Study Group. The duration of oral anticoagulant therapy after a second episode of venous thromboembolism. *N Engl J Med* 1997;**336**:393–8.

78 Urokinase Pulmonary Embolism Trial. Urokinase pulmonary embolism trial: phase I results. *JAMA* 1970;**214**:2163–72.

79 Levine M, Hirsh J, Weitz J *et al.* A randomized trial of a single bolus dosage regimen of recombinant tissue plasminogen activator in patients with acute pulmonary embolism. *Chest* 1990;**98**: 1473–9.

80 Goldhaber SZ, Haire WD, Feldstein ML *et al.* Aleptase versus heparin in acute pulmonary embolism: randomized trial assessing right-ventricular function and pulmonary perfusion. *Lancet* 1993;**341**:507–11.

81 Decousus H, for the PRECIP Group. Efficacy and safety of permanent inferior vena cava filters and of a low molecular weight heparin (Enoxaparin) in proximal deep venous thrombosis. *Haemostasis* 1996;**26**(Suppl. 3):A177.

82 Ginsberg JS, Hirsh J, Levine MN, Burrows R. Risks to the fetus of anticoagulant therapy during pregnancy. *Thromb Hemost* 1989;**61**: 197–203.

Peripheral vascular disease

60

JESPER SWEDENBORG,
JAN ÖSTERGREN

EPIDEMIOLOGY

The prevalence and incidence of lower extremity arterial occlusive disease have been examined in several studies. Large cohorts of patients have been questioned about symptoms of intermittent claudication. This has mostly been done using a questionnaire initially designed by Rose.[1] The method has an acceptable specificity but lacks sensitivity and for obvious reasons it does not detect asymptomatic arterial occlusive disease.[2] The prevalence of peripheral arterial occlusive disease varies between studies, with high figures reported from Russia and Finland.[3,4] Most studies report a prevalence of less than 5% in the age group under 50 years. The prevalence is greatly influenced by age, as pointed out in one of the major studies, the Framingham Study.[5] Other important factors are cigarette smoking and sex. Thus, non-smoking women in the age group 55–64 years showed a prevalence of 3.9% compared to smoking men in the age group 75–84 where the prevalence was 14.5%.[5]

In order to detect more specifically lower extremity arterial occlusive disease, studies have been performed measuring ankle pressure with non-invasive techniques. In general, it can be said that the prevalence of disease increases by a factor of 3 compared to studies based on questionnaires. There is a significant correlation between the ankle brachial pressure index (ABI) and the symptom of intermittent claudication, although the correlation is modest with r values between 0.1 and 0.2.[6] Based on such non-invasive methods, 11.7% of a defined population (mean age 66) had peripheral arterial disease.[7] In common with previous studies, it was also shown that there was a strong dependence of age and sex regarding the prevalence of peripheral arterial disease. Thus, assessment of peripheral arterial disease by the symptom of intermittent claudication underestimates the true prevalence[7] but the cut-off point determining what is considered to be a pathological ABI is of great importance for the estimation of the prevalence.[8]

Only a few studies have examined the incidence of peripheral arterial occlusive disease by following normal subjects and determining when claudication appears. In the Framingham Study, the incidence increases from 0.2% in 45–55-year-old men to 0.5% in 55–65-year-old men.[5]

LONG TERM OUTCOME

The natural history of patients with lower extremity peripheral arterial disease has been studied regarding both the fate of the limb and mortality. Among patients with peripheral arterial occlusive disease one of five at most will require surgical correction for their vascular disease.[9] The amputation rate is probably below 2%[5] but decreases if the patients can stop smoking.[10] Patients with peripheral arterial occlusive disease have a two- to four-fold increased risk of dying compared to the normal population. This increased risk is almost solely explained by cardiovascular disease in general and coronary artery disease in particular.[11,12] The severity of the peripheral arterial occlusive disease is also associated with the risk of dying, since the lower extremity arterial disease is a surrogate variable reflecting the severity of atherosclerosis which affects the coronary arteries. After 10 years only 52% of claudicants are still alive.[13] Smoking is also an important predictor of the risk of dying in these patient groups, which adds to the risk.[14] In patients with concomitant three vessel coronary artery disease, survival seems to be improved by coronary artery bypass grafting.[15]

The natural course of intermittent claudication is thus relatively benign in terms of limb survival, as reflected by the low risk of amputation. This may, however, partly be explained by the fact that the mortality among patients with severe disease and high risk of amputation is considerably greater than for patients with mild disease.

Key points – epidemiology and long term outcome

- The prevalence of lower extremity arterial occlusive disease is high.
- Patients with peripheral arterial occlusive disease have a high risk of dying from cardiovascular causes.
- Mortality and morbidity are increased by smoking, hypertension, and the severity of the disease.
- Intermittent claudication has a relatively benign course as reflected by the risk of amputation.

INVESTIGATION OF THE PATIENT WITH PERIPHERAL VASCULAR DISEASE

An adequate history and physical examination provide the basis for proper management of patients with peripheral vascular disease. The history should include a survey of relevant risk factors and possible symptoms of concomitant cardiovascular disease, e.g. angina pectoris.

Palpation of pulses and auscultation in the groins and over the femoral arteries may reveal signs of occlusion or stenoses in the vessels from the iliac artery down to the lower leg. The popliteal artery is best evaluated with the knee slightly elevated from the support and by pressing the tissue in the distal popliteal fossa against the tibia. Palpation at this location is especially important when a popliteal aneurysm is suspected. In cases with more severe ischemia inspection may reveal a diminished growth of hair and nails and eventually distal ischemic ulcers, often located on toes and heels. Elevation of the legs will cause a whitening of the most affected foot which, in the dependent position, typically is more red than the contralateral one due to an increase of blood in the superficial venous plexus.

Measurement of the ankle pressure is of value as a quantitative estimate of the degree of arterial insufficiency. This is easily done with a pen-Doppler detecting the pulse in either the posterior tibial or the dorsal pedal artery when a blood pressure cuff around the ankle is slowly deflated from a suprasystolic pressure. By dividing the measured value by the brachial pressure, the ABI is determined. An index below 0.9 is considered pathological. In patients with diabetes mellitus the ABI may be falsely elevated due to sclerosis of the media of the arteries which resists compression by the cuff.

Further anatomic evaluation of the arterial system is only needed when invasive procedures are indicated. Duplex sonography is usually the method of choice but in most cases has to be followed by angiography, when surgery is planned.

Key points – investigation of the vascular patient
- History and physical examination essential.
- Screen for cardiovascular risk factors.
- Measurement of ankle brachial pressure index valuable.
- Duplex sonography and angiography only when invasive procedures are considered.

INFLAMMATORY VASCULAR DISEASES – THROMBOANGIITIS OBLITERANS

Temporal arteritis, Takayashu's disease of the aortic arch, and several diseases affecting the arterioles and microcirculatory vessels have an inflammatory or immunogenic origin. In this chapter these diseases are not considered.

Thromboangiitis obliterans or Buerger's disease also has an inflammatory component although the pathophysiology is still not fully known. The major pathogenetic factor, tobacco smoke, is, however, clearly established. The patient is usually a young or middle aged man with excessive smoking habits. The disease is segmental and affects both veins and arteries, leading to recurrent thrombophlebitis and, in more severe cases, to multiple ulcerations of toes and fingers due to occlusion of distal arteries. Larger arteries are often affected which in part may be due to concomitant atherosclerotic disease.

The treatment is based on total avoidance of tobacco smoke. Treatment with prostaglandins, especially the synthetic prostacyclin analogue iloprost (see Critical ischemia below), has been shown to have positive effects on pain alleviation and healing of ulcers.[16]

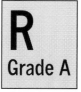

INTERMITTENT CLAUDICATION

Pathophysiology

Intermittent claudication is almost exclusively caused by atherosclerotic lesions in the arteries to the legs. The lesion causing the symptoms may be located above the inguinal ligament (the aorta, iliac artery or the common femoral artery) or below, often in the distal part of the superficial femoral artery. Combinations of series of stenoses or occlusions also involving the popliteal and lower leg vessels are not uncommon.

The evolution of the disease may be slow with a gradual onset of symptoms but in many cases the occurrence of a thrombosis in a severely stenosed area or overlying a ruptured atherosclerotic plaque may cause an acute onset of symptoms.

The most common location of pain is in the calf since the majority of vascular occlusions occur in the superficial femoral artery. When the main lesion is in the iliac region, pain and muscular dysfunction may be located in the gluteal muscles and the thigh. The symptoms are caused by a blood supply inadequate for the metabolic needs of the muscles during exercise. When an occlusion of the artery occurs gradually, collaterals, often from the deep femoral artery, may compensate for the limited arterial supply through the natural artery.

Medical therapy

GENERAL MEASURES

The aim of therapy for intermittent claudication is two-fold: to improve walking distance and thus the quality of life for the patient and to reduce risk factors associated with the disease and thereby improve the long term prognosis.

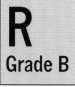

In the general management of the patient it is mandatory to screen for risk factors associated with atherosclerosis. Smoking should be stopped immediately, in which case the risk for the patient with claudication having an amputation in the future is reduced to virtually zero.[10] Hyperlipidemia and hypertension should be treated according to guidelines outlined in other sections of this book. A fear of reducing distal perfusion pressures in patients with claudication by antihypertensive treatment has sometimes hindered doctors in the adequate treatment of hypertension. Beta-blockers have been considered by some to be especially contraindicated in this situation. Controlled studies have, however, shown that treatment of claudicants with beta-blockers only reduces walking capacity marginally or not at all.[17] Therefore, if strong indications exist, such as angina pectoris or a previous myocardial infarction, beta-blockers should be used in claudicants.

If symptoms of increased ischemia of the legs occur during treatment for hypertension, this strengthens the indication for an invasive procedure in order to relieve the symptoms of leg ischemia. If this is not possible, the antihypertensive therapy should be reduced with caution.

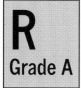

Since patients with intermittent claudication have an increased risk for major cardiovascular events due to their generalized atherosclerotic disease, antiplatelet therapy should be given prophylactically, preferably with aspirin.[18] Combination with dipyridamole may provide an additional preventive effect,[19] but so far only one study has shown an effect on major endpoints by this combination in the case of the secondary prevention of stroke.[20] As an alternative to aspirin, ticlodipine could be given since it has a preventive effect on major cardiovascular events. It has been shown to reduce overall mortality by 29% and may produce some increase in walking capacity in comparison with placebo.[21,22] Further, in 687 claudicants studied over a 7-year period ticlopidine reduced the need for vascular reconstructive surgery by 51% compared to placebo.[23] The disadvantage of this compound is the risk of side effects and the need for laboratory control of white blood cell counts. A possible future alternative to ticlodipine for patients who cannot tolerate aspirin is clopidogrel, which showed a relative risk reduction of 23.8% compared to aspirin in patients with peripheral arterial disease.[24]

EXERCISE

Patients with claudication should be instructed to walk as much as possible, even when pain occurs.[25] Training by intensive walking on a treadmill or outdoors has been shown to be as effective or even better than other programs of physical training and in most cases will improve walking capacity by 100–200%.[25] In some cases, the symptoms of claudication may even disappear completely. The optimal exercise program includes walking to near maximal pain for more than 30 minutes per session at least three times weekly over at least a 6-month period.[26]

PHARMACOLOGIC TREATMENT TO INCREASE WALKING CAPACITY

Different pharmacologic agents have been evaluated for the improvement of walking distance in addition to physical training. Most of these treatments have been inconsistent in their effect and of marginal benefit. Generally, vasodilators have not been shown to be effective. The agent most extensively studied to date has been pentoxiphylline, which is available in most countries for the treatment of intermittent claudication. The patients most likely to respond are those with a claudication history of more than 1 year and an ABI of less than 0.8.[27] In such patients the increase in walking capacity with pentoxiphylline was 99% (190 m) in comparison with 47% (95 m) on placebo.[27] Using Medicare expenditure data, pentoxiphylline is calculated to reduce average hospital costs per patient by $1173.[28] The mechanism behind the effect is believed to stem from positive effects on hemorheologic factors such as a decrease in blood viscosity and an increase of red cell deformability. A recent randomized but open study[29] indicates that prostaglandin E1 given intravenously may be more effective than pentoxiphylline (60.4% compared to 10.5% increase in walking capacity), but further studies are needed to establish the role of prostaglandins in this context.

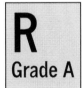

R
Grade A

> **Key points – treatment of intermittent claudication**
> - Quit smoking!
> - Intervention against other cardiovascular risk factors.
> - Regular exercise – walking until intolerable pain.
> - Antiplatelet therapy to be considered.
> - Other pharmacologic therapy is of very limited benefit.

CRITICAL ISCHEMIA

Pathophysiology

When the distal pressure in the leg is too low to provide sufficient perfusion to meet the metabolic demands of the tissue, pain will occur also in the resting situation, particularly in the supine position when there is no contribution to distal pressures from the hydrostatic forces. Subsequently, ulcers in the apical parts of the extremity may develop due to insufficient nutritional blood flow in the skin.

According to the European Consensus Document on chronic critical lower limb ischemia, it is defined as "persistently recurring rest pain requiring regular analgesia for more than 2 weeks and/or ulceration or gangrene of the foot and toes in combination with an ankle systolic pressure less than 50 mmHg". In the case of diabetes, where the measurements of ankle pressure are unreliable because of incompressible arteries, the absence of palpable pulses is sufficient.[30] This definition, however, has been criticized both because many patients with critical limb ischemia according to the above definition still have an intact lower extremity after 1 year, as exemplified by the findings in control groups of randomized trials regarding non-surgical treatment of critical limb ischemia,[31] and also because some patients who do not fit into this definition may lose their legs because of ischemia.[32]

The crucial factor regarding tissue nutrition is the flow through the capillary bed which is dependent not only on the driving pressure in the arteries but also on other factors such as blood viscosity and distribution of flow between nutritional and non-nutritional vessels, i.e. arteriovenous shunts. Intravital capillaroscopy and transcutaneous oxygen tension are methods that can assess tissue nutrition, thereby offering additional prognostic information in these patients.[30] Patients with critical ischemia should be evaluated for possible vascular reconstructive surgery or endovascular treatment (see below).

Medical treatment

When invasive procedures to restore blood flow (see below) are not possible, several therapeutic measures should be considered. Optimization of the hemodynamic situation is one aim. Heart failure and edema should be treated vigorously. Lowering the foot of the bed at night may improve distal perfusion pressure and relieve symptoms. Shoes should be well fitting to avoid the risk of pressure against the skin. Ulcers should be treated with care and dry dressings are generally preferable in order to avoid moisturizing intact skin around the ulcer area.

Though not scientifically proven in this situation, anticoagulation may be of benefit. Thus, oral anticoagulants or low molecular weight heparin should be considered as an alternative or an addition to aspirin, since in the severely ischemic leg both arterial and venous thrombi are common[33] and warfarin has been shown to lower the risk of occlusions in femoro-popliteal vein grafts.[34] Pain should be treated, usually by pharmacologic measures. Spinal cord stimulation could be utilized since this method has been shown to decrease pain, possibly in part by increasing microvascular blood flow.[35] Further long term trials are, however, needed to establish the role of this treatment modality in limb survival.

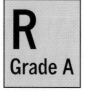

The only pharmacologic agent so far convincingly shown to have a positive influence on the prognosis of patients with critical limb ischemia is a synthetic prostacyclin (iloprost) which is given intravenously daily for a period of 2–4 weeks. In a meta-analysis, rest pain and ulcer size were found to be improved in comparison with placebo treatment and, more importantly, the probability of being alive with both legs still intact after 6 months was 65% (85 out of 130 patients) in the iloprost treated group compared to 45% (56 out of 124) in the placebo treated patients.[31] Pentoxiphylline has been shown to be of benefit in the short term as a pain reliever but no long term trials have been performed.[36]

Key points – treatment of critical ischemia

- Evaluate possibilities for revascularization.
- Optimize cardiac hemodynamics.
- Avoid hypotension – lower foot of bed at night.
- Adequate pain relief.
- Optimal local skin and wound care.
- Consider anticoagulation or antiplatelet therapy.
- Consider iloprost treatment when revascularization is not possible or has failed.

SURGICAL TREATMENT OF INTERMITTENT CLAUDICATION AND CRITICAL ISCHEMIA

Both conventional open surgery and endovascular treatment will be considered. In the latter group, percutaneous transluminal angioplasty (PTA) in combination with both thrombolysis and stenting is included. The major indications for reconstructive procedures for lower extremity ischemia are critical ischemia and claudication.

Preoperative cardiac evaluation

Since patients with peripheral vascular disease have a high frequency of cardiac comorbidity, the perioperative mortality and morbidity are dominated by cardiac problems. Many attempts have been made to identify patients with a high risk of perioperative cardiac complications. The rationale for such a strategy is to identify patients in need of coronary artery revascularization before the vascular procedure and also to provide a basis for more intensive cardiac monitoring during peripheral vascular surgery. Although not specifically designed for peripheral vascular surgery, clinical risk scores according to Goldman[37] or Detsky[38] have been used. Further tests include ambulatory ECG, dipyridamole thallium scintigraphy, ejection fraction estimation by radionuclide ventriculography and stress echocardiography. All these tests are effective in predicting perioperative cardiac mortality and morbidity but dobutamine stress echocardiography seems to be most promising in a meta-analysis.[39] Patients who have reversible defects on preoperative thallium scintigraphy are at high risk of perioperative cardiac mortality and morbidity[40] and successful coronary revascularization decreases this risk following vascular surgery.[41] Nevertheless, routine evaluation of all patients scheduled for peripheral vascular surgery with thallium scintigraphy is not warranted.[42] The reason for this is that both coronary angiography and the possible later procedure of coronary revascularization add to the risk.[43] Today, it can therefore be concluded that patients with a low risk, as reflected by either absence of angina pectoris or mild

1031

disease, do not benefit from further evaluation aiming at coronary angiography.[44] Patients with high risk according to clinical scoring systems or careful history should be evaluated with dipyridamole thallium scintigraphy or dobutamine stress echocardiography.

Open surgical vascular reconstructions

The vascular reconstructions for lower limb ischemia are mainly divided into aortoiliac and infrainguinal procedures.

SUPRAINGUINAL VASCULAR RECONSTRUCTIONS

In the aortoiliac segment, vascular reconstructive procedures were initially dominated by thromboendarterectomy (TEA), which, however, requires large dissections. After the introduction of bypass grafting with synthetic materials, TEA was largely abandoned except for short localized lesions. The results of aortobifemoral bypass using Dacron grafts for arterial occlusive disease are usually good, with 1-year patency rates in the range of 95%. The patency rates are influenced by the outflow bed so that patients with a patent superficial femoral artery (SFA) have better patency rates than those with an occluded SFA. There are no prospective randomized trials comparing TEA and aortofemoral bypass. TEA is said to have lower long term patency rates and another disadvantage is that the surgical procedure is more extensive. Aortofemoral bypass with a synthetic graft, however, has the disadvantage of risk of infection. Although this is an infrequent complication, it is associated with major morbidity and mortality since an infected graft has to be removed.

During recent years, the number of aortobifemoral reconstructions have declined due to the more frequent use of endovascular methods, particularly PTA with or without stenting. Thus, the extensive procedure of aortobifemoral bypass can be converted into a lesser procedure if at least one iliac artery can be opened with PTA. In such cases the contralateral leg can be revascularized with an extra-anatomic procedure, i.e. femorofemoral bypass. The latter procedure has good patency rates, approximately 90% at 1 year and 65% at 3 years.[45] In patients who are unfit for major surgery and where the iliac arteries cannot be opened up with endovascular procedures, another extra-anatomic bypass can be employed. In such patients axillobifemoral bypass can be used but this type of extra-anatomic bypass is a compromise since it has lower patency rates than aortobifemoral bypass.[46]

INFRAINGUINAL VASCULAR RECONSTRUCTIONS

The standard procedure for infrainguinal occlusive disease is femoropopliteal bypass or bypass to the crural arteries. The latter is often performed in diabetics since their occlusive disease is in many cases more peripherally located than in non-diabetics with atherosclerosis. The most commonly used graft material is the saphenous vein but if this is unavailable arm veins or synthetic grafts may be used. In general, it has been stated that use of autologous material is superior in infrainguinal reconstructions.[47] Some randomized studies have failed to detect a difference in long term patency between synthetic grafts and saphenous vein grafts but this has been the case for femoropopliteal bypass with the lower anastomosis above the knee. For bypass grafts with the lower anastomosis below the knee, autogenous material is clearly preferred.[48] This is particularly true when bypass procedures are done to the crural arteries where the use of synthetic grafts produces dismal results.

When using autologous vein, the original procedure implied excision and reversal of the vein so that the blood can flow freely across the valves. However, the *in situ* technique originally introduced by Hall has in recent years gained more popularity.[49] When using this technique, the saphenous vein is left in its bed, the valves are destroyed by special instruments, and tributaries are identified and tied off. Some prospective randomized trials have been performed comparing the two methods but no definitive advantage with either method has been shown.[50] Therefore, the personal preference of the surgeon often determines which method is be used. The advantage with the *in situ* method is that the larger end of the vein is anastomosed to the larger artery and the smaller end of the vein to the small distal artery. With meticulous technique, it is said that the vein is exposed to less trauma but the valve destruction definitely induces some damage to the vein.

In order to improve long term patency rates, two methods have been employed: graft surveillance and pharmacologic treatment. Postoperative surveillance of vein grafts is used by many surgeons to detect a failing graft which is defined as a graft with a developing stenosis that threatens to reduce the blood flow below a critical level. Only a few randomized studies have been done trying to prove the efficacy of a surveillance program where graft stenosis can be eliminated and the method seems to improve long term patency rates.[51] Whether a graft surveillance program which identifies and treats critical stenosis in the grafts also has a beneficial effect upon amputation rate remains to be shown, however.

Pharmacologic therapy seems to improve the patency rate for infrainguinal vascular reconstructions. Most centers use antiplatelet therapy with acetylsalicylic acid and meta-analysis has indicated that such treatment improves the patency rate.[52] Oral anticoagulants are not used as widely as antiplatelet therapy but many surgeons use them selectively for grafts where the prognosis for some reason is bad. One group in Vienna has, however, performed randomized studies and found that oral anticoagulant treatment improves the patency rate in femoropopliteal autologous vein grafts. After 48 months, they reported 96% limb salvage in patients receiving oral anticoagulants but only 76% for controls.[34] Although not a primary endpoint, survival was also reported to be improved – 72% vs 53% at 5 years.

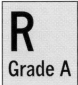

Key points – surgical treatment

- For bilateral suprainguinal occlusions, aortofemoral bypass is the standard procedure but endovascular methods are used at an increasing rate.
- For unilateral suprainguinal occlusions, femorofemoral bypass can be used.
- For infrainguinal occlusions, saphenous vein bypass is the standard procedure but synthetic grafts can be used if suitable veins are lacking.
- Bypass to infragenicular arteries using synthetic grafts produces inferior results compared to saphenous vein bypass.

Endovascular procedures

Since the introduction of transluminal dilation by Dotter, this field has grown enormously.[53] The introduction of percutaneous balloon angioplasty has resulted in widened indications for endovascular procedures, partially at the expense of open surgical reconstructions.

PERCUTANEOUS TRANSLUMINAL ANGIOPLASTY

In common with other vascular reconstructive procedures, the success rate of PTA is highly dependent upon various factors. In general, it can be said that proximal lesions, i.e. iliac lesions, have a better success rate than distal ones, i.e. femoropopliteal lesions. The chance of a successful outcome is higher for stenoses than occlusions, irrespective of the site of the lesion. In common with surgical vascular reconstructions, the outflow also determines the outcome for PTA. Thus, in cases with a good outflow the results are better than if the outflow is poor.[54] In general, it can be said that the chance of success is much higher when dilating a short iliac stenosis in a patient with patent superficial femoral and profunda femoris arteries than after dilation of a popliteal occlusion in a patient with occlusion in two of three crural arteries. The indication for the procedure has, however, to be included in this calculation. PTA of an iliac stenosis in a patient with claudication has a low risk and a high chance of success and may therefore be perfectly appropriate, even if the severity of the disease state is relatively mild as compared to a patient with critical limb ischemia and a threat of amputation. On the other hand, a patient with an occluded popliteal artery and poor leg run-off with ischemic ulceration has a strong indication for the procedure and in such a patient, it may also be perfectly appropriate to make an attempt at PTA, even though the success rate is relatively low. For patients with critical ischemia, PTA of infrapopliteal vessels has also been performed successfully and could even be used for short occlusions.[55,56]

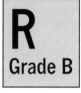

Recently, subintimal angioplasty has been advocated.[57] The method implies that a guidewire enters the subintimal space and then re-enters the vessel distal to the occlusion and the subintimal space is dilated with the balloon. In the femoropopliteal segment, occlusions longer than 20 cm can be treated whereas intraluminal angioplasty is generally not advocated for occlusions longer than a few centimeters. Patency rates of approximately 60% at 3 years for femoropopliteal occlusions have been reported after subintimal angioplasty.[58] The reported figures are patency rates for technically successful procedures but in 20% the procedure could not be performed. The method has also been used for infrapopliteal arteries.[59] Subintimal angioplasty, if proven successful, could be a future alternative to femoropopliteal bypass.

Formal comparisons in prospective randomized trials between PTA and surgery are relatively scarce. Such trials are difficult because in order for a patient to be included, the lesion has to be suitable for PTA, i.e. it should be either a stenosis or a short occlusion. Knowing that the treatment of a stenosis with PTA is relatively successful with less risk and shorter hospital stay, it is sometimes considered ethically questionable to include patients in a trial between PTA and surgery. In a comparative study between bypass surgery and PTA, primary success favored surgery while limb salvage favored PTA but the differences were not statistically significant in a relatively small trial including 263 patients with lesions in the iliac, femoral or popliteal arteries. After 4 years there was no significant difference in outcome.[60]

Randomized trials comparing angioplasty with non-surgical treatment for intermittent claudication have been performed but they are relatively small and the results are to some extent contradictory. In one study the treadmill distances improved in both groups but were superior in those undergoing an exercise program and after 6 years there was no benefit in treadmill walking distance after angioplasty.[61] In another study, an improvement was shown in ABI 6 months following angioplasty which could not be found in patients undergoing exercise programs. Significantly more patients were asymptomatic after 6 months in the angioplasty group as compared to those treated conservatively. This study, however, has a shorter follow-up and the conservative treatment was not as active as in the study where no difference could be seen between exercise program and PTA.[62] Summing up these studies, it can still be concluded that PTA is suitable for stenoses or short occlusions in claudicants but few claudicants have discrete lesions suitable for PTA.[62]

Stenting has been used at an increasing rate over the last few years. It is generally advised not to use stents in smaller arteries and this implies that stents are used relatively seldom in the femoropopliteal region. However, they are used in the iliac arteries after PTA, particularly when there is recoil or dissection. Several types of stents have been used, both self-expandable and balloon-expandable ones. Stenting below the inguinal ligament is not generally recommended.

Thrombolysis

Thrombolysis of peripheral arterial occlusive disease is recommended for acute arterial occlusions but in subacute occlusions it also has a place. Thrombolysis should be intra-arterial and preferably the thrombolytic agent should be delivered into the clot, with either an endhole catheter or a catheter with multiple side holes. Today there is a choice, essentially between three agents: streptokinase, urokinase or tissue plasminogen activator (tPA). Other agents are, however, available and some have been tried for indications other than peripheral arterial occlusive disease. Streptokinase is not generally recommended since it is a foreign protein that may induce an antibody response. Furthermore, one trial has suggested that intra-arterial tPA is superior to streptokinase for lysis of intra-arterial occlusions.[63] The dosage and rate of administration of thrombolytic agent vary between different reports and this makes comparisons difficult.

There are, however, some prospective randomized trials comparing surgery with intra-arterial thrombolytic therapy. In one study, the mean duration of ischemia was almost 2 months and patients were included if the duration was less than 6 months. Overall, the study favored surgery. Patients randomized to catheter directed thrombolysis had significantly greater ongoing or recurrent ischemia, life threatening hemorrhage and vascular complications compared with surgical patients. Stratification by duration of ischemia, however, showed that patients treated within 14 days of onset of symptoms had an amputation rate after thrombolysis of 6% compared to 18% for those undergoing surgery. Patients treated with thrombolysis in this group also had a shorter hospital stay. In patients with acute ischemia the amputation-free survival at 6 months follow-up was also better in those treated with thrombolysis.[64] Further, thrombolysis reduces the likelihood of a subsequent surgical procedure.[65]

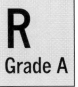

Key points – endovascular procedures

- PTA is more successful for stenoses than for occlusions.
- PTA is more successful for short than for long occlusions.
- PTA may be combined with stent if recoil occurs or if PTA produces dissection with intimal flaps.
- Thrombolysis should be performed by local intrathrombal administration of the drug.
- PTA may be preceded by thrombolysis in cases with recent occlusions.

REFERENCES

1 Rose G. The diagnosis of ischaemic heart pain and intermittent claudication in field surveys. *Bull WHO* 1962;**27**:645–58.

2 Fowkes F. The measurement of atherosclerotic peripheral arterial disease in epidemiological surveys. *Int J Epidemiol* 1988;**17**:248–54.

3 Bothig S, Metelisa V, Barth W *et al.* Prevalence of ischaemic heart disease, arterial hypertension and intermittent claudication, and distribution of risk factors among middle-aged men in Moscow and Berlin. *Cor Vasa* 1976;**18**:104–18.

4 Heliovaara M, Karvonen W, Vilhunden R, Punsar S. Smoking, carbon monoxide and atherosclerotic diseases. *Br Med J* 1978;**1**:268–70.

5 Kannel W, McGee D. Update on some epidemiological features of intermittent claudication. *J Am Geriatr Soc* 1985;**33**:13–18.

6 Feinglass J, McCarthy W, Slavensky R, Manheim L, Martin G. Effect of lower extremity blood pressure on physical functioning in patients who have intermittent claudication. *J Vasc Surg* 1996;**24**:503–12.

7 Criqui M, Fronek A, Barrett-Connor E *et al.* The prevalence of peripheral arterial disease in a defined population. *Circulation* 1985;**71**(3):510–15.

8 Hiatt W. Effect of diagnostic criteria on the prevalence of peripheral arterial disease. The San Luis Valley Diabetes Study. *Circulation* 1995;**91**:1472–79.

9 McGrath M, Graham A, Hill D *et al.* The natural history of chronic leg ischaemia. *World J Surg* 1983;**7**:314–18.

10 Jonason T, Bergstrom R. Cessation of smoking in patients with intermittent claudication: effects on the risk of peripheral vascular complications, myocardial infarction and mortality. *Acta Med Scand* 1987;**221**:253–60.

11 Criqui M, Langer R, Fronek A *et al.* Mortality over a period of 10 years in patients with peripheral arterial disease. *N Engl J Med* 1992;**326**:381–5.

12 Leng G, Fowkes F, Lee A *et al.* Use of ankle brachial pressure index to predict cardiovascular events and death: a cohort study. *Br Med J* 1996;**313**:1440–4.

13 Kallero K. Mortality and morbidity in patients with intermittent claudications defined by venous occlusion plethysmography: a ten year follow up. *J Chron Dis* 1981;**34**:445–62.

14 Reunanen A, Takkunen H, Aromaa A. Prevalence of intermittent claudication and its effect on mortality. *Acta Med Scand* 1982;**211**:249–56.

15 Rihal S, Eagle K, Mickel C *et al.* Surgical therapy for coronary artery disease among patients with combined coronary artery and peripheral vascular disease. *Circulation* 1995;**91**:46–53.

16 Fiessinger J, Schäfer M. Trial of iloprost versus aspirin treatment for critical limb ischemia of thromboangitis obliterans. *Lancet* 1990;**335**:556–7.

17 Hiatt W, Stoll S, Nies A. Effect of beta-adrenergic blockers on the peripheral circulation in patients with peripheral vascular disease. *Circulation* 1985;**72**:1226–31.

18 Antiplatelet Trialists' Collaboration. Collaborative overview of randomised trials of antiplatelet therapy. I: Prevention of death, myocardial infarction, and stroke by prolonged antiplatelet therapy in various categories of patients. *Br Med J* 1994;**308**:81–106.

19 Hess H, Mietaschik A, Deichsel G. Drug induced inhibition of platelet function delays progression of peripheral occlusive arterial disease: a prospective double blind arteriographic controlled trial. *Lancet* 1985;**i**:416–19.

20 Diener F, Coccheri S, Libretti A *et al.* European stroke prevention study 2. Dipyridamole and acetylsalicylic acid in the secondary prevention of stroke. *J Neurol Sci* 1996;**143**:1–13.

21 Balsano F, Coccheri S, Libretti A *et al.* Ticlodipine in the treatment of intermittent claudication. A 21-month double-blind trial. *J Lab Clin Med* 1989;**114**:84–91.

22 Janzon L, Bergqvist D, Boberg J *et al.* Prevention of myocardial infarction and stroke in patients with intermittent claudication: effects of ticlopidine, results from STIMS, the Swedish Ticlopidine Multicenter Study. *J Intern Med* 1990;**227, 228**:301–8, 659.

23 Bergqvist D, Almgren B, Dickinson J. Reduction of requirement for leg vascular surgery during long-term treatment of claudicant patients with

ticlopidine: results from the Swedish Ticlopidine Multicentre Study (STIMS). *Eur J Vasc Endovasc Surg* 1995;**10**:69–76.

24 Caprie Steering Committee. A randomised, blinded, trial of clopidogrel versus aspirin in patients at risk of ischemic events (CAPRIE). *Lancet* 1996;**348**:1329–39.

25 Hiatt W, Wolfel E, Meire R, Regesteiner J. Superiority of treadmill walking exercise versus strength training for patients with peripheral arterial disease. Implications for the mechanism of the training response. *Circulation* 1994;**90**: 1866–74.

26 Gardner A, Poehlman E. Exercise rehabilitation programs for the treatment of claudication pain. A meta-analysis. *JAMA* 1995;**274**:975–80.

27 Lindgärde F, Jelnes R, Björkman H *et al.* Conservative drug treatment in patients with moderately severe chronic occlusive peripheral arterial disease. *Circulation* 1989;**80**:1549–56.

28 Gillings D. Pentoxiphyllin and intermittent claudication. Review of clinical trials and cost-effectiveness analyses. *J Cardiovasc Pharmacol* 1995;**25**:S44–50.

29 Scheffler P, de la Hamette D, Gross J, Müller H, Schieffer H. Intensive vascular training in stage IIb of peripheral arterial occlusive disease. The additive effects of intravenous prostaglandin E1 or intravenous pentoxiphylline during training. *Circulation* 1994;**90**:818–22.

30 The European Working Group on Critical Leg Ischaemia. Second European consensus document on chronic critical leg ischaemia. *Circulation* 1991;**84**(4):1–22.

31 Loosemore T, Chalmers T, Dormandy J. A meta-analysis of randomized placebo control trials in Fontaine stages III and IV peripheral occlusive arterial disease. *Int Angiol* 1994;**13**:133–42.

32 Thompson M, Sayers R, Varty K *et al.* Chronic critical leg ischaemia must be redefined. *Eur J Vasc Surg* 1993;**7**:420–6.

33 Conrad M. Abnormalities of the digital vasculature as related to ulceration and gangrene. *Circulation* 1968;**49**:1196–201.

34 Kretschmer G, Herbst F, Prager M *et al.* A decade of oral anticoagulant treatment to maintain autologous vein grafts for femoropopliteal atherosclerosis. *Arch Surg* 1992;**127**:1112–15.

35 Jivegård LE, Augustinson LE, Holm J *et al.* Effects of spinal cord stimulation (SCS) in patients with inoperable severe lower limb ischemia: a prospective randomised controlled study. *Eur J Vasc Endovasc Surg* 1995;**9**(4):421–5.

36 The European Study Group. Intravenous pentoxiphylline for the treatment of chronic critical limb ischemia. *Eur J Vasc Endovasc Surg* 1995;**9**(4):426–36.

37 Goldman L, Caldera D, Nussbaum S. Multifactorial index of cardiac risk in noncardiac surgical procedures. *N Engl J Med* 1977;**297**:845–50.

38 Detsky A, Abrams H, Forbath N, Scott J, Hilliard J. Cardiac assessment for patients undergoing noncardiac surgery: a multifactorial clinical risk index. *Arch Intern Med* 1986;**146**:2131–4.

39 Mantha S, Roizen M, Barnard J *et al.* Relative effectiveness of four preoperative tests for predicting adverse cardiac outcome after vascular surgery: a meta-analysis. *Anesth Analg* 1994;**79**: 422–33.

40 Eagle K, Singer D, Brewster D *et al.* Dipyridamole-thallium scanning in patients undergoing vascular surgery. *JAMA* 1987;**257**:2185–9.

41 Hertzer N, Beven E, Young J *et al.* Coronary artery disease in peripheral vascular patients. A classification of 1000 coronary angiograms and results of surgical management. *Ann Surg* 1984; **199**:222–3.

42 Mangano D, London M, Tubau J *et al.* Dipyridamole thallium-201 scintigraphy as a preoperative screening test. *Circulation* 1991;**84**: 493–502.

43 Mason J, Owens D, Harris D *et al.* The role of coronary angiography and coronary revascularization before noncardiac vascular surgery. *JAMA* 1995;**273**:1919–25.

44 Wong T, Detsky A. Preoperative cardiac risk assessment for patients having peripheral surgery. *Ann Intern Med* 1992;**116**:743–53.

45 Mason R, Smirnov V, Newton G, Giron F. Alternative procedures to aortobifemoral bypass grafting. *J Cardiovasc Surg (Torino)* 1989;**30**: 192–7.

46 Swedenborg J, Bergmark C. Is there a place for primary axillofemoral bypass? In: Greenhalgh R, Fowkes F. Eds. *Trials and tribulations of vascular surgery.* London: WB Saunders, 1996.

47 Michaels J. Choice of material for above-knee femoropopliteal bypass graft. *Br J Surg* 1989;**76**: 7–14.

48 Veith F, Gupta S, Ascer E *et al.* Six-year prospective multicenter randomised comparison of autologous saphenous vein and expanded polytetrafluoroethylene grafts in infrainguinal arterial reconstruction. *J Vasc Surg* 1986;**3**: 104–14.

49 Hall K, Rostad H. In situ vein bypass in the treatment of femoropopliteal atherosclerotic disease. A ten year study. *Am J Surg* 1978;**136**: 158–61.

50 Moody A, Edwards P, Harris P. In situ versus reversed femoropopliteal vein grafts: long-term follow-up of a prospective, randomized trial. *Br J Surg* 1992;**79**:750–2.

51 Lundell A, Lindblad B, Bergqvist D, Hansen F. Femoropopliteal–crural graft patency is improved

by an intensive surveillance program: a prospective randomized study. *J Vasc Surg* 1996; **21**:26–33.

52 Antiplatelet Trialists' Collaboration. Collaborative overview of randomised trials of antiplatelet therapy. II: Maintenance of vascular graft or arterial patency by antiplatelet therapy. *Br Med J* 1994;**308**:159–68.

53 Dotter C, Judkins M. Transluminal treatment of arteriosclerotic obstructions. *Circulation* 1964;**30**: 654–70.

54 Johnston K, Rae M, Hogg-Johnston S *et al*. 5-year results of a prospective study of percutaneous transluminal angioplasty. *Ann Surg* 1987;**206**: 403–12.

55 Dorros G, Lewin R, Jamnadas P *et al*. Below-the-knee angioplasty: tibioperoneal vessels, the acute outcome. *Cathet Cardiovasc Diagn* 1990;**19**: 170–8.

56 Sivananthan U, Browne T, Thorley P *et al*. Percutaneous transluminal angioplasty of the tibial arteries. *Br J Surg* 1994;**81**:1282–85.

57 Bolia A, Miles K, Brennan J, Bell P. Percutaneous transluminal angioplasty of occlusions of the femoral and popliteal arteries by subintimal dissection. *Cardiovasc Intervent Radiol* 1990;**13**: 357–63.

58 London N, Srinivasan R, Naylor A *et al*. Subintimal angioplasty of femoropopliteal artery occlusions: the long-term results. *Eur J Vasc Surg* 1994;**8**: 148–55.

59 Nydahl S, London N, Bola A. Technical report: recanalisation of all three infrapopliteal arteries by subintimal angioplasty. *Clin Radiol* 1996;**51**: 366–7.

60 Wolf G. Surgery or balloon angioplasty for peripheral vascular disease: a randomized clinical trial. Principal investigators and their Associates of Veterans Administration Cooperative Study Number 199. *J Vasc Interv Radiol* 1993;**4**(5): 639–48.

61 Perkins J, Collin J, Creasy T, Fletcher E, Morris P. Exercise training versus angioplasty for stable claudication. Long and medium results of a prospective, randomised trial. *Eur J Vas Endovasc Surg* 1997; (in press).

62 Whyman M, Fowkes F, Kerracher E *et al*. Randomised controlled trial of percutaneous transluminal angioplasty for intermittent claudication. *Eur J Vasc Endovasc Surg* 1996;**12**: 167–72.

63 Berridge L, Gregson R, Hopkinson B, Makin G. Randomized trial of intra-arterial recombinant tissue plasminogen activator, intravenous recombinant tissue plasminogen activator and intra-arterial streptokinase in peripheral arterial thrombolysis. *Br J Surg* 1991;**78**:988–95.

64 The STILE Investigators. Results of a prospective randomized trial evaluating surgery versus thrombolysis for ischemia of the lower extremity. The STILE Trial. *Ann Surg* 1994;**220**(3): 251–68.

65 Weaver F, Comerota A, Youngblood M *et al*. Surgical revascularization versus thrombolysis for nonembolic lower extremity native artery occlusions: results of a prospective randomized trial. *J Vasc Surg* 1996;**24**:513–23.

Part IV
Clinical applications

ERNEST FALLEN, Editor

Introduction: clinical applications

ERNEST L. FALLEN

Evidence based on well designed randomized clinical trials not only provides a sound, rigorous approach to clinical management but often enables the practicing physician to feel secure about making critical decisions on diagnosis, prognosis, and therapeutics. However, even the most vociferous defendants of evidence based medical practice will caution against using an evidence based approach as the sole basis on which to render a clinical management decision for an individual patient. In the context of day to day practice, it is as important to know *how* to apply evidence as it is to know *what* the evidence is. It is well to bear in mind that grade A evidence from large scale clinical trials, albeit persuasive, is ultimately derived from a large population database wherein the entry criteria permit a broad mix of clinical manifestations of a unified diagnosis. The practicing physician may properly ask "where can I find my patient within this statistical data set?" In other words, how can one use the evidence derived from a large population base to guide management of a patient with a similar diagnosis but with, perhaps, a different clinical expression of the disease with or without attendant complexities? Although a specific therapeutic strategy has withstood the rigors of grade A evidence, does this mean that each and every patient with the same diagnosis would have qualified for entry into the study?

This section is an attempt to put a clinical face on the statistical bottom line. The following Case Studies represent examples of real life clinical presentations in which the therapeutic decisions based solely on evidence derived from clinical trials are either well substantiated or somewhat questionable. For each of the 11 clinical topics there are 2 case presentations from the files of distinguished consultant cardiologists. One of the cases represents a clinical scenario in which a straightforward decision can be unequivocally based on available evidence while the second case represents a challenge to incorporate external evidence with reasoned judgment, an experienced examination and a sound knowledge of cardiovascular pathophysiology.

61 Stable angina: choice of PTCA vs CABG vs drugs

Douglas A. Holder

CASE 1

While vacationing in Puerto Rico, a 51-year-old Canadian woman sustains an uncomplicated inferior myocardial infarction. Prior to discharge she undergoes coronary angiography which reveals a 90% stenosis of the mid third of a dominant right coronary artery (RCA) (Figure 61.1). Upon returning to Canada she experiences angina up to four to five times per day, relieved by one or two nitroglycerin sprays. Her risk factors include a history of smoking, a positive family history of coronary artery disease, and a total cholesterol of 5.4 mmol/l (LDL-C 4.1; HDL-C 1.2) and triglycerides 1.34 mmol/l. Her medications are diltiazem 60 mg p.o. t.i.d.; transdermal nitroglycerin 0.4 mg/h patch ON in a.m. and OFF h.s.; enteric coated aspirin 325 mg daily; salbutamol and beclomethosone dipropianate puffs. She is unable to take beta-blockers because of increased airways resistance secondary to chronic smoking.

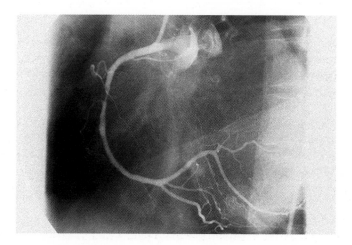

Figure 61.1 A 90% discrete stenosis in a dominant right coronary artery (RCA).

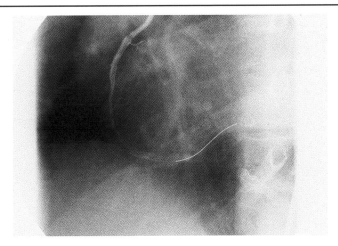

Figure 61.2 After the second balloon inflation, note the spiral dissection extending down towards the crux.

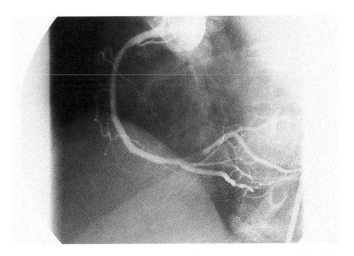

Figure 61.3 Post-stent deployment revealing adequate patency of the RCA.

A decision is made to proceed with coronary angiography with the view to revascularization. Angiographically, the dominant RCA stenosis, being severe, non-calcified and discrete, is technically suitable for percutaneous transluminal coronary angioplasty (PTCA). After the second inflation with a 2.5 mm balloon the procedure is complicated by acute closure due to a spiral dissection which extends down well below the original stenosis towards the crux (Figure 61.2). Three Palmaz–Schatz stents are deployed to tack up the intima from the distal end of the dissection back to and including the original stenosis. This results in an angiographically excellent result (Figure 61.3). The patient makes an uneventful recovery and is discharged on ticlopidine 250 mg p.o. b.i.d. in addition to her previous medications.

She is well for 2 months but then develops recurrent angina. An exercise (treadmill) thallium study is positive at $5\frac{1}{2}$ minutes with angina; 1 mm ST depression and reversible inferior wall ischemia on scanning. A repeat coronary angiogram reveals a discrete

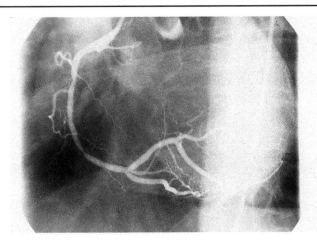

Figure 61.4 Restenosis at the juncture of the distal and middle stents 2 months post-angioplasty.

restenosis at the juncture of the distal and middle stents (Figure 61.4). The patient and her husband decide to choose coronary artery bypass surgery (CABG) rather than repeat PTCA.

Question: Is there evidence to support these therapeutic steps?

COMMENT

There were three decision points where the patient was presented with options for therapeutic interventions.

1   Evidence to recommend initial PTCA

The patient presented with postmyocardial infarction angina due to single vessel RCA stenosis. To date, randomized controlled trials (RCT) comparing CABG to medical treatment have shown no survival benefit from surgery because of the low prognostic risk associated with single vessel right coronary disease.[1,2] There have been no direct comparisons of PTCA with CABG in this subset of single vessel disease, but the recent BARI study of multivessel disease showed no survival benefit for either treatment over a 5-year follow-up period.[3] Thus, in making the therapeutic recommendation at this stage, prognosis was not the main issue. Symptom relief was.

The ACME trial compared medical treatment to PTCA for single vessel left anterior descending disease with the endpoint being anginal frequency and treadmill time at 6 months of follow-up.[4] In this trial of 107 patients, 46% of medically treated patients were free of angina compared to 64% of PTCA patients ($P = <0.01$) and there was an increase in treadmill time, 2.1 minutes over baseline in the PTCA group compared to 0.5 minutes in the medically treated group ($P = 0.0001$). However, because of restenosis, those patients assigned to PTCA had a more frequent requirement for further procedures (16 patients required PTCA; 2 required CABG). In another trial comparing medical treatment to PTCA to left internal mammary artery (LIMA) grafting for proximal single vessel left anterior descending artery stenosis $\geq 80\%$ there were no differences among the groups in mortality or infarction rates, but no patient needed further revascularization in the surgical group compared to 8/72 (11%) of those undergoing PTCA and 7/72 (10%) on medical treatment ($P = 0.019$).[5]

Acknowledging that clinical trials that specifically apply to our patient are lacking, these studies nevertheless allow us to conclude that surgery would be an acceptable choice for achieving symptomatic relief, and that PTCA is intermediate between medical treatment and surgery in achieving symptomatic relief but at a cost of a higher likelihood of further revascularization in the future. The other considerations in comparing surgery to PTCA is a higher initial mortality and morbidity with surgery, as well as the fact that the patency of a saphenous vein graft in the circulation is less than a mammary artery. The angiographic characteristics of the stenosis were consistent with a high likelihood of primary success with PTCA and if restenosis did not occur then the time when CABG might have to be done could be delayed.

2   Evidence for the decision to employ a "bail-out" stent

Acute closure due to spiral dissection is a recognized complication occurring in 1–2% of patients undergoing PTCA. The surgical mortality in the setting of an emergency operation is approximately twice the risk of an elective procedure. Although there are no RCTs comparing emergency CABG to coronary stenting for acute closure due to dissection, the prompt deployment of a stent, as opposed to simply re-ballooning, quickly repairs the dissection and relieves the ischemia.[6] However, an inability to advance and deploy the stent properly necessitates immediate CABG. In this patient, because the original stenosis had been relieved, the stents could be advanced and positioned properly so that surgery was avoided.

3   Evidence for the decision for coronary bypass surgery

Unfortunately, the patient developed restenosis within the stented segment of the RCA. This was discrete, distal to the site of the original plaque and very unlikely to dissect with repeat dilation because of the stent buttressing the vessel wall. Thus, this stenosis would have been amenable to either repeat PTCA or coronary bypass surgery (CABG). The clinical advice was to offer repeat PTCA. However, when the substance of the earlier discussion of PTCA vs medical therapy vs CABG was again reviewed, the patient and her husband opted for surgery as a more "definitive" method of dealing with her problem. In addition to this "definitive" approach, she was advised on preventive measures targeted at lowering her LDL cholesterol.

REFERENCES

1 Alderman EL, Bourassa M, Cohen LSE. Ten year follow-up of survival and myocardial infarction in the randomized Coronary Artery Surgery Study. *Circulation* 1990;82:1629.

2 European Coronary Surgery Study Group. Long-term results of prospective randomized study of coronary artery bypass surgery in stable angina pectoris. *Lancet* 1982;ii:1173.

3 The Bypass Angioplasty Revascularization Investigation (BARI) Investigators. Comparison of coronary bypass surgery with angioplasty in

patients with multivessel disease. *N Engl J Med* 1996;**335**:217–25.

4 Parisi AF, Folland ED, Hartigan P, for the Veterans Affairs ACME Investigators. A comparison of angioplasty with medical therapy in the treatment of single vessel coronary artery disease. *N Engl J Med* 1992;**326**:10.

5 Hueb WA, Bellotti G, deOliveira SA *et al.* A prospective randomized trial of medical therapy, balloon angioplasty or bypass surgery for single proximal left anterior descending coronary stenosis. *J Am Coll Cardiol* 1995;**26**:1600.

6 Lincoff AM, Topol EJ, Chapekis AT *et al.* Intracoronary stenting compared with conventional therapy for abrupt closure complicating coronary angioplasty: a matched case control study. *J Am Coll Cardiol* 1993;**21**: 866–75.

CASE 2

A 63-year-old man tells the following story. Approximately $1\frac{1}{2}$ years ago he experienced a feeling of "indigestion" while walking. This led to a symptom limited exercise test that was considered positive by ECG criteria but was not accompanied by any symptoms. His symptom of "indigestion" did not recur and he continued to pursue outdoor activities such as canoe tripping, camping and walking without limitation. Risk factors include type II diabetes mellitus and hypercholesterolemia. He is a non-smoker.

His current medications are humulin insulin 70/30; 20 units a.c. breakfast and 18 units a.c. supper, pravastatin 40 mg q.h.s. (total cholesterol now is 4.47 mmol/L; LDL 2.87; HDL 1.12; TG 1.05), acebutolol 100 mg p.o. b.i.d. and enteric coated aspirin 325 mg p.o. daily.

A stress MUGA scan reveals the following. Exercise duration 11 minutes and 31 seconds; maximum heart rate 144 per minute; maximum blood pressure 170/84 and no angina. The ECG shows 4.5 mm downsloping ST segment at maximum stress. Ejection fraction: baseline 69%; 200 kpm 73%; 400 kpm 66%; 600 kpm 61%; 800 kpm 58%; post exercise recovery 67% indicating a fall in EF at higher workloads. Left ventricular wall motion analysis demonstrated hypokinesis of the septum, posterolateral and inferior walls.

Conclusion: Silent ischemia. Suggest referral for coronary angiography. Coronary angiography reveals a normal left main coronary artery trifurcating into a left anterior descending, intermediate and circumflex branches (Figure 61.5). There is a "left main equivalent" distribution of disease with stenoses involving the LAD 75%, intermediate 90%, and circumflex 90%. The RCA is diffusely diseased with a maximal narrowing of 60% in the midthird segment. LV systolic function is normal at rest.

Question: Is conservative medical management optimal at this point?

COMMENT

Here, the decision rests, in part, on whether clear evidence is available to offer sound advice to an asymptomatic patient with objective evidence of three vessel disease and exercise induced silent ischemia. If this patient had symptoms of classical angina pectoris the therapeutic decision for recommending coronary bypass surgery (CABG) with the expectation of symptom relief and improved prognosis could be substantiated. If the

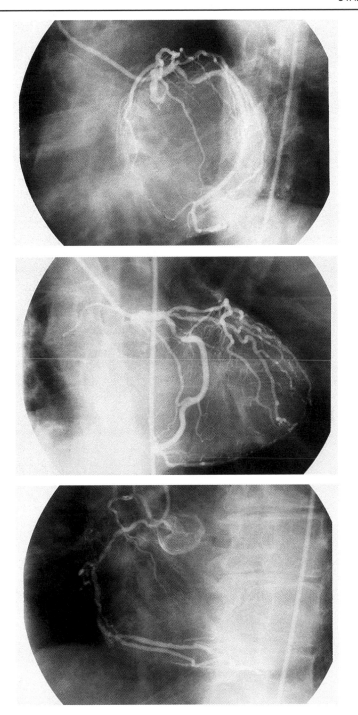

Figure 61.5 Multivessel coronary artery stenoses suggesting a "left main equivalent" with LAD 75%, intermediate 90%, and circumflex 90%. The RCA is diffusely diseased.

patient had a definite left main stenosis, or depressed LV function, the argument for CABG is strongly made because in this setting CABG improves prognosis even in the absence of symptoms.[1,2] This patient is somewhat unusual in that not only is he asymptomatic but he is capable of a good workload (800 kpm of supine bicycle exercise). However, there is convincing evidence of significant ischemia at this level of work with ST depression of 4.5 mm and a reduction in ejection fraction from 69% at rest to 58% with maximal effort. There is also evidence of LV wall motion abnormality in multiple sites consistent with the extent of coronary artery disease noted on the angiogram.

The question therefore is one of prognosis rather than symptom relief. Common sense alone argues that his myocardium would benefit from revascularization. There is evidence to suggest that the long term prognosis of patients with documented silent ischemia is similar to those with symptomatic angina pectoris,[3,4] and thus our treatment should be aimed at the coronary disease substrate, rather than the clinical chest pain syndrome. Given the left main equivalent distribution as well as the diseased RCA, this patient was referred for consideration of coronary bypass surgery. This decision is supported by evidence gleaned from a careful review of all major trials on bypass surgery for different severities of coronary artery disease.[5]

REFERENCES

1 Alderman EL, Bourassa M, Cohen LSE. Ten year follow-up of survival and myocardial infarction in the randomized Coronary Artery Surgery Study (CASS). *Circulation* 1990;**82**:1629.

2 European Coronary Surgery Study Group. Long-term results of prospective randomized study of coronary artery bypass surgery in stable angina pectoris. *Lancet* 1982;**ii**:1173.

3 Lotan C, Lokovitsky L, Gilon D *et al*. Silent myocardial ischemia during exercise testing. Does it indicate a different angiographic and prognostic syndrome? *Cardiology* 1994;**85**(6):407.

4 Marwick TH. Is silent ischemia painless because it is mild? *J Am Coll Cardiol* 1995;**25**(7): 1513–15.

5 Yusuf S, Zucker D, Peduzzi P *et al*. Effect of coronary artery bypass surgery on survival. *Lancet* 1994; **344**:563–70.

Unstable angina: management issues

62

Joseph M. Delahanty,
William B. Hood Jr

CASE 1

A 59-year-old male presents to the Emergency Ward with non-exertional precordial dull chest pain radiating to the left arm, sweating, and mild nausea. He has had similar episodes intermittently for the past 2 years, lasting up to 20 minutes, but these were usually brought on by exertion and relieved by sublingual nitroglycerin which his physician had prescribed. The episodes have become somewhat more frequent over the past month, and have sometimes occurred at rest. He has had several episodes over the past 48 hours with little or no effort.

Physical exam is within normal limits except for a blood pressure of 160/100. The initial ECG and the one taken an hour later after resolution of symptoms are shown in Figures 62.1 and 62.2.

Question: What initial and further measures should be taken in this patient?

COMMENT

In this straightforward case of unstable angina, the initial therapy is strongly guided by clear evidence from recent large scale clinical trials, while long term management requires a judicious combination of external evidence and clinical expertise. The diagnosis of coronary disease seems clearcut in this patient based on a classic description of angina pectoris. The diagnosis of unstable angina also seems secure based on the history of an escalating pattern of pain and the presence of distinctive transient ST and T wave changes on the ECG. The increased cardiac workload from mild hypertension may be responsible, in part, for exacerbating the angina.

Strong evidence exists for the use of aspirin and full dose intravenous heparin.[1,2] The use of intravenous nitroglycerin[3] in unstable angina has become widely accepted,

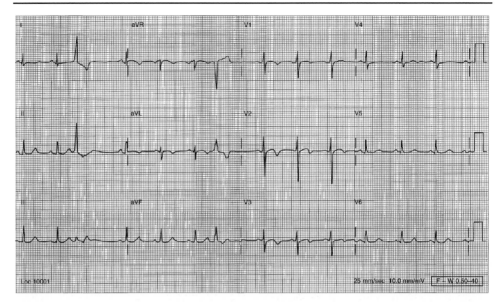

Figure 62.1 Tracing shows right precordial ST elevation with accompanying T wave inversions, compatible with anterior wall transmural ischemia. Ventricular extra systoles are also present.

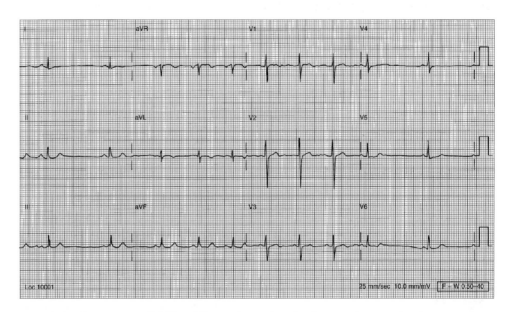

Figure 62.2 The right precordial ST and T wave changes have largely reverted to normal and ectopy is absent. However, occasional sinus pauses are noted.

although its effect on outcome events has yet to be evaluated by large scale randomized studies. Intravenous or oral beta-blocker[4] is also helpful, especially in this type of patient with hypertension and persisting pain. *Note:* In the HINT trial although the effects of beta-blockers were equivocal, there was a strong trend in favour of this therapy.

The dose and monitoring of heparin are important. In this situation full dose heparin should be given, i.e. 80 units/kg IV followed by 18 units/kg per hour. The effect should be monitored by measuring the activated partial thromboplastin time (aPTT) 6 hours after beginning therapy and after any dose change, with the aPTT maintained between 45 and 70 seconds. Recently, the use of low molecular weight heparin[5] and newer platelet inhibitors[6] has also shown promise.

This patient may be at relatively high risk and should be treated initially with oxygen.[7] *Note:* No decisive randomized trial of oxygen therapy has been carried out in either unstable angina or acute myocardial infarction. However, the use of oxygen therapy for both conditions is widely accepted. The reference suggests a beneficial effect of oxygen breathing in acute myocardial infarction.

Additional agents should be used to lower the blood pressure if required. There are no immediate indications for thrombolytic therapy,[8] however the ECG should be monitored continuously to determine whether clearcut ST segment elevation associated with continuation of pain develops. This would probably call for treatment with a thrombolytic agent or urgent cardiac catheterization with primary angioplasty if the anatomy warrants. Serial measurements of serum enzymes should also be made to detect possible myocardial necrosis.

Subsequent management would depend upon the clinical course. Refractory symptoms would mitigate in favor of early cardiac catheterization and intervention with either coronary angioplasty or bypass surgery. With resolution of symptoms and ECG changes, as occurred in the case presented, this could be done on a more elective basis. In either case, a coronary angiographic study should probably be carried out in this patient, although the evidence for revascularization vs medical therapy in asymptomatic survivors from unstable angina is not clear at this juncture.

REFERENCES

1 Theroux P, Ouimet H, McCans J *et al.* Aspirin, heparin or both to treat acute unstable angina. *N Engl J Med* 1988;**319**:1105–11.

2 The RISC Group. Risk of myocardial infarction and death during treatment with low dose aspirin and intravenous heparin in men with unstable coronary artery disease. *Lancet* 1990;**336**:827–30.

3 Conti CR. Use of nitrates in unstable angina pectoris. *Am J Cardiol* 1987;**60**:31H–34H.

4 HINT Research Group. Early treatment of unstable angina in the coronary care unit: a randomized, double-blind, placebo-controlled comparison of recurrent ischaemia in patients treated with nifedipine or metoprolol or both. *Br Heart J* 1986; **56**:400–13.

5 Cohen M, Demers C, Gurfunkel EP *et al.* A comparison of low molecular heparin with unfractionated heparin for unstable coronary artery disease. *N Engl J Med* 1997;**337**:447–52.

6 The EPILOG Investigators. Platelet glycoprotein IIb/ IIIa receptor blockade and low-dose heparin during percutaneous coronary revascularisation. *N Engl J Med* 1997;**336**:1689–96.

7 Madias JE, Hood WB Jr. Reduction of precordial ST-segment elevation in patients with anterior myocardial infarction by oxygen breathing. *Circulation* 1976;**53**(Suppl I):198–200.

8 Ambrose JA, Hjendahl-Monson C, Borrico S *et al.* Quantitative and qualitative effects of intracoronary streptokinase in unstable angina and non-Q wave infarction. *J Am Coll Cardiol* 1987;**9**: 1156–65.

CASE 2

A 63-year-old female with mild but classical effort angina that responds to sublingual nitroglycerin is seen at a routine clinic visit. She has noted a change in the pattern of her chest pain, and now experiences it on milder than usual exertion, and occasionally at rest when excited. She notes that two nitroglycerin tablets might be needed to relieve the discomfort, but it never lasts more than 5 minutes. The patient has mild diabetes

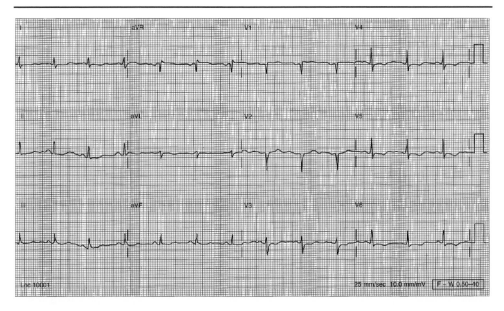

Figure 62.3 The tracing shows non-specific T wave changes, with slight T wave inversions noted particularly in the anterolateral leads.

well controlled with an oral hypoglycemic agent for 10 years. The physical exam is not remarkable except for diminished pedal pulses. The ECG is shown in Figure 62.3. It resembles earlier ECGs except that T wave abnormalities are now more apparent.

Question: How should this patient be managed?

COMMENT

This case represents a good example of how not to treat every clinical manifestation of so-called "unstable angina" as a single entity. The presence of underlying coronary disease in this patient seems unequivocal. The history has been one of exertional chest discomfort that responds well to nitroglycerin and, until recently, the pattern has been a stable one. The recent change in the pattern of pain is of some concern, but apparently it is not accompanied by striking changes in the ECG. None of the possible precipitating causes for a change in anginal pattern, such as tachycardia, hypertension, anemia, fever, or thyrotoxicosis appears to be present in this case. On the basis of her clinical syndrome, the patient was considered to have class I angina.[1] The fact that her symptoms are quite mild, do not occur at rest, and are not associated with documented ECG changes puts her at low risk for immediate serious outcomes. And yet the symptoms qualify as representing instability insofar as there has been a distinct change in pattern and exacerbation.

Based on currently published guidelines, she could be safely managed on an outpatient basis.[2] This patient might be managed medically by adding, in addition to nitroglycerin, aspirin[3] and a beta-blocker, while studying her on an outpatient basis by performing an exercise radionuclide stress test after a 48-hour period of freedom from angina. An exercise ECG alone would carry a high false positivity in view of the resting ST and T wave abnormalities. The decision about further testing, including coronary angiography, could be based upon the stress test, which may suggest a more aggressive approach if marked ST depression or limitation of exercise tolerance is observed, or if there is an exercise-induced decrease in blood pressure or a large reversible perfusion defect.

REFERENCES

1 Braunwald E. Unstable angina. A classification. *Circulation* 1989;**80**:410–14.

2 Braunwald E, Jones RH, Mark DB *et al*. Diagnosing and managing unstable angina. *Circulation* 1994;**90**:613–22.

3 Cairns JA, Gent M, Singer J *et al*. Aspirin, sulfinpyrazone or both in unstable angina. *N Engl J Med* 1985;**313**:1369–75.

63 Acute myocardial infarction: management issues

Bryan Dias,
Ernest L. Fallen

CASE 1

A 68-year-old woman with an 18-month history of chronic stable angina presents to the Emergency Room with a 2-hour history of severe retrosternal chest pain. There is associated weakness, diaphoresis, and nausea. Three applications of nitroglycerin spray 5 minutes apart failed to relieve her symptoms. She is a well controlled type II diabetic on glyburide 5 mg o.d. She also has esophageal reflux disease but clearly distinguishes her reflux symptoms from angina. There is no history of gastrointestinal bleeding.

On examination, she is pale, anxious, and diaphoretic. The blood pressure is 110/80 in both arms and the pulse is 70 and regular. Her neck veins are elevated 3 cm at 45 degrees with a sustained hepatojugular reflux. She has a soft late

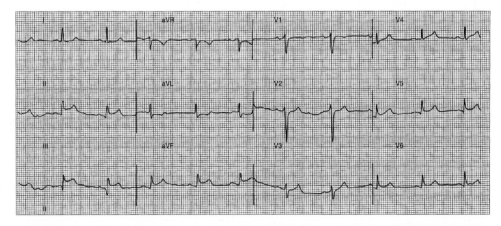

Figure 63.1 Twelve lead ECG showing hyperacute ST segment elevation in leads II, III, and AVF, signifying inferior wall ischemic injury.

crescendo apical systolic murmur. Her lungs are clear. An ECG is immediately ordered (Figure 63.1).

Question: What is the proper course of action at this juncture?

COMMENT

There is now overwhelming evidence from many major clinical trials that the early administration of thrombolytic therapy and aspirin for acute myocardial infarction substantially reduces mortality and the risk of recurrent ischemic events.[1-3] Let us examine this case and see if she fits the entrance criteria. The symptoms of prolonged chest pain unresponsive to nitroglycerin together with accompanying symptoms of nausea, weakness, and diaphoresis raise a strong suspicion of acute myocardial infarction. This is confirmed by the ECG which demonstrates significant ST segment elevation in leads II, III, AVF, V5, and V6.

With an evolving acute myocardial infarction of less than 3 hours from onset there is level A evidence that the treatment of choice is prompt coronary thrombolysis plus aspirin.[1-3] The patient is given 160 mg of enteric coated aspirin to chew while an intravenous line is inserted. In the absence of any obvious contraindication, the patient is given streptokinase intravenously as there is no evidence that rtPA (recombinant tissue plasminogen activator) is superior to the less expensive streptokinase in patients with first onset acute inferior infarction.[4,5]

The patient is monitored in the Coronary Care Unit where anxiety and relief of pain is handled by administering oxygen, intravenous nitroglycerin, and morphine as needed. She is prescribed an oral beta-blocker which will be continued indefinitely.[6-8] Because there is no major complication such as congestive heart failure or persistent pain, the patient will continue on aspirin and beta-blocker without the need for full dose heparin.[4,5,9-11] There is also no echocardiographic evidence of significant left ventricular dysfunction (estimated LV ejection fraction = 0.50) to indicate the need for an ACE inhibitor.[12]

This patient would have qualified for entry into most of the large clinical trials on thrombolysis for acute myocardial infarction. She therefore benefits by a therapeutic strategy (thrombolysis, aspirin, and beta-blocker) which in combination reduces her likelihood of a major outcome event or death by 30–40% within the first year of follow-up.

REFERENCES

1 Gruppo Italiano per lo Studiio della streptochinasi nell' Infarto Miocardico (GISSI). Effectiveness of intravenous thrombolytic treatment in acute myocardial infarction. *Lancet* 1986;i: 397–401.

2 ISIS-2 (Second International Study of Infarct Survival) Collaborative Study Group. Randomized trial of intravenous streptokinase, oral aspirin, both or neither among 17 187 cases of suspected acute myocardial infarction: ISIS-2. *Lancet* 1988; ii;349–60.

3 Fibrinolytic Therapy Trialists' (FTT) Collaborative Group. Indications for fibrinolytic therapy in suspected acute myocardial infarction: collaborative overview of early mortality and major morbidity results from all randomized trials of more than 1000 patients. *Lancet* 1994;**343**: 311–22.

4 Cairns J, Armstrong P, Belenkie I *et al.* Canadian Cardiovascular Society Consensus Conference on

Coronary Thrombolytics – 1994 Update. *Can J Cardiol* 1994;**10**:517–29.

5 Collins R, Peto R, Baigent C, Sleight P. Aspirin, heparin and fibrinolytic therapy in suspected acute myocardial infarction. *N Engl J Med* 1997; **336**:847–60.

6 Beta-Blocker Heart Attack Study Group. A randomized trial of propranolol in patients with acute myocardial infarction. *JAMA* 1982;**247**: 1707–14.

7 The Norwegian Multicentre Study Group. Six year follow-up of the Norwegian Multicentre Study on Timolol after acute myocardial infarction. *N Engl J Med* 1985;**313**:1055–8.

8 Yusuf S, Peto R, Lewis JA *et al.* Beta-blockade during and after myocardial infarction: a review of the randomised trials. *Prog Cardiovasc Dis* 1985; **27**:335–71.

9 ISIS-3. A randomised comparison of streptokinase vs tissue plasminogen activator vs anistreplase and of aspirin plus heparin vs heparin alone among 41 299 cases of suspected acute myocardial infarction. *Lancet* 1992;**339**: 753–70.

10 GISSI-2. A factorial randomised trial of alteplase vs streptokinase and heparin vs no heparin among 12 490 patients with acute myocardial infarction. *Lancet* 1990;**336**:65–71.

11 The GUSTO Investigators. An international randomised trial comparing four thrombolytic strategies for acute myocardial infarction. *N Engl J Med* 1993;**329**:673–82.

12 Syed M, Borzak S, Jafri SM *et al.* ACE inhibition after acute myocardial infarction with special reference to the Fourth International Study of Infarct Survival (ISIS-4). *Prog Cardiovasc Dis* 1996;**39**:201–6.

CASE 2

A 66-year-old man presents to the Emergency Room with severe chest pain. He has had previous coronary artery bypass graft surgeries (2 and 12 years ago) with a history of two previous myocardial infarctions (Q wave and non-Q wave) prior to his last bypass operation. For the past year his functional status has been stable, with Canadian Cardiovascular Society class I angina.

He is now seen 3 hours after the sudden onset of severe retrosternal chest pain with no relief from sublingual nitroglycerin (0.6 mg sublingual × 3). The pain is characterized as 10/10 in severity, crushing in nature, with radiation into the jaw. Associated symptoms include dyspnea, diaphoresis, and weakness. These symptoms are similar to those he had with his previous infarcts.

Examination reveals an acutely ill looking patient. He is in painful distress, pale, and diaphoretic. His blood pressure is 100/80 and equal in both arms. His pulse is 90 bpm and regular. Lung fields are clear to auscultation. His neck veins are not abnormally elevated. There are no murmurs or extra heart sounds. His ECG is shown in Figure 63.2.

Question: What action would you now take?

COMMENT

Here is an example where strict adherence to algorithms based on the results of clinical trials can be misleading. For, in this case, the widespread ST segment depression led to the diagnosis of subendocardial myocardial ischemia manifested as either unstable angina or a non-Q infarction. Thrombolysis in unstable angina or non-Q infarction has been studied but the results of these trials show a trend towards no benefit and perhaps even harm.[1,2] The patient was therefore given aspirin 325 mg and full dose intravenous heparin starting at 7 units/kg bolus and followed at 1200 units/h IV. Within the next

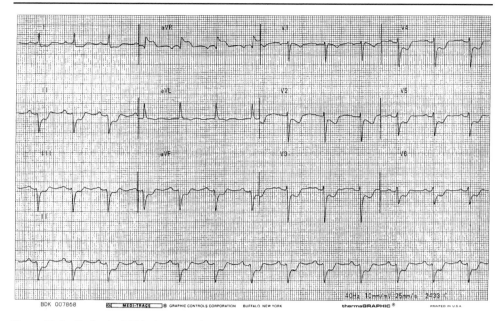

Figure 63.2 Twelve lead ECG showing widespread ST segment depression with left axis deviation. There are no Q waves nor ST segment elevations except in lead AVR.

hour neither sublingual nor intravenous nitroglycerin had any effect on the pain, which persisted at 10/10 severity. Similarly, intravenous beta-blocker (propranolol 5 mg IV) and morphine (10 mg IV over 30 minutes) had little effect. The pain remained unabated and serial ECGs showed ongoing ischemic changes but no evidence of an injury (ST elevation) pattern.

This patient received the standard treatment with aspirin and heparin because he would have qualified for entry into any of the unstable angina trials.[3,4] And yet, these measures plus intensification of antianginal therapy failed to relieve his symptoms. On careful re-review of the clinical presentation, there is a strong suspicion for an acute myocardial infarction. He had suffered two similar episodes with previous infarcts; he is acutely ill with diaphoresis, weakness, and restlessness – symptoms that are characteristic of myocardial necrosis as opposed to reduced perfusion. On reflection, the ECG changes may be construed as misleading since there is every likelihood that a thrombotic occlusion of a coronary artery is taking place. Given the nature of what sounds like an infarct process clinically, a decision was made to proceed with thrombolytic therapy. Within 45 minutes following intravenous infusion of rtPA, the pain completely abated and his ECG normalized with only persistent T wave negativity seen in the anterior leads. Subsequent investigations revealed a peak creatine kinase of 2969 with a positive MB fraction. The patient subsequently had an uneventful recovery and was discharged from hospital on day 7.

Although the evidence from large scale clinical trials would not necessarily support the routine use of thrombolytic agents based on the ECG changes seen in this case, here is an example where the symptoms, strongly suggestive of an occlusive coronary artery with myocardial necrosis, call for an intervention to restore arterial patency as promptly as possible.[5] In this regard, a case could also be made for primary angioplasty should facilities be available. However, in view of the probability of extensive three vessel coronary artery disease and multiple blocked bypass grafts, it would be more prudent to consider further invasive investigation and intervention on an elective basis.

REFERENCES

1 Freeman MR, Langer A, Wilson RF, Morgan CD, Armstrong PW. Thrombolysis in unstable angina: randomized double-blind trial of tPA and placebo. *Circulation* 1992;**85**:150–7.

2 The TIMI-IIIB Investigators. Effects of tissue plasminogen activator and a comparison of early invasive and conservative strategies in unstable angina and non-Q wave myocardial infarction. Results of the TIMI-IIIB trial. *Circulation* 1994;**89**: 1545–56.

3 Theroux P, Quimet H, McCans J *et al.* Aspirin, heparin, or both to treat unstable angina. *N Engl J Med* 1988;**319**:1105–11.

4 Cairns JA, Gent M, Singer J *et al.* Aspirin, sulfinpyrazone or both in unstable angina. Results of a Canadian multicentre trial. *N Engl J Med* 1985; **313**:1369–75.

5 The GUSTO Investigators. An international randomised trial comparing four thrombolytic strategies for acute myocardial infarction. *N Engl J Med* 1993;**329**:673–82.

Postmyocardial infarction: routine prophylaxis

64

Ernest L. Fallen

CASE 1

A 53-year-old sedentary, mildly overweight male chartered accountant, previously symptom free, was admitted to hospital 6 days ago with an acute anteroseptal myocardial infarction. He received rtPA (total dose 100 mg) and his peak creatinine kinase was 3500. The acute phase of his illness was complicated by frequent isolated ventricular ectopic beats (>10/h) and mild cardiac decompensation (Killip class 2a). His risk factors are (a) positive family history; (b) 30 pack year smoking history; (c) mild hypertension – untreated; and (d) mild obesity (Body Mass Index = 29). His lipid status is unknown.

It is now 6 days post MI and he is ready for discharge. He is free of all signs of congestive heart failure and he is not experiencing chest pain on exertion (climbing one flight of stairs). His ECG shows a sinus rhythm at 70 bpm with qS waves and T wave inversion in V1 to V3 without ST elevation. His echocardiogram reveals severe hypokinesis of the septum and apex but no other regional wall motion abnormalities. There is no LV dilation and his estimated ejection fraction is 45%. There is no valvular abnormality and no endocardial thrombus.

On physical exam he is in sinus rhythm at 70 beats per minute; blood pressure 122/80 and respiratory rate 16 breaths per minute. His lungs are clear. There is a soft S4 but no murmurs. There are good peripheral pulses. His neck veins are not elevated.

Question: What advice would you now give him?

COMMENT

Here is an example where the physician's common sense advice to an otherwise recalcitrant patient is strongly fortified by clearcut evidence that preventive strategies actually yield favourable outcomes. On paper, this is a relatively straightforward case of a man who is recovering from a first onset anteroseptal infarction. The patient is now pain free and failure free, although he exhibits mild residual left ventricular dysfunction. He has one non-modifiable risk factor (family history) and several modifiable ones (smoking, sedentary lifestyle, mild obesity, and previous hypertension). His lipid status is unknown. In actuality, it will require solid evidence to convince him that a preventive strategy of pharmacologic prophylaxis combined with risk factor modification and lifestyle changes has gone beyond mere platitudes.

Pharmacologic (secondary) prophylaxis

To reduce the risk of recurrent ischemic events and mortality he should continue to be prescribed enteric coated aspirin 325 mg a day[1] and a beta-blocker.[2,3] In view of his reduced LV function, recent findings from the ISIS-4 study[4] and the SOLVD study[5] argue in favour of prescribing an ACE inhibitor.

Risk stratification

For risk stratification he should be scheduled for a symptom-limited exercise test in about 2–4 weeks with a view to assessing his exercise capacity as well as prescribing a rational graded exercise rehabilitation program.[6,7] The exercise test is also useful to determine the presence or absence of residual ischemia.

Risk factor modification/lifestyle change

A comprehensive rehabilitation program should therefore include (a) an exercise rehabilitation program; cessation of smoking;[8] and maintenance of an ideal weight (BMI <25) through exercise combined with nutrition counseling. He should have lipid measurements (cholesterol, triglycerides, LDL-C and HDL-C) done in about 4–6 weeks. On the basis of these results efforts should be made to reduce his LDL-C to less than 2.6 mmol/l (see Chapters 13, 14 and 31).

In summary, using evidence guided recommendations[7] the patient's chance of avoiding recurrent ischemic events and returning to a satisfactory quality of life is significantly enhanced by aspirin, beta-blocker, ACE inhibitor (a lipid lowering agent if required), an exercise rehabilitation program, and cessation of smoking. Depression is a significant risk factor but it has not yet been confirmed, with certainty, that antidepressants are effective in reducing the risk of ischemic events.

REFERENCES

1 ISIS-2 (2nd International Study of Infarct Survival Collaborative Study Group). Randomized trial of intravenous streptokinase, oral aspirin, both or neither among 17 187 cases of suspected acute myocardial infarction: ISIS-2. *Lancet* 1988;**ii**: 349–60.

2 Pederson TR (for the Norwegian Multicentre Study Group). Six year follow-up of the Norwegian Multicentre Study on timolol after acute myocardial infarction. *N Engl J Med* 1985;**313**: 1055–8.

3 Yusuf S, Peto R, Lewis JA *et al.* Beta blockade during and after myocardial infarction: a review of the randomized trials. *Prog Cardiovasc Dis* 1985;**27**: 335–71.

4 ISIS-4 Study Group. A randomized factorial trial assessing early oral captopril, oral mononitrate, oral magnesium sulphate in 58 050 patients with suspected acute myocardial infarction. *Lancet* 1995;**345**:669–85.

5 The SOLVD Investigators. Effect of enalapril on survival in patients with reduced left ventricular ejection fractions and congestive heart failure. *N Engl J Med* 1991;**325**:293.

6 Oldridge NB, Guyatt GH, Fischer ME *et al.* Cardiac rehabilitation after myocardial infarction. Combined experience of randomized clinical trials. *JAMA* 1988;**260**:945–50.

7 Fallen EL, Cairns J, Dafoe W, Frasure-Smith N *et al.* Management of the post myocardial infarction patient: a consensus report – revision of the 1991 CCS guidelines. *Can J Cardiol* 1995;**11**: 477–86.

8 Mulcahy R. Influences of cigarette smoking on morbidity and mortality after myocardial infarction. *Br Heart J* 1983;**49**:410–15.

CASE 2

A 66-year-old female sustains an acute inferoposterior myocardial infarction for which she receives streptokinase (1.5 million units over 1 hour) and aspirin to chew. She makes a satisfactory recovery. The only complications are persistent but asymptomatic sinus bradycardia (45–50/min), papillary muscle dysfunction with moderate mitral regurgitation, and an estimated left ventricular ejection fraction of 0.35. There are no overt signs of heart failure or ventricular irritability. She is angina free post MI.

Her risk factors include heavy smoking (40 pack years); severe peripheral vascular disease with asymptomatic carotid bruits (80% stenosis of the right internal carotid artery), and intermittent claudication of the right leg. She has elevated triglycerides at 6.5 mmol/l. Her previous total cholesterol (3 months ago) was 5.8 mmol/l and HDL-C was 0.98. She is 22 years post hysterectomy and bilateral oophorectomy. That operation was complicated by phlebitis and a pulmonary embolus. Her only medication at the time of hospital admission was an H_2 receptor antagonist because of a history of upper gastrointestinal bleeding 12 years ago and episodic epigastric burning. There is no significant family history of heart disease. However, her mother died of breast cancer at age 65.

Physical examination at the time of hospital discharge shows a resting heart rate of 48 beats per minute. Her blood pressure is 160/85. Her urea is 9.5 and creatinine is 180. An ECG shows sinus rhythm but with a first degree atrioventricular block of 0.24 seconds.

Question: What advice would you now give her?

COMMENT

This case raises several issues regarding the risk vs benefit of routine prophylactic strategies which, for most post-MI patients, are supported by strong evidence from well designed clinical trials. For instance, one would want to be cautious about automatically prescribing a beta-blocker as she has persistent bradycardia with partial AV block, significant symptomatic peripheral vascular disease and hyperlipidemia. On the other hand, beta-blockers have been shown to be more effective in reducing mortality among post-MI patients with mild to moderate LV dysfunction.[1] Here the benefit of a beta-blocker probably outweighs the risk.

In view of her LV dysfunction, she would be a candidate for an ACE inhibitor but she is a non-diabetic with an elevated creatinine, severe vasculopathy, and persistent hypertension. It is possible, indeed likely, that her hypertension is wholly or in part renovascular in origin. As for hormone replacement therapy with estrogen the benefits as secondary prophylaxis may outweigh the risks although the patient is asking some hard questions regarding the history of breast cancer in the family and her previous history of phlebitis and pulmonary embolus. Finally, the history of gastrointestinal bleeding raises caution with respect to aspirin prophylaxis.

The clinical trials unfortunately have not provided satisfactory guidelines on how to weigh the risk vs benefit of postinfarction prophylaxis for patients with certain potential hazards such as our case here. In other words, this case does not easily qualify for entrance criteria to most of the large post-MI clinical trials. One could nevertheless proceed without denying her useful protective and rehabilitative measures. For instance, although it would be difficult for her to achieve a high level of exercise training using leg exercise, there is now evidence that a well supervised upper arm exercise program may be useful.[2] Instead of an ACE inhibitor, perhaps the combination of hydralazine and nitroglycerin[3] serve to improve circulatory function, control her hypertension, and improve her heart rate. She should continue on aspirin as long as she also continues with an H_2 blocker. As for her lipids, she probably would benefit from a fibrate rather than a statin, although there are no clinical trials that have compared the two, head to head, for this type of patient.

REFERENCES

1 Beta Blocker Heart Attack Study Group. A randomised trial of propanolol in patients with acute myocardial infarction. *JAMA* 1982;**247**: 1707–14.

2 Ghilarducci LE, Holly RG, Amsterdam EA. Effects of high resistance training in coronary artery disease. *Am J Cardiol* 1989;**64**:866–70.

3 Cohn JN, Archibald DG, Ziesche S *et al.* Effect of vasodilator therapy on mortality in chronic congestive heart failure: results of a Veterans Administration Cooperative Study. *N Engl J Med* 1986;**314**:1547–52.

Postmyocardial infarction risk factor modification: dyslipoproteinemias

65

Jacques Genest Jr

CASE 1

The patient is a 53-year-old man who presented with an acute myocardial infarction in March 1993. He was treated with thrombolytic therapy within 4.5 hours of his symptoms. He made an uneventful recovery and his predischarge stress test did not reveal ischemia at 7 METs. He was evaluated in a Cardiology–Secondary Prevention Clinic 2 months following hospital discharge. His metabolic profile at this time is shown in Table 65.1. Nutritional evaluation revealed that the patient was already following a diet with less than 10% of calories as saturated fat. A decision was made to prescribe an HMG-Co A reductase inhibitor – simvastatin 20 mg/day. A review of his metabolic profile 2 years later is also shown for comparison.

Question: Are there other clinically relevant measures that can improve both his metabolic profile and prognosis?

COMMENT

Sound preventive strategies for patients with premature coronary artery disease (CAD) are not merely intuitive but now supported by considerable evidence from large scale clinical trials. This patient, at an early age, has already suffered an acute coronary event. The metabolic disorders identified in this patient include an elevated LDL-C and a reduced HDL-C resulting in a significantly elevated total cholesterol/HDL-C ratio of 9.14. In addition, there is a family history of premature CAD, excess weight (BMI >25), a moderately elevated Lp(a) (normal range = <30 g/l), and an elevated total plasma homocysteine (tHcy) level (normal = 10 ± 2 μmol/l).

Table 65.1   Case 1: metabolic profile

Date	May 1993	May 1995
Age (yr)	52	54
Medications	Metoprolol 100 mg/d Aspirin 325/d	Aspirin 80/day Simvastatin 20 mg/d Folic acid 2.5 mg/d
Cholesterol (mmol/l)	6.76	4.19
Triglycerides (mmol/l)	2.18	0.75
HDL-C (mmol/l)	0.74	1.16
LDL-C (mmol/l)	4.51	2.69
Apo B (g/l)	1.87	
Chol/HDL-C	9.14	3.61
BP (mmHg)	110/70	120/74
BMI (kg/m^2)	27.0	26.7
Glucose (mmol/l)	4.8	5.0
Cigarette smoking	Stopped $\times$ 2 months	Stopped
Lp(a) (g/l)	30	25
Homocysteine (μmol/l)	15.96	7.5

Although dietary therapy is strongly recommended for the treatment of dyslipoproteinemias, diet alone is unlikely to decrease the LDL-C level to a target level <2.6 mmol/l.[1] The current recommendation for secondary prevention of lipoprotein disorders in high risk individuals is to initiate drug therapy concomitantly with nutritional advice.[2] These same guidelines indicate that subjects with an increased body mass index (>25 kg/m^2), especially those with abdominal obesity, are encouraged to reduce their weight by appropriate exercise combined with dietary intervention.

In this case, substantial evidence exists for the initiation of an HMG-CoA reductase inhibitor as the drug of first choice.[3,4] As for the other metabolic abnormalities, there is inconclusive evidence that altering a risk factor such as HDL-C or Lp(a) or even triglycerides by themselves prevents adverse outcome events as either a primary or secondary preventive strategy. For instance, although the patient was prescribed folic acid (2.5 mg per day) because of an elevated homocysteine level (>95th percentile for age and gender-matched subject), the effect of this treatment on cardiac events is unknown. However the use of lipid lowering drugs for the prevention of outcome events after MI has been substantiated.[3,4]

REFERENCES

1 Fodor JG for the Working Group on Hypercholesterolemia and other Dyslipidemias. Health Canada (abstract). *Can J Cardiol* 1997;**13**: 214B.

2 Fallen EL, Cairns J, Dafoe W *et al.* Management of the postmyocardial infarction patient: a consensus report – revision of the 1991 CCS guidelines. *Can J Cardiol* 1996;**11**:477–86.

3 The Scandinavian Simvastatin Survival Study Group. Randomised trial of cholesterol lowering in

4444 patients with coronary heart disease. *Lancet* 1994;**344**:1383–9.

4 Sacks FM, Pfeffer MA, Moye LA *et al.* The effect of pravastatin on coronary events after myocardial infarction in patients with average cholesterol levels. CARE Investigators. *N Engl J Med* 1996; **335**:1001–9.

CASE 2

The patient is a 60-year-old diabetic man with premature coronary artery disease (CAD) who sustained a myocardial infarction in 1984 at age 47 years. His risk factors are: (a) hypertension treated with a beta-adrenergic blocking agent; (b) former smoker; (c) a family history of premature CAD; (d) type II diabetes on oral hypoglycemics; and (e) moderate obesity. Because of persistent post-MI angina, coronary angiography was performed and he subsequently underwent quadruple coronary artery bypass surgery. He remained stable until 1993 when effort angina recurred.

He is now admitted with unstable angina and his medical therapy is increased, including the addition of insulin and pravastatin. His metabolic profile in 1993 is shown in Table 65.2, together with the changes 3 years later.

Question: What would be optimum management in this patient with a complex assortment of metabolic abnormalities?

Table 65.2 Case 2: metabolic profile

Date	March 1993	December 1996
Age (yr)	57	60
Medications	Acebutolol 100 mg b.i.d. Aspirin 325 mg o.d. Metformin 500 mg t.i.d.	Acebutolol 200 mg b.i.d. Aspirin 80 mg o.d. Nitropatch 0.4 mg/h o.d. Insulin – pravastatin 40 mg o.d.
Cholesterol (mmol/l)	6.43	5.05
Triglycerides (mmol/l)	3.11	2.02
HDL-C (mmol/l)	0.9	1.15
LDL-C (mmol/l)	4.06	2.9
Apo B (g/l)	1.87	—
Chol/HDL-C	7.14	4.39
BP (mmHg)	140/78	130/70
BMI (kg/m²)	28	28
Glucose (mmol/l)	11.8	7.3
Lp(a) (g/l)	31	NA

COMMENT

A major issue, as yet unresolved, is whether "normalization" of certain metabolic risk factors necessarily confers protection against adverse coronary events. This patient presents, in addition to adult onset diabetes, with a combination of moderate obesity (BMI 28; ideal <25), a history of hypertension, a dyslipidemia characterized by an increase in apo B lipoproteins of 1.87 (normal $= 1.2 + 0.3$ g/l), with increased triglycerides and LDL-C and reduced HDL-C. This clustering of metabolic factors is not an infrequent finding in subjects with CAD. Although certain lifestyle interventions (weight reduction, exercise, and proper diet) are essential in the proper management of these disorders, they are often not fully implemented by the patient.

The treatment of the lipoprotein disorder in this patient represents a therapeutic challenge. Management of the diabetes is essential in order to modify the hypertriglyceridemia.[1] The choice of drug therapy has not been clearly established in such individuals. Treatment with fibric acid derivatives is particularly appealing to reduce triglyceride levels, increase HDL-C levels and, in some cases, reduce LDL-C levels.[2] In addition, second generation fibrates have an advantageous profile on some homeostatic factors (such as fibrinogen).[3] The HMG-CoA reductase inhibitors have a more potent effect in reducing LDL-C levels and in improving the total cholesterol/HDL-C ratio. In the 4S and CARE studies, subgroup analyses of diabetic patients have shown that the HMG-CoA reductase inhibitors are effective in preventing cardiovascular events in diabetic subjects with a dyslipoproteinemia similar to the present case.[4,5]

Although the treatment of an elevated Lp(a) with conventional medications has not been favorable, niacin may be the preferred treatment for those with very high Lp(a) levels. However, it has yet to be determined whether reducing Lp(a) levels reduces coronary risk. The effect of beta-blockers on glycemic control or lipoprotein metabolism must play a secondary role to their clear lifesaving properties in postmyocardial infarction patients. The optimal management of subjects with multiple risk factors (obesity, insulin resistance, dyslipidemia, and hypertension) remains controversial. Just because evidence from large scale clinical trials is currently lacking for patients with this cluster of abnormalities should not be an excuse for therapeutic nihilism. Rather, an approach as outlined above makes intuitive sense where each of the abnormalities can be monitored and followed accordingly.

REFERENCES

1 Thompson GR. *A handbook of hyperlipidemia.* Whitehorse Sta. NJ: Current Science Ed. USA, 1994.

2 Bruckert E, De Gennes JL, Malbecq W, Baigts F. Comparison of the efficacy of simvastatin and standard fibrate therapy in the treatment of primary hypercholesterolemia and combined hyperlipidemia. *Clin Cardiol* 1995;**18**: 621–9.

3 Ernst E, Resch KL. Therapeutic interventions to lower plasma fibrinogen concentrations. *Eur Heart J* 1995;**16A**:47–52.

4 The Scandinavian Simvastatin Survival Study Group. Randomised trial of cholesterol lowering in 4444 patients with coronary heart disease. *Lancet* 1994;**344**:1383–9.

5 Sacks FM, Pfeffer MA, Moye LA *et al.* The effect of pravastatin on coronary events after myocardial infarction in patients with average cholesterol levels. CARE Investigators. *N Engl J Med* 1996; **335**:1001–9.

Peripheral vascular disease with suspect coronary artery disease: management issues

66

PETER C. SPITTELL

CASE 1

Over the past several years, a 74-year-old man has noticed progressive left leg discomfort with walking. Standing still provides complete relief. His walking distance had gradually decreased to less than one block in the past year. He is a non-smoker, non-diabetic, and has no prior cardiac history. His medications include captopril and dyazide for hypertension.

On examination, his blood pressure is 140/80 mmHg (both arms), and his resting pulse is 65 bpm and regular. There is a right carotid bruit and reduced femoral pulses with bilateral bruits. Pulses are non-palpable below the femoral level on the left. On the right, the popliteal and posterior tibial pulses are mildly reduced and the dorsalis pedis pulse is absent. Elevation pallor is grade III (pallor is less than 30 seconds) on the left and grade O (no pallor in 60 seconds) on the right. The remainder of the physical examination is normal.

A resting ECG reveals normal sinus rhythm with a non-specific T wave abnormality. The chest radiograph is normal. Routine hematology and chemistry values are normal.

The resting ankle:brachial systolic pressure indexes (ABI, normal >0.9) are 1.0 on the right, 0.6 on the left. After walking 124 yards (113 meters) on a treadmill (10% incline, 1.5 mph) and developing left hip, thigh, and calf claudication, his post-exercise ABIs are 0.3 on the right and 0.2 on the left, consistent with moderate (right) and moderately severe (left) peripheral arterial occlusive disease, respectively.

Carotid ultrasound demonstrates a large amount of atheromatous plaque in the right carotid bulb associated with a 70–99% stenosis.

Question: What would be the most appropriate management at this point?

COMMENT

Here, one seeks evidence to guide the management of an elderly patient with extensive peripheral vascular disease who may or may not have concomitant coronary artery disease. The finding of an asymptomatic high grade carotid stenosis (>60%) warrants consideration of prophylactic carotid endarterectomy if the patient's general health is good. A 60% diameter reducing stenosis (carotid ultrasound) is considered as an indication for surgical intervention in asymptomatic patients who are in a low risk surgical category: using a ratio of 3.2 for the peak systolic velocity at the site of narrowing divided by that from the carotid artery, a sensitivity of 92% and a specificity of 86% can be achieved. This gives a positive predictive value of 85%, a negative predictive value of 93% and an overall accuracy of 89%.[1] The evidence shows that carotid endarterectomy in patients with an asymptomatic carotid stenosis >60% in severity, significantly reduces the risk of ipsilateral stroke, perioperative stroke, or death; when compared to medical therapy alone.[2]

In view of the patient's age and widespread peripheral vascular disease it is prudent to assess the patient's perioperative cardiac risk. A dobutamine stress echocardiography was performed and was negative for ischemia. This test is associated with a high negative predictive value.[3]

The patient underwent right carotid endarterectomy without complication. Postoperatively, following a discussion with the patient regarding the natural history of intermittent claudication and indications for restoration of pulsatile flow,[4] he elected a conservative treatment program which included aspirin 325 mg/day, a walking program for intermittent claudication, and foot care and protection.

REFERENCES

1 Edwards JM *et al.* Duplex ultrasound criteria for determining >50% and <60% internal carotid artery stenosis: implications for screening examinations. Noninvasive vascular laboratory and vascular imaging In: Young JR, Olin JW, Bartholomew JR, eds. *Peripheral vascular diseases,* 2nd edn. St Louis: Mosby, 1996, p 45.

2 Executive Committee for the Asymptomatic Carotid Atherosclerosis (ACAS) Study. Endarterectomy for asymptomatic carotid artery stenosis. *JAMA* 1995; 273:1421–8.

3 Eichelberger JP, Schwarz KQ, Black ER, Green R, Ouriel K. Predictive value of dobutamine echocardiography before non-cardiac vascular surgery. *Am J Cardiol* 1993; 72:602–7.

4 McDaniel MD, Cronenwett JL. Basic data related to the natural history of intermittent claudication. *Ann Vasc Surg* 1989;3:273–7.

CASE 2

A 52-year-old man presents with progressive exertional right calf discomfort over the past year. Standing still provides complete relief of the discomfort, but his walking distance has gradually shortened to one block. He notes similar, less severe discomfort in the left calf. His claudication is severely limiting his lifestyle.

He is taking amlodipine for systemic hypertension, has smoked tobacco for the past 34 years and has a history of hyperlipidemia treated by diet. Blood glucose is normal. He denies a history of angina pectoris or diabetes mellitus.

On examination his blood pressure is 140/90 mmHg (both arms), resting pulse is 85 bpm and regular. A grade 1/4 systolic murmur at the cardiac apex and a right carotid bruit are present. A small abdominal aortic aneurysm is also palpable. The popliteal, posterior tibial, and dorsalis pedis pulses are absent on the right. On the left, the popliteal and posterior tibial pulses are moderately reduced. The dorsalis pedis pulse is absent. Elevation pallor is grade III (pallor in less than 30 seconds), grade I (pallor in less than 60 seconds), on the right and left, respectively.

A resting ECG shows normal sinus rhythm without other abnormalities. Routine hematology and chemistry values are normal.

Resting ankle:brachial systolic pressure index (ABI) is 0.5 on the right and 0.6 on the left (ABI normal >0.9). After walking 282 yards (258 meters) on a treadmill (10% incline, 2 mph) and developing right calf claudication, his post-exercise ABIs are 0.2 on the right, 0.7 on the left, consistent with severe peripheral arterial occlusive disease on the right and mild disease on the left.

Carotid ultrasound reveals a right external carotid artery stenosis with mild atherosclerotic disease in the right carotid bulb, but is otherwise normal. Abdominal ultrasound confirms a small abdominal aortic aneurysm (2.5 cm).

After a discussion of peripheral arterial occlusive disease with the patient, including its natural history, prognosis, treatment, and goals of treatment, he elects to pursue restoration of pulsatile flow.

Question: How would you proceed at this point?

COMMENT

This case is somewhat more complex insofar as there is more suspicion of concomitant coronary artery disease. And so, with the decision to pursue vascular surgery, an assessment of the patient's perioperative cardiac risk is warranted.[1] Although he has no history of angina pectoris, he has a number of cardiovascular risk factors (male gender, tobacco, hypertension, hyperlipidemia). Furthermore, his intermittent claudication limits his activity and may prevent him from experiencing exertional angina. To further assess his perioperative cardiac risk, dobutamine stress echocardiography was performed and demonstrated normal left ventricular size and function, but was positive for ischemia (new regional wall motion abnormalities in the mid and apical anterior wall). A positive dobutamine stress echocardiogram has a positive predictive value of 35% for a perioperative cardiac event. When ischemia occurs at a significantly lower heart rate during dobutamine stress (<70% of the age-corrected maximal heart rate) the positive predictive value increases to 53%.[2]

Medical therapy was elected (suspect single vessel disease with normal left ventricular function), and it was felt safe to proceed with peripheral revascularization. Peripheral angiography demonstrated a high grade stenosis involving a short segment of the distal right superficial femoral artery. Percutaneous transluminal angioplasty of the stenosis was performed. Although no well designed large scale clinical trial has yet been done to determine the efficacy of percutaneous angioplasty for this type of patient, percutaneous angioplasty was nonetheless felt to be indicated because the prognosis for limb loss in patients with intermittent claudication is related mostly to the severity of disease, as assessed by ankle pressure measurements, at the time of study entry.[3] After the procedure, a normal dorsalis pedis pulse was restored on the right. Intermittent claudication completely resolved following the procedure. He was placed on aspirin (325 mg/d), advised to discontinue tobacco, and instructed in foot care and protection. Amlodipine was continued for treatment of his hypertension, and the importance of adequate control of hypertension was discussed. Ultrasound of the abdominal aorta in one year was recommended to re-evaluate his abdominal aortic aneurysm. Additional instruction on dietary therapy for hyperlipidemia was given and a follow-up lipid profile was arranged in 3 months.

REFERENCES

1 Eagle KA, Brundage BH, Chaitman BR *et al.* Guidelines for perioperative cardiovascular evaluation for noncardiac surgery. ACC/AHA Task Force report. *Circulation* 1996;**93**: 1278–317.

2 Poldermans D, Arnese M, Fioretti PM *et al.* Improved cardiac risk stratification in major vascular surgery with dobutamine stress echocardiography. *J Am Coll Cardiol* 1995;**26**: 648–53.

3 McDaniel MD, Cronenwelt JL. Basic data related to the natural history of intermittent claudication. *Ann Vasc Surg* 1989;**3**:271–7.

Congestive heart failure: management issues

67

HERBERT J. LEVINE

CASE 1

A 50-year-old male with a history of chronic alcoholism presents with a 1-year history of congestive heart failure characterized by effort dyspnea and dependent edema. An echocardiogram 6 months ago revealed a dilated, hypokinetic left ventricle with an estimated ejection fraction of 0.25 and mild to moderate mitral regurgitation. He was treated with digoxin 0.25 mg od and furosemide 40 mg. He was also started on an ACE inhibitor which had to be discontinued because of a troublesome dry cough.

He now comes to your office complaining of increasing dyspnea on exertion, a recumbent cough and worsening of his edema. Examination reveals a displaced apex beat, a sinus tachycardia of 100 beats/min, bibasilar pulmonary râles, an S3 gallop rhythm and 2–3 + pretibial edema.

Question: How would you proceed with management of this patient?

COMMENT

The objectives of management are relief of symptoms, improvement in functional capacity and prolongation of useful life. To achieve all three goals in this patient clinical expertise and a sound understanding of circulatory pathophysiology is now aided by external evidence from several well conducted clinical trials. In this particular case, the diagnosis of congestive heart failure is clearly established and there is convincing clinical and laboratory evidence for combined left ventricular systolic and diastolic dysfunction.

The patient is already on digoxin, which should be continued according to the recent DIG trial which demonstrated that digoxin is probably the only inotropic agent that does not shorten survival while improving the patient's wellbeing and reducing the need for hospitalization.[1] One should optimize the inotropic support of the ventricle by checking the serum digoxin level to be sure the level is in the therapeutic range.[2] To effect afterload and preload reduction of the ventricle while improving both quality and prolongation of life the optimum treatment is an ACE inhibitor.[3,4] Although side effects (the non-productive cough) of an ACE inhibitor were not well tolerated in this patient, there is evidence that much of the benefit of these drugs can be achieved by use of the angiotensin-2 receptor blocker losartin, without the side effect of cough[5,6] or, alternatively, by the combination of hydralazine and nitrate therapy.[7]

For treatment of the congestive symptoms (diastolic dysfunction), more aggressive diuretic therapy is warranted, as well as careful attention to the dietary history with emphasis on salt restriction and abstinence from alcohol. One could begin by increasing the morning dose of furosemide and if the diuretic threshold is not easily reached, the next step would be to add a second diuretic (i.e. a thiazide, metolazone or spironolactone). Although the need for a diuretic is intuitive in this patient, who has developed an edematous state, there are no definitive large scale placebo controlled trials on diuretic therapy for advanced congestive heart failure. Nitrate therapy, too, may be useful to reduce both systemic arterial and pulmonary venous pressures, although again, besides the benefit of combined isosorbide dinitrate-hydralazine in the V-Heft II trial,[7] the use of nitrates alone in the management of congestive heart failure has not been clearly documented.

REFERENCES

1 The Digitalis Investigation Group (DIG). The effect of digoxin on mortality and morbidity in patients with heart failure. N Engl J Med 1997;**336**: 525–33.

2 Guyatt GH, Sullivan MJJ, Fallen EL et al. A controlled trial of digoxin in congestive heart failure. Am J Cardiol 1988;**61**:371–5.

3 The SOLVD Investigators. Effect of enalapril on survival in patients with reduced left ventricular ejection fraction and congestive heart failure. N Engl J Med 199;**325**:293–302.

4 The CONSENSUS Trial Study Group. Effects of enalapril on mortality in severe congestive heart failure. N Engl J Med 1987;**316**:1429–35.

5 Crozier I et al. Losartin in heart failure: hemodynamic effects and tolerability. Circulation 1995;**91**:691–7.

6 Dickstein K et al. Comparison of the effects of losartin and enalapril on clinical status and exercise performance in patients with moderate or severe congestive heart failure. J Am Coll Cardiol 1995;**26**:438–45.

7 Cohn JN et al. A comparison of enalapril with hydralazine-isosorbide dinitrate in the treatment of chronic congestive heart failure. N Engl J Med 1991;**325**:303–10.

CASE 2

A 56-year-old woman with a bicuspid aortic valve recently developed subacute bacterial endocarditis due to *Streptococcus viridans* which was treated successfully with antibiotic therapy. She was left, however, with substantial aortic regurgitation. She now presents, one year later, with signs and symptoms of congestive heart failure with effort dyspnea and mild pedal edema. Echocardiography reveals severe (3–4+) aortic regurgitation, a dilated left ventricle, normal end-systolic volume, and a normal ejection fraction of 55%. Aortic valve replacement is recommended, but the patient adamantly refuses surgery.

Question: How would you manage this patient?

COMMENT

This patient fits a specific category which does not readily qualify for entry criteria of most heart failure clinical trials. Namely, a case of severe congestive symptoms, a volume overloaded state, and compensated LV function all on a background of a mechanical (hydraulic) abnormality. She also has isolated diastolic dysfunction, that is, congestive heart failure with normal systolic function (her end-systolic volume is normal). In the presence of a normal ejection fraction, digoxin therapy is probably not indicated, although in the DIG study an ancillary group of patients with EF >0.45 (492 patients randomized) enjoyed the same qualitative benefit as the main group.[1] Ordinarily, there would be little reason to employ afterload reduction in patients with isolated diastolic dysfunction. But in this case, evidence exists that the use of long term vasoactive (afterload reducing) drugs is helpful in peripherally unloading the left ventricle, thereby reducing the degree of aortic valve regurgitant flow, ventricular volumes, and wall stress.[2] My own choice would be an ACE inhibitor. The major therapeutic agent for treatment of the congestive symptoms (as with other patients with diastolic dysfunction) would be diuretic therapy. This is a rational choice based on clinical observation and sound hemodynamic principles, although no large scale RCTs have been reported so far to confirm this option.

While this regimen may be successful in ameliorating symptoms and perhaps delaying the need for surgery, efforts to convince the patient of the need for surgery should continue, particularly if serial echocardiography or radionuclide studies indicate a decrease in systolic ventricular function manifested by a progressive rise in the end-systolic dimension.

REFERENCES

1 The Digitalis Investigation Group (DIG). The effect of digoxin on mortality and morbidity in patients with heart failure. *N Engl J Med* 1997;**336**: 525–33.

2 Levine HJ, Gaasch WH. Vasoactive drugs in chronic regurgitant lesions of the mitral and aortic valves. *J Am Coll Cardiol* 1996;**28**:1083–91.

68 Atrial fibrillation: management issues

MICHAEL D. KLEIN

CASE 1

A 56-year-old professor who has been followed for 5 years with annual health examinations requests an expedited office visit because of an episode of palpitations and diminished exercise endurance. Review of his prior medical records indicates a patrilineal history of late life hypertension, excellent personal health habits including regular recreational exercise, borderline hypertension (avg BP 144/90 mmHg), and a LV–S_4 on cardiac auscultation. Owing to his reluctance to take medicine regularly, no antihypertensive medication has been initiated. On the present examination he acknowledges some concern about faculty downsizing at his University. His BP is 148/92. Auscultation reveals a variable intensity S_1 without an S_3 or heart murmurs. Thyroid exam is normal and thyroid chemistries show a total T_4 of 7.5 µg/dl, a total T_3 of 1.3 ng/ml and a TSH of 4.2. His ECG documents the presence of atrial fibrillation, a ventricular response rate of 96, and borderline voltage for left ventricular hypertrophy.

Question: What action should be taken now?

COMMENT

In this case, evidence is sought to address two clinical questions: (a) is this man a candidate for lifelong oral anticoagulant therapy and (b) should he be cardioverted and maintained in sinus rhythm or should he be left in atrial fibrillation using drug treatment to control his ventricular rate?

The immediate concern is treatment of the atrial fibrillation, the cause of which probably relates to mild hypertension and some work-related stress. Hypertension-induced mild left ventricular hypertrophy can reduce diastolic distensibility and alter the left ventricular inflow velocity profile with consequent episodic left atrial hypertension and the spawning of atrial ectopic beats triggering atrial fibrillation.[1] Atrial fibrillation is associated with thrombus formation, especially in the left atrial appendage,[2] and thereby an enhanced risk for thromboembolic stroke, particularly when atrial fibrillation converts back to sinus rhythm. Anticoagulation with warfarin to an INR of 2.0–3.0 should be instituted to minimize the risk of thromboembolic stroke.[3] Then, drug therapy to treat hypertension and, hopefully, restore sinus rhythm could be initiated, although restoration of sinus rhythm pharmacologically is not terribly effective. A beta-adrenergic blocker would be an excellent first choice because of both its antihypertensive action as well as heart rate control which is undermined by atrial fibrillation. Digoxin, which sensitizes the heart to parasympathetic restraint, can synergize with the beta-blocker in slowing the heart rate. Non-dihydropyridine calcium-channel blocker drugs offer an alternative to beta-blocker therapy, especially in patients prone to hyperactive airways symptoms.

While these measures are being accomplished, an echocardiogram should be obtained to evaluate left ventricular wall thickness, cardiac chamber size, myocardial and valvular function, as well as unlikely associated causes of atrial fibrillation, such as atrial tumors or non-dilated cardiomyopathy. Left atrial size and left ventricular systolic function can be quantified, refining the clinical appraisal of thromboembolic stroke risk.[4,5] A transesophageal echocardiogram (TEE) provides a clearer view of the left atrial appendage and quantification of appendicular inflow and outflow velocity enhancing clot identification, and possibly improving stroke risk estimate.[6] But, from a cost-effective viewpoint, since the patient is already anticoagulated, a transthoracic echocardiogram (TTE) offers almost the same amount of laboratory information in estimating stroke risk. A TEE would be useful, however, to exclude left atrial thrombus if early cardioversion is elected before or after only several days of anticoagulation.

Follow-up

The TTE showed an increased LV posterior wall thickness (12 mm), normal LV size, and systolic function (LVEF 60%), borderline left atrial enlargement (42 mm) without indwelling clot or tumor. At follow-up office visit, the BP is 138/88 mmHg and sinus rhythm happened to be restored while on digoxin and beta-blocker therapy. Should this not have been the case, electroversion or primary antiarrhythmic drug therapy with class IC or III agents such as propafenone or sotalol could have been considered. Electroversion is preferable, as it is quicker, can be accomplished during a several hour hospital stay without overnight admission, and avoid possible proarrhythmic hazards and other related adverse side effects associated with primary antiarrhythmic agents.[7]

With restoration and persistence of sinus rhythm consideration can be given to replacing warfarin with aspirin for long term antistroke prophylaxis. Satisfactory drug control of hypertension, the absence of diabetes, the absence of recent congestive heart failure or prior thrombotic stroke, bespeak a low clinical risk profile for atrial fibrillation related stroke in this patient.[4,5] Minimal left atrial enlargement with normal left ventricular systolic function reinforce the low stroke estimate.[8] Moreover population studies show that the attributable risk of stroke for atrial fibrillation is very low for patients in the sixth decade.[9] Finally, the atrial fibrillation randomized clinical trials indicating a superior antistroke benefit for warfarin vs aspirin have included very few patients in the sixth decade. Hence, long term antithrombotic aspirin therapy in this particular case might prudently be given and avoid both the cost and time required for monthly INR checks.

REFERENCES

1 Ganau A, Devereux RB, Roman MJ *et al.* Patterns of left ventricular hypertrophy and geometric remodelling in essential hypertension. *J Am Coll Cardiol* 1992;**19**:1550–7.

2 Aberg H. Atrial fibrillation. A study of atrial thrombosis and system embolism in a necropsy material. *Acta Med Scand* 1996;**195**:373–9.

3 Laupacis A, Alberg G, Dalen J, Dunn M, Feinberg W, Jacobson A. Antithrombotic therapy in atrial fibrillation. *Chest* 1995;**108**(Suppl):352S–359S.

4 Stroke Prevention in Atrial Fibrillation Investigators. Prevention of thromboembolism in atrial fibrillation: I. Clinical features of patients at risk. *Ann Intern Med* 1992;**116**:1–5.

5 Stroke Prevention in Atrial Fibrillation Investigators. Predictors of thromboembolism in atrial fibrillation: II. Echocardiographic features of patients at risk. *Ann Intern Med* 1992;**116**:6–12.

6 Atrial Fibrillation Investigators. Atrial fibrillation: risk factors for embolization and efficacy of antithrombotic therapy. *Arch Inten Med* 1994;**154**: 1149–57.

7 Middlekauf HR, Stevenson WG, Gornbein JA. Antiarrhythmic prophylaxis versus warfarin anticoagulation to prevent thromboembolic events among patients with atrial fibrillation. A decision analysis. *Arch Intern Med* 1995;**155**:913–20.

8 Vaziri SM, Larson MG, Benjamin EJ, Levy D. Echocardiographic predictors of non-rheumatic atrial fibrillation: the Framingham Study. *Circulation* 1994;**89**:724–30.

9 Wolf PA, Abbott RD, Cannel WB. Atrial fibrillation as an independent risk factor for stroke: the Framingham Study. *Stroke* 1991;**22**:983–8.

CASE 2

A 68-year-old female calls for an office appointment because of a 1-week history of palpitations and fatigue, especially notable on exertion. Atrial fibrillation is documented on exam and confirmed by ECG which shows a ventricular response rate of 105 bpm at rest, QRS duration of 80 msec, QRS axis of $-30°$, and no ventricular ectopy. Review of past medical history indicates a bleeding duodenal ulcer 30 years previously without recurrence, seasonal hay fever and asthma, an apical mid-systolic murmur attributed to mitral valve prolapse, and mild anxiety concerning her personal health.

Treatment options are discussed with the patient, including anticoagulation and cardioversion with drugs or electricity versus attempted symptom alleviation with heart rate control. Her apprehension regarding anticoagulants and concerns about possible side effects of antiarrhythmic drugs results in a drug treatment plan to slow the heart rate. The non-dihydropyridine calcium-channel blocker diltiazem is selected in preference to a beta-blocker because of the predisposition to asthma.[1] Digoxin is also given for its procholinergic effect, with prolongation of AV nodal refractoriness.

When seen again 2 weeks later, her atrial fibrillation is still present, albeit with a slower resting ventricular response of 85 bpm. Palpitations are much reduced in frequency but exertional fatigue persists. A Holter ambulatory ECG was done several days earlier and showed atrial fibrillation with minimal, mean, and maximal ventricular rates of 70, 105, and 148 bpm respectively. After further discussion concerning the difficulty of heart rate control in atrial fibrillation,[2] and the need for chronic and often high dose drug therapy, she accedes to anticoagulation with subsequent electrical cardioversion.

Warfarin therapy is initiated, adjusted to an INR of 2.0–3.0 and maintained in that range for three weeks[3] with the aid of an anticoagulation clinic. A transesophageal echocardiogram (TEE) prior to electroversion is proposed to exclude atrial appendicular thrombus[4] but the patient demurs. (The patient was probably right in view of the fact that there was no need for urgent as opposed to elective cardioversion.)

After 3 weeks of diltiazem and warfarin, the patient is successfully cardioverted to sinus rhythm using a 50 Joule countershock. Warfarin is continued for 4 weeks, thereafter, to provide for an interval of gradual return of atrial contractility and minimize the potential for post-countershock thromboembolism, especially in view of the lack of prior TEE studies. Anticoagulation with warfarin is adjusted to an INR of 2.0–3.0 and is continued.

COMMENT

Several confounding variables and the patient's concerns raise several issues when seeking best available evidence to guide therapy in this case. Atrial fibrillation results in a loss of heart rate control. Heart rate may only be moderately elevated at rest but rises precipitously with exercise or emotional excitement. In the absence of heart failure, several drugs are available to effect heart rate slowing by increasing AV nodal refractoriness. Digoxin can slow the resting ventricular response rate but has not been successful in re-establishing sinus rhythm in randomized clinical trials.[5,6] Diltiazem was added because of its negative dromotropic action on AV nodal tissue, which facilitates ventricular rate slowing during exertion. In this case a combination of digoxin and diltiazem was selected because of their synergistic action to slow conduction through the AV node.

After several weeks of therapy, the resting heart rate was slower and the patient calmer. Her persistent fatigue was probably related to some fall in her left ventricular stroke output associated with loss of left atrial contribution to left ventricular diastolic filling. Or, possibly, to a still brisk heart rate acceleration with exertion. The patient was more willing to accept electrical cardioversion once she saw that drugs had not restored sinus rhythm. Similarly, her concerns regarding long term anticoagulation were allayed after it was pointed out to her that adjusted dose warfarin was about four times more effective than aspirin plus low dose warfarin in reducing stroke risk in atrial fibrillation patients.[7]

The importance of maintaining the INR between 2.0 and 3.0 was also stressed in case control studies which have indicated that the risk of thromboembolic stroke associated with non-valvular atrial fibrillation increased at lower INR with an adjusted odds ratio of 2.0 (95% CI 1.6–2.4) at an INR of 1.7 and 3.3 (95% CI 2.4–4.6) at an INR of 1.5.[8]

Follow-up

When seen a month later, she had maintained sinus rhythm but with rare atrial premature beats. If atrial fibrillation had recrudesced, then anticoagulation would be continued and antiarrhythmic therapy could be instituted with an oral Class Ic or Class III agent such as flecainide, propafenone or amiodarone. Cardioversion could then be repeated under cover of antiarrhythmic and anticoagulant therapy and consideration should be given to long term antiarrhythmic drug therapy to prevent atrial fibrillation recurrence.

The patient was maintained in sinus rhythm on daily warfarin. Digoxin and diltiazem were discontinued since there is no randomized trial data to indicate that they would maintain sinus rhythm indefinitely. The benefits of sinus rhythm versus effective ventricular rate control in atrial fibrillation is currently being appraised in the randomized clinical trial, Affirm.[9]

REFERENCES

1 Prystowsky EN, Benson DW Jr, Hart RG *et al.* Management of patients with atrial fibrillation. A statement for health care professionals. From the AHA Subcommittee on Electrocardiography and Electrophysiology. *Circulation* 1996;**93**:1262–77.

2 Falk RH. Pharmacologic control of heart rate in atrial fibrillation. *Cardiol Clin* 1996;**14**:521–36.

3 Laupacis A, Albers G, Dalen J *et al.* Antithrombotic therapy in atrial fibrillation. *Chest* 1995;**108**: 352S–359S.

4 Klein AL, Grimm RA, Black IW *et al.* Cardioversion guided by transesophageal echocardiography. The ACUTE Pilot Study. A randomized, controlled trial. *Ann Intern Med* 1997;**126**:200–9.

5 Jordaens L, Trouerback J, Calle P *et al.* Conversion of atrial fibrillation to sinus rhythm and rate control by digoxin in comparison to placebo. *Eur Heart J* 1997;**18**:643–8.

6 The Digitalis in Acute Atrial Fibrillation (DAAF) trial group. Intravenous digoxin in acute atrial fibrillation. Results of a randomized, placebo-controlled multicentre trial in 239 patients. *Eur J Cardiol* 1997;**18**:649–54.

7 Stroke Prevention in Atrial Fibrillation Investigators. Adjusted-dose warfarin versus low-intensity fixed-dose warfarin plus aspirin for high-risk patients with atrial fibrillation: Stroke Prevention in Atrial Fibrillation III randomized clinical trial. *Lancet* 1996;**348**:633–8.

8 Hylek EM, Skates SJ, Sheehan MA, Singer DE. AV analysis of the lowest effective intensity of prophylactic anticoagulation with nonrheumatic atrial fibrillation. *N Engl J Med* 1996;**335**:540–6.

9 The Planning and Steering Committees of the Affirm study for the NHLBI Affirm Investigators. Atrial fibrillation follow-up investigation of rhythm management – The Affirm study design. *Am J Cardiol* 1997;**79**:1198–202.

Ventricular dysrhythmias: pharmacology vs non-pharmacology treatment

69

L. BRENT MITCHELL

CASE 1

At the age of 60 years, Mr D presents a therapeutic choice in the management of a patient who has had ventricular tachycardia (VT). Two years previously he had experienced an acute anterolateral myocardial infarction but did not receive thrombolysis. When post-MI angina continued, he underwent cardiac catheterization which demonstrated three vessel coronary artery disease and compromised LV function. Accordingly, he underwent three vessel coronary artery bypass surgery. Thereafter, Mr D was free of any potential cardiovascular symptoms until now, when he presents to the Emergency Department after the sudden onset, while performing minor car maintenance, of presyncope followed by diaphoresis and dyspnea. He is found to have VT at a rate of 175 beats per minute with a right bundle branch "block" pattern, a left axis deviation QRS morphology and 2:1 retrograde VA block (Figure 69.1). His systolic BP is 85 mmHg. Under general anesthesia this rhythm is cardioverted with a 50 Joule QRS synchronous D/C shock to another VT with a right bundle branch "block" configuration and right axis deviation QRS morphology (Figure 69.2). A second 200 Joule QRS synchronous D/C shock restores normal sinus rhythm. His initial postconversion evaluation reveals no transient or reversible causes of VT (such as acute myocardial infarction, electrolyte disturbance or proarrhythmic drug effect).

On a treadmill exercise test Mr D exercises for 4 minutes, reaching stage II of the standard Bruce protocol. The endpoint was dyspnea at a maximum heart rate of 153 beats per minute (target heart rate = 136 beats per minute). The blood pressure response is flat. There is no evidence of reversible myocardial ischemia or exercise-related arrhythmia. A 24-hour ambulatory ECG shows sinus rhythm within the physiologic rate range and only rare isolated premature ventricular beats (two on the 24 hour recording). A cardiac catheterization demonstrates patent coronary bypass grafts and no new native coronary artery lesions. His left ventricular angiogram reveals an anteroapical LV aneurysm.

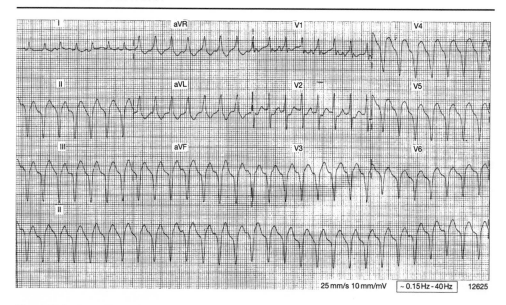

Figure 69.1 Presenting ventricular tachycardia of right bundle "block" pattern with left axis deviation QRS morphology and 2:1 retrograde VA block.

A catheter electrophysiologic study shows normal sinus nodal, atrial, and AV nodal electrophysiology. The HV interval is prolonged to 60 msec. Programmed ventricular stimulation induces sustained VT (Figure 69.3) that matches the initial presenting VT and could be pace terminated. The mechanism of the VT is not bundle branch re-entry. Intravenous procainamide is administered (total dose 1 gm). Thereafter, VT is no longer inducible.

Question: What treatment, if any, should now be applied?

COMMENT

For this case, current available "best" evidence does not define a single preferred therapeutic approach This 60-year-old male presents with hypotensive VT in the setting of stable atherosclerotic heart disease on the background of a previous anterolateral wall myocardial infarction and a left ventricular aneurysm. After ruling out a transient or reversible cause for his VT and optimizing the therapy of underlying structural heart disease, an electrophysiologic study demonstrated the persistence of a substrate for VT that was suppressed by intravenous procainamide.

Viable alternatives for the treatment of this man's high future risk of VT recurrence include (a) standard antiarrhythmic drug therapy individualized by the Holter monitoring approach; or (b) the electrophysiologic study approach; or (c) empiric amiodarone therapy; or (d) implantation of a tiered-therapy implantable cardioverter defibrillator (ICD); or (e) surgical/transcatheter ablative therapy. In addition, grade B evidence supports the concomitant use of ancillary beta-blocker therapy where possible.[1]

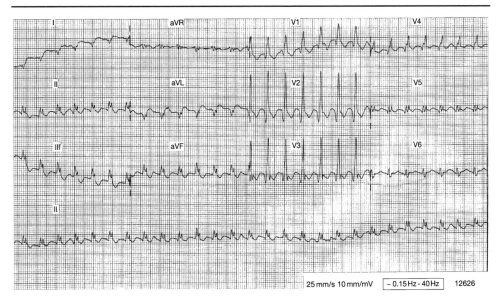

Figure 69.2 Ventricular tachycardia with right bundle branch "block" configuration and right axis deviation QRS morphology after low energy cardioversion.

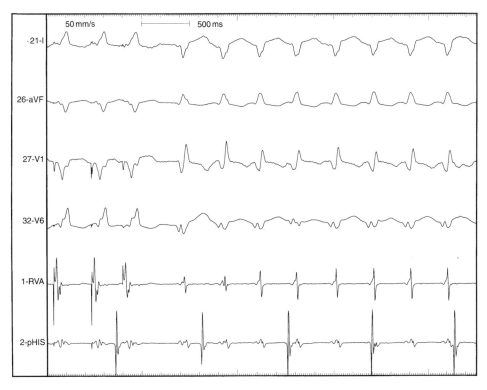

Figure 69.3 Ventricular tachycardia of right bundle branch "block" configuration and right axis deviation QRS morphology induced by program stimulation.

Mr D's clinical circumstance is a frequent clinical scenario, and such patients have been the most commonly recruited subjects of clinical trials evaluating treatment for life-threatening VT. Nevertheless, there is still uncertainty as to the most appropriate initial form of therapy. Randomized clinical trials relative to the treatment of this patient population include the Calgary study;[2] ESVEM: Electrophysiologic Study vs Electrocardiographic Monitoring Study;[3] CASCADE: Cardiac Arrest in Seattle: Conventional vs Amiodarone Drug Evaluation;[4] the Antiarrhythmics vs Implantable Defibrillator (AVID) trial;[5] the ongoing Cardiac Arrest Study Hamburg (CASH) study;[6] and the Canadian Implantable Defibrillator Study (CIDS).[7] It should be noted that each of these trials compares one therapy to another therapy. To date, ethical considerations have precluded comparisons of one form of therapy to no therapy.

Both the Calgary study and the ESVEM trial compared the long term outcome of patients treated with standard antiarrhythmic drug therapy selected by the Holter monitoring approach to that selected by the electrophysiologic study approach. In a small population of drug-naive patients with inducible VT, the Calgary study reported superiority of therapy selected by the electrophysiologic study approach. Furthermore, such therapy was associated with low VT recurrence and sudden death probabilities in the Calgary trial. In contrast, in a larger population of drug-resistant patients with either inducible VT or VF, the ESVEM trial reported equivalence of therapy selected by either of the approaches. Furthermore, such therapy was associated with a high VT/VF recurrence rate in the ESVEM trial. Mr D's clinical situation was most comparable to the patients in the Calgary trial who had arrhythmia substrates for which the electrophysiologic study performs best (inducible VT in the setting of stable atherosclerotic heart disease). Furthermore, Mr D did not have sufficient spontaneous ventricular arrhythmia on his Holter monitor as to provide an index to guide the Holter monitoring approach. Accordingly, Mr D had standard antiarrhythmic drug therapy – procainamide in this case – selected by the electrophysiologic study approach.

Empiric amiodarone therapy was considered. The most impressive data supporting the use of empiric amiodarone in a patient such as Mr D emerges not from randomized clinical trials but rather from descriptions of excellent long term outcomes of patients who had failed other therapy and then received empiric amiodarone. Some would argue that CASCADE demonstrated the superiority of empiric amiodarone over standard antiarrhythmic drug therapy in this setting. However, we must recall that CASCADE included only patients with out-of-hospital VF cardiac arrests. Furthermore, in CASCADE, empiric amiodarone appeared superior to antiarrhythmic therapy selected by either the electrophysiologic study approach or the Holter monitoring approach (rather than the better of these two approaches). Finally, many of the patients in the standard antiarrhythmic therapy limb of CASCADE received therapy that was predicted to be (and presumably was) ineffective. Nevertheless, this report and the concerns regarding the inefficacy of standard antiarrhythmic therapy in the ESVEM trial have allowed empiric amiodarone to emerge as the "gold standard" pharmacologic therapy to which ICD therapy is being compared in ongoing trials. Accordingly, this therapeutic choice would also have been appropriate.

Electrosurgery/transcatheter ablation therapy was considered. Ablative therapies have had their greatest success in patients with atherosclerotic heart disease and previous myocardial infarction. This is particularly true if another indication exists for open heart surgery such as a need for a coronary revascularization procedure. Nevertheless, this approach exposes the patient to an important surgical mortality and may not be appropriate for patients with a single episode of VT who do not need coronary revascularization and have other therapeutic alternatives. Of course had the electrophysiologic study demonstrated a VT that required the participation of the right bundle branch (bundle branch re-entry), then ablation of the right bundle branch would have been a preferred form of therapy.

The use of an implantable automatic cardioverter defibrillator (ICD) was considered. Once reserved for patients with VT/VF resistant to other therapy, the long term results of ICD therapy have been impressive. Furthermore, the Data and Safety Monitoring Board of the AVID trial recently recommended that the study be terminated after slightly more than 1000 patients had been enrolled as a statistically significant advantage had emerged relative to all-cause mortality in favour of the ICD over antiarrhythmic drug therapy, consisting of empiric amiodarone for the vast majority of patients with a few patients having received sotalol, that was predicted to be effective by either the electrophysiologic study approach or the Holter monitoring approach. However, preliminary costing analysis has suggested that the ICD may not be an economically competitive strategy with a cost per year of life saved of approximately $130 000. Nevertheless, patients such as Mr D frequently receive an ICD. Of note, the results of the Multicenter Automatic Defibrillator Implantation Trial (MADIT),[8] which suggested the superiority of ICD therapy over "conventional" therapy, are not relevant to patients such as Mr D. All the patients enrolled in MADIT had demonstrated drug-resistant VT by virtue of continued VT induction after the administration of IV procainamide.

Outcome

Mr D had therapy initiated with oral procainamide. On Procan-SR 1000 mg q 6 hours, his procainamide level was 26 µmol/l (therapeutic range 17–43 µmol/l) and his NAPA level was 19 µmol/l. A drug assessment electrophysiologic study was performed and no VT/VF was inducible. In follow-up, Mr D's procainamide dosage has been altered to maintain the procainamide/NAPA levels that were predicted to be effective, requiring dosages as high as 1250 mg q 6 hours and as low as 750 mg q 6 hours. He has now been receiving this therapy for 6 years without arrhythmia recurrence.

REFERENCES

1 Szabo BM, Crijns HJGM, Wiesfeld ACP *et al.* Predictors of mortality in patients with sustained ventricular tachycardias or ventricular fibrillation and depressed left ventricular function: importance of beta blockade. *Am Heart J* 1995;**130**:281–6.

2 Mitchell LB, Duff HJ, Manyari DE, Wyse DG. A randomized clinical trial of the noninvasive and invasive approaches to drug therapy of ventricular tachycardia. *N Engl J Med* 1987;**317**:1681–7.

3 Mason JW, Electrophysiologic Study versus Electrocardiographic Monitoring Investigators. A comparison of electrophysiologic testing with Holter monitoring to predict antiarrhythmic drug efficacy for ventricular tachyarrhythmias. *N Engl J Med* 1993;**329**:445–51.

4 The CASADE Investigators. Randomized antiarrhythmic drug therapy in survivors of cardiac arrest (the CASADE study). *Am J Cardiol* 1993;**72**: 280–7.

5 AVID Investigators. Antiarrhythmics versus Implantable Defibrillator (AVID): rationale, design and methods. *Am J Cardiol* 1995;**75**:470–5.

6 Siebels J, Cappato R, Ruppel R *et al.*, CASH Investigators. ICD versus drugs in cardiac arrest survivors: preliminary results of the cardiac arrest study Hamburg. *PACE* 1993;**16**:552–8.

7 Connolly SJ, Gent M, Roberts RS *et al.*, CIDS Investigators. Canadian Implantable Defibrillator Study (CIDS): study design and organization. *Am J Cardiol* 1993;**72**:103F–108F.

8 Moss AJ, Hall J, Cannom DS, Doubert JP *et al.* Multicenter Automatic Defibrillator Implantation Trial Investigators (MADIT). Improved survival with an implanted defibrillator in patients with coronary disease at high risk for ventricular arrhythmia. *N Engl J Med* 1996;**335**:1933–40.

CASE 2

Miss M presents a therapeutic choice in the management of a propensity to ventricular tachycardia (VT) at the age of 17 years. When Miss M was 3 years old her father died suddenly during sleep at the age of 28 years. The father's autopsy documented the presence of a right ventricular cardiomyopathy. When Miss M was 13 years of age her sister died suddenly during sleep at the age of 18 years. The sister's autopsy documented the presence of a right ventricular cardiomyopathy. Understandably, Miss M's mother became alarmed and Miss M was referred for her initial evaluation. That evaluation included clinical examination, a 2D echocardiographic examination, a biventricular radionuclide angiogram, a Holter monitoring examination, and a treadmill exercise test. All were entirely normal. Over the next three years, annual clinical examinations, Holter monitoring examinations, and echocardiographic examinations remained normal. However, her annual evaluation at the age of 17 years included a Holter examination showing frequent ventricular premature beats (14 VPB/hour) that were complex to the level of four beat salvos of consecutive ventricular beats. Accordingly, a search for evidence of right ventricular structural heart disease and for a propensity to ventricular tachyarrhythmia was undertaken.

An echocardiographic examination shows questionable right ventricular enlargement. A biventricular radionuclide angiogram shows normal right and left ventricular size and function at rest but the right ventricle becomes mildly and diffusely hypokinetic with supine bicycle exercise. Cardiac catheterization is performed and the right ventricular angiogram demonstrates two dyskinetic right ventricular segments. A treadmill exercise test precipitates a ventricular triplet. Finally, a transvenous catheter electrophysiologic study is performed. Triple ventricular extra stimuli applied during right ventricular pacing at a rate of 150 bpm initiates a polymorphic VT that then stabilizes into sustained monomorphic VT at a rate of 230 bpm. The monomorphic VT has a left bundle branch "block" configuration and normal frontal plane QRS axis morphology.

Question: What treatment, if any, should now be applied?

COMMENT

Although rare, there is persuasive evidence in the literature that should help guide therapy for this high risk state. The studies performed in this 17-year-old female indicate both structural right ventricular disease and a propensity to VT with a QRS morphology consistent with a right ventricular "origin". One must conclude that Miss M has developed the same arrhythmogenic right ventricular dysplasia (ARVD) that had affected her father and her sister. The natural history of this disorder as defined by her father and her sister strongly suggests that Miss M is at high risk of sudden death. In this setting, Miss M's viable therapeutic alternatives include individualized antiarrhythmic drug therapy selected by (a) the Holter monitoring approach or (b) the electrophysiologic study approach; or (c) empiric amiodarone; or (d) electrosurgery/transcatheter ablation; or (e) placement of an implantable automatic cardioverter defibrillator (ICD).

Miss M's clinical circumstance is unusual and has not been the subject of specific randomized clinical trials. The closest patient population studied to date is that of the

Multicenter Automatic Defibrillator Implantation Trial (MADIT),[1] which suggested that early use of an ICD was superior to "conventional" therapy. However, the study population of MADIT (patients with remote myocardial infarction, compromised left ventricular function, and inducible sustained VT/VF that could not be suppressed by intravenous procainamide) was unrelated to that of Miss M. Accordingly, a therapeutic decision was made without definitive clinical trial data.

Individualized antiarrhythmic drug therapy was considered. Both approaches to individualized antiarrhythmic drug therapy have been validated in patient populations dominated by atherosclerotic heart disease. Furthermore, such therapy is more prone to failure when the underlying structural heart disease is cardiomyopathic rather than atherosclerotic. Nevertheless, the factor that most recommended an alternative approach was that if a spontaneous episode of VT/VF subsequently occurred, it would be impossible to distinguish between a failure of drug therapy to prevent an episode of VT/VF that was inevitable and a proarrhythmic drug response that precipitated an episode of VT/VF that was not otherwise going to occur.

Empiric beta-blocker therapy was considered. Steinbeck et al.[2] have published evidence suggesting that empiric beta-blocking therapy is as effective as antiarrythmic drug therapy selected by the electrophysiologic approach for the prevention of VT/VF. Careful scrutiny of their results shows that empiric beta-blocking therapy is actually more effective than is standard drug therapy predicted to be ineffective by the electrophysiologic study approach, but is less effective than is a standard drug therapy predicted to be effective by the electrophysiologic study approach. Nevertheless grade B evidence supports the concomitant use of ancillary beta-blocking therapy where possible.[3]

Empiric amiodarone was considered. Empiric amiodarone has prophylactic efficacy in patient populations at high risk of VT/VF who have not yet experienced a spontaneous VT/VF episode. Such trials include that of Grupo de Estudio de la Sobrevida en la Insuficiencia Cardiaca en Argentina (GESICA),[4] CHF-STAT,[5] the Canadian Amiodarone Myocardial Infarction Arrhythmia Trial (CAMIAT),[6] and the European Myocardial Infarct Amiodarone Trial (EMIAT).[7] Furthermore, GESICA and CHF-STAT suggested that empiric amiodarone is particularly effective when the underlying structural heart disease is cardiomyopathic rather than atherosclerotic. Finally, the proarrhythmic potential of amiodarone is very low (approximately 1%), rendering the probability of a future need to distinguish drug failure from proarrhythmia vanishingly small. Nevertheless, the factor that most recommended an alternative approach was the expected adverse effect profile of amiodarone in one so young who might require therapy for more than 50 years.

Electrosurgery/transcatheter ablation therapy was considered. Ablative therapies have had their greatest success in patients with atherosclerotic heart disease and previous myocardial infarction.[8] The probability of long term success is compromised in patients with a cardiomyopathy, especially when the natural history of that cardiomyopathy is progression with new lesion formation. Although a right ventricular disconnection electrosurgical procedure has been developed for the treatment of patients with arrhythmogenic right ventricular dysplasia, the long term consequences of right ventricular failure are frequently devastating. Nevertheless, the factor that most recommended an alternative approach was consideration of the surgical risk in a person who has not yet had a spontaneous episode of VT/VF.

These considerations favored the implantation of an ICD. ICD therapy provides excellent protection from sudden death in patients whose structural heart disease is atherosclerotic or cardiomyopathic.[9] Furthermore, the proarrhythmia potential of an

ICD is low, thereby reducing concern of a future need to distinguish between therapeutic failure and therapy-related proarrhythmia. Finally, the availability of single lead transvenous ICD conformations allows the therapy to be instituted with a low risk surgical procedure.

Outcome

Miss M had her ICD implanted when she was 17 years of age. The procedure was uncomplicated and her convalescence was unremarkable. Three years later, her ICD reached end of battery life indicators. During these years she did not have a spontaneous episode of VT/VF and had received no therapies from her device. A new ICD impulse generator was implanted when Miss M was 20 years of age. One year later, 4 years after her initial presentation, Miss M was playing baseball (at bat) when she suddenly felt marked presyncope followed by a shock from her ICD. She then felt well and completed her turn at bat. Subsequent interrogation of her ICD showed that the pre-event rhythm was sinus tachycardia at 162 beats per minute that gave way to a ventricular tachycardia at 300 beats per minute. These rhythm assessments were augmented by the availability of ICD-stored intracardiac electrograms. She is presently undergoing genetic counseling relative to her desire to conceive a child – evidence of a satisfactory quality of life.

REFERENCES

1 Moss AJ, Hall J, Cannom DS et al. Multicenter Automatic Defibrillator Implantation Trial Investigators. Improved survival with an implanted defibrillator in patients with coronary disease at high risk for ventricular arrhythmia. N Engl J Med 1996;335:1933–40.

2 Steinbeck G, Anderson D, Bach P et al. A comparison of electrophysiologically guided antiarrythmic drug therapy with beta blocker therapy in patients with symptomatic sustained ventricular arrythmias. N Engl J Med 1992;327:987–92.

3 Szabo BM, Crijns HJGM, Weisfeld ACP et al. Predictors of mortality in patients with sustained ventricular tachycardias or ventricular fibrillation and depressed left ventricular function: importance of beta blockade. Am Heart J 1995;130:281–6.

4 Doval HC, Nul DR, Grancelli HO et al. GESICA Investigators. Randomized trial of low-dose amiodarone in severe congestive heart failure. Lancet 1994;344:493–8.

5 Singh SN, Fletcher RD, Fisher SG et al, CHF-STAT Investigators. Amiodarone in patients with congestive heart failure and asymptomatic ventricular arrhythmia. N Engl J Med 1995;333:77–82.

6 Cairns JA, Connolly SJ, Roberts R, Gent M, CAMIAT (Canadian Amiodarone Myocardial Infarction Arrhythmia Trial) Investigators. Randomized trial of outcome after myocardial infarction in patients with frequent or repetitive ventricular premature depolarizations: CAMIAT. Lancet 1997;349:675–82.

7 Julian DG, Camm AJ, Frangin G et al, EMIAT Investigators. Randomized trial of effect of amiodarone on mortality in patients with left ventricular dysfunction after recent myocardial infarction: EMIAT. Lancet 1997;349:667–74.

8 Levy S. Non-medical therapy of ventricular tachyarrhythmias. Eur Heart J 1989;10(Suppl E):48–52.

9 Gillis AM. The current status of the implantable cardioverter defibrillator. Ann Rev Med 1996;47:85–93.

Bradyarrhythmias: choice of pacemaker

70

JOHN A. BOONE

CASE 1

A 66-year-old man had a VVIR pacemaker implanted because of syncope due to complete heart block. He was previously well except for one documented and, possibly, a second undocumented episode of atrial fibrillation. An ECG taken prior to pacemaker insertion showed sinus bradycardia. When he presented with transient complete heart block it was believed he would do well with VVIR pacing. However, he now presents with a form of "pacemaker syndrome" characterized by a combination of fatigue and the presence of cannon A waves due to intermittent VA conduction (Figure 70.1). Furthermore, episodes of paroxysmal atrial fibrillation became more frequent and, interestingly, he was less symptomatic when in atrial fibrillation, presumably due to the

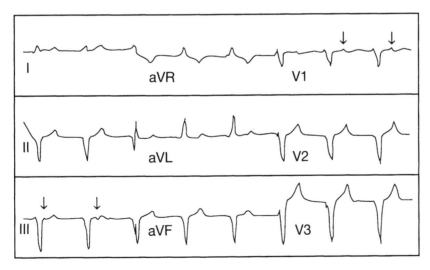

Figure 70.1 VVI pacing with ventriculoatrial dissociation (arrows).

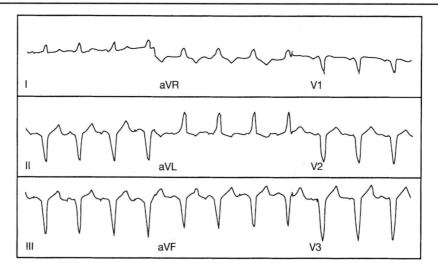

Figure 70.2 Following implantation of DDDR pacemaker.

absence of cannon waves. He was anticoagulated with warfarin. As he was in sinus rhythm more often than in atrial fibrillation, and as he was symptomatic with asynchronous pacing, the VVIR pacemaker was removed and his pacing was "upgraded" to DDDR pacing (Figure 70.2).

Question: Should this patient have had a DDD type pacemaker inserted from the start?

COMMENT

With established symptoms of syncope in the presence of documented complete heart block there is little doubt about the need for pacemaker implant for this patient. Rather, one seeks evidence to support the choice of the optimum pacemaker mode. The treatment of symptomatic acquired complete heart block by cardiac pacing became established practice in the 1960s. Following the introduction of permanent cardiac pacing – initially VOO followed by VVI (see Chapter 38 for description of pacemakers) – published experience clearly documented that patients with complete heart block and syncope had an improved survival.[1-3]

Although one might have felt intuitively that "physiological" pacing was indicated from the start in this patient, trials that randomized patients to receive either single chamber or dual chamber pacemakers are recent or only now in progress. For instance, several studies have demonstrated a benefit of atrial synchrony over VVI pacing[4-7] in evaluating cardiac output, exercise capacity, and feeling of wellbeing. But the increase in cardiac output with exercise is mostly achieved by an increase in heart rate rather than by AV synchrony.[8-10] It was on this basis, namely, to enable adequate tracking of patient's physical activity, that VVIR pacing was originally chosen in this patient.

However, factors other than exercise capacity may determine suitability of a particular pacing mode, as exemplified by this patient, wherein VVI pacing caused a form of pacemaker syndrome, i.e. a clinical state wherein stroke volume is reduced by virtue of asynchrony between atrial transport function and ventricular systole. The incidence of pacemaker syndrome in VVI pacing is not known but estimates vary from 0.1% to 5%.[11,12]

Other benefits attributed to DDD pacing include prevention of atrial fibrillation, prevention of embolic stroke and other systemic emboli as well as protection from congestive heart failure and early mortality. The data suggesting these benefits are mostly from studies that are retrospective and non-randomized so far.[13,14] However, when these data are used to calculate annual event rates, there is a two-thirds risk reduction for atrial fibrillation and a one-third reduction for death in patients who have received DDD pacing. One prospective randomized trial that compared atrial to ventricular pacing found significantly less atrial fibrillation and thromboemboli in the atrial paced patients compared with those receiving ventricular pacing, but there was no significant difference in congestive heart failure or mortality.[15] The current prospective randomized trials may or may not confirm these findings.

REFERENCES

1 Friedberg CK, Donoso E, Stein WB. Nonsurgical acquired heartblock. *Ann NY Acad Sci* 1964;**111**: 833–47.

2 Donmoyer TL, DeSanctis RW, Austen WG. Experience with implantable pacemakers using myocardial electrodes in the management of heartblock. *Ann Thorac Surg* 1967;**3**:213–27.

3 Edhag O, Swahn A. Prognosis of patients with complete heartblock or arrhythmic syncope who are not treated with artificial pacemakers: a long-term follow-up study of 101 patients. *Acta Med Scand* 1976;**200**:457–63.

4 Kristensson E, Arnman P, Smedgard P, Ryden L. Physiological versus single rate ventricular pacing: a double-blind cross-over study. *PACE* 1985;**8**:73–84.

5 Perrins EJ, Morley CA, Chan SL, Sutton R. Randomized control trial of physiological and ventricular pacing. *Br Heart J* 1983;**50**:112–17.

6 Yee R, Benditt DG, Kostuk WJ *et al*. Comparative functional effects of chronic ventricular demand and atrial synchronous ventricular inhibited pacing. *PACE* 1984;**7**:23–8.

7 Rediker DE, Eagle KA, Homma S *et al*. Clinical and hemodynamic comparison of VVI versus DDD pacing in patients with DDD pacemakers. *Am J Cardiol* 1988;**61**:323–9.

8 Fananapazir L, Bennett DH, Monks P. Atrial synchronized ventricular pacing: contribution of the chronotropic response to improved exercise performance. *PACE* 1983;**6**:601–8.

9 Ehrsson SK. Influence of heart rate and atrioventricular synchronization on maximal work tolerance in patients treated with artificial pacemakers. *Acta Med Scand* 1983;**214**:311–15.

10 McMeekin JD, Lautner D, Hanson S, Gulamhusein SS. Importance of heart rate response during exercise in patients using atrial ventricular synchronous and ventricular pacemakers. *PACE* 1990;**13**:59–68.

11 Rosenqvist M, Brandt J, Schuller H. Long-term pacing in sinus node disease: the effects of stimulation mode on cardiovascular morbidity and mortality. *Am Heart J* 1988;**1126**:16–22.

12 Santini M, Alexidou G, Ansalone G *et al*. Relation of prognosis of sick-sinus syndrome to age, conduction defects and modes of permanent cardiac pacing. *Am J Cardiol* 1990;**65**:729–35.

13 Hesselson AB, Parsonnet V, Bernstein AD, Bonavita GJ. Deleterious effects of long-term single chamber ventricular pacing in patients with sick-sinus syndrome: the hidden benefits of dual chamber pacing. *J Am Coll Cardiol* 1992;**19**: 1542–9.

14 Andersen HR, Thuesen L, Bagger JP, Vesterlund T, Thomsen PEB. Prospective randomized trial of atrial versus ventricular pacing in sick-sinus syndrome. *Lancet* 1994;**344**:1524–8.

15 Connolly SJ, Gent M, Roberts RS, Dorian P *et al*. CIDS Investigators (Canadian implantable defibrillator study): study designs and organization. *Am J Cardiol* 1993;**72**:103F–108F.

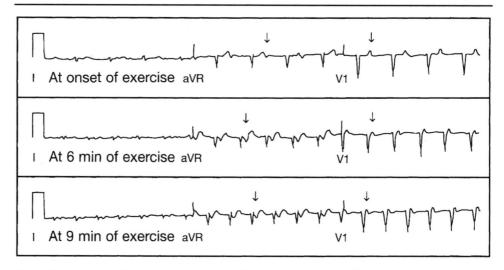

Figure 70.3 Exercise ECG prior to pacemaker implant. Arrows indicate P waves. Note the almost fixed first degree block such that at the peak of exercise, atria and ventricles depolarize spontaneously.

CASE 2

A 30-year-old woman complains of sudden shortness of breath and exhaustion occurring during moderate to severe exertion. She is fine at the beginning of exercise, but if she continues she feels as if she had "hit a brick wall". She is a member of a woman's softball team and the example she gives is when she hits what she believes to be a home-run she would run past first base without difficulty, but beyond that she would suddenly be incapable of running and would barely make it to second base. On one occasion she lost consciousness during exertion. Her history otherwise is unremarkable and clinical examination is completely normal. The ECG shows sinus rhythm with a first degree AV block and a PR interval of 0.38 seconds. An echocardiogram is normal. An exercise stress test is performed according to the Bruce protocol. Upon completion of Stage III her heart rate reaches 166 beats per minute with a PR interval of 0.34 seconds (Figure 70.3). The P waves are superimposed on the terminal portion of the QRS. At this point she experiences sudden exhaustion and the test is terminated.

Question: What advice would you now give her?

COMMENT

In this rather unusual circumstance, a search for evidence from clinical trials to guide therapy would be better served by reliance on clinical judgment and a sound knowledge of electromechanical physiology. This woman's symptoms were the result of an almost fixed first degree AV block, such that with exercise atrial contraction would frequently occur against closed AV valves during the period of ventricular contraction. The consequence of this is that the atria "empty" in a retrograde fashion during atrial systole (producing the equivalent of "cannon waves") resulting in severely reduced filling

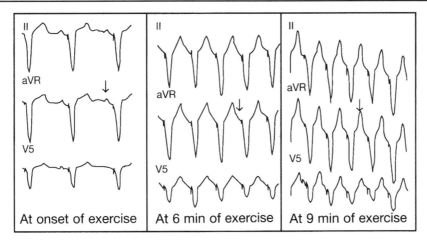

Figure 70.4 Exercise ECG after DDD pacemaker implant. Arrows indicate P waves. Note the DDD pacemaker mode maintains a physiologic AV interval.

volumes. The result is a reduced stroke volume and a fall in cardiac output during heart rate acceleration.

This patient received implantation of a DDD pacemaker with a good clinical result. The device was programmed to a nominal AV delay of 200 msec, thus permitting normal ventricular filling. A repeat exercise test demonstrated a ventricular pacing "tracking" sinus rhythm with a more physiologic PR interval (Figure 70.4).

The original published ACC/AHA Task Force guidelines for the implantation of cardiac pacemakers in 1991 state there is no evidence to support pacemaker implantation in patients with isolated first degree AV block and thus assign this condition to a class III recommendation (i.e. there is general agreement that pacemakers are not necessary). The revised guidelines, however,[1] acknowledge the usefulness of pacemaker implantation for patients with symptomatic first degree AV block. This wise decision is largely based on physiologic need substantiated by the comparison of atrioventricular vs ventricular pacemaker activity on cardiac function as well as the relative low prevalence of these types of cases in the population. This physically active patient clearly benefited from the pacemaker.

REFERENCE

1 Barold SS. ACC/AHA guidelines for implantation
  of cardiac pacemakers. *PACE* 1993;**16**:1221.

71 Valvular heart disease: timing of surgery

Adrian P. Banning
Brian Gribbin

CASE 1

A 74-year-old man is referred to the Cardiology Clinic with a 3-month history of worsening breathlessness. Three years earlier he was referred for cardiology review after a systolic murmur had been detected at a routine medical examination. At that time, he was asymptomatic despite an active lifestyle and Doppler echocardiography that had shown evidence of a calcified aortic valve with a peak Doppler instantaneous gradient of 70 mmHg (mean gradient 40 mmHg), left ventricular hypertrophy, and dynamic left ventricular systolic function. In the absence of symptoms, he was advised to avoid sudden or strenuous exercise and the need for endocarditis prophylaxis. A 6-month follow-up appointment was arranged for clinical assessment and repeat Doppler echocardiography. Subsequently he defaulted from all medical follow-up. He now presents with severe exertional dyspnea, orthopnea, and paroxysmal nocturnal dyspnea. He has no risk factors for coronary artery disease and there is no history of exertional chest pain or presyncope. Examination reveals a slow upstroke carotid pulse, blood pressure of 115/75, elevated venous pressure, sustained left ventricular impulse, soft aortic closure sound, and an ejection systolic murmur. Examination of the lungs reveals a right-sided pleural effusion and bibasal crepitations.

An ECG shows sinus rhythm with voltage criteria of severe left ventricular hypertrophy and a left ventricular strain pattern (Figure 71.1). Doppler echocardiography demonstrates a hypertrophied, dilated left ventricle with severe global impairment of systolic function and an ejection fraction estimated at 0.20. There is evidence of moderate mitral regurgitation. The aortic valve is heavily calcified with restricted opening and a Doppler peak gradient of 40 mmHg (mean gradient 32 mmHg). The continuity equation measures the aortic valve area at 0.5 cm.^{2}

Question: Was the initial management of this man appropriate, and what is the appropriate management now?

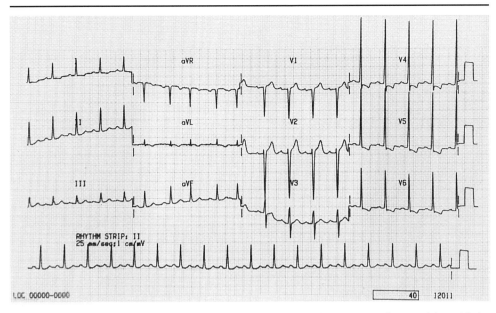

Figure 71.1 Case 1. A 12 lead ECG showing sinus rhythm with voltage criteria of severe left ventricular hypertrophy and a left ventricular strain pattern.

COMMENT

This case presents two major issues calling for evidence to support the correct timing of surgical intervention for aortic stenosis: (a) the asymptomatic patient with severe aortic stenosis; (b) the symptomatic patient with severe aortic stenosis but with a reduced transvalvular gradient presumably due to impaired left ventricular function.

The incidence of sudden death is increased in patients with severe aortic stenosis. Fortunately, this rarely occurs without premonitory symptoms, and in elderly patients particularly, the risk of sudden death in an asymptomatic patient is less than the risk of valve replacement. Thus, following careful clinical and echocardiographic assessment, asymptomatic elderly patients with severe aortic stenosis can be managed conservatively with regular but close outpatient review at least every 6 months.[1] However, any genuine deterioration in exercise capacity must be declared and followed by early surgical assessment.[2]

Aortic valve replacement should always be considered in symptomatic patients as their mortality rates with medical management are 50% at 3 years and 90% at 10 years.[3,4] Survival curves have shown that the interval from onset of symptoms to death is approximately 2 years in patients with heart failure, 3 years in patients with syncope, and 5 years in patients with angina.[5,6] Despite the increased incidence of sudden death, the principal cause of death is progressive heart failure.

In the absence of a myocardial infarct or atrial fibrillation, the concomitant development of severe heart failure with a fall in the Doppler peak instantaneous gradient (from 70 mmHg to 40 mmHg) indicates critical aortic stenosis in this patient. Although left ventricular function is poor, valve replacement surgery is the treatment of choice, the alternative of balloon valvoplasty being only a temporary remedy.[7] Poor preoperative left ventricular function should never be a contraindication to valve replacement surgery, although those in congestive cardiac failure face an increased perioperative risk,[8] as do those with coronary artery disease.[9] However, the majority of surviving patients will experience functional improvement and a reduction in their NYHA classification.[9] Mitral insufficiency secondary to dilation of the left ventricle is common in patients with "end stage" aortic stenosis. Following successful aortic valve replacement, the degree of mitral regurgitation can be expected to improve and mitral valve surgery is rarely necessary unless the mitral valve is structurally abnormal or the mitral regurgitation is severe.

When 2D echocardiography shows a heavily calcified aortic valve with restricted opening and impaired left ventricular function, peak instantaneous gradients of less than 50 mmHg should be regarded as indicating significant stenosis until proved otherwise. Applying the Continuity Equation to measure the aortic valve area is recommended[10,11] and cardiac catheterization need only be performed when coronary arteriography is necessary[12] and in those few patients in whom doubt remains despite careful echocardiographic assessment.

REFERENCES

1 Selzer A. Changing aspect of the natural history of valvular aortic stenosis. N Engl J Med 1987; 317:91–8.

2 Otto CM, Burwash IG, Legget ME et al. Prospective study of asymptomatic valvular aortic stenosis: clinical, echocardiographic and exercise predictors of outcome. Circulation 1997;95: 2262–70.

3 Frank S, Johnson A, Ross J Jr. Natural history of valvular aortic stenosis. Br Heart J 1973;35:41–6.

4 Rapaport E. Natural history of aortic and mitral valve disease. Am J Cardiol 1975;35:221–7.

5 Ross J, Braunwald E. Aortic stenosis. Circulation 1968;38(Suppl 5):V61–V67.

6 Olesen KH, Warburg E. Isolated aortic stenosis – the late prognosis. Acta Med Scand 1958;160: 437–46.

7 Bernard Y, Etievent J, Mourand JL et al. Long-term results of percutaneous aortic valvuloplasty compared with aortic valve replacement in patients more than 75 years old. J Am Coll Cardiol 1992;20:796–801.

8 Obadia JF, Eker A, Rescigno G et al. Valvular replacement for aortic stenosis in NYHA class III and IV. Early and long term results. J Cardiovasc Surg 1995;36:251–6.

9 Connoly HM, Oh JK, Orszniak TA et al. Aortic valve replacement for aortic stenosis with severe left ventricular dysfunction: prognostic indicators. Circulation 1997;95:2395–400.

10 Richards KL, Cannon RS, Miller JF, Crawford MH. Calculation of aortic valve area by Doppler echocardiography: a direct application of the continuity equation. Circulation 1986;73:964–9.

11 Zoghbi WA, Farmer KL, Soto JG, Nelson JG, Quinones MA. Accurate noninvasive quantification of stenotic aortic valve area by Doppler echocardiography. Circulation 1986;73: 452–9.

12 Hall RJC, Kadushi OA, Evemy K. Need for cardiac catheterization in assessment of patients for valve surgery. Br Heart J 1983;49:268–75.

CASE 2

A 32-year-old man with no previous medical history presents with severe exertional breathlessness and some orthopnea. Examination reveals a collapsing pulse, a blood pressure in the right arm of 120/45 mmHg, a volume overloaded and laterally displaced apex, an early diastolic murmur, and a third heart sound. Femoral pulses and distal lower limb pulses are barely palpable.

Transthoracic echocardiography demonstrates a dilated left ventricle (LVEDD 7.9 cm, LVESD 5.9 cm) with severe global impairment of systolic function and an ejection fraction estimated at less than 0.2. The aortic valve is lightly calcified, bicuspid, and there is a broad jet of severe aortic reflux. Doppler interrogation of the descending aorta confirms coarctation with an estimated gradient of 30 mmHg. Magnetic resonance

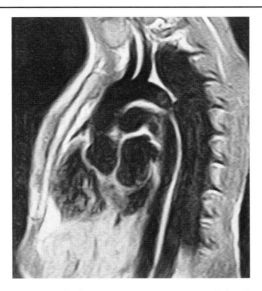

Figure 71.2 Case 2. Sagittal T1-weighted magnetic resonance image of the descending aorta. There is a concentric narrowing of the upper descending aorta which does not involve the left subclavian artery.

imaging (Figure 71.2) confirms a normal ascending aorta, coarctation in the upper descending aorta distal to the left subclavian artery, and some enlargement of the left internal mammary artery.

Question: What are the pharmacological and surgical management options for this man?

COMMENT

Here is a therapeutic challenge where one must strengthen what little external evidence exists with a combination of clinical judgment, experience, and a sound knowledge of cardiovascular pathophysiology. There are two issues to address: the aortic valve disease and the coarctation of the aorta.

A bicuspid aortic valve is commonly associated with coarctation of the aorta. When the valvular disease is significant, aortic stenosis is more common than aortic insufficiency, although a combination may occur. Coarctation results in a high vascular resistance and, when present, the combination of coarctation and dominant aortic regurgitation results in both a large volume and pressure load on the left ventricle.

The insidious onset of severe aortic insufficiency may be well tolerated for many years. In asymptomatic patients with isolated aortic insufficiency, vasodilation using nifedipine has been shown to lengthen the period before valve replacement is necessary.[1] In a patient with coarctation of the aorta, the elevated fixed afterload is unlikely to respond to vasodilator treatment and distal perfusion could be compromised. Treatment with nifedipine is also best avoided in patients with impaired left ventricular function.

When patients with aortic insufficiency do develop symptoms this is usually a reflection of left ventricular dysfunction and valve replacement is advised.[2] When left ventricular dysfunction is mild and prompt surgery is performed, the benefits of surgery are maximal.

However, if surgery is delayed until symptoms or left ventricular dysfunction are established, the prognostic and symptomatic benefits of surgery can be limited.[2] Therefore, evidence of significant left ventricular dilation (end-systolic dimension >5.5 cm)[3,4] or a reduction in the resting left ventricular ejection fraction[5] is usually considered sufficient reason to recommend valve replacement, even in the absence of symptoms.

In this patient, recovery of left ventricular function following valve surgery is likely to be limited if the coarctation is significantly obstructive. Doppler assessment of the severity of the coarctation is complicated by the valvar and myocardial dysfunction but a gradient of 30 mmHg suggests significant but not critical obstruction. In adults, severe aortic coarctation is usually accompanied by increased collateral flow through enlarged branches of subclavian arteries. The presence of an enlarged internal mammary artery in this patient also suggests that the coarctation is likely to be hemodynamically significant. The risk of paraplegia during surgical repair of aortic coarctation is low, but this is enhanced when clamping of the left subclavian artery is necessary. As the coarctation does not involve the left subclavian artery in this patient, the risk of coarctation surgery is predominantly determined by his left ventricular impairment.

Combined surgery attempting to replace the aortic valve and repair the coarctation could be considered as a single procedure. In practice, surgery could not be performed easily through the same incision (left thoracotomy for the upper descending aorta and median sternotomy for the aortic valve) and a protracted procedure could have a detrimental effect on the already compromised left ventricle.

If expertise is available, balloon dilation of the coarctation is an alternative, but in the absence of this expertise, initial surgical repair of the coarctation is probably the initial management of choice,[6] although no well conducted comparative studies are available. Reducing afterload in this way together with the introduction of an ACE inhibitor is likely to reduce the degree of aortic regurgitation and improve left ventricular function. Subsequent aortic valve replacement could then be performed at a reduced risk. If following successful coarctation surgery the left ventricle remains severely compromised, cardiac transplantation could be considered.

REFERENCES

1 Scognamigilo R, Rahimitoola SH, Fasoli G, Nistri S, Dalla Volta S. Nifedipine in asymptomatic patients with severe aortic regurgitation and normal left ventricular function. *N Engl J Med* 1994;**331**: 689–94.

2 Bonow RO, Rosing DR, Kent KM, Epstein SE. Timing of operation for aortic regurgitation. *Am J Cardiol* 1982;**50**:325–36.

3 Stone PH, Clark RD, Goldschlager N, Selzer A, Cohn K. Determinants of prognosis of patients with aortic regurgitation who undergo aortic valve replacement. *J Am Coll Cardiol* 1984;**3**: 1118–26.

4 Henry WL, Bonow RO, Borer JS *et al.* Observations on the optimum time for operative intervention for aortic regurgitation: 1. Evaluation of the results of aortic valve replacement in symptomatic patients. *Circulation* 1980;**61**:471–83.

5 Bonow RO. Radionuclide angiography in the management of asymptomatic aortic regurgitation. *Circulation* 1991;**84**(Suppl I):296–302.

6 Cohen M, Fuster V, Steele PM, Driscoll D, McGoon DC. Coarctation of the aorta. Long-term follow-up and prediction of outcome after surgical correction. *Circulation* 1989;**80**:840–5.

Index